T. Ruzicka · J. Ring · B. Przybilla (Eds.)

Handbook of Atopic Eczema

With 152 Figures and 95 Tables

Springer-Verlag Berlin Heidelberg New York London Paris
Tokyo Hong Kong Barcelona Budapest

PD Dr. Thomas Ruzicka
Dermatologische Klinik und Poliklinik der Universität München
Frauenlobstr. 9–11, 8000 München 2, FRG

Prof. Dr. Dr. Johannes Ring
Hautklinik, Universitätskrankenhaus Eppendorf
Martinistr. 52, 2000 Hamburg 20, FRG

PD Dr. Bernhard Przybilla
Dermatologische Klinik und Poliklinik der Universität München
Frauenlobstr. 9–11, 8000 München 2, FRG

ISBN 3-540-52992-6 Springer Verlag Berlin Heidelberg New York
ISBN 0-387-52992-6 Springer Verlag New York Berlin Heidelberg

Library of Congress Cataloging-in-Publication Data

Handbook of atopic eczema / T. Ruzicka, J. Ring, B. Przybilla (eds.).
p. cm.
Includes index.
ISBN 3-540-52992-6 (alk. paper) : — ISBN 0-387-52992-6
(alk. paper)
Atopic dermatitis — Handbooks, manuals, etc. I. Ruzicka, Thomas. II. Ring Johannes, 1945– .
III. Przybilla, Bernhard, 1949– .
[DNLM: 1. Dermatitis, Atopic. WR 160 H236]
RC593.A8H36 1991
616.97'3—dc20
DNLM/DLC 991-5077
for Library of Congress CIP

Typesetting: SatzStudio Pfeifer, Gräfelfing
Printing and binding: Appl, Wemding
2119/3335-543210 – Printed on acid-free paper

Foreword

Atopic eczema is one of the most common dermatologic conditions. According to recent data, up to 10 % of all children may be affected. Particularly in its severe form, atopic eczema is a distressing and even disabling disease. Even the far more frequent minor forms may pose problems because of their chronicity or the unpredictable tendency for relapse. Atopic eczema must therefore be regarded as a major health problem, and it is one that is today drawing mounting attention, not only from the medical community, but increasingly from the nonmedical public as well.

Since atopic eczema first emerged as a disease entity in the early decades of this century, it has been the subject of both extensive research and intense scientific controversies. The recent development of sophisticated research tools has also stimulated profound investigations of atopic eczema.

Altough the etiopathogenesis of the disease has not yet been fully elucidated, the large body of data already available provides important clues for both our understanding of the disease and for daily patient care. This **Handbook of Atopic Eczema** aims to put together current knowledge on this multifacted disease in the most comprehensive way. This volume covers the whole range of relevant information. Since each topic is dealt with by authors expert in that particular field, the up-to-date knowledge provided is not only extensive but also critical. I believe that this **Handbook of Atopic Eczema** will not only enhance our ability to treat our patients, but will also stimulate our efforts to fully understand this enigmatic disease.

Munich, Spring 1991

Prof. Dr. Dr. h.c.mult. O. Braun-Falco

Contents

List of Contributors

Aalberse, R. C.
Central Laboratory of the Netherlands Red Cross Blood Transfusion Service and Laboratory for Clinical and Experimental Immunology, University of Amsterdam, Plesmanlaan 125
1006 AD Amsterdam, The Netherlands

Abeck, D.
Hautklinik, Universitätskrankenhaus Eppendorf, Martinistr. 52, 2000 Hamburg 20, FRG

Benyon, R. C.
Department of Microbiology and Infectious Diseases, Faculty of Medicine, The University of Calgary Health Sciences Centre, 3330 Hospital Drive N. W., Calgary, Alberta T2N 4N1, Canada

Bernhisel-Broadbent, J.
Department of Pediatrics, Division of Immunology, The Johns Hopkins University Medical School, The Johns Hopkins Hospital, 600 N. Wolfe Street, Baltimore, MD 21205, USA

Bieber, T.
Dermatologische Klinik und Poliklinik der Ludwig-Maximilians-Universität
Frauenlobstraße 9–11, 8000 München 2, FRG

Björkstén, B.
Department of Pediatrics, Faculty of Health Sciences and University Hospital
581 85 Linköping, Sweden

Borelli, S.
Dermatologische Klinik und Poliklinik der Technischen Universität München
Biedersteinerstraße 29, 8000 München 40, FRG

Bosse, K.
Hautklinik und Poliklinik, Universität Göttingen, von-Siebold-Straße 3, 3400 Göttingen, FRG

Braun-Falco, O.
Dermatologische Klinik und Poliklinik der Ludwig-Maximilians-Universität
Frauenlobstraße 9–11, 8000 München 2, FRG

Bruijnzeel, P.
Swiss Institute of Allergy and Asthma Research, Obere Straße 22, 7270 Davos, Switzerland

Bruijnzeel-Koomen, C.
Swiss Institute of Allergy and Asthma Research, Obere Straße 22, 7270 Davos, Switzerland

Businco, L.
Division of Allergy and Clinical Immunology,
Department of Pediatrics, Universität "La Sapienza", Medical School, Viale Regina Elena 324, 00161 Rome, Italy

Cantani, A.
Division of Allergy and Clinical Immunology,
Department of Pediatrics, University "La Sapienza", Medical School, Viale Regina Elena 324, 000161 Rome, Italy

Chan, S. Ch.
Department of Dermatology L468, The Oregon Health Sciences University, 3181 S. W. Sam Jackson Park Road, Portland, OR 97201, USA

Chapman, M. D.
Division of Allergy and Clinical Immunology, Department of Medicine, University of Virginia, Box 225, Charlottesville, VA 22908, USA

Church, M. K.
Clinical Pharmacology Group, University of Southampton, Centre Block, Southampton General Hospital, Tremona Road, Southampton SO9 4XY, UK

Cotterill, J. A.
Department of Dermatology, The General Infirmary at Leeds, Great George Street, Leeds LS1 3EX, UK

Czarnetzki, B. M.
Hautklinik und Poliklinik und Asthma-Poliklinik, Universitätsklinikum Rudolf-Virchow Standort Charlottenburg, Augustenburger Platz 1, 1000 Berlin 65, FRG

Dahl, M. V.
Department of Dermatology, University of Minnesota Medical School, Delaware Street S. E., 420, Minneapolis, MN 55455, USA

Deuell, B.
Division of Allergy and Clinical Immunology, Department of Medicine, University of Virginia, Box 225, Charlottesville, VA 22908, USA

Eckert, F.
Dermatologische Klinik und Poliklinik der Ludwig-Maximilians-Universität, Frauenlobstraße 9–11, 8000 München 2, FRG

Fritsch, P.
Universitätsklinik für Dermatologie und Venerologie, Anichstraße 35, 6020 Innsbruck, Austria

Giannetti, A.
Istituto di Clinical Dermatologica, Università degli Studi di Modena, Via del Pozzo, 71, 41100 Modena, Italy

Gloor, M.
Hautklinik, Städtisches Klinikum, Moltkestraße 18, 7500 Karlsruhe 1, FRG

Goerz, G.
Hautklinik, Universität Düsseldorf, Moorenstraße 5, 4000 Düsseldorf 1, FRG

Gollhausen, R.
Gröbenriederstr. 6a, 8060 Dachau, FRG

Hägermark, Ö.
Department of Dermatology, Karolinska Sjukhuset, 104 01 Stockholm 60, Sweden

Hanifin, J. M.
Department of Dermatology L468, The Oregon Health Sciences University, 3181 S. W. Sam Jackson Park Road, Portland, OR 97201, USA

Heymann, P. W.
Division of Allergy and Clinical Immunology, Department of Medicine, University of Virginia, Box 225, Charlottesville, VA 22908, USA

Hintner, H.
Universitätsklinik für Dermatologie und Venerologie, Anichstraße 35, 6020 Innsbruck, Austria

Hornstein, O. P.
Dermatologische Klinik und Poliklinik, Universität Erlangen-Nürnberg, Hartmannstraße 14, 8520 Erlangen, FRG

Kapp, A.
Funktionsbereich Allergologie/Immundiagnostik, Hautklinik, Klinikum der Universität Freiburg, Hauptstraße 7, 7800 Freiburg, FRG

Korting, H. C.
Dermatologische Klinik und Poliklinik der Ludwig-Maximilians-Universität, Frauenlobstraße 9–11, 8000 München 2, FRG

Kunz, B.
Hôpital Necker, Enfants malades, Unité de Dermatologie, 149 rue de Sèvres , 75743 Paris Cedex 15, France

Lehmann, P.
Hautklinik, Universität Düsseldorf, Moorenstraße 5, 4000 Düsseldorf 1, FRG

Marghescu, S.
Hautklinik Linden, Medizinische Hochschule Hannover, Ricklinger Straße 5, 3000 Hannover 91, FRG

Melnik, B. C.
Hautklinik, Universität Düsseldorf, Moorenstraße 5, 4000 Düsseldorf 1, FRG

Merk, H.
Klinik für Dermatologie und Venerologie der Universität zu Köln, Joseph-Stelzmann-Straße 9, 5000 Köln 41, FRG

Mitchell, B.
Division of Allergy and Clinical Immunology, Department of Medicine, University of Virginia, Box 225, Charlottesville, VA 2908, USA

Morison, W. L.
The Johns Hopkins Medical Institutions, 600 N. Wolfe Street, Baltimore, MD 21205, USA

Mudde, G.
Swiss Institute of Allergy and Asthma Research, Obere Straße 22, 7270 Davos, Switzerland

Neumann, Ch.
Hautklinik Linden, Medizinische Hochschule Hannover, Ricklinger Straße 5, 3000 Hannover 91, FRG

Platts-Mills, T. A. E.
Division of Allergy and Clinical Immunology, Department of Medicine, University of Virginia, Box 225, Charlottesville, VA 22908, USA

Prinz, J. C.
Dermatologische Klinik und Poliklinik der Ludwig-Maximilians-Universität, Frauenlobstraße 9–11, 8000 München 2, FRG

Przybilla, B.
Dermatologische Klinik und Poliklinik der Ludwig-Maximilians-Universität, Frauenlobstraße 9–11, 8000 München 2, FRG

Rieber, E. P.
Institut für Immunologie, Universität München, Goethestraße 31, 8000 München 2, FRG

Riedel, F.
Zentrum für Kinderheilkunde, Philipps-Universität, Deutschhausstraße 12, 3550 Marburg, FRG

Ring, J.
Hautklinik, Universitäts-Krankenhaus Eppendorf, Martinistraße 52, 2000 Hamburg 20, FRG

Ruzicka, T.
Dermatologische Klinik und Poliklinik der Ludwig-Maximilians-Universität, Frauenlobstraße 9–11, 8000 München 2, FRG

Ryan, T. J.
Department of Dermatology, The Slade Hospital, Headington, Oxford OX3 7JH, UK

Rystedt, I.
Division of Occupational Dermatology, National Institute of Occupational Health and Karolinska Hospital, 1721 84 Solna, Sweden

Sampson, H. A.
Department of Pediatrics, Division of Immunology, The Johns Hopkins University Medical School, The Johns Hopkins Hospital, 600 N. Wolfe Street, Baltimore, MD 21205, USA

Saurat, J.-H.
Clinique de Dermatologie, Hôpital Cantonal Universitaire de Genève, 24, rue Micheli-du-Crest, 1211 Genève 4, Switzerland

Schmied, C.
Clinique de Dermatologie, Hôpital Cantonal Universitaire de Genève, 24, rue Micheli-du-Crest, 1211 Genève 4, Switzerland

Schmutzler, W.
Institut für Pharmakologie und Toxikologie I, Medizinische Fakultät der RWTH Aachen, 5100 Aachen, FRG

Schultz Larsen, F.
Dronningensgade 72, 7000 Frederica, Denmark

Seidenari, S.
Istituto di Clinica Dermatologica, Università degli Studi di Modena, Via del Pozzo, 71, 41100 Modena, Italy

Steiger, T.
Dermatologische Klinik und Poliklinik der Technischen Universität München, Biedersteinerstraße 29, 8000 München 40, FRG

Strannegård, I.-L.
Department of Pediatrics, University of Göteborg, Göteborg, Sweden

Strannegård, Ö.
Department of Virology, Central Microbiological Laboratory, The Stockholm County Council, P. O. Box 70470, 107 26 Stockholm, Sweden

Thoma, K.
Institut für Pharmazie und Lebensmittelchemie, Ludwig-Maximilians-Universität, Sophienstraße 10, 8000 München 2, FRG

Uehara, M.
Department of Dermatology, Shiga University of Medical Science, Seta, Tsukinowa-cho, Otsu 520–21, Japan

Vickers, C. F. H.
Department of Dermatology, The University of Liverpool, Royal Liverpool Hospital, Prescot Street, Liverpool L69 3BX, UK

Vieluf, D.
Abteilung für Allergologie, Hautklinik, Universitäts-Krankenhaus Eppendorf, Martinistraße 52, 2000 Hamburg 20, FRG

Willemse, T.
Department of Clinical Sciences of Companion Animals, Dermatology Section, University of Utrecht, Yalelaan 8, 3584 CM Utrecht, The Netherlands

Wüthrich, B.
Allergiestation, Dermatologische Klinik, Universitätsspital Zürich, Gloriastraße 31, 8091 Zürich, Switzerland

Zachariae, H.
Department of Dermatology, University of Aarhus, Marselisborg Hospital, 8000 Arhus C, Denmark

Clinical Aspects of Atopic Eczema

Atopy: Condition, Disease, or Syndrome?

Ring, J.

History

The term "atopy"is relatively new, although it is derived from the ancient Greek. The American allergists Coca and Cooke [7] wanted to describe a strange, abnormal type of hypersensitivity against environmental substances which was observed only in humans and tended to occur within families without obvious prior sensitization. They wanted to differentiate this type of hypersensitivity from other forms such as anaphylaxis [30] and asked the philologist Perry, from Columbia University, for help. This is in contrast to many other famous physicians who felt confident enough to create their own words from ancient languages, sometimes linguistically not very correct but yet successful. For example, the term "anaphylaxis", referring to a lack of protection, should have been, in correct Greek, "aphylaxis". However, for reasons of rhythm or out of lack of knowledge of Greek. Richet, who later won the Nobel Prize, preferred "anaphylaxis" [30]. Perry came up with the term "atopy", meaning not in the right place or strange [7].

Since that time almost 70 years have passed. Yet, the term "atopy" is still controversially discussed and even strictly avoided by some authors. Nonetheless, the clinical conditions described by this name are old and have been well-known for thousands of years. This is clear from the classical medical literature, where we find descriptions of asthma, eczema, and rhinitis (catarrhus) [36]. Similar descriptions can be found in Chinese medical literature from the Sui dynasty (581-618 A. D.) i.e., *On Etiologies of Diseases* by Chao Yuan Fang, volumes 35 and 50. (K. Kang and J. Hanifin, personal communication).

The first documented atopic individual most likely was Emperor Augustus, who suffered from extremely itchy skin, seasonal rhinitis, and tightness of the chest (Suetonius: *Vita Caesarum*) [32]. His grandson, Emperor Claudius, suffered from symptoms of rhinoconjunctivitis. Together with Augustus' great grandnephew, Britannicus, who supposedly suffered from horse dander allergy, one can safely state that we find the first family history of atopy in the Julian-Claudian family of emperors (and this with an almost equal accuracy of methodology of family history taking as is done today in most of offices or clinics) [32].

From the beginning of the modern history of atopy a difficulty in defining this condition has been that many authors have tried to describe a clinical condition and an etiopathophysiological mechanism at the very same time.

Table 1 gives a short review of the historical milestones relevant to the discovery of the pathophysiology of atopy.

By 1925, the presence of "reaginic antibodies", transferable by serum as had been shown by Prausnitz and Küstner [27] was included by Coca [6] in his new definition of atopy. In the following we want to differentiate between the clinical aspects and findings and the etiopathophysiological concepts of atopy.

A common characteristic of all atopic diseases is a hypersensitivity of skin and mucous membranes, that is, at the sites where the reaction of an individual with his environment takes place [33].

Table 1. Historical milestones in the discovery of the etiopathophysiology of atopy

Observation	*Investigator(s)*	*Date*
Pollen skin and provocation test	Blackley	1870
Neurodermite diffuse	Brocq	1891
Prurigo diathésique	Besnier	1892
Anaphylaxis	Richet, Portier	1902
Allergy	von Pirquet	1906
Hyposensitization	Noon and Freeman	1911
Familial occurrence	Cooke	1916
Transferable hypersensitivity	Prausnitz and Küstner	1921
Atopy	Coca and Cooke	1923
Reagins in atopy	Coca, Groove	1925
Bronchial hyperreactivity	Tiffeneau	1945
Vegetative dysregulation	Korting	1954
Genetic relations	Schnyder	1960
Type I reaction	Coombs, Gell	1963
Immunoglobulin E	Ishizaka K. and T.	1966
	Johansson	1967
Beta blockade	Szentivanyi	1968
Fc_ε receptor I	Metzger	1977
Releasibility	Conroy et al.	1977
Fc_ε receptor II	Spiegelberg et al.	1978
IgE binding factor	Ishizaka et al.	1981
Interleukin 4	Coffmann	1987

Clinical Aspects

There is general agreement that atopic eczema, extrinsic allergic bronchial asthma, and allergic rhinoconjunctivitis (hay fever) are the three most important atopic diseases. Yet, atopy cannot be confined to these three diseases; we need only to think of allergic gastrointestinal conditions such as food anaphylaxis!

At the center of the controversy regarding the term atopy we find the atopic skin disease called atopic eczema with its numerous synonyms. The term "atopic eczema" seems to us the most modest, since it only describes eczema occurring in atopic individuals and does not imply mechanisms (e.g., neurological) or sources of elicitation (e.g., endogenous). In the USA the term "atopic dermatitis" is prevalent. This leaves open the debate regarding the difference between eczema and dermatitis, two terms not very well-defined in the dermatological literature [1, 13, 21]. The criticism becomes even more understandable if one confines the definition of eczema to a spongiosiform dermatitis, which in many cases of atopic eczema is not present. We want to define eczema according to the tradition of von Hebra and Miescher [13, 21, 33]: We consider it a noncontagious epidermodermititis with typical clinical (itch, erythema, papule, seropapule, vesicle, squames, crusts, lichenification, in the sense of a synchronous or metachronous polymorphy) and dermato-histological (spongiosis, akanthosis, parakeratosis, lymphocytic infiltrates, and exocytosis) findings, mostly due to a hypersensitivity. Over time the clinical morphology of this skin disease can significantly change in an individual, changing from more eczematous to lichenified and finally pruriginous skin lesions.

Apart from the typical eczematous lesions, the skin also exhibits minor changes which do not or only slightly represent an illness and which are therefore called either stigmata or minimal variants (see the chapters by Przybilla and Wüthrich et al., this volume). It is questionable whether nickel allergy can be regarded as a stigma of atopic eczema [10].

The primary lesion of atopic eczema, whether it is an erythema, a papule, a seropapule, a vesicle, or simply itch, remains unknown. We join a respected tradition, that of French dermatology, German literature, and the Bible, when we say "in the beginning, there was the itch!" [31].

Allergic Rhinoconjunctivitis

Allergic rhinoconjunctivitis or, better, rhinoconjunctivopathia, is accompanied by several clinical symptoms which are physiologically well known under certain conditions (sneezing, secretion, etc.). In massive manifestation, however, these symptoms can be present as disease [22]. Rhinitis often goes along with conjunctivitis, to the extent that the term "rhinoconjunctivitis" has gained clinical acceptance.

Allergic rhinitis can be distinguished from infectious rhinitis, by the nature of the secretion (putrid, milky in infectious and aqueous, clear in noninfectious rhinitis [22]. However, not all cases of noninfectious rhinitis are allergic in origin. A remarkable percentage remains in which hyperreactivity of the nasal mucous membranes seems to be the prominent feature without obvious immunological sensitization. These conditions are called vasomotor rhinitis and can be further differentiated according to the number of eosinophils in the secretion [22, 23].

Bronchial Asthma

Asthma is a mostly reversible airway obstruction on the basis of bronchial hyperreactivity. This is probably one of the most widely accepted current definitions of this condition [2, 11, 17].

Bronchial asthma occurs in 2%–4% of the population and can be classified in different ways, according to either the eliciting stimulus, the reactivity of the patient, or the underlying disease [11, 33). Most commonly, bronchial asthma is classified according to patho-

Table 2. Classification of bronchial asthma

Allergic, extrinsic (IgE-mediated)
Physical, irritative, chemical
Intrinsic (cryptogenic)
Special features
Infection triggered
Psychogenic
Analgesic idiosyncrasy
Pharmacological effects (beta blockers, etc.)
Exercise induced

physiological aspects (Table 2). The frequent differentiation between extrinsic (allergic) and intrinsic (nonallergic) asthma is not quite satisfactory since the term "intrinsic" is not well-defined. Mostly, so-called infectious – allergic or otherwise unclear conditions have been so described. It would be better to talk about cryptogenic asthma, since the possible elicitors or causes are just not well-known [11].

Many patients with atopic eczema also suffer from bronchial asthma. Some studies report a high percentage of patients with provocable bronchoconstriction by nonspecific stimuli (e.g., exercise) who were otherwise asymptomatic and suffered only from skin symptoms of atopic eczema [28].

Genetic studies have shown clearly that the three atopic diseases are closely connected within families [38]. Although there is a genetic component determining the specific organ manifestation, there is also a strong interrelationship and a slightly different distribution of these three diseases in children vs adults (Fig. 1).

In some patients with atopic eczema, the skin lesions seem to disappear when the asthma deteriorates and vice versa. These "alternate" courses were first described by Brocq in 1927 [*alternance morbide*) [4].

In our own investigation, only 10% of patients with atopic eczema exhibited alternate course disease. Some patients, however, clearly showed a coincident exacerbation of both skin lesions and respiratory symptoms during allergen exposure.

Orogastrointestinal symptoms

Quite a number of patients with atopic eczema complain about symptoms in the oropharyngeal mucosa after eating certain foods, especially fruits. The problem of food allergy in atopic eczema will be discussed separately in this volume.

Etiopathophysiological Aspects

A common characteristic of atopic diseases is the familial occurrence, first scientifically recognized by Besnier [3] who classified the prurigo diathésique, asthma, hay fever, and gastrointestinal disturbances found within families. Later on this pattern of occurrence gave rise to the definition of atopy by Coca and Cooke [7]. Schnyder found a strong correlation between the three atopic diseases in the Zurich population, with a prevalence of 9%–12%. Twin studies [38] showed a significantly elevated rate of concordance (60%–79% in homozygous vs ca. 30% in heterozygous twins).

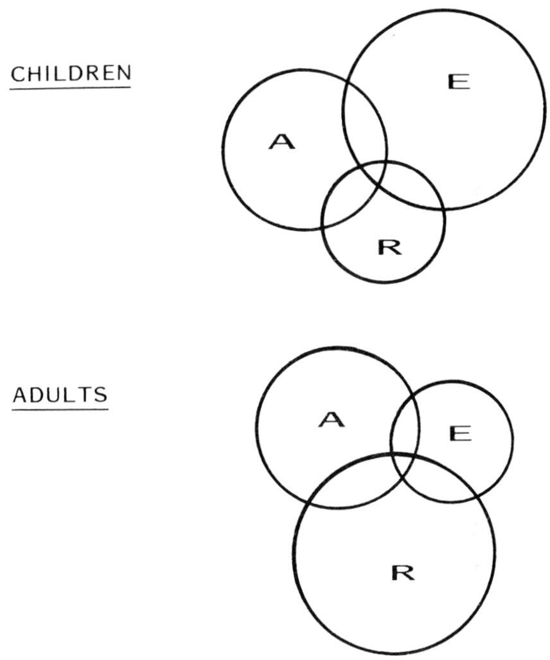

Fig. 1. Distribution of atopic eczema (E), bronchial asthma (A) and allergic rhinoconjunctivitis (R) in Swedish schoolchildren and adults (According to [29])

Atopy and IgE

Increased IgE production is one of the hallmarks of atopic disease. Yet, the simple equation "atopy equals IgE"is incorrect and definitions such as "atopy is associated with but not necessarily caused by IgE antibodies" remain doubtful.

Atopy is only one of many conditions leading to increased IgE production. The origin of this increased IgE production is still largely obscure, although we know that T cells seem to play a role via certain cytokines, such as interleukin-4. The possible influence of environmental factors (e.g., pollution, viral infection, mode of allergen contact) is a current focus of research. Nonetheless, atopy is more than IgE, since it also comprises an altered nonspecific reactivity together with specific IgE production (Fig. 2). One has to be reminded of the statement of Pepys [25] that every individual can, under certain conditions, produce IgE antibodies, but while nonatopics do this only under very potent and

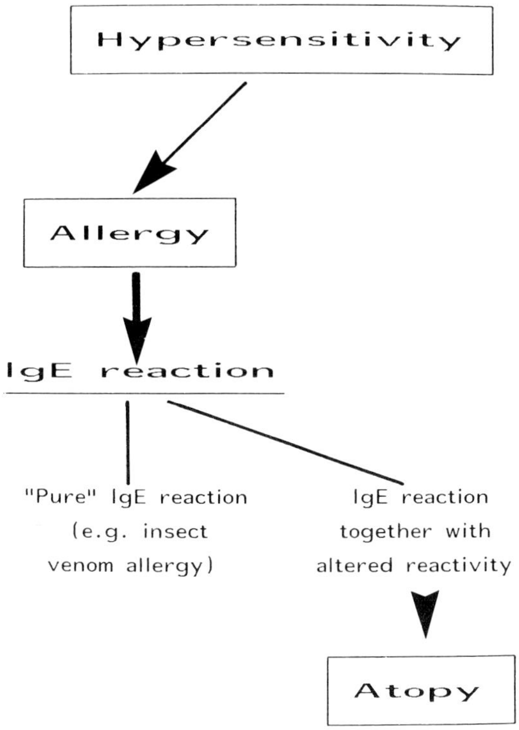

Fig. 2. Classification of atopy within different forms of hypersensitivity reactions

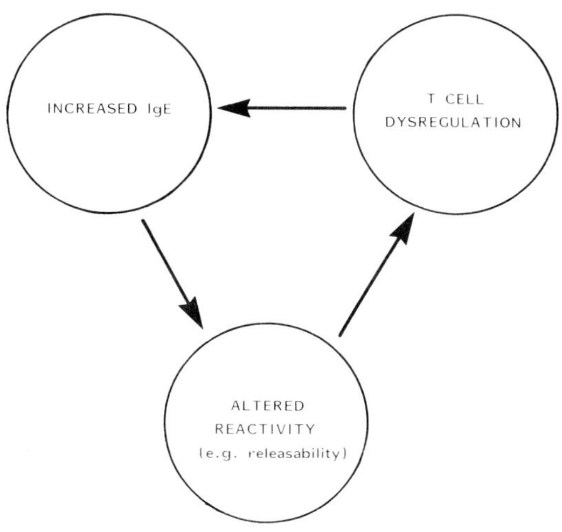

Fig. 3. The hypothetical vicious circle of atopy

Table 3. Atopic diseases and nonatopic differential diagnoses

IgE mediated	*Disease*	*Relevant allergy not detectable*
Extrinsic allergic	Asthma	Intrinsic (cryptogenic)
Allergic	Rhinitis	Vasomotor
Allergic (type I)	Conjunctivitis	Keratoconjunctivitis vernalis?
Extrinsic	Atopic eczema	Intrinsic (cryptogenic)

peculiar allergen exposure conditions, atopics readily respond with IgE antibody production even to moderate allergen exposure.

Apart from increased IgE production, one finds an altered nonspecific reactivity, manifesting as, among others, increased α-adrenergic and cholinergic reactivity together with a β-adrenergic hyporesponsiveness [12, 24, 31, 40]. Since vasoactive mediators, such as histamine or prostaglandin E2, also have an inhibiting influence upon lymphocyte function, one might consider a possible hypothetical vicious circle of atopy in which altered reactivity, T cell dysregulation, and increased IgE production each reinforce the next (Fig. 3).

Like many other biological phenomena, atopy is not an all-or-nothing response. There are marginal conditions difficult to classify, such as urticaria or positive skin prick tests to common environmental allergens. Therefore, some authors use the terms "latent atopy" or "degrees of atopicness."

Atopic diseases should be classified as type I according to the classification of Coombs and Gell [9], with the exception of atopic eczema, in which type IV (lymphocytic inflammatory infiltrates) reactions might also be important.

It is evident that allergic reactions play a role in some patients but not necessarily in all. In many patients different factors such as a disturbance of skin function, infection, and psychosocial interactions, are relevant.

Thus, one could classify all the atopic diseases according to the relative role of immunological sensitization, on the one hand, and nonspecific, altered reactivity on the other (Table 3]. In Fig. 4 a Gaussian distribution of atopic diseases is shown. Where there is an overlap between the parameters IgE production and altered reactivity, we find the classic atopic diseases. On the left and right sides the curve tends to become increasingly indistinct. These areas include people with latent atopy, e.g., positive skin tests without clinical symptoms.

Atopy can be classified according to different criteria, depending upon whether one primarily regards the clinical disease (asthma, rhinoconjunctivitis, eczema, etc.), other clinical features (e.g., stigmata), family history, immunological disturbances (IgE production), or the nonspecific altered reactivity (increased releasability of mediator secreting cells and bronchial, nasal, and skin hyperreactivity).

On the basis of our considerations we define **atopy** as **familial hypersensitivity of skin and mucous membranes against environmental substances, associated with increased IgE production and/or altered nonspecific reactivity** [31, 33].

To answer the question asked in the title of this chapter: Atopy is primarily a *condition* of hyper-

Fig. 4. Gaussian distribution of atopic diseases and conditions according to IgE production and altered reactivity

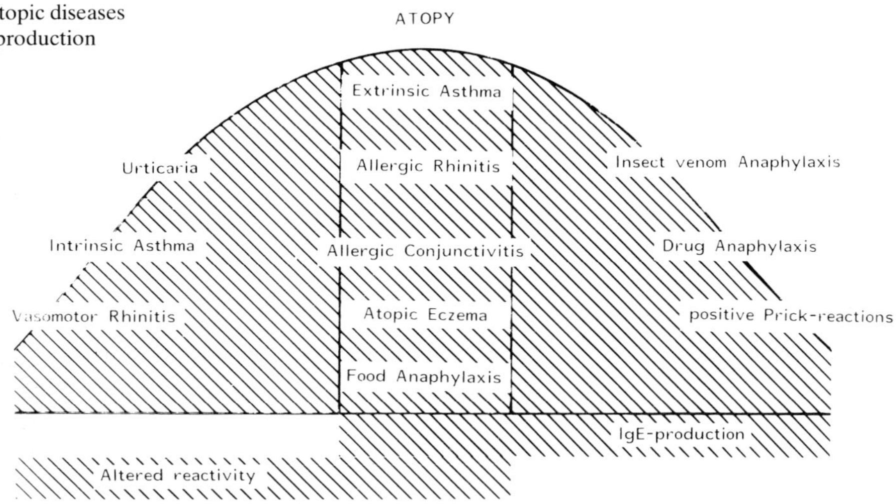

sensitivity which can lead to a *disease* (namely, an atopic disease such as atopic eczema, allergic bronchial asthma, or hay fever) and in many cases to a "*syndrome*" of different diseases (including respiratory, gastrointestinal, and skin symptoms).

References

1. Ackermann AB, Ragaz A (1984) A plea to expunge the word "eczema" from the lexicon of dermatology and dermatopathology. Am J Dermatopathol 4: 315
2. Baur X (1986) Asthma, Alveolitis, Aspergillose. Charakterisierung ursächlicher Allergene. Springer, Berlin Heidelberg New York
3. Besnier E (1892) Première note et observations preliminaires pour servir d'introduction à l'étude diathésique. Ann Dermatol Syphiligr 4: 634
4. Brocq L (1927) Conception générale des dermatoses, nouvelle note sur leur classification. Ann Dermatol Syphilol 8: 65
5. Brocq L, Jacquet L (1891) Notes pour servir a l'histoire des néurodermites: du lichen circumscriptus des anciens auteurs, ou lichen simplex chronique de M. le Dr. E. Vidal. Ann Dermatol Syphiligr 2: 97, 193
6. Coca AF (1925) Zur Frage der Identität der anaphylaktischen und der atopischen Überempfindlichkeit. Med Klin 21: 57
7. Coca AF, Cooke RA (1923) On classification of the phenomena of hypersensitiveness. J Immunol 6: 63
8. Conroy MC, Adkinson NF, Lichtenstein LM (1977) Measurement of IgE in human basophils; relation to serum IgE and anti-IgE-induced histamine release. J Immunol 118: 1317–1324
9. Coombs RRA, Gell PGH (1963) The classification of allergic reactions underlying disease. In: Gell PGH, Coombs RRA (eds) Clinical aspects of immunology. Davis, Philadelphia, p 317
10. Diepgen TL, Fartasch M, Hornstein OP (1989) Evaluation and relevance of atopic basic and minor features in patients with atopic eczema and in the general population. Acta Derm Venereol (Stockh) 144: 50–54
11. Fuchs E, Schultze-Werninghaus G (1986) Asthma bronchiale. Wander, Nürnberg (Themen der Medizin, vol 7)
12. Hanifin JM (1982) Atopic eczema. J Am Acad Dermatol 8: 1–13
13. Hebra F (1860) Acute Exantheme und Hautkrankheiten. In: Virchow R (ed) Handbuch der speciellen Pathologie und Therapie, vol 3. Erlangen, p 209
14. Ishizaka K, Ishizaka T (1967) Identification of γE antibodies as carrier of reaginic activity. J Immunol 99: 1187–1198
15. Jacquet L (1904) La pratique dermatologique. In: Besnier E, Brocq L, Jacquet L (eds) La pratique dermatologique, vol 5. Masson, Paris, p 341
16. Johansson SGO (1967) Raised levels of a new immunoglobulin (IgND) in asthma. Lancet 2: 951
17. Kay AB, Austen KF, Lichtenstein LM (eds) (1984) Asthma. Physiology, immunopharmacology and treatment. Academic Press, London
18. Korting GW (1954) Zur Pathogenese des endogenen Ekzems. Thieme, Stuttgart
19. Kunz B, Ring J, Überla K (1989) Frequency of atopic diseases and allergic sensitization in pre-school children in different parts of Bavaria. Allergologie [Suppl 1] 12: 44
20. Middleton E, Reed CE, Ellis EF (eds) (1988) Allergy. Principles and practice, 3rd edn. Mosby, St Louis
21. Miescher G (1962) Ekzem. In: Marchionini A (ed) Handbuch der Haut- und Geschlechtskrankheiten. Ergänzungswerk, vol 2/1. Springer, Berlin Heidelberg, p 1
22. Mygind N (1986) Essential allergy. Blackwell, Oxford
23. Naclerio RM, Proud D, Togias AG, Adkinson NF Jr, Meyers DA, Kagey-Sobotka A, Plaut M, Norman PS, Lichtenstein LM (1985) Inflammatory mediators in late antigen-induced rhinitis. N Engl J Med 313: 65–70
24. Nadel JA (ed) (1980) Physiology and pharmacology of the airways. Dekker, New York
25. Pepys J (1975) Atopy. In: Gell PG, Coombs RA, Lachmann PF (eds) Clinical aspects of immunology, 3rd Edn. Blackwell, Oxford, p 877

26. Pirquet C von (1906) Allergie. Münch Med Wochenschr 30:1457–1458
27. Prausnitz C, Küstner H (1921) Studien über die Überempfindlichkeit. Zentralbl Bakteriol, I Orig. 86:160
28. Price JF, Cogswell JJ, Joseph MC, Cochrane GM (1976) Exercise-induced bronchoconstriction, skin sensitivity and serum IgE in children with eczema. Arch Dis Child 51: 912
29. Rajka G (1990) Essential aspects of atopic eczema. Springer, Berlin Heidelberg New York
30. Richet C (1904) De l'anaphylaxie ou sensibilité croissante des organismes à des doses successives de poison. Arch Fisiol 1: 129
31. Ring J (1983) Was ist Atopie? In: Braun-Falco O, Burg G (eds) Fortschritte der praktischen Dermatologie und Venerologie, vol 10. Springer, Berlin Heidelberg New York, pp 103–111
32. Ring J (1985) Erstbeschreibung einer "atopischen Familienanamnese" im Julisch-Claudischen Kaiserhaus: Augustus, Claudius, Britannicus. Hautarzt 36:470
33. Ring J (1988) Angewandte Allergologie, 2nd edn. MMV-Vieweg, München
34. Rost GA, Marchionini A (1932) Asthma-Ekzem, Asthma-Prurigo und Neurodermitis als allergische Hautkrankheiten. Würzb Abh Gesamtgeb Prakt Med 27: 10
35. Saurat JH, Woodley H, Helfer N (1985) Cutaneous symptoms in primary immunodeficiencies. Curr Probl Dermatol 13:50
36. Schadewaldt H (1980–1984) Geschichte der Allergie, 4 vols. Dustri, München
37. Schnyder UW, Borelli S (1962) Neurodermitis constitutionalis sive atopica. In: Miescher G, Storck H (eds) Entzündliche Dermatosen I. Springer, Berlin Heidelberg New York, p 228 (Handbuch der Haut- und Geschlechtskrankheiten, vol 2/1)
38. Schultz-Larsen F (1985) Atopic eczema. Etiological studies based on a twin population. Legeforeningens, Copenhagen
39. Spiegelberg HL, Boltz-Nitulescu G, Plummer JM, Melewicz FM (1983) Characterization of the IgE Fc receptors on monocytes and macrophages. Fed Proc 43:124–128
40. Szentivanyi A (1968) The beta adrenergic theory of the atopic abnormality in asthma. J Allergy 42: 203–232
41. Tiffeneau R, Beauvallet M (1945) Production exclusive d'effets pulmonaires locaux par inhalation d'aérosol d'acétylcholine. Son utilisation comme teste d'insuffisance respiratoire. Sem Hop Paris 21:154–166
42. Willan R (1808) On cutaneous diseases. Johnson, London
43. Wise F, Sulzberger MB (1933) Editors remarks. In: Yearbook of dermatology and syphilology. Year Book Medical, Chicago
44. Wüthrich B (1983) Neurodermitis atopica sive constitutionalis. Ein pathogenetisches Modell aus der Sicht des Allergologen. Aktuel Dermatol 9:1–7

Epidemiology of Atopic Eczema

C. Schmied and J.-H. Saurat

Introduction

Epidemiology is the study of the relationships existing between diseases and certain factors intervening in the appearance, distribution and evolution of these diseases, whether these factors depend on the individual or on his environment. When applied to atopic eczema (AE), epidemiology should provide information in the following fields:

- Prevalence of the disease
- Genetic and environmental factors
- Natural history
- Prognosis
- Risk factors and detection methods
- Environmental and occupational consequences
- Definition of subgroups.

With regard to AE, epidemiology comes up against two difficulties.

The first is the indispensable prerequisite of any epidemiological study to establish a precise definition of the disease involved which must serve as a common reference to different investigators. Due to its complexity, AE is a disease that defies attempts at definition. Clinically, there is no specific primitive lesion, and the cutaneous picture changes depending on the age of the patient. AE does not have a unique biological marker or pathognomonic histological image, rather, its pathogenesis is multifactorial and intricate. This explains the confusion of certain epidemiological results, as the studies do not always refer to the same disease. The establishment in 1980 by Hanifin and Rajka of diagnostic criteria for AE is a milestone in the attempt to clarify the situation [1].

The second difficulty in studying the epidemiology of AE is that much of the available epidemiological data concerning AE are based on retrospective studies which are sometimes outdated; prospective studies are the exception. The biases inherent in retrospective studies are many and well known. Let us take as an example the retrospective evaluation of the prevalence of AE. Over the years, both the medical infrastructure and the interest in nonlethal infantile diseases have increased, contributing to a misleading increase in the number of reported cases of AE [2]. The epidemiological information now available to us should be looked upon as an achievement in the progression of knowledge about AE, but not as a final result.

Prevalence of the Disease

AE is a widely prevalent disease, as it affects on average 5% of children in the West [3, 4]. Table 1 gives the figures found in some recent works.

The prevalence of AE is subject to variations depending on certain parameters: sex, age, race, and climatic and geographic conditions. AE affects both sexes almost equally; the proportion between men and women is 1.2/1 [8]. It is during early infancy that boys seem to be more often affected [9]. In addition AE is much more prevalent in children than in adults; even in adults, AE is clearly predominant in younger persons [3, 4, 5]. Concerning possible risks linked to race, Caucasians seem particularly susceptible, but the data are fragmentary and at times contradictory. Some researchers found that the incidence of AE was higher among black children [7, 10], whereas others did not report the same findings [11]. Lastly, AE is a disease that is widely spread throughout the world, since it is to be found in the five continents. AE seems more prevalent in overcrowded urban areas, and in cold or temperate

Table 1. Prevalence of AE

Study	*Prevalence of AD*	*Reference*
National census of dermatological diseases in the United States	0.7%–2.4% of the population; maximal figures concerning the youngest individuals	[5]
Swedish schoolchildren, age 7	active or subsided 8%	[6]
Department of pediatric dermatology, Los Angeles	22% of the children	[7]

climates; it is rarer in rural, tropical and underdeveloped areas [12]. However, these variations are not accepted by all investigators [13].

Not only is AE not a rare disease; its frequency seems to be increasing. In recording the different cases of "childhood eczema" in various regions of Great Britain (England, Scotland and Wales) since the Second World War, a work published in 1984 [2] noted an increase in the prevalence of this disease. In 1946, 5% of children were affected. This figure rose to 7% in 1958 and reached 12% in 1970. Although this proportion seems high, a second paper published in 1986 [14] found virtually the same result in studying the prevalence of AE among Danish twins. Among twins born between 1960 and 1964, the prevalence of AE was 3%; between 1965 and 1969 it increased to 5%; and between 1970 and 1974 it rose to 10%. However discussed above, and in the opinion of the authors of these studies, the real value of these figures is uncertain since these percentages may reflect either a real increase in the prevalence of AE, or an evolution in the method of recording cases. Prospective studies based on the strictest diagnostic criteria will make it possible to decide between these two possibilities. If the increase in the number of AE cases is confirmed, it will be up to epidemiologists to try to explain this rise by looking into the influence of unknown or heretofore neglected environmental factors. These factors include the extreme example of HIV, as it has been reported that the AE rate is much higher in children with AIDS [15].

Genetic and Environmental Factors

The etiology of AE is multifactorial and its complex pathogenesis is still poorly understood. Nonetheless, this disease generally corresponds to the resultant of two main parameters: an "intrinsic" parameter, or genetic heritage and an "extrinsic" parameter, or environmental factors capable of modulating the expression of the genetic heritage to a certain extent. *Genetically*, the family nature of AE is well established, but the precise mode of genetic transmission is not known. According to a series of studies in 15–30% of the cases, no family history of atopy was found [8, 16, 17]. Nonetheless, AE is very frequent (86%) in pairs of monozygotic twins, whereas it is to be found in only 21% of dizygotic twins, a figure no different from that found in cases of non-twin brothers and sisters [14]. Correlation tests with the HLA system provided no significant conclusions [18].

A dominant autosomal monogenic transmission with weak penetration and/or a recessive autosomal transmission have been proposed, but could not be upheld. Instead, more recent suggestions of a variable polygenic transmission make it possible to account for the variety of immunological and biochemical anomalies detected in AE [19–21].

Many *environmental factors*, often intricate, influence the phenotypic expression of AE and act as indicators of the genetic predisposition. These factors include:

1. *Non specific irritants* 'physical or chemical' such as repeated exposure to a cold, desicating climate, or repeated use of industrial or household detergents.
2. *Secondary infection* of eczematous lesions, especially by *Staphylococcous aureus*, which easily colonizes the skin of AE sufferers and maintains cutaneous inflammation [22].
3. *Allergens*, consisting of several groups:
   a) Simple chemical substances, such as metals (e.g. nickel), or haptens of topical drugs causing allergic contact dermatitis. It was believed for a long time that AE subjects escaped such sensitization due to a cellular immunity deficit. However, it is now recognized that such a sensitization can very well trigger outbreaks of AE, especially in adults [23].
   b) Microbes, especially *Staphylococcus aureus*, now believed to be capable of maintaining eczematous lesions not only through its infecting power but also through the allergic reaction it provokes [24].
   c) Inhalant allergens, house dust mites, pollens, animal hairs, and dander: these have attracted renewed interest, for the following reasons: (1) Inhalant allergens seem capable of penetrating transcutaneously; (2) when applied to the skin of AE sufferers, these inhalant allergens can induce eczematous lesions [25, 26]; and (3) IgE can be found on the surface of epidermal Langerhans cells, but only in the epidermis of patients with atopic eczema [27]. If some of this IgE turned out to be specific to the inhalant allergens, its strategic disposition on the surface of those Langerhans cells holding the antigen could help the triggering, by these very same inhalant allergens, of an immunological reaction which is in itself a breeder of inflammatory cutaneous lesions [28].
   d) Alimentary allergens. Although they are too often implicated in outbreaks or maintenance of AE, food allergens probably do play a part in AE, especially with certain children. Proof of their responsibility which can only be affirmed by double-blind oral provocation tests still remains hard to establish [29].

4. *Psychological stress*, readily mentioned by many investigators and, above all, by patients as an aggravating factor in AE. However, there are too few studies available to evaluate objectively the impact of psychic inputs [30, 31].
5. *Climatic and geographic elements* (referred to above). It should be stressed that the influence of certain environmental factors on outbreaks of AE is highly variable from one person to the next and thereby difficult to foresee. In a study dealing with 300 cases of children with AE living in Towns [16], a stay by the sea improved 68% of the cases, but aggravated 24% of them; a stay in the mountains improved 30% of the cases, but worsened 8%. Variations linked to the susceptibility of the genetically predisposed and variations in the intensity of exposure to different environmental agents may combine to explain these individual differences.

Natural History

One characteristic trait of AE is the variation in clinical manifestations, both in morphology and distribution, depending on the age of the patient. One of the tasks of epidemiological analysis is to spot the elements that contribute to that variation. A good deal of work remains to be done in this field. Recent studies have, nonetheless, sought to elucidate two major aspects of AE development: age at onset and age at "cure."

Age at Onset

A prospective study in Paris, covering about 500 cases of infantile AE [17], provided data concerning the age at onset of AE (Table 2). This study brings out the following points concerning age at onset and factors triggering AE:

1. The average at the onset of AE is between the 6 and 7 months.
2. Contrary to what has been taught for a long time, AE often begins during the first 3 months of life. It is in this age sector that over a third of the cases occur, but lesions can also be found at birth.
3. Consistent with other data found in the literature [8], most cases occur during the first year. There are, however, cases of AE starting later in childhood, adolescence, and even, although in less than 2% of the cases, after age 20 [8]. These late-onset forms pose problems of differential diagnosis with diseases such as contact dermatitis or cutaneous lymphoma.
4. In a little over one-half of the cases, the parents of AE patients do not find a precipitating agent. When they do find such an agent, it may be a change in diet (27%), a dental problem (18%), a bout of diarrhea (14%), or even a change of domicile (10%). However, as the authors point out, these events are routine in a child's life and their real importance in triggering AE remains doubtful.

Table 2. Age at the onset of AE [17]

Age	%
0– 3 months	38
3– 6 months	26
6–12 months	16
12–24 months	9
2– 3 years	6
3– 6 years	1.3
>6 years	1.6

Duration of the Disease and Age at Cure

Available data are fragmentary and inconclusive. Since AE is a chronic disease where phases of upsurge alternate with periods of remission it is difficult to determine when a patient is finally cured. Moreover, long-term prospective studies are lacking or are tainted with sources of error. This was the case of the only study, partly prospective, carried out over 20 years and which followed 2000 children [32]. This study reported very optimistic results: 90% cure in a 15-year follow-up. Some investigators [19] feel that there was an element of bias in this figure as it included children with dermatological conditions more benign than AE e.g., seborrheic dermatitis.

Despite these difficulties and shortcomings, in the vast majority of cases the infant's AE enters a prolonged remission phase, even though the duration of the first outbreak varies greatly from one individual to the next [3]. The Parisian prospective study mentioned above [17] reported that, out of 200 infants with AE, one-quarter benefited from a remission of over 2 years beginning at age 3. If the remission was not complete, AE persisted and its intensity and extent were usually proportional to its initial gravity. If remission was total, it was not necessarily definitive, as generally discrete, lichenified lesions sometimes reappeared at school age. This study found no precise correlation between the age at the onset of AE and the length of its evolution.

Concerning the persistence of AE in adults, the best documented and most recent study followed the cases of nearly 1000 individuals, aged 24–44, who had AE in childhood [33]. Some 62% of patients with serious infantile AE (having required hospitalization), and 40% of patients with moderate AE (treated as outpatients), still presented skin troubles, mostly on their hands. One surprising epidemiological finding concerning the persistence of AE into adulthood appeared recently. Subjects who had AE during childhood found their disease reappearing or worsening if they developed AIDS. At present, there is no definitive explanation of this phenomenon, but it may possibly be linked to an imbalance in the secretion of different cytokines, including a drop in the secretion of interferon-γ [34].

Prognosis

In this important field, the studies [17, 32, 33, 35, 36] do not provide sufficiently precise data to establish the prognosis of an individual patient. Nonetheless, there are some criteria that could lead one to fear a lengthy disease evolution for some individuals. Overlooking some differences, the criteria for a poor prognosis are:

1. Severity of AE during childhood
2. Family history of AE
3. Association with allergic rhinitis or asthma (serious childhood AE seems to favor the early development of asthma [17])
4. A late onset (after 2 years) of dermatosis
5. Atypical distribution of the lesions relative to age, with early flexural extension
6. Involvement of the hands which are often resistant to treatment and a potentially serious handicap in the everyday and occupational life of adult patients
7. Persistence of xerosis into adulthood

Risk Factors and Detection Methods

These are of prime interest to parents concerned with the future of an atopic child, and to the public health services, since preventive measures against AE depend, to a large extent, on the information available on the risks of an unexpected appearance of this disease.

Clinically, two elements may be taken into account in trying to detect infants likely to get AE: family background and personal atopic stigmata [20]. A family background of atopy is the most reliable element with respect to risk factors. In a family, the higher the number of atopics, the greater is the risk of atopy in descendants. Thus, the risk rises to 60% if one of the parents is atopic, 80% if both parents are atopic, and even higher if there is an atopic brother or sister. Regarding personal atopic stigmata, to the best of our knowledge, there is no systematic study of cutaneous signs enabling one to foretell the unexpected appearance of AE in infants. However, a recent study of the Hanifin group [37], using as a basis the severity of diaper dermatitis, suggested the following elements in order of severity of risk: AE, diarrhea, and antibiotics. In children with AE, diaper rash occurs more frequently with cloth diapers than with cellular core or absorbent gel diapers, a relationship that was not found among the control subjects. Along with the dermatological anomalies, other manifestations foreshadowed the risk of AE, such as a fit of asthma, a possible prelude to the onset of AE.

On the biological level, neonatal detection of children at risk remains difficult. There are diagnostic markers, some of which are sensitive and specific, but they are unfortunately not yet available for routine use.

The different biological features of AE include:

1. Eosinophilia, at over 400 cells/mm^3. However, this is no longer generally accepted as a criterion due to its lack of specificity [20].
2. An increase in the serum level of IgE in umbilical cord blood; this IgE comes from the fetus, which produces it starting from the 11th week of gestation. To have significance, the rise must be greater than the value of the geometrical mean corresponding to the child's age plus two standard deviations, that is, greater than 1.3 units/ml as measured with the PRIST (paper radioimmunosorbent test). However, the increase in the serum level of IgE is not an infallible marker as its specificity varies between 75% and 90%, and its sensitivity between 50% and 80% [20, 38, 39]. Using the RAST (radioallergosorbent test) method, it is possible to detect IgE specifically directed against certain allergens. The value to be

accorded to the presence of these antibodies does not seem to be greater than that of the total IgE serum level.

3. An increase in leukocyte cyclic adenosine monophosphate phosphodiesterase (cAMP PDE) is found in the cord blood of children of atopic parents. This could constitute a reliable and early marker of atopy. Measured in the blood of 82 umbilical cords, the activity of cAMP PDE was distinctly higher in babies having a family history of atopy; moreover, there was a clear correlation between this parameter and the appearance during the first 18 months of life of cutaneous signs of atopy [40].
4. A decrease in the amount and function of T lymphocyte suppressor cells, together with an increase in the ratio of OKT4 to OKT8, constitutes a promising marker in neonatal detection of AE [41].
Detection of the last two features, (3 and 4), although methodologically difficult is of such importance that one must hope that they may quickly benefit from progress in biotechnology so as to become available for general use.

Environmental and Occupational Consequences

One only has to consider the multiple impacts of AE – medical, economic, social, and occupational – to become convinced of the necessity for preventive measures and the urgent need to apply them.

In the medical field, a recent paper [7] noted that 22% of patients in a pediatric dermatology consultation had AE, and that this diagnosis was by far the most frequent, exceeding impetigo by a factor of 3. The latter was second in frequency and sometimes grafts itself onto a case of AE.

From the socio-occupational perspective, the influence of AE is considerable and is mainly explained by contact dermatitis, to which one is exposed by having AE. One recent report [42] noted that in South Carolina: (a) over 80% of cases of contact dermatitis occurred in an atopic context; (b) the risk of developing such a condition increased by a factor of 13 in atopic subjects; (c) the severity of contact dermatitis was greater if it existed in an atopic background. Thus, through an increased susceptibility to contact dermatitis, atopy leads to absenteeism and, therefore, substantial social costs.

Contact dermatitis appears mostly as hand eczema. In a study covering over 500 patients with AE in childhood, Rystedt [43] noted that later on they developed hand eczema 4–5 times more often than nonatopic persons. Cronin [44] found atopy in about 75% of cases of hand eczema. Agrub [45] recorded AE in almost 20% of the 800 cases of hand eczema examined. It has also been shown that over 30% of AE cases start on the hands, and that over 70% of AE sufferers have involvement of the hands [18]. It is therefore easy to understand the damaging effect of an exposure to physicochemical agents and the importancc of protective measures in the private environment of the patient as well as in his workplace. An immense information effort – which should benefit parents, young children, and especially adolescents who must choose an occupation – is needed to make these measures effective. There are occupations which AE sufferers must forgo provided, of course, they have received prior counselling. These include the most highly exposed occupations such as barbers, mechanics and building, chemical industry, pharmaceutical and food workers.

Definition of Subgroups

One of the most striking characteristics of AE is the heterogeneity of its genetic transmission, clinical expression, evaluation and relationship with the environment. One of the most pressing tasks of epidemiologists is to recognize subgroups of patients which would constitute more homogeneous study populations. Clinical, biological, therapeutic, and of course, epidemiological studies would be greatly facilitated, as would be obtaining results that are more precise, – and above all more coherent – than they are at present. It still remains to define parameters making it possible to identify such subgroups. Some appear evident such as late onset, absence of associated respiratory problems, absence of a rise in the serum level of IgE, and weak release of histamine in vitro, whereas others are still to be determined.

References

1. Hanifin JM, Rajka G (1980) Diagnostic features of atopic eczema. Acta Derm Venereol [suppl] (Stockh) 92: 44–47
2. Taylor B, Wadsworth J, Wadsworth M, Peckham C (1984) Changes in the reported prevalence of childhood eczema since the 1939–45 war. Lancet ii: 1255–1257
3. Saurat J-H (1987) Dermatite atopique de l'enfant. Ann Nestle 45: 9–25
4. Rajka G (1986) Natural history and clinical manifestations of atopic eczema. Clin. Rev. Allergy 4: 3–26
5. Johnson ML (1977) Prevalence of dermatologic disease among persons 1–74 years of age: United States. Advance data from vital and health statistics of the National Center for Health Statistics, No 4
6. Kjellman NIM (1977) Atopic disease in seven-year-old children. Acta Paediatr. Scand. 66: 465–471
7. Schachner L, Ling NS, Press S (1983) A statistical analysis of a pediatric dermatology clinic. Pediatr. Dermatol 1: 157–164
8. Rajka G (1975) Atopic eczema. Saunders, London
9. van Neste D, Lachapelle JM (1986) Dermatite atopique. In: Saurat J-H et al. (eds) Précis de dermatologie et de vénéréologie. Masson, Paris, pp 40–45
10. Castellar C, Brum Negreiros E (1961) Atopic dermatitis. Clinical study of 214 cases. J. Pediatr. (Rio) 26: 149
11. Wingert WA, Friedman DB, Larson WR (1986) The demographical and ecological characteristics of a large urban pediatric outpatient population and implications for improving community pediatric care. Am. J. Public Health 58: 859–876
12. Davis RH, Sarkany I (1961) Atopic eczema in European and Negro West Indian infants in London. Br. J. Dermatol 73: 410–414
13. Rajka G (1986) Atopic eczema. Correlation of environmental factors with frequency. Int J Dermatol 25: 301–304
14. Shultz-Larsen F, Holm NV, Henningsen K (1986) Atopic eczema. A genetic-epidemiologic study in a population based twin sample. J. Am. Acad. Dermatol 15: 487–494
15. Scott GB, Buck BE, Leterman JG, Bloom FL, Parks WP (1984) Acquired immunodeficiency syndrome in infants. N Engl J Med 310: 76–81
16. Queille C, Saurat J-H (1981) Dermatite atopique (eczéma constitutionnel). Etude informatisée de 300 observations. In: Journées parisiennes de pédiatrie. Flammarion Médecine-Science, Paris, pp 293–301
17. Queille-Roussel C, Raynaud F, Saurat J-H (1985) A prospective computerized study of 500 cases of atopic eczema in childhood. I. Initial analyses of 250 parameters. Acta Derm Venereol [Suppl] (Stockh) 114: 87–92
18. Schultz-Larsen F, Grunnet N (1987) Genetic investigations in atopic eczema. Tissue Antigens 29: 1–6
19. Hanifin JM (1987) Epidemiology of atopic eczema. Monogr Allergy 21: 116–131
20. Kjellman NIM (1982) Prediction and prevention of atopic allergy. Allergy 37: 463–473
21. Marsh DG, Meyers DA, Bias WB (1981) The epidemiology and genetics of atopic allergy. N Engl J Med 305: 1551–1559
22. Leyden JJ, Maples RR, Klingman AM (1974) *Staphylococcus aureus* in the lesions of atopic eczema. Br J Dermatol 99: 525–530
23. Marghescu S (1985) Patch test reactions in atopic patients. Acta Derm Venereol [Suppl] (Stockh) 114: 113–116
24. Hauser C (1986) The role of *Staphylococcus aureus* in atopic eczema. Int J Dermatol 25: 573–574
25. Mitchell EB, Crow J, Chapman MD, Jouhal SS, Pope FM, Platts Mills TAE (1982) Basophils in allergen-induced patch test sites in atopic eczema. Lancet i: 127–130
26. Norris PG, Schofield O, Camp RDR (1988) A study of the role of house dust mite in atopic eczema. Br J Dermatol 118: 435–440
27. Bruynzeel-Koomen C, van Wichen DF, Toonstra J, Berrens L, Bruynzeel PLB (1986) The presence of IgE molecules on epidermal Langerhans cells in patients with atopic eczema. Arch Dermatol Res 278: 199–205
28 Schmied C, Saurat JH (1989) Pneumallergènes et dermatite atopique: noveaux concepts. Rev Eur Dermatol MST 1: 393–401
29. Caputo RV, Frieden I, Krafchick BR et al (1986) Diet and atopic eczema. J Am Acad Dermatol 15: 543–545
30. Hanifin JM (1986) Pharmacology of atopic eczema. Clin Rev Allergy 4: 43–65
31. Saurat J-H (1986) Peau et psyché. In: Saurat J-H, Grosshans E, Laugier P, Lachapelle JM (1986) Précis de dermatologie et de vénéréologie. Masson, Paris, pp 597–601
32. Vickers CFH (1980) The natural history of atopic eczema. Acta Derm Venereol [Suppl] (Stockh) 92: 113–115
33. Rystedt I (1985) Prognostic factors in atopic eczema. Acta Derm Venereol (Stockh) 65: 206–213
34. Parkin JM, Eales LJ, Galazka AR, Pinching AJ (1987) Atopic manifestations in the acquired immune deficiency syndrome: response to recombinant interferon gamma. Br Med J 294: 1185–1186
35. van Hecke E, Leys G (1981) Evolution of atopic eczema. Dermatologica 163: 370–375
36. Wütrich B, Schudel P (1982) Atopic eczema after the childhood phase. Ann Hautkr 58: 1012–1023
37. Seymour JL, Keswick BH, Milligan MC, Jordan WP, Hanifin JM (1987) Clinical and microbial effects of cloth, cellulose core and cellulose core/absorbent gel diapers in atopic eczema. Pediatrician 14 (Suppl 1): 39–43
38. Gordon RR, Noble DA, Ward MA, Allen R (1982) Immunoglobulin E and the eczema-asthma syndrome in early childhood. Lancet i: 72–74
39. Leung DJM, Geha RS (1986) Immunoregulatory abnormalities in atopic eczema. Clin Rev Allergy 4: 67–86
40. Heskel NS, Chan SC, Thiel ML, Stevens SR, Casperson LS, Hanifin JM (1984) Elevated umbilical cord blood leukocyte cyclic adenosine monophosphatephosphodiesterase activity in children with atopic parents. J Am Acad Dermatol 11: 422–426
41. Chandra RK, Baker M (1983) Numerical and functional deficiency of suppressor T cells precedes development of atopic eczema. Lancet ii: 1393–1394
42. Keil JE, Shmunes E (1983) The epidemiology of work-related skin disease in South Carolina. J Am Acad Dermatol 119: 650–654
43. Rystedt I. (1985) Work-related hand eczema in atopics. Contact Dermatitis 12: 164–171
44. Cronin E (1985) Clinical patterns of hand eczema in women. Contact Dermatitis 13: 153–161
45. Agrup G (1969) Hand eczema and other hand dermatoses in south Sweden. Acta Derm Venereol [Suppl] (Stockh) 61: 49

Genetic Aspects of Atopic Eczema

F. Schultz Larsen

Introduction

Because of advances in medicine, diseases due to infections and nutritional deficiences are, with few exceptions, being increasingly controlled in developed countries. These environmental diseases are being replaced by others which are entirely, or at least partly, genetically determined such as atopic eczema. Since the classic study of Cooke and Van der Veer [16] in 1916, it has been known that allergy runs in families. Furthermore, it has been convincingly substantiated that such family aggregation is caused by common genes rather than by a common family environment. However, the exact mechanism involved in the genetic basis of allergy has so far escaped precise characterization. In this review, particular attention has been paid to studies of atopic eczema in twins. The textbook of Vogel and Motulsky [82] should be consulted for definitions and genetic concepts.

Historical Perspective

Atopic eczema is now a common disease; however, the clinical manifestations of the disease are so varied that only a trained dermatologist is able to diagnose all such cases. This multi-faceted clinical picture contributes to the difficulty in establishing diagnostic guidelines for atopic eczema and is one of the reasons why so few genetic studies have been published. A second problem is related to the definition of atopy. The modern concept of atopy as a group of diseases comprising atopic eczema, bronchial asthma, and allergic rhinitis was not generally accepted until the 1960s, although it was already proposed and used by Sulzberger and Goodman [77] in 1936. Previously, the atopic diathesis was often widened to include urticaria, gastrointestinal disturbances, sinusitis, and otitis media. Even though such cases of atopy may exist, their inclusion often obscured the results of many earlier investigations. A third problem is associated with the family history of atopy. Some of the genetic analyses are based on the antecedent family history no matter how remote. For example, in some studies, the history was said to be positive and bilateral even if the only affected individuals were the maternal grandfather and the paternal great uncle.

The first part of this historical review will present some of the important stages in the recognition of the genetic basis of atopy in general; the second part will specifically explore studies directed towards examining the inheritance of atopic eczema.

The earliest comprehensive publication dates back to the study of Cooke and Van der Veer [16] in 1916. In a monumental study which fills no less than 105 pages in the first volume of the *Journal of Immunology*, the familial aggregation of atopy, especially bronchial asthma, was underlined. The work was founded on 504 probands with bronchial asthma, allergic rhinitis, urticaria, Quincke's edema, and gastrointestinal reactions, and a control group of 76 nonallergic subjects. They found a positive family history in 48% of the probands compared with only 14% in the control group. The authors concluded that these allergic diseases were inherited as a Mendelian autosomal dominant trait, and that almost 75% of children with a bilateral family history developed allergy compared to nearly 50% with a unilateral family history.

In 1920 Adkinson [1] investigated the families of 400 asthmatics. Besides bronchial asthma and hay fever, the positive family history included cases with urticaria and different types of eczema. Most of the family histories were best explained on the basis of a recessive mode of inheritance. In the 1920s and 1930s the one-gene hypothesis alternated between dominant and recessive models, which included partial or incomplete dominant and recessive heredity. In 1936 Wiener et al. [83] put forward the theory that the inheritance of atopy (at that time still only bronchial asthma and allergic rhinitis) was recessive since it developed before puberty in the homozygote and after 16 years of age following stress in a small proportion of heterozygotes. Thus, the majority of heterozygotes were carriers without manifest atopy. The theory was attractive because it allowed explanation of the apparent skipping of one generation that was occasionally observed in affected families. However, subsequent works were unable to demonstrate a correlation between family disposition and the age of onset of atopy, and during 1940–1950 a great deal of skepticism existed about the heredity concept in atopy [62]. Thus, there were good reasons for reinvestigating the heredity of allergic diseases.

One of the most important subsequent research efforts into the genetic basis of atopy was published by Schwartz [72] in 1952. The study population consisted of 191 asthmatic probands, 50 probands with baker's asthma, and 200 control probands from hospitals in the Copenhagen area. Based on the proband technique of Weinberg, identical diagnostic criteria and identification methods were used for each group. Records were obtained from parents, grandparents, parents' siblings, and probands' siblings and children – a total of 3815 relatives. Bronchial asthma, hay fever, vasomotor rhinitis, and atopic eczema occurred with a far higher frequency in relatives of asthma probands than in relatives of controls. There was no difference in the frequency of migraine, gastrointestinal allergy, epilepsy, urticaria, Quincke's edema, ichthyosis, or psoriasis. A not often cited but equally well-performed study is that of Edgren [22]. The results demonstrated, by comparison with a well-defined control group, that there was an increased frequency of bronchial asthma and allergic rhinitis in a group who previously suffered from atopic eczema. It is remarkable that both Edgren [22] and Schwartz [72] personally visited and interviewed all the accessible living relatives of study participants.

In 1960 Schnyder [64] published an extensive study of allergy, one of the objects of which was to elucidate genetic factors in atopy based on a population study, a family study, and a twin study. The population investigated was found by mailing questionnaires to every 15th taxpayer in Zürich. The response rate was 53% (8246 of 15431 mailed questionnaires), and about two-thirds originated from men between the ages of 20 and 80 years. The family investigation was based on 361 consecutive cases of bronchial asthma, allergic rhinitis, and/or atopic eczema from the departments of dermatology and pediatric allergy. The population findings were used for comparison. Schnyder concluded that bronchial asthma, allergic rhinitis, and atopic eczema (childhood phase and adult phase) were genetically linked, and that the family history of respiratory atopy in probands with atopic eczema was significantly lower than in probands with respiratory atopy. In addition he found that the female sex (119:65 or 1.83:1) predominated in atopic eczema (childhood phase and adult phase); the other findings remain highly debatable. Both Schwartz [72] and Schnyder [64] suggested that the mode of inheritance was most probably by a single, autosomal dominant gene with reduced penetrance.

In a comprehensive German textbook on human genetics Vogel and Dorn [81] showed, on the basis of pooled data from Schwartz [72] and Dorn [20], that organ-specific factors are involved in atopy. That is to say that among first-degree relatives of asthmatics, respiratory atopy is much more frequent than atopic eczema, whereas among relatives of atopic eczema probands, involvement of the skin prevails. This concept of "end-organ sensitivity" in atopy was already considered by Clarke et al. [15] in 1928 and has recently been confirmed by several investigators [21, 40, 66].

Finally, in the 1960s, most researchers realized that the available data strongly indicated atopy as being polygenic and multifactorially determined, which means that several genes (polygenic) as well as genetic and nongenetic factors (multifactorial) determine the expression of the disease [3, 23, 44]. In addition, within this polygenic and multifactorial genetic system there are genetic factors which increase the liability to atopy and which act side by side with other genetic factors that influence specific organ manifestation.

So far, most studies have dealt with the genetics of atopy in general. Unfortunately, much less attention has been focused on atopic eczema in particular and several of the publications cited below served other main purposes than that of studying the heredity of atopic eczema. Furthermore, a detailed definition of the genetic backgrund and age composition of the probands and their families is often lacking in these studies.

Sulzberger and Goodman [77] based some of their earliest findings on "more than 50 cases of typical adult atopic eczema." In more than 50% of these cases, "one or more members of the family have or have had one or more of the atopic diseases" (Table 1). In the late 1930s casuistic reports underlining the occurrence of atopic eczema in subsequent generations were published [36].

Table 1. Atopic heredity in atopic dermatitis

Study	Positive heredity of atopy
Sulzberger and Goodman [77]	50%
Nexmand [58]	43%
Kochs [41]	38%
Baer [4]	62%
Hellerström and Lidman [33]	78%
Dorn [19]	63%
Rajka [60]	68%
Schnyder [64]	67%
Dorn [20]	83%
Uehara [85]	62%

On the basis of a thorough review of hospital records from Copenhagen, Nexmand [58] described the course, clinical aspects, significance of airborne allergens, intracutaneous testing, and value of treatments available at that time. In relation to the occurrence of family allergy, 43% (of 100 patients) reported bronchial asthma, allergic rhinitis, and "eczema" in the family (Table 1).

In 1951 Kochs [41] published an extensive discussion of the many facets of the diagnosis and nature of atopic eczema. However, there were only few details concerning the 221 probands followed since 1937–1938. Of these 38% had bronchial asthma and/or atopic eczema among first-degree and second-degree relatives (Table 1). Thus, allergic rhinitis was omitted from the definition of atopic disorders, and it is also not quite clear if the infantile phase of atopic eczema was included. The study also demonstrated a female preponderance (123:98 or 1.26:1), and that atopic eczema was more frequent among siblings than among parents. The paper presented a total of 28 pedigrees, on the basis of which it was suggested that a single-gene theory could not explain all of the familial patterns of inheritance. Kochs therefore postulated two independent heredity factors: a dominant atopic gene which could be expressed as atopic eczema, bronchial asthma or, rarely, hay fever, and a dominantly inherited, decreased function of the sebaceous glands.

A series of 311 inpatients from the Karolinska Institute in Stockholm was the background for studies of the different aspects of the pathogenesis of atopic eczema [33] (Table 1). The concept of atopic eczema as a "sensitization machine" was introduced, and "only 69 patients did not mention familial occurrence of asthma, hay fever, allergic rhinitis and prurigo Besnier."

In Berlin, Dorn [19] observed 154 inpatients with atopic eczema, and in 97 (63%) of the probands there was a family history of atopic disorders including migraine (Table 1). An accompanying pedigree chart of family P. illustrated "just as in many other cases" that "in a certain proportion of cases it is a matter of irregular dominant inheritance."

An extensive hospital series of 1200 inpatients from Stockholm formed the groundwork of Rajka's [60] many profound studies. A positive atopic heredity was reported in 68% of those with pure atopic eczema, i.e., those without complicating respiratory manifestations (Table 1). This figure included parents, siblings, and "other relatives." Rajka found it improbable that atopic eczema was recessively inherited as several nonatopic children were observed in families where both parents had atopic diseases. Furthermore, the finding of allergic offspring in families where both parents were unaffected argued against a dominant mode of inheritance, unless the penetrance were reduced. Later on, Rajka concluded that atopic eczema is determined by both genetic and environmental factors [61].

In the aforementioned large-scale study of Schnyder [64], the family study dealt with 117 probands with atopic eczema of which 78 (67%) had a family history of atopy which included affected first-degree and second-degree relatives and some of the brothers and sisters of the grandparents (Table 1). Like Rajka, [61] Schnyder did not find any genetic influence on the age of onset and the severity of atopic eczema.

The last extensive family study, which primarily concentrated on atopic eczema from a genetic point of view, came from a hospital clinic in Berlin and constituted an extension of a previously published report [19, 20]. The population comprised 235 probands who were compared with 250 control families (Table 1). There were few details on the ascertainment of the probands and the controls. The families of 196 probands (83%) contained relatives (not otherwise stated) with atopic diseases including migraine and urticaria. Dorn personally examined 1470 relatives of the probands and found that 23% had atopic eczema, 4% had bronchial asthma and 3% had hay fever. It was concluded that the pedigrees of the families were compatible with both an irregular dominant inheritance and a multifactorial inheritance with a threshold, as suggested for respiratory atopy [3].

What lessons are to be learnt from the literature? Uncertainty in the classification of atopic eczema and atopy in the family members included are characteristic features of many of the investigations. However, it seems permissible to conclude that, among inpatients with atopic eczema, about 50%–67% had a single or double parental history of atopy (atopic eczema, bronchial asthma, allergic rhinitis). In addition, the studies indicated that this percentage was higher when siblings were included, especially if the brothers and sisters were examined after the period of manifestation of all the atopic disorders. There is no population-based study on the subject; it can be assumed, however, that the frequency of parental atopy in unselected, nonhospital-based probands is less than the percentage given above.

The genetic mode of atopy inheritance is uncertain. Most of the latest evidence supports a polygenic multifactorial model rather than a single autosomal dominant gene with reduced penetrance. The following aspects favor a multifactorial mechanism: (a) penetrance is reduced to less than 50% in population-based cases of atopic eczema; (b) atopic eczema is a very common disease and has become still more common during less than one generation [71, 79]; (c) as cases of discordant monozygotic twins definitely exist, the disease must be susceptible to influence from exogenous factors [66];

(d) at present it seems unlikely that a single basic biochemical or immunological defect which fits a simple understanding of the disease will be found.

Several criteria have been developed to support the concept of a multifactorial model in combination with a threshold effect [82]. However, most of these criteria presuppose that the prevalence of the disease is constant, just as genetic heterogeneity could be a confounding feature. The multifactorial model implies that the frequency among first-degree relatives is approximately equal to $\sqrt{q}$, where q is the frequency in the general population [23]. Our own study population (born between 1960 and 1974) showed a joint frequency of 67/1126 = 0.06 ($\sqrt{0.06}$ = 0.24). This fits well with the reported cases of atopic eczema in the probands' siblings, namely 16/65 = 0.25 [71].

Nonetheless, the evidence for a multifactorial model of atopy remains circumstantial [54] and additional investigations should be done. The multifactorial model might be further supported by the demonstration that the frequency of the disease is higher in siblings of probands with a single parental history of atopic eczema than in siblings of probands with a negative parental history. Thus, for now we have to rely on the aforementioned, rather indirect, evidence in favor of the polygenic and multifactorially determined mode of inheritance.

Despite our incomplete data, clinicians have a need to supply their patients counseling that provides empirical risk data for atopic eczema appearing in the family (Table 2). These figures, although rough, are based upon the most valid and recent Scandinavian publications. In Table 3, the background prevalence of atopy in the parental generation of mainly 7-year-old school children in Denmark and Sweden in the 1970s is shown. However, in family counseling situations the figures should be accompanied by an explanation of the difficulties in achieving more precise data from a large enough series of population-based patients followed up over a sufficiently large period of time. Changes in the prevalence of atopy, and especially atopic eczema, in the general public have not diminished that difficulty.

Twin Studies

When the mode of inheritance is not simple Mendelian, classical twin studies are an accessible and efficient method of estimating the weight of genetic influence on a given disease. However, the validity of the outcome of these studies presupposes that the twin series is representative and that the diagnosis of zygosity is reliable. In the following review of twin studies, special

Table 2. Empirical risk figures for atopic eczema

Family history of atopy	Percentage risk
Double parental history	50–75
Single parental history	25–30
Negative parental history and one affected child	20–25
Negative parental history	10–15

1. If the parents both have or have had atopic eczema, the risk figure is skewed to the higher value.
2. If the parents both have or have had respiratory atopy, the risk for atopic eczema is skewed to the lower value.
3. If the affected parents or children have or have had combined atopy (i. e., both respiratory atopy and atopic eczema), the risk is skewed to the higher value.
4. If the respiratory atopy (in noncombined atopy) in question is allergic rhinitis only, the risk is skewed to the lower value; with a double parental history of allergic rhinitis the risk of atopic eczema might not be higher than 30%–40%.

Table 3. Parental history of atopy in Scandinavian population studies

Study	Single parental history of atopy (%)	Double parenteral history of atopy (%)
Kjellman [40]	22	3
Schultz Larsen [66]	17	1
Storm et al. [76]	26	3

Table 4. Twin literature on atopic eczema

	Number of monozygotic twin pairs		Number of dizygotic twin pairs	
	Concordant	Discordant	Concordant	Discordant
Schmidt-Kehl [63]	1	0	0	0
Mayr [50]	1	0	0	0
Bueno [10)	1	0	0	0
Spaich and Ostertag [75]	1	0	0	2
Buffum and Feinberg [11]	2	1	0	0
Criep [17]	1	0	0	0
Melsom [51]	0	2	0	0
Kochs [41]	0	0	2	1
Illig [37]	1	0	0	0
Höcker [34]	1	0	0	0
Bowen [9]	0	3	0	0
Frain-Bell and Koblenzer [25]	1	0	0	0
Rajka [60]	2	3	6	3
Schnyder [64]	2	2	0	1
Dorn [20, Vogel and Dorn [81]	1	6	0	0
Niermann [57]	5	0	3	10
Lynfield [46]	1	1	0	2

attention will be given to the diagnosis of atopic eczema and the common problems concerning the identification of twins, concordance rates, and the determination of zygosity.

The first case report was published by Schmidt-Kehl in 1933 (Table 4) [63]. This communication, on the occurrence of allergic diseases in two families, noted that one of the families included a monozygotic twin pair in which both partners suffered from mild eczema. No further information was given. The concomitant course of typical atopic eczema in the members of a monozygotic twin pair was described in a thoroughly prepared report from 1935 [50]. The twins, followed up from 1 to 21 years of age, still had characteristic dermatologic features at the time of investigation. The diagnosis of zygosity was made by taking many anthropological measurements. A less detailed report dealing with a concordant monozygotic twin pair was published in Spanish [10]; no statement was given about the criteria for determination of zygosity.

The oldest unselected twin series with atopic eczema dates back to 1936, when 2500 twins in Germany replied to a mailed questionnaire about allergy which was said to have been explained in simple language [75]. The method of identification of the twins was not given. Among the 1250 pairs of twins (age 3–79 years), there were 113 pairs where one or both partners gave positive answers. Following the mailing of a more detailed questionnaire and a subsequent clinical examination, nine pairs of twins were diagnosed as suffering from various skin diseases. This group contained one concordant monozygotic pair and two discordant dizygotic pairs of twins where the diagnosis of atopic eczema appears reasonably certain. No mention was made of the criteria for determination of zygosity.

A short report from 1940 deals with intracutaneous testing in three monozygotic twin pairs with bronchial asthma and atopic eczema [11]. The clinical description of the skin disease was very superficial and, except for the designation "identical twins," no data were given on the diagnosis of zygosity.

An American study published in 1942 discussed the clinical course in seven monozygotic twin pairs suffering from allergic diseases [17]. One of the pairs was concordant with regard to atopic eczema since the age of 3 years. The clinical features were carefully delineated. The diagnosis of zygosity rested upon the fact that the twins "look exactly alike."

In 1945 Melsom [51] diagnosed two discordant monozygotic twin pairs out of 22 pairs of identical twins in a clinical investigation from the Department of Dermatology in Oslo. In one of the pairs the affected partner had mild itching eczema every winter on the back of the foot. The clinical details are convincingly described in the second pair of twins. The diagnosis of zygosity was based on clinical resemblance between the partners: "identical hair, ears, eyes, teeth, nose and mouth facial form."

The extensive German publication by Kochs [41] contained a few data on three dizygotic pairs of twins of which the author had investigated two pairs which were both concordant. However, the pedigree of one of the families showed that one of the partners was 21 and the other 23 years of age! There was no information on the diagnosis of zygosity. In a work on skin reactivity in atopics following local application of nicotinic acid esters, the patients included a concordant monozygotic pair of twins in which the partners had both atopic eczema and ichthyosis [37].

In 1953 Höcker [34] published a careful study of a concordant monozygotic twin pair where both partners were followed up from the age of 9 months by repeated visits to the Department of Dermatology in Munich. A complete description of the anthropologic methods used was given, and the diagnosis of zygosity was determined by detection of identical genetic markers with regard to the AB0 and Rhesus systems.

Bowen [9] observed 59 monozygotic atopic twin pairs over a period of 15 years. The ages of the twins ranged from 8 weeks to 56 years. The diagnosis of zygosity was based on the similarity between twin partners and confirmed by the obstetric records which showed them to be monoplacental. Three pairs of twins were discordant with regard to "infantile eczema."

In a summary from a society meeting, a short case report was given on a 14-month-old monozygotic twin pair in which both partners had shown eczematous skin changes since the age of 6 weeks [25]. In both cases the eczema started behind the ears with subsequent spreading to the face, body, and extremities. There were no details about the diagnosis of zygosity.

Among the hospital subjects studied by Rajka [60], there were 14 pairs of twins suffering from atopic eczema. The age of the twins varied from 10 to 49 years, the average being 24 years. The pairwise concordance rate was higher in the dizygotic than in the monozygotic twin pairs, namely 40% for monozygotic and 67% for dizygotic twin pairs. The diagnosis of zygosity was established in the "usual manner."

The monograph by Schnyder [64] was partly based on a twin series compiled in different ways. A total of 22 pairs of twins with atopy were identified through the family study. The population study supplied information regarding an additional 46 pairs, thus a total of 68 pairs of twins were identified, but 33 pairs were excluded because the twin partner was either dead or had emigrated. Of the remaining 13 pairs, seven had contacted the author due to the public interest the investigation aroused in Zürich.

The pairwise concordance rate of atopic eczema was 50% for monozygotic and 0% for dizygotic pairs of twins (Table 4). The diagnosis of zygosity was made on the basis of Siemens' polysymptomatic method [73] and blood typing, presumably the AB0 and Rhesus systems.

In the family study of Dorn [20], eight pairs of twins were reported. The same material was discussed in a chapter on skin diseases in a comprehensive German textbook of genetics [81], although mention is only made of seven monozygotic pairs, of which one pair was concordant and six were disconcordant. One of the authors had examined three of the pairs himself, while reliable information was said to be available about the others. No information was provided as to the criteria for determination of zygosity.

Niermann [57] published a thesis in 1964 on skin diseases in twins which had been identified in two ways: (1) The questioning of all patients at the University Hospital in Münster, FRG, as to whether they were twins; this resulted in 468 twin pairs. (2) All the persons in the regional Register of Tuberculosis and Cancer were questioned to determine the number of twins; a further 85 twin pairs were identified. Some of the twin partners, however, had either died or emigrated, and thus, out of 553 twin pairs, an examination of both partners was possible in only 370 of them. The determination of zygosity relied on Siemens' polysymptomatic method [73], and it was not entirely clear whether the infantile phase was included in the definition of atopic eczema, which was diagnosed in 18 twin pairs; the pairwise concordance rate for monozygotic twins was 100% and 23% for dizygotic twins (Table 4). In 1974 a study was reported from the National Research Council Twin Register, which stores medical data on all male American citizens who served in the Armed Forces, mainly during World War II [46]. Although it was possible to identify 16000 pairs in which both partners were alive, only seven pairs of twins within an accessible distance of the author were willing to participate. The results are given in Table 4. The case history for the discordant monozygotic pair was convincingly stated, while the history of the concordant monozygotic pair "seemed to be that of dyshidrosis." No clinical information was supplied about the two discordant dizygotic pairs or the remaining unaffected pairs of twins. The determination of zygosity relied on seven blood type systems and on finger prints.

The most extensive investigation of atopic diseases in twins was based on a mailed questionnaire study from the Swedish Twin Register [21]. The twin register covers all twin pairs born in Sweden during the period 1886–1925 with both partners alive in 1961. In 1967 a questionnaire was sent to all the unbroken, like-sexed pairs of twins. Of these, 75% or about 7000 pairs completed and returned the questionnaire, which contained a number of questions designed to evaluate the type of zygosity by means of the similarity method [12]. In relation to atopic eczema the following questions were asked (numbered as on the form):

4. Did you have eczema when your were a baby?
   No ...
   Yes ...
6. Do you know the name of the skin condition you have or have had?
   e) Yes, eczema at the knee or elbow fold
   g) Yes, other, namely ...

An affirmative answer was given by 350 twins (2.5%): 280 gave a positive answer to question 4, although only 70 twins answered "Yes" to 6e and 6g. The pairwise concordance rate was 15% for monozygotic and 5% for dizygotic twin pairs. The difference was statistically significant with a χ^2 value of 10.83. The number of concordant and discordant pairs was not given.

This historical survey of twin studies has provided an opportunity to emphasize some general problems in twin studies. Uncertainty in the classification of the disease and of zygosity is evident in several of the investigations. The case reports were often published for the sake of curiosity value rather than for their scientific value. It is surprising that none of them contained a detailed and profound analysis of discordant monozygotic pairs of twins. Representativeness is of crucial importance in twin studies; representative twin series is defined as a series of twins in which the distribution of the type of zygosity and the concordance-discordance status is the same as in the twin population for the disease under consideration. In the study of Schnyder [64] the self-reported twins and the twins identified by the familial study may introduce a degree of selection which cannot be evaluated. The consecutive, patient-based series of twins of Niermann [57] might be representative if all the patients had been classified correctly as either being a twin or a nontwin individual. In fact, a twinning ratio of 553:33956 = 0.02 was found, which is in agreement with the expected value. However, in the twin series there was a predominance of females (64%) which exceeded that of the background population (54%). In addition, the distribution of like-sexed dizygotic and unlike-sexed twin pairs did not fit with the distribution expected from Weinberg's difference method (expected number of like-sexed dizygotic pairs = 2 x number of unlike-sexed pairs; actual data 142 vs 2x 129). The result of the Swedish twin study [21] gave surprisingly low pairwise concordance rate for both monozygotic and dizygotic twin pairs. A possible explanation might include: (1) no validation of the consequences of the 25% nonresponders resulting in presumably missing data; (2) no sufficient evaluation of replies to the vague question 4, the answers to which may merely reflect skin problems in childhood; (3) recall bias in twins 42–81 years of age and (4) the fact that this mailed questionnaire study served purposes other than the study of atopy and included more than 200 questions about general health.

Since valid criticism can be directed against the twin studies referred to above, we initiated a Danish population-based twin study. The object was to identify all living twins restricted to a well-defined geographical area (the county of Fyn) and to a limited age group (birth cohort 1960–1974) suitable for the study of atopic eczema [66, 68, 71]. The strategy for establishing the actual twin series rested upon the data content of the Danish identification number system. By means of demographic data and the follow-up of a relevant birth cohort, it was recognized that the identification system implied a deficiency of about 3%–4% of twin pairs where both partners were alive. The compilation of probands was achieved by a short and simple one page mailed questionnaire and an accompanying letter defining atopic eczema in common language. The response rate surpassed 98%, and an evaluation of the question of atopic eczema revealed very few false-negative answers. In the subsequent clinical examination of the affirmative responders, attention was primarily directed to the diagnosis of atopic eczema. The criteria [29, 30] were adapted to the special clinical situation which allowed us to interview both the twins and the parents at the same time. In doubtful cases the twins were classified as possible atopic eczema and were not included in the calculations. The diagnosis of zygosity was confirmed by an extensive system of polymorphic genetic markers [67]. The number of concordant and discordant twin pairs and the derived concordance rates are given in Table 5. This twin study demonstrated that the genetic component has a far greater influence on the phenotypic expression of atopic eczema than presumed from the Swedish twin study [21]. The risk of developing the disease in a monozygotic twin having a twin partner with atopic eczema (0.86) differs significantly from the risk run by dizygotic twin partners (0.21) and other siblings (0.25). Thus, there can be no doubt that genetic susceptibility plays a decisive role in the development of atopic eczema.

Table 5. Number of concordant and discordant twin pairs with atopic eczema and the concordance rates for the two types of zygosity

	Zygosity Monozygous	Dizygous
Concordant twin pairs	17 (32)	4 (6)
Discordant twin pairs	5 (5)	22 (22)
Pairwise concordance rate	0.77*	0.15
Proband concordance rate	0.86	0.21

Number of probands in parentheses
$^*\chi^2 = 18.54$, $p < 0.001$

Table 6. The number of siblings with and without atopic eczema of concordant and discordant monozygotic pairs of twins

	Number of siblings of: concordant monozygotic twin pairs	discordant monozygotic twin pairs
With atopic eczema	6*	0
Without atopic eczema	11	6
Total	17	6

* Fisher's exact test (1-tailed): $p = 0.12$.

Genetic heterogeneity within a disease entity means that identical or almost identical clinical manifestations (phenotypes) are caused by different genotypes. If atopic eczema was caused by one and the same genotype, one would expect that the occurrence of the disease to be the same in siblings to concordant and discordant monozygotic twin pairs [69]. As illustrated in Table 6, application of this twin-family method reveals a tendency of single-born siblings of discordant monozygotic twin pairs not to have the disease, although available data are unable to confirm this statement at an acceptable level of significance.

Human Leucocyte Antigen (HLA) System

As a majority of HLA-associated diseases are characterized by abnormal immunity, it has been of obvious interest to study the distribution of HLA antigens in atopic eczema. Many of the basic features of the genetics of the HLA system have been explored during the past two decades. Population and family studies have shown that the HLA haplotype is inherited in a codominant fashion and behaves in accordance with Mendelian principles. The HLA complex is located on the short arm of chromosome 6, which also carries other well-defined genetic markers. Humans have four loci with well-established relative chromosomal positions: HLA-A, HLA-B, HLA-C, and HLA-D, with the centromeric limit being the HLA-D locus. Each of the four loci has a series of alleles which determines the corresponding gene products (HLA antigens) on the cell membrane.

The extent of polymorphism varies among different genes. Currently, approximately 20 A, 40 B, 8 C, and 12 D alleles have been defined. However, there are strong indications that undetected alleles, especially of HLA-C and HLA-D genes, remain. The HLA frequencies vary over a broad range in different ethnic populations. The HLA complex reveals linkage disequilibrium, and certain haplotypes such as A1, B8, Dw3/DR3 are strikingly common in Caucasians. The mechanism for this nonrandom gametic association has been the subject of speculation. The most favored explanation of the presumed survival advantage attributed to certain HLA-haplotypes is that the phenomenon represents an augmented resistance to certain infectious diseases, especially to those which are prevalent in the environment.

In the first publication on HLA antigens in atopic eczema, by Krain and Terasaki [42] in 1973, reported an enhanced frequency of HLA-A3 and HLA-A9 in a group comprising 45 patients and 870 controls. This association could not be detected in later French studies of a limited study population of 30 patients and 27 controls, rather, HLA-B35 was significantly increased with the disease [18, 27]. However, a simultaneous, but less detailed study reported no difference in the antigen frequency of 26 HLA types in 103 patients with atopic eczema [65]. Similar negative observations have been made in the Japanese population [59] and, recently, in a population-based nonethnically mixed group of 68 Caucasians with atopic eczema [67]. Thorough evaluation of earlier positive studies disclose that no regard had been taken to the number of antigens studied when calculating the level of significance, i.e., without correction for mass significance. The calculated p values in all the positive studies were not below the level of 0.01, which is considered necessary in order to demonstrate an association between an HLA antigen and a disease. Other sources of bias may be attributed to stratification effects owing to data collected from ethnically mixed groups and hospital-based control subjects in which the tested individuals had been HLA-typed due to suspected HLA-associated diseases.

Some early studies reported an augmented prevalence of the HLA-A1, B8 haplotype in childhood asthma [80], and in 1977 Turner et al. [80a] undertook an investigation of HLA-A1, B8 in combined atopy. They found an increased frequency in 18 patients with combined atopy characterized by bronchial asthma, allergic rhinitis, and atopic eczema. Later works were unable to confirm this finding either in 43 cases of combined atopy [78] or in an atopic eczema group consisting of 61 patients with pure atopic eczema and seven with combined atopy [67]. In the only existing report on HLA-DR antigens, Svejgaard et al. [78] mentioned a strikingly low frequency of HLA-DR7 in 34 cases of both pure atopic eczema and combined atopy. However, the decrease was not statistically significant even before correcting for the number of studied antigens.

Thus, population studies in the field of HLA and atopic eczema have not provided any conclusive observations, nor have the few family studies [47, 68], although the last-mentioned study revealed an astonishing, but possibly coincidental, linkage between haplotype A2, Bw35, Cw2 and atopic eczema in five family members in three generations. However, in light of recent findings, family studies of extended haplotypes might be a fruitful area of research.

Immunogenetics

Two important discoveries in the 1960s changed the approach to studying the genetics of atopy: the new immunoglobulin class IgE and the demonstration of immune response genes in inbred strains of mice [38, 45]. In accordance with this progress, we have to consider two broad classes of immunogenetic control in atopy: (1) the regulation of the biosynthesis and metabolism of IgE class antibodies and (2) the effect of specific immune response genes, although a complete discussion of this complex area of research is far beyond the scope of this chapter.

Bazarel et al. [5] were the first to explore the genetics of IgE by measuring serum IgE levels in infants and their mothers. By ranking the values of IgE, the study revealed an apparent relationship of IgE levels both to family history and to the allergic symptoms reported in the 6-month-old infants. They postulated that the IgE level was controlled by two alleles at a single locus. The genetic basis of IgE expression was supported by a subsequent study in adult twins and twin children estimating the heritability to be 0.59 in adults and 0.79 in children [6]. Although some criticism can be raised against the calculation of genetic variance and heritability according to the now rarely employed Holzinger's index [13, 14, 39], it is remarkable that the intrapair variance of log IgE levels in adult monozygotic and dizygotic twin pairs is of exactly the same magnitude as was found later on in a nonatopic control group [66].

There is no agreement on how to analyze and present quantitative twin data; however, some of the simplifying prerequisite assumptions of heritability estimates have been enumerated [13, 82]. These include: (1) The effect of environment is similar for the two types of twins. This is one of the most troublesome assumptions in twin research as higher common environmental covariance in monozygotic than in dizygotic twin pairs results in overestimation of genetic variance. (2) There is no interaction between genotype and environment. If such a genotypic-environmental covariance exists, it could influence twin partners differently in dizygotic twin pairs thereby inducing a further degree of overestimation in the calculation of genetic variance. (3) The trait under study is continuously distributed without variance due to dominance or epistasis. (4) Computation of the heritability requires knowledge of the total population variance for the trait under consideration. These obstacles in the computations of heritability estimates have not been considered thoroughly in several twin studies on IgE expression [2, 6, 35, 43, 74, 84]. The studies indicate that the level of IgE in peripheral blood is partly genetically determined and that the heritability index is around 0.60–0.70. In light of the aforementioned reservations, this estimate is probably biased upwards. Thus, in an attempt to overcome some of these problems, the serum IgE level was measured in a nonatopic control group of twins [66]. The study showed that genetic variance comprised about 50% of the total phenotypic variance of IgE. Furthermore, an analysis of variance of IgE indicated a greater environmental covariance in monozygotic than in dizygotic twin pairs and that dominance variance plays a role in the regulation of IgE. The data did not indicate the presence of genotypic-environmental interaction in serum IgE.

Two family studies [7, 28] have confirmed that genetic factors are operative in the regulation of IgE. By segregation analysis the heritability was calculated to 0.44 and 0.40, respectively. The population study of Billewicz et al. [7], from two villages in Gambia, provided an outcome that was comparable to those of twin studies [66]. Despite differences in race and the mode of analysis, the genetic variance and the phenotypic variance of IgE exhibited almost identical results in the two investigations.

The twin studies and the family studies clearly demonstrate that a strictly environmental hypothesis can be rejected. However, no definite conclusions have been reached as to the mode of inheritance of IgE. Marsh et al. [49] provided the first segregation analysis, based on 28 mainly Maryland families having a total of 108 children. At least one of the children in each family was allergic to pollens. The parents were classified into different mating types with regard to IgE levels (high x high, high x low, low x low) and their offspring were also classified as having either high or low IgE levels. The IgE value that best discriminated between allergic and nonallergic individuals was used as a cutoff point between high and low serum IgE. The analyses provided evidence for a major IgE-regulating gene (*R*/*r*) with hyper-IgE production (high serum IgE level) being inherited as an autosomal recessive trait. Gerrard et al. [26] studied 173 white Canadian families, 145 randomly selected and 29 with a high prevalence of atopy. The computer-assisted complex segregation analyses of Morton and MacLean [56] supported the hypothesis of a major IgE locus, as well as a significant polygenic influence for IgE regulation. The gene frequency for the *r* allele was 0.49 in Saskatchewan, which was in close agreement with the value of 0.52 obtained by Marsh and his coworkers [49] in Baltimore. However, subsequent studies of three large allergic families [8], 23 randomly selected Amish families [52], and five Mormon pedigrees [32] failed to prove the existence of a major IgE-regulating locus. The latter studies used complex segregation analyses according to the method of Elston and Stewart [24]. Mendelian, polygenic, sporadic, and mixed models (major gene plus a polygenic component) were fitted to the data. In the work of Blumenthal et al. [8] the same model did not give the best fit for each pedigree, thus suggesting genetic heterogeneity, and in the Mormon study a mixed model with a major gene and a polygenic component did not fit the data significantly better than did a polygenic model alone [32]. In an extension of the last-mentioned investigation, Meyers et al. [53] performed a linkage study between 21 polymorphisms including HLA-A, HLA-B, and the postulated IgE-regulating gene, with negative results. Recently, Meyers et al. [55] conducted a new study of IgE levels in 42 nuclear families selected through a member working in a large corporation in Baltimore. Segregation analysis (including a mixed model described by Hasstedt [31]) of these fairly randomly ascertained families once more indicated the existence of a major recessive high IgE gene, but in addition like previous researchers [8, 32, 52], they observed significant polygenic control over IgE production.

The specific immune response, as measured by the radioallergosorbent test (RAST) and skin testing, has been studied in twins [35, 84]. However, because of the previously discussed problems and limitations in twin research, the results are difficult to interpret. The investigations indicated that sensitivity to antigens, as opposed to the IgE level, may be influenced more by the environment than by genetic factors. It is also possible that the detrimental effect of certain antigens, e. g., house dust may involve a greater genetic component in the diseased individual than does the susceptibility to certain other antigens, for example, pollens.

In summary, genetic analyses of total IgE and the

specific IgE response to certain antigens represent an extremely difficult task to accomplish. The strategy for future studies must include randomly ascertained nonethnically mixed probands taking due regard to age, sex, smoking habits, the presumed period of minimal antigenic stimulation, and perhaps other confounding variables. However, the sophisticated computer programs used necessitate cautiousness about the conclusions as only small changes in the data could change the outcome. Thus, less technical approaches to data processing would be highly desirable. For now, it is apparent from the literature that about 50% of the variation in serum IgE can be attributed to genetic variation. Furthermore, in keeping with the indication of dominance variance from twin studies [66], it seems that this genetic component could be explained by a Mendelian component (with high IgE being recessively inherited) that may act on a polygenic background. However, another interpretation might be that a major gene is operative in some families, but not in others, and careful consideration of genetic heterogeneity in IgE regulation appears essential.

In continuation of the mouse studies of the 1960s [38, 45], research into the area of immune response (Ir) genes in humans has been closely linked to the science of immunology. As in all rapidly developing areas of research, new techniques and terminology form an almost insurmountable barrier for those who are not specialists in the field. A comprehensive and challenging review has recently been published [48], and some of the features should be recounted. Recent developments indicate that the HLA-D region in humans contains the Ir genes. Immune-associated (Ia) molecules, or class II antigens (designed DR, DQ, and DP), are a set of Ir genes expressed on antigen-presenting cells which interact with specific receptors on subsets of T lymphocytes. That is, a response occurs only if the antigen is presented in the context of a specific class II antigen. Current thinking suggests the following steps: (1) "processing" of the antigen by the antigen-presenting cell with subsequent presentation of the antigen (or antigen fragment), together with a Ia molecule, to a specific receptor on a helper T cell (with secondary interleukin-1 mediated clonal expansion of the T cell involved); (2) interaction of the antigen with an immunoglobulin-like receptor on a B cell that has affinity for the specific antigen (or antigen fragment) followed by processing and presentation of the antigen to the expanding population of antigen-specific T cells; (3) clonal expansion of the B cells involved leading to formation of plasma cells and specific antibody production, including IgE and IgG4.

Recently Marsh and Bias [48] postulated that during normal exposure to, for example, pollens only certain (antigenic) fragments of the antigen will be processed by the antigen-presenting cell, and that sometimes only a few peptides on the antigens can be expected to contain the immunoreactive sites that bind both to T cell receptors and the Ia molecule.

From this concept of the T-cell-dependent humoral immune response, one might predict that it would be relatively simple to show linkage between a specific immune response and a particular familial HLA haplotype. This, however, has not been the case, and accordingly it has been suggested that the lack of success in observing genetic linkage in family studies may result from: (1) a failure of certain family members to process the correct HLA haplotype containing the appropriate Ir gene, (2) the involvement of different HLA-linked Ir genes on different haplotypes, (3) a decisive role of as yet unidentified non-HLA-linked Ir genes, or (4) a not yet understood interaction with anti-idiotype antibodies. Finally, there are other HLA-linked loci coded on the short arm of chromosome 6 such as C2, C4a, C4b, GLO, and PGM3. Together with the HLA system they form so-called extended haplotypes. Thus far, the genetics of atopy, including atopic eczema, has not been analyzed as a function of such extended haplotypes. It remains possible that discrepancies in the HLA studies on the immune response are due to a hitherto undetected segregation of certain Ir gene containing extended haplotypes.

Conclusions and Closing Remarks

First, it should be stated that the study of the genetics of atopic eczema is in its infancy. Part of the explanation for this might be related to selected or incompletely defined study subjects. With the recently proposed diagnostic guidelines [29, 30], these obstacles should be surmounted, but the criteria cannot said to be adequate for studies dependent on anamnestic data. Secondly, it is highly probable that strong genetic components are operative in atopic eczema. Moreover, there is a growing body of evidence favoring the concept that atopic eczema, like many other common diseases, is multifactorial in nature. It is particularly worth emphasizing the potential role of one or a few major genes in many supposedly multifactorial traits. The identification of such major genes clearly ought to have high priority, and obviously the gene that determines IgE production must be one of the candidates. Thirdly, there is some indication of genetic heterogeneity within atopic eczema. This implies that still undetected subgroups of atopic eczema may be inherited by different genetic mechanisms or they may not be genetic at all. Thus, another research effort should be directed towards the elaboration of certain marker profiles that will aid in identifying those subgroups. Finally, in the more distant future, one could hope that a more complete understanding of the genetic control of the immune response and how it works in respiratory atopy will help us to gain more insight into the genetics of atopic eczema.

References

1. Adkinson J (1920) The behaviour of bronchial asthma as an inherited character. Genetics 5: 363–418
2. Al-Agidi S (1980) Serum immunoglobin levels in Iraqi twins. Hum Biol 52: 393–399
3. Arsdel PP van, Motulsk AG (1959) Frequency and heritability of asthma and allergic rhinitis in college students. Acta Genet (Basel) 9: 101–114
4. Baer RL (1955) The development of the concept of atopic dermatitis. Am Pract Dig Treat 6: 1074–1078
5. Bazarel M, Orgel HA, Hamburger RN (1971) IgE levels in normal infants and mothers and an inheritance hyphothesis. J Immunol 107: 794–801
6. Bazarel M, Orgel HA, Hamburger RN (1974) Genetics of IgE and allergy: serum IgE levels in twins. J Allergy Clin Immunol 54: 288–304
7. Billewicz WZ, McGregor IA, Roberts DF, Rowe DS, Wilson RJM (1974) Family studies in immunoglobulin levels. Clin Exp Immunol 16: 13–22
8. Blumenthal MN, Namboodiri K, Mendell N, Gleich G, Elston RC, Yunis (1981) Genetic transmission of serum IgE levels. Am J Med Genet 10: 219–228
9. Bowen R (1953) Allergy in identical twins. J Allergy 24: 236–244
10. Bueno LE (1935) Eczema verdadero en dos gemelos. Acta Derm Sifiliogr 27: 579–583
11. Buffum WP, Feinberg B (1940) Bronchial asthma in three pairs of identical twins. J Allergy Clin Immunol 11: 604–606
12. Cederlöf R, Friberg L, Johnsson E, Kaij L (1961) Studies of similarity diagnosis in twins with the aid of mailed questionnaires. Acta Genet (Basel) 11: 338–362
13. Christian JC (1979) Testing twin means and estimating genetic variance. Basic methodology for the analysis of quantitative twin data. Acta Genet Med Gemellol (Roma) 28: 35–40
14. Christian JC, Kang KW, Norton JA (1974) Choice of an estimate of genetic variance from twin data. Am J Hum Genet 26: 154–161
15. Clarke JA, Donnally HH, Coca AF (1928) Studies in specific hypersensitivenss. XXXII. On the influence of heredity in atopy. J Immunol 15: 9–11
16. Cooke RA, van der Veer A (1916) Human sensitization. J Immunol 1: 201–305
17. Criep LH (1942) Allergy in identical twins. J Allergy 13: 591–598
18. Desmons F, Delmas-Marsalet Y, Goudemand J (1976) HLA antigens in atopic dermatitis. Allergol Immunopathol (Madr) 4: 29–38
19. Dorn H (1957) Erbbiologische Betrachtungen zum Allergieproblem. Z Haut Geschlechtskr 23: 5–10
20. Dorn H (1961) Neurodermitis vom humangenetischen Standpunkt. Acta Allergol 16: 451–462
21. Edfors-Lubs M-L (1971) Allergy in 7000 twin pairs. Acta Allergol 26: 249–285
22. Edgren G (1943) Prognose und Erblichkeitsmomente bei Ekzema Infantum. Eine Klinisch-statistische Untersuchung von Allergieerscheinungen. Acta Paediatr Scand [Suppl 2] 30: 1–204
23. Edwards JH (1960) The stimulation of Mendelism. Acta Genet (Basel) 10: 63–70
24. Elston RC, Steward J (1971) A general model for the genetic analysis of pedigree data. Hum Hered 21: 523–542
25. Frain-Bell W, Koblenzer P (1960) Eczema in identical twins. Br J Dermatol 72: 165
26. Gerrard JW, Rao DC, Morton NE (1978) A genetic study of immunoglobulin E. Am J Hum Genet 30: 46–58
27. Goudemand J, Defrenne C, Desmons F (1977) HLA antigens and atopic dermatitis. Monogr Allerg 11: 24–29
28. Grundbacher FJ (1975) Causes of variation in serum IgE levels in normal populations. J Allergy Clin Immunol 56: 104–111
29. Hanifin JM, Lobitz WC (1977) Newer concepts of atopic dermatitis. Arch Dermatol 113: 663–670
30. Hanifin JM, Rajka G (1980) Diagnostic features of atopic dermatitis. Acta Derm Venereol [Suppl] (Stockh) 92: 44–47
31. Hasstedt SJ (1982) A mixed-model likelihood approximation on large pedigree. Comput Biomed Res 15: 295–307
32. Hasstedt SJ, Meyers DA, Marsh DG (1983) Inheritance of immunoglobulin E: genetic model fitting. Am J Med Genet 14: 61–66
33. Hellerström S, Lidman H (1956) Studies of Besnier's prurigo (atopic dermatitis) Acta Derm Venereol (Stockh) 36: 11–22
34. Höcker H (1953) Konkordantes Auftreten eines exsudativen Ekzematoids bei eineiigen weiblichen Zwillingen. Hautarzt 4: 21–24
35. Hopp RJ, Bewtra SAK, Watt GD, Nair NM, Townley RG (1984) Genetic analysis of allergic disease in twins. J Allergy Clin Immunol 73: 265–270
36. Hruszek H (1938) Zur Frage der Erblichkeit des Ekzems, insbesondere der Neurodermitis. Dermatol Wochenschr 106: 239–240
37. Illig L (1952) Die Reaktion der Haut des Neurodermitikers auf zwei nikotinsäuresterhaltige Reizstoffe. Dermatol Wochenschr 126: 753–55
38. Ishizaka K, Ishizaka T, Hornbrook MM (1966) Physicochemical properties of reaginic antibodies. V. Correlation of reaginic activity with γE antibody. J Immunol 97: 840–853
39. Kang KW, Corey LA, Evans MM, Christian JC, Norton JA (1977) Dominance and environmental variances: Their effect on heritabilities estimated from twin data. Hum Hered 27: 9–21
40. Kjellman N-IM (1977) Atopic disease in seven-year-old children. Acta Paediatr Scand 66: 465–471

41. Kochs AG (1951) Untersuchungen zur Konstitutions- und Erblichkeitsfrage bei der atopischen Dermatitis (Neurodermitis). Arch Dermatol Syphilol 193: 363–405
42. Krain LS, Terasaki PI (1973) HLA types in atopic dermatitis. Lancet i: 1059–1060
43. Lee SK, Metrakos JD, Tanaka KR, Heiner DC (1980) Genetic influence on serum IgD levels. Pediatr Res 14: 60–63
44. Leigh D, Marley E (1967) Bronchial asthma. A genetic, population and psychiatric study. Pergamon, Oxford
45. Levine BB, Ojeda A, Benacerraf B (1963) Studies on artificial antigens. III. The genetic control of the immune response to hapten-poly-L-lysine conjugates in guinea pigs. J Exp Med 118: 953–957
46. Lynfield YL (1974) Skin diseases in twins. Arch Dermatol 110: 722–724
47. MacKie RM, Dick HM (1979) A study of HLA antigen distribution in families with atopic dermatitis. Allergy 34: 19–23
48. Marsh DG, Bias WB (1988) The genetics of atopic allergy. In: Samter M, Talmage DW, Frank MM, Austen KF, Claman HN (eds) Immunological diseases, 4rd edn. Little, Brown, Boston, pp 1027–1045
49. Marsh DG, Bias WB, Ishizaka K (1974) Genetic control of basal serum immunoglobulin E level and its effect on specific reaginic sensitivity. Proc Natl Acad Sci USA 71: 3588–3592
50. Mayr JK (1935) Zur Vererbbarkeit des Ekzems. Arch Dermatol Syphilol 171: 612–621
51. Melsom R (1945) Dermatological investigations on 22 pairs of identical twins. Acta Derm Venereol (Stockh) 25: 29–47
52. Meyers DA, Beaty TH, Freidhoff LR, Marsh DG (1987) Inheritance of total IgE (basal levels) in man. Am J Hum Genet 41: 51–62
53. Meyers DA, Bias WB, Marsh DG (1982) A genetic study of total IgE in the Amish. Hum Hered 32: 15–23
54. Meyers DA, Freidhoff LR, Marsh DG (1986) Predicting skin-sensitivity and total serum IgE levels in family members. J Allergy Clin Immunol 77: 608–616
55. Meyers DA, Hasstedt SJ, Marsh DG (1983) The inheritance of immunoglobulin E: linkage analysis. Am J Med Genet 16: 575–582
56. Morton NE, MacLean CJ (1974) Analysis of family resemblance. III. Complex segregation of quantitative traits. Am J Hum Genet 26: 489–503
57. Niermann H (1964) Zwillingsdermatologie. Springer, Berlin Heidelberg New York
58. Nexmand PH (1948) Clinical studies of Besnier's prurigo. Thesis, University of Copenhagen, Rosenkilde and Bagger, Copenhagen
59. Ohikido M, Ozawa A, Matsuo I, Niizuma K, Nakano M, Tsuji I, Nose Y, Ito M, Kato S, Yamamoto K (1977) HLA antigens and susceptibility to atopic dermatitis. Monogr Allergy 11: 36–43
60. Rajka G (1960) Prurigo Besnier (atopic dermatitis) with special reference to the role of allergic factors. I. The influence of atopic hereditary factors. Acta Derm Venereol 40: 285–306
61. Rajka G (1975) Atopic dermatitis. Saunders, London
62. Ratner B, Silberman D (1953) Critical analysis of the hereditary concept of allergy. J Allergy 24: 371–378
63. Schmidt-Kehl L (1933) Über den Vererbungsmodus bei den allergischen Krankheiten. Arch Rassen Gesellschaftsbiol 27: 175–179
64. Schnyder UW (1960) Neurodermitis – Asthma – Rhinitis. Eine genetisch-allergologische Studie. Acta Genet Stat Med 10 (Suppl 18): 1–106
65. Scholtz S, Ziegler E, Wünster H, Braun-Falco O, Albert ED (1977) HLA family studies in patients with atopic dermatitis. Monogr Allergy 11: 44
66. Schultz Larsen F (1985) Atopic dermatitis. Etiological studies based on a twin population. Thesis, University of Odense, Lægeforeningen, Copenhagen
67. Schultz Larsen F, Grunnet N (1987) Genetic investigations in atopic dermatitis. Tissue Antigens 29: 1–6
68. Schultz Larsen F, Holm NV (1983) Evaluation of an identification method of twin pairs based on the personal numbering system in Denmark. Dan Med Bull 30: 424–427
69. Schultz Larsen F, Holm NV (1985) Genetic heterogeneity in atopic dermatitis elucidated by a twin-family study. Ann Allergy 55: 266
70. Schultz Larsen F, Grunnet N, Vase P (1980) HLA antigens in atopic dermatitis. A family study. Dermatologica 160: 17–20
71. Schultz Larsen F, Holm NV, Henningsen K (1986) Atopic dermatitis. A genetic-epidemiologic study in a population-based twin sample. J Am Acad Dermatol 15: 487–494
72. Schwartz M (1952) Heredity in bronchial asthma. Thesis, University of Copenhagen, Munksgård, Copenhagen
73. Siemens HW (1924) Die Zwillingspathologie. Springer, Berlin
74. Sistonen P, Johnsson V, Koskenvuo M, Aho K (1980) Serum IgE levels in twins. Hum Hered 30: 155–58
75. Spaich D, Ostertag M (1936) Untersuchungen über allergische Erkrankungen bei Zwillingen. Z Menschl Vererbungs-Konstitutionslehre 19: 731–752
76. Storm K, Haahr J, Kjellman N-IM, Østerballe O (1986) Forekomsten af asthma allergisk rhinitis, atopisk dermatitis og urticaria hos en årgang af danske børn. Ugeskr Læger 148: 3295–3299
77. Sulzberger MB, Goodman J (1936) The relative importance of specific skin hypersensitivity in adult atopic dermatitis. JAMA 106: 1000–1003
78. Svejgaard E, Jakobsen B, Svejgaard A (1985) Studies of HLA-ABC and DR antigens in pure atopic dermatitis and atopic dermatitis combined with allergic respiratory disease. Acta Derm Venereol [Suppl] (Stockh) 114: 72–76
79. Taylor B, Wadsworth M, Wadswoth J, Peckham C (1984) Changes in the reported prevalence of childhood eczema since 1939–45 war. Lancet ii: 1255–1258
80. Thorsby E, Engeset A, Lie SO (1971) HL-A antigens and susceptibility to diseases. A study of patients with acute lymphoblastic leukaemia, Hodgkin's disease, and childhood asthma. Tissue Antigens 1: 147–152
80a. Turner MW, Brostoff J, Wells RS, Stokes CR, Soothill JF (1977) HLA in eczema and hay fever. Clin Exp Immunol 27: 43–47
81. Vogel F, Dorn H (1964) Atopische Hauterkrankungen. Atopische Dermatitis. In: Becker PE (ed) Humangenetik, vol 4. Thieme, Stuttgart, pp 418–428
82. Vogel F, Motulsky AG (1986) Human genetics. Problems and approaches. Springer, Berlin Heidelberg New York
83. Wiener AS, Zieve I, Fries JH (1936) The inheritance of allergic disease. Ann Eugener 7: 141–162
84. Wüthrich B, Baumann E, Fries RA, Schnyder UW (1981) Total and specific IgE (RAST) in atopic twins. Clin Allergy 11: 147–154
85. Uehara M (1982) Reduced histamine reaction in atopic dermatitis. Arch Dermatol 118: 244–245

Clinical Symptoms of Atopic Eczema

H. Merk

The clinical symptoms of atopic eczema may be precipitated at any time in a patient's lifetime, although in most cases first signs and symptoms appear during childhood. Most patients have a personal or family history of asthma, hay fever, or eczema. At least 5% of all children are affected at some time and although a late onset is possible, it is rare. In a study performed with a group of 121 patients the average age of the patients at first manifestation of the disease was 5.5 months and the prognosis of atopic eczema turned out to be worse if the disease had begun within the first 6 months after birth, if it occurred in firstborn or only children, or if the patients had a history of allergies of the respiratory tract [19]. The data on prognosis vary greatly in the literature. In a prospective study of about 2000 children, 87% of the patients had a significant improvement of the disease after 5–20 years.

The main signs and symptoms of atopic eczema are dry skin, itching, and eczematous inflammation. Lichenification and eczematous lesions in the antecubital and popliteal areas are the most typical signs of atopic eczema, apart from infantile onset, and allow a first view diagnosis. Minor atopic features including perlèche, Dennie-Morgan infraorbital fold, hyperlinear palms, nickel sensitivity, Hertoghe sign, pityriasis alba, periauricular fissures, follicular accentuations, nipple dermatitis, and ichthyosis are most important for the diagnosis of minor forms of atopic eczema and will be discussed in detail in another chapter of this volume. Although the major features of atopic eczema are most familiar and there is no difficulty in recognizing them, there is no specific histologic or laboratory marker for diagnosing the majority of clinical signs and symptoms of this multifaceted disease. Its diagnosis is therefore entirely dependent upon the history of the patients and their family and the composition of the signs and symptoms of the disease. Furthermore, the physical findings will hint at the pathophysiological characteristics of atopic eczema and have a major impact on therapeutic decisions.

The clinical signs and symptoms of atopic eczema, differ according to the period of the patient's life in which onset occurs. The very early infantile phase usually starts around 3 months of age, but may also start even earlier in the 2nd week after birth, although this is uncommon. Apart from this, there is also a childhood, an adolescent, and finally an adult phase.

In the infantile phase, the face, the extremities – especially the extensor aspect –, and finally the trunk are involved. The early infantile phase is characterized by erythematous, squamous inflammation which may worsen to the point of exudation, a feature which is much more often observed in the early infantile phase than in the late infantile phase. In late infantile phase impetiginized, vesicular, nummular, papulovesicular, infiltrated, eczema-like, and especially lichen-like symptoms become more and more prominent. In early

Fig. 1. Eczematous inflammation on the face in the early childhood phase of atopic eczema

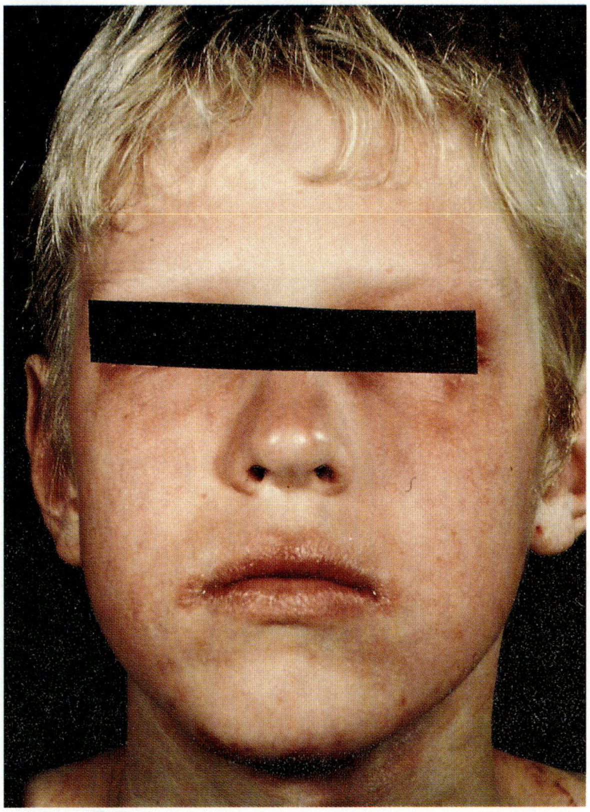

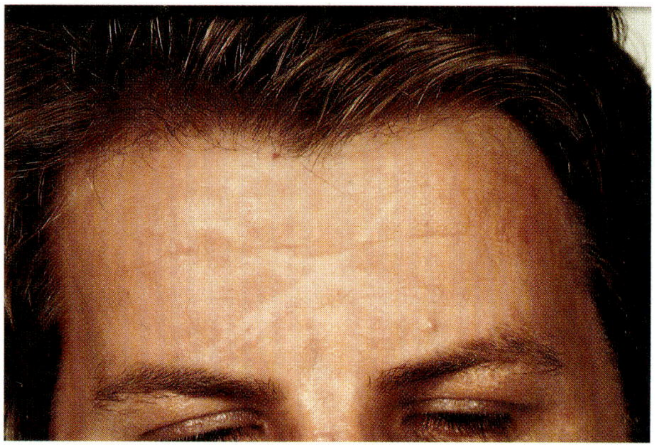

Fig. 2. White dermographism

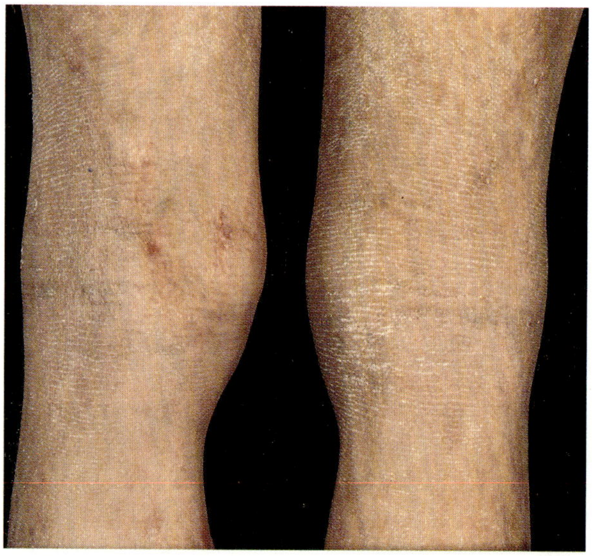

Fig. 3. Patchy pityriasiform lichenoid eczema

Fig. 4. Atopic hand eczema

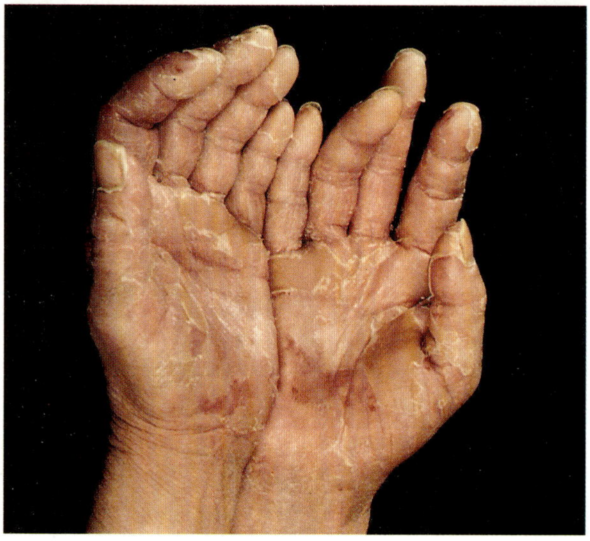

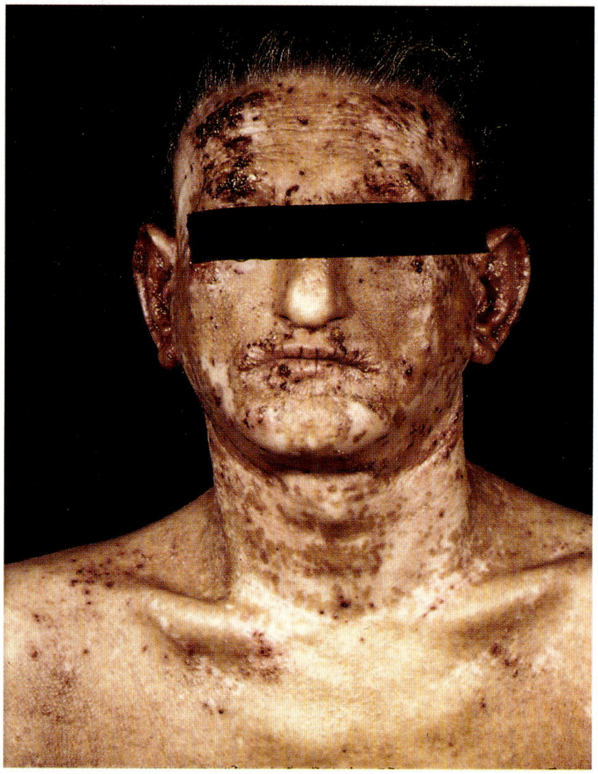

Fig. 5. Severe infection with *Staphylococcus aureus* in a patient with hyper IgE syndrome

onset eczematous lesions of the face, scalp, and extensor aspect are typical, whereas in late infantile onset and in the adolescent and adult phases usually other areas are involved, such as dry lichenified flexural lesions, or hand eczema.

In order to distinguish atopic eczema from infantile seborrheic dermatitis, the location of the lesions has been proposed to be most useful. In atopic eczema an increased incidence of lesions on the forearm and shins was found, unlike in seborrheic dermatitis, in which the

Table 1. Features of hyperimmunoglobulin E syndrome and atopic eczema (From Leung & Geha [10])

Feature	Hyperimmuno-globulin E syndrome	Atopic eczema
Age of onset	1–8 weeks	older than 2 months
IgE level	extremely high	normal to very high
Eosinophilia	frequent	frequent
Keratoconjunctivitis	infrequent	infrequent
Dermatitis	atypical eczema	typical eczema
S. aureus infection	deep seated (sepsis)	superficial (skin)
Other infection	frequent	rare
Respiratory allergy	not common	common
Coarse facies	common rare	
Frequency of occurrence	very rare	common

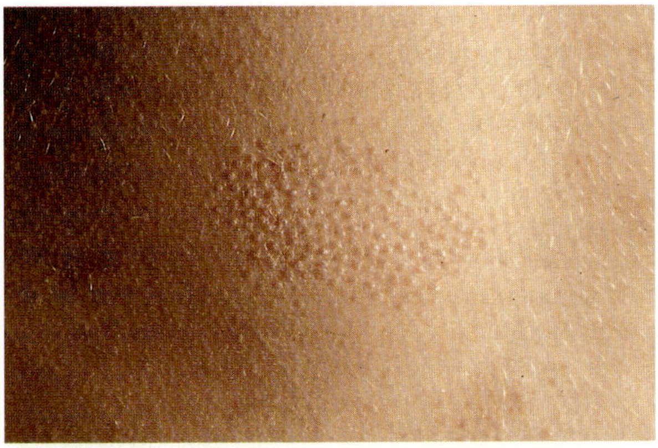

Fig. 6. Kaposi's varicelliform eruption (Herpes virus)

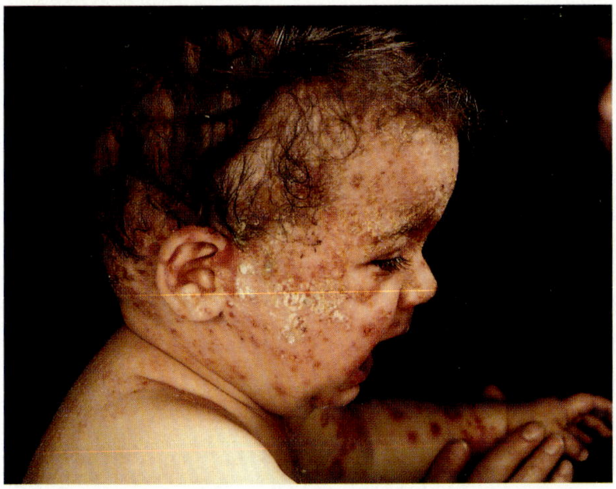

Fig. 7. Eczematous inflammation on the face of a child with superinfection of *Staphylococcus aureus*

axillae were most often affected [1]. Features which may be used to distinguish atopic eczema from hyperimmunoglobulin E (hyper IgE) syndrome are presented in Table 1.

Dry skin is very often seen in patients with atopic eczema. The clinical condition is characterized by a rough, finely scaling, noninflamed skin surface. Seen under the scanning electron microscope, this roughness corresponds to a change in the skin surface, from regular major and minor furrows into a coarse and irregular pattern. This change is the result of reduced sebum secretion, the composition of which is also changed – increased cholesterol, decreased squalene and unsaturated fatty acids –, and this leads to increased epidermal water loss. Abnormalities of sweat secretion – increased sensitivity and productivity – might be the expression of an endogenous β-receptor blockade. The dry skin condition worsens in a cold environment with reduced humidity, especially in winter and after bathing.

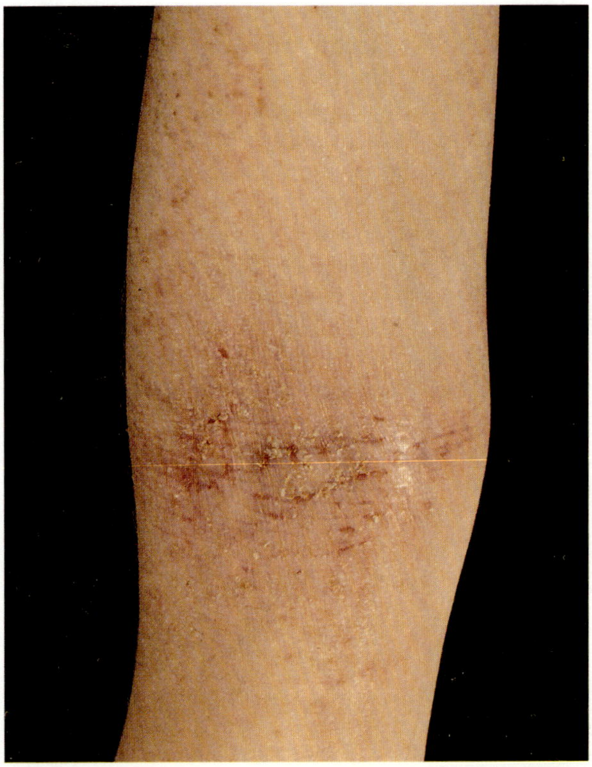

Fig. 8. Dry skin

Fig. 9. Periorbital eczema in a patient with atopic eczema

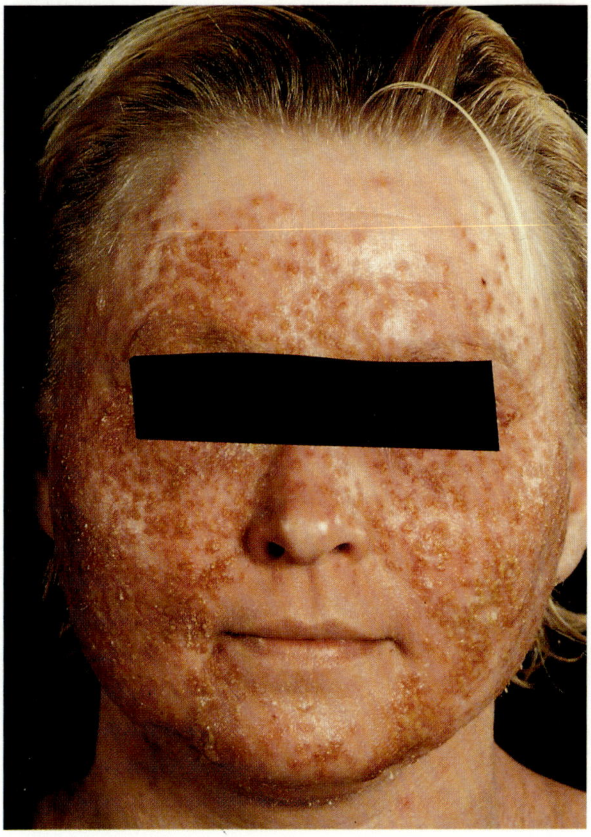

Other pharmacophysiological alterations in atopic eczema are also heralded by clinical signs and symptoms, especially the altered vascular reaction in white dermatographism, the chemical dermatographism which occurs after topical application of niacin, the delayed blanching reaction after intradermal injection of acetylcholine-like drugs, and wheals induced by reduced histamine.

Itching is a major problem in atopic eczema, because scratching is one factor which leads to eczematous lesions, lichenification, pigment change, and sometimes scarring. Without itching there can be no atopic eczema. Itching may result in prurigo, which is characterized by groups of several small papules with excoriated surfaces in areas of the body which can be reached by the hands. The pathophysiology of itching is not very well understood. In atopic eczema one cause at least is an increased level of histamine. It has been shown, for example, that children with food allergies reacted with itching as the first symptoms after food challenge, which is paralleled by an increased histamine level in the plasma, followed afterwards by erythema and then eczematous lesions [2]. Apart from allergic reactions, stress may be another factor which leads to increased histamine release. The itching threshold is lower in individuals with atopic eczema and the itching sensation is prolonged. Itching as an intolerant reaction to wool is especially typical for atopic eczema.

The face is mainly affected during the infantile phase of atopic eczema. In other phases the perioral area, the lips, and the periocular area are the sites of predilection. Lichenification occurs especially in the periocular area and the eyelids, and together with the dry skin and white dermographism due to pathological vascular reactivity produces the typical "facies atopica".

References

1. Aly RA, Maibach HI, Shinefield HR (1977) Microbial flora of atopic dermatitis. Arch Dermatol 113: 780–782
2. Amlot PL, Kemeney DM, Zachary C, Parkes P, Lessof MH (1987) Oral allergy syndrome (OAS): symptoms of IgE-mediated hypersensitivity to foods. Clin Allergy 17: 33–42
3. Costa C, Rilliet A, Nicolet M, Saurat J-H (1989) Scoring atopic dermatitis: the simpler the better? Acta Derm Venereol 69: 41–45
4. Hanifin JM, Portland OR (1982) Atopic dermatitis. J Am Acad Dermatol 6: 1–13
5. Hanifin JM (1984) Basic and clinical aspects of atopic dermatitis. Ann Allergy 52: 386–393
6. Hauser C, Wuethrich B, Matter L, Wilhelm JA, Sonnabend W, Schopfer K (1985) *Staphylococcus aureus* skin colonization in atopic dermatitis patients. Dermatologica 170: 35–39
7. Hauser C, Wuethrich B, Matter L, Wilhelm JA, Schopfer K (1985) Immune response to *Staphylococcus aureus* in atopic dermatitis. Dermatologica 170: 114–120
8. Herzberg J (1972) Wenig bekannte Ausdrucksformen der Neurodermitits. Arch Derm Forsch 244: 350–352
9. Huber A, Fartasch M, Diepgen TL, Bäurle G, Hornstein OP (1987) Auftreten von Kontaktallergien beim atopischen Ekzem. Dermatoses 35: 119–123
10. Leung DYM, Geha RS (1988) Clinical and immunologic aspects of the hyperimmunoglobulin E syndrome. Hematol Oncol Clin North Am 2: 81–100
11. Linde YW (1989) Dry skin in atopic eczema. Acta Derm Venereol 69: 311–314
12. Linde YW, Bengtsson A, Loden M (1989) Dry skin in atopic eczema II. A surface profilometry study. Acta Derm Venereol 69: 315–319
13. Ring J (1983) Was ist Atopie? Fortschr Prakt Dermatol Venerol 10: 103–111
14. Ring J, Sedlmeier F, von der Helm D, Mayr T, Walz U, Ibel H, Riepel H, Przybilla B, Reimann H.-J., Dorsch W (1986) Histamine and allergic diseases. In: Ring J, Burg G (eds) New trends in allergy. Springer, Berlin Heidelberg New York Tokyo, pp. 44–77
15. Sampson HA, Broadbent KR, Broadbent JB (1989) Spontaneous release of histamine from basophils and histamine-releasing factor in patients with atopic eczema and food hypersensitivity. N Engl J Med 321: 228–232
16. Wüthrich B (1975) Zur Immunpathologie der Neurodermitis constitutionalis. Huber, Basel
17. Wüthrich B (1986) Die trockene Haut bei Neurodermitis atopica, Schweiz Rundschau Med (Praxis) 75: 193–200
18. Wüthrich B, Schudel P (1982) Die Neurodermitis atopica nach dem Kleinkindesalter. H+G 58: 1013–1023

Stigmata of the Atopic Constitution

B. Przybilla

Atopy is a constitutional state defined by the genetically determined disposition to develop atopic eczema, allergic rhinoconjunctivitis, and/or allergic asthma. Up to now, no definite marker has been available which would allow one to decide with certainty whether atopy is present or absent in a given individual. This hampers not only the recognition of atopy in persons without manifest symptoms, but even the diagnostic classification of overt disease: It may not be possible to diagnose a condition as atopic when considering only its immediate symptomatology; this holds true particularly for the diagnosis of atopic eczema. Thus, in order to establish the presence of an atopic disposition or of an atopic disease, it is necessary to look for features known to be characteristically related to atopy.

Features of Atopy

There are numerous features which are characteristic, yet mostly nonspecific indicators of atopy. With regard to the diagnosis of atopic eczema, the criteria established by Hanifin and Rajka [18], based on previous suggestions of these authors [17, 51], are those most often referred to. Similarly, these and additional clues to atopy have been recognized by many others (Table 1). In principle, information on the "atopy status" can be obtained from the patient history, physical findings, and skin or laboratory tests.

History

The problem of the interpretation of subjective complaints is well-known. Anamnestic data on previous, objective clinical findings may be reported by the patient or information may be obtained from medical records. This makes a difference with regard to reliability. Furthermore, as the patient's knowledge of his or her childhood diseases or the health state of family members is not based on the patient's direct observations, the interpretation of a history must always be cautious. In particular, a history negative for atopic symptoms cannot be considered as definitely diagnostic, whereas a positive history of clear-cut atopic disease, particularly when obtained from medical records, provides valuable clues.

Physical Findings

Physical features related to atopy fall into three categories.

Clinical Manifestations of Atopic Diseases. By definition, the presence of allergic rhinoconjunctivitis or asthma due to common inhalant allergens, or characteristic atopic eczema lead to a definite diagnosis of atopy. However, atopic respiratory diseases cannot be diagnosed without allergy testing and the clinical presentation of atopic eczema is by no means always clear-cut.

Besides full-blown atopic eczema, there are minor disease manifestations (Table 1). Many of them, such as non-specific hand dermatitis, nipple eczema, cheilitis, and infraauricular fissuring, have been referred to as indicators of atopic eczema. Indeed, their presence can support the diagnosis. However, these disease manifestations are actually atopic eczema and thus do not provide additional independent clues with regard to the presence of atopy in a given individual.

Secondary to atopic disease, physical sequelae may occur which also can be considered markers (Table 1). These include reticulate pigmentation of the neck, pityriasis alba, polished nails due to atopic eczema, transverse nasal creases, facial deformities, and facial mannerisms due to respiratory atopic disease.

Associated Diseases. A heterogeneous group of diseases has been found to be related to atopy. Basically,

Table 1. Features of atopy
(compiled from [2, 4–10, 15–31, 33–41, 43–46, 48–52, 54–56, 58, 60–62, 64–67, 69–71, 75, 76])

Anamnestic Data

Atopic diseases (atopic eczema, allergic rhinoconjunctivitis, allergic asthma):
- Personal history
- Family history

Eczema with the following characteristics:
- Pruritus
- Early age of onset
- Chronically relapsing course
- Seasonal variation
- Influenced by environmental or emotional factors, or infections

Nonspecific hand dermatitis
Food intolerance
Allergic (contact) urticaria
Cutaneous infections
Itch when sweating
Light sensitivity
Irritation from textiles
- Wool intolerance
- Intolerance of occlusive clothing

Solvent intolerance

Physical Findings

Atopic eczema: manifestations and sequelae
Full-blown typical atopic eczema (age-dependent)
(Infantile) seborrheic atopic eczema
Patchy pityriasiform lichenoid eczema
Nummular atopic eczema
Prurigo variant of atopic eczema
Pityriasis alba
Widespread skin infection
Atopic hand eczema
Dyshidrotic eczema (pompholyx)
Pulpitis sicca
Nipple eczema
Cheilitis
Perlèche (angular cheilitis)
Median fissuring of the lower lip
Retroauricular intertrigo
Infraauricular fissuring
Anterior neck folds
Linear grooves
Polished nails
Pigmentary changes
- Depigmentation
- Hyperpigmentation

Atopic respiratory disease: manifestations and sequelae
Manifest allergic rhinitis, conjunctivitis or asthma (due to common aeroallergens)
Facial mannerisms ("allergic salute", nose or mouth wrinkling)
Transverse nasal crease
Mouth breathing
Gingival hyperplasia
Furrowed mouth syndrome
Hypertrophy of the tonsils
Granular pharyngitis
Facial deformities (e.g., longer face, flattened malar eminences, pinched nostrils, raised upper lip, overbite)
Thoracic deformities (pectus carinatum/excavatum)
Pulmonary emphysema

Associated conditions
Ichthyosis vulgaris
Keratosis pilaris
Lingua geographica
Juvenile plantar dermatosis
Keratosis punctata
Lichen striatus
Cataract
Keratoconus

Constitutional stigmata of atopy
Dry skin
Hyperlinearity of the palms/soles
Infraorbital fold
White dermographism
Facial pallor
Orbital darkening
Hertoghe's sign
Low hairline

Skin and Laboratory Test Findings

Immediate type (type I) skin test reactions to common allergens
Specific IgE antibodies to common allergens
Elevated serum level of total IgE
Abnormal vascular reactions (e.g., delayed blanch to cholinergic stimulation, white reaction to nicotinic acid esters)
Depressed cellular immunity
Nickel contact sensitivity

these conditions cannot be interpreted as direct manifestations or sequelae of atopic diseases. Among them, some are amenable to physical examination,' e.g., ichthyosis vulgaris, lingua geographica, keratoconus, and cataract. Some more examples are given in Table 1.

Stigmata of the Atopic Constitution. Only those features of atopy which are not directly associated with morbidity, that is, which are not manifestations or consequences of atopic or associated disease, should be regarded as true constitutional stigmata. Furthermore, they should be observable without any technical devices. The features listed in Table 1 meet these criteria and are discussed below.

Skin and Laboratory Testing

An increased serum level of total IgE, the demonstration of specific IgE antibodies, or positive skin tests to common environmental allergens are referred to most often as being indicative of atopy. The diagnostic relevance of these findings is discussed elsewhere in this volume. Some other pertinent tests are included in Table 1.

Constitutional Stigmata of Atopy

Dry Skin

Dry skin (xerosis, sebostasis) (Fig. 1) is a hallmark of the patient with atopic eczema [4, 6, 8, 16–18, 24, 27–31, 33, 46, 51, 52, 54, 56]. Clinically it is characterized by a skin surface which is rough to touch, noninflamed, and sometimes slightly scaly. This description meets the concept of both the physician and the patient.

However, dry skin has been regarded a mismoner, as the cause underlying this feature apparently is not a lack of water, at least not in the outermost layers of the skin [47]. Thus, it was proposed that the designation "rough skin" would be more appropriate [47]. Indeed, a recent study, in which a profilometry method was employed, demonstrated quantitatively an increased roughness of dry skin in atopic eczema [72]. Nonetheless, as there is a long tradition of using the term "dry skin", it seems doubtful whether this can be replaced with ease by "rough skin." Furthermore, the latter term may be mistaken for keratosis follicularis by the patients.

When looking for dry skin it has to be taken into account that its occurrence is influenced by exogenous factors, e.g., season of the year or individual skin care measures. This, as well as subjective interpretation, can lead to divergencies between history and clinical findings [62, 71]. Also, localized and "generalized" dry skin have been distinguished [68].

It is beyond the scope of this chapter to deal in detail with the etiology of dry skin; therefore, only the relation of dry skin to eczema and ichthyosis vulgaris will be considered. Biopsies taken from dry, clinically non-inflamed skin in patients suffering from atopic eczema have been reported to exhibit the histological picture of mild eczema [14, 66, 68]. From this it was concluded that dry skin is a minor disease manifestation of atopic eczema. However, these results were not confirmed by other

Fig. 1. Dry skin

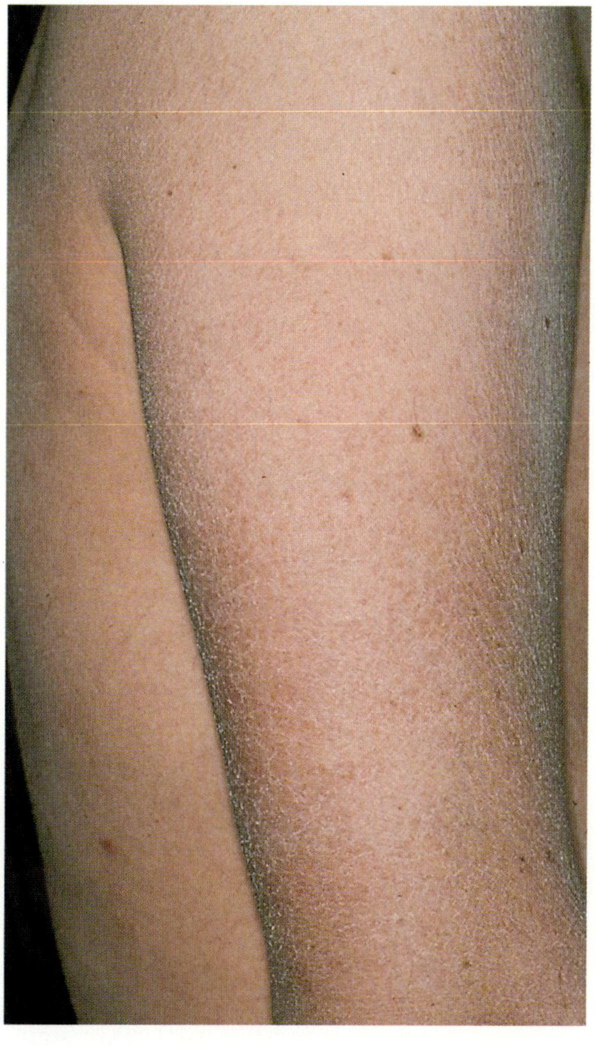

investigators, who found histologically eczematous changes in less than 10% of biopsies taken from the dry skin of atopic eczema patients [12, 13]. Thus, present knowledge does not allow us to reach definite conclusions with regard to the cause of dry skin. In particular, it cannot be regarded simply as a subclinical variant of eczema, although minor disease manifestations may present as dry skin. Presumably, the causes leading to the clinical impression of dry skin are heterogeneous.

Another concept is that dry skin, if it is not eczema, may actually be autosomal dominant ichthyosis vulgaris, which was reported in up to 30% of atopic eczema patients [66, 68]. These studies do not sufficiently substantiate such an association, as the diagnosis of ichthyosis vulgaris was based merely on clinical findings (ichthyotic scaling, hyperlinearity of the palms) and light microscopical features, such as an absent or reduced granular layer [66, 68]. However, ultrastructural studies of dry skin in atopic eczema have disclosed that concomitant ichthyosis vulgaris, proven by the presence of abnormal keratohyaline granules, is a rare occurrence, found in only 4% of patients [12, 13]. The aforementioned features should thus be regarded as related to atopic eczema *and* ichthyosis vulgaris [13]. In order to prevent misunderstandings, "ichthyosis vulgaris" should not be used to describe ichthyosiform scaling in atopic eczema patients.

The prevalence of dry skin has been studied by several investigators (Table 2). In patients with atopic eczema dry skin was present in 48%–98%, whereas it was seen in only 14%–34% of the controls. Dry skin evidently is linked to atopic eczema.

Table 2. Prevalence of dry skin

Study	Patients with atopic eczema Total (*n*)	Dry skin (%)	Controls[a] Total (*n*)	Dry skin (%)	*P*	Remarks
Uehara and Miyauchi 1984 [68]	436	31	–	–		
	303	63	–	–		Localized dry skin (<70% of body surface)
	without "ichthyosis vulgaris"	4				Generalized dry skin (>70% of body surface)
Svensson et al. 1985 [62]	47	98	47	53	<0.001	By history
		98		34		Clinical findings
Kang and Tian 1987 [26]	372	65	213	18	<0.01	
Diepgen et al. 1989 [10]	110	96	527	25	<0.01	
Werner Linde 1989 [71]	50	84	50	36	<0.01	Patients' opinion
		48		14	<0.01	Clinical findings
Our patients [49]	34	74	23	31	<0.01	Any skin dryness (mild, moderate or prominent)[b]
		50		0		Moderate or prominent dryness of the skin

[a]See Table 9.
[b]See Table 10.

Hyperlinearity of the Palms or Soles

Hyperlinearity of the palms (Fig. 2) is a feature of atopic eczema referred to frequently [4, 6, 16–18, 31, 33, 46, 51, 54], whereas hyperlinearity of the soles is mentioned

Fig. 2. Palmar hyperlinearity

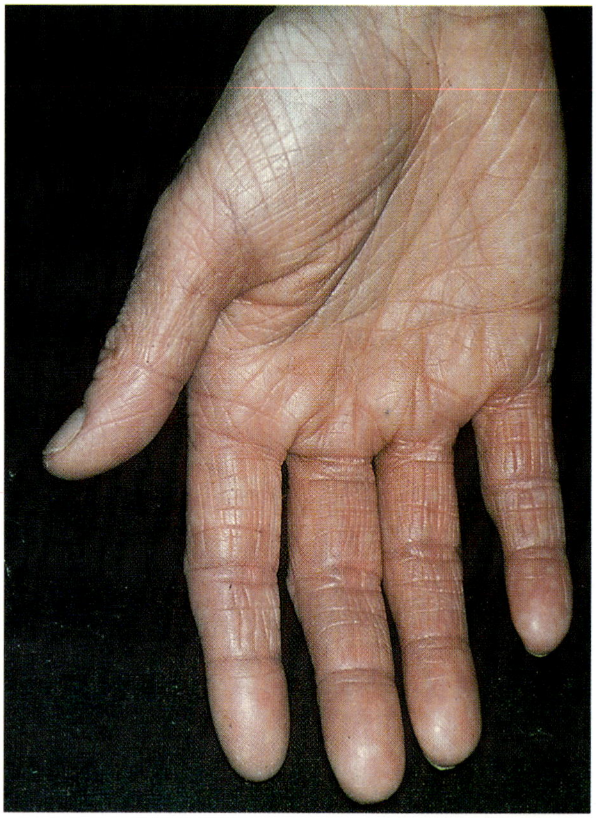

only rarely [46, 54]. The meaning of "hyperlinearity" seems self-evident, but it has not yet been defined clearly. Palmar creases can be divided into three groups: major, minor, and secondary [57].

The major and minor (primary) creases represent defined skin markings [57], the term "secondary crease" describes any visible palmar lines other than the primary ones [57]. Systems for quantitative evaluation of palmar creases have been devised using either five or three grades of intensity [57, 63]. These refer particularly to the area of the palms which is traversed by secondary creases. Furthermore, the density and depth of creases can be evaluated. Imprints are the best method to visualize crease patterns, although the palms and soles of only a few patients with atopic eczema have been assessed by this method [21]. For clinical purposes such a procedure evidently is too sophisticated and the overall impression of "hyperlinearity" usually is considered.

The expression of palmar markings may be influenced by environmental factors (particularly manual work, chemical, and thermal factors) and age [21]. Furthermore, there may be differences between the right and left side [21].

As with dry skin, the relation of palmar hyperlinearity to autosomal dominant ichthyosis vulgaris has been a matter of discussion. It has been suggested that hyperlinearity in patients with atopic eczema is indicative of concomitant ichthyosis vulgaris [32, 42, 66–68]. This view has been doubted by others for clinical reasons [23, 60]. Recently, it has been shown by ultrastructural analysis that abnormal keratohyaline granules, proving autosomal dominant ichthyosis vulgaris, are demonstrable only in a minority (2/17) of atopic eczema patients with hyperlinearity of the palms [13]. This trait thus seems to be common to both ichthyosis vulgaris and atopic eczema [13].

Studies on the prevalence of hyperlinearity are summarized in Table 3. The wide range of 28%–88% given for its prevalence presumably is due to the particular interpretation of "hyperlinear," as exclusion of minor intensity grades changes the frequency rates fundamentally (Table 3 [21, 49]). Generally, palmar/plantar hyperlinearity was significantly more frequent in patients than in controls. Only in a single study could no such difference be found [42], and this may have been due to the exclusion of atopic eczema patients with concomitant "frank ichthyosis," diagnosed evidently on the basis of clinical findings. Thus, particularly atopic eczema patients with "ichthyotic" hyperlinearity may have been omitted.

Table 3. Prevalence of hyperlinearity of the palms or soles

Study	Patients with atopic eczema Total (*n*)	Patients with atopic eczema Hyperlinearity (%)	Controls[a] Total (*n*)	Controls[a] Hyperlinearity (%)	*P*	Remarks
Hirth et al. 1971 [21]	17	65	300	31	ng	Creases of left palm: Intensity grade III or IV
		24		1		Intensity grade IV
	17	65	300	29	ng	Creases of left sole: Intensity grade III or IV
		18		5		Intensity grade IV
Leutgeb et al. 1972 [32]	130	29	–	–		Hyperlinear palms
Uehara and Hayashi 1981 [67]	178	28	–	–		Hyperlinear palms
Høyer et al. 1982 [23]	40	37	–	–		Hyperlinear palms
Smith 1984 [60]	59	44	–	–		Hyperlinear palms
Mevorah et al. 1985 [42]	61[b]	33	247	22	ns	Hyperlinear palms or soles
Kang and Tian 1987 [26]	372	49	213	9	<0.01	Hyperlinear palms
Diepgen et al. 1989 [10]	110	49	527	6	<0.01	Hyperlinear palms
Our patients [49)	34	88	23	48	<0.01	Any hyperlinearity of the palms (mild, moderate or prominent)[c]
		64		18		Moderate or prominent hyperlinearity of the palms
	34	74	23	30	<0.01	Any hyperlinearity of the soles (mild, moderate or prominent)[c]
		44		8		Moderate or prominent hyperlinearity of the soles

ns = not significant; ng = not given

[a]See Table 9. [b]Patients with both atopic eczema and "frank ichthyosis" were excluded. [c] See Table 10.

Infraorbital Fold

Infraorbital fold (Fig. 3) has been included in most descriptions of atopic eczema [4, 6, 8, 16–18, 28, 31, 33, 46, 51, 52, 54]. Morgan [44] was the first to report this sign. He referred to Dennie, who had considered a "definite wrinkle just beneath the margin of the lower lid of both eyes" to be pathognomonic for allergy, especially eczema, hay fever, and asthma. Accordingly, this feature has been linked to the names of Morgan and Dennie (e.g. Dennie-Morgan infraorbital fold, Morgan's fold, Dennie's fold). It has also been described as being similar to a Mongolian fold [51].

There may be single or double folds. Usually, the wrinkle is present on both eyelids, but occasionally a unilateral manifestation is seen [43, 65]. The original definition, as given above [44], has been modified by some authors who regard the sign as being present only if there is a definite double fold [39] or if one or more creases, outlining skin folds and starting at the inner canthus, extend laterally at least beyond an imaginary perpendicular line through the pupil [43]. When creases are considered, the physiologic sulcus palpebralis inferior must not be mistaken for the stigma.

Infraorbital folds seem to be more prevalent in younger than in older individuals [39, 62]. According to Morgan, the wrinkle "is retained throughout life" [44], but long-term follow-up of patients with this sign has not yet been performed.

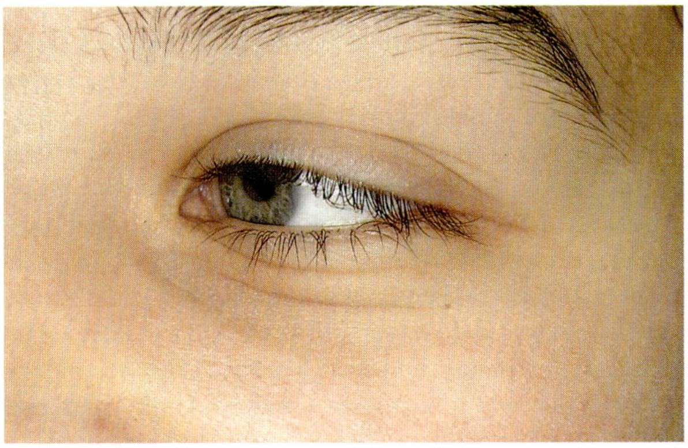

Fig. 3. Infraorbital fold

It has been claimed that infraorbital folds are strongly related to eyelid eczema: Uehara [65] found this feature in 83% of atopic eczema patients with lower eyelid dermatitis, but in only 7% of patients who lacked inflammation of this site. Furthermore, he reported that there were infraorbital folds in 8 of 11 nonatopic patients with allergic contact dermatitis of the lower eyelids [65]. No other study systematically addressing this issue has yet been published. However, as infraorbital folds are not infrequent in subjects without eczema [62], it is evident that by no means are all folds due to inflammation. However, a preexistent infraorbital fold may be accentuated by intermittent eczema and thus

Table 4. Prevalence of infraorbital fold

Study	Patients with atopic eczema		Controls[a]		*P*	Remarks
	Total (*n*)	Infraorbital fold (%)	Total (*n*)	Infraorbital fold (%)		
Holzegel 1977 [22]	120	85	–	–		
Meenan 1980 [39]	100	9	100	2	ng	Only definite double folds were considered
Meenan 1981 [40]	148	12	168	1	ng	Only definite and obvious folds were considered
Uehara 1981 [65]	300	25	300	2	ng	
Svensson et al. 1985 [62]	47	60	47	38	<0.05	
Mevorah et al. 1988 [43]	105	51	113	51	ns	Folds going laterally beyond a vertical line through the pupil were considered
Diepgen et al. 1989 [10]	110	57	527	17	<0.01	
Our patients [49]	34	82	23	13	<0.01	Any infraorbital folds (mild, moderate or prominent)[b]
		59		4		Moderate or prominent infraorbital folds

ns, not significant; ng, not given

[a] See Table 9.

[b] See Table 10.

become more prominent [22]. We have seen infraorbital folds in patients with atopic eczema as frequently as in subjects with respiratory atopic diseases without a history of eczema [49]. An obligatory association between infraorbital folds and dermatitis localized to the eyelids is not probable.

The percentage of atopic eczema patients exhibiting infraorbital folds was found to be 50%–60% in most studies (Table 4). Higher values probably are attributable to the inclusion of marginal manifestations of this sign, as exemplified by our own findings (see Table 4). The low prevalence (9%–12%) reported by Meenan [39, 40] is probably due to the consideration of only major expressions of this feature. As infraorbital folds were less prevalent and, if present at all, strongly related to eyelid dermatitis in Uehara's Japanese patients, ethnical differences with regard to the expression of this sign seem probable. This is further supported by the report of Kang and Tian [26] who did not see "meaningful infraorbitalfolds" in Chinese individuals. Surprisingly high frequencies of infraorbital folds in two of the control groups 38% [62] or 51% [43]) cannot be explained easily, they may be related to the inclusion criteria or to ethnic variations. With the exception of one study [43], the prevalence of infraorbital folds is significantly different between patients and controls (Table 4); thus, this feature can be regarded as a marker of atopy.

White dermographism

White dermographism [Fig. 4) is among the features of atopic eczema cited most often [4, 5, 8, 16–18, 24, 27–31, 33, 46, 51, 52, 54, 56, 61]. According to Korting [29] it was first described by Marey in 1858. Whereas firm stroking of normal skin with a blunt instrument leads to a partially or fully developed triple response of Lewis (red, more or less urticarial "line" with reflex erythema) in the majority of the population [74], white dermographism (white line) develops instead in some individuals. This

Fig. 4. White dermographism

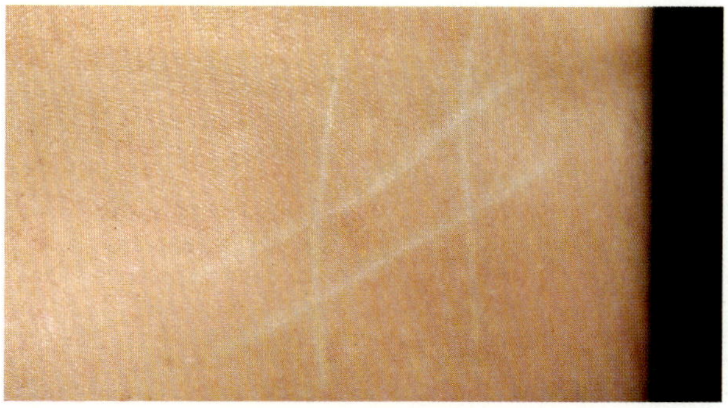

white reaction replaces the initially mechanically provoked red line about 15–60 s after stroking [5, 15, 74]. Thus, the reaction must not be read earlier. Generally, dermographism is assessed qualitatively by using an instrument easily available, such as a paper clip or a tongue depressor. For quantitative studies various other instruments have been devised [11, 53, 59].

The elicitation of white dermographism depends on a number of factors. The reaction has been said to occur more easily on the lower than on the upper half of the body [5] or on the arms, legs, and neck rather than on the abdomen and trunk [53]. Its occurrence may also be restricted to some localized skin sites [29]. Even slight stroking can elicit white dermographism [73] and, with too strong a stimulus, a red line with a white halo may develop instead [53]. White dermographism has been found to occur with greater ease in individuals up to 30 years of age rather than in older ones [11]. During infancy the ability to develop white dermographism on eczematous skin is reduced but increases up until the age of 1 year [1]. In patients with atopic eczema, the occurrence of white dermographism on skin appearing clinically normal is positively related to disease severity [55, 76].

The pathophysiologic aspects of abnormal vascular reactivity in atopic eczema are reviewed elsewhere in this volume. Here, only the relation of white dermographism to eczema itself will be briefly considered. For more than 60 years it has been known that white dermographism can be elicited almost regularly in the diseased skin of patients with atopic eczema [55]. However, this reaction can also be elicited in lesions of other chronic inflammatory dermatoses [53, 73]. A study of 100 patients with atopic eczema disclosed white dermographism on lichenified skin in 86%, on dry and rough skin in 76%, and on normal appearing skin in only 1% [69]. As histologic examination of biopsies taken from dry and rough skin revealed eczematous changes, it was concluded that white dermographism in atopic eczema patients is a secondary phenomenon related to inflammation. Nonetheless, since white dermographism is more frequent in atopic lesions compared to other types of eczema [26, 69] (Table 5), the atopic state may predispose one to this form of reaction. Furthermore, the observation of white dermographism on the normal skin of individuals without atopic eczema (see Table 5) argues against the concept that white dermographism is only secondary to inflammatory skin changes. Assumedly, white dermographism can have different causes, some of which may concur in the lesioned skin of patients with atopic eczema (skin inflammation plus atopic state).

With regard to the reported prevalence of white dermographism in atopic eczema patients, there are large differences between various studies (Table 5). This

Table 5. Prevalence of white dermographism[a]

Study	Patients with atopic eczema Total (*n*)	White dermo-graphism (%)	Controls[b] Total (*n*)	White dermo-graphism (%)	*P*	Test site
Rajka 1960 [50]	100	81	40	10	ng	Diseased skin (atopic eczema patients)
Yoshida et al. 1974 [76]	46	74	–	–		Healthy skin
Uehara and Ofuji 1977 [69]	100	86	20	18	ng	Lichenified skin
		76		–		Dry and rough skin
		1		0		Normal skin
Svensson et al. 1985 [62]	47	100	47	100		Normal skin of the foreleg
Kang and Tian 1987 [26]	230	60	32	34	<0.05	Lesioned skin
Mevorah et al. 1988 [43]	103	42	111	14	<0.005	Uninvolved skin (usually on the forehead)
Our patients [49]	34	38	23	4	<0.01	Clinically normal skin (usually on the upper back)

ng, not given
[a] Studies indicating the condition of the test site and not using a test apparatus.
[b] See Table 9.

holds true particularly for reactions obtained on normal looking skin. These differences are probably due to varying test modalities. Thus, in one study, testing was done on the legs, and white dermographism was obtained in 100% of patients and controls [62]. In all other studies, including a control group, there were higher prevalence rates of white dermographism in atopic eczema patients (Table 5).

Facial Pallor

Facial pallor is generally regarded as a characteristic feature of atopic eczema [4, 8, 16–18, 33, 46, 51, 52, 54, 56]. Just like white dermographism, this diffuse paleness is atrributable to an abnormal vascular reactivity with a tendency towards vasoconstriction of small blood vessels. Beyond the clinical impression, facial pallor can be recognized more distinctly by comparing a skin area rendered anemic by pressure of a glass spatula to the natural skin color. Maximum pallor is characterized by the finding of no difference in response to this maneuver. Patchy pale areas on the face may also occur due to rubbing in patients with white dermographism [16], and flushing or erythema can alternate with pallor [16, 17, 51]. Facial pallor (erythema) was found to be more frequent in younger than in older patients [26, 62].

Only a few studies deal with the prevalence of facial pallor (Table 6). It seems to be present definitely in about 50%–60% of Caucasian patients [49, 62], whereas in China the frequency rate was only 22% [11]. This could point to ethnical variations. Regardless of this, in all studies the prevalence of facial pallor was found to be significantly higher in patients than in controls.

Table 6. Prevalence of facial pallor

Study	Patients with atopic eczema Total (*n*)	Facial pallor (%)	Controls[a] Total (*n*)	Facial pallor (%)	*P*	Remarks
Svensson et al. 1985 [62]	47	64	47	32	<0.001	Facial pallor/erythema considered
Kang and Tian [26]	372	22	213	4	<0.01	
Our patients [49]	34	85	23	13	<0.01	Any facial pallor (mild, moderate, prominent)[b]
		47		4		Moderate or prominent facial pallor

[a] See Table 9.
[b] See Table 10.

Orbital Darkening

Orbital darkening (Fig. 5) is regarded as a feature of both atopic eczema [16–18, 52, 54] and allergic nasal disease [34–37, 41]. Also known as allergic shiner this sign is characterized by a brownish to greyish or bluish discoloration of the orbital region particularly in its lower half. Sometimes there is also slight edema. Altogether, this gives the patient a tired look [33]. Orbital darkening was found to be correlated to young age [62].

Orbital darkening in patients with atopic eczema has been interpreted as secondary hyperpigmentation following chronic inflammation [16]. Thus, it could be caused by atopic eyelid eczema, conjunctivitis leading to skin irritation, or a combination of both. Another mechanism has been suggested for orbital darkening associated with perennial rhinitis. Persistent edema of the mucous membranes of the nasal cavities and perhaps also allergic spasm of the musculus tarsalis would impede venous bloodflow from the orbital region, thus causing edema and discoloration [34, 35]. Both proposed mechanisms, alone or in combination, can explain the occurrence of orbital darkening in a number of patients, and in either case it would be a sequela of disease. However, it is a common clinical observation that orbital darkening may also be seen in atopic patients who never had eczema of the eyelids or manifest respiratory disease.

The results of studies on the prevalence of orbital darkening are summarized in Table 7. As can be seen, this feature is quite frequent in atopic eczema patients. When compared to controls, there were significant differences in the prevalence rates of two studies [26, 49], but not in another one [62]. The reason for this discrepancy is not evident.

Hertoghe's Sign

Hertoghe's sign (Fig. 6), the thinning or complete absence of the eyebrows in their lateral aspects, is mentioned rarely in the English literature [16, 51], but elsewhere it has attracted some attention [6, 27, 29, 30, 52, 54]. Hertoghe, who first described this feature at the turn of the century, found it to be related to hypothyroidism [29].

The occurrence of rarefied eyebrows in patients with atopic eczema has been attributed to different causes. Whereas some have interpreted the feature as secondary to rubbing of the skin [16, 70], others have suggested that

Table 7. Prevalence of orbital darkening

Study	Patients with atopic eczema Total (n)	Orbital darkening (%)	Controls[a] Total (n)	Orbital darkening (%)	P	Remarks
Svensson et al. 1985 [62]	47	47	47	32	ns	
Kang and Tian 1987 [26]	372	55	213	7	<0.01	
Our patients [49]	34	85	23	26	<0.01	Any periorbital darkening (mild, moderate or prominent)[b]
		41		0		Moderate or prominent orbital darkening

ns, not significant
[a] See Table 9.
[b] See Table 10.

Fig. 5. Orbital darkening

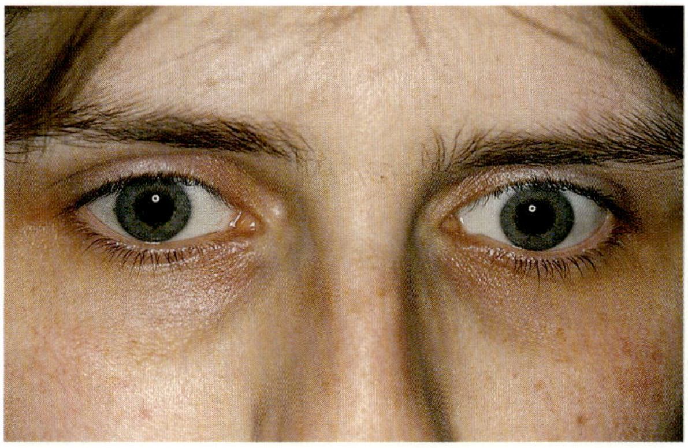

Fig. 6. Hertoghe's sign

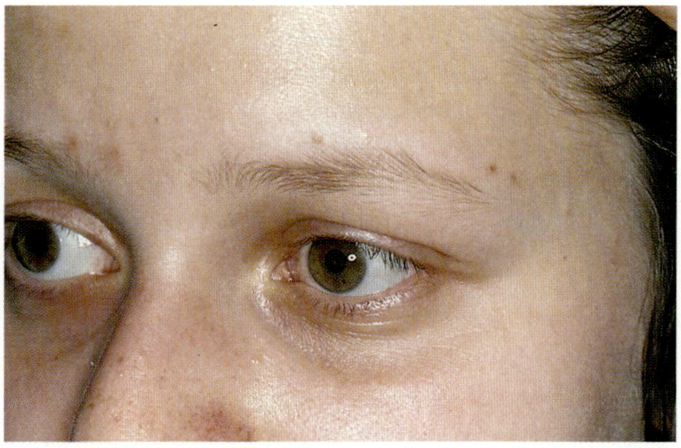

Table 8. Prevalence of Hertoghe's sign

Study	Patients with atopic eczema		Controls[a]		P	Remarks
	Total (n)	Hertoghe's sign (%)	Total (n)	Hertoghe's sign (%)		
Diepgen et al. 1989 [10]	110	39	527	1	<0.01	
Our patients [49]	34	68	23	44	<0.01	Any Hertoghe's sign (mild, moderate, prominent)[b]
		35		14		Moderate or prominent Hertoghe's sign

[a] See Table 9.
[b] See Table 10.

it is not induced mechanically, but related to disturbances of the autonomic nervous system [29]. There are no data available which would allow one to decide this issue. Generally, it seems probable that rubbing or scratching of atopic skin in the eyebrow region may mechanically cause loss of the brows. Nevertheless, there are individuals who exhibit typical Hertoghe's sign without any manifest or previous eczema or other inflammatory skin disease of the face. It has been proposed to term rarefied eyebrows secondary to mechanical injury "pseudo" Hertoghe's sign in order to delineate them from "true" Hertoghe's sign [29]. However, in the individual patient with atopic eczema it will be difficult or impossible to differentiate in this way. It seems appropriate to use the term "Hertoghe's sign" as a descriptive one devoid of pathogenetic implications.

Data on the prevalence of Hertoghe's sign are scarce (Table 8). The values found by Diepgen et al. [10] and by us in atopic eczema patients are in good accordance, when considering the rates after omitting our patients with only slight expression of the sign. The large difference of prevalence seen in controls may be related to our small sample size. This also may explain the lack of a significant difference of prevalence between controls and atopic eczema patients in our study.

Low Hairline

A low hairline (Fig. 7) in the frontal and temporal region, as a stigma of patients with atopic eczema, has been reported only by a few authors [6, 27, 29, 54]. The term "fur hat-like hairline" describes this feature in plain words [30]. Often a low hairline is most prominent in the temporal region, where there may be, between the scalp and the margin of the eyebrows, not only a reduced distance, but even a definite connection by some terminal hairs. Rarefied lateral eyebrows, that is Hertoghe's sign, do not preclude this feature.

In the pertinent literature figures were not available on the prevalence of a low hairline. We found a low hairline, defined as a distance of ≤3 cm between scalp and margin of the eyebrows, in 88% of 34 atopic eczema patients and in 52% of 23 controls ([49]; for definition of controls see Table 9; $p<0.01$, chi-square test). The difference was more prominent when only scalp-to-eyebrow distances ≤1.5 cm or direct transitions from scalp hairs to eyebrows (65% or 47%, respectively, in atopic eczema patients; 26% or 9%, respectively, in controls) were considered. Thus, a low temporal hairline is significantly related to atopic eczema.

Fig. 7. Low hairline

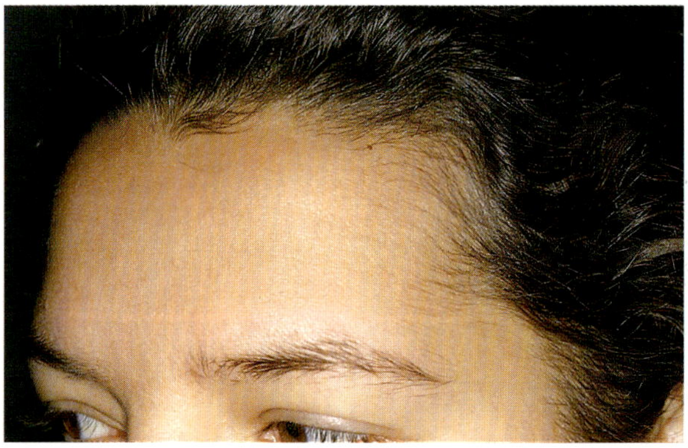

Are Constitutional Stigmata Markers of Atopy?

It is apparent that the stigmata reviewed are nonspecific with regard to atopic eczema, as they may also be found in other conditions (e. g., hyperlinearity of the palms or dry skin in autosomal dominant ichthyosis vulgaris) or in controls. However, although in different studies the prevalence rates found for certain stigmata varied considerably, there was, with a few exceptions, a significant association between these features and atopic eczema.

Some features (dry skin, infraorbital fold, white dermographism, orbital darkening, Hertoghe's sign) have been said to be direct manifestations or sequelae of atopic eczema itself. These then would not fulfil the criteria proposed for "true" constitutional stigmata. The interpretation of some features as secondary to disease is correct apparently in certain, but evidently not in all cases. The rather frequent occurrence of some stigmata in controls points to their manifestation in the absence of eczema. One could try to discriminate between primary or "true" stigmata and secondary or "pseudo" stigmata, as has been proposed for Hertoghe's sign [29]. Such a differentiation, however, would not only be difficult or even impossible practically, it would also be misleading. Secondary changes are not necessarily just phenocopies, they may represent provoked manifestations under conditions of a given liability. This is exemplified by white dermographism, which is more frequent in the lichenified skin of atopic than of nonatopic eczema [69].

So far, constitutional stigmata have been discussed mainly in relation to atopic eczema. The question arises as to their prevalence in respiratory atopic disease. In the pertinent literature there are only scarce quantitative data on this issue. White dermographism was reported to occur in 10% of patients with asthma and/or atopic rhinitis compared to 81% with the lesioned skin of atopic eczema [50]. In another study [62] there was a significant correlation between the absence of orbital darkening and allergic rhinitis or asthma, respectively, which contrasts with other opinions [34–37, 41, 54]. Furthermore, the same authors found an association between asthma and the absence of an intraorbital fold [62].

We have evaluated the prevalence of the constitutional stigmata discussed in this chapter in 16 patients with allergic rhinoconjunctivitis and/or asthma without any present or previous atopic eczema. The findings were compared to those obtained in our atopic eczema patients and controls (Tables 2 to 8). With the exception of Hertoghe's sign, dry skin and white dermographism, all other features were significantly more frequent in patients with respiratory atopic disease than in controls; except for dry skin, individuals with atopic eczema or respiratory atopic disease did not differ significantly with regard to any of the other stigmata investigated [49]. This suggests that most of these stigmata are related to the atopic state and not only to atopic eczema. Therefore, patients with atopic respiratory disease should be omitted from control groups in studies on the prevalence of stigmata in atopic eczema, which was not done in all comparative studies (Table 9). Furthermore, by testing with common aeroallergens it will be possible to also identify atopic subjects who lack or do not consciously perceive manifest symptoms.

Table 9. Studies[a] on the prevalence of constitutional atopy stigmata in atopic eczema patients: Selection criteria for controls with regard to disease and/or atopy

Study		Selection criteria for controls
Rajka 1960	[50]	Patients with asthma bronchiale and/or atopic rhinitis
Hirth et al. 1971	[21]	Persons without skin disease
Uehara and Ofuji 1977	[69]	Patients with contact dermatitis
Meenan 1980, 1981	[39, 40]	Children suffering from warts and with no history of atopy
Uehara 1981	[65]	Persons with no personal or family history of atopy
Mevorah et al. 1985	[42]	Patients with dermatoses other than ichthyosis or atopic eczema and without a past history of atopic eczema or a known family history of ichthyosis or scaling
Svensson et al. 1985	[62]	Patients without a present eczematous dermatitis or previous medical care for such a disease
Kang and Tian 1987	[26]	*Assessment of white dermographism:* Patients with chronic eczema without atopy *Assessment of other stigmata:* Dermatological patients without atopy
Mevorah et al. 1988	[43]	Individuals without a personal or family (close relatives) history of eczema, asthma, or allergic rhinitis
Diepgen et al. 1989	[10]	Persons without present or previous flexural eczema
Werner Linde 1989	[71]	Persons from the venereal disease outpatient clinics without atopy
Our study	[49]	Individuals without a personal or family history of atopic eczema, allergic rhinitis, or asthma and with negative prick test reactions to common aeroallergens (grass pollen, cat epithelia, housedust mite)

[a] For results see Tables 2–8.

Table 10. Assessment of constitutional stigmata of atopy

Stigma	Parameter	Grading[a]			
Dry skin	Clinical impression obtained by evaluation of the entire skin surface	Absent	Mild	Moderate	Prominent
Hyperlinearity of palms or soles	Clinical impression	Absent	Mild	Moderate	Prominent
Infraorbital fold	Fold starting at the inner corner of the eye and running laterally	Absent	Mild: Underlining at most of the medial half of the palpebral fissure	Moderate: Underlining at most of the whole palpebral fissure	Prominent: Running beyond the palpebral fissure
White dermographism	Testing on clinically normal skin (preferrably on the upper back) with a blunt instrument	Red dermographism	White dermographism		Red dermographism with a white halo
Facial pallor	Clinical impression	Absent	Mild	Moderate	Prominent
Orbital darkening	Clinical impression	Absent	Mild	Moderate	Prominent
Hertoghe's sign	Lateral thinning/ absence of the eyebrows extending medially	Absent	Mild: Thinning/absence extending not beyond the lateral corner of the palpebral fissure	Moderate: Thinning/ absence involving the eyebrow above the lateral quarter of the palpebral fissure	Prominent: Thinning/absence extending to the eyebrow above the medial three quarters of the palpebral fissure
Low hairline	Lowest distance between scalp hairs and the margin of the eyebrows	Absent: >3.0 cm	Mild: 1.6 cm–3.0 cm	Moderate: up to 1.5 cm	Prominent: Direct transition from scalp hair to eyebrows

[a] External influences (e. g., the use of emollients on dry skin, the effect of eyebrow plucking on Hertoghe's sign) have to be considered.

The Relevance of Constitutional Stigmata

There are not yet any test methods which would allow one to establish the presence of an atopic state precisely. Accordingly, in the absence of manifest atopic disease, the individual with an atopic disposition cannot be identified. In this respect the assessment of constitutional stigmata of atopy, together with other pertinent features, may aid considerably, e.g., in counseling individuals at the start of an occupational career in order to prevent the provocation of an atopic disease. Furthermore, identification of presumably atopic individuals ("silent atopy") will allow their exclusion from control groups in studies on atopic diseases. Markers of atopy certainly also corroborate the clinical diagnosis of manifest atopic disease – but they do not prove it! The use of atopic stigmata for such purposes is hampered by their nonspecificity. As exemplified by our own data (see Tables 2 to 8) specifity increases when slightly expressed stigmata are not considered. Practically, only in the presence of several clear-cut features should atopy be presumed.

In order to discriminate between atopic eczema patients and nonaffected individuals computed score systems have been designed which take into account various markers [10, 62]. The evaluation of a given individual by such a system allows one to decide whether his or her status is similar to the selection criteria of the reference group, and possibly if there is a risk of developing the group-specific disease symptoms. No direct conclusions can be drawn with regard to parameters not pertinent to the reference group. For example, a score system useful in characterizing patients with flexural eczema cannot be applied to assessing directly the risk of developing atopic hand eczema.

The assessment of atopic stigmata is also useful if possible pathogenetic relationships between atopy and diseases other than the classic atopic ones are examined. When investigating a possible association between polymorphous light eruption and atopy, we found no difference between patients and controls without light hypersensitivity with regard to the frequency of either a history of atopic diseases or of positive skin prick test reactions to common aeroallergens; however, in patients with polymorphous light eruption there was a significantly increased prevalence of dry skin, palmar hyperlinearity, facial pallor, orbital darkening, and a low temporal hairline [3]. Thus, not the atopic state as such, but rather a subgroup of features connects atopy and polymorphous light eruption. This leads to interesting pathogenetic considerations, which have to be assessed by further investigation.

The evaluation of constitutional atopy stigmata can be used for both clinical purposes and for research. However, further studies are needed to demonstrate their value more precisely. Particularly, the expression of stigmata should be assessed with regard to possibly modifying parameters (e.g., disease activity, environment, age, ethnic background). In this regard, it is of importance that stigmata are defined clearly and by reproducible criteria. Furthermore, as the expression of most features is variable, it seems advantageous to discriminate between different grades of intensity in order to enhance accuracy. A proposal for a classification of constitutional atopy stigmata is given in Table 10.

Acknowledgement

The author wants to thank Mr. P. Bilek, photographer, for skillful photography

References

1. Aizawa H, Tagami H (1989) Inability to produce white dermographism in the early stage of infantile eczema. Pediatr Dermatol 6: 6–9
2. Anderson WA, Elam MD, Clark Lambert W (1984) Keratosis punctata and atopy. Report of 31 cases with a prospective study of prevalence. Arch Dermatol 120: 884–890
3. Bieber K, Przybilla B, Ring J, Moosburner M (1989) Polymorphous light eruption (PLE): relationship to atopy and skin reactivity to sequels of mast cell activation (Abstr). Arch Dermatol Res 281: 124
4. Blaylock WK (1976) Atopic dermatitis: diagnosis and pathobiology. J Allergy Clin Immunol 57: 62–79
5. Borelli S, Schnyder UW (1962) Neurodermitis constitutionalis sive atopica. II. Ätiologie, Pathophysiologie, Pathogenese, Therapie. In: Miescher G, Storck H (eds) Entzündliche Dermatosen I. Springer, Berlin Göttingen Heidelberg, pp 254–319 (Handbuch der Haut- und Geschlechtskrankheiten, vol 2/1)
6. Braun-Falco O, Plewig G, Wolff HH (1984) Dermatologie und Venerologie. Springer, Berlin Heidelberg New York
7. Bresolin D, Shapiro GG, Shapiro PA, Dassel SW, Furukawa CT, Pierson WE, Chapko M, Warren Bierman C (1984) Facial characteristics of children who breathe through the mouth. Pediatrics 73: 622–625
8. Champion RH, Parish WE (1986) Atopic dermatitis. In: Rook A, Wilkinson DS, Ebling FJG, Champion RH, Burton JL (eds) Textbook of dermatology, 4th edn. Blackwell, Oxford, pp 419–434
9. Cusumano D, Berman B, Bershad S (1983) Dermatoglyphic patterns in patients with atopic dermatitis. J Am Acad Dermatol 8: 207–210
10. Diepgen TL, Fartasch M, Hornstein OP (1989) Evaluation

and relevance of atopic basic and minor features in patients with atopic dermatitis and in the general population. Acta Derm Venereol [Suppl] (Stockh) 144: 50–54
11. Ebbecke U (1917) Die lokale vasomotorische Reaktion (LVR) der Haut und der inneren Organe. Arch Gesamte Physiol 169: 1–81
12. Fartasch M, Haneke E, Anton-Lamprecht I (1987) Ultrastructural study of the occurrence of autosomal dominant ichthyosis vulgaris in atopic eczema. Arch Dermatol Res 279: 270–272
13. Fartasch M, Diepgen TL, Hornstein OP (1989) Atopic dermatitis – ichthyosis vulgaris – hyperlinear palms – an ultrastructural study. Dermatologica 178: 202–205
14. Finlay AY, Nicholls S, King CS, Marks R (1980) The "dry" non-eczematous skin associated with atopic eczema. Br J Dermatol 102: 249–256
15. Grosshans E, Woehl M (1982) Troubles vasomoteurs, sudoraux et sébacés de l'éczéma constitutionnel. Ann. Dermatol Venereol 109: 151–162
16. Hanifin JM (1988) Atopic dermatitis. In: Middleton E, Reed CE, Ellis EF, Adkinson NF, Yunginger JW (eds) Allergy. Principles and practice, 3rd edn. Mosby, St Louis, pp 1403–1428
17. Hanifin JM, Lobitz WC (1977) Newer concepts of atopic dermatitis. Arch Dermatol 113: 663–670
18. Hanifin JM, Rajka G (1980) Diagnostic features of atopic dermatitis. Acta Derm Venereol [Suppl] (Stockh) 92: 44–47
19. Hellerström S, Rajka G (1967) Clinical aspects of atopic dermatitis. Acta Derm Venereol (Stockh) 47: 75–82
20. Herzberg J (1973) Wenig bekannte Formen der Neurodermitis. Hautarzt 24: 47–51
21. Hirth L, Schöpf E, Benkmann HG, Goedde H W (1971) Untersuchungen der Hautfurchen bei Patienten mit endogenem Ekzem mit einem Beitrag zur Technik der Daktyloskopie. Anthropol Anz 33: 26–38
22. Holzegel K (1977) Unterlidfalte beim endogenen Ekzem. Hautarzt 28: 45
23. Høyer H, Agdal N, Munkvad M (1982) Palmar hyperlinearity in atopic dermatitis. Acta Derm Venereol (Stockh) 62: 346–348
24. Ingram JT (1955) Besnier's prurigo: an ectodermal defect. Br J Dermatol 67: 43–49
25. Jones SK, English JSC, Forsyth A, MacKie RM (1987) Juvenile plantar dermatosis – an 8-year follow-up of 102 patients. Clin Exp Dermatol 12: 5–7
26. Kang K, Tian R (1987) Atopic dermatitis. An evaluation of clinical and laboratory findings. Int J Dermatol 26: 27–32
27. Keining E, Braun-Falco O (1969) Dermatologie und Venerologie. Lehmanns, Munich
28. Kierland RR (1955) Certain stigmata associated with atopic dermatitis. In: Baer RL (ed) Atopic dermatitis. Lippincott, Philadelphia, pp 43–55
29. Korting GW (1954) Zur Pathogenese des endogenen Ekzems. Thieme, Stuttgart
30. Korting GW (1959) Das endogene Ekzem. In: Gottron HA, Schönfeld W (eds) Dermatologie und Venerologie, vol 3/1. Thieme, Stuttgart, pp 549–593
31. Leung DYM, Rhodes AR, Geha RS (1987) Atopic dermatitis. In: Fitzpatrick TB, Eisen AZ, Wolff K, Freedberg IM, Austen KF (eds) Dermatology in general medicine, 3rd edn. McGraw-Hill, New York, pp 1385–1408
32. Leutgeb C, Bandmann HJ, Breit R (1972) Handlinienmuster, Ichthyosis vulgaris und Dermatitis atopica. Arch Dermatol Forsch 244: 354–356
33. Lobitz WC, Dobson RL (1956) Physical and physiological clues for diagnosing eczema. JAMA 161: 1226–1229
34. Marks MB (1963) Significance of discoloration in the lower orbitopalpebral grooves in allergic children (allergic shiners). Ann Allergy 21: 26–32
35. Marks MB (1966) Allergic shiners. Dark circles under the eyes in children. Clin Pediatr 5: 655–658
36. Marks MB (1967) Physical signs of allergy of the respiratory tract in children. Ann Allergy 25: 310–317
37. Marks MB (1973) Unusual signs of respiratory tract allergy. Ann Allergy 31: 611–617
38. Marks R, Simons MJ (1979) Geographic tongue – a manifestation of atopy. Br J Dermatol 101: 159–162
39. Meenan FOC (1980) The significance of Morgan's fold in children with atopic dermatitis. Acta Derm Venereol [Suppl] (Stockh) 92: 42–43
40. Meenan FOC (1981) Further observations of the Dennie-Morgan fold. Ir J Med Sci 150: 89–92
41. Meltzer EO, Schatz M, Zeiger RS (1988) Allergic and nonallergic rhinitis. In: Middleton E, Reed CE, Ellis EF, Adkinson NF, Yunginger JW (eds) Allergy. Principles and practice, 3rd edn. Mosby, St Louis, pp 1253–1289
42. Mevorah B, Marazzi A, Frenk E (1985) The prevalence of accentuated palmoplantar markings and keratosis pilaris in atopic dermatitis, autosomal dominant ichthyosis and control dermatological patients. Br J Dermatol 112: 679–685
43. Mevorah B, Frenk E, Witlisbach V, Carrel CF (1988) Minor clinical features of atopic dermatitis. Evaluation of their diagnostic significance. Dermatologica 177: 360-364
44. Morgan DB (1948) A suggestive sign of allergy. Arch Dermatol 57: 1050
45. Myers WA (1960) the "nasal crease". A physical sign of allergic rhinitis. JAMA 174: 1204–1206
46. Norins AL (1971) Atopic dermatitis. Pediatr Clin North Am 18: 801–838
47. Piérard GE (1989) What do you mean by dry skin? Dermatologica 179: 1–2
48. Podmore P, Burrows D, Eedy DJ, Stanford CF (1986) Seborrhoeic eczema – a disease entity or a clinical variant of atopic eczema? Br J Dermatol 115: 341–350
49. Przybilla B, Enders F, Ring J, Winklmann H (1991) Stigmata of atopic constitution in patients with atopic eczema or atopic respiratory disease. Acta Derm Venereol (Stockh) (in press)
50. Rajka G (1960) Prurigo Besnier (atopic dermatitis) with special reference to the role of allergic factors. I. The influence of atopic hereditary factors. Acta Derm Venereol (Stockh) 40: 285–306
51. Rajka G (1975) Atopic dermatitis. Saunders, London
52. Rajka G (1989) Essential aspects of atopic dermatitis. Springer, Berlin Heidelberg New York
53. Reed WB, Kierland RR, Code CF (1958) Vascular reactions in chronically inflamed skin. I. Mechanical stimuli to the skin; inhibition of white dermographism. Arch Dermatol 77: 91–96
54. Ring J (1988) Angewandte Allergologie. MMV-Medizin, Munich
55. Rost GA (1929) Allergische Disposition und Status exsudativus. Klin Wochenschr 8: 2009–2013
56. Rost GA, Marchionini A (1932) Asthma-Ekzem, Asthma-Prurigo und Neurodermitis als allergische Hautkrankheiten. Würzburger Abh Gesamtgeb Med 27: 337–400
57. Schaumann B, Alter M (1976) Dermatoglyphics in medical disorders. Springer, Berlin Heidelberg New York

58. Schnyder UW, Borelli S (1962) Neurodermitis constitutionalis sive atopica. I. Nomenklatur, klinische Symptomatologie. In: Miescher G, Storck H (eds) Entzündliche Dermatosen I. Springer, Berlin Göttingen Heidelberg (Handbuch der Haut- und Geschlechtskrankheiten, vol 2/1)
59. Schönberger A, Langenstein B, Heyer G, Hornstein OP (1988) Quantifizierte Bestimmung des Dermographismus bei Patienten mit atopischem Ekzem. Hautarzt 39: 72–76
60. Smith DA (1984) Hyperlinear palms in atopic dermatitis: a manifestation of ichthyosis vulgaris? Cutis 34: 49–51
61. Solomon LM (1985) Atopic dermatitis. In: Moschella SL, Hurley HJ (eds) Dermatology, 2nd edn. Saunders, Philadelphia, pp 334–353
62. Svensson Å, Edman B, Möller H (1985) A diagnostic tool for atopic dermatitis based on clinical criteria. Acta Derm Venereol [Suppl] (Stockh) 114: 33–40
63. Tillner I (1956) Über zwei Merkmale der Handfurchung und ihre Anwendbarkeit in der erbbiologischen Vaterschaftsbegutachtung. Anthropol Anz 20: 79–94
64. Toda KI, Okamoto H, Horio T (1986) Lichen striatus. Int J Dermatol 25: 584–585
65. Uehara M (1981) Infraorbital fold in atopic dermatitis. Arch Dermatol 117: 627–629
66. Uehara M (1985) Clinical and histological features of dry skin in atopic dermatitis. Acta Derm Venereol (Stockh) 114: 82–86
67. Uehara M, Hayashi S (1981) Hyperlinear palms. Association with ichthyosis and atopic dermatitis. Arch Dermatol 117: 490–491
68. Uehara M, Miyauchi H (1984) The morphologic characteristics of dry skin in atopic dermatitis. Arch Dermatol 120: 1186–1190
69. Uehara M, Ofuji S (1977) Abnormal vascular reactions in atopic dermatitis. Arch Dermatol 113: 627–629
70. Urbach E (1935) Klinik und Therapie der allergischen Krankheiten. Maudrich, Vienna
71. Werner Linde Y (1989) "Dry" skin in atopic dermatitis. I. A clinical study. Acta Derm Venereol (Stockh) 69: 311–314
72. Werner Linde Y, Bengtsson A, Lodén M (1989) "Dry" skin in atopic dermatitis. II. A surface profilometry study. Acta Derm Venereol (Stockh) 69: 315–319
73. Whitfield A (1938) On the white reaction (white line) in dermatology. Br J Dermatol 50: 71–82
74. Wong RC, Fairley JA, Ellis CN (1984) Dermographism: a review. J Am Acad Dermatol 11: 643–652
75. Wüthrich B, Schnyder UW (1981) Eine wenig bekannte Ausdrucksform der Neurodermitis atopica im Kindesalter: Das Patchy pityriasiform lichenoid eczema ("Kitamura-Takahashi-Sasagawa"). Aktuel Dermatol 7: 85–87
76. Yoshida K, Mizuno N, Tada T (1974) Serum IgE level and white dermographism in atopic dermatitis, atopic skin, and infantile eczema. J Dermatol 1: 152–156

Minimal Forms of Atopic Eczema

B. Wüthrich

The description of the atypical forms of atopic eczema can be attributed primarily to French authors in the middle of the 1960s and the beginning of the 1970s [2, 3, 30, 37, 38]. In the German-speaking sphere, special credit is due to Herzberg [12–14] for having alluded to atopic eczema found usually in two but occasionally even in three and four generations of patients, based on his clinical observations and skin reaction studies. These special forms and minimal variants may occur alone, together, or alternate with the more typical eczematoid, lichenoid, pruriginous, and seborrheic forms whose occurrence is related to age, individual predisposition, and disease duration – indicative of their status as atopic skin manifestations. When occurring alone, their classification as a minimal form of atopic eczema may be disputable, especially in the "intrinsic type," in which no demonstrable sensitization to atopic allergens exists [47, 49, 50]. Thus, the diagnosis can only be finally accepted on the basis of a family and personal history, progress monitoring, further clinical features related to other stigmata of the atopic constitution, positive skin reaction (e.g. white dermatographism), and histology. The special forms of presentation attract attention because they are clinical and morphological variants, and because of their particular sites of location, such as the eyelids, lips, nipples, vulva, fingerpads and toes [22].

The Follicular Variant or Patchy Pityriasiform Lichenoid Eczema

Patchy pityriasiform lichenoid eczema is a dry, only slightly irritating, follicular form of atopic eczema occurring in childhood. Its first description is attributable to Kitamura [17]. In a 1966 paper published in *Hautarzt*, he mentioned that, as far back as 1950, together with Takahashi and Sasagawa, he had described a plaque-shaped, lichenoid, scaly eczema as an independent "dry" type of childhood eczema. This type, evidently common in Japan, was allocated by Sasagawa in 1967 to the group of atopic forms. Histologically, these itchy "chicken-skin spots" exhibit a spongiosis of the follicular epithelium and an intra- and perifollicular lymphohistiocytic infiltration [33, 51], which indicates the eczematous nature of this condition (Figs. 1 and 2).

Thus, clinically there are partly confluent areas with densely juxtaposed, mildly bran-like, scaly, nonhyperkeratotic, skin-colored papules (Figs. 3 and 4). They are found, with a generally dry integument, especially on the trunk but also on the nape of the neck and the extensor aspects of the knees. Pruritus is usually present, though not always severe. Mildly scaly depigmented areas, rather like a pityriasis alba [45, 46] and isolated, frequently asymmetric, typical lichenified foci on the backs of the hands or elbows are also occasionally present. In our series, a discrete perennial or seasonal allergic rhinitis was frequently associated. Progression of the disease is observed particularly in winter, whereas summer visits to the seaside usually lead to improvement or healing of the rash. Ofuji and Uehara [28] also found, in 96% of their patients with atopic eczema, similar itchy follicular papules, particularly on the lateral parts of the trunk. They suggested that these lesions probably constitute the primary efflorescence of atopic eczema.

Differential diagnosis requires distinction from suprafollicular keratosis, follicular hyperkeratoses in the context of an autosomal dominant ichtyosis vulgaris [24], lichen planopilaris, lichen nitidus, and the various lichenoid id reactions, e.g., mykid or Gianotti-Crosti syndrome [9, 10].

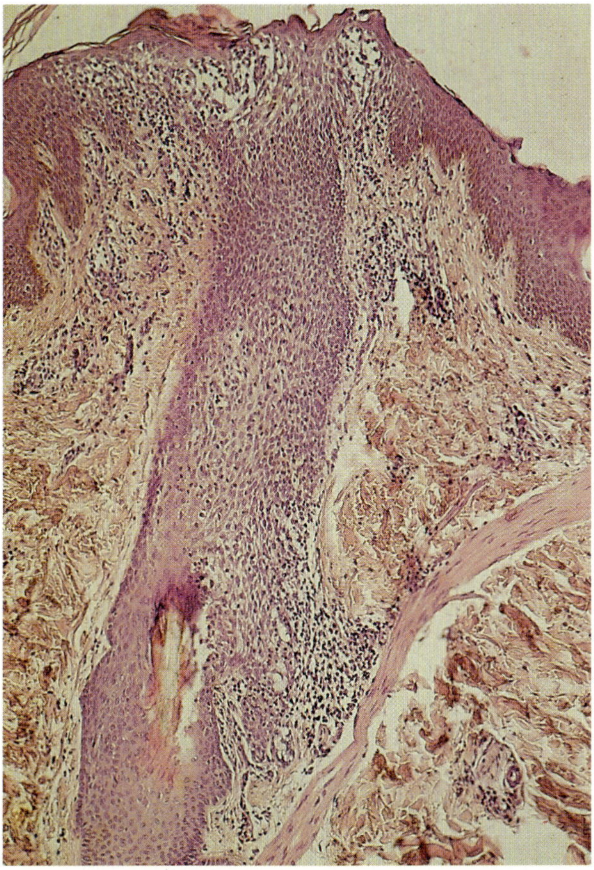

Fig. 1. Follicular form of atopic eczema in a 10-year-old girl. Histologic findings: follicular papule with spongiosis of the epidermis and lymphohystiocytic intra- and perifollicular infiltration.

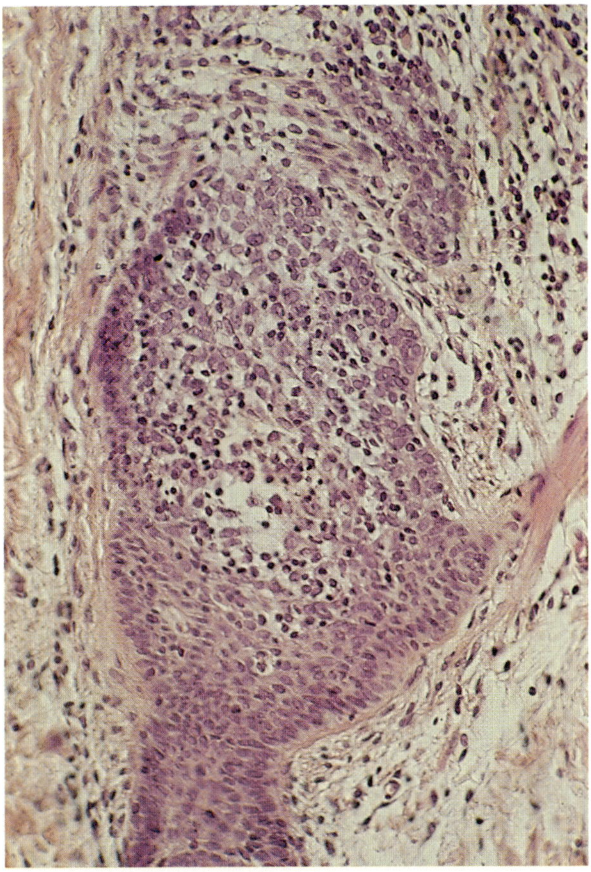

Fig. 2. Histologic findings: spongiosis of follicular epithelium with lymphohistiocytic infiltration (same patient as in Fig. 1)

Fig. 3. Follicular form of atopic eczema. Clinically: plaque-shaped "chicken-skin spots" on infrascapular region of back. (1-year-old boy, dark skinned)

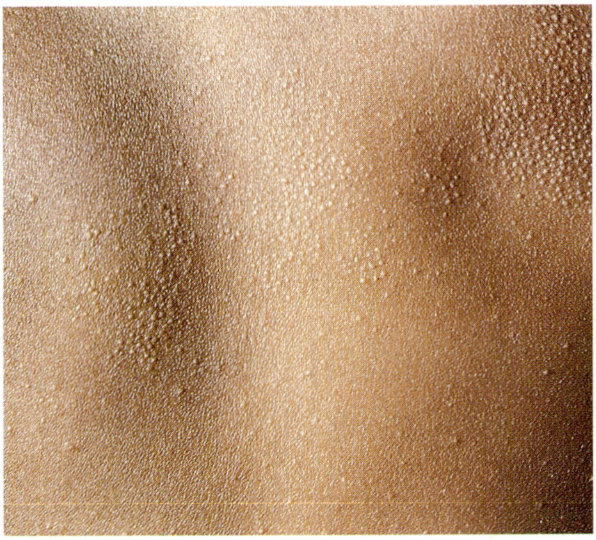

Fig. 4. Follicular form of atopic eczema. Clinically: closely packed, skin-colored follicular papules (1-year-old boy)

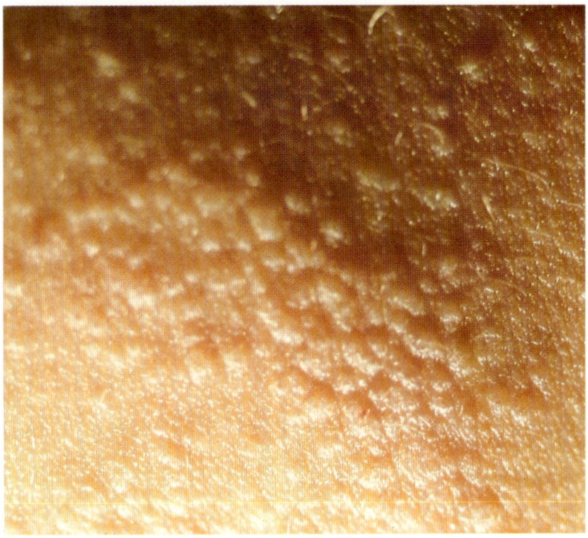

The Papular Variants of Atopic Eczema

Similar differential diagnostic considerations apply to the papular variants of atopic eczema, mostly found on the extensor aspects of the knees, but occasionally also of the elbows and backs of the hands. The clinical picture corresponds to those designated in the literature as juvenile papular dermatitis [4, 32], frictional lichenoid eruption in children [44], or dermatite du toboggan [6, 18] (Figs. 5 and 6).

We have assigned these acro-localized, small papular lesions to atopic eczema based on family and personal history, demonstration of specific IgEs to inhaled or nutrient allergens, and the eczematoid histologic picture (Fig. 7), which distinguishes these lesions from those hitherto described in juvenile papular dermatitis [48]. In contrast to the follicular variants, the papular forms appear mainly in the spring and summer, often in association with a pollinosis. This is pathogenetically suggestive of an inhaled precipitant as a "hay fever equivalent" [50] in addition to a mechanical component (friction, chafing).

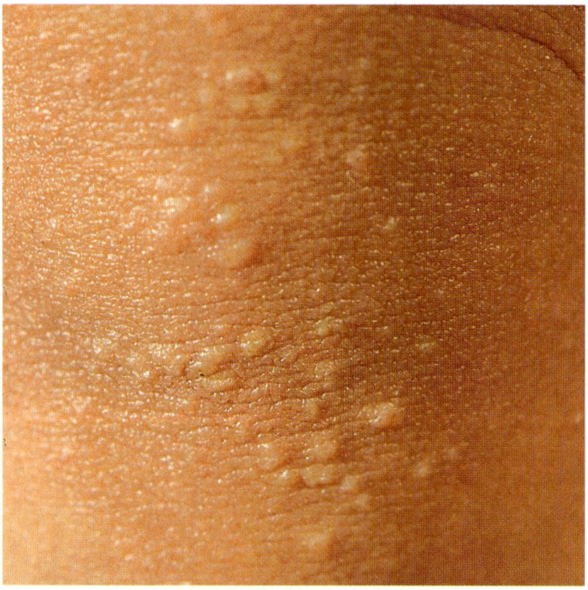

Fig. 5. Papular form of atopic eczema. Clinically: disseminated flat papules on extensor aspect of knees (5-year-old girl with mild rhinitis pollinosa)

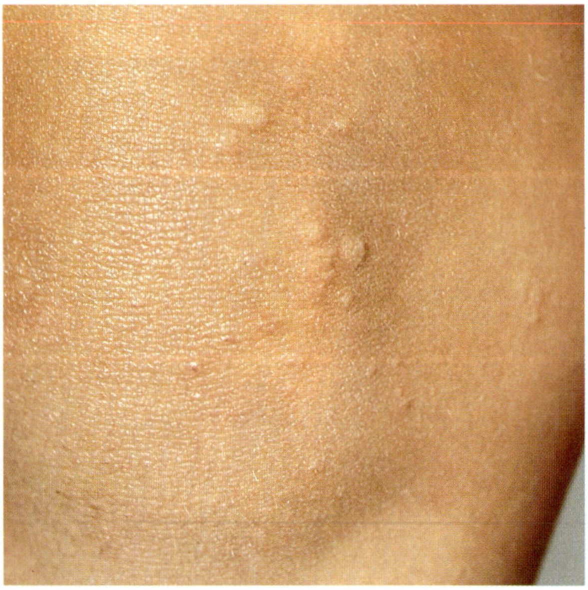

Fig. 6. Papular form of atopic eczema. Clinically: several itchy papules together with follicular variants on extensor aspect of knees (7-year-old boy)

Fig. 7. Papular form of atopic eczema. Histologic findings in papule of right knee: eczematoid dermatitis (same patient as in Fig. 5)

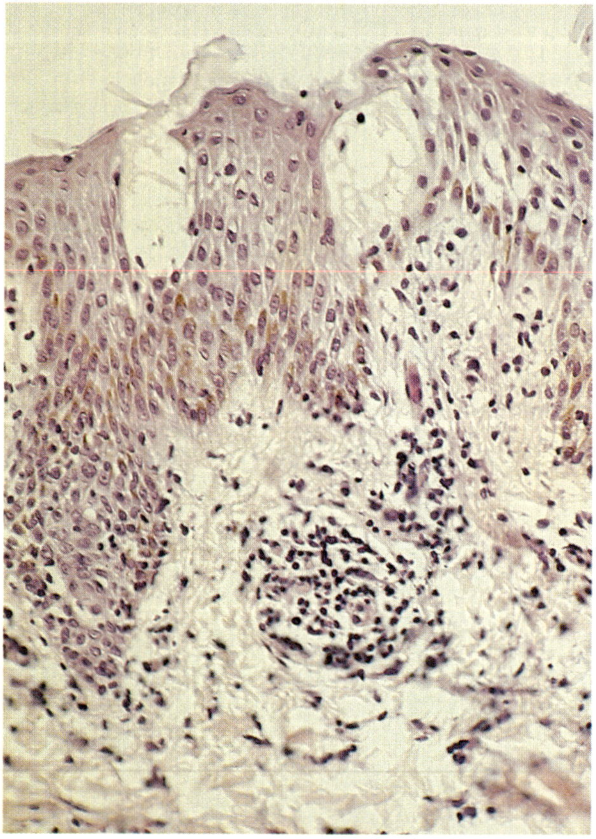

Localized Minimal Variants of Atopic Eczema

Such localized variants ("les petits signes cliniques du terrain atopique;" [30]) include:

- Exfoliating cheilitis with perlèche (Fig. 8)
- Retroauricular intertrigo or earlobe rhagades (Fig. 9)
- Rhagades of the nasal orifices, often with chronic nasal obstruction as the expression of a perennial allergic rhinitis (Fig. 10)
- Lower lid eczema, frequently occurring in the spring as a pollinosis equivalent [36, 50] (Fig. 11)
- Nipple eczema (Fig. 12)
- Tylotic, rhagadiform, fingerpad eczema (pulpite digitale keratosique craquelée récidivante or pulpite sèche) (Figs. 13 and 14)
- Similar manifestations on the toes ("atopic feet" or "juvenile plantar dermatosis"; see below) (Figs. 15 and 16)

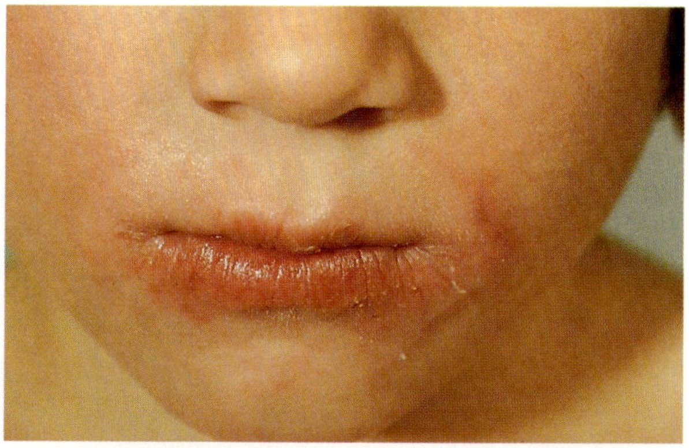

Fig. 8. Exfoliative cheilitis with perleche (6-year-old boy)

Fig. 9. Retroauricular rhagades (9-year-old boy)

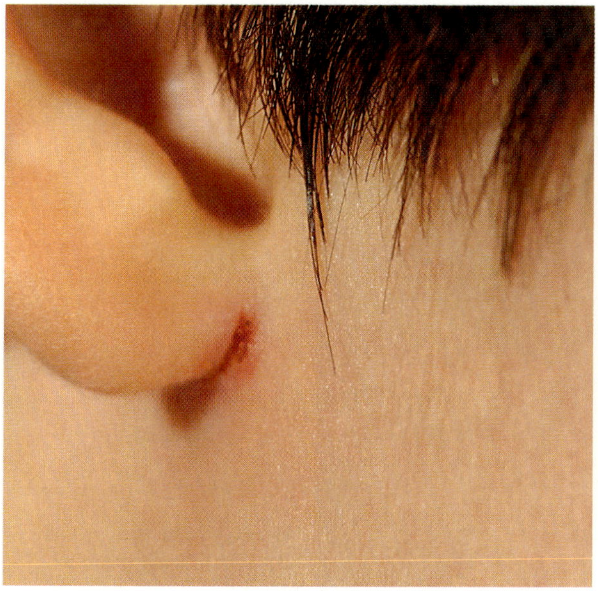

Fig. 10. Rhagades at both nasal orifices (right more than left) in chronic allergic rhinopathy (same patient as in Fig. 9)

Fig. 11. Atopic eyelid eczema, bilateral, "pollinosis equivalent" (31-year-old woman with grass pollen allergy)

Fig. 12. Nipple eczema (23-year-old woman)

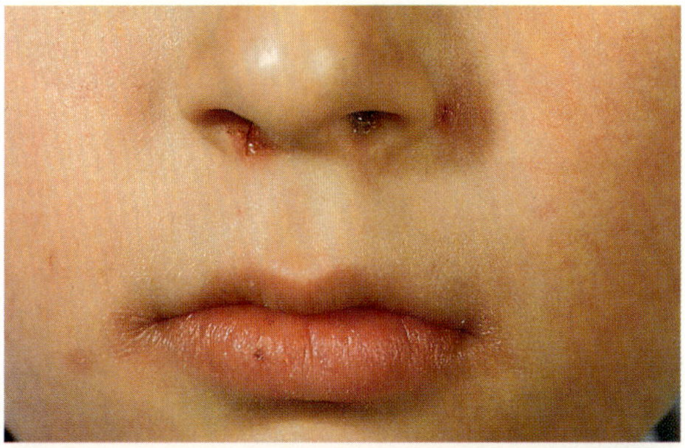

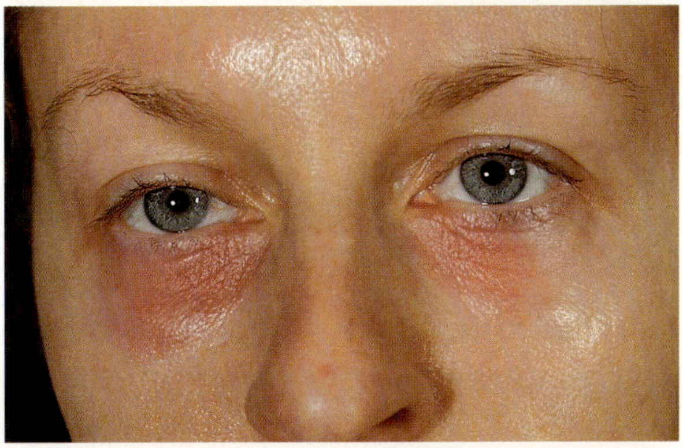

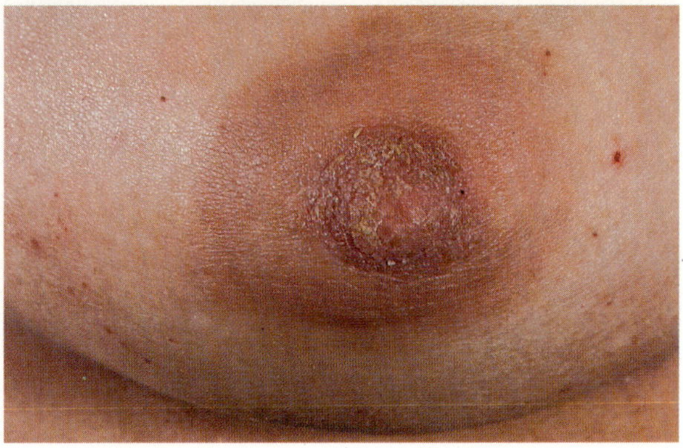

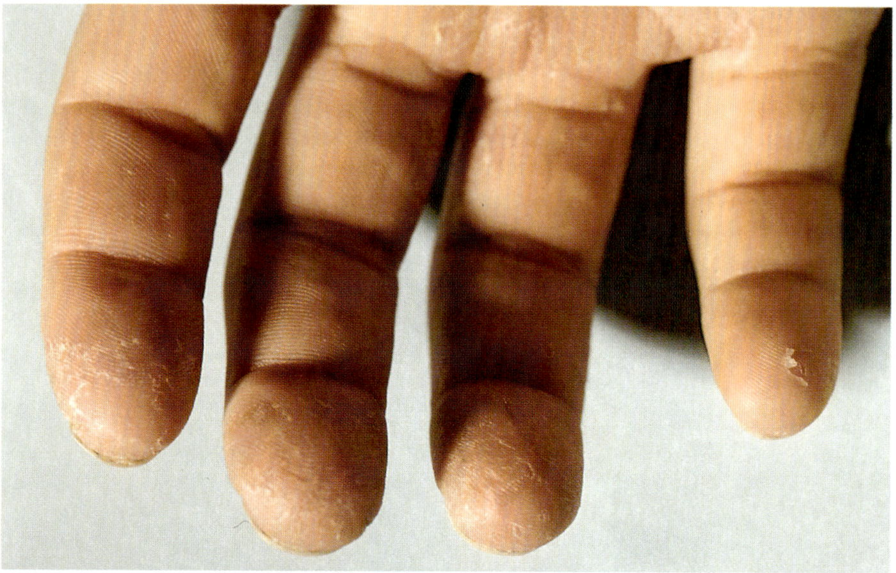

Fig. 13. Tylotic, rhagadiform, fingerpad eczema (10-year-old boy)

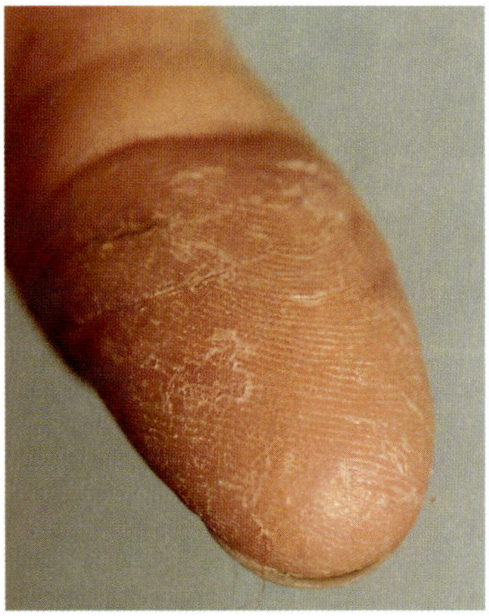

Fig. 14. Rosette-shaped scaling similar to a lamellosis sicca with painful rhagades (same patient as in Fig. 13)

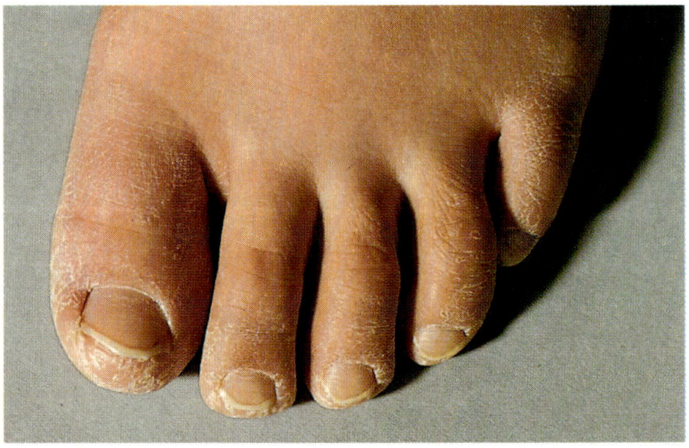

Fig. 15. Atopic toes, dorsal aspect (same patient as in Figs. 13 and 14)

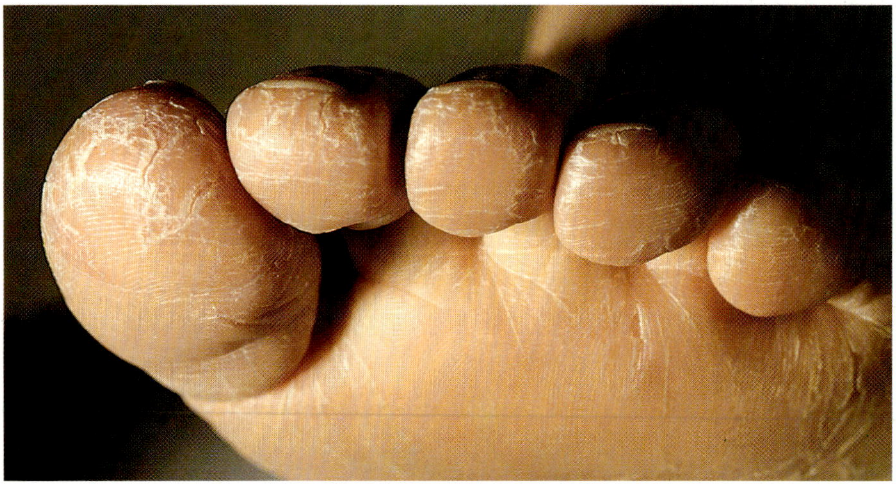

Fig. 16. Atopic toes, plantar aspect (same patient as in Fig. 13)

According to Herzberg [13], over 70% of patients with pulpite sèche are women, in whom the role of skin traumatization in influencing localization is emphasized by the fact that the pads of the first to third fingers are initially affected and those of the fourth and fifth fingers only later. Furthermore in right-handed persons the right hand is more often affected than is the left. Apart from the clinical signs of a pale erythema, insignificant edema, keratosis, scaling, and fissuring, concomitant pain leads subjectively to impairment of function in the involved hand. Herzberg also mentioned, as a practical sign, that delicate materials such as nylon stockings are torn by the sharp edges of the fissures when being put on and taken off!

The allocation of these localized variants to atopic eczema obviously postulates negative epicutaneous testing to possible contact allergens (perioral group, shoe eczema group, etc.). In a prospective study of 105 patients with typical atopic eczema (average age 8.5 years) and 113 controls without atopy (average age 16 years), Mevorah et al. [25] came to the conclusion that retroauricular rhagades, cheilitis, nipple eczema, and pityriasis alba are undoubtedly statistically highly significant ($p < 0.005$) as regards diagnostic importance in atopic eczema, but that Dennie-Morgan infraorbital creases [27, 39] and anterior neck creases are not. Also controversial is the allocation to atopy of the "dirty neck" sign, a reticular pigmentation of the neck which makes it appear unwashed [5], and the correlation between either "geographic tongue" [23, 40] or dandruff [19] and atopy.

Juvenile Plantar Dermatosis

This disease concerns a painful variant of atopic eczema, frequently occurring in children. It is chiefly observed on the anterior part of the sole of the foot and is characterized by erythema, hyperkeratosis, and rhagades (Figs. 17 and 18). Histologically, there is an eczematoid dermatitis (Fig. 18). As early as 1966, Racouchot [30] had explicitly alluded to its relationship to the group of atopic forms: "La kératose plantaire et les fissures hivernales des bords des talons sont à retenir," and in 1968 Silvers and Glickman [34] gave a thorough description of the special features of atopic eczema of the feet in children. In 1972 this affection became well known due to a publication of Moller [26] who proposed the name of "atopic

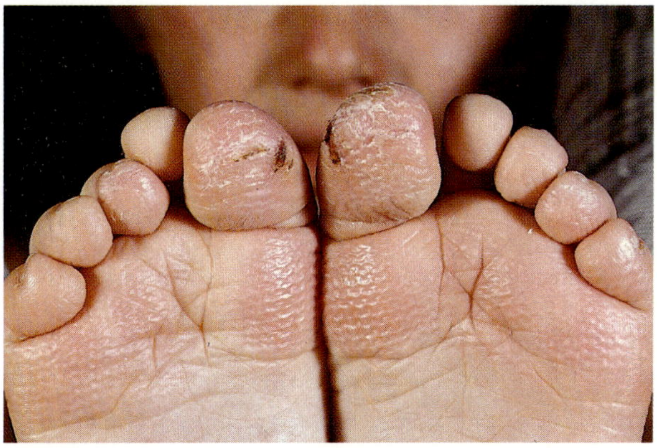

Fig. 17. Tylotic, rhagadiform eczema of tips of toes, often misdiagnosed as foot mycosis (mycoid form of atopic eczema (4-year-old boy)

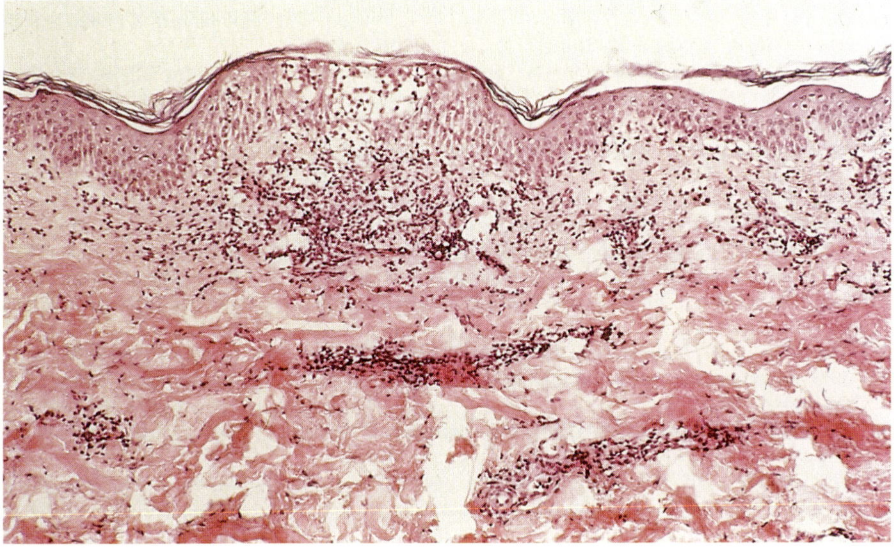

Fig. 18. Atopic toes. Histologic findings: eczematoid dermatitis with spongiosis and lymphohistiocytic infiltration (subepidermal and perivascular)

winter feet." However, it also occurs in the summer months, so that in practice it is often misdiagnosed as a foot mycosis and thus erroneously treated with antimycotics (see [13]).

Whereas, in 1978, Verbov [41] as well as Hambly and Wilkinson [11] also described "forefoot eczema" in the context of an atopy, Mackie and Husain, in 1976, considered "juvenile plantar dermatosis" to be a new entity since only 9 of the 102 children they studied had a manifest atopy [20]. They attributed the cause to nylon socks. Subsequently, other terms were proposed such as "dermatitis plantaris sicca" [8, 16], "peridigital dermatitis" [7], or "wet and dry foot syndrome" [35], but the term most commonly used today is the simple descriptive "juvenile plantar dermatosis" (JPD). Although association with atopy has been found by various authors, ranging from 50.3% of patients [42] to 61% [1], 68% [11], ad 74% [43]. Young in 1986 [48], like Mackie and Husain [20] earlier, found no preponderance of atopy. Rajka [31] suggested distinguishing between an "atopy-associated" and a "nonatopic" variant. In both types, along with a possible constitutional weakness of the skin, various other endogenous and exogenous factors have been discussed as pathogenetic, such as frequently repeated microtraumata ("frictional contact dermatitis"), a clammy microclimate due to the wearing of synthetic socks and high shoes, or a contact allergy to parts of shoes. In a recently published paper, Pirkl et al. [29] suggest broad-spectrum epicutaneous testing in JPD in the following circumstances:

- The appeareance of a JPD after wearing newly bought shoes
- Characteristic JPD which spreads secondarily over the heels or dorsum of the foot or toes or the outer border of the foot
- Severe JPD with primary involvement of the heels.

If the rare cases of allergic contact eczema are excluded, follow-up studies have-shown that complete recovery may be expected with puberty in the majority of patients after a course of 7–8 years on average [15, 21, 42].

References

1. Asthton RE, Griffith WAD (1986) Juvenile plantar dermatosis – atopy or footwear? Clin Exp Dermatol 11: 529–534
2. Bazex A, Salvador R, Dupré A, Christol B (1965) Eczéma nummulaire: ses rapports avec l'eczéma atopique. Bull Soc Dermatol Syphiligr 72: 432
3. Bazex A, Dupré A, Christol B (1966) Aspects morphologiques atypiques de l'eczéma atopique. Rev Med 1: 62
4. Bork K, Hoede N (1978) Juvenile papulöse Dermatitis. Hautarzt 290: 216–219
5. Colver GB, Mortimer PS, Millard PR, et al. (1987) The "dirty neck" – a reticulate pigmentation in atopics. Clin Exp Dermatol 12: 1–4
6. Dupré MMA, Christol B, Bonafe JL, et al. (1974) La dermite du toboggan (variant de "frictional lichenoid eruption in children"). Bull Soc Fr Dermatol Syphiligr 81: 203–205
7. Enta T (1980) Peridigital dermatitis in children. Int J Dermatol 19: 390–391
8. Friis B (1974) Dermatitis plantaris sicca bei Kindern. Dermatol Monatsschr 160: 614–620
9. Gianotti F (1976) Die infantilen papulösen Akrodermatitiden. Die Akrodermatitis papulosa und das infantile papulovesikulöse akrolokalisierte Syndrom. Hautarzt 27: 467–472
10. Gianotti F (1979) Papular acrodermatitis of childhood and other papulovesicular acro-located syndromes. Br J Dermatol 100: 49–58
11. Hambly EM, Wilkinson DS (1978) Sur quelques formes atypiques d'eczéma chez l'enfant. Ann Dermatol Venereol 105: 369–371
12. Herzberg (1972) Wenig bekannte Ausdrucksformen der Neurodermitis. Arch Dermatol Forsch 244: 350–352
13. Herzberg J (1973) Wenig bekannte Formen der Neurodermitis. Hautarzt 24: 47–51
14. Herzberg J (1976) Besondere Manifestationsformen der Neurodermitis diffusa (atopische Dermatitis). In: Braun-Falco O, Marghescu S (eds) Fortschritte der praktischen Dermatologie und Venerologie. Springer, Berlin Heidelberg New York, pp 19–24
15. Jones SK, English JSC, Forsyth A, Mackie RM (1987) Juvenile plantar dermatosis – an 8-year follow-up of 102 patients. Clin Exp Dermatol 12: 5–7
16. Kint A, van Hecke E, Leys G (1982) Dermatitis plantaris sicca. Dermatologica 165: 500–509
17. Kitamura K (1966) Zur Frage des Kinderekzems. Hautarzt 17: 53–55
18. Laurent MMR, Agache P (1975) Dermite lichénoide de friction (dermite des toboggans). Bull Soc Fr Dermatol Syphiligr 82: 220–221
19. Lindmaier A, Lindemayr H, Schmidt JB (1987) Kopfschuppen – ein atopisches Stigma? Hautarzt 38: 138–141
20. Mackie RM, Husain SL (1976) Juvenile plantar dermatosis: a new entity? Clin Exp Dermatol 1: 253–260
21. Maleville J, Marsan PH, Coindre MCL, et al. (1984) Une dermatose infantile peu connue: la pulpite sèche de l'avant-pied ou dermatose plantaire juvénile. A propos de 68 cas. Sem Hop Paris 60: 2401–2404
22. Marghescu S (1990) Besondere Manifestationsformen des atopischen Ekzems. In: Braun-Falco O, Ring J (eds) Fortschritte der praktischen Dermatologie und Venerologie, vol 12. Springer, Berlin Heidelberg New York, pp 99–102
23. Marks S, Simons MJ (1979) Geographic tongue – a manifestation of atopy. Br J Dermatol 101: 159–162
24. Mevorah B, Marazzi A, Frenk E (1985) The prevalence of

accentuated palmoplantar markings and keratosis pilaris in atopic dermatitis, autosomal dominant ichthyosis and control dermatological patients. Br J Dermatol 112: 679–685
25. Mevorah B, Frenk E, Wietlisbach V, Carrel CF (1988) Minor clinical features of atopic dermatitis. Evaluation of their diagnostic significance. Dermatologica 177: 360–364
26. Moller H (1972) Atopic winter feet in children. Acta Derm Venereol (Stockh) 52: 401–405
27. Morgan DB (1948) A suggestive sign of allergy. Arch Dermatol Syphitol 57: 1050
28. Ofuji S, Uehara M (1973) Follicular eruption of atopic dermatitis. Arch Dermatol 107: 54–55
29. Pirkl S, Tennstedt D, Egger S, Lachapelle JM (1990) Juvenile plantar dermatosis: wann sind Epikutantestungen indiziert? Hautarzt 41: 22–26
30. Racouchot MJ (1966) Les petits signes cliniques du terrain eczémateux. Bull Soc Dermatol Syphiligr 73: 531–535
31. Rajka G (1989) On definition and framework of atopic dermatitis. Acta Derm Venereol (Stockh) Suppl 144: 10–12
32. Rook A (1978) Juvenile papular dermatitis. In: Rook A, Wilkinson DS, Ebling FJG (eds) Textbook of dermatology, vol 1, 3rd edn. Blackwell, Oxford, pp 676
33. Sasagawa S (1967) Studies on the dry form of eczema in childhood – patchy pityriasiform lichenoid eczema (Kitamura-Taahashi-Sasagawa) Jpn J Dermatol 77: 62–87
34. Silvers SH, Glickman FS (1968) Atopy and eczema of the feet in children. Am J Dis Child 116: 400–401
35. Steck WD (1983) Juvenile plantar dermatosis: The "wet and dry foot syndrome". Cleve Clin Q 50: 145–149
36. Storck H (1960) Neurodermitis disseminata mit Verschlimmerung im Sommer, Aufflammen nach Inhalation von Pollenallergenen. Dermatologica 121: 150–151
37. Temime P, Oddoze L (1970) La chéilite exfoliatrice et la pulpite digitale keratosique craquelée récidivante peuvent être des manifestations atopiques. Bull Soc Dermatol Syphiligr 77: 150–156
38. Temime P, Bazex A, de Graciansky P, et al. (1972) The atypical cutaneous manifestations of atopy. Excerpta Med Int Congr Ser 251: 147
39. Uehara M (1981) Infraorbital fold in atopic dermatitis. Arch Dermatol 117: 627–629
40. Ullmann W (1981) Korrelation zwischen Exfoliatio linguae areata und Atopie. Hautarzt 32: 629–631
41. Verbov J (1978) Atopic eczema localized to the forefoot. An unrecognized entity. Practitioner 220 (1313): 465–466
42. Verbov J (1989) Juvenile plantar dermatosis (JPD). Acta Derm Venereol (Stockh) 144: 153–154
43. Voss Jepsen L (1978) Dermatitis plantaris sicca: a retrospective study of children with recurrent dermatitis of the feet. Acta Derm Venereol (Stockh) 59: 257–259
44. Waisman M, Gables C, Sutton RL (1966) Frictional lichenoid eruption in children. Arch Dermatol 94: 592–593
45. Watkins CDB (1961) Pityriasis alba: a form of atopic dermatitis. Arch Dermatol 83: 915–919
46. Wolf R, Sandbank M, Krakowski A (1983) Extensive pityriasis alba and atopic dermatitis. Br J Dermatol 84: 247
47. Wüthrich B (1983a) Neurodermitis atopica sive constitutionalis. Ein pathogenetisches Modell aus der Sicht des Allergologen. Aktuel Dermatol 9: 1–7
48. Wüthrich B (1983b) Papulöse Neurodermitis atopica: eine besondere Form der juvenilen papulösen Dermatitis? Dermatologica 167: 196
49. Wüthrich B (1987) Neurodermitis atopica (atopische Dermatitis). In: Fuchs E, Schuld KH (eds) Manuale allergologicum. Dustri, Deisenhofen, pp V1–V34
50. Wüthrich B (1989) Atopic dermatitis flare provoked by inhalant allergens. Dermatologica 178: 51–53
51. Wüthrich B, Schnyder UW (1981) Eine wenig bekannte Ausdrucksform der Neurodermitits atopica im Kindesalter: Das Patchy Pityriasiform Lichenoid Eczema ("Kitamura-Takahashi-Sasagawa"). Aktuel Dermatol 7: 85–87
52. Young E (1986) Forefoot eczema – further studies and a review. Clin Exp Dermatol 11: 523–528

Complications and Diseases Associated with Atopic Eczema

D. Vieluf and T. Ruzicka

Introduction

Numerous factors lead to great difficulties in assessing the possible complications and diseases associated with atopic eczema (AE) [122, 248]. A major problem is correct diagnosis of AE, which has only recently been subjected to a certain standardization [29, 67a, 121, 123, 124, 125, 126, 128, 166a, 212, 273, 306a, 347]. A survey of the innumerable case reports and review articles dealing with this topic is hampered by the variable definition of AE and by imprecise description of skin lesions, particularly in the nondermatological literature, making proper classification impossible. Exact epidemiological data concerning the prevalence of atopic diseases are rare (see chapter by Schmied and Saurat, this volume). Thus, it is even more difficult to assess the frequency of diseases associated with AE, and to answer the question whether the association is incidental, rare, frequent, or constant. In addition, epidemiological studies and case reports mostly do not address the question of the causal relation between the underlying AE and the reported association. Despite these shortcomings, we will attempt to review diseases associated with AE and, if possible, discuss current ideas on causes and pathogenesis. We will omit from this review disorders dealt with in other chapters of this book (e. g. allergic contact eczema, food hypersensitivity, occupational aspects, psychosomatic abnormalities, severe immunodeficiency syndromes, side effects of glucocorticosteroids).

Complications of Atopic Eczema

General Remarks

As yet, it is still controversial whether the increased susceptibility and severity of different viral, mycotic, and bacterial skin infections in AE is a direct consequence of defective cell-mediated immunity and/or other immunological abnormalities [29, 113, 121, 123, 145, 172, 218, 252, 265, 267, 273] (see chapters by Strannegard and Strannegard and by Fritsch and Hintner, this volume), or is due to a defective barrier function of the skin (see chapters by Melnik and Gollhausen, this volume). In addition, eczematous skin with crusted erosions and excoriations may provide a favorable milieu for the growth and multiplication of infectious agents [130, 194]. Finally, prolonged topical or systemic glucocorticosteroid treatment may enhance the susceptibility of the skin to specific viral or bacterial infections due to its immunosuppressive effects. Prolonged antibiotic treatment is likely to favor the emergence of pathogenic microbial agents [57, 194, 252].

Bacterial Infections

The skin of atopic patients shows a high rate of colonization with coagulase-positive *Staphylococcus aureus* [7, 8, 25, 57, 60, 123, 127, 130, 135, 140, 140a, 146, 191, 194, 227, 258, 273, 295, 339] (see chapter by Abeck and Ruzicka, this volume). This is predominantly seen on lesional skin with excoriations and fissures in infants and children [123]. Extensive serous weeping and/or honey-colored crusting, especially in the presence of lymphadenopathy, indicates infection with *Staphylococcus aureus* [60, 125, 146, 227, 295]. Though bullous impetigo may also occur in atopic children [295] (Fig. 1), staphylococcal scalded skin syndrome (SSSS) is exceedingly rare despite the regular colonization with staphylococci. This is due to the absence of epidermolytic toxin-producing strains [7, 8]. Other clinical manifestations besides impetignization may include folliculitis [339] and small pruritic pustules not always confined to follicles which may precede exacerbations of AE [57, 124, 130, 146, 252, 295, 339]. Staphylolococcal infection may provoke intense pruritus and scratching, hence crusted erosions are more frequently encountered than pustular lesions [130, 146]. Deeper tissue involvement such as furuncles, carbuncles, abscesses, erysipelas and systemic signs of infec-

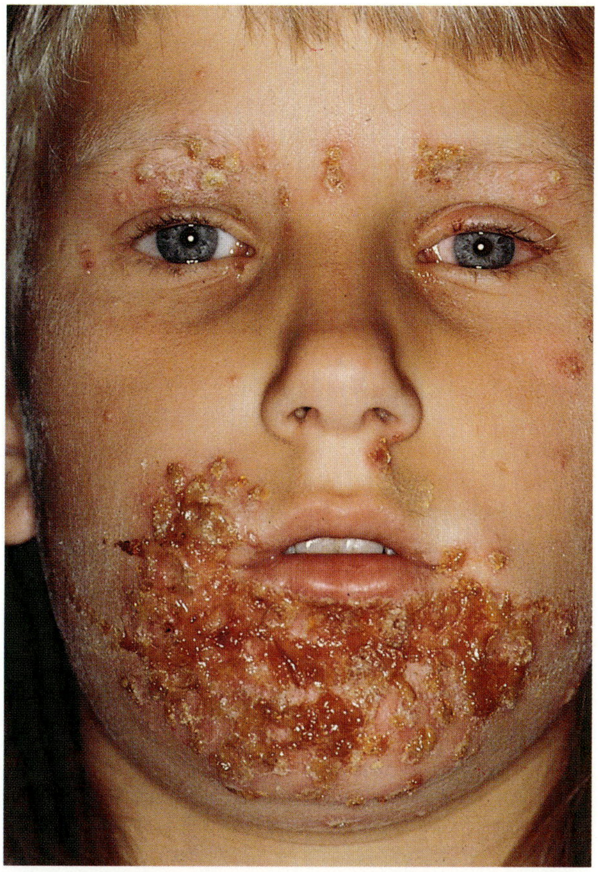

Fig. 1. Bullous impetigo in a child with atopic eczema

tion such as fever and leukocytosis are rather uncommon [124, 130, 184, 227, 252]. Their occurrence should alert one to the possibility of a hyper-IgE-syndrome (see chapter by Fritsch and Hintner, this volume). The presence of crusted vesicles should initiate the search for viral, particularly herpetic, superinfection [125, 191]. Superinfection of eczematous skin lesions with β-hemolytic streptococci is a rare event [57, 130, 146, 191, 227, 233, 252].

In three children with severe atopic eczema, osteomyelitis of the distal phalanges has recently been described. One case of olecranon bursitis has also been mentioned in the literature [31]. The pathogenetic concepts relating to staphylococcal infection and AE are summarized by Abeck and Ruzicka elsewhere in this volume.

Mycotic Infections

Dermatophytic infections of the skin, hair, or nails show a variety of clinical manifestations ranging from acute discrete or intensely inflammatory skin lesions to chronic recalcitrant ones [302]. In the general population, dermatophytoses are among the most frequently occurring skin disorders (USA: 3.8% of the population, with 35%–45% of all clinical manifestations comprising tinea pedum) [303]. Males are more often affected (6.8%) than females (1.1%). Infections in children are rare (0.04%–1.4%, males more than females) [304].

The susceptibility to dermatophyte infections is probably influenced by sex, age, and a variety of local factors such as skin disorders accompanied by increased keratinization (e. g., ichthyoses), dryness of the skin, defects of the epidermal barrier function, humidity, and maceration facilitating the colonization by the fungus [302]. Besides these individual factors, environmental circumstances are also of importance (footwear, profession, sports, etc.) [302, 304]. Atopy, defined as AE, allergic rhinitis, or exogenous allergic bronchial asthma, or as a familial predisposition to these disorders, has been shown in several studies to be associated with a predisposition to acquiring persistent extensive, usually superficial, infections with *Trichophyton rubrum*, predominantly on feet, hands, and nails.

Recent epidemiological studies have confirmed the increased susceptibility to infections with *Trichophyton rubrum* and enhanced risk for persistant infections in atopic individuals [129, 164–166, 302–304].

In the atopic population, intradermal tests have shown diminished delayed type skin reactivity to *Trichophyton* antigens (especially *Trichophyton rubrum* antigens). Most patients with AE showed a lack of delayed response, despite the frequent occurrence of immediate-type reactions to trichophytin [129, 142, 164, 165, 166, 253, 302, 304, 305]. This may be a sign of cross-reactivity to mold antigens [253]. Atopic respiratory disease seemed to be a more important predisposing factor than AE [164, 166]. The lack of a pronounced inflammatory component is a regular conspicuous finding in chronic dermatophyte infections in atopic individuals. Despite the frequency of superficial mycoses, widespread or severe infection rarely occurs [302, 304, 305].

Atopic Eczema and Pityrosporum Infection

Pityrosporum orbiculare (P. ovale) is a saprophytic lipophilic yeast belonging to the normal microbial flora of human skin. Under certain circumstances it may become pathogenic and cause skin disorders such as Pityriasis versicolor, *Pityrosporum folliculitis, Papillomatose confluente et réticulée*, etc. [35, 49, 270, 329].

Pityrosporum species may be involved in the so-called head, neck, and shoulder dermatitis (HNS dermatitis). The patients show highly pruritic, intensely inflammatory eczematous skin lesions localized to head, neck, and shoulders. In these patients, *Pityrosporum* species have been isolated from skin lesions. Most interestingly, strong immediate skin reactivity, positive radioallergosorbent tests (RAST), and histamine release could be demonstrated using *Pityrosporum* extracts. It is assumed that in atopic individuals colonization of the skin with *Pityrosporum* species causes IgE-mediated sensitization, leading to flare up of AE. An additional hint to the causal relationship between HNS dermatitis and *Pityrosporum* species is the response to local or systemic antimycotic treatment with imidazole derivatives, but relapses occur after weeks to months [49, 269, 309a, 329, 348].

Other yeasts such as *Candida albicans* have been discussed as flare factors in AE [211], but conclusive scientific evidence for their pathogenetic importance is lacking.

Viral Infections

Ever since the description of Kaposi's varicelliform eruption (pustulosis vacciniformis acuta) in 1887 [167], numerous publications have underlined the increased susceptibility of AE patients to unusually severe cutaneous infections with vaccinia and, later on, herpes simplex virus (HSV) [30, 33, 35, 45, 52, 108, 128, 139, 146, 181, 191, 193, 217, 227, 252, 338].

Although Kaposi is generally accepted as the first describer of the varicelliform eruption in eczema vaccinatum, it was Martin in 1882, who attributed this disease to smallpox vaccination [52].

That HSV could cause a clinically similar eruption and illness in patients with AE was not recognized until Esser and Seidenberg isolated and identified it during a small epidemic of such cases in an infants' ward in 1941 [52]. Kaposi's varicelliform eruption due to Coxsackie virus A16 is a rarity [33].

Viral infections in AE may range from harmless problems such as increased incidence of warts and mollusca contagiosa to potentially life-threatening disseminated infections such as eczema herpeticum or vaccinatum. Although exact epidemiological data are lacking, available evidence suggests a slightly higher incidence of HSV 1 and 2 infections, mollusca contagiosa, and, to a lesser degree, common warts in the atopic population compared with nonatopics [33, 56, 62, 108, 128, 233, 252, 280, 293].

Eczema Herpeticum

Eczema herpeticum is a form of disseminated cutaneous HSV type 1 or 2 infection [143]. HSV is a karyotropic DNA virus belonging, together with zoster, Epstein-Barr and cytomegalovirus to the Herpesvirus group. The severity of HSV-induced infections varies from localized and mild transient mucocutaneous lesions to widespread and fulminant, potentially life-threatening, disease [30, 35, 61, 62, 139, 181, 191, 193, 217, 252, 257, 270, 280, 345].

Eczema herpeticum complicates AE mostly in children and young adults [33, 35, 62, 181, 191, 252, 270, 280, 345]. It is characterized by the appearance of initially discrete localized clusters of tiny pruritic superficial vesicles and vesiculopustules which may disseminate over a large skin surface area (Fig. 2 a–c). They often erupt in crops on erythematous and edematous skin. Individual lesions pass almost simultaneously through developmental stages characterized by vesicles with or without umbilication, pustulation, and crust formation. In severe cases, hemorrhagic and eroded lesions can be observed. Typical locations include face, neck, shoulders, upper trunk, and abdomen, with a symmetrical distribution. The eruption is often accompanied by constitutional

Fig. 2a. Eczema herpeticum with widespread monomorphous dissemination of crusted vesicles in a patient with atopic eczema. **b.** Detail of **a. c.** Close up view of umbilicated vesicles. **d.** Tzanck smear of vesicle fluid (courtesy of Dr. B. Gizycki-Nienhaus, Department of Dermatology, University of Munich). **e.** Electron microscopic detection (negative staining technique) of herpes simplex virus in vesicle fluid (courtesy of Dr. W. Stolz, Department of Dermatology, University of Munich).

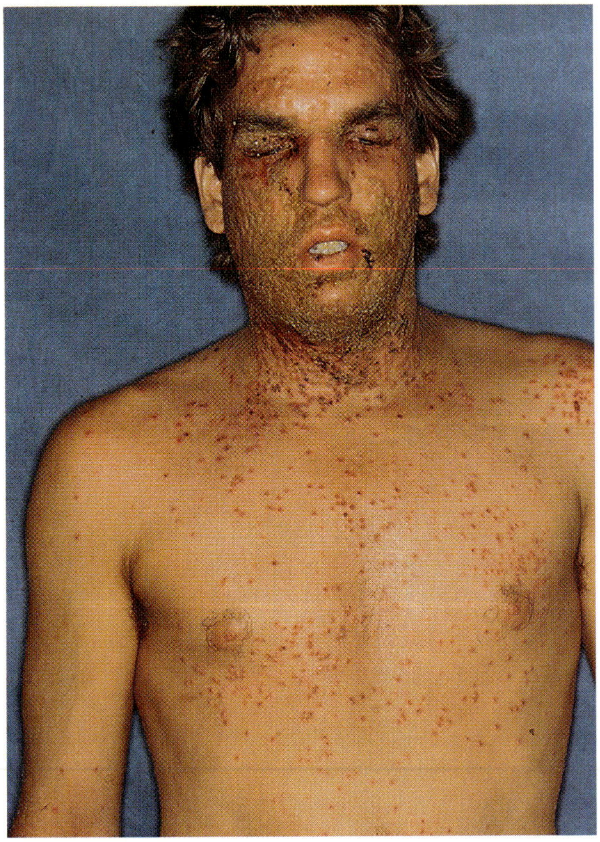

a

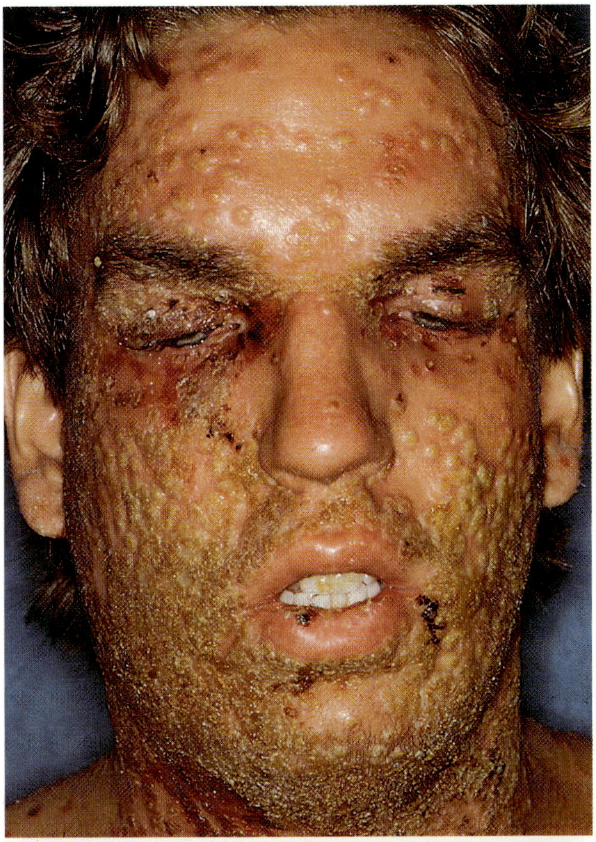
b

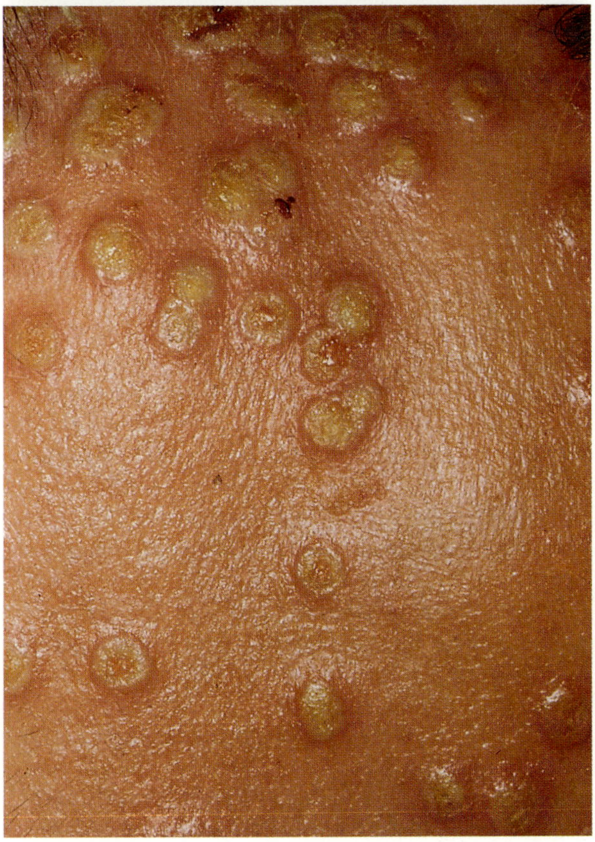
c

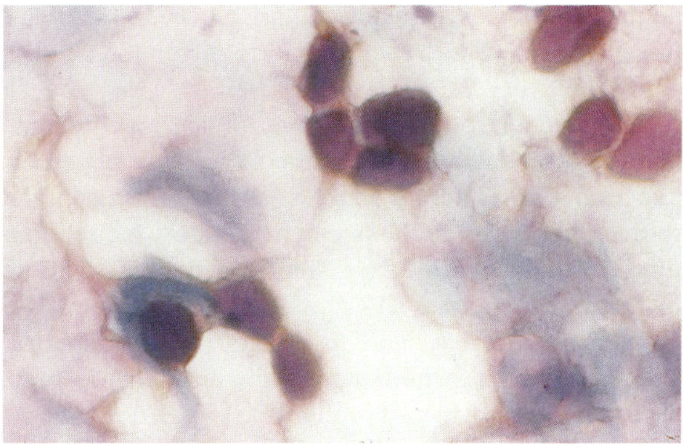
d

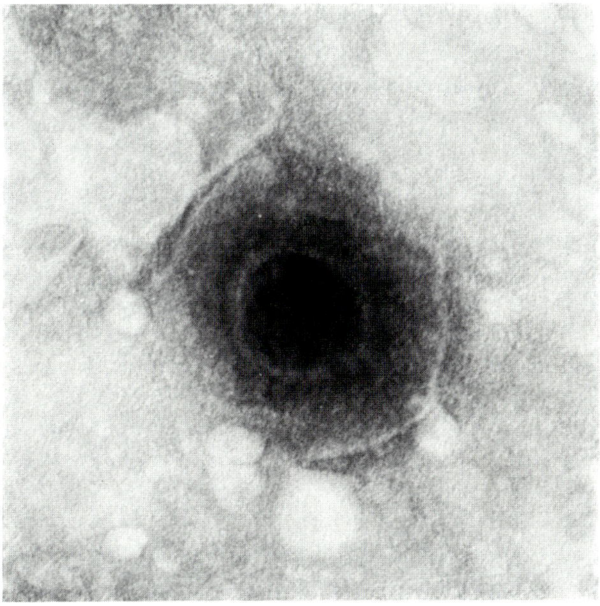
e

symptoms like fever, headaches, malaise, regional or generalized lymphadenopathy, and, often, exacerbation of AE. Secondary bacterial infection may occur. New corps of lesions may continue to appear for several days, but usually the disease subsides after an average duration of 16 days [33, 35, 87, 123, 161, 181, 191, 193, 217, 227, 252, 270, 338].

The diagnosis of eczema herpeticum is frequently delayed because lesions initially may resemble acute exacerbation of AE or bacterial superinfection with *Staphylococcus aureus* and occassionally β-hemolytic streptococci, and are frequently excoriated due to pruritus and scratching [35, 62, 161, 181, 191, 227, 252, 270, 338].

Usually eczema herpeticum occurs in patients with active severe and persistent AE, often after prolonged topical or systemic glucocortisteroid use. Sometimes, however, even patients in clinical remission or exhibiting minimal atopic skin manifestations such as keratosis follicularis may develop eczema herpeticum [33, 35, 61, 62, 181, 191, 193, 270, 322, 345].

The infection route in eczema herpeticum is often via heteroinoculation from a close contact with a herpes infection such as herpes simplex labialis, but a contact source of HSV cannot be traced in all cases. Incubation time is estimated at 2–7 days. Alternatively, reactivation of latent endogenous HSV infection and spread via autoinoculation may lead to disseminated cutaneous disease. In young children, eczema herpeticum may occur as a consequence of primary HSV infection such as gingivostomatitis herpetica. Male children are more often affected than female. Dissemination of the virus may occur cutaneously or systematically via viremia [33, 35, 181, 191, 193, 227, 270, 338].

Eczema herpeticum, particularly if it occurs in the setting of a primary herpetic infection, may occasionally run a serious or even lethal course with internal organ involvement, leading to meningoencephalitis or bronchopneumonia, less frequently to herpes sepsis, hepatitis, colitis, etc. Morbidity and mortality depend upon the extent of internal organ and skin involvement, secondary bacterial infection, and the age and immune status of the patient (prognosis is poorer in young children and immuno-compromised individuals). Further complications may include gingivostomatitis herpetica and dendritic keratitis with ulcerations. A careful ophthalmologic examination should be initiated in patients with eczema herpeticum to exclude herpetic keratoconjunctivitis. Recurrent disease may occur and tends to be milder and of shorter duration. Recurrences are frequently limited to areas of eczema and usually lack internal organ involvement [33, 45, 61, 62, 139, 193, 227, 257, 338].

Diagnosis of eczema herpeticum is based upon the clinical picture of an explosive development of a vesiculopustular eruption at the same stage of development occurring in the setting of AE. Diagnosis can be strengthened by cytological examination of a Tzanck smear (Fig. 2 d) showing ballooning degeneration, multinucleate giant cells, and intranuclear inclusion bodies. Rapid diagnosis is possible with electron-microscopic (negative staining) (Fig. 2 e) or immunofluorescent demonstration of HSV.

Therapy. The prognosis of eczema herpeticum has improved dramatically since the advent of effective antiviral agents. Fever and general symptoms rapidly disappear after initiation of intravenous acyclovir therapy (5–20 mg/kg body weight every 8 h) [61, 62, 84, 161, 307, 310, 311, 345]. In addition to antiviral therapy, avoidance of secondary bacterial infections should be achieved by adequate local treatment with antiseptic wet compresses or lotions with, for example quinolone derivatives. In the case of bacterial superinfection, topical and systemic antibiotic treatment should be instituted. Parenteral administration of γ-globulins may be useful in selected cases.

Eczema Vaccinatum

Until recently, poxvirus officinalis vaccination has been required by law in most countries of the world in children and travelers. The first vaccination had to be performed during the first year of life, the second by the age of 12. AE, even quiescent, is considered to be an absolute contraindication to vaccination due to the risk of eczema vaccinatum. Exceptionally, vaccinations were given after contact with a known or suspected case of smallpox or to people travelling to endemic smallpox areas. Under these circumstances, vaccination was recommended to be carried out under concomitant protection with antivaccinal hyperimmunoglobulin.

Epidemiological data estimating the risk of eczema vaccinatum in atopic individuals vary according to patient selection [52, 78, 328]. Data from Great Britain suggested that one in 20 000 individuals developed eczema vaccinatum after primary vaccination, with a mortality rate of 6% [52]. Following an outbreak of smallpox in Stockholm in 1963, 309 persons with AE were vaccinated. In these individuals there was an exacerbation of skin disease in 36 cases and satellite or secondary vaccinial lesions in 27 cases [78]. Patients with severe and persistent AE and those requiring topical or systemic glucocorticosteroid treatment were at particular risk of developing eczema vaccinatum, but sometimes even individuals with mild disease or in clinical remission were affected [35, 52, 78, 181, 191, 217, 270].

Besides autoinoculation, mostly after the first vaccination, heteroinoculation from a vaccinated family member or close contact with other vaccinated individuals could also cause eczema vaccinatum. Thus, children with AE had to be kept isolated from recently vaccinated persons. In patients with AE, poxvirus officinalis may disseminate either via the cutaneous route or systemically via a viremia phase. The incubation time of eczema vaccinatum is 5–12 days. The disease affects males more frequently than females (ratio 2 : 1) [52, 227]. The severity of eczema vaccinatum varies from localized and mild to fulminant, generalized, potentially life-threatening disease. The clinical picture may be indistinguishable from eczema herpeticum, though vesicles and pustules tend to be larger with thicker walls, show a more pronounced umbilication, and are multilocular.

High fever, occurring 2–3 days after eruption of

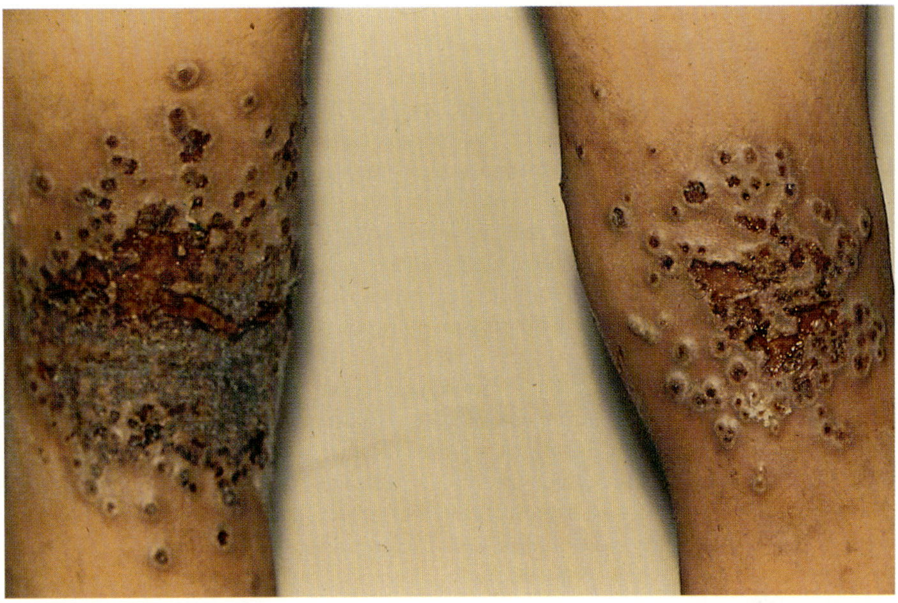

Fig. 3. Eczema vaccinatum.

vesicles, secondary bacterial infection, prominent regional and sometimes general lymphadenopathy, and flare-up of the eczema may be observed. In uncomplicated cases, defervescence occurred within about 10 days, and the sometimes hemorrhagic vesicles dried up and healed, partly with scarring (Fig. 3). Dissemination of virus with organ involvement could lead to a fatal outcome [35, 52, 181, 191, 227, 270].

Eczema vaccinatum may be clinically indistinguishable from eczema herpeticum (see above); further differential diagnostic considerations include variola vera, modified smallpox, and varicella as well as disseminated coxsackie virus A16 infection. Initial lesions of eczema vaccinatum may be difficult to distinguish from acute vesicular exacerbation of AE or bacterial superinfection.

Diagnosis and differentiation from eczema herpeticum can easily be recognized by the typical history of vaccination or contact with a vaccinated person and electron-microscopic examination of vesicle fluid. Tzanck smears and histological examination may also aid in diagnosis.

Molluscum Contagiosum

Mollusca contagiosa are a common viral infection, especially in children with AE. Predilection sites are the flexures, most commonly the axillae, neck, and lateral aspects of the trunk. Rarely, dissemination occurs with development of eczema molluscatum, an unsightly but rather harmless complication of AE (Fig. 4). The risk for developing dissemination of mollusca contagiosa in-

Fig. 4. Eczema molluscatum: dissemination of mollusca contagiosa on preexisting flexural eczema.

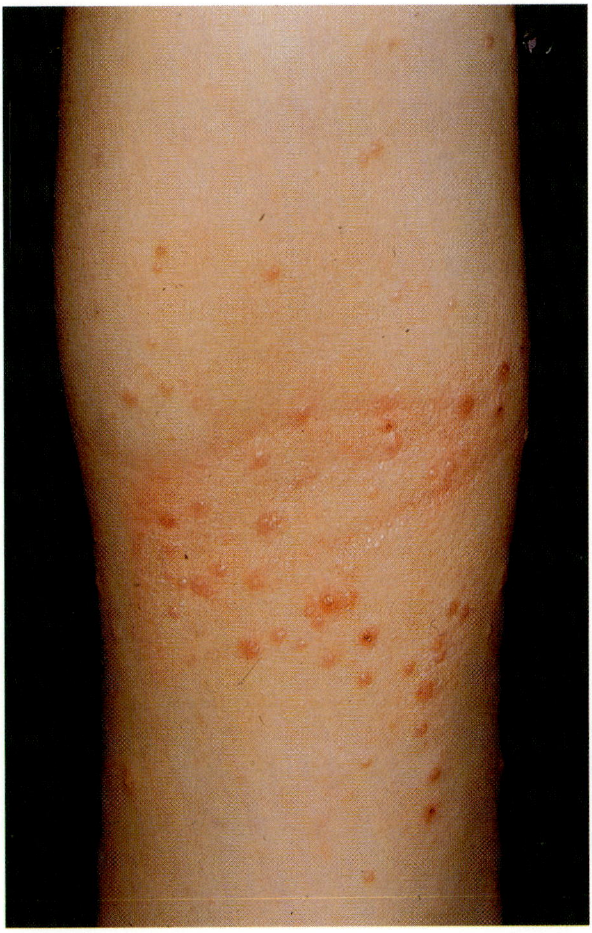

creases with long-lasting use of glucocorticosteroids [108, 227, 241, 281, 293, 344].

The molluscum contagiosum virus is a strongly epidermotropic DNA poxvirus 240 x 320 nm in size. The incubation period ranges from weeks to months. The spread of infection occurs directly from person to person or indirectly via bedding, clothes, towels, etc.

The typical skin lesions are shining, whitish to yellowish or pink, hemispherical, umbilicated papules with a smooth, dome-shaped surface. A thick greasy material can be expressed from the central depression by squeezing the papules.

Initial mollusca contagiosa lack the central porus and may be difficult to distinguish from eczematous papules or milia. In atopic children, mollusca contagiosa may cause pruritus and a patchy eczema around the lesions. Mollusca contagiosa tend to be superinfected and after a variable duration (mostly 6–9 months, sometimes persisting for up to 5 years) show spontaneous inflammatory changes resulting in suppuration, crusting, and eventual destruction of the lesion [35, 181, 191, 217, 270].

Rarely, pediculated tumors or mollusca contagiosa gigantea may occur (Fig. 5) [281, 344].

Due to the viral infection an increased epidermal proliferation occurs, producing lobulated tumors with fibrous septa. The infected epidermal cells undergo necrobiotic changes and appear as so-called molluscum bodies (hyaline bodies up to 25 μm in diameter) containing masses of viral material in the cytoplasm (Fig. 6). Numerous mollusum bodies are present near the surface at the center of the lesion [181, 217, 270].

The treatment of choice is mechanical expression of the contents by squeezing the papules with specially formed tweezers and subsequent application of antiseptics. If, in children, the number of lesions is very large, e.g., in eczema molluscatum, local anesthetic creams or general anesthesia may be necessary. Alternatively, several treatments with cryotherapy may be necessary. Alternatively, several treatments with cryotherapy at intervals of 2–3 weeks may lead to involution of lesions.

Especially in young children, for whom the recommended treatment modalities may be painful or

Fig. 5. Mollusca contagiosa gigantea

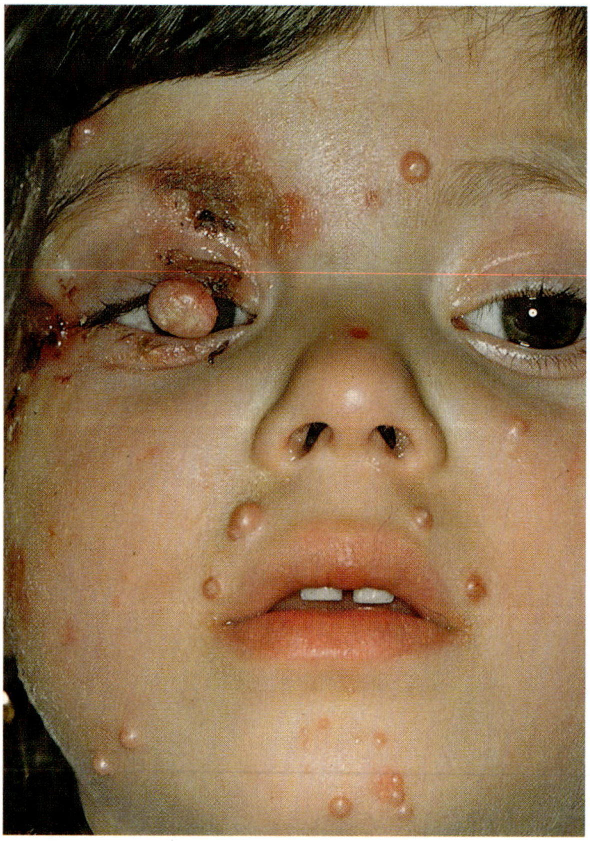

Fig. 6. Molluscum bodies in exprimate of a molluscum contagiosum (courtesy of Dr. B. Gizycki-Nienhaus, Department of Dermatology, University of Munich)

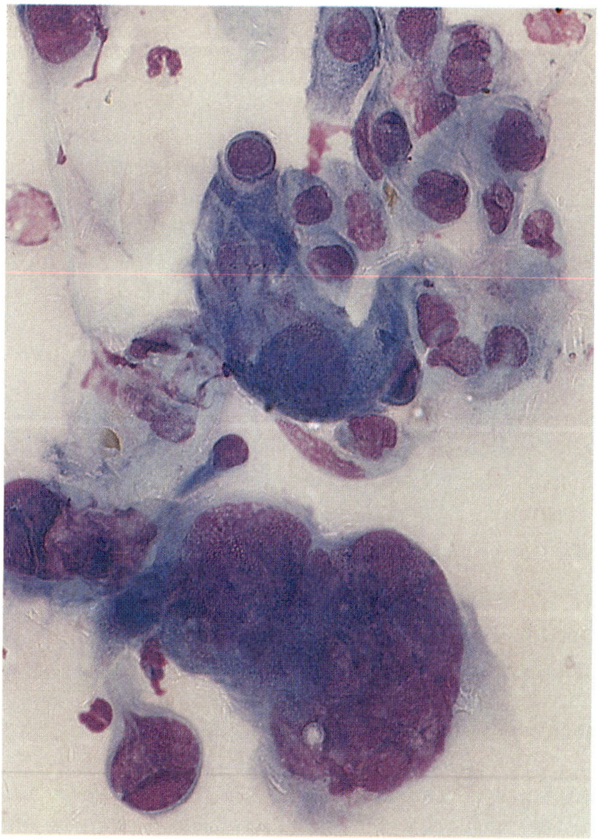

frightening, application of salicylic acid-containing plaster or local antiseptics may represent alternative treatment choices.

Other Viral Diseases

Cutaneous Viral Diseases. *Bowenoid papulosis* of the genitalia associated with HPV type 16 occurred in a 2-year old boy with extensive AE. The mother gave a history of genital warts prior to delivery. The child's skin lesions resolved spontaneously [36].

A 16-month-old-child with generalized AE developed a disseminated *orf infection* after close contact with infected lambs. The lesions developed particularly in eczematous excoriated skin pretreated with glucocorticoisteroids and resembled clinically granuloma pyogenicum with multiple satellite lesions [72].

Although Strannegard et al. recently reported on a significantly increased frequency of *zoster* in individuals with AE as compared to nonatopic controls, the incidence of varicella zoster virus infections does not seem to be markedly increased in patients with AE. However, the course of varicella or zoster may be more severe in the presence of active eczematous skin lesions [181, 227, 270, 321].

Extracutaneous Viral Diseases. Reports of an increased frequency of extracutaneous viral diseases support the assumption of a general immune dysfunction as one of the causes of the enhanced susceptibility to infections in AE [95, 274, 275, 276, 299, 300]. In a retrospective study of almost 1000 patients, Strannegard et al. showed that recurrent upper respiratory tract infections were more common in children with past or present history of AE, particularly in those with severe AE, than in nonatopic controls [275, 300]. In a further study, a remarkable correlation between the activity and severity of AE and the incidence of recurrent viral infections of the respiratory tract was found. However, even patients with AE in remission for more than 1 year reported a higher incidence of recurrent viral infections [275, 300].

Serological studies revealed a higher prevalence of elevated Epstein-Barr virus antibodies in AE patients, irrespective of age, and simultaneous bronchial asthma or hay fever than in nonatopic controls. Epstein-Barr virus, a polyclonal B-cell activator, may also play a pathogenetic role in the development of atopic diseases in genetically predisposed individuals. In the early phase of mononucleosis, raised IgE levels may be found [231, 274, 275, 299, 300].

Parainfluenza, respiratory syncytial virus, and cytomegalovirus may lead to provocation of atopic diseases including eczema [276].

Of interest are recent observations of AE in adults infected with the human imunodeficiency virus (HIV) [195, 270]. In children with AIDS [283a], as well as in HIV-seropositive hemophiliacs [17], genetically predisposed patients, HIV infection led to exacerbation of atopic manifestations, whereas patients without a prior history of atopic disease did not develop atopic symptoms [111]. One of our patients developed severe AE with eczema herpeticum for the first time at the age of 23, 2 years after contracting HIV-1 infection as a result of intravenous drug abuse. Another patient with previously mild AE and hemophilia showed a severe aggravation of his disease after HIV infection from factor VIII concentrate. The question whether atopic individuals are more highly susceptible to HIV infection than nonatopic ones should be of great interest in further investigations.

By contrast, improvement or healing of skin lesions in patients with AE about 3 weeks following measles infection has been reported by Boner et al. The improvement paralleled the short-term suppression of cell-mediated immunity, as evident by tuberculin anergy [32]. Nephrosis [32], sometimes possibly associated with atopic disease, hyper-IgE syndrome [36a] and alopecia areata [235] have also been reported to improve following measles vaccination and natural measles infection.

Parasitic Disorders

Infestation with *Acarus siro* var. *hominis* may provoke juvenile AE. Children with AE infected with scabies mites often develop severe pruritus with exacerbation of eczema and secondary skin infections which often persist despite eradication of the mites. In addition, even short-term treatment with antiparasitic preparations may cause irritation of atopic skin and contribute to the aggravation of AE.

A high incidence of atopy was found among patients with scabies, raising the possibility of enhanced susceptibility to infection with *Acarus siro* in this population. The patients exhibited immediate-type reactivity to scabies mite antigens on skin and serological testing, which may be caused by cross allergy to pyroglyphid mite species (e.g., *Dermatophagoides pteronyssinus* and *D. farinae*). Atopic individuals were found to develop more serious scabies infections than nonatopic ones [82, 83, 84, 146].

Common Warts

Common clinical experience suggests that viral warts are encountered more frequently and in higher numbers in atopic individuals, particularly children. Patients with AE have an increased susceptibility to spreading recalcitrant infections with human papilloma virus which are prone to be more resistent to therapy than usual [33, 108, 227, 252]. However, most recent reviews and standard texts (e.g. Jablonska, Rook) provide no information on atopy as a predisposing factor for common and genital warts [147, 159, 270, 285]. Epidemiological studies of warts in the atopic population and of atopy in wart patients are rare. The data of Bonifazi et al. [33] suggest a slight correlation between warts and atopy in children. Gianetti [108] reports an incidence of atopic disease in children with warts of 13.2%, which does not differ from that in healthy children. Among children with atopic eczema a slightly increased incidence of warts was found (17%) [33]. Currie et al. [56] also reported an increased incidence of warts among children with AE. In rare cases, a massive dissemination of warts can occur in AE patients (Fig. 7), leading to the picture of eczema verrucatum [196, 344]. Clearly, further epidemiological studies are needed to clarify the correlation between atopic eczema and viral warts.

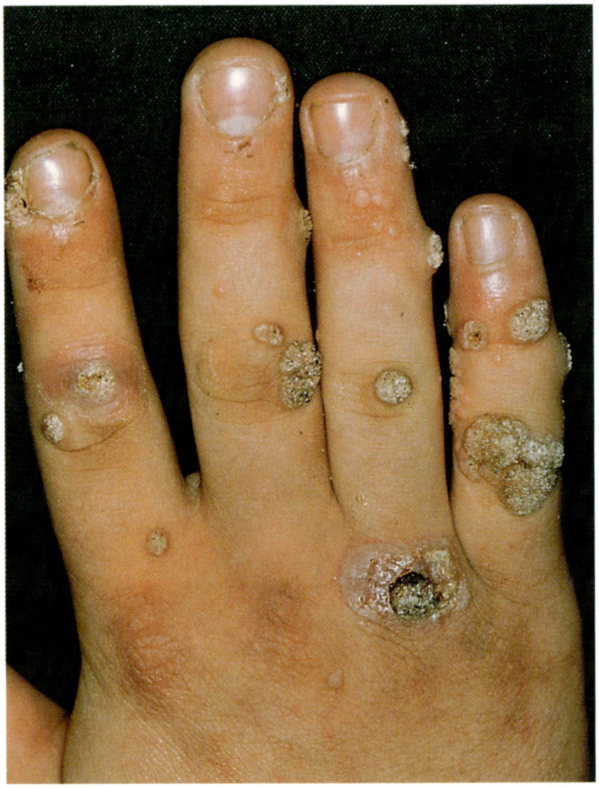

Fig. 7. Disseminated warts in a child with mild atopic eczema

"Exfoliative Erythroderma"

Exfoliative erythroderma is characterized by generalized redness, infiltration, and scaling of skin accompanied by systemic toxicity, lymphadenopathy, and fever (Fig. 8). Prominent blood eosinophilia may be observed. It often results from exacerbation of a preexisting dermatosis, in 4%–14% of cases from AE. Exfoliative erythroderma in patients with AE may be related to withdrawal of systemic corticosteroids used to control severe disease, to widespread superinfection, or to generalized contact irritant reactions.

The disease may be lifethreatening due to cardiac failure, systemic infection, severe pruritus, heat loss, protein depletion, etc [3, 136, 181, 191, 228].

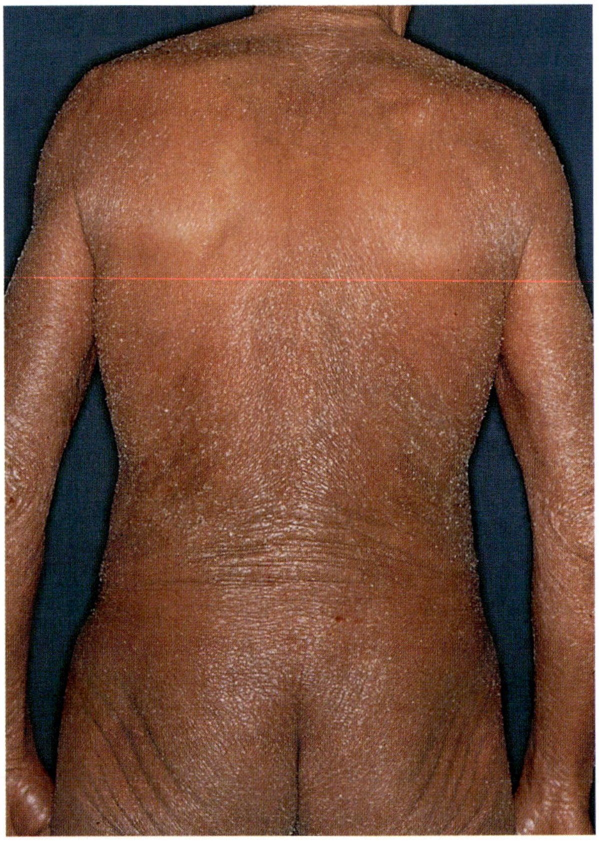

a

▸ **Fig. 8a–c.** Exfoliative erythroderma with lymphadenopathy in a patient with atopic eczema with massive hyperimmunoglobulinemia E. No unequivocal evidence of Sézary syndrome was found.

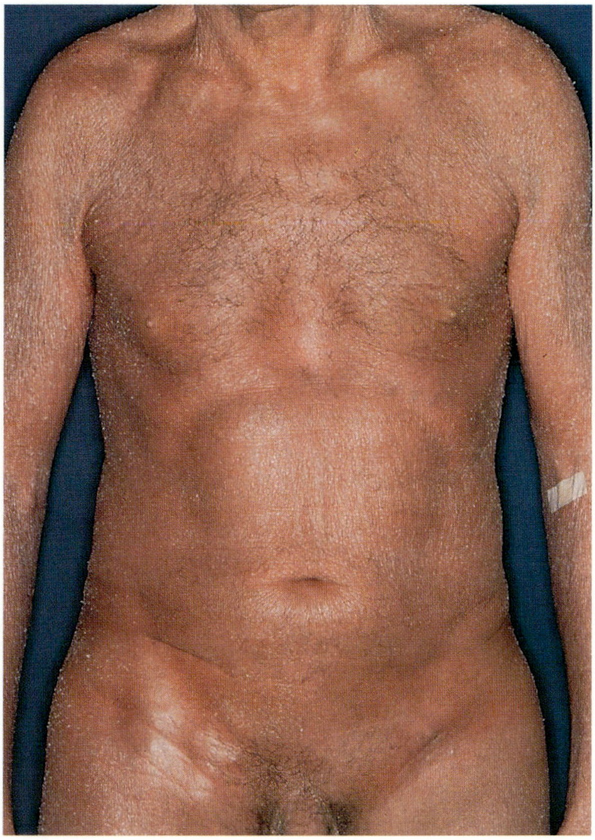

8 b

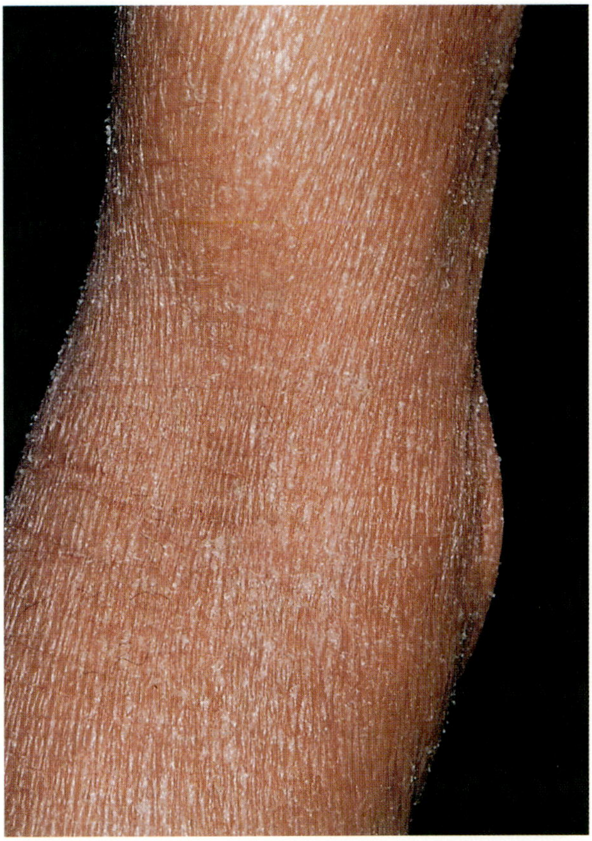

8 c

Associated Ocular Diseases

Depending on selection criteria, up to 40% of patients [103] with AE may show conjunctival or ocular diseases like blepharoconjunctivitis, atopic or vernal keratoconjunctivitis, ocular herpes simplex infections, keratoconus, cataracts, or retinal detachment [65, 96].

Atopic eczema may be associated with seasonal or perennial allergic conjunctivitis or rhinoconjunctivitits (see chapter by Ring, this volume) as well as with atopic keratoconjunctivitis [96].

In blepharoconjunctivitis, the periorbital skin and the eyelids may show mild dryness and scaling, erytemhematous, edematous, and exudative or crusted lesions, sometimes associated with severe lichenification (Fig. 9) [306]. Secondary staphylococcal impetiginization may occur. There may be hyperemia, chemosis, filamentous exudate, thickening of the bulbar and palpebral conjunctiva, or a giant papillary hypertrophy on the palpebral conjunctiva. The tarsal conjunctiva is thickened, hypertrophic, and milky opaque and causes burning, prickling, and itching sensations [96, 103]. While allergic conjunctivitis is a common association of AE, atopic or vernal keratoconjunctivitis represent rare but more serious ocular disorders and are difficult to treat. Atopic keratoconjunctivitis may persist for months to years and in severe cases the patients show extreme photophobia and lacrimation as well as conjunctival redness accom-

Fig. 9. *Lichénification géante* of the eylids in chronic atopic blepharitis

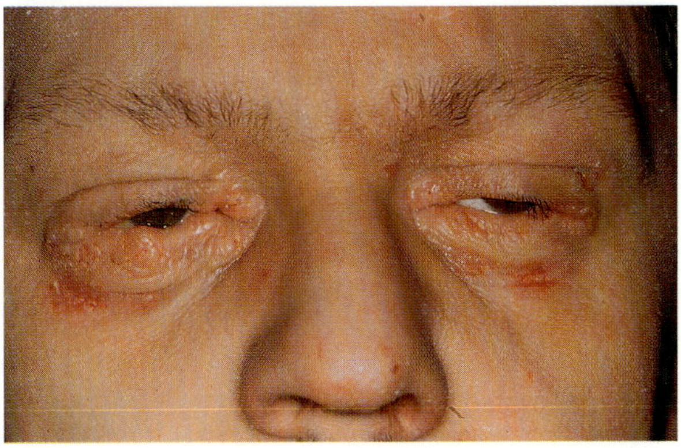

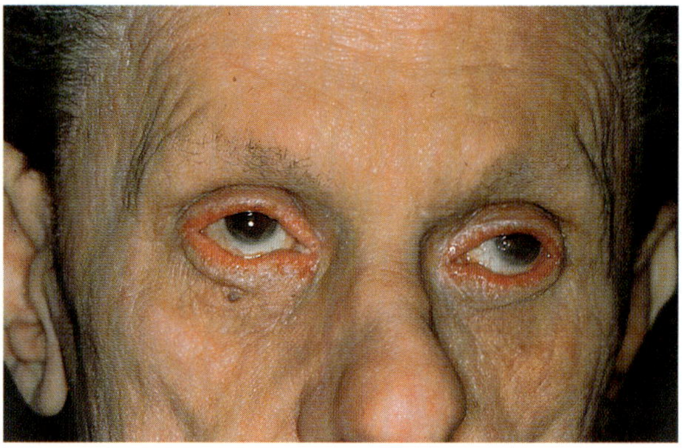

Fig. 10. Blepharoconjunctivitis with ectropion formation

panied by ocular irritation, itching, and discharge. In rare cases additional conjunctival scarring or lichenification of the skin of the eyelids may lead to ectropion and constant tearing by shortening of the inferior fornix with symblepharon formation, punctal eversion, and stenosis (Fig. 10). In severe cases of atopic and vernal keratoconjunctivitis, corneal scarring, vascularization, and loss of vision have been described. Conjunctival changes may parallel flare-up of eczema. Short-term treatment with topical glucocorticosteroids and cromolyn eyedrops is useful [96, 103, 114, 149, 162, 168, 186, 238, 263, 266].

Vernal keratoconjunctivitis occurs mainly in children (in males more often than females) and young adults (peak incidence 11–13 years) and is rare after the age of 30 (male to female ratio 1 : 1 after age of 20). The patients frequently have a personal or family history of atopic diseases [6, 92, 96, 103, 114, 149, 162, 168, 186, 238, 263, 266]. Vernal keratoconjunctivitis is characterized by a granular appearance, bilaterally mainly of the upper palpebral conjunctiva with giant polygonal papillae, resulting in a cobblestone-like surface, or by gelatinous swellings at the limbus (more common among dark-skinned races). Secondary corneal findings are superficial erosions or ulcers and plaque-like deposits in the anterior cornea [6, 96, 103, 278]. The patients' complaints include burning, extreme itching, photophobia, lacrimation and mucous discharge. Climatic factors may play a role in the pathogenesis of vernal keratoconjunctivitis, since the disease seems to be more common in warm climates than in temperate or cold zones. Allergic (sensitivity to pollens, house dust mites, cat dander) or physical factros may also contribute to the pathogenesis of the disease [6, 18, 22, 92, 96, 278]. Vernal keratokonjunctivitis is usually a self-limited disorder, disappearing after 5–10 years. Short-term topical and sometimes systemic administration of glucocorticosteroids may be useful to influence the inflammatory changes. In addition, topical cromolyn, vasoconstrictors, cold compresses, ice packs, and climatotherapy may be indicated in selected cases [75, 92, 96, 103, 154, 173, 308].

Keratoconus is an unusual cone-shaped ectasia of the cornea that is sometimes associated with AE (first described by Hilgartner et al. [23, 96, 104]. Copeman reported that AE was present in 16% of patients with keratoconus [51]. Gasset reported on a significant incrase in the prevalence of keratoconus in patients with asthma and/or hay fever, but there was no difference in the incidence of AE compared to the control group [104]. Other studies revealed only rare or no cases of keratoconus associated with AE [9, 38, 180, 189]. It has been suggested that excessive eye rubbing in combination with a thinned and weakened cornea may lead to the development of keratoconus [96, 105]. Keratoconus may occur in severe cases of AE and is rarely apparent before puberty [38, 74, 101, 103, 104, 168, 189, 197, 238, 250, 256, 294].

Itch-induced rubbing of the eyes has also been reported to be responsible for some cases of retinal detachment, but its association with AE is uncertain [9, 50, 53, 137, 153, 156, 168, 170, 175, 220, 226, 238, 325].

The association between cataracts and AE was first described by Andogsky in 1914 [13]. He reported the bilateral development of cataracts accompanying dermatitis in a youth. In 1921 Davis reported a 15-year-old patient suffering from neurodermatitis and asthma who rapidly developed bilateral cataracts. Further publications appearing before the introduction of glucocorticosteroids in the 1950's supported the possible relationship between cataract in young patients and eczema [21, 37, 50, 54]. AE is the most common skin disease associated with cataracts. On the other hand, the incidence of cataracts among patients with AE is not exactly known, but the disease is uncommon. In selected populations with widespread severe AE involving mainly facial skin, the incidence of atopic cataracts has been reported to range between 0,4% and 33% [38, 232, 238, 282, 318]. In a recent study of 51 AE patients, however, not a single case was identified [46]. Atopic cataracts may appear already in early childhood or before the age of 30, with the peak incidence between 15 and 25 years after an average duration of AE of 5–10 years. In most cases, cataracts are subclinical and cause no visual disturbance [9, 21, 38, 42, 46, 53, 79, 103, 105, 168, 169, 197, 220, 221, 232, 238, 277, 282, 325].

In slit lamp studies two types of cataracts associated with AE have been discerned: anterior and posterior subcapsular cataracts. The cataracts are frequently bilateral (50%–70%) and the posterior subcapsular cataract is more frequent than the anterior. While the anterior subcapsular cataract seems to be specific to AE, it is well known that posterior subcapsular cataracts in AE are indistinguishable from those induced by glucocorticosteroids [71, 238, 266]. Anterior and posterior subcapsular cataracts are probably both the result of similar pathological mechanisms. The ectodermal origin of the skin and the lens invites speculations that there may be common factors in the pathogenesis of skin and lens changes [53, 79, 109]. A significant use of steroids has been noted in both types of atopic cataracts. This, however, was probably related to the severity of the skin disease rather than the use of steroids. No correlation was made between the use of steroids and the development or type of cataract [103, 232, 238, 282]. On the other hand, was suggested extensive use of systemic and potent topical glucocorticosteroids, especially in the periorbital region, has been implicated in increasing the risk of formation of posterior subcapsular cataracts and increased ocular pressure [42, 103, 230, 232, 238, 271, 282, 288, 352]. In a further study, it appeared questionable whether the use of steroids contributed to the development of the posterior subcapsular cataracts in AE. The complication appeared to be associated with but not necessarily caused by steroids [103, 232]. Furthermore, enhanced susceptibility to HSV infections like keratoconjunctivitis may cause scarring of the cornea [74]. No strict dose-effect relation has been found, and individual susceptibility appears the most important factor in the development of corticosteroid-induced posterior subcapsular cataract [42, 282, 291]. Psoralen and ultraviolet A (PUVA) therapy has also been reported in association with cataract development [55, 117, 120, 297, 346].

Associated Gastrointestinal Disorders

In up to 20% of patients with *gluten-sensitive enteropathy (GSE)*, scaly skin lesions on the hands, forearms, legs, and face, resembling AE, have been described. The intensity of the skin disease varies with the severity of GSE. It may show an improvement on a gluten-free diet and a relapse after reinstitution of gluten-containing food [97, 112, 148]. Other or no changes of the mucosa of the small bowel in AE have been reported by different authors [26, 34, 70, 80, 144, 177, 204, 206, 243, 319].

A higher than expected association between dermatitis herpetiformis Duhring, GSE, and AE has been reported by Davies and Buckley and coworkers [39, 64]. However, Leroy et al. reported about the association of AE with bullous linear IgA dermatosis with normal gastrointestinal function [190].

In *eosinophilic gastroenteritis*, predominantly in patients with primary mucosal involvement, allergic factors have been demonstrated. The exact incidence of AE in this disorder is not known. Associated histories and features of atopic diseases like bronchial asthma, allergic rhinitis, and AE, as well as elevated total or food-antigen-specific serum IgE and food hypersensitivity reactions suggest an atopic nature to this disorder in at least a subgroup of patients. Disruption of the integrity of the lamina propria with a slight villous atrophy or loss of villi, eosinophilic infiltration and edema of the lamina propria may cause malabsorption, protein-losing enteropathy, gastrointestinal blood loss, and possibly growth retardation and nutritional deficiencies. Small intestinal permeability to potential dietary allergens (e.g., with large molecular weight) may be increased in some patients with AE as compared to noneczematous subjects [15, 24, 26, 34, 43, 70, 80, 85, 100, 144, 160, 171, 177, 203, 204, 206, 243, 247, 331, 332, 349].

An increased incidence of atopy has been found by some authors in *inflammatory bowel disease* but has not been confirmed by others [210, 216, 268]. In some patients with ulcerative colitis or ileitis terminalis, atopy and hypersensitivity reactions may be of possible pathogenic significance. However, in a study of 39 patients with ulcerative colitis and 35 patients with Crohn's disease no atopic eczema and no differences in the frequency of personal or family history of atopy or in serum IgE levels were found. The patrents however, showed significantly more positive prick test reactions to food allergens [210]. The assumption that hypersensitivity reactions may play a role in the pathogenesis of inflammatory bowel disease is based on three clinical studies showing that sodium cromoglycate was of some benefit in patients with colitis and on reports of increased numbers of eosinophils and plasma cells staining for IgE and elevated histamine content in rectal mucosa [210, 268].

Another study showed that a history of asthma, hay fever, and flexural eczema was significantly more common in adults and children with *coeliac disease* than in normal controls. In addition, first degree relatives of patients with adult coeliac disease had an increased incidence of atopic disorders [148, 324].

Gastric hyposecretion and epithelial degeneration in the first year of life has been observed in atopic patients, and it has been suggested that this may promote the passage of unchanged food or bacterial antigens through the jejunal mucosa [177].

Two case reports discussed a possible relationship between AE and lymphangiectasia of small intestine [76, 262]. Dent and Garrets found eczema in six patients with hypocalcaemia, steatorrhea and hypothyroidism [67]. In patients with various widespread skin diseases including AE, a so-called dermatogenic enteropathy has been described which is assumed to be secondary to the dermatosis. The enteropathy resulting in steatorrhea rapidly disappears after successful treatment of the underlying skin disease [99, 112, 160, 202, 204, 205, 290].

The reported possible association of AE with intestinal abnormalities (malabsorption, gluten sensitive enteropathy, subtotal villous atrophy etc.) and the success of specific therapeutic interventions are interesting features justifying further investigations of intestinal function in patients with severe AE.

Cystic Fibrosis

Since the report by Lowe in 1949 about the increased prevalence of atopic diseases in patients with cystic fibrosis (CF), a number of publications have confirmed and others have disputed this association [150, 309, 314, 334, 336]. The occurrence of allergies and atopic diseases is increased in homozygotes as well as heterozygotes for CF [39, 334]. The reason for the increased prevalence of atopy, especially respiratory allergy, in CF is unknown. Increased antigen access or genetic linkage between atopy and CF have been discussed. It is obvious that abnormal mucosal permeability, defective secretory IgA, or failure of antigen clearance at mucosal surfaces may be responsible for this relationship. Representative figures in patients with CF range from 11% to 49% for the incidence of respiratory allergy or other atopic diseases (AE 8%–13%) and 26%–62% for a positive family history of atopic diseases (significantly increased compared to controls). Immediate skin reactivity to various aeroallergens (especially molds and house dust mites) was present in 43%–88% of patients with CF. No relationship has been found between atopy and severity of CF [150, 308, 314, 334, 336].

Steroid-Responsive Nephrotic Syndrome

In some atopic patients with steroid-responsive (sensitive) nephrotic syndrome (SRNS; minimal change nephrosis, polycyclic or recurrent nephrotic syndrome) proteinuria and edema appeared to be exacerbated by allergic reactions to aeroallergens (like pollen and house dust mites) [134, 261, 313, 341, 343] or food antigens (predominantly cow's milk proteins) [90, 279, 335]. The incidence of atopic diseases (40%–70%) and increased total and allergen specific serum IgE levels (70%–100%) is greater in children with SRNS and their first degree relatives than in controls [90, 116, 209, 234, 238, 316, 335]. The association was stronger in HLA-B12-positive patients [316]. The relative risk of developing SRNS in patients with HLA-B12 and atopy has been reported to be 13 as compared to controls with neither factor [313]. Mouzon-Cambon reported a correlation between SRNS and HLA-DR7 predominantly in patients with associated allergic disorders [219]. Relapses of SRNS may follow allergen exposure and infections, particularly of the upper respiratory tract [134, 209, 261, 279, 335, 341, 343]. The beneficial effects of antiallergic therapy (like allergen avoidance, specific immunotherapy, etc.) on the course of SRNS is uncertain (209, 264, 279]. However, Sandberg et al. found a decrease of proteinuria in four of six patients with SRNS and cow's milk allergy, while on an elimination diet and exacerbation of the disease after oral challenge with cow's milk [279].

In atopic patients with seasonal SRNS, remission may be induced by steroids or measle infection [209, 313]. Trompeter et al. reported a greater tendency to relapse in patients with a history of eczema than in those with other atopic diseases [316].

Poststreptococcal glomerulonephritis may be a rare consequence of superinfection of AE with β-hemolytic streptococci [248]. However, Steiner reported an uncertain coincidence of various types of glomerulonephritis and AE [296]. Kay found only one case of glomerulonephritis in 137 adult patients with long-lasting AE [172].

Metabolic Disorders

Eczematous skin lesions have been described in a variety of hereditary or nutritional metabolic disorders. Differentiation of the dermatitis from AE has to be considered. Coincidence of AE and metabolic disorders is possible, but due to the rarity of these disorders, the causal relationship remains doubtful [157, 181, 191, 272, 340].

In *biotin-responsive multiple carboxylase deficiency,* skin lesions have been classified as localized or widespread, atopic eczema-like erythematous dermatitis, frequently superinfected with *Candida albicans*. There is also some similarity in appearance to the periorificial dermatitis of acrodermatitis enteropathica [157, 340].

In 19%–50% of cases, patients with *phenylketonuria* show eczematous skin lesions indistinguishable from AE (clinically, histologically and immunologically) during the first year of life [88]. The intensity of skin lesions paralleled the serum level of phenylalanine. The skin lesions clear with appropriate dietary therapy. The proportion of patients with AE having phenylketonuria is unknown but seems to be very low. However, almost half of 21 patients with phenylketonuria showed positive prick test reactions to common allergens [88, 89, 157, 163, 315, 326, 340].

Three of 22 patients with *Hurler's syndrome* (a hereditary defect in mucopolysaccharide metabolism) seen by Peterson had typical AE, but it is doubtful from the small number of observations whether the incidence is higher than expected for the general population [119, 245]. An eczematous pellagra-like dermatitis (with erythema and scaling) which may be aggravated by exposure to sunlight is one of the early symptoms of *Hartnup's disease* (a hereditary aminoaciduria) [157, 192, 340].

Infants with *essential fatty acid deficiency* are usually quite ill and show a periorificial dermatitis and a scaly dermatosis [132, 340].

Prolidase deficiency is a rare autosomal recessive disorder characterized, among other things, by chronic dermatitis with erythematous and crusted lesions on the face, palms, and soles, ecchymosas, or a fine purpuric rash [157, 284, 340].

Snyderman et al. [292] found in five of six infants below 3 months of age, that a diet *deficient in histidine* resulted in a papular and scaly nonpruritic dermatitis within 3–4 days. Lesions were localized predominantly on the face. Any relation to AE was not studied. Reintroduction of histidine led to rapid clearing of lesions after 24–48 h. In older infants, skin lesions could not be provoked by this deficiency [292]. On the other hand, *histidinemia* may also be associated with atopy or AE, although exact data are lacking (107, 158, 214]. Finally, in a study by Zaslow, all 12 patients with atopy showed normal histidine serum levels [351].

Cutaneous Lymphomas

Mycosis fungoides, Sézary's syndrome, and Hodgkin's disease may initially present with eczematous skin lesions and develop thickening and lichenification of the skin as well as pruritic papules and plaques. Differentiation from AE may be difficult. Some reports suggest that cutaneous T-cell lymphomas can be associated with an atopic diathesis and some authors discuss a possible relationship between AE and Sèzary's syndrome or mycosis fungoides. This assumption is based on preexisting AE in some patients with cutaneous lymphomas, the progression of generalized "atopic erythroderma" into Sézary's syndrome, and the high IgE levels in patients with cutaneous T-cell lymphomas and Hodgkin's disease with or without a personal or family history of atopy [11, 73, 251, 255, 330, 342]. Regarding other hematological malignancies, no association with atopy was seen in the study of 229 patients with chronic leukemias reported by McCormack [207]. The incidence of atopy in patients with Hodgkin's disease and other lymphomas did not differ from controls in a study by Amlot [10]. However, anecdotal reports hint at possible relations between atopy and cutaneous lymphomas. For example, Zarafonetis reported a single case of "reticulum cell sarcoma" complicating severe AE [350].

Lange-Vejlsgaard reported on a 13-year-old child with AE who developed a fatal cutaneous T-cell lymphoma [187]. A patient seen by Abel et al. [1] who had received long-term corticosteroid therapy showed an association between adult-onset asthma and AE-like skin lesions, markedly elevated IgE, and the development of tumor-stage mycosis fungoides. The eczematous skin lesions may have been initial specific infiltration of mycosis fungoides in which the diagnosis was overlooked due to topical or systemic treatment with glucocorticosteroids [1].

Anhidrotic Congenital Ectodermal Dysplasia

In seven patients with anhidrotic congenital ectodermal dysplasia (ACED), Vanselow et al. found an increased prevalence of atopic diseases and positive prick test reactions to common aeroallergens: bronchial asthma in four patients, allergic rhinitis in three and AE in three [320]. In addition, other publications have reported an association of ACED with AE, asthma, and a positive family history of atopy [77, 260].

Growth Impairment

In a recent study in Manchester [59, 183] concerning growth in 89 children aged 1–16 years with severe or intractable AE (chronic AE for at least 1 year, more than 5% of skin surface affected), standing height was compared to national standards. Short stature, defined as a standing height below the third centile when corrected for mid-parenteral height, was found in 22% of these children. Significantly reduced sitting height and delayed skeletal maturity scores were also found in both boys and girls [59]. Impaired growth was particularly associated with widespread eczema but also with bronchial asthma (which is a known cause of impaired growth) and the use of potent topical glucocorticosteroids [44, 59, 86, 141, 161, 183, 225]. The cause of growth impairment in AE is not known in most cases but treatment with potent topical or systemic glucocorticosteroids, coexisting bronchial asthma, gastrointestinal abnormalities like malabsorption, or inappropriate dietary restrictions causing malnutrition may contribute to growth impairment [58, 59, 63, 183]. In a 10-month-old infant suffering from extensive AE, large amounts of albumin were lost through the skin, leading to a failure to thrive, hypoalbuminemia, and edema. Treatment with steroids resulted in a dramatic clearing of dermatitis and subsequent correction of his hypoalbuminemia, edema and anemia [2, 312]. Lack of sleep and vitamin D deficiency (due to avoidance of sun exposure?) may be further factors. The growth impairment seems to be a temporary growth delay, but if the short stature is caused by glucocorticosteroid treatment or if severe AE persists, permanent growth failure may occur [59, 183]. Longitudinal studies will provide further information concerning growth impairment in AE.

Psoriasis

The coincidence of the common skin diseases AE and psoriasis should not be a rare event. Among 1065 patients with psoriasis, Welp et al. found 18 with simultaneous AE, which is in keeping with the statistical probability [337]. A similar frequency (9 cases of AE in 390 psoriatic patients, 2.3%) was determined by Geyer et al. [106]. Studies by Cristophers and Henseler [47] and Knopf et al. [176], however, showed that the coincidence is rather below the expected frequency [176]. Garofalo showed that the incidence of atopy is significantly higher in inverted psoriasis than in stable plaque-type psoriasis and 4 times higher than in the psoriatic group as a whole and in healthy children. In this study, no patient showed both skin diseases simultaneously [102].

Photosensitivity

Although sunlight and therapeutic UV irradiation improve AE in many patients [12, 81, 131, 258], in a proportion of them, estimated at about 10%, AE may deteriorate. The UVB portion of the spectrum may be responsible for aggravation of eczema [246]. Although sunlight may improve or provoke AE [84, 91, 133, 213, 252, 298], the importance of UV irradiation in this effect is unclear, since improvement or aggravation may be explained by a host of unrelated circumstantial factors (relative humidity, scratching, infrared irradiation, pollen exposure, psychological factors, skin care, associated polymorphous light eruption or photoallergy, etc.) [68, 191, 252].

Drug Sensitivity

The relationship between atopy and drug sensitivity is a highly controversial field. The clinical expression of adverse drug reactions like drug allergy appears to be influenced by several different individual risk factors, and also by genetic factors including atopy [301]. Among atopic individuals those with bronchial asthma may be at particular risk [14]. It has therefore been discussed by some authors [5, 254, 301] that drug reactions of the anaphylactic type may possibly be more common and more severe in atopic patients due to their increased liability to produce antibodies on exposure to antigens. Others have not accepted this [118]. In addition, it was reported that atopic persons may also be at increased risk of developing severe, anaphylactoid, IgE-independent reactions to radiocontrast media [14]. An explanation may be the enhanced releasability of inflammatory mediators in atopic subjects. Although the assumption is made by many authors that the allergic/atopic diathesis predisposes individuals to allergic reaction to drugs, the contested association between atopy and drug reactions must be clarified in systematic epidemiological investigations.

Insect Venom Allergy

Atopic individuals were presumed to be at particular risk of developing insect venom allergy [152, 287]. Some recent comprehensive studies, however, have shown that the incidene of atopy or atopic diseases was about the same in subjects with insect venom allergy as in the normal population, whereas others support a certain correlation between venom allergy and atopy. Investigations of Przybilla et al. [249] on the relation of atopy and insect venom allergy showed that atopic patients with positive prick test reactions to common aeroallegens (*Dermatophagoides pteronyssinus*, cat dander, grass pollen) more often had lower hymenoptera venom prick test thresholds than patients without skin reactivity to these aeroallergens. Furthermore, atopic patients with high total serum IgE levels may have higher hymenoptera venom-specific IgE concentrations than patients with normal or slightly elevated total serum IgE. These observations have to be taken into consideration in judging diagnostic criteria for insect venom allergy in atopic patients [249a, 249b]. Miyauchi et al. reported that 47% of bee keepers with honeybee venom allergy are atopic as compared to 13% of other subjects allergic to bee venom [215]. Atopic bee keepers may become sensitized more easily via inhalation of bee antigens or frequent stings. Müller reported that atopic individuals develop insect venom allergy earlier and need fewer stings to become sensitized than normal ones [215]. Overall, the data suggest that insect venom allergy occurs, if at all, only somewhat more often in atopic than in nonatopic populations.

Congenital Perceptive Hearing Loss

Hearing loss has been associated with atopy in some families [14, 178, 189]. A familial aggregation of atypical AE (atypical in age of onset and distribution) and congenital perceptive hearing loss has been described in three of four siblings [178]. In another family, two brothers suffered from bilateral perceptive cochlear hearing loss, AE, and mild palmoplantar keratoderma. There was a predisposition to atopic diseases in the maternal family and palmoplantar keratoderma as a dominant trait in the paternal family [94]. In addition, Seinedari et al. reported an association of Waardenburg-Klein syndrome and AE [286].

Vitiligo

It is a common clinical impression that an atopic diathesis, though not necessarily AE, is often present in patients presenting with vitiligo [93, 200, 237]. Kierland asserted that vitiligo is seen more frequently in patients with AE [174] but the correlation between the two diseases is not substantiated by epidemiological investigations. In most vitiligo series the occurrence of AE and other atopic manifestations have not specifically been assessed [179, 236]. When they do coincide AE often involves not the vitiliginous but the surrounding skin [200].

Hair Anomalies

Alopecia areata seems to be associated with atopy, particularly in childhood. There are, however, only few recent comprehensive statistical studies comparing these patients to a normal population with regard to the possible link between alopecia areata and AE. Furthermore, there is some evidence that in atopic patients with alopecia areata the prognosis with regard to hair regrowth is worse than in nonatopic patients (Fig. 11). In a large North American series, eczema and/or asthma were present in 18% of children and 9% of adults with alopecia areata; in children with alopecia areata totalis the incidence reached 23% [222]. Ikeda (Japan 1965) found 10% of patients with alopecia areata to be atopic [155] and Penders (Holland 1968), 52.4% [242]. In a Danish study, the incidence of atopic eczema in patients with alopecia areata was only 1% [110]. The discrepancies may be due to differences in diagnostic criteria and patient selection [66, 98, 110, 155, 222, 242, 244, 283].

Braun-Falco et al. reported on the coincidence of uncombable hair with hair shaft changes (longitudinal grooves, angular or kidney-shaped cross sections) and pili torti, progressive alopecia areata, and AE in six members of one family [35a]. A further report mentions uncombable hair and teeth anomalies in association with ichthyosis vulgaris and AE [185].

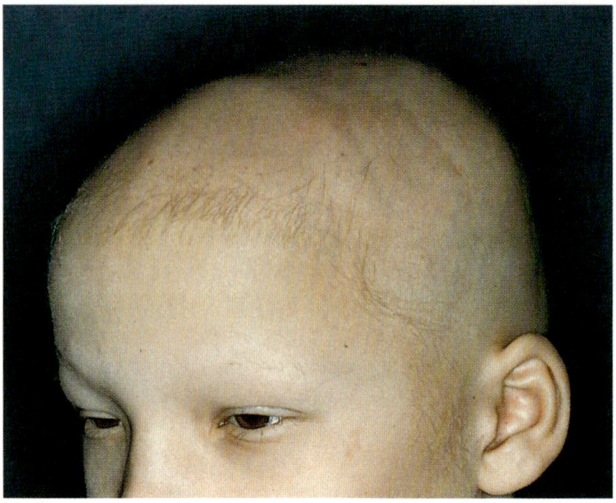

Fig. 11. Alopecia areata fere totalis in an atopic child

Netherton's Syndrome

Atopic eczema-like skin changes are also present in Netherton's syndrome, an autosomal recessive disorder characterized by trichorrhexis invaginata, bamboo hairs, ichthyosis linearis circumflexa, and eczematous lesions [40, 115, 182, 184].

The association of Siemens syndrome (keratosis follicularis decalvans) with atopy has also been described in one patient [248].

Down's Syndrome

Trisomy 21 or Down's syndrome, frequently exhibiting cellular immunodeficiency, may be associated in 25%–56% of cases with atopy. Less frequently, autoimmune phenomena such as alopecia areata, vitiligo, and Hashimoto thyreoiditis with antithyreoideal antibodies occur [41, 245]. During a course of treatment with a topical immunomodulator, rapid regrowth of hair following an attack of measles was reported in an 11-year-old child suffering from Down's syndrome and alopecia areata totalis [235].

Sudden Infant Death Syndrome

In rare cases of sudden infant death syndrome (SIDS), atopy has been implicated as a possible cause [239]. The assumption is supported by a strong family history of atopic disease in a retrospective study of SIDS and by the high incidence of specific IgE antibodies to *Dermatophagoides pteronyssinus*, *Aspergillus fumigatus*, and bovine β-lactoglobulin [224, 317]. Another study failed to support the interrelation of atopy and SIDS [333]. A further explanation may be allergy to environmental antigens such as cow's milk, A hypothetical mechanism postulates an anaphylactoid reaction to the inhalation of cow's milk proteins regurgitated from the stomach during sleep [239].

Dubowitz Syndrome

Since the first description by Dubowitz in 1965 [69], the association of low birth weight dwarfism, distinct facial dysplasia, and other associated anomalies as well eczematous skin lesions has been frequently described. In one of our own cases, a 2-year-old boy with Dubowitz syndrome showed features of classical AE [327].

Eczematous Skin Lesions in X-Linked Immunodeficiency with Hyperimmunoglobulinemia M Syndrome

Atopic eczema-like skin lesions are common and nonspecific skin manifestations of many primary immunodeficiency syndromes (see chapter by Fritsch and Hintner, this volume). Other symptoms of atopy such as rhinitis or bronchial asthma are usually absent. Immunodeficiency with hyperimmunoglobulinemia M is a defined primary immunodeficiency syndrome characterized by the absence of or low serum levels of IgG and IgA together with normal to elevated IgM levels and normal T-cell functions. We reported a 3½-year-old boy with a typical hyper-IgM syndrome associated with AE but in most of the cases of hyper-IgM syndrome, hitherto described skin involvement has not been analyzed in detail [327a].

Cutaneous Amyloidosis

Several reports, mostly from Japan, attest to the association of AE and macular amyloidosis of the skin. In some series up to 25% of patients with amyloidosis showed evidence of AE [28, 201]. Rippled pigmentation of the neck is a special manifestation usually reported as a characteristic of macular amyloidosis in Japan [151, 201, 208]. Manabe et al. [208] showed, however, that in a certain proportion of adults, ripple pigmentation was associated with AE. Amyloid deposits in primary cutaneous amyloidosis may be derived from epidermal keratin [138]. Long-term irritation of the skin such as the chronic scratching in AE may result in amyloid formation in predisposed individuals [201]. Therefore, AE may be one of the underlying disorders causing cutaneous amyloidosis [273a]. Shanon [289] analyzed 13 patients with papular amyloidosis and identified AE, as the cause in nine of them. In our experience [273a], in adult patients of European origin, amyloidosis may complicate chronic AE (Fig. 12). More frequently, however, patients with macular amyloidosis of the upper back were misdiagnosed as AE and treated for long periods of time. Until the correct diagnosis was established by biopsy with specific histological staining methods.

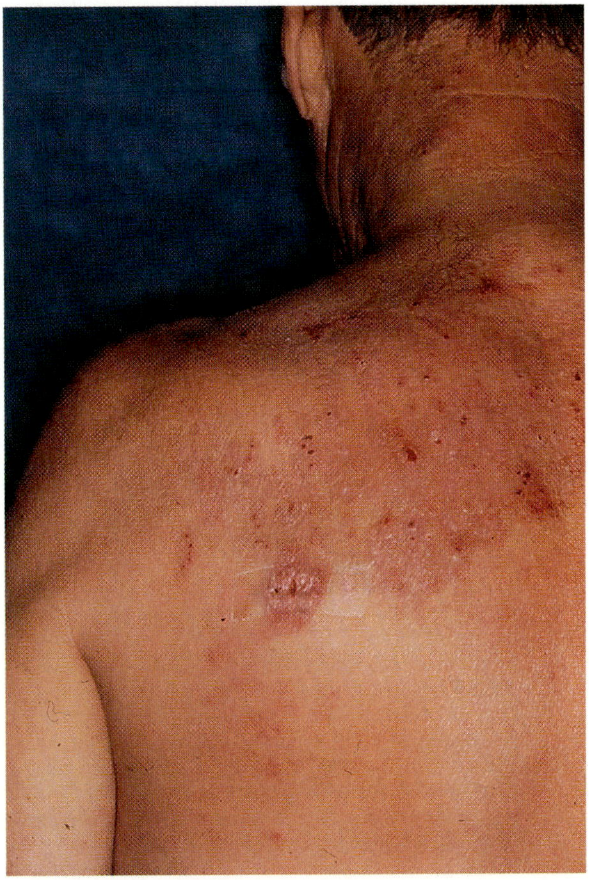

Fig. 12. Macular amyloidosis developing on the basis of chronic atopic eczema

Gynecological Diseases

Nichols et al. [229] reported an increased incidence of atopic diseases in patients with endometriosis. Two other publications reported the association of atopy and persistent lactation [199, 323].

Pityriasis Rosea

Chuang et al. [48] and Bjönberg et al. [27] reported an increased incidence of atopy in patients with pityriasis rosea.

References

1. Abel EA, Nickoloff BJ, Shelby DM, Watson W, Wood GS (1988) Tumor stage mycosis fungoides in a patient treated with long-term corticosteroids for asthma and atopic-like dermatitis. J Dermatol Surg Oncol 12: 1089–1093
2. Abrahamov A, Schifmann R, Goldstein R, Tal Y, Freier S (1986) Growth failure due to protein loss in dermatitis. Eur J Pediatr 145: 223–226
3. Abrahams I, McCarthy JT, Sanders SS (1963) 101 cases of exfoliative dermatitis. Arch Dermatol 87: 96–101
4. Abramson S, Dahl MV, Walsh G, Blumenthal NN, Douglas SD, Quie PG (1982) Antistaphylococcal IgE levels in patients with atopic dermatitis. J Am Acad Dermatol 7: 105–110
5. Adkinson NF jr (1984) Risk factors for drug allergy. J Allergy Clin Immunol 74: 567–572
6. Allansmith MR, Hahn GS, Simon MA (1976) Tissue, tear, serum IgE concentrations in vernal conjunctivitis. Am J Ophthalmol 81: 506–511
7. Aly R (1980) Bacteriology of atopic dermatitis. Acta Dermatol Venereol Suppl 92: 16–18
8. Aly R, Maibach HI, Shinefield HR (1977) Microbial flora of atopic dermatitis. Arch Dermatol 113: 780–782
9. Amemiya T, Matsuda H, Uehara M (1980) Ocular findings in atopic dermatitis with special reference to the clinical features of atopic cataract. Ophthalmologica 180: 129–132
10. Amlot PL, Green LA (1978): Atopy and immunoglobulin E concentrations in Hodgkin's disease and other lymphomas. Br Med J 1: 327–329
11. Amlot PL, Slaney J (1981): Hypergammaglobulinemia E in Hodgkin's disease and its relationship to atopy or a familial predisposition to atopy. Int Arch Allergy Appl Immunol 64: 138–145
12. Anderson TF, Waldinger TP, Voorhees JJ (1984) UVB phototherapy: an overview. Arch Dermatol 120: 1502–1507
13. Andogsky H (1914) Cataracta dermatogenes. Klin Mbl Augenh 52: 824–831
14. Ansel G, Tweedic MCK, West CR (1980) The current status of reactions to intravenous contrast media. Invest Radiol 15: 32–39
15. Aoki T, Funai T, Kojima M, Adachi J, Okano M (1989) Absorption of egg antigens by the gut observed by oral Prausnitz-Küstner (Walzer) reaction in atopic dermatitis. Acta Derm Venereol Suppl 144: 100–104
16. Balfour-Lynn L (1986) Growth and childhood asthma. Arch Dis Child 61: 1049–1055
17. Ball LM, Harper JI (1987) Atopic eczema in HIV-seropositive haemophiliacs. Lancet II: 627–628
18. Ballow M, Mendelson L (1980) Specific immunoglobulin E antibodies in tear secretions of patients with vernal conjunctivitis. J Allergy Clin Immunol 66: 112–118
19. Balyeat RM (1937) Complete retinal detachment (both eyes) with special reference to allergy as a possible primary etiologic factor. Am J Ophthalmol 20: 580–583
20. Barnetson R, Hardie RA, Merret TG (1981) Late onset atopic eczema and multiple food allergies after infectious mononucleosis. Br Med J 283: 1086–1087
21. Beetham WP (1940) Atopic cataracts. Arch Ophth 24: 21–37
22. Beigelman MV (1950) Vernal conjunctivitis. Los Angeles, University of Southern California Press, p 278
23. Bereston ES, Baer RL (1942) Keratoconus associated with atopic dermatitis: report of 2 cases. Arch Dermat Syph 46: 358–361
24. Bernard A (1953) Eczéma et gastrite hypertrophique. J Sc Méd Lille 71: 219–222
25. Bibel DJ, Greenberg JH, Cook JL (1977) Staphylococcus aureus and the microbial ecology of atopic dermatitis. Can J Microbiol 23: 1062–1068
26. Bjarnason J, Goolamali SK, Levi AJ, Peters TJ (1985) Intestinal permeability in patients with atopic eczema. Br J Dermatol 112: 291–297
27. Björnberg A, Hellgren L (1962) Pityriasis rosea. A statistical, clinical and laboratory investigation of 826 patients and matched healthy controls. Acta Derm Venereol 42 (Suppl 50): 1
28. Black MM, Jones EW (1971) Macular amyloidosis. A study of 21 cases with special reference to the role of epidermis in its histogenesis. Br J Dermatol 84: 199–209
29. Blaylock WK (1976) Atopic dermatitis: diagnosis and pathobiology. J Allergy Clin Immunol 57: 62–79
30. Böhm C, Johne HO (1956) Zur Kasuistik des Eczema herpeticatum (herptiforme) Kaposi. Hautarzt 7: 213–216
31. Boiko S, Kaufman RA, Lucky AW (1988) Osteomyelitis of the distal phalanges in three children with severe atopic dermatitis. Arch Dermatol 124: 418–423
32. Boner AL, Valletta EA, Bellanti JA (1985) Improvement of atopic dermatitis following natural measles virus infection. Four case reports. Ann Allergy 55: 605–608
33. Bonifazi E, Garofalo L, Pisani V, Meneghini CL (1985) Role of some infectious agents in atopic dermatitis. Acta Derm Venereol Suppl 114: 98–100
34. Braathen LR, Baklien K, Hovig T, Fausa O, Brandtzaeg P (1979) Immunological, histological and electron microscopical investigations of the gut in atopic dermatitis. Acta Derm Venereol Suppl 92: 78–80
35. Braun-Falco O, Plewig G, Wolff H (1984) Dermatologie und Venereologie, 3rd ed. Springer, Berlin Heidelberg New York

35a Braun-Falco O, Ryckmanns F, Heilgemeir GP, Ring J (1982) Zum Syndrom: Unkämmbare Haare. Beobachtungen von sechs Mitgliedern einer Familie mit Pili canaliculi, verbunden mit Pili torti, progredienter Alopezie, atopischem Ekzem und Hamartomen. Hautarzt 33: 366–372

36. Breneman DL, Lucky AW, Ostrow RS, Faras AJ, Volger C, Jenski LJ (1985) Bowenoid papulosis of the genitalia associated with human papilloma virus DNA type 16 in an infant with atopic dermatitis. Pediatr Dermatol 2: 297–301
36a. Bröcker EB (1990) Hyper IgE-Syndrom: Remission nach Maserninfektion. Allergologie 13: 65
37. Brunsting LA (1936) Atopic dermatitis (disseminated neurodermatitis) of young adults: analysis of precipitating factors in 101 cases and report of 10 cases with associated juvenile cataract. Arch Dermatol Syph 34: 935–957
38. Brunsting LA, Reed WB, Bair HL (1955) Occurrence of cataracts and keratoconus with atopic dermatitis. Arch Dermatol 72: 237–241
39. Buckley DB, English J, Molloy W, Doyle CT, Conelton MJ (1983) Dermatitis herpetiformis: a review of 119 cases. Clin Exp Dermatol 8: 477–487
40. Caputo R, Vanotti P, Bertani E (1984) Netherton's syndrome in two adult brothers. Arch Dermatol 120: 220–222
41. Carter DM, Jegasothy RV (1976) Alopecia areata and Down syndrome. Arch Derm 112: 1397–1399
42. Castrow FF (1981) Atopic cataracts versus steroid cataracts. J Am Acad Dermatol 5: 64–66
43. Cello JP (1979) Eosinophilic gastroenteritis – a complex disease entity. Am J Med 67: 1097–1104
44. Chang KC, Miklich DR, Barwise G, Chai H, Miles-Lawrence R (1982) Linear growth of chronic asthmatic children: the effects of the disease and various forms of steroid therapy. Clin Allergy 12: 369–378
45. Chen YP, Wu YC (1986) Eczema herpeticum in three siblings: clinical features and acyclovir treatment. J Dermatol 13: 334–338
46. Christensen JD (1980) Frequency of cataract in atopic dermatitis. Acta Derm Venereol 61: 76–77
47. Christophers E, Henseler T (1987) Contrasting disease patterns in psoriasis and atopic dermatitis. Arch Dermatol Res (Suppl) 279: 48–51
48. Chuang T et al (1982) Pityriasis rosea in Rochester, Minnesota, 1969 to 1978. A 10-year epidemiologic study. J Am Acad Dermatol 7: 80
49. Clemmensen OJ, Hjorth N (1983) Treatment of dermatitis of the head and neck with ketokonazole in patients with type I sensitivity to Pityrosporon orbiculare. Semin Dermatol 2: 26–29
50. Coles RS, Laval J (1952) Retinal detachments occurring in cataract associated with Neurodermatitis. AMA Arch Ophth 48: 30–39
51. Copeman PWM (1965) Eczema and keratoconus. Br Med J 2: 977
52. Copeman PWM, Wallace HJ (1964) Eczema vaccinatum. Br Med J 2: 906–908
53. Cordes FC, Cordero-Moreno R (1946) Atopic cataracts. Report of four cases. Am J Ophthal 29: 402–407
54. Cowan A, Klauder JV (1950) Frequency of occurrence of cataract in atopic dermatitis. Arch Ophth 43: 759–768
55. Cox NH, Jones SK, Downey DJ, Tuyp EJ, Jay JL, Moseley H, Mackie RM (1987) Cutaneous and ocular side-effects of oral photochemotherapy: results of a 8 year follow up study. Br J Dermatol 116: 145–152
52. Currie JM, Wright RC, Miller OG (1971) The frequency of warts in atopic patients. Cutis 8: 243–245
57. Dahl MV (1983) Staphylococcus aureus and atopic dermatitis. Arch Dermatol 119: 840–846
58. David TJ (1985) The overworked or fraudulent diagnosis of food allergy and food intolerance in children. J Roy Soc Med 78 (Supll 5): 21–31
59. David TJ (1989) Short stature in children with atopic eczema. Acta Derm Venereol Suppl 144: 41–44
60. David TJ, Cambridge GC (1986) Bacterial infection and atopic eczema. Arch Dis Child 61: 20–23
61. David TJ, Lakhani PK, Haeney MR (1984) Severe atopic eczema, recurrent pneumococcal meningitis and recurrent eczema herpeticum. J R Soc Med 77: 696–697
62. David TJ, Longson M (1985) Herpes simplex infections in atopic eczema. Arch Dis Child 60: 338–343
63. David TJ, Waddington E, Stanton RJH (1984) Nutritional hazards of elimination diets in children with atopic eczema. Arch Dis Child 59: 323–325
64. Davies MG, Fifield P, Marks R (1979) Atopic disease and dermatitis herpetiformis. Br J Dermatol 101: 429–434
65. Davis WT (1921) The relation of the eye and certain skin diseases. South Med J 14: 237–241
66. de Weert J, Timmerman L, Kint A (1984) Alopecia areata and atopy. Dermatologica 168: 224–229
67. Dent GE, Garrets M (1960) Skin changes in hypocalcemia. Lancet 1: 142–146
67a. Diepgen TL, Fartasch M, Hornstein OP (1989) Evaluation and relevance of atopic basic and minor features in patients with atopic dermatitis and in the general population. Acta Derm Venereol Suppl 144: 50–54
68. Draelos ZK, Hansen RC (1985) Polymorphic light eruption in childhood. Clin Pediatr 24: 692–695
69. Dubowitz V (1965) Familial low birth weight dwarfism with an unusual facies and skin eruption. J Med Genet 2: 12–17
70. DuMont GCL, Beach RC, Menzies IS (1984) Gastrointestinal permeability in food-allergic eczematous children. Clin Allergy 14: 55–59
71. Dunand P, Chai H, Weltman D (1975) Posterior polar cataracts and steroid therapy in children. J Allergy Clin Immunol 55: 123
72. Dupré AS, Christol B, Bonafe JL, Lassere J (1981) Orf and atopic dermatitis. Br J Dermatol 105: 103–104
73. Dworin M, Diamond HD, Craver LF (1955): Hodgkin's disease and allergy. Cancer 8: 128–131
74. Easty D, Entwhistle C, Funk A, Witcher J (1975) Herpes simplex keratitis and keratoconus in the atopic patients. Trans Ophthalmol Soc UK 95: 267–276
75. Easty D, Rice NSC, Jones BR (1971) Disodium cromoglycate (Intal) in the treatment of vernal keratoconjunctivitis. Trans Ophthalmol Soc UK 91: 491
76. Eisenberg BC (1976) Congenital lymphangiectasia and atopy. Ann Allergy 36: 342–350
77. Ellis J, Dawber RPR (1980) Ectodermal dysplasia syndrome: a family study. Clin Exp Dermatol 5: 295–304
78. Eriksson G, Forsbeck M (1963) The assessment and the vaccination of patients with cutaneous disorders. Acta Med Scand (Suppl) 464: 147
79. Fagerholm P, Plamquist BM, Philipson B (1984) Atopic cataract: Changes in the lens epithelium and subcapsular cortex. Graefes Arch Clin Exp Ophthalmol 221: 149–152
80. Fairris GM, Hamilton I, Cunliffe WJ, Axon ATR (1984) Intestinal permeability in adults with atopic eczema. Br J Dermatol 111: 711
81. Falk ES (1985) UV-light therapies in atopic dermatitis. Photodermatol 2: 241–246
82. Falk ES, Bolle R (1980) IgE antibodies to house dust mite in patients with scabies. Br J Dermatol 103: 283–288
83. Falk ES, Bolle R (1983) In vivo demonstration of specific immediate hypersensitivity to scabies mite. Br J Dermatol 103: 367–373
84. Falk ES, Dale S, Bolle R, Haneberg B (1981) Antigens

common to scabies and house dust mites. Allergy 36: 233–238
85. Fälth-Magnusson K, Kjellman NIM, Magnusson KE, Sundqvist I (1984) Intestinal permeability in healthy and allergic children before and after sodium cromoglycate treatment assessed with different-size polyehtylenglycols (PEG 400 and PEG 1000). Clin Allergy 14: 277–286
86. Ferguson AC, Murray AB, Tze WJ (1982) Short stature and delayed skeletal maturation in children with allergic disease. J Allergy Clin Immunol 69: 461–466
87. Fernon MJ, Guillet G, Maleville J (1980) Pustulose de Kaposi-Juliusberg et eczéma atopique: Mise au point clinique et immunopathologique: A propos de trois observations recentes. Ann Pediatr 27: 451–456
88. Fisch RO, Tsai MY, Gentry WC (1981) Studies of phenylketonurics with dermatitis. J Am Acad Dermatol 4: 284–290
89. Fleisher TL, Zeligman I (1960) Cutaneous findings in phenylketonuria. Arch Derm 81: 893–903
90. Fontana VJ, Spain WC, Desanctis AG (1956) The role of allergy in nephrosis. NY State J Med 56: 3907–3910
91. Frain-Bell W, Scatchard M (1971) The association of photosensitivity and atopy in child. Br J Dermatol 85: 105–110
92. Frankland AW, Easty D (1971) Vernal Keratoconjunctivitis: An atopic disease. Trans Ophthalmol Soc UK 91: 479–482
93. Fregert J, Möller H, Rorsman H (1959) Observations on vitiligo in a patient with atopic dermatitis. Acta Derm Venereol 39: 225–229
94. Frentz G, Everberg G, Wulf HC (1976) Congenital perceptive hearing loss and atopic dermatitis. Acta Otolaryngol 82: 242–244
95. Frick OL, Asthon FA, Mills J (1977) Virus infection associated with onset of allergic sensitization in infants. Ann Allergy 38: 449
96. Friedländer MH (1988) Ocular Allergy. In: Middleton E, Reed CE, Ellis EF (eds) Allergy: Principle and practice, 3rd edn., Mosby, St. Louis
97. Friedman M, Hare PJ (1965) Gluten-sensitive enteropathy and eczema. Lancet 1: 521–524
98. Fritsch-Kieffer MG (1980) Immunopathologie et immunotherapie de la pelade. Thesis, Strasbourg
99. Fry L, McMinn RMH, Shuster S (1966) The small intestine in skin diseases. Arch Derm 93: 647–653
100. Fry L, Shuster S, McMinn RMH (1965) D-Xylose absorption in patients with eczema. Br Med J 1: 967–968
101. Galin MA, Berger R (1958) Atopy and keratococuns. Am J Ophth 45: 904–906
102. Garofalo L, Pisani V, Mazzotta F, Bonifazi E (1989) Psoriasis in atopic children. Acta Derm Venereol Suppl 146: 63–65
103. Garrity JA, Liesegang TJ (1984) Ocular complications of atopic dermatitis. Can J Ophthalmol 19: 21–24
104. Gasset AR, Hinson WA, Frias IL (1978) Keratoconus and atopic diseases. Ann Ophthalmol 10: 991–994
105. Gault N (1933) Cataracte neurodermitique. Bull Soc d'Ophth de Paris 3: 280–284
106. Geyer A, Knopf B, Roth H, Barta U: Gemeinsames Auftreten von Psoriasis und atopischen Erkrankungen im Rahmen einer klinischen Studie. (cited in 176)
107. Ghadimi HK (1981) Histidinemia. Am J Dis Child 135: 210–211
108. Gianetti A (1987) Viral skin diseases in atopic dermatitis. In: Happle R, Grosshans E (eds) Pediatric Dermatology. Springer, Berlin Heidelberg, pp 110–113
109. Gingrich RE, Fusano RM (1964) The lens and the skin. In: Common antigens of the skin and crystalline lens. J Invest Derm 43: 235–236
110. Gip L, Lodin A, Molin L (1969): Alopécia. areato. Acto Devm Venercol 49: 180–188
111. Gottlieb MS, Mildvan D, Quinn TC, Jeffries DJ, Pinching AJ, Weiss RA (1987) Current topics in AIDS. Wiley, Chichester, pp 255–257
112. Graciansky P de, Bernier JJ, Bégniél JC, Daniel F, Larrègue M (1967) Eczéma constitutionnel et atteinte de l'intestin grele. Bull Soc Fr Derm Syph 74: 318–319
113. Graham-Brown RAC (1988) Atopic dermatitis. Sem Dermatol 7: 37–42
114. Grayson M (1979) Diseases of the cornea. Mosby, St. Louis
115. Greene SL, Muller SA (1985) Netherton's Syndrome. Report of a case and review of the literature. J Am Acad Dermatol 13: 329–337
116. Groskong T, Mendelson L, Mandoza S (1973) Serum IgE in patients with minimal change nephrotic syndrome. J Pediatr 83: 767
117. Gupta AK, Anderson TF (1987) Psoralen photochemotherapy. J Am Acad Dermatol 17: 703–734
118. Haddi E, Charpin D, Tafforeau M, Kulling G, Lauteaume A, Kleisbauer JP, Vervleot D (1990) Atopy and systemic reactions to drugs. Allergy 45: 236–239
119. Hambrich GW jr., Schrie HG (1962) Studies of the skin in Hurler's Syndrome. Arch Dermatol 88: 455–471
120. Hammershog O, Jessen F (1982) A retrospective study of cataract formation in 96 patients treated with PUVA, Acta Derm Venereol 62: 444–446
121. Hanifin JM (1982) Atopic dermatitis. J Am Acad Dermatol 6: 1–13
122. Hanifin JM (1983) Atopic dermatitis. Special clinical complications. Postgrad Med J 74: 183–193, 196–199
123. Hanifin JM (1983) Clinical and basic aspects of atopic dermatitis. Sem Dermatol 2: 5–19
124. Hanifin JM (1984) Atopic dermatitis. J Allergy Clin Immunol 73: 211–222
125. Hanifin JM (1988) Atopic eczema. In Middleton E, Reed CE, Ellis EF (eds) Allergy: Principles and practice, 3rd edn. Mosby, St. Louis
126. Hanifin JM, Cooper KD, Roth HL (1986) Atopy and atopic dermatitis. J Am Acad Dermatol 15: 703–706
127. Hanifin JM, Homburger HA (1986) Staphylococcal colonization, infection and atopic dermatitis – association not etiology. J Allergy Clin Immunol 78: 563–565
128. Hanifin JM, Lobitz WC (1977) Newer concepts of atopic dermatitis. Arch Dermatol 113: 663–670
128a. Hanifin JM, Rajka G (1980) Diagnostic features of atopic dermatitis. Acta Derm Venereol Suppl 92: 44–47
129. Hanifin JM, Ray LF, Lobitz WC jr. (1974) Immunological reactivity in dermatophytosis. Br J Dermatol 90: 1–8
130. Hanifin JM, Rogge JL (1977) Staphylococcal infections in patients with atopic dermatitis. Arch Dermatol 113: 1383–1386
131. Hannuksela M, Karvonen J, Husa M, Jokela R, Katajamäki L, Leppisaari M (1985) Ultraviolet light therapy in atopic dermatitis. Acta Derm Venereol (Suppl) 114: 137–139
132. Hansen AE (1963) Role of linoleic acid in infant nutrition. Clinical and chemical study of 428 infants fed on mixtures varying in kind and amount of fat. Pediatrics 31 (Suppl): 171–192
133. Harber LC, Bickers DR (1981) Photosensitivity diseases. Principles of diagnosis and treatment. Saunders, New York
134. Hardwicke J, Soothill JF, Squire JR, Holti G (1959)

Nephrotic syndrome with pollenhypersensitivity. Lancet 1: 500–502

135. Hare R, Cooke EM (1961) Self-contamination of patients with staphylococcal infections. Br Med J 2: 333–336
136. Hasan T, Jansen CT (1983) Erythroderma: a follow up of fifty cases. J Am Acad Dermatol 8: 836–840
137. Hashii R, Uyama M (1972) Cataract and retinal detachment asscociated with atopic dermatitis. Report of a case. Jap J Clin Ophthal 26: 35–40
138. Hashimoto K, Kobayashi H (1980) Amyloidogenesis in primary skin amyloidoses. In: Glenner GG et al. (eds) Amyloid and amyloidosis. Excerpta Medica, Amsterdam, pp 426–435
139. Hata S (1985) Recurrent eczema herpeticum in an adult. J Dermatol 12: 372–374
140. Hauser C (1986) The role of staphylococcus aureus in atopic dermatitis. Int J Dermatol 25: 573–574

140a. Hauser C, Wuethrich B, Matter L, Wilhelm JA, Sonnabend W, Schopfer K (1985) Staphylococcus aureus skin colonization in atopic dermatitis patients. Dermatologica 170: 35–39

141. Hauspie R, Susanne C, Alexander F (1977) Maturational delay and temporal growth retardation in asthmatic boys. J Allergy Clin Immunol 59: 200–206
142. Hay RJ, Brostoff J (1977) Immune responses in patients with chronic Trichophyton rubrum infections. Clin Exp Dermatol 2: 373–380
143. Hazen PG, Eppes B (1977) Eczema herpeticum caused by Herpes virus type 2. Arch Dermatol 113: 1085–1086
144. Heine W, Richter I, Tessmann D, Heise H (1976) Partielle Zottenatrophie mit entzündlichen Veränderungen der Dünndarmschleimhaut beim konstitutionellen Ekzem und seborrhoischen Ekzem des Säuglings. Kinderarztl Prax 44: 399–402
145. Henocq E, Hewitt B, Guerin B (1982) Staphylococcal and human dander IgE antibodies in superinfected atopic dermatitis. Clin Allergy 12: 113–120
146. Heskel N, Lobitz WC Jr (1983) Atopic dermatitis in children: clinical features and management. Sem Dermatol 2: 39–44
147. Highet AS (1988) Viral warts. Sem Dermatol 7: 53–57
148. Hodgson HJF, Davies RJ, Gent AE, Hodson ME (1976) Atopic disorders and adult coelic a disease. Lancet 2: 115–117
149. Hogan MJ (1953) Atopic Keratoconjunctivitis. Am J Ophthalmol 36: 937–947
150. Holzer FJ, Olinsky A, Phelan PD (1981) Variability of airways hyperreactivity and allergy in cystic fibrosis. Arch Dis Childh 56: 455–459
151. Hori Y, Kobori T (1981) Macular amyloidosis: clinical and pathological studies. In: Fitzpatrick TB (ed) Biology and diseases of dermal pigmentation. University of Tokyo Press, Tokyo, pp 299–309
152. Huber P, Schmid P, Hoigné R, Müller U (1983) Atopie und generalisierte allergische Reaktionen auf Insektenstiche. Schweiz Med Wschr 113: 1863–1865
153. Hurlbut WB, Domonkos AN (1961) Cataract and retinal detachment associated with atopic dermatitis. Arch Ophth 52: 852–857
154. Hyams SW, Bialik M, Neumann E (1975) Clinical trial of topical disodium cromoglycate in vernal keratoconjunctivitis. J Pediatr Ophthalmol 12: 116–118
155. Ikeda T (1965) A new classification of alopecia areata. Dermatologica 131: 421–445
156. Ingram RM (1965) Retinal detachment associated with atopic dermatitis and cataract. Br J Ophthalmol 49: 96–97
157. Irons M, Levy HL (1986) Metabolic syndromes with dermatologic manifestations. Clin Rev Allergy 4: 101–124
158. Ito F, Aoki K, Eto Y (1981) Histidinemia. Biochemical parameters for diagnosis. Am J Dis Child 135: 227–229
159. Jablonska S (1984) Wart Viruses: Human Papillomaviruses. Sem Dermatol 3: 120–129
160. Jackson PG, Baker RWR, Lessof MH, Ferrett J, MacDonald DM (1981) Intestinal permeability in patients with eczema and food allergy. Lancet 1: 1285–1286
161. Jawitz JC, Hines HC, Moshell AN (1985) Treatment of eczema herpeticum with systemic acyclovir. Arch Dermatol 121: 274–275
162. Jay JL (1981) Clinical factors and diagnosis of atopic keratoconjunctivitis and the effect of treatment with sodium cromoglycate. Br J Ophthal 60: 335–340
163. Jervis GA (1937) Phenylpyruvic oligophrenia: introductory study of 50 cases of mental deficiency associated with excretion of phenylpyruvic acid. Arch Neurol Psychiatr 38: 944–963
164. Jones HE (1980) The atopic-chronic-dermatophytosis syndrome. Acta Derm Venereol Suppl 92: 81–85
165. Jones HE, Reinhardt JH, Rinaldi MG (1973) A clinical, mycological, and immunological survey for dermatophytosis. Arch Dermatol 108: 61
166. Kaaman T (1985) Skin reactivity in atopic patients with dermatophytosis. Mykosen 28: 183–190

166a. Kang K, Tian R (1987) Atopic dermatitis. An evaluation of clinical and laboratory findings. Int J Dermatol 26: 27–32

167. Kaposi M (1887) Pathologie und Therapie der Hautkrankheiten. Urban und Schwarzenberg, Berlin, p 483
168. Karel I, Myska V, Kvicalova E (1965) Ophthalmological changes in atopic dermatitis. Acta Derm Venereol 45: 381–386
169. Katavisto M (1949) Prurigo diathésique Besnier and cataract. Acta Ophth 27: 581–589
170. Katsura H, Hida T (1984) Atopic dermatitis. Retinal detachment associated with atopic dermatitis. Retina 4: 148–151
171. Katz AJ, Twarog FJ, Zeiger RS, Falckhuk ZM (1984) Milk-sensitive and eosinophilic gastroenteropathy – similar clinical features with contrasting mechanisms and clinical course. J Allergy Clin Immunol 74: 72–78
172. Kaye J (1977) Atopic dermatitis: an immunologic disease complex and its therapy. Ann Allergy 38: 345–352
173. Kazden JJ, Crawford JS, Langer H, MacDonald AL (1976) Sodium cromoglycate (Intal) in the treatment of vernal keratoconjunctivitis and allergic conjunctivitis. Can J Ophthalmol 11: 300–303
174. Kierland RR (1955) Certain stigmata associated with atopic dermatitis. In: Baer RL (ed) Atopic dermatitis. New York University Press, New York.
175. Kleerberger F (1962) Demonstration of atopic cataract with retinal detachment. Klin Mbl Augenklinik 140: 734
176. Knopf B, Wollina U, Broening TC (1989) Kombination von Psoriasis vulgaris und atopischem Ekzem. Akt Dermatol 15: 177–178
177. Kokkonen J, Similä S, Herva R (1980) Gastrointestinal findings in atopic children. Eur J Pediatr 134: 249–254
178. Konigsmark BW, Hollander MB, Berlin CI (1988) Familial neural hearing loss and atopic dermatitis. JAMA 204: 953–957
179. Koranne RV, Sachdeva KG (1988) Vitiligo. Int J Dermatol 27: 676–681
180. Kornerup T, Lodin A (1959) Ocular changes in 100 cases of

Besnier's prurigo (Atopic dermatitis). Acta Ophthalmol 37: 508–521
181. Krafchik BR (1988) Eczematous dermatitis. In: Schachner LA, Hansen RC (eds) Pediatric dermatology. Churchill-Livingstone, New York, pp 695–724
182. Krafchik BR, Toole JW (1983) What is Netherton's syndrome? Int J Dermatol 22: 459–462
183. Kristmundsdottir F, David TJ (1987) Growth impairment in children with atopic eczema. J Roy Soc Med 80: 9–12
184. Kuebler HC, Kuehn W, Rummel HH, Kaufmann J, Kaufmann M (1987) Zur Karzinomentstehung (Vulvakarzinom) beim Netherton-Syndrom (Ichthyosis, Haaranomalien, atopische Diathese). Geburtshilfe Frauenheilk 47: 742–744
185. Kuhlwein A, Wasilew SW, Schuette B (1982) Cheveux incoiffables mit Kuticulasspornen und Zahnanomalien bei Ichthyosis vulgaris und atopic dermatitis. Z Hautkr 57: 1421–1429
186. Kunz R, Fellinger C (1985) Dokumentation des klinischen Bildes der Keratoconjunctivitis atopica bei Neurodermitis constitutionalis. Klin Monatsbl Augenheilk 187: 366–368
187. Lange-Vejlsgaard G, Ralfkiaer E, Larsen JK, O'Connor N, Thomsen K (1989) Fatal cutaneous T-cell lymphoma in a child with atopic dermatitis. J Am Acad Dermatol 20: 954–958
188. Larsen-Schultz F, Vase P, Schmidt H (1978) Atopic dermatitis and congenital deafness. Br J Dermatol 99: 325–328
189. Lemke L, Jütte A (1966) Augenbefall bei Neurodermatitis disseminata. Derm Wschr 152: 921–927
190. Leroy D, Michel M, Leport Y, Deschamp P (1988) Association d'un eczéma atopique, d'une dermatose bulleuse à IgA linéaire et d'une grele crouteuse. Ann Dermatol Venereol 107: 933–936
191. Leung DYM, Rhodes AR, Geha RS (1987) Atopic dermatitis. In: Fitzpatrick TB, Eisen AZ, Wolff K, Freedberg JM, Austen KF (eds) Dermatology in general medicine. McGraw-Hill, USA, pp 1385–1408
192. Levy HL (1977) Hartnup disease. In: Goldensohn ES, Appel SH (eds) Scientific approaches to clinical neurology. Lea and Febiger, Philadelphia, p 75
193. Leyden JJ, Baker DA (1979) Localized Herpes simplex infection in atopic dermatitis. Arch Dermatol 115: 311–312
194. Leyden JJ, Marples RR, Kligman AM (1974) Staphylococcus aureus in the lesions of atopic dermatitis. Br J Dermatol 90: 525–530
195. Lin RY (1988) Chronic diffuse dermatitis and hyper IgE in HIV infection. Acta Derm Venereol 68: 486–491
196. Lipman BL (1983) Atopic dermatitis in an infant complicated by generalized verrucae vulgares. Ann Allergy 51: 33–34
197. Longmore L (1970) Atopic dermatitis, cataract and keratoconus. Aust J Dermatol 11: 139–141
198. Lowe CU, May CD, Reed SC (1949) Fibrosis of the pancreas in infants and children. Am J Dis Child 78: 349–374
199. MacDonald CT, Lerner AB (1966) Atopic dermatitis and persistent lactation. Arch Dermatol 93: 174–176
200. Mac Millan A, Rook A (1971) Vitiligo with a raised rim in atopic subjects. Br J Dermatol 85: 491
201. Manabe T, Inagaki Y, Nakagawa S, Miyoshi K, Ueki H (1987) Ripple pigmentation of the neck in atopic dermatitis. Am J Dermatopathol 9: 301–307
202. Marks J (1968) Systemic effects of skin disease with particular reference to the small intestine. Thesis, University of Oxford
203. Marks S, Shuster S (1970) Small-intestinal mucosal abnormalities in various skin diseases – fact or fancy? Gut 11: 281–291
204. Marks J, Shuster S (1971) Intestinal malabsorption and the skin. Gut 12: 938–947
205. Matuchansky C, Certin M, Bognel JC, Bognel C, Modigliani R, Daniel F, Galian A, Civatte J, Bernier JJ (1974) Dermatoses chronique et absorption intestinale. Étude anatomofonctionelle de l'intestin grele dans 35 observations. Ann Med Interne 125: 253–259
206. McCalla R, Savilahti E, Perkkiö, Kuitunen P, Backman A (1980) Morphology of the jejunum in children with eczema due to food allergy. Allergy 35: 563–571
207. McCormick DP, Ammann AJ, Ishizaka K, Miller DG, Hong R (1971) A study of allergy in patients with malignant lymphoma and chronic lymphocytic leukemia. Cancer 27: 93–99
208. McDonald DM, Fergin PE, Black MM (1980) Localized cutaneous amyloidosis. In: Glenner GG et al. (eds) Amyloid and amyloidosis. Excerpta Medica, Amsterdam, pp 239–242
209. Meadow SR, Sarsfield JK (1981) Steroid responsive nephrotic syndrome and allergy: clinical studies. Arch Dis Child 56: 509–516
210. Mee AS, Brown D, Jewell DP (1979) Atopy in inflammatory bowel disease. Scand J Gastroenterol 14: 743–746
211. Menzel I (1984) Zur Provokation der Dermatitis atopica durch intestinale Candidamykose. Z Hautkr 59: 1463–1468
212. Mevorah B, Frenk E, Wietlisbach V, Carrel CF (1988) Minor clinical features of atopic dermatitis. Dermatologica 177: 360–364
213. Midelfart K, Stenvold SE, Volden G (1985) Combined UVB and UVA phototherapy of atopic eczema. Dermatologica 171: 95–98
214. Minnesota Dermatological Society (1968) Histidinemia and atopic dermatitis. Arch Dermatol 98: 317–319
215. Miyachi S, Lessof MH, Kemeny DM, Green IA (1979) Comparison of the atopic background between allergic and non-allergic beekeepers. Int Arch Allergy Appl Immunol 58: 160–166
216. Morris T, Rhodes J (1979) Ulcerative colitis: is it an allergic disorder? In: Pepys J, Edwards AM (eds) The mast cell. Pitman, London
217. Moschella SL, Hurley HJ (eds) (1958) Dermatology, 2nd edn. Saunders, Philadelphia
218. Motala C, Potter PC, Weinberg EG, Malherbe D, Hughes J (1986) Antistaphylococcus aureus specific IgE in atopic dermatitis. J Allergy Clin Immunol 78: 583–589
219. Mouzon Cambon A, Ohayou E, Bouissou F, Barthe P (1980) HLA DR typing in children with glomerular diseases. Lancet 2: 868
220. Mukai K (1966) A case of atopic dermatitis with cataract and retinal detachment. Jap Rev Clin Ophthal 60: 1043
221. Muller SA, Brunsting LA (1963) Cataracts associated with dermatologic disorder. Arch Dermatol 88: 330–339
222. Muller SA, Winkelmann RK (1963) Alopecia areata. An evaluation of 736 patients. Arch Dermatol 88: 290–297
224. Mulvey PM (1972) Cot death survey. Anaphylaxis and the house dust mite. Med J Aust: 1240–1244
225. Murray AB, Fraser BM, Hardwick DF, Pirie GE (1976) Chronic asthma and growth failure in children. Lancet 2: 197–198
226. Mylius K (1949) Doppelseitige spontane Netzhautablösung bei 2 Jugendlichen, seit Jahren an Neurodermitis

disseminata leidenden Patienten. Klin Mbl Augenheilk 115: 247–250

227. Neubert U, Wolff HH (1982) Komplikationen bei atopischem Ekzem. Allergologie 5: 52–57
228. Nicolis GD, Helwig EB (1973) Exfoliative dermatitis: a clinicopathologic study of 135 cases. Arch Dermatol 108: 788–797
229. Nichols TR, Lamb K, Arkins JA (1987) The association of atopic diseases with endometriosis. Ann Allergy 59: 360–363
230. Nielsen NV, Sorensen PN (1978) Glaucoma induced by application of corticosteroids to the periorbital region. Arch Dermatol 114: 953–954
231. Nordbring F, Johannson SGO, Espmark A (1972) Raised serum levels of IgE in infectious mononucleosis. Scand J Infect Dis 4: 119–124
232. Norris PG, Rivers JK (1987) Screening for cataracts in patients with severe atopic eczema. Clin Exp Dermatol 12: 21–22
233. Oakes RC, Cox AD, Burgdorf WHC (1983) Atopic dermatitis. Clin Pediat 22: 467–475
234. Ohnishi M, Kimura K, Matsumoto T, Sakamoto F, Yamaguchi M, Kadowaki J (1978) Idiopathic nephrotic syndrome and atopic features. In: Proceedings of the fourteenth annual meeting of the Japanese Society of Pediatric Nephrology, 1978, Abstract 97
235. Orecchia G (1987) Alopecia areata and measles. J Am Acad Dermatol 17: 840–841
236. Ortonne JP, Perrot H, Thivolet J (1976) Étude clinique et statistique d'une population de 100 vitiligos: facteurs étiologiques et étude clinique. Associations fonctionelles. Sem Hop Paris 52: 679–686
237. Ortonne JP, Perrot H, Thivolet J (1976) Étude clinique et statistique d'une population de 100 vitiligos. Sem Hop Paris 52: 475–481
238. Oshinskie L, Haine C (1982) Atopic dermatitis and its ophthalmic complications. J Am Optom Assoc 53: 889–894
239. Parish WE, Barrett AM, Coombs RRA, Gunther M, Camps FE (1960) Hypersensitivity to milk and sudden death in infancy. Lancet II: 1106–1110
240. Parkin JM, Eales LJ, Galazka AR, Pinching AJ (1987) Atopic manifestations in AIDS: response to recombinant gamma interferon. Br Med J 294: 1185–1186
241. Pauly CR, Artis WM, Jones HE (1978) Atopic dermatitis, impaired cellular immunity and molluscum contagiosum. Arch Dermatol 114: 391–393
242. Penders AJM (1968) Alopecia areata and atopy. Dermatologica 136: 395–399
243. Perkkio M (1980) Immunohistochemical study of intestinal biopsies fro children with atopic eczema due to food allergy. Allergy 35: 573–580
244. Perret CM, Steijlen PU, Happle R (1990) Alopecia areata. J Dermatol 29: 83–88
245. Peterson RDA (1965) Immunologic responses in infantile eczema. J Pediatr 66: 224–234
246. Pigatto PD, Altomare G, Polenghi MM, Roveroni S, Menni S, Docchio F (1986) Atopy and photosensitivity in children. Photodermatol 3: 303
247. Pike MG, Haddle RJ, Boulton P, Turner MW, Atherton DJ (1986) Increased intestinal permeability in atopic eczema. J Invest Dermatol 86: 101–104
248. Prigent F, Civatte J (1982) Atopie et syndrome associés. Ann Dermatol Venereol 109: 341–353
249. Przybilla B, Ring J, Grießhammer B (1987) Atopy and hymenoptera venom allergy (HVA). J Allergy Clin Immunol 79: 233

249a. Przybilla B, Ring J (1986) Hyposensibilisierungsbehandlung der Hymenopterengiftallergie: Aspekte der Indikationsstellung und Dosierung. Allergologie 9: 2–10

249b. Przybilla B, Ring J, Grießhammer B (1989) Diagnostische Befunde bei Hymenopterengiftallergie. Allergologie 12: 192–202

250. Rahi A, Davies P, Ruben M (1977) Keratokonus and coexisting atopic disease. Br J Ophthalmol 61: 761–764
251. Rajka G (1983) Atopic dermatitis and Hodgkin's disease. Acta Derm Venereol 63: 176
252. Rajka G (1989) Essential aspects of atopic dermatitis. Berlin, Springer
253. Rajka G, Barlinn C (1979) On the significance of the trichophytin reactivity in atopic dermatitis. Acta Derm Venereol 59: 45–47
254. Rajka G, Skog E (1965) On the relation between drug allergy and atopy. Acta Allergol 20: 387–394
255. Rajka G, Winkelmann RK (1984) Atopic dermatitis and Sézary syndrome. Arch Dermatol 120: 83–84
256. Rao M, Victoria MS, Jabbar H, Steiner P (1981) Atopic dermatitis, asthma and eye changes in children. J Asthma 18: 47–48
257. Räsänen L, Lehto M, Reunala T, Jansen C, Lehtinen M, Leinikki P (1987) Langerhans cell and T-lymphocyte functions in patients with atopic dermatitis with disseminated cutaneous herpes simplex virus infection. J Invest Dermatol 89: 15–18
258. Rasmussen JE (1989) Management of atopic dermatitis. Allergy 44 Suppl 9: 108–113
259. Reed WB, Epstein WL, Boder E, Sedgwick R (1966) Cutaneous manifestations of ataxia-teleangiectasia. JAMA 195: 746–753
260. Reed WB, Lopez DA, Landing B (1970) Clinical spectrum of anhidrotic ectodermal dysplasia. Arch Dermatol 102: 134–143
261. Reeves WG, Cameron JS, Johannson SGO, Ogg CS, Peters DK, Weller RO (1975) Seasonal nephrotic syndrome. Description and immunologic findings. Clin Allergy 5: 121–137
262. Revuz J, Delebarre P, Modigliani P, Touraine R (1976) Eczéma atopique, déficit immunitaire mixte, hyperplasie lymphoide du gréle. Bull Soc Fr Derm Syph 83: 154–157
263. Rice NSC, Easty D, Garner A, Jones BR, Tripathi R (1971) Vernal kerato-conjunctivitis and its management. Trans Ophthalmol Soc UK 91: 483–489
264. Richards W, Olsen D, Church JA (1977) Improvement of idiopathic nephrotic syndrome following allergy therapy. Ann Allergy 39: 332–334
265. Ring J (1982) Atopisches Ekzem. Dtsch Med Wschr 107: 483–485
266. Ring J (1988) Angewandte Allergologie. MMV Medizin Verlag, Munich
267. Ring J, Dorsch W (1985) Altered releasability of vasoactive mediator secreting cells in atopic eczema. Acta Derm Venereol Suppl 114: 9–23
268. Roberts DL, Rhodes J, Heatley RV, Newcombe RG (1978) Atopic features in ulcerative colitis. Lancet 1: 1262
269. Rokugo M, Tagami H, Usaba Y, Tomita Y (1990) Contact sensitivity to pityrosporum ovale in patients with atopic dermatitis. Arch Dermatol 126: 627–632
270. Rook A, Wilkinson DS, Ebling FJG, Champion RH, Barton JL (eds) (1986) Textbook of dermatology, 4th edn. Blackwell, Oxford
271. Rooklin AR (1979) Posterior subcapsular cataracts in steroid-requiring asthmatic children. J Allergy Clin Immunol 63: 383–386

272. Rostenberg A jr., Solomon LM (1968) Infantile eczema and systemic disease. Arch Dermatol 98: 41–46
273. Roth HL (1987) Atopic dermatitis revisited. Int J Dermatol 26: 139–149
273a. Ruzicka T, Donhauser G, Linke RP, Landthaler M, Bieber T (1990) Kutane Amyloidosen. Hautarzt 41: 245–255
274. Rystedt I, Strannegard IL, Strannegard O (1984) Increased serum levels of antibodies to Epstein-Barr virus in adults with history of atopic dermatitis. Int Arch Allergy Appl Immunol 75: 179–183
275. Rystedt I, Strannegard IL, Strannegard O (1986) Recurrent viral infections in patients with past or present atopic dermatitis. Br J Dermatol 114: 575–582
276. Rystedt I, Strannegard IL, Strannegard O (1989) Infections as contributing factors to atopic dermatitis. Allergy 44 (Suppl 9): 79–83
277. Sack SS (1947) Atopic cataract: report of a case with tabulated summary of previously reported cases. Ann Allergy 5: 353–363
278. Sampolinsky D, Samra Z, Zavaro A, Barishak Y (1984) Allergen-specific immunoglobulin E antibodies in tears and serum of vernal conjunctivitis patients. Int Arch Allergy Appl Immunol 75: 317–321
279. Sandberg DH, McIntosh RM, Bernstein CW, Carr R, Strauss J (1977) Severe steroid responsive nephrosis associated with hypersensitivity. Lancet I: 388–391
280. Sanderson IR, Brueton LA, Savage MO, Harper JI (1987) Eczema herpeticum – a potentially fatal disease. Br Med J 294: 693–694
281. Schaarschmidt S (1983) Pendelnde Mollusca contagiosa bei einer Patientin mit endogenem Ekzem. Z Hautkr 58: 343–345
282. Schmutz JL, Weber M, Beurey J (1989) Cataracte et dermatologie. Ann Dermatol Venereol 116: 133–139
283. Schulz-Kopetz M, Weigl-Jakobi J, Einsiedel E, Korting GW (1981) Zur Alopecia areata im Kindesalter. Akt Dermatol 7: 1–5
283a. Scott BG, Buck BE, Leterman JG, Bloom FL, Parks WP (1984) Acquired immunodeficiency syndrome in infants. N Engl J Med 310: 76–81
284. Scriver CR et al (1983) Disorders of proline and hydroxyproline metabolism. In: Stanbury JB et al (eds) The metabolic basis of inherited disease, 5th edn. McGraw-Hill, New York, p 360
285. Sehgal VN, Koranne RV, Srivastava SB (1989) Genital warts. Int J Dermatol 28: 75–85
286. Seinedari S, Gianetti A, Di Silverio A (1979) Sindrome di Waardenburg-Klein e atopia: observazioni su 7 casi familiari. G Ital Dermatol Minerva Dermatol 114: 565–568
287. Settipane GA, Klein DE, Boyd GK (1978) Relationship of atopy and anaphylactic sensitization: a bee sting allergy model. Clin Allergy 8: 259–265
288. Sevel D (1977) Lenticular complications of long-term steroid therapy in children with asthma and eczema. J Allergy Clin Immunol 60: 215–217
289. Shanon J (1970) Cutaneous amyloidosis associated with atopic disorders. Dermatologica 141: 297–302
290. Shuster S, Marks J (1965) Dermatogenic enteropathy: A new cause of steatorrhoea. Lancet 1: 1367–1368
291. Skalka HW, Prehal JT (1980) Effect of corticosteroids on cataract formation. Arch Ophthalmol 98: 1773–1777
292. Snyderman SE (1965) An eczematoid dermatitis in histidine deficiency. J Pediatr 66: 212–215
293. Solomon LM, Telner P (1966) Eruptive molluscum contagiosum in atopic dermatitis. Can Med Assoc 95: 978–979
294. Spencer WH, Fisher JJ (1959) The association of keratoconus with atopic dermatitis. Am J Ophthal 47: 332–334
295. Stalder JF, Sourisse M (1989) La dermatite atopique et l'infection staphylococcique. Ann Dermatol Venereol 116: 341–345
296. Steiner K (1952) Glomerulonephritis associated with atopic dermatitis. N Engl J Med 247: 201–204
297. Stern RS, Parrish JA, Fitzpatrick TB (1985) Ocular findings in patients treated with PUVA. J Invest Dermatol 85: 269–273
298. Stevanovic DV (1960) Apparent light sensibility in atopic subjects. Acta Derm Venereol (Stockh) 40: 220–227
299. Strannegard IL, Strannegard O (1981) Epstein-Barr Virus antibodies in children with atopic disease. Int Arch Allergy Appl Immunol 64: 314–319
300. Strannegard O, Strannegard IL, Rysted I (1985) Viral infections in atopic dermatitis. Acta Derm Venereol Suppl 114: 121–124
301. Sullivan TJ (1988) Drug Allergy. In: Middleton E, Reed CE, Ellis EF (eds) Allergy: Principle and practice, 3rd edn. Mosby, St. Louis
302. Svejgaard E (1985) Immunologic investigations of dermatophytes and dermatophytosis. Sem Dermatol 4: 201–221
303. Svejgaard E, Albrechtsen B, Baastrup N (1983) The occurrence of tinea of the feet in 15-year old schoolchildren. Mykosen 26: 450–454
304. Svejgaard E, Christophersen J, Jelsdorf HM (1986) Tinea pedis and erythrasma in danish recruits. J Am Acad Dermatol 14: 993–999
305. Svejgaard E, Faergeman J, Jemec G, Kieffer M, Ottevanger V (1989) Recent investigations on the relationship between fungal skin diseases and atopic dermatitis. Acta Derm Venereol Suppl 144: 140–142
306. Svennsson A, Möller H (1986) Eyelid dermatitis: the role of atopy and contact allergy. Contact Dermatitis 15: 178–182
306a. Svensson A, Edman B, Möller H (1985) A diagnostic tool for atopic dermatitis based on clinical criteria. Acta Derm Venereol Suppl 144: 33–40
307. Swart RNJ, Vermeer BJ, van Der Meer JWM, Enschede FAJ, Versteeg J (1983) Treatment of eczema herpeticum with acyclovir. Arch Dermatol 119: 13–16
308. Tabbara KF, Arafat NT (1977) Cromolyn effects on vernal keratoconjunctivitis in children. Arch Ophthalmol 95: 2184
309. Tacier-Eugster H, Wüthrich B, Meyer H (1980) Atopic allergy serum IgE and RAST specific IgE antibodies with cystic fibrosis. Helv Ped Acta 35: 31–37
309a. Tagami H, Rokugo M, Usuba Y, Tomita Y (1990) Contact sensitivity to Pityrosporum ovale in patients with atopic dermatitis. Allergologie 13: 240
310. Taieb A, Dubiau JM, Guillet G, Duboz A, Maleville J (1984) Un cas de pustulose de Kaposi-Juliusberg (eczema herpeticum du nourisson), traité per acyclovir. Ann Dermatol Venereol 111: 173–175
311. Taieb A, Fontan I, Maleville J (1985) Acyclovir therapy for eczema herpeticum in infants. Arch Dermatol 121: 1380–1381
312. Tarnow-Mordi WO, Moss C, Ross K (1984) Failure to thrive owing to inappropriate diet free of gluten and cow's milk. Br Med J 289: 1113–1114
313. Thomson PD, Barrat TM, Stokes CR, Turner MW,

Soothill JF (1976) HLA antigens and atopic features in steroid responsive nephrotic syndrome of children. Lancet II: 765–768

314. Tobin MJ, Maguire O, Reen D, Tempany E, Fitzgerald MX (1980) Atopy and bronchial reactivity in older patients with cystic fibrosis. Thorax 35: 807–813

315. Tourian AY, Sidbury IB (1983) Phenylketonuria and hyperphenylalaninemia. In: Stanbury JB et al (eds) The metabolic basis of inherited Disease, 5th edn. McGraw-Hill, New York, p 270

316. Trompeter RS, Barrat TM, Kay R, Turner MW, Soothill JF (1980) HLA, atopy and cylcophosphamide in steroid responsive childhood nephrotic syndrome. Kidney Int 17: 113–117

317. Turner KJ, Baldo BA, Hilton JMN (1975) IgE antibodies to Dermatophagoides pteronyssinus (house dust mite), Aspergillus fumigatus and β-lactoglobulin in sudden infant death syndrome. Br Med J: 357–360

318. Uehara M, Amemiya T, Arai M (1985) Atopic cataracts in a Japanese population. Dermatologica 170: 180

319. Ukabam SO, Mann RJ, Cooper BT (1984) Small intestinal permeability to sugars in patients with atopic eczema. Br J Dermatol 110: 649–652

320. Vanselow NA, Yamate M, Adams MS, Callies Q, Arbor A (1970) The increased prevalence of atopic diseases in anhidrotic congenital ectodermal dysplasia. J Allergy 45: 302–309

321. Verbov J, Hart A (1986) Severe varicella in a child with atopic eczema and ichthyosis. Practitioner 230: 15–16

322 Verbov J, Munro DD, Miller A (1972) Recurrent eczema herpeticum associated with ichthyosis vulgaris. Br J Dermatol 86: 638–640

323. Verbov JL (1967) Atopic dermatitis and persistent lactation. Br J Dermatol 79: 726–727

324. Verkasalo M, Tillikainen A, Kuitunen P, Savilahti E, Backman A (1983) HLA antigens and atopy in children with coeliac disease. Gut 24: 306–310

325. Vetter G (1957) Eine weitere Beobachtung von doppelseitiger Amotio bei Cataracta syndermatotica bilateralis. Klin Mbl Augenheilk 130: 264–265

326. Vickers CFH (1964) Eczema and phenylketonuria. Trans St John's Hospital 50: 56–57

327. Vieluf D, Korting HC, Braun-Falco O, Walther JU (1990) Dubowitz syndrome: atopic dermatitis, low birth weight dwarfism and facial dysmorphism. Dermatologica 180: 247–249

327a. Vieluf D, Korting HC, Braun-Falco O, Belohradsky BH (1989) Eczematous skin lesions in X-linked immunodeficiency with hyper-IgM. In: Fritsch P, Schuler G, Hintner H (eds) Immunodeficiency and skin. Curr Probl Dermatol, Basel, Karger, Vol 18, pp 60–65

328. Waddington E, Bray PT, Evans AD, Richards IDG (1964) Cutaneous complications of mass vaccination against small pox in South Wales 1962. Trans St John's Hosp Dermatol Soc 50: 22

329. Waersted A, Hjorth N (1985) Pityrosporon orbiculare – a pathogenic factor in atopic dermatitis of the face, scalp and neck? Acta Derm Venereol Suppl 114: 146–148

330. Waldmann TA, Bull JM, Bruce RM, Broder S, Jost MC, Balestra ST, Suer ME (1974) Serum IgE levels in patients with neoplastic disease. J Immunol 113: 379–386

331. Waldmann TA, Wochner RD, Laster L, Gordon RS (1967) Allergic gastroenteropathy – a cause of excessive gastrointestinal protein loss. New Engl J Med 276: 761–769

332. Walsh WE (1979) Atopic dermatitis associated with citric and malic acid intolerance. Minn Med 62: 637–639

333. Warnasuriya N, Downham MAPS, Skelton A, Turner MW, Soothill JF (1980) Atopy in patients of children dying with sudden infant death syndrome. Arch Dis Child 55: 876–878

334. Warner JO, Taylor BW, Norman AP, Soothill JF (1976) Association of cystic fibrosis with allergy. Arch Dis Child 51: 507–511

335. Warren R, Olsen D, Church JA (1973) Improvmeent of idiopathic nephrotic syndrome following allergy therapy. Ann Allergy 39: 332–333

336. Warren CPW, Tai E, Batten JC, Hutchcroft BJ, Pepys J (1975) Cystic fibrosis – immunological reactions to A. fumigatus and common allergens. Clin Allergy 5: 1–12

337. Welp K, Gieler U, Ständer M, Friederich HC (1989) Koinzidenz von Psoriasis vulgaris und atopischer Dermatitis. Hautarzt 40: 496–500

338. Wheeler CE, Abele DC (1966) Eczema herpeticum, primary and recurrent. Arch Dermatol 93: 162–171

339. White MI, Noble WC (1986) Consequences of colonization and infection by staphylococcus aureus in atopic dermatitis. Clin Exp Dermatol 11: 34–40

340. Williams ML, Packman S, Cowan MJ (1983) Alopecia and periorificial dermatitis in biotin-responsive multiple carboxylase deficiency. J Am Acad Dermatol 9: 97–103

341. Williamson DAJ (1970) Nephrotic syndrome associated with inhaled antigens. Lancet I: 778

342. Winkelmann RK, Rajka G (1983) Atopic dermatitis and Hodgkin's disease. Acta Derm Venereol 63: 176–177

343. Wittig HJ, Goldman AS (1970) Nephrotic syndrome associated with inhaled allergens. Lancet I: 542–543

344. Wolff HH (1977) Eczema herpeticatum, Eczema vaccinatum, Eczema verrucatum, Eczema molluscatum. Hautarzt 28: 98–99

345. Woolfson H (1984) Oral acyclovir in eczema herpeticum. Br Med J 288: 531–532

346. Wooty-Wong RC, Wong JM, Anderson TF, Lerman S (1985) Lenticular psoralen photoproducts and cataracts of a PUVA-treated psoriatic patient. Arch Dermatol 121: 1307–1308

347. Wüthrich B (1987) Atopische Dermatitis. Tägl Prax 28: 85–98

348. Young E, Koers WJ (1989) Intracutaneous tests with pityrosporon extract in atopic dermatitis. Acta Derm Venereol Suppl 144: 122–124

349. Zachary CB, Baker RW, Lessoff MH, MacDonalds DM (1982) Increased intestinal peremeability in atopic eczema – polyethylenglycol used as a probe molecule. Br J Dermatol Suppl 22: 14–15

350. Zarafonetis CJD (1961) Reticulum cell sarcoma complicating atopic dermatitis. Cancer 14: 5–12

351. Zaslow L, Derbes VI (1970) Serum histidine levels in atopic dermatitis patients. South Med J 63: 1000

352. Zugerman C (1976) Glaucoma from topically applied steroids. Arch Derm 112: 1326

Natural History of Atopic Eczema

C. F. H. Vickers

Infantile atopic eczema is still a very real problem for the dermatologist and primary care physician alike, despite the addition of more useful topical steroids and systemic antihistamines to the older regimes of tars, cooling lotions and bandages, all of which remain part of our armamentarium. That the natural history of atopic eczema in children was favourable was first stated by Sulzberger [1], but the published literature is at variance with this. The paediatrician Sedlis [2] commented on the unsatisfactory information on this subject, noting that it all came from retrospective studies. The earliest papers on this subject were from Germany. Boddin [3] found a persistence rate of 57% at 15–20 years, but the total series involved only 33 patients.

A more confusing study was that of Edgren [4] who followed a group of sufferers and stated that of those reaching 25 years of age 30% still had some form of allergic disease, though it is not clear what is meant by allergic disease. In the UK, Purdy [5] attempted a retrospective survey of 329 patients but obtained only a 30% reply rate. He found that 20% still had troublesome eczema at 15–20 years of age and another 30%, some problems. Vowles, Appley and Warin [6], Meenan [7] and Burrows and Penman [8] all added fuel to the fire, suggesting a poor prognosis, but all reported on series of children admitted to hospital and thus inevitably those which were either the worst patients or perhaps the most deprived. Again in Germany, Berlinghof [9] in a postal survey with a very low return stated that 56% of patients still had allergic disease but not how many had persistent eczema. In the USA, Roth and Kierland [10] and Stifler [11] in small series found poor clearance rates at 20 years, averaging 20%–30%. The method of referal of patients to the institutions reporting inevitably leads to these being the most severe or intractable patients. Rajka [12] states that one of the major difficulties is the definition of atopic eczema, which is by no means clear cut. He also found in his series that the prognosis was not very favourable, but he made the telling comment that only 2% of his patients were over 45 years of age. Again by the nature of Rajka's interest he may have seen only severe or problem patients. Musgrave and Morgan [13] conducted a 15–17 year follow-up on 99 patients who had suffered from infantile eczema. The persistence of the eczema and the occurrence of related conditions were noted. The persistence of eczema was shown to be greater in those patients with a positive family history of eczema and in those who had developed asthma or hay fever. An attempt was made to see whether or not the persistence of eczema was affected by the position of the child in the family, and some factors provoking relapses were noted. The evidence, therefore, seemed to be against Sulzberger. There were, however, others who did not believe the published evidence, and in 1958 the late Dr. I. B. Sneddon suggested that a retrospective survey of children with atopic eczema in Sheffield (UK) be made. There were three reasons for this: first, a diagnostic index for outpatients exists from 1946; second, the population is fairly static; third, under the National Health Service, it is easier to trace those patients who leave the area via the local Executive Committee. Accordingly a survey was undertaken.

Methods I

The diagnostic index yielded the names of 218 children suffering from infantile eczema who first attended the Department between 1947 and 1952, were under 2 years of age when first seen and had developed the disease within 1 year of first attendance. The two dermatologists making the original diagnoses believed like Ingram that only one form of infantile eczema exists, though they recognise a seborrhoeic pattern of infantile eczema. The parents were then contacted by letter. When the letters were returned "gone away", patients were traced with the help of the local practitioners and the NHS executive committees; some were traced as far as the antipodes. Those who were too far away for personal interview were either interviewed by their general practitioners with a questionnaire or sent a questionnaire to answer. Those patients seen personally were interviewed at length (the older children both with and without their patients) on all points thought likely to influence the prognosis, regularity of therapy, use of bandages, antihistamines, etc., normality of life allowed and school achievement.

Severity of Eczema

Whilst it was easy to assess the severity of the eczema present at follow-up (account being taken of the parent or child's comment, "this is a good day", "this is a bad day", "this is average"), to assess the severity of the eczema in retrospect was more difficult, but the following criteria were applied after interviewing the parents and studying the clinical notes mainly made by two senior clinicians (Dr. H. R. Vickers and Dr. I. B. Sneddon):

Mild. Those children who developed lesions on the face and scalp only, with only transient lesions on the trunk and limbs, and never requiring very active treatment.

Moderate. Those children with more extensive eczema, often with many exuding areas (this was before topical steroids).

Severe. Those children with more extensive eczema. All children admitted to hospital were not necessarily placed in the severe group as several were admitted for other reasons (poor home conditions, parenteral illness, eczema herpeticum and eczema vaccinatum).

Criteria at follow-up:

Mild. Those children with minimal lesions; fissures below the ears in cold or very occasional (less than once a month) patches of eczema on face or flexures, requiring no treatment.

Moderate. Those children with few lesions on face or flexures which required treatment on a regular basis.

Severe. Those children with extensive active eczema requiring regular treatment, often under hospital care.

Results I

Of the 218 children in the series, 209 (91%) were traced. Of these 175 (74.4%) were seen personally, the remainder either being seen by their general practitioners or answering questionnaires.

Length of follow-up ranged from 7.5 to 12.75 years (mean 10.7); the average age at review was 9.7 years. There were 114 boys (55%) and 94 girls (45%): 18 were considered to have the seborrhoeic pattern of eczema, 4 were found to have coincident psoriasis, 3 tinea pedis and 1 recurrent herpes simplex. Seven (4%) were or had been enuritic, and eight (4%) exhibited behaviour problems (three of these children were clear). The incidence of enuresis was half that in a control series of 200 children with warts, while that of behaviour disorders was twice that of controls.

Prognosis

Criteria applied for complete clearance were strict. Of the 26 children in the mild group the parents were unaware of the presence of eczema. In 16 the only sign was the atopic ear crack.

Of the 18 children with the seborrhoeic pattern of eczema, 10 were clear, 2 had mild eczema, 4 moderate and 2 severe. At follow-up, therefore, only a little over half of this admittedly small group as clear, and there seemed to be evidence that this is one pattern of atopic eczema.

It is interesting to note the different prognosis in those parents replying to the first letter (131). Some 77 (58.7%) were clear whilst of the remaining 77 whom it took several attempts to contact, 73 (92.4%) were clear. Thus, the overall clearance rate was found at an average age of 9.7 years. The improved clearance rate found after the first attempt to contact patients may have been because those who replied to the first had the hope that children with persistent eczema might be offered new advances in therapy. Certainly, it seems to suggest that previous retrospective surveys which gave clearance rates very near to those derived from the first follow-up letter might have yielded different results if a more persistent follow-up had been attempted.

Factors Influencing the Prognosis

There was a suggestion that an onset of eczema later than 2 years of age had a worse outlook than onset under 6 months, but the numbers were small. Infant feeding appeared to have no influence, coexisting asthma occurred twice as frequently in the non-clearers as the clearers. The most striking fact involved the children who had been admitted. Excluding those admitted with secondary viral infections, there were 18 children admitted because of the severity of their eczema. Of these only 4 were completely clear (22.2%), a figure comparing well with other inpatient retrospective studies.

As a result of many discussions and much encouragement from Dr. Ian Sneddon and Dr. Marion Sulzberger, I decided that the only way to settle this whole issue was to set up a prospective survey of alle new patients attending my outpatient clinics with infantile atopic eczema. This was started in 1958, but there was a gap in collecting, and the series that will be reported here started in 1964 in Liverpool and Southport and continued until 1981, when 200 patients had been documented. It is hoped to complete documentation on 1000 of these at 20 years but with the more mobile English population today it is proving difficult to keep track of the patients collected since 1975.

Methods II

The patients were consecutive new patients attending my outpatient clinics with infantile atopic eczema. All had suffered from the disease for less than 6 months. The diagnostic techniques of Rajka [14] were applied (retrospectively to some of the earlier patients), but this only resulted in the loss of 11 patients from the early part of the series.

The patients were mostly seen at regular intervals until clearance and then major reviews were made in 1975, 1978 and 1982. The final review is underway now, and the results reported here are those of 1982.

A total of 2000 children entered the study between 1964 and 1980, at the last major review. The follow-up rate at 20 years was 91%, and it is expected that many more will still be traced at the final follow up in 1990–1991. The follow-up rate at 5 years was almost 100%.

Results II

The most important part of this study has been to establish the actual clearance rate, which has been shown to be 88.6% completely clear for more than 3 years at 20 years; this takes into account a pubertal recurrence rate of 4.5% after preliminary clearance at an earlier age.

Many factors which might influence the prognosis were considered. Age of onset was found to be highly significant; onset at less than 6 months of age corresponded to a clearance rate of 94.5% at 20 years and that after 2 years of age to a clearance rate of only 50%. Numbers in the late onset group were relatively small (48) compared with onset before 6 months of age (1253).

The other highly significant finding was the influence of the reversed (inverted pattern) with knees and elbows involved, rather than, or in addition to, antecubital and popliteal fossae. In these patients the clearance rate at 20 years was only 64%. Again, numbers (64) were small, but the results obviously significant. A separate study of 100 adult (persistent) atopic sufferers showed that 90% had either late onset, reversed pattern or both thus confirming the follow-up results.

Another adverse factor is the presence of hand eczema in the young child, though this does not have a very significant effect on prognosis on its own; it is often associated with late onset or reversed pattern.

Factors not influencing the prognosis include severity at onset, a family history of severe or persistent disease, the type of infant feeding, the presence of discoid lesions or the presence of proven food allergies. The presence of associated asthma and/or allergies to animals have not yet been assessed, but data should be forthcoming at the next review.

Discussion

It is clear from these results that the suggestions of Sneddon and Sulzberger that a prospective survey would be able to throw a better light on the factual prognosis of infantile atopic eczema were correct. Clearance rates are high, and indeed if they were not, our adult clinics would be full of little else than adult atopics, in view of the disease's frequency among young children, estimated as high as 5% in some Western countries and Japan. The fallacies of retrospective surveys with low follow-up rates were exposed in the Sheffield study as were those of studies investigating only inpatients.

There are several important points to be made. Perhaps most important of all, there is no definitive age at which clearance can be expected but merely an increasing incidence of clearance, even into the early teenage period, though after that there is less chance of real clearance. Next, some idea of the well-known pubertal recurrence rate has been determined; this is something that the next full assessment may clarify even further. The importance of recognising the bad prognostic effects of late onset and reversed (inverse) patterns need to be stressed to the physician though not, I believe, to the patient, with whom a confident attitude should always be taken. The adverse influence on prognosis of a strong family history was perhaps expected, but the lack of correlation of severity in different generations needs to be stressed, especially to the persistent adult atopic patient seeking genetic advice.

The major difficulty in assessing the significance of these results hinges around the argument whether active and effective treatment of children with atopic eczema by active and interested dermatologisits may of itself influence the prognosis. All the cohort reported were seen within 6 months of diagnosis and have been under active care until clearance. It is my opinion that active and aggressive treatment of these children probably does modify the prognosis, in that by suppressing itch and thus scratch, the skin may go into remission earlier. There is no way unfortunately to prove this fact, though there is much suggestive evidence.

The anecdotal evidence from general practitioners is that an even higher proportion of children with very mild eczema clear without needing hospital referral. In a personal communication McArthur (1980) said that of 100 new patients seen in one general practice with infantile eczema, only 10 were referred to hospital, the others clearing in a few months. Whether all these children would have satisfied the criteria of Rajka could not be established partly because of their very early clearance.

References

1. Sulzberger MB (1940) Dermatogie allergy. Thomas, Springfield
2. Sedlis E (1965) Conference on infantile eczema. Pediatr 66: 158
3. Boddin M (1930) Beitrag zur Klinik des neurogenen Ekzems im Kindesalter. Med Klin 26: 270–272
4. Edgren G (1943) Prognose und Erblichkeitsmomente bei Ekzema Infantum. Acta Paediatr [Suppl II] 30:
5. Purdy MJ(1953) The long term prognosis in infantile eczema. Br Med J i: 1366–1368
6. Vowles M, Warin RP, Appley J (1955) Infantile eczema: observations on natural history and prognosis. Br J Dermatol 67: 53–57
7. Meenan FOC (1959) Prognosis in infantile eczema. Ir J Med Sci 398: 79–81
8. Burrows D, Penman RWB (1960) Prognosis of the eczema-asthma syndrome. Br Med J ii: 825–827
9. Berlinghoff W (1961) Die Prognose des Säuglingsekzems. Dtsch Gesundheitsw 16: 110–112
10. Roth HL, Kierland RR (1964) The natural history of atopic dermatitis. Arch Dermatol 89: 209–211
11. Stifler WC (1965) Conference on infantile eczema – a 21 year follow-up of infantile eczema. J Pediatr 66: 166–169
12. Rajka G (1961) Prurigo Besnier (atopic dermatitis) with special reference to the role of allergic factors. Acta Derm Venereol 41: 363–368
13. Musgrave K, Morgan JK (1976) Infantile eczema – a long-term follow-up study. Br J Dermatol 95: 365–369
14. Rajka G (1975) Diagnosis of atopic children in atopic dermatitis. Saunders, Philadelphia

Dry Skin and Inflammation

M. Uehara

Introduction

Many patients with atopic eczema have dry skin, even on areas apparently unaffected by the dermatitis [15, 22]. The dry skin shows various physiological abnormalities [10, 12, 29], suggesting that it is different in nature from the skin of normal people. Thus, there has been a common belief among dermatologists that the uninvolved skin of atopic eczema patients is generally dry. The term atopic skin, which originally meant the "uninvolved" skin of these patients, is often used as a synonym of dry skin [4, 19].

Recently, however, considerable doubt has been cast on this widespread assumption that the skin of patients with atopic eczema shows general dryness and abnormal physiology. Evidence has accumulated that the dry skin often seen in these patients is a mild eczematous lesion of the disease or a manifestation of concomitant ichthyosis vulgaris [9, 44].

This chapter will discuss arguments for and against the concept that the skin of atopic eczema patients reveals physical and physiological abnormalities.

The General Dry Skin Theory

The arguments in favour of the general dryness and abnormal physiology of atopic skin may be summarised as follows:

1. Many patients with atopic eczema have general dry skin which exhibits keratosis pilaris-like follicular papules [19, 22]. The palms of these patients are also dry and contain an increased number of fine lines and markings (hyperlinear palms, or atopic palms) [5, 22].
2. Skin surface lipids are decreased in the dry skin of patients with atopic eczema [23]. The skin lipids in the dry skin are deficient in constituents derived from the sebaceous glands [1, 27].
3. Sebaceous glands in the dry skin are reduced in number and size as compared with those found in the skin of normal subjects [39, 55].
4. Transepidermal water loss, which is considered to be a parameter reflecting the functional state of the epidermal diffusion barrier, is increased in the dry skin of atopic eczema [28, 52]. The water binding capacity of the stratum corneum, which also is said to be closely related to its functional integrity, is reduced in the dry skin [53]. These findings may suggest a defect in the epidermal barrier function of the dry skin of this condition.
5. The skin of atopic eczema patients is more readily damaged by soaps and other irritants than the skin of normal persons [2, 6, 32]. The atopic skin also shows a high incidence of pustular patch test reactions to heavy metals [38], which probably represent some form of irritation.
6. The cutaneous vessels of patients with atopic eczema tend to react abnormally to mechanical and pharmacologic stimuli. In normal people, firm stroking of the skin results in a red line, while in atopic skin the line is first red and then white (white dermographism) [22, 25]. Epicutaneous absorption of nicotinic acid esters normally produces erythema but yields an anaemic reaction in atopic skin [17, 35]. Intracutaneous injection of methacholine chloride is normally followed by reddening, while atopic skin exhibits blanching around the wheal (delayed blanch) [21, 30]. When histamine phosphate is injected into the skin of atopic eczema patients, it causes a diminished erythema compared with control subjects [7, 31].
7. The skin of patients with atopic eczema is in a state of "itchy skin" [5]. Skin tests with pruritogenic stimuli show that atopic skin itches more readily and for a longer time than does normal skin [3, 14, 26].

Comment

In view of these abnormal findings, it seems rather natural to assume that the "uninvolved" skin of patients with atopic eczema is abnormal. Indeed, many authors from various countries of the world [12, 13, 18, 37, 40] have regarded the dryness of skin as an excellent diagnostic sign of atopic eczema.

Heterogeneity of Dry Skin

On the other hand, it is well-known that dry skin in patients with atopic eczema fluctuates with the disease severity; during remissions it may not be detectable [11, 34]. It is also known that there are some patients with atopic eczema who have perfectly normal, smooth skin except where lichenified lesions are present [16, 47]. These clinical facts throw strong doubt on the popular concept that patients with atopic eczema inherently have general dry skin.

Several investigators [9, 45] have demonstrated that the dry skin of atopic eczema histologically shows a mild eczematous change. Others [39, 55] found atrophy of sebaceous glands in the dry skin. These data would suggest that the dry skin is in a pathologic state and not an "uninvolved" skin.

Furthermore, it is worthwhile noting that ichthyosis vulgaris is an important complication of atopic eczema [29]. Ichthyosis vulgaris is characterised by generalised dry skin, hyperlinear palms [49] and atrophy of sebaceous glands [8, 50]. It is then likely that the primary characteristics of the dry skin in atopic eczema are often modified by the concomitant ichthyosis vulgaris.

In order to see clinical, histological and immunohistological features of dry skin in patients with atopic eczema who do not have ichthyosis vulgaris, recent studies [42, 44] examined a large number of patients with the disease. The examinations were performed during the winter when dry skin becomes most prominent. The results of these studies are summarised as follows:

Clinical Features of Dry Skin

Prevalence of Ichthyosis Vulgaris in Patients with Atopic Eczema

Skin signs of ichthyosis vulgaris (i.e. small polygonal scales symmetrically distributed on the extensor limbs and hyperlinearity of the palms) were present in approximately 30% of patients with atopic eczema who were observed during the winter. It should be noted that the 30% prevalence of ichthyosis vulgaris in these patients may be higher than the prevalence of ichthyosis vulgaris in patients with atopic eczema in general. It has been reported previously that ichthyosis vulgaris occurs in 2%–10% of patients with atopic eczema in general [29].

Clinical Features of "Uninvolved" Skin of Patients with Atopic Eczema Alone

In patients with atopic eczema who did not have ichthyosis vulgaris, the uninvolved skin was not homogeneous. Generalised dry skin (covering 70% or more of the body surface) occurred in approximately 5%, partial dry skin (i.e. coexistence of dry skin and normal-

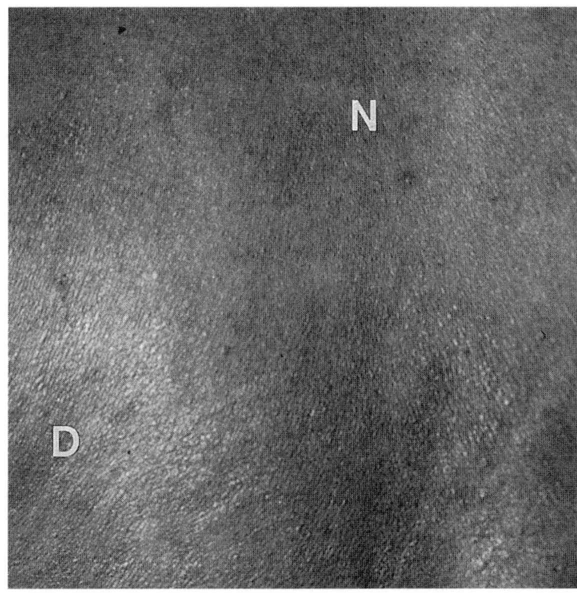

Fig. 1. Lower part of back of an 18-year-old patient with atopic eczema alone, showing coexistence of dry skin (*D*) and normal-appearing skin (*N*)

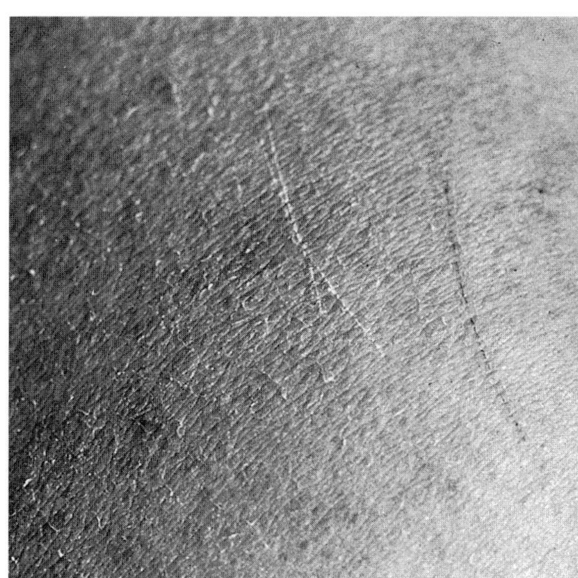

▶ **Fig. 2.** Lower part of back of a 22-year-old patient with atopic eczema and ichthyosis vulgaris. Dryness of skin is more intense than that seen in pure atopic eczema (see Fig. 1)

appearing skin) in 65%, and normal-appearing skin alone in 30%.

This clinical picture was very different from that seen in patients suffering also from ichthyosis vulgaris. In the dry skin of patients with atopic eczema alone, the degree of dryness usually was mild (Fig. 1), while in the dry skin of patients with atopic eczema and ichthyosis vulgaris, severe dryness was common (Fig. 2).

Comment

These clinical data show that generalised dry skin is observed in only a small number of patients with atopic eczema who do not have ichthyosis vulgaris. The majority of patients with solely atopic eczema have partial dry skin or normal-appearing skin alone.

The frequent occurrence of general dry skin in patients with atopic eczema in previous reports [15, 22, 29] might be due to a material including both patients with and without ichthyosis vulgaris.

Histological Features of Dry Skin

Dry Skin in Patients with Atopic Eczema Alone

Mild eczematous changes were regularly observed in the dry skin of patients with atopic eczema who did not have ichthyosis vulgaris (Fig. 3). The epidermis showed patchy parakeratosis, slight acanthosis and focal spongiosis with exocytosis of mononuclear cells. Hair follicles in the dry skin often had an eczematous change, which resembled the "follicular lesion" [24, 54, 56] of the disease. The dermis showed mononuclear cell infiltrates around the superficial blood vessels. Sebaceous glands consistently exhibited normal development.

Dry Skin in Patients with Atopic Eczema and Ichthyosis Vulgaris

The histological pictures of dry skin in patients with atopic eczema who simultaneously had ichthyosis vulgaris were essentially those of ichthyosis vulgaris (Fig. 4).

Fig. 3. Biopsy specimen from dry skin on lateral buttock of a 16-year-old patient with atopic eczema alone, showing parakeratosis, spongiosis, slight infiltrate of mononuclear cells and normally developed sebaceous glands

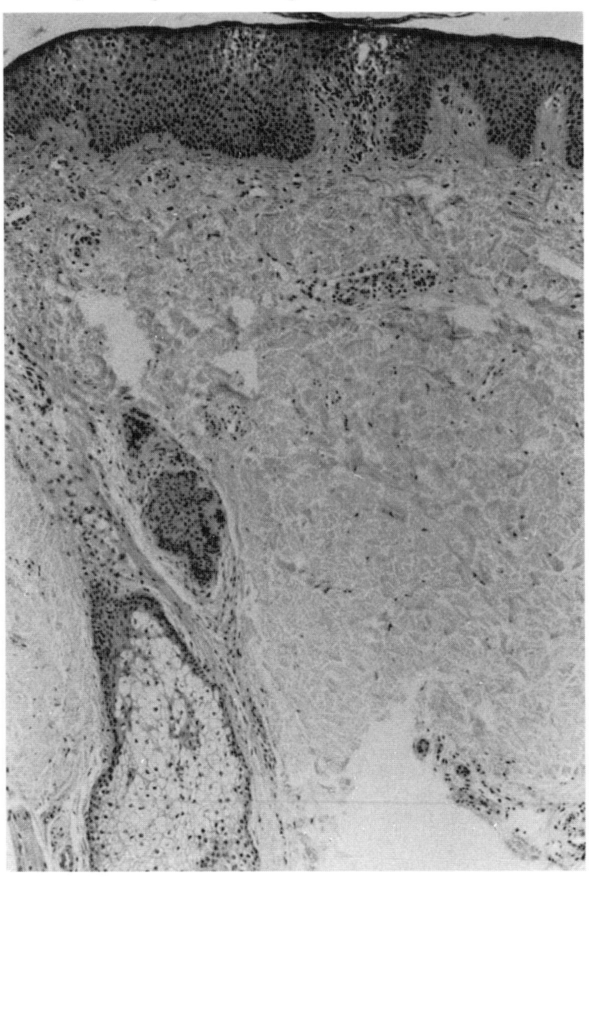

Fig. 4. Biopsy specimen from dry skin on lateral buttock of a 18-year-old patient with atopic eczema and ichthyosis vulgaris. Note hyperkeratosis, reduced thickness of the granular layer and atrophic sebaceous glands

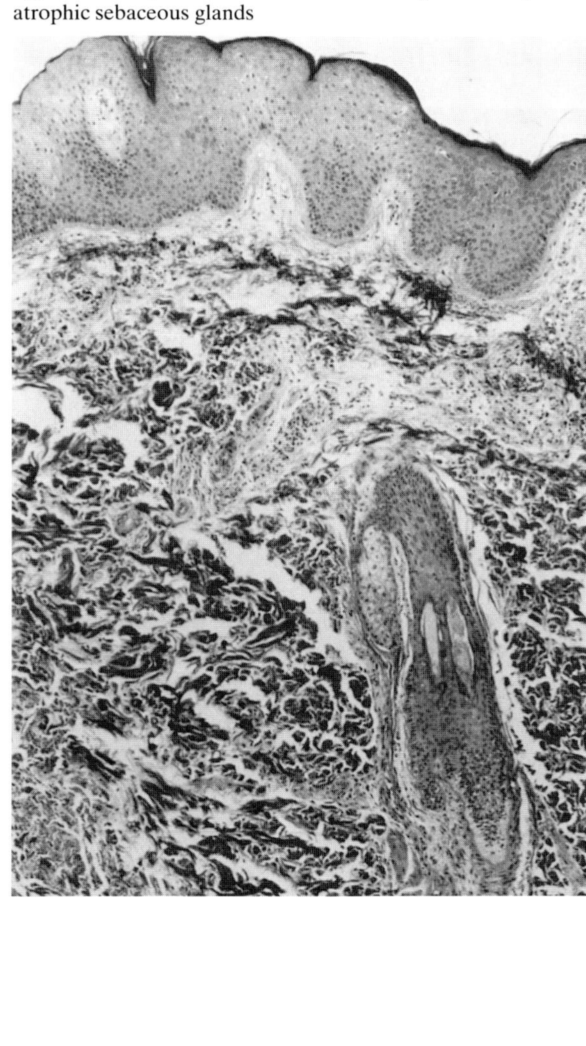

There was a moderate degree of hyperkeratosis with a thin or absent granular layer. Sebaceous glands were remarkably atrophic. The ichthyotic changes were frequently superimposed on the mild eczematous changes described above.

Normal-Appearing Skin in Patients with Atopic Eczema Alone

There were no pathological findings except for a mild perivascular infiltrate of mononuclear cells which were occasionally seen in the upper dermis (Fig. 5). Sebaceous glands were normally developed.

Comment

The results of these studies make it clear that the dry skin often seen in patients with atopic eczema is heterogeneous in nature. It may be a mild eczematous lesion, a manifestation of concomitant ichthyosis vulgaris or a mixture of both.

Previous reports [39, 55] found atrophy of sebaceous glands in dry or uninvolved skin of patients with atopic eczema. It is not clear, however, whether the patients in these previous reports suffered from atopic eczema alone or whether they had both atopic eczema and ichthyosis vulgaris. The decrease of sebaceous lipids [1, 23, 27] often seen in the dry skin of atopic eczema might also be due to the frequent concomitance of ichthyosis vulgaris.

The increased transepidermal water loss [28, 52] and the decreased water-binding capacity [53] of the stratum corneum in atopic skin may be due to the eczematous changes of dry skin or the concomitant ichthyosis

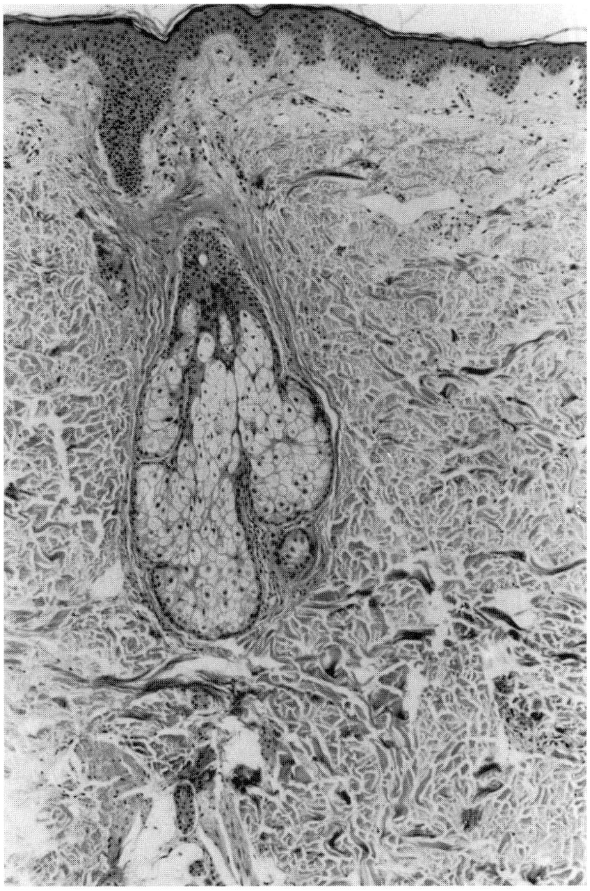

Fig. 5. Biopsy specimen from normal-appearing skin on lateral buttock of a 16-year-old patient with atopic eczema alone. No pathological changes except for slight infiltrate of mononuclear cells. Sebaceous glands are normally developed

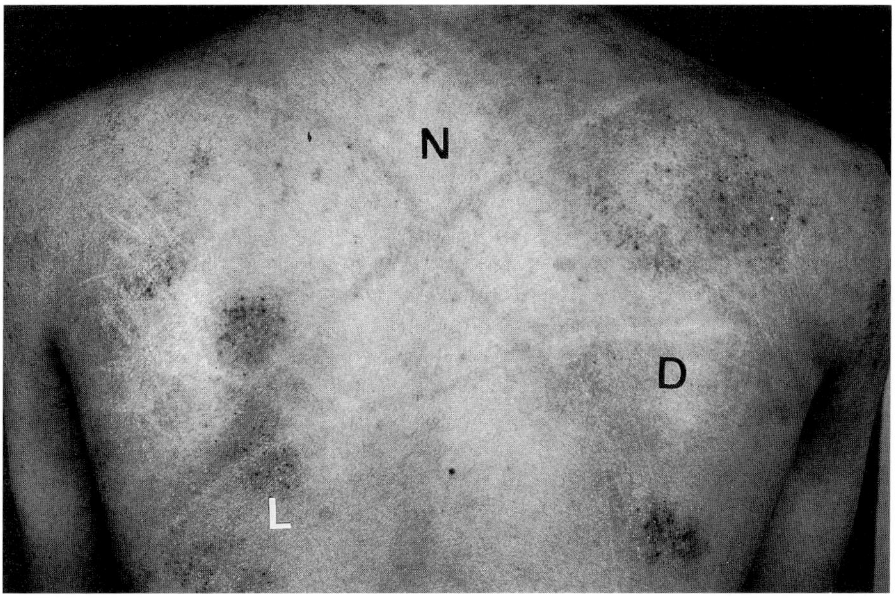

Fig. 6. Vascular reactions to mechanical stroking on back of a 17-year-old patient with atopic eczema, showing white dermographism in lichenified lesion (*L*) and dry skin (*D*), but normal red response in normal-appearing skin (*N*)

vulgaris. A recent study has demonstrated that the water content of the stratum corneum is decreased in dry skin of patients with atopic eczema, while normal-appearing skin of these patients has a normal water content [51].

Pustular patch test reactions to heavy metals were thought to be one of the common hallmarks of atopic skin [5, 22]. But it is now known that the pustular patch test reactions do not occur in normal-appearing skin of patients with atopic eczema, whereas the pustular reactions are consistently produced in the dry skin with follicular eczema of these patients [48].

Recent reports [41, 45, 46] have demonstrated that abnormal responses of cutaneous vessels to mechanical and pharmacological stimuli (white dermographism, pale reaction to nicotinic acid esters, delayed blanch with methacholine chloride and reduced reaction to histamine) commonly occur in areas of dry skin and slightly lichenified patches of patients with atopic eczema, while normal vascular responses are observed in the normal-appearing skin of these patients (Fig 6). Thus, it is likely that the abnormal vascular reactions often seen in patients with atopic eczema may all be phenomena occurring secondarily to the eczematous inflammatory process.

The state of "itchy skin" frequently seen in patients with atopic eczema [3, 14, 26] may also be at least partly due to the mild eczematous change of dry skin. It is known that around a point of itching (e. g. eczematous change of the dry skin), a widespread area develops which does not itch spontaneously but responds by itching to light friction and other nonadequate stimuli ("itchy skin") [33].

In summary, although a large variety of physical and physiological abnormalities were reported to occur in the "uninvolved" skin of patients with atopic eczema, it is now clear that most of these abnormalities are (a) manifestations of concomitant ichthyosis vulgaris or (b) secondary phenomena due to the mild eczematous "dry skin" of atopic eczema.

Immunohistological Features of the Dry Skin

Using monoclonal antibodies, recent studies [42, 43] examined the phenotypic characteristics of the mononuclear cell infiltrate in the dry skin of patients with atopic eczema who did not have ichthyosis vulgaris. The majority of infiltrating lymphocytes in dry skin were stained with monoclonal antibodies Leu-1 and Leu-3a, indicating that they were T helper/inducer cells. Only a small proportion of infiltrating lymphocytes reacted with Leu-2a antibody, which defines T suppressor/cytotoxic cells. Langerhans cells, as defined by reactivity with OKT-6 antibody, were increased in the slightly acanthotic epidermis and in the dermal infiltrate.

Comment

The distribution of infiltrating T-cell subsets and Langerhans cells in the dry skin of atopic eczema is compatible with the observations in lichenified lesions of the disease [20, 36]. Thus, the immunohistological findings provide further evidence that dry skin in patients with solely atopic eczema is a mild eczematous lesion of this disorder.

References

1. Abe T, Ohkido M, Yamamoto K (1978) Studies on skin surface barrier function – skin surface lipids and transepidermal water loss in atopic skin during childhood. J Dermatol 5: 223–229
2. Allison JH, Bettley FR (1958) Investigations into cantharidin blisters raised on apparently normal skin in normal and abnormal subjects. Br J Dermatol 70: 331–339
3. Arthur RP, Shelley WB (1958) The nature of itching in dermatitic skin. Ann Intern Med 49: 900–908
4. Blaylock WK (1976) Atopic dermatitis: diagnosis and pathology. J Allergy Clin Immunol 57: 62–79
5. Chenowith BR, Lobitz WC, Dobson RL (1974) Atopic dermatitis. In: Demis DJ, Crounse RG, Dobson RL, McGuire J (eds) Clinical dermatology. Harper and Row, New York, unit 13-2, pp 1–29
6. Cronin E (1980) Contact dermatitis. Churchill Livingstone, Edinburgh, pp 22–23
7. Eyster WH, Roth GM, Kierland RR (1952) Studies on the peripheral vascular physiology of patients with atopic dermatitis. J Invest Dermatol 18: 37–46
8. Feinstein A, Ackerman AB, Ziprkowski L (1970) Histology of autosomal dominant ichthyosis vulgaris and X-linked ichthyosis. Arch Dermatol 101: 524–527
9. Finlay AY, Nichols S, King CS, Marks R (1980) The 'dry' non-eczematous skin associated with atopic eczema. Br J Dermatol 102: 249–256
10. Hanifin JM (1983) Clinical and basic aspects of atopic dermatitis. Semin Dermatol 2: 5–19
11. Hanifin JM, Dahl MV (1983) Some aspects of atopic dermatitis. Arch Dermatol 119: 237–242
12. Hanifin JM, Lobitz WC (1977) Newer concepts of atopic dermatitis. Arch Dermatol 13: 663–670
13. Hanifin JM, Rajka G (1980) Diagnostic features of atopic dermatitis. Acta Derm Venereol [Suppl] (Stockh) 92: 44–47
14. Harnack K (1980) Experimental itch as a diagnostic method. Acta Derm Venereol [Suppl] (Stockh) 92: 40–41
15. Hill LW, Sulzberger MB (1935) Evolution of atopic dermatitis. Arch Dermatol 32: 451–463
16. Hill LW, Wheatley VR (1965) Secretions of the skin in eczema. J Pediatr 66: 200–202

17. Illig L (1952) Die Reaktion der Haut des Neurodermitikers auf zwei nikotinsäureesterhaltige Reizstoffe. Dermatol Wochenschr 126: 753–763
18. Kang K, Tian R (1987) Atopic dermatitis: an evaluation of clinical and laboratory findings. Int J Dermatol 26: 27–32
19. Kierland RR (1955) Certain stigmata associated with atopic dermatitis. In: Baer RL (ed) Atopic dermatitis. Lippincott, Philadelphia, pp 43–55
20. Leung DYM, Bhan AK, Schneeberger EE, Geha RS (1983) Characterization of the mononuclear cell infiltrate in atopic dermatitis using monoclonal antibodies. J Allergy Clin Immunol 71: 47–56
21. Lobitz WC, Campbell CJ (1953) Physiological studies in atopic dermatitis (disseminated neurodermatitis): 1. The local cutaneous response to intradermally injected acetylcholine and epinephrine. Arch Dermatol 67: 575–589
22. Lobitz WC, Dobson RL (1956) Physical and physiological clues for diagnosing eczema. JAMA 161: 1226–1229
23. Mustakallio KK, Kiistala U, Piha HJ, Nieminen E (1967) Epidermal lipids in Besnier's prurigo (atopic eczema). Ann Med Exp Fenn 45: 323–325
24. Ofuji S, Uehara M (1973) Follicular eruptions of atopic dermatitis. Arch Dermatol 107: 54–55
25. Rajka G (1960) Prurigo Besnier (atopic dermatitis) with special reference to the role of allergic factors: 1. The influence of atopic hereditary factors. Acta Derm Venereol (Stockh) 40: 285–306
26. Rajka G (1968) Itch duration in the uninvolved skin of atopic dermatitis (prurigo Besnier). Acta Derm Venereol (Stockh) 48: 320–321
27. Rajka G (1974a) Surface lipid estimation on the back of the hands in atopic dermatitis. Arch Dermatol Forsch 251: 43–48
28. Rajka G (1974b) Transepidermal water loss on the hands in atopic dermatitis. Arch Dermatol Forsch 251: 111–115
29. Rajka G (1975) Atopic dermatitis. Saunders, Philadelphia, pp 4–35
30. Ramsay C (1969) Vascular changes accompanying white dermographism and delayed blanch in atopic dermatitis. Br J Dermatol 81: 37–43
31. Reed WB, Kierland RR, Code CF (1958) Vascular reactions in chronically inflamed skin: III. Action of histamine, the histamine releaser 48–80, and monoethanolamine nicotinate (Nicamin). Arch Dermatol 77: 263–268
32. Rostenberg A, Sulzberger MB (1937) Some results of patch tests; a comparison and discussion of cutaneous reactions to about five hundred different substances, as elicited by over ten thousand tests in approximately one thousand patients. Arch Dermatol 35: 433–454
33. Rothman S (1954) Physiology and biochemistry of the skin. University of Chicago Press, Chicago, pp 120–152
34. Sasagawa S (1967) Studies on the dry form of eczema in childhood. Jpn J Dermatol 77: 62–87
35. Schultz H, Zachariae H (1972) The Trafuril test in recurrent juvenile eczema of hands and feet. Acta Derm Venereol (Stockh) 52: 398–400
36. Sillevis Smitt JH, Bos JD, Hulsebosch HJ, Krieg SR (1986) In situ immunophenotyping of antigen presenting cells and T cell subsets in atopic dermatitis. Clin Exp Dermatol 11: 159–168
37. Sulzberger MB (1971) Atopic dermatitis, part III. In: Fitzpatrick T, Arndt KA, Clark WH (eds) Dermatology in general medicine. McGraw-Hill, New York, pp 687–697
38. Sulzberger MB, Goodman J (1936) The relative importance of specific skin hypersensitivity in adult atopic dermatitis. JAMA 106: 1000–1003
39. Sulzberger MB, Hermann F, Morrill SD, Pascher F, Miller K (1959) Studies of sweat, lipids, and histopathology in children with "dry skin" (xerosis). Int Arch Allergy 14: 129–143
40. Svensson Å, Edman B, Möller (1985) A diagnostic tool for atopic dermatitis based on clinical criteria. Acta Derm Venereol [Suppl] (Stockh) 114: 33–40
41. Uehara M (1982) Reduced histamine reaction in atopic dermatitis. Arch Dermatol 118: 244–245
42. Uehara M (1985) Clinical and histological features of dry skin in atopic dermatitis. Acta Derm Venereol [Suppl] (Stockh) 114: 82–86
43. Uehara M (1986) Dry skin (sebostasis) and inflammation: heterogeneity of "dry skin" in atopic dermatitis. In: Ring J, Burg G (eds) New trends in allergy II. Springer, Berlin Heidelberg New York, pp 135–144
44. Uehara M, Miyauchi H (1984) The morphologic characteristics of dry skin in atopic dermatitis. Arch Dermatol 120: 1186–1190
45. Uehara M, Ofuji S (1977) Abnormal vascular reactions in atopic dermatitis. Arch Dermatol 113: 627–629
46. Uehara M, Ofuji S (1978) Delayed blanch reaction in atopic dermatitis. Arch Dermatol 114: 1098–1099
47. Uehara M, Ofuji S (1980) Atopic dermatitis: a discussion of theories concerning its pathogenesis. J Dermatol 7: 231–238
48. Uehara M, Takahashi C, Ofuji S (1975) Pustular patch test reactions in atopic dermatitis. Arch Dermatol 111: 1154–1157
49. Wells RS, Kerr CB (1966a) Clinical features of autosomal dominant and sex-linked ichthyosis in an English population. Br Med J 1: 947–950
50. Wells RS, Kerr CB (1966b) The histology of ichthyosis. J Invest Dermatol 46: 530–535
51. Werner Y (1986) The water content of the stratum corneum in patients with atopic dermatitis. Acta Derm Venereol (Stockh) 66: 281–284
52. Werner Y, Lindberg M (1985) Transepidermal water loss in dry and clinically normal skin in patients with atopic dermatitis. Acta Derm Venereol (Stockh) 65: 102–105
53. Werner Y, Lindberg M, Forslind B (1982) The water-binding capacity of stratum corneum in dry non-eczematous skin of atopic eczema. Acta Derm Venereol (Stockh) 62: 334–337
54. White CR (1983) Histopathology of atopic dermatitis. Semin Dermatol 2: 34–38
55. Wirth H, Gloor M, Stoika D (1981) Sebaceous glands in uninvolved skin of patients suffering from atopic dermatitis. Arch Dermatol Res 270: 167–169
56. Wüthrich B, Schnyder UW (1981) Eine wenig bekannte Ausdrucksform der Neurodermitis atopica im Kindesalter: das patchy pityriasiform lichenoid eczema (Kitamura-Takahashi-Sasagawa). Aktuel Dermatol 7: 85–87

Occupational Aspects of Atopic Eczema with Emphasis on Atopic Hand Eczema

I. Rystedt

Introduction

Dermatitis of various types has become the most common occupational disease in the industrialised world [1, 2]. The hands are affected in the majority of those who contract occupational dermatitis [3–5]. "Wet work" and exposure to irritants and sensitisers often represent eliciting factors [3].

Before 1980, only a few studies had been published on atopic patients in risk occupations [6–8]. During recent years, however, investigations of employees in various industries and other places of work including domestic activities have shown that there is a significant relationship between atopic eczema and occupational skin disease [1, 9–18]. Adults with current widespread atopic eczema constitute a small but, from an occupational point of view, important group. Their problems have actually been very little elucidated. Instead, the interest has been focussed on work-related hand eczema in atopic patients [11, 13, 15–16]. In two large scale studies from Finland and Sweden, respectively, atopic patients engaged in hospital work were investigated [19–20]. A third investigation, also Swedish, comprises a long-term follow-up of atopic patients with emphasis on the occupational aspects of atopic hand eczema [21].

Occupational Aspects of Widespread Atopic Eczema

Atopic eczema in adulthood often appears spontaneously and quite unexpectedly, seemingly unrelated to occupation and home environment. On the other hand, environment conditions often elicit or worsen existing eczema in the atopic patient. A great occupational handicap for adult patients with persistent atopic eczema is the disease itself [6]. This means that the distress due to intense itching and the resulting excoriation sometimes forces them to lose time from their job or education, or that the emotional stress which follows itching makes it impossible for them to continue their work. Frequent hospitalisation may even cause dismissal.

Triggering factors which aggravate itching in atopic eczema patients include exposure to dust, perspiration during work, change of environmental temperature, climatic changes, dampness and low humidity [6, 21–24]. Water, soap and other external irritants may also provoke or aggravate the atopic eczema.

Occupational Aspects of Atopic Hand Eczema

It is generally agreed that the atopic skin has a reduced resistance to irritants [25–27] and that consequently individuals with a history of or with current atopic eczema have a tendency to develop an irritant, often work-related, contact dermatitis on an atopic base, often localised to the hands [28–30]. In fact, the most common localisation of atopic eczema in adults is the hands [9, 24, 31–34].

Hand eczema often causes important medical, social and economic problems. The work-related implications of hand eczema are therefore the most important in the relationship between atopy and occupational skin disease and will consequently be emphasised in the following.

Aetiology of Hand Eczema

The prevalence of hand eczema in southern Sweden has been estimated at approximately 2% [5]. The aetiology is always multifactorial, and the relative importance of exogenous and endogenous factors is difficult to measure in the individual case [35–37]. Neither of these factors seems to lead to a specific pattern or typical clinical distribution of the hand eczema [24, 38]. Only looking at the hands of the patient does not, therefore, give any guidance as regards the cause of the eczema [38]. Consequently, it is most often impossible to distinguish between an irritant contact dermatitis on an atopic base, seemingly caused by exogenous factors, and an atopic hand eczema mainly elicited by endogenous factors.

Despite these difficulties it is for medico-legal reasons sometimes important to try to establish the balance between endogenous and exogenous factors, e.g. in cases of retirement brought on by occupational damage to the skin the clinical assessment may have far-reaching economic consequences for the individual in question. Furthermore, the healing of the eczema can be expected to be faster and often more complete, by special treatment or a change of job, if the eczema is of exogenous origin. This will be further elaborated upon in the following.

In general, from a practical, occupational point of view it is, however, more important to establish how common and how serious hand eczema is in atopic patients compared with non-atopic persons, to try to find out who is most at risk of developing hand eczema and finally to investigate the work implications of atopic hand eczema.

Frequency of Atopic Hand Eczema

It is widely held that exposure to irritants is the most common cause of hand eczema in atopic patients as well as in non-atopic persons. Because the former are thought to have a reduced resistance to irritants, the effects of such substances are assumed to be more pronounced in them [10–11, 26–27].

According to recent investigations, exogenous factors as a cause of hand eczema should not be underestimated as dermatitis of the hands is more common both in atopic patients and non-atopic persons among those exposed than among those not exposed to irritants in their work or home environment [15, 21]. There do not, however, seem to be indications that exposure to irritants is the main cause of hand eczema in the majority of people with a history of atopic dermatitis [21, 39]. Since no reliable tests are available to determine whether an irritant is relevant in an individual case, determination of the role of irritants in hand eczema and in particular in atopic hand eczema must be based on clinical assessment. It is, however, obvious and has been shown, i.e. in the previously mentioned three Scandinavian investigations, that hand eczema is more common in individuals with a history of atopic eczema than in non-atopic persons [11, 13, 24]. The differences reported, however, vary widely, the prevalence of hand eczema in people with past or present atopic eczema being from two [11, 13] to up to as much as ten times higher than in non-atopic persons [21, 24]. One explanation for these discrepancies is that the frequency of hand eczema in adult life proves to be much lower in people with a childhood history of mild to moderate rather than severe atopic eczema [21, 24].

Another explanation is connected with the observation that the difference in frequency of hand eczema between people with and without a history of atopic eczema is much greater at the actual time of an investigation than when measured over longer periods [21]. The most likely explanation for this is, in its turn, that the hand eczema seems to be more protracted and shows more frequent recurrences in people with past or present atopic eczema than in unaffected people [21].

People with a history of respiratory allergy (atopic mucosal symptoms) without simultaneous atopic eczema have a lower incidence of hand eczema than people with childhood atopic eczema [11, 13, 24]. Neither are they significantly more prone to develop hand eczema than non-atopic persons. In people with respiratory allergy and in non-atopic people, however, the simultaneous presence of dry/itchy skin [21] in combination with white dermographism and facial pallor (called atopic skin diathesis) [11] markedly increase the incidence of hand eczema.

Severity of Atopic Hand Eczema

In comparison with non-atopic persons, hand eczema in people with a childhood history of atopic eczema is more intense [13], recurs, as previously mentioned, more often and appears over lengthier periods [21]. This is manifested by higher figures for medical consultations, longer periods of sick-leave and more frequent use of corticosteroids [13, 21, 24].

Severe hand eczema is, however, rather unusual in both atopic and non-atopic people [24].

Atopic Hand Eczema in Various Occupations

Irritant Contact Dermatitis

Irritant contact dermatitis is usually used as a comprehensive term for dermatitis for which exogenous factors are assumed to be the dominant cause. Even though only a few investigations concerning mainly irritant hand eczema among people with a history of atopic eczema in various occupations have been carried out [11, 13, 15, 16, 40], it is well-known and has also been shown that, among others, wet jobs including exposure to tensides and food-handling are hazardous to the hands. Examples of risk occupations are:

Hairdresser	Domestic worker
Nurse's assistant	Motor mechanic
Other nursing staff	Farmer
Laboratory assistant	Painter
Dentist	Printer
Cleaner	Metal worker
Food-handler	Restaurant (kitchen) worker

The investigations concerned with atopic patients engaged in hospital "wet work" showed very high frequencies of hand eczema among kitchen workers, cleaners and assistant nurses [11, 13, 19–20, 40]. In the long-term follow-up of atopic children, the highest rate of hand eczema was found among food-handlers, hairdressers, assistant nurses, other nursing staff and domestic workers [15]. The high frequency of hand eczema among food-handlers may be partly of irritant origin, partly caused by delayed hypersensitivity and partly due to the fact that hand eczema in such workers is often caused by type I reactions giving rise to contact urticaria followed by protein contact dermatitis [41].

In most studies of hand eczema there is a female predominance both among atopic and non-atopic persons [5, 24, 42–43] which seems to be most pronounced in groups of women exposed to irritants [21]. One reason is probably that women are often exposed to irritants both occupationally and domestically. According to several researchers, female skin is also more reactive or irritable than male skin [44–45]. A hormonal factor might also be involved.

From a medico-legal aspect it is important to point out that apart from occupational domestic exposure to irritants, domestic factors at home prove to be of significant importance for the development of hand eczema [13, 15, 21]. One of the dominating risk occupations is that of housewife [13, 15, 21, 46]. A highly significant difference in the prevalence of hand eczema has been found between women exposed and not exposed to irritants at home, irrespective of occupational exposure [15]. Furthermore, the observations that the incidence of hand eczema increases with an increasing number of children [21] and is more common in women with children under 4 years of age [13] coborate these findings.

In considering the effect of irritants on the skin it should be noted that roughly ¼ of high-risk workers with a history of atopic eczema never develop hand eczema, probably due to better "skin quality" [11, 13, 15]; compare section on Risk individuals and risk occupations below.

Allergic Contact Dermatitis

The prevalence of contact sensitivity among patients with atopic eczema has been reported to vary between 15% and 35% [5, 9, 33, 47–50]. Differences with regard to materials and number of allergens used in the patch tests in all probability explain the wide range. In addition, false-positive irritant test reactions, especially of the follicular type, which are common in patients with atopic eczema, in some cases may have caused confusion and been mistaken for positive patch tests [51, 52].

Because contact allergens are believed to penetrate traumatised skin more readily than intact skin [3, 37], the risk of developing contact sensitivity might be expected to be high in patients with current atopic eczema and especially in patients with severe atopic eczema. Although, however, in some investigations atopic patients have been found to be sensitised more often to balsam of Peru, fragrances and nickel than are non-atopic persons [49, 50, 53], contact allergy does not in general seem to be significantly more common in the former [49, 50]. A clinical investigation by Jones et al. [54] has indicated that, because of reduced cell-mediated immunity, patients with active atopic eczema are less likely to develop contact sensitivity that non-atopic persons. In patients with current atopic eczema the risk of becoming sensitised due to increased permeability of the skin in all probability is counteracted by a depressed cell-mediated immunity. The result of these counteracting factors seems to be a sensitisation rate similar to that of non-atopic persons.

The allergic contact dermatitis that develops in atopic patients in association with exposure to a known allergen may boost an existing dermatitis but has, most often, nothing to do with or is of marginal significance for persistent or recurrent atopic eczema [21]. Also, when consideration is taken only of hand eczema in atopic patients, contact sensitivity seems to be largely a contributory factor in the aetiology [9]. Neither the frequency nor the severity of hand eczema among atopic patients has been shown to be greater in sensitised than in non-sensitised people [50]. Even though, however, most atopic patients are unable to correlate current episodes of hand eczema to any obvious exposure to allergens to which they react, hybrid forms of dermatitis with coexisting atopic hand eczema and allergic contact dermatitis occur [55]. In patients with active dermatitis working in an environment in which potent allergens, e.g. nickel, are frequent, sensitisation may cause a severe occupational hindrance. Hairdressers, employees in hospital "wet work" and food-handlers are examples of such professions.

Contact Urticaria and Protein Contact Dermatitis

The vesicular eruptions and the wheal-and-flare response in protein contact dermatitis and contact urticaria, respectively, are both immediate hypersensitivity reactions which may be IgE-mediated [56].

There is conflicting evidence concerning a possible relationship between contact urticaria of the immunological type and atopy. In a recent investigation however, an overrepresentation of atopy has been found among patients with IgE-mediated rubber latex sensitivity [57]. Contact urticaria to cobalt, common in hard metal workers, has also been found to be of the IgE-mediated type [60]. A lot of food substances, among others lettuce and endive, may also produce an immunologic contact urticaria [58, 59]. A current irritant dermatitis on an atopic base may be the prerequisite for contact urticaria.

As the role of IgE-mediated allergy in atopic eczema is unclear, an immunological connection between contact urticaria and protein contact dermatitis, on the one side, and atopic eczema, on the other, has not been stated [56]. Nor is it clear whether protein contact dermatitis is more common among atopic eczema patients than among non-atopic persons [9, 41]. It is, however, a rational concept that eczematous atopic skin, with its impaired barrier to penetration, may be more susceptible both to contact allergy of the delayed type and to contact urticaria and protein contact dermatitis than healthy skin. Relatively large molecules, like those of protein, presumably can pass through damaged better than through undamaged epidermis. However, even after the apparent cure of an eczema, previously affected areas may remain in a state of continuous increased responsiveness compared with unaffected skin, reacting with an immediate type response when repeatedly encountering the aetiologic stimulus. Consequently, the identified hypersensitivity of immediate type in e. g. food-handlers may either be primarily responsible for the dermatitis or contribute secondarily to the flare of a preexisting atopic eczema. An overrepresentation of protein contact dermatitis in atopic eczema patients might therefore be possible.

The work of preparing food carries, as previously mentioned, a high occupational risk. Occupational dermatitis in this trade is often of mixed irritant and allergic origin. The type I – sensitivity causing protein contact dermatitis has been found to be common among kitchen workers, who nearly all complain that their dermatitis is aggravated by contact with fish and certain vegetables [41].

Contact with animal hair seems to be a major cause of protein contact dermatitis in veterinary surgeons [61].

Risk Individuals and Risk Occupations

An increased transepidermal water loss (TEWL) [62] and a decreased ability of the stratum corneum to bind water [63] indicate that in patients with atopic eczema there is an early defect in the skin barrier function which seems to cause a constitutional vulnerability of the skin that varies from individual to individual. As a consequence, a reduced resistence to irritants seems to appear. Due to unidentified endogenous factors, many atopic patients, however, also seem to develop hand eczema independently of exposure to irritants [20, 21, 39]. Such exposure often increases the risk of getting hand eczema or worsens an already existing hand eczema, especially in atopic patients with pronounced constitutional skin vulnerability.

Taken as a group, patients with a history of atopic eczema in childhood run a higher risk of developing hand eczema than non-atopic persons and consequently, in this context, are *risk individuals*. However, people with past or present atopic eczema are not at all a uniform group and can be separated into sub-groups. It may be of crucial importance for a young atopic adolescent about to choose his or her first job to know to which sub-group he or she belongs and then to evaluate the possible risk of developing hand eczema and/or worsening a persistent atopic hand eczema. According to recent investigations, it is possible to distinguish *high- and low-risk individuals* among atopic patients by assessment of some appropriate strong predictors.

Very strong predictors are, according to the previously mentioned Swedish follow-up study of 1177 atopic children [39], eczematous hand involvement of atopic eczema in childhood, persistent eczema on parts of the body other than the hands and persistent dry/itchy skin, with the first being the predominant one. In atopic patients without eczematous hand involvement in childhood, severe (widespread) childhood dermatitis is a fairly strong predictor. Weak predictors for hand eczema seem to be female sex, family history of atopic eczema and associated respiratory allergy [39].

In a group of people with all three strongest predictors, 90% of those who during some period had been engaged, in "wet work" developed hand eczema as adults. The corresponding figure for those without any of the strong predictors was only 13% [21]. The stronger and the more numerous the risk factors are, the higher is the consequent risk of hand eczema appearing. Previous hand eczema is always a very strong risk factor.

For a high-risk individual the choice of occupation is sometimes of limited importance as he or she may already have developed or later will develop hand eczema independently of the job chosen. Even so, it is very important to point out that frequent exposure to water in combination with some chemicals, especially tensides, often worsens an existing hand eczema, which can make the patient incapable of working. Many of the individuals who are constitutionally more moderately burdened with fewer numbers of predictors as signs of a less pronounced skin fragility will probably manage in dry work, while work involving frequent exposure to irritants may elicit hand eczema. People without any or with a few weak risk factors do not, however, seem to develop hand eczema to a higher extent than non-atopic persons.

People with a history of childhood respiratory allergy are risk individuals only if they have dry/itchy skin in addition to asthma/rhinitis. This is in accordance with dry/itchy skin being a strong predictor for hand eczema. Also among non-atopic persons, there is a group of individuals with dry/itchy skin who carry an increased risk of developing hand eczema.

For atopic risk individuals it is always important to consider risk levels of different jobs. Jobs that incur exposure to irritants are always *risk occupations*. As previously mentioned, high-risk occupations seem to be particularly characterised by exposure to tensides in typical wet jobs. Food-handling, involving skin contact with various food substances and certain irritants, ladies' hairdressing and nursing, involving "wet work" with exposure to tensides, are high-risk occupations as are cleaning and domestic "wet work". The last is often an additional aggravating factor in women with occupational exposure to irritants but can also when excessive in this context be looked upon as a high-risk occupation in itself.

Even though the frequency of hand eczema in atopic patients does not seem to be higher in sensitised than in nonsensitised persons, occupations in which potent allergens are present can sometimes be risk occupations for atopic patients with an already existing hand eczema. The traumatised skin may in these persons predispose to the development of a contact sensitivity, which may further aggravate the eczema and diminish the possibility of the person going on working in the same profession.

Skin Care Programme

As atopic eczema patients regularly develop persistent hand eruptions when exposed to irritants which would produce only a transitory dermatitis in a normal individual, a disciplined skin care programme is clearly indicated beside the usual topical treatment. In some patients the hands must be protected from every possible contactant. This may involve relinquishing favourite hobbies and a complete alteration in life style. All this can be achieved only by meticulously detailed instructions to the patient, who in some cases can no longer shampoo her own hair or use oven cleaners barehanded. The patient must recognise that all which was handled before with impunity is now a serious potential risk. Good hand protection includes the wearing of two pairs of gloves, a light cotton one and a plastic covering one, for all work. The cotton one must be removed very often and replaced with a clean dry one. Intensive skin protection is necessary for a period of at least 6 months before the hands return to their normal status. With certain individuals, such as hairdressers and mechanics, such total protection is not feasible, and a sick-leave period away from work is mandatory if they do not wish to suffer from years of dermatitis.

Change of Occupation

In spite of fully satisfactory treatment and protection, some atopic patients do not heal and therefore have to change occupation because of eczema. People with a history of atopic eczema are forced to change jobs because of hand eczema to a somewhat greater extent than non-atopic persons, which is probably mainly due to their higher incidence of hand eczema [15–16]. Aggravation of hand eczema by exposure to irritants is often the main reason for change of job, but also heat, humidity, cold, dust and dryness can sometimes force people with generalised atopic eczema to change job. In many cases, social, economic and labour market factors contribute to the decision, especially in those instances when the eczema is of a relatively mild nature [15]. Common jobs that people with a history of atopic eczema frequently are unable to cope with are ladies' hairdressing, food-handling, cleaning, printing, metalwork, assistant nursing, motor mechanical work, hotel and restaurant work, farming and forestry work.

The value of a change of occupation for patients who have contracted eczema at work has been discussed in many papers. Some authors consider a change of job to be of value [64–65], while others have expressed doubt [66]. After perusal of 10 years of patient records at a department of occupational dermatology in southern Sweden [3], it appeared, as in several other studies [67–68], that no difference in prognosis as regards complete healing of the dermatitis after change of job existed between patients who had changed jobs and those who went on working in their original occupations. In the Swedish follow-up study of atopic patients, the healing rate of hand eczema after change of occupation was no higher than about 20% [15]. The beneficial effect was less marked in atopic than in non-atopic persons, in all probability due to a more complex aetiological pattern of hand eczema in patients with a history of childhood atopic eczema. However, a change to clean dry work had improved the course of the hand lesions in the majority of atopic patients, giving them an opportunity to work which otherwise might not have been possible at all [29].

Vocational Guidance

The practical work implications of atopic eczema, especially hand eczema, in atopic patients are extensive. Vocational guidance is therefore important. It is, however, obvious that no general simple rules can be given for this guidance as the individual variations are innumerable. The general knowledge about risk groups and risk occupations does not allow full advice to a specific individual. In the first place it is necessary to find out to what extent an atopic person is a risk individual. It is also important to study the characteristics of the specific job in question.

In addition, the assumptions and starting points for advice must vary, depending on whether the recipient is an adolescent aiming at special training, a trained experienced person planning to take up a particular job or simply someone having trouble in his present occupation because of eczema. As a general rule, however, it is of importance that the fullest possible information about the risk of developing or worsening an already existing eczema is given in every case. There are not only dermatological aspects to be addressed. Personal ambition and motivation as well as social, educational, economic and other factors must also be taken into consideration when different job problems are discussed.

Keeping the above remarks in mind, the following outlines for individuals with a history of atopic eczema may be suggested:

- In order to avoid worsening of the eczema, people with current widespread atopic eczema should be advised against heavy or high temperature jobs which can cause excessive sweating, stress, dirty or dusty jobs, jobs involving great variations of temperature, and environments with potent allergens which can cause contact allergy.
- With regard to the risk of acquiring hand eczema, high-risk individuals among atopic adolescents should avoid all sorts of risk occupations involving exposure to irritants. There should be no restrictions for the atopic patients who do not run a higher risk of developing hand eczema than non-atopic persons. The large group of atopic adolescents between these two extremes should be warned against high-risk occupations. Also, experienced atopic individuals should be advised against employment in risk occupations if they have a current atopic hand eczema or a history of such eczema. Such individuals with a history of atopic eczema, but without past or present hand eczema, should not be advised against risk occupations, but a careful regular follow-up over at least 1 year after employment in a risk occupation, especially a high-risk occupation, is recommended.
- Advice to change job in the first place because of hand eczema should be given with caution. It must be considered very important to inform high-risk individuals with severe hand eczema that the dermatitis may not disappear in a "safer" job but in all probability improve, this being the only way for the patient to work at all. In atopic patients with moderate or mild hand eczema, medical reasons for a change of job should be weighed against social reasons before a decision is taken. A good skin care programme might be helpful in controlling the hand eczema, thus enabling the patient to continue in the chosen job.

The recommendations above are mainly based on statistical data from recent epidemiological studies. As previously mentioned large individual variations occur. It is therefore important once more to emphasise that it is very difficult to predict whether an individual will develop hand eczema or not. In most situations it is with few exceptions preferable – when it seems necessary – to try to advise the person against a job than to prohibit him from taking it. Exceptions are people with active hand eczema who apply for work in medical service involving direct future contact with patients and people who work in the food trade. As the damaged skin in atopic eczema is often colonised by *Staphylococcus aureus*, the risk of transmitting staphylococci [69] as well as the risk the patient takes of being barred from work for long periods should always be considered.

References

1. Shmunes E, Keil JE (1983) Occupational dermatoses in South Carolina: a descriptive analysis of cost variables. J Am Acad Dermatol 9: 861–866
2. Keczkes K, Bhate SM, Wyatt EM (1983) The outcome of primary irritant hand dermatitis. Br J Dermatol 109: 665–668
3. Fregert S (1975) Occupational dermatitis in a 10-year material. Contact Dermatitis 1: 96–107
4. Malten KE, Fregert S, Bandmann HJ, Calnan CD, Cronin E, Hjorth N, Magnusson B, Maibach HI, Meneghini CL, Pirilä V, Wilkinson DS (1971) Occupational dermatitis in five European dermatological departments. Berufsdermatosen 19: 1–15
5. Agrup G (1969) Hand eczema and other hand dermatoses in South Sweden. Acta Derm Venereol [Suppl] (Stockh) 61: 1–91
6. Nexmand PH (1958) Occupational problems for patients with Besnier's prurigo. In: Occupational allergy. Stenfert, Kroese, Leiden, pp 66–70
7. Wilkinson DS, Hambly EM (1978) Prognosis of hand eczema in hairdressing apprentices. Contact Dermatitis 4: 63
8. Cronin E, Kullavanijaya P (1979) Hand dermatitis in hairdressers. Acta Derm Venereol [Suppl] (Stockh) 85(59): 47–50
9. Forsbeck M, Skog E, Asbrink E (1983) Atopic hand dermatitis: A comparison with atopic dermatitis without hand involvement, especially with respect to influence of work and development of contact sensitization. Acta Derm Venereol (Stockh) 63: 9–13
10. Högberg M, Wahlberg JE (1980) Health screening for occupational dermatoses in house painters. Contact Dermatitis 6: 100–106
11. Lammintausta K, Kalimo K (1981) Atopy and hand dermatitis in hospital wet work. Contact Dermatitis 7: 301–308
12. Shmunes E, Keil JE (1984) The role of atopy in occupational dermatoses. Contact Dermatitis 11: 174–178
13. Nilsson E, Mikaelsson B, Andersson S (1985) Atopy occupation and domestic work as risk factors for hand eczema in hospital workers. Contact Dermatitis 13: 216–223
14. Lammintausta SK, Kalimo K, Aantaa S (1985) Course of hand dermatitis in hospital workers. Contact Dermatitis 8: 327–332
15. Rystedt I (1985) Work-related hand eczema in atopics. Contact Dermatitis 12: 164–171
16. Rystedt I (1985) Atopic background in patients with occupational hand eczema. Contact Dermatitis 12: 247–254
17. Fisher T, Rystedt I (1985) Hand eczema among hard metal workers. Am J Ind Med 8: 381–394
18. Van der Burg CKH, Bruynzeel DP, Vreeburg KJJ, von Blomberg BME, Scheper RJ (1986) Hand eczema in hairdressers and nurses: a prospective study. Evaluation of atopy and nickel hypersensitivity at the start of apprenticeship. Contact Dermatitis 12: 275–279
19. Lammintausta K (1982) Risk factors for hand dermatitis in wet work. Atopy and contact sensitivity in hospital workers. Thesis, Turku, Finland
20. Nilsson E (1986) Individual and environmental risk factors for hand eczema in hospital workers. Thesis, Umeå University, Sweden
21. Rystedt I (1985) Hand eczema and long-term prognosis in atopic dermatitis. Acta Derm Venereol [Suppl] (Stockh) 117: 1–59
22. Rajka G (1967) Occupational choice for persons with common chronic dermatoses and pathological skin function. Acta Derm Venereol (Stockh) 47: 15–19
23. Rycroft RJ, Smith WDL (1980) Low humidity occupational dermatoses. Contact Dermatitis 6: 488–492
24. Rystedt I (1985) Hand eczema in patients with history of atopic manifestations in childhood. Acta Derm Venereol (Stockh) 65: 305–312
25. Blaylock WK (1976) Atopic dermatitis: diagnosis and pathobiology. J Allergy Clin Immunol 57: 62–79
26. Hanifin JM (1984) Atopic dermatitis. J Allergy Clin Immunol 73(2): 211–222
27. Epstein E (1984) Hand dermatitis: practical management and current concepts. J Am Acad Dermatol 10: 395–424
28. Hanifin JM, Rajka G (1980) Diagnostic features of atopic dermatitis. Acta Derm Venereol [Suppl] (Stockh) 92: 44–47
29. Hanifin JM, Lobitz WC (1977) Newer concepts of atopic dermatitis. Arch Dermatol 113: 663–6870
30. Hjort N, Fregert S (1979) Contact dermatitis. In: Rook R, Wilkinson DS, Ebling FSG (eds) Textbook of dermatology, 3rd edn. Blackwell Scientific, Oxford, pp 363–441
31 Bandmann H-J, Agathos M (1980) Die atopische Handdermatitis. Derm Beruf Umwelt 28: 110–113
32. Breit R, Leutgeb C, Bandmann H-J (1972) Zum neurodermititischen Handekzem. Arch Dermatol Forsch 244: 353–354
33. Cronin E, Bandmann H-J, Calnan CD, Fregert S, Hjort N, Magnusson B, Maibach HI, Malten K, Meneghini CL, Pirilä V, Wilkinson DS (1970) Contact dermatitis in the atopic. Acta Derm Venereol (Stockh) 50: 183–187
34. Wilkinson DS, Bandmann HJ, Calnan CD, Cronin E, Fregert S, Hjoirt N, Magnusson B, Maibach HI, Malten KE, Meneghini CL, Pirilä V (1970) The role of contact allergy in hand eczema. Trans St John's Hosp Dermatol Soc 56: 19–25
35. Calnan CD (1968) Eczema for me. Trans St John's Hosp Dermatol Soc 54: 54–64
36. Calnan CD (1968) Studies in contact dermatitis. XXII. Chronicity. Trans St John's Hosp Dermatol Soc 54: 170–177
37. Wilkinson DS (1971) Contact dermatitis of the hands. Trans St John's Hosp Dermatol Soc 58: 163–171
38. Cronin E (1985) Clinical patterns of hand eczema in women. Contact Dermatitis 13: 153–161
39. Rystedt I (1985) Factors influencing the occurrence of hand eczema in adults with a history of atopic dermatitis in childhood. Contact Dermatitis 12: 185–191
40. Lammintausta K (1983) Hand dermatitis in different hospital workers, who perform wet work. Derm Beruf Umwelt 31: 14–19
41. Hjort N, Roed-Petersen J (1976) Occupational protein contact dermatitis in foodhandlers. Contact Dermatitis 2: 28–42
42. Coenraads PJ, Nater JP, van der Lende R (1983) Prevalence of eczema and other dermatoses of the hands and arms in the Netherlands. Association with age and occupation. Clin Exp Dermatol 8: 495–503
43. Lantinga H, Nater JP, Coenraads PJ (1984) Prevalence, incidence and course of eczema on the hands and forearms in a sample of the general population. Contact Dermatitis 10: 135–159
44. Wagner G, Pürschel W (1962) Klinisch-analytische Studie zum Neurodermitis Problem. Dermatologica 125: 1–32
45. Mathias CGT, Maibach HI (1978) Dermatoxicology mono-

graphs I. Cutaneous irritation: factors influencing the response to irritants. Clin Toxicol 13: 333–346
46. Glickman FS, Silvers SH (1967) Hand eczema and atopy in housewives. Arch Dermatol 95: 487–489
47. Rudzki E, Grzywa Z (1975) Contact sensitivity in atopic dermatitis. Contact Dermatitis 1: 285–287
48. Bandmann H-J, Breit R, Lautgeb Chr (1972) Kontaktallergie und Dermatitis atopica. Arch Invest Dermatol 244: 332–339
49. Lammintausta K, Kalimo K, Havu VK (1982) Contact allergy in atopics, who perform wet work in hospital. Derm Beruf Umwelt 30: 184–189
50. Rystedt I (1985) Contact sensitivity in adults with atopic dermatitis in childhood. Contact Dermatitis 13: 1–8
51. Fischer T, Rystedt I (1985) False positive follicular and common irritant patch test reactions to metal salts. Contact Dermatitis 12: 93–98
52. Rajka G (1975) Atopic dermatitis. Saunders, London
53. Huber von A, Fartasch M, Diepgen TL, Bäurle G, Hornstein OP (1987) Auftreten von Kontaktallergien beim atopischen Ekzem. Zusammenhänge mit gleichzeitig gefundenen atopischen Merkmalen. Derm Beruf Umwelt 35: 119–123
54. Jones HE, Lewis CW, McMartin MSL (1973) Allergic contact sensitivity in atopic dermatitis. Arch Dermatol 107: 217–222
55. Malten KE (1968) The occurrence of hybrids between contact allergic eczema and atopic dermatitis (and vice versa) and their significance. Dermatologica 136: 404–406
56. von Krogh G, Maibach HI (1981) The contact urticaria syndrome – an updated review. J Am Acad Dermatol 5: 328–342
57. Wrangsjö K, Wahlberg JE, Axelsson IGK (1988) IgE-mediated allergy to natural rubber in 30 patients with contact urticaria. Contact Dermatitis 19: 264–271
58. Krook G (1977) Occupational dermatitis from *Lactuca sativa* (lettuce) and *Chicorium* (endive). Simultaneous occurrence of immediate and delayed allergy as a cause of contact dermatitis. Contact Dermatitis 3: 27–36
59. Maibach HI (1976) Immediate hypersensitivity in hand dermatitis. Role of food-contact dermatitis. Arch Dermatol 112: 1289–1291
60. Smith JD, Odom RB, Maibach HI (1975) Contact urticaria to cobalt chloride. Arch Dermatol 111: 1610–1611
61. Hjort N, Roed-Pedersen J (1976) Occupational protein contact dermatitis in veterinary surgeons. Contact Dermatitis 2: 28–42
62. Werner Y, Lindberg M (1985) Transepidermal water loss in dry and clinically normal skin in patients with atopic dermatitis. Acta Derm Venereol (Stockh) 65: 102–105
63. Werner Y (1986) The water content of the stratum corneum in patients with atopic dermatitis. Acta Derm Venereol (Stockh) 66: 281–284
64. Rajka G (1966) Katamnestische Untersuchungen beruflicher chemisch-allergische Kontaktekzeme. Acta Allergol 136: 236–256
65. Peters K (1968) Über das Schicksal der Patienten mit Gewerbeekzem. Dermatologica 136: 236–256
66. Neumann YB (1966) Rehabiliation problems in occupational skin diseases. Proceedings of the International Congress of Occupational Health, pp 7–10
67. Hellier FF (1962) Rehabilitation of skin patients (I). Symposium Dermatologorum de morbis cutaneis. Professionalibus Pragae 2: 345–346
68. Meneghini CL, Rantuccio F, Coqqa G (1967) The persistence and recurrence of contact eczema: clinical experimental observations (XIII). Congressus Internationalis Dermatologiae, pp 249–252
69. Selwyn S (1965) Mechanism and prevention of cross infection in dermatology wards. J Hyg 63: 59–71

Allergic Contact Eczema and Atopic Eczema

Ch. Neumann and S. Marghescu

Immunological Findings

Allergic Contact Eczema

Since Landsteiner and Chase used cell transfer experiments to demonstrate that the potential of eliciting allergic contact eczema resides in the mononuclear cell fraction of leucocytes, one must regard the allergic contact eczema as a manifestation of delayed-type hypersensitivity (DTH) [1, 2]. Later on, several other groups showed that the induction and elicitation of allergic contact eczema requires a complex interaction of multiple components. Various T-lymphocyte subpopulations and their products react with antigen-presenting cells which express HLA II antigens on their surface. In the epidermis, these are the Langerhans cells [3]. The sensitization phase includes the generation of T-helper and various types of regulatory T-suppressor lymphocytes which are specifically sensitized by percutaneously penetrating molecules of low molecular weight [4, 5]. The specificity is carried by CD4+ T-helper cells, as proven for nickel sensitivity [6]. After sensitization has occurred, any further cutaneous contact with the allergen will provoke the manifestation of an allergic contact eczema [7]. Immunologically, this represents the effector phase of cell-mediated immunity (CMI). Several investigators suggest a biphasic development of allergic contact eczema and consider the first part a mandatory prerequisite of the second. Within 4 h after contact with antigen, basophils which have been activated by T-cell factors invade the skin [8]. This specific "cutaneous basophil hypersensitivity" [9] is followed by an invasion with mononuclear cells, the vast majority of which are T cells without antigen specificity. It appears that a single antigen-specific helper cell is sufficient to initiate this late classic effector phase [10]. During this late phase of allergic contact eczema the kinetics of emigration and the phenotypic composition of the infiltrating cells cannot be distinguished from an irritant dermatitis [11].

It was possible to demonstrate by experiments on different strains of guinea pigs that the susceptibility for developing DTH to certain contact allergens is genetically controlled [12]. In humans this question has rarely been investigated, but preliminary results seem to support the findings obtained in guinea pigs [13]. Probably more important than the genetical determination of the individual to become sensitized, are the physicochemical properties of the sensitizing molecule. Some contact allergens such as 1,3-dinitro-4-chlorobenzene (DNCB) will almost inevitably lead to contact allergy while others, even after repeated applications, will only sensitize a small cohort of individuals.

Atopic Eczema

In contrast to allergic contact eczema, the pathogenesis of atopic eczema is still widely unknown, despite the fact that the term "atopic eczema" used by Wise and Sulzberger links the immunological basis of atopy to the skin manifestations of these patients [14]. Up to the present time the significance of immunological mechanisms leading to the manifestation of dermatitis remains unclear. The concept of an immunological basis for atopic eczema was originally suggested by the observation that 75% of patients with this disorder have a personal or family history of other atopic diseases such as allergic asthma and rhinitis [15]. McDevitt reviewed the evidence for specific immune response genes in families with various manifestations of atopy [16]. A recent population-based twin study confirms the importance of genetic factors in atopic eczema [90].

Interest in the role of immunology in atopic eczema was revived when Ishizaka and co-workers were able to classify reaginic antibodies to IgE class of immunoglobulins [17] and when Juhlin et al. reported the presence of increased serum levels of IgE in many patients with atopic eczema [18]. Subsequently, other investigators conformed that up to 80% of patients with atopic eczema may have elevated serum IgE levels [19]. The regulation of IgE in the mouse and with some certainty also in humans strictly controlled by T cells. In both systems there is evidence that suppression of IgE synthesis is mediated by the T8+ (CD8) suppressor/cytotoxic T-cell subset [20–22]. This suggests a distinct T-cell defect in atopic individuals. More recently, it has become clear that the lymphokine IL-4 and possibly soluble Fc_{ε} receptor are essential factors stimulating in vitro-induced IgE synthesis [23–25]. One can hypothesise that the findings reported here may be related to elevated serum IgE levels in atopic disorders.

A causal role of IgE for the manifestation of allergic asthma and rhinitis has now been established. However, its importance for the manifestation of the dermatitis remains speculative. Morphologically, atopic eczema represents an eczematous infiltration with various cellular elements. Mononuclear cells are probably primarily responsible for the epidermal damage [26]. It is unclear how IgE participates in the pathogenesis of the cellular infiltration of the skin. Interesting recent observations indicate that antigen-presenting epidermal cells in biopsies of atopic eczema bear Fc_{ε} receptors which are occupied by IgE [27, 28]. This phenomenon, which positively correlates with serum IgE levels, may provide a clue to the role of IgE in atopic eczema.

In addition to the described dysregulation in the atopic humoral immune system, 80% of patients with atopic eczema manifest various abnormalities of cellular immunity [29]. Increased susceptibility to herpes virus, human papillomaviruses, vaccinia and certain bacterial and dermatophyte infections is often seen. Decreased delayed skin test responses to candidal, streptococcal and trichophytal antigens have also been noticed [30–32]. Reactions to PPD-tuberculin injected intracutaneously appeared to be significantly reduced in those patients with high serum IgE levels [32, 33]. As will be discussed later, the development of allergic contact eczema may also be reduced [33, 34]. In general, the observed immunological defects are mild and in many instances were shown to fluctuate with the severity of the dermatitis and with actual IgE levels.

Over the past decade much experimental effort has been devoted to the detection of the basic immunological defects which are presumably responsible for the observed deviations in vivo. Quantitative enumeration of rosette-forming T cells revealed a decrease of 30%–50% in the majority of patients with atopic eczema [35, 36]. Using monoclonal antibodies to cell surface antigens, several investigators reported a decreased proportion of circulating T3+ (CD3) and T8+ suppressor cells [37, 38]. In contrast, atopic patients with allergic rhinitis and asthma showed normal quantities of T-cell subpopulations in their peripheral blood. It should be noted, however, that patients with atopic eczema do not exhibit a global suppressor cell defect. Their concanavalin A-inducible suppressor cell activity was in the normal range [39].

Contradictory results were obtained for antigen-or mitogen-induced T-lymphocyte proliferation in atopic eczema. More consistently, the autologous mixed lymphocyte reaction was found to be impaired [40–42]. According to newer concepts, the autologous cell reaction represents an immune circuit that leads to activation of effector cells of the helper, suppressor and cytotoxic types [43]. Several authors concluded that a defective autologous cell reaction might be responsible for some of the immunoregulatory abnormalities observed in patients with atopic eczema [31, 40]. Leung et al. reported that T4+ (CD4) inducer T cells in patients with atopic eczema had failed to generate T8+ cytotoxic lymphocytes [44] and that this deficiency caused the impairment of the autologous lymphocyte reaction. Whether this defective T4+ subset is identical to the T4+ suppressor-inducer cell described more recently by Morimoto et al. [45] remains open.

It is beyond the scope of this review to discuss all the cellular deviations described to date in patients with atopic eczema, but one more finding deserves further discussion. The cytokine IL-1 contributes to T-cell activation. It possesses chemotactic activity for leucocytes and has a multitude of additional biologic activities [46]. It appears that in atopic eczema the production of this cytokine by blood monocytes and also epidermal cells is impaired [31, 47]. Räsänen et al. were capable of restoring the defective autologous mixed reaction of atopics by supplementation with IL-1. Therefore, dysregulation of IL-1 may contribute to the subtle cellular defects observed in some diseased individuals. Moreover, since IL-4 is known to play a unique role in the regulation of IgE synthesis, it seems even more warranted to study the secretion pattern of this lymphokine by T cells of atopic patients.

Clinical Studies on the Relationship of Allergic Contact Eczema and Atopic Eczema

General Considerations

The question whether or not allergic contact eczema and atopy are related to one another has become a matter of continuous debate because of its great practical importance. Even before detailed knowledge on the basic mechanisms of cellular immunology was available, much clinical work had concentrated on the capability of patients with atopic eczema to develop allergic contact eczema. Does pre-existing chronic atopic eczema influence the development of a delayed-type reaction? If CMI is impaired, this does not necessarily imply that the atopic individual will also acquire less contact allergy in his lifetime. The chronically damaged skin may facilitate sensitization to standard environmental sensitizers and thus compensate for endogenous cell-mediated defects [48, 49].

Principally two types of studies emerge from the literature: a prospective and a retrospective type. As the former type implies active sensitization of atopic and healthy individuals, only small cohorts of patients have been studied. This limits the significance of these studies. The second type suffers from one or another of the following drawbacks. On clinical grounds the patient selection was biased towards allergic contact eczema. Probably this has led to overestimation of the incidence of contact sensitivity in atopic eczema. Rarely, non-atopic and non-eczematous controls were tested in the same study, and consequently a comparison of contact sensitivity in the normal and the atopic population was not possible. Age and sex matching were often inadequate. Also, the comparability of these studies is limited by the fact that the definition of the atopic state was not uniform, and standardized criteria such as proposed by Hanifin and Rajka [52] for atopic eczema had not been applied. Another important point is the subjective evaluation of the patch test itself. As it is well accepted that patients with atopic eczema are more prone to skin irritation, positive patch test reactions in these patients have to be interpreted very cautiously [53, 54]. In most studies, the criteria separating a toxic from a true allergic reaction are not precisely stated. Last but not least, in several studies it cannot be clearly distinguished between the number of positive patients and the number of positive patch tests. This may have a definite impact on the interpretation of the results.

Experimental Contact Sensitization of Patients with Atopic Eczema

In the prospective type of studies patients with atopic eczema were exposed to a strong contact allergen to which they previously had not been sensitized. After several weeks the degree of sensitization was re-evaluated with the aid of patch tests. Ideally, an age- and sex-matched control group was subjected to the same procedure. With this method DNCB, which is otherwise known to sensitize 90% of normal individuals following exposure, was found to be less potent in some patients with atopic eczema. Palacios et al. showed that 30 of 39 atopic patients, 9 of 10 patients with nummular eczema and 13 of 15 patients with psoriasis vulgaris reacted positively [34]. The results of this work are of questionable significance because the atopics and the controls came from different ethnical groups. Forsbeck reported a reduced incidence of sensitization in patients with severe atopic eczema in a group of 85 patients sensitized to DNCB and parantitroso-dimethylaniline [33]. Interestingly, the degree of impairment was dependent on the serum IgE level. Only 18% of patients with a serum IgE >1000 U/ml became sensitized compared with 42% with a serum IgE <1000 U/ml. The impact of this work is limited by the fact that no controls without atopic eczema had been sensitized to DNCB.

Another paper postulating the reduced capability of patients with atopic eczema to mediate allergic contact sensitivity was presented by Jones et al. [50]. They investigated allergic contact sensitivity to *Rhus* in 171 American patients, 40 of whom had atopic eczema. Patch tests with *Rhus* oleoresin were positive in 61% of controls but in only 15% of atopics. This reduction of naturally acquired allergic sensitivity to *Rhus* might be the result of a more cautious behaviour of atopic individuals towards environmental contactants. However, a second *Rhus* patch test performed on the primarily non-sensitive individuals revealed that only 6% of atopic patients compared with 31% of the controls had become sensitized by the first patch test. This seems to indicate a true deficiency of some patients with atopic eczema to develop cellular immunity against the *Rhus* allergen. As early as 1960 Skog had reported on sensitization with 3-*n*-pentadecylcatechol (which is known to sensitize a great majority of individuals previously not exposed to *Rhus*). In his study marked differences could only be detected when atopic patients were evaluated according to the severity of their dermatitis. Then it became apparent that individuals with severe dermatitis were less frequently sensitized by the same procedure [51].

In summary, some patients with atopic eczema do not become sensitized to contactants under experimental conditions, which might reflect impaired CMI. The degree of impairment appears to correlate with the severity of the atopic eczema and the level of serum IgE. A cautious interpretation of these results is warranted as the total number of patients included in the studies described was small, calling for further confirmation of these findings. Moreover, it must be taken into consideration that the observed defect may not be primary but rather secondary to the high levels of IgE in these patients.

Acquired Contact Sensitization in Patients with Atopic Eczema

The retrospective type of studies compares the incidence of contact allergies in patients with and without an atopic background based on the analysis of patch tests. Undoubtedly, employing this study design it cannot be avoided that the results are influenced by a multitude of factors, leading to conflicting conclusions.

Despite the shortcomings, some of these studies on the incidence of contact allergy will be discussed in detail as a few conclusions can apparently be drawn. As will be shown below, the most important finding is the lack of convincing differences in patients with atopic eczema and those with other endogenous eczemas.

Routine patch testing by Rostenberg and Sulzberger in 1937 produced a higher incidence of reactions in patients with contact dermatitis than in any other group of dermatoses including atopic eczema [55]. Unfortunately, this paper was later on often incorrectly quoted as evidence for a decreased incidence of contact allergy in patients with atopic eczema. In fact in this study the reactions in patients with atopic eczema did not differ significantly from those in patients with other dermatoses than allergic contact eczema.

Another early report by Skog and Thyresson comparing a total of more than 3287 patch-tested patients with different types of eczema arrives at the conclusion that atopic patients are not particularly prone to developing contact dermatitis. Nineteen of 126 patients with atopic eczema and 17% with several other types of endogenous eczema showed contact sensitivity [56].

In 1970 a large series of patients was investigated by the International Contact Dermatitis Research Group, as a multicenter study of eight European contact dermatitis clinics [57]. This study included 4000 patients, all of which were subjected to patch tests with an identical series of 20 standard allergens. Of this group 233 had atopic eczema as a primary diagnosis. It was found that the atopic patients were as likely to develop allergic contact dermatitis as patients with seborrhoeic or nummular eczema [26%, 22%, 19%).

More recently Marghescu, investigating an equally large cohort, reported on patch test reactions in 4609 patients with different types of dermatitis, 129 of which were atopic [58]. Of the patients with contact dermatitis 57.9% showed a positive reaction, as did 39.5% of those with atopic eczema and 44.9% of those with dyshidrotic hand dermatitis. In part these patients may have also been atopic.

Thus in the most pertinent contributions advocating for a "normal" rate of contact sensitivity in atopic eczema, the incidence ranged from 16% to 26% to 39.5%. It was as high as 40.4% in another large study by the Belgian Contact Dermatitis Group published by Blondeel et al. [59].

Eczema is very often associated with the atopic state when it presents as a dyshidrotic vesicular eruption confined to the hands. Bandmann and co-workers even concluded from their work that eczema of the hands is the most frequent "mani"festation of atopy. They registered symptoms of dyshidrotic eczema in 44% of their atopic patients [60, 61]. More recently, Bäuerle et al. found that 63% of their 683 patients with hand eczema (all types) without a history of occupational provocation displayed features of atopy [62]. In the large clientele with eczema investigated by Agrup, 19% were considered to be atopic [63]. Schwanitz studied 58 patients with the dyshidrotic type of hand eczema and found 59% of his patients to have associated atopy [64]. The prevalence of atopy as based on the history of hay fever, eczema, wool intolerance and asthma was as high as 82% in another study dealing with 134 patients who had been compensated for work-related contact dermatitis of the hands [65]. Also, 82% of 50 housewives with hand eczema had a personal or family history of atopy compared with 28% of normal controls [66]. The incidence of atopy in the normal population is estimated to range from 10% to 20% depending on the criteria used for the definition of the atopic state [67]. In the material of Bäuerle 39% of patients with proven contact sensitization and hand eczema displayed three criteria of atopy. In the same study a comparably high incidence of atopy (34%) was found in a similar number of 164 patients with irritant hand eczema. Also Schwanitz and Agrup found a similar degree of allergic sensitization in their patients with atopic and non-atopic hand eczema. Thus, the studies on hand eczema provide evidence that there are no significant differences in the frequencies of positive patch tests between the atopic, the irritant, the nummular and the unclassifiable types.

These retrospective studies are not valid for establishing the incidence of contact eczema in atopics as compared with the normal population since the control group in these cases was naturally already highly selected for contact eczema. The proper control group would have been a non-selected, non-atopic population. For the same reason these studies also do not allow conclusions to be drawn concerning an impaired immune system in atopic individuals. They indicate rather that patients with atopic eczema can acquire contact allergy to a substantial degree.

Sensitization to Individual Allergens in Patients with Atopic Eczema

Nickel and Topicals

It is widely suspected that damaged (irritated) skin is more susceptible to contact allergy [49, 68, 69]. Therefore, some authors suspect a high rate of sensitization in patients with atopic eczema against individual allergens, e.g. topicals to which patients are amply exposed, as well as ubiquitous contact allergens such as nickel. In fact, some earlier investigators even declared nickel allergy to be a phenotypic property of atopic eczema [70, 71].

The normal population exhibitis a high frequency of nickel sensitivity, particularly among women. Of 1158 volunteers 9% of the women [72] and more recently 14% of German preschoolgirls were found to be sensitive [73]. In the USA the incidence of nickel sensitivity in contact allergic patients was 11% [74].

To investigate the relationship between nickel allergy and atopy several authors have assessed the incidence of atopic stigmata in nickel-sensitive subjects. Calnan and Caron stated that atopic signs and symptoms are not more frequent in nickel contact allergic patients than in a normal unselected population, ranging between 10% and 20% [75, 76], Caron, using the method of postal questionnaire, found 11% of 37 patients with proven nickel contact dermatitis to have both a personal and a family history of atopy. An investigation of 100 nickel hypersensitive patients by Malten concluded that 18% would have to be classified as atopic [77]. Both researchers concluded that the incidence of atopy was not higher in these nickel-sensitive patients compared with the general population. By using IgE as a parameter of atopy Wahlberg and Skog found only 4 of a total of 47 patients with nickel allergy to have elevated IgE levels. Only 9% of these patients evidenced overt atopic disease [78]. Prystowski showed that ear piercing increased the frequency of nickel sensitivity to a similar degree in patients with non-atopic as well as atopic skin [72].

Vice versa, while looking for the incidence of nickel allergy in atopic patients, a large number of investigators came to the conclusion that there was no significant difference when comparing patients with atopic eczema and other types of eczema. In atopic eczema the incidence of nickel sensitization ranged between 7.8% and 12.9%, with a clear preponderance of women and an increase in recent years [58, 59, 79]. In addition, in several of the studies cited, sensitization to dichromate and cobalt showed a similar incidence in atopic and non-atopic individuals. Schwanitz in agreement with Breit [80] reported that in vesicular hand eczema sensitization against metal salts occurred at about the same rate in non-atopic as in atopic patients. Also, contrary to what might have been suspected, in most studies there was no higher rate of sensitization to balsams (6.5% versus 6.7% in non-atopic individuals in Blondeel's study; 15.7% versus 19.7% in non-atopic women in Cronin's study; and 2.3% versus 5.6% of all patients tested in Marghescu's study).

In view of the relatively high incidence of positive patch test reactions to metal salts in atopic individuals (sometimes with an equally high frequency as in allergic contact eczema), one must be aware of the widely accepted fact that the atopic subject may often show a follicular or pustular non-allergic reaction when patch-tested with metal salts [53, 69, 81]. In a careful study retesting a major part of his patients, Wilson was able to prove that follicular reaction against nickel, arsenic, mercury and dichromate was often unspecific [82]. Only one of the eight patients with a positive reaction to nickel sulphate showed clinical evidence of nickel sensitivity. Also, in non-atopic subjects weak and moderately strong positive patch test reactions to metal salts may be of an irritant nature [54]. Unfortunately, most of the large studies discussed earlier do not clearly differentiate between true allergic and irritant reactions. Therefore, the real incidence of nickel sensitivity may be smaller than discussed above.

There are a few studies reporting an increased rate of contact sensitivity in atopic patients. Epstein and Mohajerin reported that 28 of 100 patients with atopic eczema reacted mainly to drugs compared with 9 of 100 with psoriasis and none of 20 with acne [83]. In another report on 120 patients sensitive to neomycin, the author classified 75% of this group as atopic [84]. These results are unusual as many other studies could either not confirm the predominance of sensitization to neomycin (and some other topical drugs) or, if present at all, the difference was much less distinctive [58, 59, 85].

Probably a sampling effect of patients accounted for these great differences in results. In fact, the work of Magnusson et al. clearly shows that the frequency of positive reactions to various substances is greatly influenced by sex distribution and localization of the eczema. These authors also suspected significant differences in the composition of the patient population of various clinics. It is easily conceivable that the proportion of atopic patients presenting predominantly with eczema of the hands influenced the prevalence of contact sensitivity in atopic eczema in one or the other study.

In summary, these results show that patients with atopic eczema definitely can become sensitized to standard antigens at about the same rate as patients with other "endogenous" eczemas. There also appears to be no consistent difference in the sensitization rate to individual allergens such as balsams and other topicals and metal salts.

Inhalant Allergens

Is there a pathogenetic role for inhalant proteinaceous allergens in atopic eczema? This question is as old as the term atopic eczema itself and has been answered differently at various times. The opinion that allergens and especially inhalant allergens are a major causal factor was outlined elegantly by Tuft in 1949 [86]. He reported on a series of 54 patients of whom 46 where sensitive to extracts of floor dust made from their own houses, two patients being "cured" be cleaning their houses.

After this early enthusiasm scepticism about the role of allergens in atopic eczema grew. The following observations were used as major arguments against a causal role: Desensitization is not a consistently effective treatment for atopic eczema. Injections of allergens into the skin of allergic individuals give rise to wheal and flare reactions without any indication that this procedure causes eczema. Patients with atopic eczema often also suffer from an inhalant allergy. Consequently, the observed high levels of IgE antibodies to dust allergens were explained by the co-existing inhalant allergy rather than being related to the dermatitis.

With the ability to measure specific IgE levels it has become clear that there is a proportion of patients with atopic eczema who never have asthma, and these too may have very high levels of IgE antibodies to house dust mite antigen. Thus, the levels of IgE antibodies to inhalant allergens cannot be explained by concomitant asthma but rather reflect allergy to mite antigen in patients with atopic eczema. As these patients are continuously exposed to house dust in their environment, Platts-Mills et al. posed the question, what is the effect of large quantities of allergen applied directly to the skin by a patch test? Because most allergens have a molecular weight larger than 10 000 dalton and are water soluble the authors mildly abraded the skin to remove the keratinized layer before applying the allergen on a pad of gauze for 48 h. These patch tests performed with 5 μg proteinaceous antigen of the house dust mite were able to elicit an eczematous reaction in a subgroup of patients [87]. Microscopic investigation of the reaction revealed a cellular infiltrate in these patch test lesions similar to that observed by Dvorak et al. in the cutaneous basophil hypersensitivity reaction [9]. This latter is a form of DTH which, as reported by several researchers, preceeds a classic DTH lesion. Platts-Mills et al. felt that this type of experiment provided strong although circumstantial evidence that inhalant allergens such as house dust may play a role in the pathogenesis of the dermatitis of atopic patients.

More recently, Reitamo used birch pollen and dust mite antigen at a 500-fold concentration of that employed in the prick test and produced 9 positive eczematous patch test reactions in 17 patients with atopic eczema [88]. Most of these patients had positive prick test reactions to birch pollen and house dust mite antigen. These authors performed immunohistopathological investigations on the positive lesions and could show that the epicutaneously applied protein allergens had elicited spongiosis, microvesiculation and infiltration of T lymphocytes in a manner very similar to a classic DTH reaction. In contrast to Platts-Mills, they did not find a predominance of basophils in the biopsies, which might be explained by different developmental stages of the skin lesions. Thus, it appears that in certain patients with atopic eczema a proteinaceous inhalant allergen when applied epicutaneously may elicit an eczematous reaction in the skin which more or less resembles that observed in classical DTH. As favoured by Reitamo and Platts-Mills, these allergens may be capable of primarily eliciting the eczematous reaction of atopic eczema. Alternatively, as stressed by others, they may act as secondary agents which are only effective on irritated skin [53, 89].

In fact, much more work is necessary to confirm the concept of exogenous contact with inhalant allergens either causing or precipitating atopic eczema. It has to be clarified whether specific IgE bound to Langerhans cells in the epidermis may play a role in presenting these antigens. Last but not least, it must be ascertained whether the observed epicutaneous reaction really represents an immunological effector phase or an irritant reaction. In view of the attractive hypothesis that a DTH reaction to contact with inhalant allergens may precipitate atopic eczema, further experimental efforts seem to be justified. Once a causal role for atopens has been established, new concepts for specific desensitization of patients with atopic eczema will be required.

Conclusions

Allergic contact eczema and atopic eczema both seem to represent effector phases of DTH of the skin. While allergic contact eczema is caused by a defined allergen, the evidence for an allergen eliciting atopic eczema is at most circumstantial at present. Moreover, it remains speculative how the observed dysregulation in antibody production contributes to the manifestation of atopic eczema. In vitro investigations on the blood leukocytes and skin of patients with atopic eczema have shown subtle deviations in cellular immune pathways. The evidence for a reduced ability of patients with atopic eczema to develop DTH to contact allergens is however weak. The prospective studies performed are few, and the number of patients investigated is small. Large retrospective studies on the other hand have shown that atopic patients are as likely to develop allergic contact dermatitis as patients with seborrhoeic or nummular eczema. From the practical standpoint this means that allergic contact eczema has to be suspected in atopic eczema whenever it takes an unfavourable course.

References

1. Landsteiner K, Chase MW (1942) Experiments on transfer of cutaneous sensitivity to simple compounds. Proc Soc Exp Biol Med 49: 688–690
2. Baer RL (1986) The mechanism of allergic contact hypersensitivity. In: Fisher AA (ed) Contact dermatitis, 3rd edn. Lea and Febiger, Philadelphia, pp 1–8
3. Stingl G, Katz SI, Clement L, Green I, Shevach EM (1978) Immunologic functions of Ia-bearing epidermal Langerhans cells. J Immunol 121: 2005–2013
4. Polak L (1978) Recent trends in the immunology of contact sensitivity. 1. Contact Dermatitis 4: 249–255
5. Polak L (1978) Recent trends in the immunology of contact sensitivity. 2. Contact Dermatitis 4: 259–263
6. Silvennoinen-Kassinen S, Jakkula H, Karvonen J (1986) Helper cells (Leu-3a+) carry the specificity of nickel sensitivity reaction in vitro in humans. J Invest Dermatol 86: 18–20
7. Knop J (1985) Immunologische Grundlagen des allergischen Kontakt-Ekzems. Hautarzt 35: 617–622
8. Askenase PW, van Loveren H (1983) Delayed-type hypersensitivity: activation of mast cells by antigen-specific T-cell factors initiates the cascade of cellular interactions. Immunol Today 4: 259–264
9. Dvorak HF, Dvorak AM, Simpson BA, Richerson HB, Leskowitz S, Karnovsky MJ (1970) Specificity of basophils and lymphocytes in cutaneous basophil hypersensitivity. J Immunol 114: 507–511
10. Marchal G, Seman M, Milon G, Trufa-Bachi P, Zilberfarb V (1982) Local adoptive transfer of skin delayed-type hypersensitivity initiated by a single T lymphocyte. J Immunol 129: 954–958
11. Willis CM, Young E, Brandon DR, Wilkinson JD (1986) Immunopathological and ultrastructural findings in human allergic and irritant contact dermatitis. Br J Dermatol 115: 305–316
12. Levine BB, Ojeda A, Benacerraf B (1963) Studies on artificial antigens. III. The genetic control of the immune response to hapten-polyl-l-lysine conjugates in guinea pigs. J Exp Med 118: 953–957
13. Walker FB, Smith PD, Maibach HI (1967) Genetic factors in human allergic contact dermatitis. Int Arch Allergy Appl Immunol 32: 453–462
14. Wise F, Sulzberger MB (1933) Editorial remarks. In: Yearbook of dermatology and syphilology. Yearbook Medical, Chicago, p 59
15. Rajka G (1975) Atopic dermatitis. In: Rook A (ed) Major problems in dermatology. Saunders, London, pp 2–14
16. McDevitt HO (1976) Genetic considerations in atopic and other dermatologic conditions. J Invest Dermatol 67: 320–326
17. Ishizaka K, Ishizaka T (1967) Identification of E antibodies as a carrier of reaginic activity. J Immunol 99: 1187–1198
18. Juhlin L, Johannson SGO, Bennich H, Högman C, Thyresson N (1969) Immunoglobulin E in dermatoses: levels in atopic dermatitis and urticaria. Arch Dermatol 100: 12–16
19. Gurevitch AW, Heiner DC, Reisner RM (1973) IgE in atopic dermatitis and other common dermatoses. Arch Dermatol 107: 712–715
20. Ishizaka K (1976) Cellular events in the IgE antibody response. Adv Immunol 23: 1–75
21. Tada T (1975) Regulation of reaginic antibody formation in animals. Prog Allergy 19: 122–126
22. Geha RS, Reinherz EL, Leung D, McKee KT, Schlossman S, Rosen FS (1981) Deficiency of suppressor T cells in the hyperimmunoglobulin E syndrome. J Clin Invest 67: 783–791
23. Pene J, Rousset F, Briere F, Chretien I, Paliard X, Banchereau J, Spits H, De Vries JE (1988) IgE production by normal human B cells induced by alloreactive cell clones is mediated by Il-4 and suppressed by IFN-g. J Immunol 141: 1218–1224
24. Del Prete G, Maggi E, Parronchi P, Chretien I, Tiri A, Macchia D, Ricci M, Banchereau J, De Vries J, Romagnani S (1988) Il-4 is an essential factor for the IgE synthesis induced in vitro by human T cell clones and their supernatants. J Immunol 140: 4193–4198
25. Sarfati M, Rector E, Wong K, Rubio-Trujillo M, Sehon AH, Delespesse G (1984) In vitro synthesis of IgE by human lymphocytes. II. Enhancement of the spontaneous IgE synthesis of IgE binding factors secreted by RPMI 8866 lymphoblastoid B cells. Immunology 53: 197–202
26. Tong AKF, Mihm MC Jr. (1986) The pathology of atopic dermatitis. Clin Rev Allergy 4: 27–42
27. Brynzeel-Koomen C, vanWichen DF, Toonstra J, Berrens L, Brynzeel PLB (1986) The presence of IgE molecules on epidermal Langerhans cells in patients with atopic dermatitis. Arch Dermatol Res 278: 199–205
28. Barker JWN, Alegre VA, MacDonald DM (1988) Surface-

bound immunoglobulin E on antigen-presenting cells in cutaneous tissue of atopic dermatitis. J Invest Dermatol 90: 117–121
29. Hanifin JM, Lobitz WC Jr (1977) Newer concepts of atopic dermatitis. Arch Dermatol 113: 663–670
30. Jones HE, Reinhardt JH, Rinaldi M (1973) A clinical, mycologic and immunologic survey on dermatophytosis. Arch Dermatol 108: 61–65
31. Räsänen L, Lehto M, Reunala T, Jansen C, Lehtinen M, Leinikki P (1987) Langerhans cell- and T-lymphocyte functions in patients with atopic dermatitis with disseminated cutaneous herpes simplex virus infections. J Invest Dermatol 89: 15–18
32. Rajka G (1967) Delayed dermal and epidermal reactivity in topic dermatitis (prurigo Besnier). I. Delayed reactivity to bacterial and mold allergens. Acta Derm Venereol (Stockh) 47: 158–162
33. Forsbeck M, Hovmark A, Skog E (1976) Patch testing, tuberculin testing and sensitization with dinitro chlorobenzene and nitrosodimethylanilini of patients with atopic dermatitis. Acta Derm Venereol (Stockh) 56: 135–138
34. Palacios J, Fuller EW, Blaylock WK (1966) Immunologcal capabilities of patients with atopic dermatitis. J Invest Dermatol 487: 484–490
35. Byrom NA, Timlin DA (1979) Immune status in atopic eczema: a survey, Br J Dermatol 100: 491–498
36. Schöpf E (1974) Störung zellvermittelter Immunreaktionen bei Neurodermitis atopica. Dermatologica 149: 210–219
37. Leung DYM, Rhodes AR, Geha RS (1981) Enumeration of T cell subsets in atopic dermatitis using monoclonal antibodies. J Allergy Clin Immunol 67: 450–455
38. Fulton R, Thivolet J, Garcier F, Gaucherand M (1981) Les sous populations de lymphocytes T helper et suppressor studies par les anticorps monoclonaux dans diversies dermatoses. Ann Dermatol Venereol 108: 243–250
39. Schuster DL, Person D, Bonjiovanni B, Levisas AI (1979) Suppressor cell function in atopic dermatitis associated with elevated immunoglobulin E. J Allergy Clin Immunol 64: 139–145
40. Leung DYM, Saryan YA, Frankel R, Lareau, Geha RS (1983) Impairment of the autologous mixed lymphocyte reaction in atopic dermatitis. J Clin Invest 72: 1482–1486
41. Bovbjerg DH, Wang VA, Schwab R, Lebenger KS, Siskind GW, Weksler ME (1985) Lymphocyte transformation induced by autologous cells XVII. Lower autologous mixed lymphocyte reaction in subjects with a history of hay fever. Int Arch Allergy Appl Immunol 78: 332–334
42. Dirienzo W, Bagnasco M, Caria M, Chimini G, Ciprandi G, Ferrini S, Canonica GW (1984) Activation of T lymphocytes and autologous mixed lymphocyte reaction in allergic patients. Allergy 53: 272–277
43. Smolen JS, Chused TM, Novotny EA, Steinberg AD (1982) The human autologous mixed lymphocyte reaction. J Immunol 129: 1050–1053
44. Leung DYM, Wood SN, Dubey D, Rhodes AR, Geha RS (1983) Cellular basis of defective cell-mediated lympholysis in atopic dermatitis. J Immunol 130: 1687–1692
45. Morimoto C, Letvin NL, Distaso JA, Aldrich WR, Schlossman SF (1985) The isolation and characterization of the human suppressor T cell subset. J Immunol 134: 1508–1515
46. Sauder DN (1984) Epidermal cytokines: properties of epidermal cell thymocyte-activating factor (ETAF). Lymphokine Res 3: 145–151
47. Mizoguchi M, Furusawa S, Okitsu S, Yoshino K (1985) Macrophage-derived interleukin-1 activity in atopic dermatitis (abstract). J Invest Dermatol [Suppl] 85: 155s–160s
48. Stüttgen G (1977) Die Ekzemgenese aus pathophysiologischer Sicht. Z Hautkr [Suppl 2] 52: 8–15
49. Frosch PJ (1985) Hautirritation und empfindliche Haut. Grosse, Berlin
50. Jones HE, Lewis CW, McMarlin SL (1973) Allergic contact sensitivity in atopic dermatitis. Arch Dermatol 107: 217–222
51. Skog E (1960) Primary irritant and allergic eczematous reactions induced in patients with different dermatoses. Acta Derm Venereol (Stockh) 40: 307–316
52. Hanifin JM‹ Rajka G (1980) Diagnostic features of atopic dermatitis. Acta Derm Venereol [Suppl] (Stockh) 92: 44–47
53. Fisher AA (1986) Contact dermatitis in atopic individuals. In: Fisher AA (ed) Contact dermatitis, 3rd edn. Lea and Febiger, Philadelphia, p 133
54. Fischer T, Rystedt I (1985) False-positive, follicular and irritant patch test reactions to metal salts. Contact Dermatitis 12: 93–98
55. Rostenberg A Jr, Sulzberger MB (1937) Some results of patch tests: compilation and discussion of cutaneous reactions to about 500 different substances as elicited by over 10 000 tests in approximately 1000 patients. Arch Dermatol Syph 35: 433–454
56. Skog E, Thyresson N (1953) The occupational significance of some common contact allergens. Acta Derm Venereol (Stockh) 33: 65–74
57. Cronin E, Bandmann H-J, Calnan CD, Fregert S, Hjorth N, Magnusson B, Maibach HI, Malten K, Meneghini CL, Pirilä V, Wilkinson DS (1970) Contact dermatitis in the atopic. Acta Derm Venereol (Stockh) 50: 183–187
58. Marghescu S (1985) Patch test reactions in atopic patients. Acta Derm Venereol (Stockh) 114: 113–116
59. Blondeel A, Achten G, Dooms-Goossens A, Buekens P, Buekens P, Broeck W, Oleffe J (1987) Atopie et allergie de contact. Ann Dermatol Venereol 114: 203–209
60. Bandmann H-J, Agathos M (1980) Die atopische Handdermatitis. Dermatosen 28: 110–113
61. Breit R, Leutgeb C, Bandmann H-J (1972) Zum neurodermitischen Handekzem. Arch Dermatol Forsch 244: 353–354
62. Bäurle G, Hornstein OP, Diepgen TL (1985) Professionelle Handekzeme und Atopie. Dermatosen 33: 161–165
63. Agrub G (1969) Hand eczema and other hand dermatoses in south Sweden. Acta Derm Venereol [Suppl 61] 49: 1–91
64. Schwanitz H-J (1988) Atopic palmoplantar eczema. Springer, Berlin Heidelberg New York
65. Shumunes E, Keil J (1984) The role of atopy in occupational dermatoses. Contact Dermatitis 11: 174–178
66. Glickman FS, Silvers SH (1967) Hand eczema and atopy in housewives. Arch Dermatol 95: 487–489
67. Carr RD, Berke M, Becker SW (1964) Incidence of atopy in the general population. Arch Dermatol 89: 87–92
68. Foussereau J, Cavelier C (1978) Toxische Dermatitis und Pseudo-Kontaktallergie. Dermatosen 26: 156–161
69. Fisher AA (1986) The role of patch testing. In: Fisher AA (ed) Contact dermatitis, 3rd edn. Lea and Febiger, Philadelphia, p 11
70. Blaylock WK (1976) Atopic dermatitis: diagnosis and pathobiology. J Allergy Clin Immunol 57: 62–79
71. Dobson R (1963) Discussion on Vandenberg and Epstein: experimental nickel contact sensitization. J Invest Dermatol 41: 416
72. Prystowsky SD, Allen AM, Odon RB, Akers WA (1979) Allergic contact hypersensitivity to nickel, neomycin,

ethylenediamine and benzocaine. Arch Dermatol 115: 959–962
73. Kunz B, Ring J, Überla K (1990) Frequency of contact dermatitis and contact sensitization in preschool children (abstract). Arch Dermatol Res 281: 544
74. North American Contact Dermatitis Group (1973) Epidemiology of contact dermatitis in North America 1972. Arch Dermatol 108: 537–540
75. Calnan CD (1956) Nickel dermatitis. Br J Dermatol 68: 229–236
76. Caron GA (1964) Nickel sensitivity and atopy. Br J Dermatol 76: 384–387
77. Malten KE (1971) Nickel-allergic contact dermatitis. Dermatologica 142: 113–116
78. Wahlberg JE, Skog E (1971) Nickel allergy and atopy. Threshold of nickel sensitivity and immunoglobulin E determination. Br J Dermatol 85: 97–104
79. Pürschel W, Ditrich O (1989) Neurodermitis atopica und Kontaktallergie. Allergologie 12: 203–208
80. Breit R (1981) Positive Epicutantestreaktionen bei Dermatitis atopica. Hautarzt [Suppl V] 32: 147–148
81. Wahlberg JE, Maibach HJ (1981) Sterile cutaneous pustules: a manifestation of primary irritancy. Identification of contact pustulogens. J Invest Dermatol 76: 381–383
82. Wilson HTH (1955) Standard patch tests in eczema and dermatitis. Br J Dermatol 67: 291–298
83. Epstein S, Mohajerin AH (1964) Incidence of contact sensitivity in atopic dermatitis. Arch Dermatol 90: 284–287
84. Epstein S (1965) Neomycin sensitivity and atopy. Dermatologica 130: 280–286
85. Magnusson B, Fregert S, Hjorth N, Hovding G, Pirilä V, Skog E (1969) Routine patch testing. 5th report by the Scandinavian Committee for Standardisation of Routine Patch Testing. Acta Derm Venereol (Stockh) 49: 556–563
86. Tuft LA (1949) Importance of inhalant allergens in atopic dermatitis. J Invest Dermatol 12: 211–219
87. Platts-Mills TAE, Mitchell EB, Rowntree S, Chapman MD, Wilkins SR (1983) The role of dust mite allergens in atopic dermatitis. Clin Exp Dermatol 8: 233–247
88. Reitamo S, Visa K, Kähönen K, Käyhkö, Stubb S, Salo OP (1986) Eczematous reactions in atopic patients caused by epicutaneous testing with inhalant allergens. Br J Dermatol 114: 303–309
89. Strauss JS, Kligman AM (1956) The relationship of atopic allergy and dermatitis. Arch Dermatol 75: 806–811
90. Schultz Larsen F, Holm NV, Henningsen K (1986) Atopic dermatitis. A genetic-epidemiologic study in a population-based twin sample. J Am Acad Dermatol 15: 487–494

Immunodeficiency Syndromes and Atopic Eczema

P. Fritsch and H. Hintner

Introduction

"Eczemas" are a not infrequently associated symptom of primary immunodeficiencies (PID). Morphologically, these dermatitic lesions are of varied appearance, often fairly indistinctive and difficult to classify. They have been referred to as "eczematoid", "nummular", "seborrhoeic", "resembling atopic eczema" or atopic eczema (AE). This latter point has aroused considerable interest in the past few decades because of the known abnormalities of the humoral and cell-mediated immune system in AE. If some PID are indeed linked to *unequivocal* AE – a question far from trivial – they might provide useful clues to the pathogenesis of AE. Only recently, Saurat et al. [43, 44, 45] reviewed this subject. They were the first to apply the clinical criteria of AE as formulated by Hanifin and Rajka [16] to the eczemas of PID: Wiskott-Aldrich syndrome met these criteria, but for other PID the evidence was incomplete at best or unconvincing.

Obviously, any definitive conclusion on this subject is hampered by the paucity of cases reported and by the often rather vague description of skin signs, which make retrospective evaluation doubtful. In this review, we wish to address again the following questions: Which PID syndromes are in a significant proportion of cases accompanied by eczematous lesions, and which of these are clearly AE? Is there any obvious common immunologic denominator among these syndromes and AE?

Primary and Secondary Immune Deficiencies

Immunodeficiency disorders are conventionally classified into primary and secondary types. PID occur with low incidence but are of high diversity. Only a limited number of these disorders have been defined at the molecular level [6, 42]. They are developmental or genetic disorders due to one or a few distinct abnormalities of the immune system, often accompanied by secondary adaptive phenomena. Any element of the major components of the immune system (humoral, cell-mediated, phagocytic and the complement system) can be involved (Table 1), the resulting disorders ranging from fatal disturbances to mere laboratory anomalies, which may go unnoticed.

Secondary, i.e. acquired, disorders with impairment of the immune system, in contrast, are very common and constitute a major health threat in both the Third World countries (hypoalimentation, endemic infectious diseases, parasitic infestations) and the Western world (old age, disturbances of metabolism like diabetes, renal insufficieny, alcoholism, neoplastic diseases). Viral infections are a prominent cause of immunosuppression, the most drastic example being the pandemic of the acquired immunodeficiency syndrome (AIDS). In the past decade, iatrogenic immunodeficiency states have substantially gained in importance in the context of cytostatic medication and organ transplantation. In many secondary immune deficiencies, T-cell suppression plays a pivotal role. As a rule, the immune abnormalities are more complex than in PID and less clearly defined but often potentially reversible.

The impairment of host defense mechanisms results in infections as the hallmark of immunodeficiency disorders. Infections are more frequent, more severe and prone to recurrence in immunocompromised individuals; they present under unusual clinical appearances and take unusual courses. The spectrum of pathogens involved is more diverse than in the normal host and includes opportunistic agents. It appears that specific classes of causative organisms and specific disease manifestations (Table 2) are related to specific immune defects. The organ systems most commonly involved are those with direct contact with the environment, i.e. skin, respiratory and gastrointestinal tracts. As the second major feature of immunodeficiency disorders, defects of immune surveillance lead to an increased incidence of tumors, frequently of the lymphoreticular system, skin, gut or the central nervous system. Finally, as a consequence of immunological imbalance, immunodeficiency syndromes are often complicated by autoimmune processes, such as lupus erythematosus,

Table 1. Classification of primary immunodeficiency disease (adapted from WHO Report 1983, [54])

Primary specific immunodeficiencies	Complement deficiencies	Defects of phagocytic function
A. Predominant antibody defects 1 X-linked agammaglobulinaemia 2 X-linked hypogammaglobulinaemia with growth hormone deficiency 3 Autosomal recessive agammaglobulinaemia 4 Immunoglobulin deficiency with increased IgM (and IgG) 5 IgA deficiency 6 Selective deficiency of other immunoglobulin isotypes 7 K chain deficiency 8 Antibody deficiency with normal γ-globulin levels or hypergammaglobulinaemia 9 Immunodeficiency with thymoma 10 Transient hypogammaglobulinaemia of infancy 11 Common variable immunodeficiency with predominant B-cell defect (a–d) Various defects of B-cell maturation leading to low B-cell number and/or abnormal proportion of B-cell subtypes 12 Common variable immunodeficiency with predominant immunoregulatory T-cell disorders (a) Deficiency of helper T cells (b) Presence of activated suppressor T cells 13 Common variable immunodeficiency with autoantibodies to B or T cells B. Predominant defects of cell-mediated immunity 14 Combined immunodeficiency with predominant T-cell defect 15 Purine-nucleoside phosphorylase deficiency 16 Severe combined immunodeficiency with adenosine deaminase deficiency 17 Severe combined immunodeficiency (a) Reticular dysgenesis (b) Low T- and B-cell numbers (c) Low T-cell and normal B-cell numbers (Swiss) (d) Bare lymphocyte syndrome C. Immunodeficiency associated with other defects 18 Transcobalamin 2 deficiency 19 Wiskott-Aldrich syndrome 20 Ataxia telangiectasia 21 Third and fourth pouch/arch (DiGeorge's) syndrome	Deficiencies of single complement components (Clq, Clr, C4, C2, C3, C5–C9), Cl inhibitor and C3b inactivator deficiency	A. Defects of mobility and adherence Actin dysfunction Chediak-Higashi syndrome Shwachman disease GP110 deficiency B. Defective endocytosis and killing GP150 deficiency Chronic granulomatous disease X-linked Autosomal recessive 6-PD deficiency myeloperoxidase deficiency

rheumatoid arthritis- and dermatomyositis-like conditions [45, 48].

Cutaneous signs occur frequently in primary and secondary immunodeficiencies, conforming to the pattern outlined above [2, 32, 41, 45, 52]. Skin infections are one of the predominant features. Aggressive and recurrent pyodermas and abscesses by gram-positive and gram-negative organisms arise in immunoglobulin-deficiency syndromes; extensive and aggressive mycotic and viral infections in defects of cell-mediated immunity; epidermodysplasia-like eruptions of viral warts; necrotising and generalised herpes simplex and herpes zoster; extensive dermatomycoses and candidiasis; and a vast number of unusual opportunistic infections, like cutaneous cryptococcosis, histoplasmosis and infections with other rare fungi or with algae or protozoa. Skin tumors are observed with an unusual incidence: squamous cell carcinomas both from sites of chronic actinic damage and viral papillomas, melanoma, Kaposi's sarcoma – up to the advent of AIDS considered an odd rarity – and lymphomas of the skin [17, 46]. They all prove considerably more aggressive than in the immunocompetent host.

As a final category, the skin expresses a spectrum of

additional signs in immunodeficiency disorders which are not so obviously or not linked at all to the immune defect proper but may be of considerable diagnostic importance [2, 41, 45, 52, 53]. For example, pityrosporum tends to proliferate in some of these syndromes and gives rise to "seborrhoeic dermatitis"; Epstein-Barr virus (EBV)-infection leads to the expression of "hairy leukoplakia" in AIDS patients; pigment abnormalities in the Chédiak-Higashi syndrome; teleangiectasias in ataxia teleangiectatica, ichthyosis and developmental defects in a variety of hereditary syndromes associated with immune defects. As one of these less distinctive symptoms, PID may be associated with "eczemas".

The "Immune Defect" in Atopic Eczema

Clinical and laboratory features indicate that host defense is impaired in AE, and that abnormalities of the cell- and antibody-mediated immunity play a role in its pathogenesis [23]: AE patients are heavily colonised by saprophytic and pathogenic skin flora, even if no signs of infection are manifest; they suffer from an increased susceptibility to bacterial (*Staphylococcus aureus*), viral (herpes viruses, vaccinia, human papillomavirus, molluscum contagiosum [28]) and fungal (*Candida*, dermatophytes) infections. On the other hand, the susceptibility of AE patients to sensitisation with specific contact allergens (e. G. DNCB) is decreased, and delayed-type hypersensitivity skin tests (candidal, streptococcal, fungal and other antigens) are frequently hypo- or non-reactive. This reaction pattern is obviously linked to the low T3+ cell (T3 = common T-cell antigen) and T8+ (suppressor/cytotoxic) cell numbers in the majority of AE patients; an additional defect of the T4+ (helper/inducer) T-cell subset may be conducive to the lack of a normal T8+ cytotoxic T cell function. Dysfunction of IgE suppressor T cells is the likely cause of serum IgE elevation, which represents the major serological alteration in many AE patients. Hypergammaglobulinemia E is reflected by a high incidence of positive skin tests and radioallergoabsorbent (RAST) tests reactive to a variety of common environmental, food and other antigens, both of which may or may not be of clinical significance in a given case. The pivotal role of impaired T-cell function in the pathogenesis of AE is also suggested by the observation that thymopentin, a synthetic analogue of thymopoietin, may restore T-cell function in AE and lead to clinical improvement [15, 21].

These major immunological alterations are supplemented by a number of less consistent minor features suggesting that the pathogenesis of AE is more complex and may be heterogenous. Several important questions are as yet unsettled, e.g. the impact of feedback mechanisms of histamine and other mediators on T-cell function.

Table 2. Specific defects in host defense that predispose patients to infections with selective groups of pathogens (adapted from Peterson [34])

Host defence abnormality	Major pathogens
Agammaglobulinaemia	*Streptococcus pneumoniae, Haemophilus influenzae, Neisseria meningitidis*, ECHO viruses
Complement deficiency	
Cl, 2, 3, or 4, factor B	*Streptococcus pneumoniae, Staphylococcus aureus, Strept. pyogenes*, aerobic gram-negative bacili, *N. meningitidis*, H. influenzae
C5, 6, 7, or 8	*N. meningitidis, N. gonorrhoeae*
Splenectomy (or hyposplenism)	*Strept. pneumoniae, H. influenzae, N. meningitidis*
Neutrophil disorders	
Chemotactic dysfunction	*Staph. aureus, H. influenzae, Candida, Cryptococcus*
Microbicidal dysfunction	*Staph. aureus, Pseudomonas sp., Serratia, Aspergillus, Candida*
Granulocytopenia	*Escherichia coli, Pseudomonas aeruginosa, Klebsiella pneumoniae, Staph. aureus, Staph. epidermidis, Corynebacterium* sp., *Aspergillus, Candida*
Cell-mediated immune disorders	Mycobacteria, *Nocardia, Listeria, Legionella, Pneumocystis, Toxoplasma*, herpes viruses, fungi

Eczemas in Primary Immunodeficiency Disorders

A number of non-specific causes could account for the higher than average incidence of unspecified "eczemas" in PID: a more abundant and more diverse skin flora, particularly of *Pityrosporum ovale* (seborrhoeic dermatitis), autosensitisation processes, metabolic disturbances due to catabolism, malabsorption, chronic illness and wasting, irritative dermatitis due to environmental factors in the course of episodes of infection, fever, sweating and perifocal skin irritation in pyodermas. Finally, most individuals with PID are infants or children, whose propensity for skin irritation and dermatitis per se is commonplace. We feel that most eczemas in PID ought to be viewed with this background in mind. A specific association of eczemas with PID should be suspected only if eczemas are a constant or at least much more frequent symptom than in the general population, and if there is evidence that the course of the eczemas may parallel the general course of the disease.

Table 3 gives a list of those PID in which "eczemas" have been described [45]. Fairly often, these eczemas had features of seborrhoeic or another non-specific type of dermatitis but not of AE. It appears that these eczemas do not constitute a constant or major symptom in any of these latter syndromes. Moreover, these PID are very heterogenous and do not share a common immunologic denominator.

The situation is different with AE-like eczemas in PID. AE appears to be a regular feature in three types of PID and may perhaps be occasionally encountered in a few others.

Table 3. Primary Immunodeficiencies associated with eczemas [45]

Wiskott-Aldrich syndrome[a]
Selective IgA deficiency[a]
Selective IgM deficiency[b]
Hyper IgE syndrome[a]
X-linked agammaglobulinaemia[b]
X-linked immunodeficiency with hyper-IgM[b]
Ataxia teleangiectatica[b]
Severe combined immunodeficiency
Primary neutropenias
Tuftsin deficiency
Shwachman syndrome[b]
Chronic granulomatous disease[b]
Biotin-dependent multiple carboxylase deficiency
C5 dysfunction

[a] associated with atopic eczema
[b] occasional association with atopic eczema claimed in some reports

PIDs Frequently Associated with AE

Wiskott-Aldrich Syndrome

Wiskott-Aldrich syndrome (WAS) is a rare (4 of 10^6 living newborns) and serious X-linked recessive disorder, characterised by the triad of severe, intractable AE, thrombocytopenic purpura and susceptibility to infections. Mean survival time is 6.5 years [33].

Clinical Features. The presenting sign is a severely pruritic, therapy-resistant dermatitis of early onset (within the 2nd month after birth). Purpuric eruptions and bleeding tendency (such as bloody diarrhoea) may be present even before the onset of the eczema. A characteristic sign is linear haemorrhage within scratch marks [45]. The bleeding tendency often improves when the child gets older. Susceptibility to infections usually becomes apparent at the age of 5–6 months, when maternal antibodies are lost. Main complications are infections of the respiratory tract, meningitis and otitis, the major causative organism being gram-positive and gram-negative cocci, *Haemophilus influenzae* and *Escherichia coli*. Infections may further deteriorate thrombopenia and lead to episodes of bleeding. Parallel to progressive impairment of T-cell function (vide infra), susceptibility to viral and opportunistic infections increases at pre-school and school age, resulting in significant morbidity – severe herpes virus infections, extensive viral warts and, occasionally, *Pneumocystis carinii* pneumonia. There is an increased incidence of non-Hodgkin's lymphomas, particularly of the central nervous system (relative risk approximately 100x).

Immunological Abnormalities. The basic defect of WAS is still unknown; it may be linked to a defect of the major membrane glycoprotein of platelets and T cells, sialophorin [30]. Abnormalities pertain to both humoral and cell-mediated immunity as well as to the monocyte-macrophage system. While IgG is normal, IgA and IgE are high, and IgM is absent or low (as are isohaemagglutinins). There is no humoral response to polysaccharides and various protein antigens. Immunoglobulins may be synthesised and metabolised at a higher rate than normal [7]. B- and T-cell numbers and functions appear normal initially but deteriorate progressively during childhood. T cells are reactive to mitogens, but their response to antigens becomes progressively impaired. Skin tests to the usual recall antigens are negative: attempts at sensitisation with DNCB are unsuccesful. Monocytes become unresponsive to chemotactic stimuli, probably due to the effect of a specific lymphocyte product [6].

Eczema in WAS. The eczema found is clinically indistinguishable from AE; other manifestations of atopy, like rhinitis, conjunctivitis or asthma, are notably absent. According to Saurat [44], the eczema of WAS fulfils the criteria of AE as put forward by Hanifin and Rajka [16] and thus "should not be considered different from AE".

Is the Eczema of WAS Causally Related to the Underlying Immune Defect? The eczema of WAS is not only a constant feature of the syndrome but also regresses dramatically when the immune defect is corrected by successful bone marrow grafting [4, 5, 12, 22, 26, 29].

In more than ten patients hitherto so treated, not only the eczema dissolved completely and lastingly, but also, interestingly, the characteristic lack-lustre appearance of the skin, so typical for AE, returned to normal [43].

Selective IgA Deficiency

Selective IgA deficiency (S-IgA-Def) is the most common form of PID (prevalence 1 in 500–700 in the general population). It occurs in females twice as often as in males, is likely to be heterogenous in nature and spans a wide spectrum of clinical expressions ranging from apparent health to significant morbidity. The relatively benign character of S-IgA-Def is underscored by the estimates of the time elapsing between onset of symptoms and diagnosis, which ranges between 0.5 and 6 years [37]. Also, many individuals with S-IgA-Def have an unimpaired lifespan.

Clinical Features. Symptoms are highly diverse. Presenting signs are usually recurrent, and sometimes severe infections, particularly of the upper and lower respiratory and gastrointestinal tracts, the major pathogens being gram-positive cocci, *H. influenzae* and *E. coli*. The gastrointestinal tract is a site of additional complaints, like colicky pains, vomiting, diarrhoea, steatorrhoea and malabsorption. Further associated features are an increased incidence of autoimmune diseases (rheumatoid arthritis and lupus erythematosus) and neoplasms of the lymphoreticular and gastrointestinal system. A major feature of S-IgA-Def is the high incidence of atopic diseases (vide infra).

Immunological Abnormalities. Severe and partial S-IgA-Def are conveniently distinguished, the first being defined as IgA levels below 5 mg/dl *plus absence* of secretory IgA, the latter as IgA levels above 5 mg/dl but lower than 2 standard deviations of normal, *plus presence* of secretory IgA. This distinction, although based on clinical grounds and not accounting for pathogenetic heterogeneity, is useful because only *severe* S-IgA-Def appears to be a truly genetically determined defect, which persists throughout life [35, 37]. Partial S-IgA-Def may rather be regarded as a delay in maturation, which, as a rule, reverts to normal by adolescence in approximately half of the individuals affected. Obviously, in severe S-IgA-Def incidence and severity of complications are higher.

IgG and IgM are usually normal, but IgG subclasses (IgG_2, IgG_4) may be deficient [25, 27]. In these patients, infectious complications tend to be more pronounced. IgE is elevated in 30% of affected individuals, as are eosinophils in differential white blood count.

The pathogenesis of S-IgA-Def is as yet unclear, but several aspects point to heterogeneity. Various modes of transmission have been reported, although most cases appear to arise sporadically. In several instances, defects of chromosome 14 have been reported [24]. B and T lymphocytes are normal in number and function; IgA B cells, however, appear to be arrested at an early stage of maturation and fail to differentiate into plasma cells [10]. Although no consistent T-cell defect has hitherto been demonstrated, subtly defective immunoregulation by T cells appears to be a major pathogenic feature [3, 37, 50].

S-IgA-Def and Atopy. In a large series of IgA-deficient children, Plebani et al. [37] found clinically manifest atopic symptoms in 25% on average (32% in severe and 18% in partial S-IgA-Def). Atopic manifestations included allergic rhinitis, asthma, urticaria and atopic eczema. Eczema was much less frequent an atopic symptom than rhinitis and asthma (1:2.5 in severe and 1:5 in partial S-IgA-Def). Association with atopic symptoms was clearly linked to the presence of elevated IgE: more than 50% of affected individuals *with* signs of atopy had high IgE, as compared with less than 20% in patients *without*. Interestingly, this relationship was approximately equal in both severe and partial S-IgA-Def. It is thus doubtful whether the severity of the IgA defect has a significant influence on the incidence and severity of atopy [36, 37].

Eczema in S-IgA-Def. Any eczema found is simply labeled as "AE" by most investigators. It must be pointed out, however, that no systematic analysis according to the criteria of Hanifin and Rajka [16] has been carried out as yet.

Hyper IgE Syndrome (Job's Syndrome, Buckley's Syndrome)

Hyper IgE syndrome (Hyper-IgE-S) is a blurred generalising designation lacking a broadly accepted definition, which historically developed by the lumping of similar but not identical entities characterised by (at times dramatically) elevated IgE, infections of the skin and internal organs and eczema.

Terminology. Hyper-IgE-S was first described in 1966 as Job's syndrome by Davis et al. [11] in a pair of sisters, who besides hyperextensible joints and nail dystrophy had recurrent "cold" subcutaneous staphylococcal abscesses with little inflammation but no eczema. Later reports added a defect in leucocyte chemotaxis, recurrent otitis media and "dermatitis". In the report of Paslin and Norman the skin changes of a patient with Job's syndrome were described as typical atopic eczema [31].

Buckley et al. [8, 9] expanded the syndrome by adding the feature of excessively high IgE levels in a series of 20 cases. All patients had pruritic "eczematoid dermatitis" which did *not* correspond to AE. This view is still maintained by several authorities [6]. In subsequent years, approximately 150 case reports were added under the term Hyper-IgE-S; many of these had AE-like eczemas, and by 1977, AE was listed as a major dermatological sign of Hyper-IgE-S by Weston [53], which was later carried on in several reviews on the subject [40, 45]. Obviously, Job's and Buckley's syndromes, once at least clinically if not pathogenetically well characterised, began to overlap with excessive but genuine AE and a variety of similar, less defined states of immunodeficiency with high IgE.

In a recent review, Ring and Landthaler [40] split Hyper-IgE-S into at least five pathogenetically diverse entities: severe AE, Buckley's and Job's syndrome, lymphocyte malignancy, parasite infection and idiopathic hyper-IgE-emia.

Clinical features. Disregarding its pathogenetic diversity, the following features are generally attributed to Hyper-IgE-S: the incidence is approximately 1/500 000; there is no sex prevalence and no association with HLA antigens. Most cases appear to be sporadic although both autosomal dominant and autosomal recessive modes of inheritance have been found. Onset of symptoms is usually in infancy. Major complaints are pyodermas and staphylococcal subcutaneous "cold" abscesses of the skin as well as of internal organs (liver, kidneys, lungs); *H. influenzae*, pneumococi and gram-negative enterobacteria come second in frequency. A wide range of other infections (viral and mycotic skin infections, sinusitis, otitis media, osteomyelitis, etc.) and non-infectious complications (coarse facial features, nail dystrophy, urticaria, ichthyosis, incontinentia pigmenti, etc.) have been described. As a rare but interesting finding, Hyper-IgE-S may be associated with mucocutaneous candidiasis. Prognosis is generally considered good, although few long-term observations have been published. In occasional instances, overwhelming infection causes a fatal outcome.

Immunological Features. A large number but no consistent abnormalities have been found, besides elevation of IgE. In some patients, polyclonal increase of all Ig classes has been observed; others have reduced T-cell counts, poor or absent responses to antigenic stimulation in vitro, and weak or absent mixed lymphocyte reactions, while reacting normally to mitogens. In these patients, cutaneous anergy to the usual recall antigens may be present, while immediate-type skin reactions are frequently strongly expressed; T suppressor cell activity is deficient in a large number of cases [13]. In a substantial number of patients, a defect of neutrophil chemotaxis is detected. It has been hypothesised that high levels of histamine impair both T-cell function as well as neutrophil chemotaxis.

Eczema in Hyper-IgE-S. Clearly, a significant number of patients with severe AE has been lumped together with Hyper-IgE-S. The question remains whether those patients, who suffer from the entities originally described by Buckley's and Job's syndrome, may develop AE according to the criteria of Hanifin and Rajka or whether they just have "eczematous dermatitis" as originally proposed [8]. This problem can only be sorted out once the various entitites of Hyper-IgE-S are defined at a molecular level, and more patients become available for analysis. Retrospective evaluation will certainly fail to elucidate this matter.

PIDs Occasionally or Possibly Associated with AE

X-linked Agammaglobulinaemia (Bruton)

This is a severe PID of low incidence (1 in 1 000 000) and unknown cause; it is characterised by subtotal to total absence of circulating Ig of all classes due to a maturation defect of pre-B cells into immature B cells. Cell-mediated immunity appears unimpaired. Clinical features are bacterial (gram-positive) infections, diarrhoea, malabsorption and rheumatoid arthritis- and dermatomyositis-like syndromes. More than half of the boys affected die before the age of 2 years.

Eczema is *not* a regular feature of X-linked agammaglobulinaemia [6, 41, 45]. Atopic diathesis has been reported as a minor symptom [6], usually manifesting as rhinitis or asthma; it is unclear whether the exceptional cases of eczema fulfil the diagnostic criteria of AE.

Selective IgM Deficiency

Another rare PID, this is characterised by (subtotal) absence of IgM and normal levels of the other Ig. In milder forms, recurrent gram-positive infections predominate; severe deficiency often leads to fatal meningococcal septicaemia and, according to some reports, may be associated with AE [19, 20, 45]. Again, the diagnostic criteria of AE have not been applied to these eczemas.

X-linked Immunodeficiency with Hyper IgM.

This is a less infrequent (~ 120 reported cases [1]) PID probably of heterogenous pathogenesis and poor pro gnosis. It is characterised by decreased IgG and IgA levels, accompanied by increased IgM and, occasionally, thrombo- and neutropenia. Clinical symptoms are recurrent, severe, gram-positive infections, hepatosplenomegaly, autoimmune syndromes and lymphomas [6, 45].

Eczemas are *not* a regular feature of X-linked immunodeficiency with hyper IgM. Two doubtful cases of AE have been reported in the earlier literature [1, 14]; a full-blown case of AE fulfilling the classification criteria has recently been presented by Vieluf et al. [49].

Ataxia Teleangiectatica

This not so uncommon (1 in 40 000) autosomal-recessive syndrome of defective DNA repair involves complex neurological, vascular, endocrine and immunological aspects. The main features are cerebellar ataxia, excessively increased incidence of tumours, particularly lymphomas (relative risk 1200x), and recurrent severe infections, predominantly of the upper and lower respiratory tract. It is characterised by humoral (low IgA, frequently low IgE) and cell-mediated (low T4/T8 ratio) immune abnormalities [51].

Skin symptoms are manifold in AT; they consist of the diagnostic sign of widespread teleangiectases, recurrent pyodermas, poikiloderma, epitheliomas and progeric skin changes. Eczemas are a not uncommon occurrence in AT; they are often of the seborrhoeic or nummular variety [38, 45, 53]. The presence of AE has repeatedly been claimed; in these instances, eczema may be accompanied by dry skin and keratosis pilaris but *not* by atopic rhinitis and asthma. Since no evaluation according to the diagnostic criteria of AE has been performed, the type of these eczemas is unclear.

Other Disorders

In at least two other forms of PID, chronic granulomatous disease and Shwachman syndrome, single observations of an apparent association with AE have been reported [45, 53]. Again, this association must be regarded with caution.

In another set of genetic disorders, which exhibit mild immunodeficiency as a minor associated symptom, AE-like eruptions may be present. The most prominent example is Netherton's syndrome (ichthyosis linearis circumflexa, trichorrhexis invaginata and atopy). Afflicted individuals often develop rhinitis and asthma along with clinically typical atopic eczema, which blends however with the ichthyotic lesions. Many of these patients obviously suffer from a mild immunodeficiency; in a series of three patients, we observed extensive viral warts resembling epidermodysplasia verruciformis, pyodermas and, in one case, the development of a very aggressive squamous cell carcinoma in adolescent years [18].

Is AE a Feature of Acquired Immunodeficiencies?

In contrast to PID, AE has never been implicated as a marker of acquired immunodeficiency disorders, although non-specific dermatitic skin lesions are a commonplace occurrence in marasmus, alcoholism, malabsorption syndromes, starvation and other conditions of impaired immunocompetence. That immunosuppression per se does not result in the flare-up of latent atopy is obvious from everyday clinical experience. In contrast, active immunosuppression can be used as a last therapeutic resort in desperate cases of AE [23]. The lack of association of acquired immunodeficiencies with AE is further illustrated by the clinical findings in HIV infection.

In HIV-infected individuals, skin manifestations – mostly infectious – are frequent and often a warning sign of impending AIDS. Obviously, this preferential involvement is related to the impairment of the skin immune surveillance function (skin associated lymphoid tissues = SALT; skin immune system = SIS) as discussed by Stingl and co-workers [47]. It is all the more surprising that AE is not among the skin disorders frequently found in HIV-infected persons [32, 52]. In contrast, it is our impression and that of others that AE, like other type I hypersensitivity reactions, is less common in HIV-infected individuals than in the general population [39]. This is particularly interesting since polyclonal antibody hyperproduction is a feature of early HIV immune impairment.

Comments and Conclusions

In recent years, it has become an almost commonplace statement that AE is a frequent and characteristic symptom of PID. Although AE is found in some PID more often than in others, and is absent in quite a few, it was broadly accepted that AE is a feature common to numerous entities of widely different pathogenesis. This view certainly cannot be fully maintained if the literature is critically surveyed.

The difficulties of retrospective analysis have been mentioned above. The vague descriptions of eczematous skin lesions contained in the literature more often than not preclude their unequivocal classification as AE, even if the authors use terms like "resembling AE". If we intend to identify meaningful links between AE and PID, the following conditions ought to be met: the PID in question should not be too rare an occurrence in order to exclude statistical error; AE incidence in the PID in question should be well above the incidence in immunocompetent children (e.g. 20% or higher); the clinical criteria of Hanifin and Rajka should be met in direct physical examinations. If patients are not available due to the rarity of the syndrome, the minimum conditions are sufficiently detailed clinical descriptions in the case reports.

Applying these criteria, there is no justification to postulate specific linkages to AE in any of the entities listed under PIDs occasionally or possibly associated with AE. Pending further prospective studies, there is little evidence to suggest that full-blown AE is associated with any of these syndromes in more than a haphazard fashion.

In only three PID is a regular association with AE obvious: WAS, S-IgA-Def and Hyper-IgE-S. In these entities, the scenarios of immunological abnormalities are strikingly similar to each other and to the scenario of AE: elevated IgE levels, subtle or more complex T (suppressor)-cell defects, eosinophilia and defects of neutrophil chemotaxis. This conclusion does not support the view that AE is a non-discriminating skin symptom grafted onto a variety of PID with vastly discrepant underlying pathomechanisms. It rather suggests that AE is dependent on a specific immunological setting. The expectations that investigations of these PID may help to define this specific setting better appear well founded.

It has been claimed that AE may be an associated feature of PID in which IgE is *not* synthesised (X-linked agammaglobulinaemia) or are only present at normal or sub-normal levels (AT, X-linked immunodeficiency with hyper IgM). These would, of course, be interesting observations. The literature does not provide sufficient evidence, however, that in these particular cases the eczema actually qualified as AE or that IgE levels were *not* elevated (in many case reports, particularly of the not so recent literature, IgE levels are not given). A recent report of a patient with X-linked immunodeficiency with hyper IgM by Vieluf et al. [49] may be a case in point: this patient had full-blown AE meeting all diagnostic criteria, but he also had – an exceptional finding in this syndrome – elevated IgE.

References

1. Ackerman BD (1964) Dysgammaglobulinemia: report of a case with a family history of a congenital gammaglobulin disorder. Pediatrics 34: 211–219
2. Amman AJ (1987) Cutaneous manifestations of immunodeficiency disorders. In: Fitzpatrick TB, Eisen AZ, Wolff K, Freedberg IM, Austen KF (eds) Dermatology in general medicine, 3rd edn. McGraw-Hill, New York, pp 2507–2522
3. Atwater JS, Tomasi TB (1978) Suppressor cells and IgA deficiency. Clin Immunol Immunopathol 9: 379–384
4. August CS, Hathaway WE, Githens JH, Pearlman D, McIntosh K, Favara B (1973) Improved platelet function following bone marrow transplantation in an infant with the Wiskott-Aldrich syndrome. J Pediatr 82: 58–63
5. Bach FH, Albertini RJ, Joo P, Anderson JL, Bortin MM (1968) Bone-marrow transplantation in a patient with the Wiskott-Aldrich syndrome. Lancet II: 1364–1366
6. Belohradsky BH (1986) Primäre Immundefekte. Klinik, Immunologie und Genetik. Kohlhammer, Stuttgart
7. Blaese RM, Strober W, Levy AL, Waldmann TA (1971) Hypercatabolism of IgG, IgA, IgM, and albumin in the Wiskott-Aldrich syndrome: a unique disorder of serum protein metabolism. J Clin Invest 50: 2331–2338
8. Buckley RH, Becker WG (1978) Abnormalities in the regulation of human IgE synthesis. Immunol Rev 41: 288–314
9. Buckley RH, Wray BB, Belmaker EZ (1972) Extreme hyperimmunoglobulinemia E and undue susceptibility to infection. Pediatrics 49: 59–70
10. Conley ME, Cooper MA (1981) Immature IgA B cells in IgA-deficient patients. N Engl J Med 305: 495–497
11. Davis SD, Schaller J, Wedgewood RJ (1966) Job's syndrome: recurrent "cold" staphylococcal abscesses. Lancet i: 1013–1015
12. Fisher A, Durandy A, Bordigoni P, Virelizier JL (1984) Traitement du syndrome de Wiskott-Aldrich par graffe de moëlle allogénique. Arch Fr Pediatr 41: 611–616
13. Geha RS, Reinherz E, Leung D, McKee KT, Schlossman S,

Rosen FS (1981) Deficiency of suppressor T cells in the hyperimmunoglobulin E syndrome. J Clin Invest 68: 783–791
14. Goldman AS, Ritzmann SE, Houston EW, Sidwell S, Bratcher R, Levin WC (19687) Dysgammaglobulinemic antibody deficiency syndrome. J Pediatr 70: 16–27
15. Haneke E (1989) Thymopentin in dermatology. Curr Probl Dermatol 18: 283–289
16. Hanifin JM, Rajka G (1980) Diagnostic features of atopic dermatitis. Acta Derm Venereol [Suppl] (Stockh) 92: 44–47
17. Hintner H, Fritsch P (1989) Skin neoplasia in the immunodeficient host. The clinical spectrum: Kaposi's sarcoma, lymphoma, skin cancer and melanoma. Curr Probl Dermatol 18: 210–217
18. Hintner H, Jaschke E, Fritsch P (1980) Netherton-Syndrom: Abwehrschwäche, generalisierte Verrukose und Karzinogenese. Hautarzt 31: 428–432
19. Hobbs JR (1975) IgM deficiency. Birth Defects 11: 112–116
20. Hobbs JR, Milner RDG, Watt PJ (1967) Gamma-M deficiency predisposing to meningococcal septicaemia. Br Med J 4: 583–586
21. Kang K, Cooper KD, Hanifin JR (1983) Thymopoietin pentapeptide (TP-S) improves clinical parameters and lymphocyte subpopulations in atopic dermatitis. J Am Acad Dermatol 8: 372–377
22. Kapoor N, Kirkpatrick D, Blaese RM, Hilgartner MH, Chaganti RSK, Good RA, O'Reilly RJ (1981) Reconstitution of normal megakaryocytopoiesis and immunologic functions in Wiskott-Aldrich syndrome by marrow transplantation following myeloablation and immunosuppression with busulfan and cyclophosphamide. Blood 57: 692–696
23. Leung DYM, Rhodes AR, Geha RS (1987) Atopic dermatitis. In: Fitzpatrick TB, Eisen AZ, Wolff K, Freedberg IM, Austen KF (eds) Dermatology in general medicine, 3rd edn. McGraw-Hill, New York, pp 1385–1408
24. Migone N, Oliviero S, De Lange G, Delacroix DL, Boschis D, Altruda F, Silengo L, De Marchi M, Carbonara AD (1984) Multiple gene deletions within the human immunoglobulin heavy chain cluster. Proc Natl Acad Sci USA 81: 5811–5815
25. Morell A, Muehlheim E, Schaad U, Skvaril F, Rossi E (1986) Susceptibility to infections in children with selective IgA and IgA-IgG subclass deficiency. Eur J Pediatr 145: 199–203
26. Ochs HD, Lum LG, Johnson FL, Schiffman G, Wedgewood RJ, Storb R (1982) Bone marrow transplantation in the Wiskott-Aldrich syndrome. Transplantation 34: 284–287
27. Oxelius VA, Laurell AB, Lindquist B, Golebiowska H, Axelson U, Bjorkander J, Hanson LA (1981) IgG subclasses in selective IgA deficiency. N Engl J Med 304: 1476–1477
28. Panly CR, Artis WM, Jones HE (1978) Atopic dermatitis, impaired cellular immunity, and molluscum contagiosum. Arch Dermatol 114: 391–393
29. Parkman R, Rappeport J, Geha R, Belli J, Cassady R, Levey R, Nathan DG, Rosen FS (1978) Complete correction of the Wiskott-Aldrich syndrome by allogeneic bone-marrow transplantation. N Engl J Med 298: 921–927
30. Parkman R, Remold-O'Donnell E, Kenney DM, Perrine S, Rosen FS (1981) Surface protein abnormalities in lymphocytes and platelets from patients with Wiskott-Aldrich syndrome. Lancet II: 1387–1389
31. Paslin D, Norman ME (1977) Atopic dermatitis and impaired neutrophil chemotaxis in Job's syndrome. Arch Dermatol 113: 801–805
32. Penneys NS, Hicks B (1985) Unusual cutaneous lesions associated with acquired immunodeficiency syndrome. J Am Acad Dermatol 13: 845–852
33. Perry GS, Spector BD, Schuman LM, Mandel JS, Anderson VE, McHugh RB, Hanson MR, Fahlstrom SM, Krivit W, Kersey JH (1980) The Wiskott-Aldrich syndrome in the United States and Canada (1892–1979). J Pediatr 97: 72–78
34. Peterson PK (1984) Host defense abnormalities predisposing the patient to infection. Am J Med 76: 2–10
35. Plebani A, Ugazio AG, Monafo V, Burgio GR (1986) Clinical heterogeneity and reversibility of selective immunoglobulin A deficiency in 80 children. Lancet I: 829–831
36. Plebani A, Monafo V, Ugazio AG, Monti C, Avanzini MA, Massimi P, Burgio GR (1987) Comparison of the frequency of atopic diseases in children with severe and partial IgA deficiency. Int Arch Allergy Appl Immunol 82: 485–486
37. Plebani A, Ugazio AG, Monafo V (1989) Selective IgA-deficiency: an update. Curr Probl Dermatol 18: 66–78
38. Reed WB, Epstein WL, Broder E, Sedgwick R (1966) Cutaneous manifestations of ataxia telangiectasica. JAMA 195: 746–753
39. Ring J, Kraus K, Fröschl M, Brunner R, Przybilla B, Burg G, Braun-Falco O (1987) AIDS, HIV-Infektion und allergische Reaktionen. AIFO 2: 643–646
40. Ring J, Landthaler M (1989) Hyper IgE-syndromes. Curr Probl Dermatol 18: 79–88
41. Rosen FS (1976) The primary immunodeficiencies: dermatologic manifestations. J Invest Dermatol 67: 402–411
42. Rosen FS, Cooper MD, Wedgewood RJP (1984) The primary immunodeficiencies, parts I and II. N Engl J Med 311: 235–242, 300–310
43. Saurat J-H (1987) Atopic dermatitis-like eruptions in primary immunodeficiencies. In: Happle R, Grosshans E (eds) Pediatric dermatology. Advances in diagnosis and treatment. Springer, Berlin Heidelberg New York, pp 96–100
44. Saurat J-H (1985) Eczema in primary immune deficiencies. Clues to the pathogenesis of atopic dermatitis with special reference of the Wiskott-Aldrich syndrome. Acta Derm Venereol (Stockh) 114: 125–128
45. Saurat J-H, Woodley D, Helfer N (1985) Cutaneous symptoms in primary immunodeficiencies. Curr Probl Dermatol 13: 50–91
46. Spector BD, Perry GS, Kersey JH (1978) Genetically determined immunodeficiency diseases (GDID) and malignancy: report from the Immunodeficiency-Cancer Registry. Clin Immunol Immunopathol 11: 12–29
47. Stingl G, Rappersberger K, Guggenberger K, Tschachler E, Wolff K (1989) SIS during HIV-infection. In: Bos J (ed) skin immune system (SIS) Boha Raton, FL, pp 343–355.
48. Tappeiner G (1982) Disease states in genetic complement deficiencies. Int J Dermatol 21: 175–191
49. Vieluf D, Korting HC, Belohradsky BH (1989) Eczematous skin lesions in X-linked immunodeficiency with Hyper-IgM. Curr Probl Dermatol 18: 60–65
50. Waldmann TA, Broder S, Krakauer R, Durm M, Meade B, Goldman C (1976) Defect in IgA secretions and in IgA suppressor cells in patients with selective IgA deficiency. Trans Assoc Am Physicians 89: 215–224
51. Waldmann TA, Broder S, Goldman CK, Frost K, Korsmeyer SJ, Medici MA (1983) Disorders of B-cells and

helper T-cells in the pathogenesis of the immunoglobulin deficiency of patients with ataxia teleangiectasia. J Clin Invest 71: 282–295
52. Warner LC, Fisher BK (1986) Cutaneous manifestations of the acquired immunodeficiency syndrome. Int J Dermatol 25: 337–350
53. Weston WL (1977) Cutaneous manifestations of defective host defenses. Pediatr Clin North Am 24: 295–407
54. WHO Scientific Group on Immunodeficiency (1983) Meeting Report. Primary Immunodeficiency diseases. Clin Immunol Immunopathol 28: 450–463

Atopic Eczema as a Psychosomatic Disease: A Model for Integrated Treatment

K. Bosse

Reviewing the long and varied history of atopic eczema, it can be seen again and again that extreme changes of opinion have led to very different concepts of the disease at different times. At one time the morphologic description, and at other times organic and functional aspects of the disease would be emphasized. In the past 20 years there has been renewed and increased interest in the functional aspects of the atopic disease process, such as the psychosocial circumstances, and this has become increasingly important for some dermatologic and psychosomatic units.

Our own interest should be seen in the context of this development. Since the early 1970s, we have been gathering relevant observations, evaluating them critically, and using the interpretations increasingly for therapeutic purposes.

An Initial Assessment

It is a surprising phenomenon that very many people concerned with the disease have suspected a connection between psyche and soma in atopic eczema, although no one has been able to prove the part played by the psyche in a strict sense. Nevertheless, its role is obvious. During consultation, patients often ask "Could it be psychological?" or prevent psychological interpretation defensively by saying "Everything's perfectly all right with me ... ." When giving their history, patients may unsuspectingly remark "Whenever ..., then I'm poorly well." Even in the older literature, many attempts to assign a specific personality structure to the atopic eczema patient, or at least his mother, can be found. And if, for instance, such observations led to concepts of "hostility" or "overprotectiveness" on the part of the mother, or of the sick child having a strikingly hyperactive and tense personality, little consideration was given to whether this was the cause or the effect. The mother overburdened by the chronically sick child, the disappointed parents, the mutual accusations of guilt between the parents, or the constant torment of itching for the patient were accorded little attention in causal relationship.

The nursing staff at children's hospitals remark that the atmosphere among children with atopic eczema is "different." Teachers at school or nursery school find these children "gifted" and "ambitious" but often lacking concentration. Observant relatives point out that there is tension in the parent's relationship, thoughtful parents in their turn refer to the child's place within the family as a late arrival or even as only child. In addition to these statements, it can be observed that nearly all those concerned tend to ascribe the disease (and the therapeutic consequences) to an external cause such as allergy, nutrition, chemicals in the environment, or stress. In this way, individual approaches to the connection between atopic eczema and the psyche are greatly prejudiced in one way or another.

Alert assessment shows that the experiences of those affected may be supplemented by a large number of reproducible observations. Such observations relate primarily to the temporal correlation of improvement or a new episode of eczema with desired or undesired psychosocial events in the broadest sense such as improvement experienced in the relaxed environment of a successful vacation, admission to hospital, or during treatment in a health resort away from home, and the reverse of this experience on discharge. To take one example, the physician may witness the appearance or disappearance of the patient's pruritus according to whether the consultation was stressful or confrontational. Such experiences led us to include psychosocial factors in our concept of the disease and its treatment as well as overall care in the conventional dermatologic and allergologic manner, and to take relevant training into account appropriately when selecting staff. Putting the psychosocial viewpoint into practice brings with it the need for special attention to the physician patient relationship and the patients coping with the disease. The physician's role in all this is a complicated one, since he must pay attention to and structure his relationship with the patient more consciously and read between the lines to gain nonverbal information while studying the disease. We see the physician-patient dialogue in this as centered round the rule: those who only ask receive only answers.

The Physician-Patient Relationship During Outpatient treatment

The relationship of the physician to the patient with chronic skin disease is influenced in a particular way by the concept of disease and treatment held by those involved. If compatible concepts of disease and therapy in the somatically or psychosomatically oriented sense coincide during the first consultations, and if the physician gives his opposite number the chance – or the patient himself takes the opportunity – to gain information, then an essential prerequisite is created for the future development of the physician-patient relationship and the desired success of future treatment in these first discussions. The necessary reciprocal agreement about the practicable therapeutic measures required is facilitated by this prerequisite.

Cooperation becomes more difficult if physician and patient hold fundamentally different or even opposed and more or less mutually exclusive views. If this happens, difficulties are even created by the numerous somatically orientated disease concepts (allergy, pseudoallergy, environment, nutrition) and the resulting therapeutic expectations of the patient with atopic eczema (local treatment with or without cortisone, homeopathy, diet, natural remedies) as well as the aims of treatment (cure, improvement, freedom from symptoms). However, treatment is hampered still more by contradictory views of the involvement of psychological factors, which are still mostly considered in terms of precipitating stress and thereby delegated to external factors.

Cooperation becomes particularly difficult if, in addition to somatic treatment, the patient feigns willingness to trace the psychological causes within himself in order to accomodate the physician, the relatives, the referring physician who has carried out the preliminary treatment, or indeed even the psychologist, using some such words as "I will do all I'm supposed to do" or "I've come to you because Mr X has recommended you." In such a case a mere well-meaning declaration of intent does not indicate a serious readiness and capacity to engage in a long-term undertaking like psychosomatic treatment with its complex causal network. If the physician, in these first discussions, perceives a discrepancy between his own views and those of the patient as far as the genesis and/or treatment of the atopic eczema is concerned, he should not at this point succumb to the temptation to make short work of correcting the patient's ideas by virtue of his more advanced knowledge without even giving the patient a chance to develop his own ideas. Furthermore, it is important not to disappoint the patient's hopes by what may be taken as a rejection, i.e., an abrupt disavowal of his often one-sided or quite erroneous ideas. It usually suffices at the beginning to point out that a number of factors are involved in the origin of an exacerbation, and that any concept taking account of only one factor is inadequate. Hence the necessity, in the individual case, to explain what factors may be of importance in the current episode. The basic introductory exchange of ideas provides the physician with the possibility of hearing from the patient whether the latter has his own explanation for his current state, under what conditions the deterioration became evident, or, conversely, under what circumstances the last improvement occurred (holiday, events at home or at work).

In any event, the dermatologist with psychosomatic interests is also aware that, unlike the psychotherapist, he has a longer time period available during which he can treat the somatic symptoms, while adopting a wait-and-see attitude before making the attempt to pass from the somatically oriented plane to that of psychological discussions. The decision to do so presupposes a relatively stable physician-patient relationship as well as suitable existing circumstances, i.e. plenty of time and quiet for both speakers. The move may be initiated by the patient's use of a catchphrase ("Whenever ...") or by a question ("Could it possibly be psychological?") or by a remark of the physician ("Have you ever wondered whether ...?" or "In some patients ...").

If the patient enters into such an exchange, it then becomes important to mete out the information in such a way that the new topic can be further expanded by mutual consent without the risk of provoking an abrupt interruption by making excessive demands on the patient. This phase of the physician-patient relationship still constitutes a type of experimental phase for both interlocutors. The experiment attempts, by means of increasing loading, to explore the tolerance of the relationship without altogether relinquishing the possibility of retreating to the somatic terrain.

The physician in charge of treatment must put the somatic criteria on the line but respect the patients limits in such a discussion. The limits are represented in the patient with atopic eczema scratching when it itches and the specific vascular reaction. In order of appearance, the itch-scratch sequence usually occurs first. If the conversation generally or specifically involves topics which are critical for the patient, the latter reacts with cautious – and initially apparently casual – rubbing e.g., over the bend of the elbow and forearm or the side of the nostril, finally with increasingly uninhibited scratching of the entire body. Mitigation or abandonment of the explosive topic immediately results in a reduced need to scratch in adults. For small children, the analogue to the critical topic of conversation in adult patients is often the fact that the mother, father, or both parents form the focus of the discussion. The increasingly insecure child finally begins severe scratching, occasionally announcing "If you don't ... I'll start scratching.«

In disciplined adults who do not allow themselves to scratch the physician may observe an external warning sign, the sudden appearance of circumoral or nasal pallor, which can also be made to regress very rapidly, i. e., within minutes, by verbalizing the fact or changing the subject. If this warning sign is not respected, the patient may actually refuse to continue with the session and might well be horrified at the idea of a further medical session or a visit to the psychologist in the near future. This procedure of taking things to the limit must be consciously controlled by the physician. The limit will not necessarily be consciously perceived by the patient, who in this phase of the discussion of his illness experiences the change from the somatically oriented plane of discussion to the emotional plane for the first time.

As trust grows between physician and patient, and with increasing self-awareness on the part of the patient, the ability of the patient to bear stress also grows continuously.

In the first phase when the patient is becoming aware of the psychosomatic process, the phenomena mentioned above also serve to provide the patient with convincing evidence of the correlation between the somatic process in the skin and emotional stress, e. g., in front of a mirror. An approximation of the different concepts of disease ad therapy can be introduced in this way. This simultaneously implies an important step in bringing the patient and the psychosomatically oriented physician closer together.

Aspects of Coping in Patients with Atopic Eczema

On the cognitive plane, the causal attribution of disease to fashionable concepts such as genetics, stress, allergy, chemicals in the environment is popular, usually without going into detail. The therapeutic concepts to which the patient readily submits (tests, diet programs, "healthy living") then correspond to this. The whole emphasis is on the search for external factors and corresponding disease concepts. Even those patients inclined to a partially or predominantly psychogenic concept of the disease are often induced thereby to adopt a more somatic concept of treatment (Meinhold 1987) without thinking about contradicting, or even thinking along the lines "As long as I have such bad skin, I cannot feel well or have any joy in life."

On the emotional plane, resignation, loneliness and helplessness are common. Rage at the disease, which is perceived as a millstone round the neck with its restrictive consequences on private and professional contacts, occasionally outweighs the grief and vexation at being a martyr to the constant itching and disfiguring appearance. If the disease cannot be accepted, this may be reworked into accusation or even rejection of society and the environment without leading to mobilization of the patient's intrinsic forces. On the behavioral plane, these more usually exhibited emotional but unconstructive attitudes extraordinarily often stand in opposition to a compensatory ambitious striving for performance at school and work, which fits well with the tendency to withdraw into more or less marked social isolation. This also applies to leisure activities, in which a solitary hobby (music, painting, chess) rather than a communicative one (sport, games) is pursued with intensity. The restriction on communication caused by the disease and the consequent impairment of social competence mutually interact in a vicious circle.

An allied form of coping with disease observed in patients with chronically disfiguring skin diseases such as atopic eczema and psoriasis vulgaris is withdrawal from intimate relations. The resigned withdrawal of the patient with eczema may be founded on the actual behavior of the partner who is unaffected by skin disease, but it may also be the expression of an insinuation by the skin sufferer against the partner ("... the way I look, he can't want me any more ...").

A withdrawal associated with gain from the disease is what may be regarded as a special variant of this distancing in which the eczema patient who has an inadequately developed ability to communicate, more or less consciously exploits his disease, for instance, with the aid of his (not strictly necessary) bandages, to ward off his partner before he has even expressed a desire for physical nearness.

Other forms of disease gain for the atopic eczema patient not infrequently relate to participation in school sports or undesired occupational activities, as well as abuse of claims to stay at health resorts or of invalid status. A widespread childhood form of the atopic eczematic's realization of the disease gain is blackmail of the parents, along the lines of "If you don't ... I shall scratch." This often involves the wish to come into the parents' bed at night, and then has serious consequences for all concerned if the parents always indulge this wish. On the one hand, there is the negative conditioning of the child, which promotes a learning process that favors scratching and hence the eczema. On the other hand, the child thereby prevents the parents' essential night's rest, possibly up to their total exhaustion. Relief is occasionally possible by the parents' supplying the devotion the child requires in the evening before going to sleep (stories, reading aloud, singing, caressess).

Guilt feelings, associated with pain or rage, towards the healthy partner or similarly affected children, as well as an attribution of guilt by the patient to the parents, are assigned simultaneously in both the cognitive and the emotional spheres.

Disease, disability, associated pruritus, compensation, substitution, secondary gain from the disease in the family, school and occupation: all these burning problems of coping with the disease call for intensive analysis in discussions between the physician, the patient and his family.

Types of Medical Dialogue with the Atopic Eczema Patient

The First Consultation

The collection of "hard data" to confirm the diagnosis – skin findings, family history, onset, most important site, pruritus, previous treatment – together with the accompanying nonverbally mediated information, usually affords an entry into an extended, informative medical consultation. Emphasis has already been put on the necessary medical reserve towards the potential in this situation for the physician, which is not always one offered by the patient preoccupied with his skin condition. Apart from external circumstances which influence the quality of the first dialogue, the patient's expectations should largely determine the course of this initial discussion, the physician functioning chiefly as open to questions, as observer and listener, once the hard data have been discussed. Here, the balancing act, necessary for practical reasons, between time-saving, directed questioning, and an exclusively nondirective dialogue, not usually feasible for the physician, constitutes a difficult problem. A serviceable compromise is to put forward several alternatives to the patient in the course of his enquiries ("Does it itch more at night, in the evening, or during the day ... more at work, in your spare time, on holiday?" etc.), or even to ask short questions arising from the actual situation ("Have you noticed that you have just begun to scratch yourself – does that also happen in other situations?" or "When was it recently clearly worse, or clearly better?"). It is not just the quality (the "dosage") of the content of the dialogue – insofar as it covers the somatic aspect of the reply to concrete questions posed by the patient – that must be handled very warily by the physician. This is also the case regarding the thematic diversity and duration of the initial dialogue, even if the patient or the child's parents are inquisitive and their questions and remarks neverending. A "less is more" approach is useful, i.e., a restriction of the detailed discussion to limited aspects which arise from the questions, and which offer a continuation in further consultation. Points left undecided stimulate the patients or those accompanying them to their own afterthoughts and motivate them for the next dialogue ("Next time we ought to go over that point again. You might wish to think about it once more.").

The nondirective atmosphere of the discussion, the scrupulous observation of every sign of resistance, the restriction as to content, and finally the acknowledgement of priority of the patient or parents in the choice of topic (e.g., pruritus) – all these characterize the initial dialogue of the psychosomatically oriented physician and establish the basis for the quality of the subsequent consultations and the nature of the future physician-patient relationship.

Structuring the extended Medical Dialogue

Many factors that escape assessment usually restrict one's ability to plan the duration and content of an extended dialogue (some 30 min) between the physician and the patient with atopic eczema. The patient's expectations of the physician and the current stress on the patient due to pruritus and pain limit his readiness for an open discussion. The involvement of the physician in his daily round of duties, which must allow for the often unpredictable demands of other patients, influences his decision to engage in dialogue at the psychological level. However, such an extended dialogue with the patient is occasionally necessary before the patient is even prepared for a discussion with the psychologist. To what extent, however, is it possible to plan in advance for such a contingency? The following can be done in advance:

- A general estimate can be made of the necessity, possibility and willingness of the doctor and patient to undertake such an extended dialogue.
- The content of such a discussion can be loosely prestructured with questions such as:

- What do you know about your disease?
- What does the pruritus mean to you?
- What do you hope to gain from your visit to me in the discussion hour?

Another possibility in prestructuring is that in which the patient takes home with him from the consultation room questions that remain undecided, and which can again become the subject of discussion when raised by the physician, for example:

- Guilt feelings of the parents towards the sick child (heredity, "failure")
- Significance of the pruritus for the parents or spouse of the patient (annoyance, impatience)
- Secondary gain from the disease through the chronic eczema (protection from partner's demands, etc.)

An extended dialogue between physician and patient is not necessary for every idea and should be conducted only under favorable conditions. The need for this may arise during either ambulant or hospital treatment, and it is naturally easier to satisfy in the latter circumstance. This type of discussion is not a substitute for discussion with the psychologist.

The Decision on Inpatient Treatment

Admission of the patient with atopic eczema to an inpatient center for psychosomatically oriented dermatological treatment calls for a preliminary talk with the patient, pointing out the differences from exclusively conventional treatment in the classical dermatologic sense. These differences relate to:

- The target ideas of physician and patient
- The place of corticosteroid treatment and the assessment of topical dermatologic treatment as a partial feature
- The readiness on the part of the patient and the doctors involved to take part in extended medical discussion
- Reduction of external contacts (visits, telephone, occupational activity) for a period of relative seclusion at the beginning of treatment
- The possibility of relaxation in the group as a therapeutic element
- The possibility of psychological attention in individual discussions
- Further care after inpatient stay

The physician can propose such treatment if during ambulant preliminary treatment he feels that the patient is becoming aware of the relationship between psychological and somatic processes.

The mere recruitment into an integrative dermatologic-psychosomatic course of treatment by the specialist – i.e., simple referral, without appropriate preparation by the referring or admitting physician or by an experienced psychologist – usually ends in disappointment for both physician and patient. In this case, securing merely the motivation and sensitization of the patient requires a period of several weeks at the center, even in the most favorable case, to prepare the patient for targeted treatment in a second or third inpatient stay in the event of a recurrence. Even the most assiduous preliminary discussion with the patient is not always followed by successful cooperation with the dermatologist during psychosomatically oriented inpatient treatment, as both the self-assessment of the patient and his assessment by the admitting physician are always burdened by some residual insecurity. But other individuals who are close to the patient can influence them, and this may compensate for the patient's more intermittent responsiveness to the physician.

Similar considerations apply if the patient – at the suggestion of the physician in charge of his case or of the nursing staff or under the influence of other patients – breaks off the current conventional treatment by a change of ward and thereby of staff in the hope of another, more successful treatment in the psychosomatically oriented department. The change to a new hospital team for "difficult" patients, i.e., those with a difficult relationship to the medical or nursing staff, always brings with it the chance of a new start for all concerned. However, this also means that there usually remains insufficient time to carry out an integrated treatment, in our sense of the term, since the patient has then already used up part of the length of his stay. The motives for such a change tend to be dissatisfaction with the atmosphere in the ward or lack of success in treatment hitherto – i.e., a deficit – rather than an intention now to submit to extended treatment. The patient's demands and expectations are usually small in proportion to the preparedness required for a new disease or treatment concept. The offer of a later readmission for treatment under new conditions is usually a better recommendation for the patient than a change of ward or physician during the current inpatient stay.

Integrating Inpatient Treatment

The purposes of the physician and those of the patient in deciding on inpatient treatment do not overlap entirely despite an appropriate preliminary discussion. For the referring physician and for the patient, the preeminent aspect of the situation is the inadequacy of ambulant treatment hitherto; this frequently has led to dissatisfaction with the physician previously in charge and has disappointed the patient's hopes for a (miracle) cure. The expectations of the admitting, psychosomatically oriented physician, on the other hand, relate rather to a new orientation on the part of the patient regarding the concept of improvement, i. e., freedom from symptoms instead of cure, and to an increasing awareness by the patient of the relationship between the somatic process in his skin and his mental state. Finally, he also hopes for an increasingly critical self-responsibility of the patient for treatment of his skin and his own inner situation. In the ideal case, the originally passive and orally oriented patient who expects the attainment of his unfulfillable (because unrealistic) wishes would come to accept a new concept of his disease and its treatment, develop more realistic expectations for his future, and improve his ability to live with his skin condition and to shape his life. In this ideal case, the patient would also be satisfied with the accompanying improvement in his skin condition. A discussion of these objectives under the catchphrase of "inpatient treatment as learning process" means measuring the patient's improvement in terms of his insight into his illness; this applies both to the preliminary discussion on admission and, with increasing specificity, during inpatient stay.

The place assigned to conventional local and drug treatment of the atopic eczematic patient also undergoes important extension under a psychosomatically integrative approach. In terms of local treatment, the dermatologic aspects (application of ointments, hydration, anti-inflammatory and antimicrobial agents) are supplemented by the factor of touching and being touched. This therapeutic use of bodily contact stems in part from the exciting findings of behavioral research in a study of the relationship of rhesus monkey mothers to their children (Harlow et al. 1959). This study showed that for the young animals skin contact to the mother plays a very important role compared to the feeding activity and that lack of contact leads to behavioral disturbances of the later adult mother animals towards the next generation as well as to self-manipulation of their skin by the animals involved. These findings are of particular interest for the analytic concept of atopic eczema as the expression of a disturbance of early childhood against the background of a given genetic disposition.

The behavior of the patient himself, and perhaps of his mother, also indicates the importance of contact. A sick child for example, may resist rubbing treatment by the mother because it allegedly hurts, while at the same time accepting and asking for stroking local treatment by the nursing staff, to which he responds like a purring cat. The resulting jealousy on the part of the mother is most easily dispelled if she is given the opportunity in the consulting room to compare the rubbing-in and the stroking-in treatments on her own body. A relaxed discussion between the nursing staff and the mother may then elicit the fact that the mother – herself possibly affected by eczema as a child – may never have experienced the pleasure of being stroked and may even now have no relationship to her own skin. She is thereby blocked in developing positive feelings towards skin contact even though she dutifully carries out the daily treatment of the child. The child in turn is well aware of the difference between the services wrung from an exhausted mother and the comforting devotion of a good nurse's care. A psychological or psychotherapeutic working-through of the deficits in the experience of mother and child necessarily ranges widely over the causes; this can benefit each. The introduction to (self-)treatment through skilled nursing care as a model can come to resemble a focusing behavior therapy, especially since the opportunity presents itself for an accompanying relaxed atmosphere of conversation pointedly among women (mothers).

The medical consequences of the therapeutic use of touching can extend further. Prescription of a protective or healing "stroking ointment" provides the child with the daily experience of physical attention in the form of skin contact from the parents, even if the state of the child's skin is such as not to invite spontaneous stroking from the mother (or father). The relaxing effect on the skin of a local substance (even one lacking an active agent) and of treatment with a grease, cream, or paste suited to the site (combined with other relaxing measures; see below) may by itself lead to significant improvement. In particular, if the introductory use of paraffin pastes is conceded as basic, the employment of corticosteroids is not usually necessary, and the cortisone-free treatment desired by many today is usually possible without difficulty. We do not recommend to patients the local use of corticosteroids for symptomatic treatment as a part of routine management but only for temporary use in actual crisis situations. One possible disadvantage of such symptom-oriented treatment is the loss of motivation by the patient for a comprehensive discussion of the disease from the psychosomatic aspect. This aspect should be discussed beforehand with the patient, who is usually anxious only about the – avoidable – somatic side effects of corticosteroid treatment.

Local agents can be supplemented by the administration of psychotropic drugs, although these are often refused by the patients. It has proved useful to give neuroleptics in low doses, or antihistamine agents with sedative, neuroleptic, or anxiolytic effects at the beginning of treatment. We do not use preparations containing diazepam despite their excellent effect in atopic eczema because of the risk of addiction.

The relaxing effect promotes not only the subjective well-being of the patient but also the desirable phase of relaxation and regression in preparation for treatment in the hospital. Even without additional local treatment, this has an extraordinarily positive effect on the skin symptoms and eventually increases the patient's readiness and capacity for discussion. In eczematic adults, a minimal dosage of neuroleptics over a period of some 14 days has also proved useful for the critical period between discharge from hospital and return to work.

In addition, we provide the atopic eczematic patient with the opportunity of learning relaxation techniques in a group even during the introductory phase. Besides its actual effect, this also encourages an atmosphere of open discussion within the group and in relation to the exercise leader; this can be of value in subsequent psychotherapeutically oriented discussions. Participation is voluntary and is occasionally declined.

A further important feature of our hospital treatment is the reduction of external contacts (visits, telephone calls, occupational activities) during the introductory phase for some 8–10 days. Many patients find this so difficult to accept that it cannot be enforced. The resulting regression of the patient is medically intended, temporary and deliberately measured out. This is particularly the case if the patient succumbs to an extreme, "malignant" form of regression, wanting only to be comforted and cared for like a small child. We see in this form of immoderate regression an undesirable flight from reality – "I can forget everything here." Similar to the opposite form – an overstructuring of the hospital day by the patient by means of diversions of every kind. Either mode of behavior may easily lead very rapidly to freedom from symptoms and to enthusiasm on the part of both physician and patient. However, this reaction is associated with a poor prognosis: as soon as the protection of the hospital is abandoned (and often even on the notification of possible discharge) the patient is overtaken by the reality that he has hitherto successfully repressed and suffers a recurrence immediately on return home from the hospital, sanatorium, or successful holiday.

Rapid symptomatic improvement tends to demotivate the patient in accepting the parasomatic aspect of his disease and in actively dealing with it with the help of physicians and psychologists. Rapid symptomatic improvement through mere destressing influences the ultimate prognosis unfavorably in the long run. The prophecy of an immediate recurrence, the offer of renewed treatment using all the therapeutic facilities of the hospital, and the patient's own wretched experience after discharge permit, in the most favorable case, a second treatment under better preconditions and without loss of prestige for the patient.

The completion of further treatment phases with a view to increasing self-responsibility, confrontation, and preparation for discharge (Bosse 1985) is therefore extremely important despite improvement in the skin condition. Understandably, it is not always accepted by the patient. Even during the initial relaxation/regression phase, the patient is offered supplementary medical, informative, and supportive discussion in preparation for the more searching discussion with the psychotherapist.

A renewed exacerbation of the eczema requiring a further period of hospital treatment (revolving-door effect) may affect patients after a stay in hospital for skin disease, after climatic cures, or after successful holidays. In the search for an effective prophylaxis against such recurrence, we began from the assumption that the patient's temporary freedom from symptoms is due among other things to the destressing psychosocial climate, and that after discharge (or even in anticipation of it) this is replaced by the eczema-favoring psychosocial home setting. Our own studies (Hünecke et al. 1990) under hospital conditions confirm that desired or undesired psychosocial events are very closely related in time to a corresponding alteration in somatic and psychologic status. These findings of our own, the observation of the revolving-door effect and of the strikingly common "destressing improvement" on admission to hospital without changes in other essential parameters, and the predischarge deterioration have increasingly prompted us during the past 10 years to seek a training program as prophylaxis against recurrence. Initially this was also considered a diagnostic measure. The patient is offered a short period of leave at home after the relaxation phase, i.e., during the 2nd or 3rd week, with psychological briefing in a detailed discussion before and after. A controlled assessment of these patients showed that the deterioration in the skin state precipitated by a short leave of 1 night at home was largely predictable and diminished with repeated short-leave periods. Patients who accepted regular dialogues with a hospital psychologist profited more from this technique than those who declined such talks (Rowold et al. 1990).

In a modification of this technique, and as long as the

mother is accommodated at the hospital as an accompanying person, it may be desirable for children to be visited at hospital by siblings, not otherwise permitted on grounds of infection, as a therapeutic preparation for discharge. At such visits the mother has an opportunity to train the family in matters of sibling rivalry under the guidance of psychologists and nursing staff. We do not advise admission of the mother as a matter of principle. In our opinion, a totally exhausted mother tends to be a stressful factor for the child and his skin condition. A temporary separation constitutes an advantageous relaxation for both parties, which can be used simultaneously for talks with the parents. However, well before discharge, the parents must take up contact again with the child and acquaint themselves with the child's skin (see above). As such a temporary separation of mother and child does not usually correspond to parents' expectations, it requires an intensive discussion between physician and parents. The argument is based mainly on ensuring rest for the mother.

This therapeutic intercourse with the atopic eczematic patient allows the development of an atmosphere peculiar to the ward and one which is characterized by a special relationship among physicians, nursing staff, psychologists, and patients, as well as among the patients themselves. This is marked by openness in discussion, care, and empathy, but also by criticism and rejection. The atopic eczematic patient learns to relate his own experience of illness in intensive meetings with other patients in a circle of patients and healthy individuals. The therapeutic effect of this hospital ward atmosphere can be regarded as a training model of a minisociety.

Continuity in medical and nursing staff is a beneficial contribution to the ward atmosphere, and changes in personnel should be kept to a minimum. This also applies to temporary changes due to holiday replacements and the performance of night duties, leading to free days which as far as possible should not be covered by staff strange to the ward.

The collaboration and reciprocal information of the permanent personnel is promoted by weekly team meetings in which the permanent nursing staff, physicians, and psychologists discuss problem patients in working parties similar to Balint groups and problems among coworkers. Here it becomes evident which staff members are most important to an individual patient, and these are opportunities for discussion of how to deal with patient and the resistance of nursing or medical staff, and for verbalization of complaints by individual team members or by a group, and for settling organizational problems.

Psychological Dialogue as a Component of Integrating Treatment

Apart from the occasional extended medical discussions during outpatient and inpatient care of the atopic eczema patient, the motivated patient has the opportunity of dialogue with the psychologist. If the patient so desires, this can take place even during the 1st week of inpatient stay; however, from the medical side it usually occurs only from the 2nd week as an optional offer or arises in the context of regular training in relaxation (autogenous training, training in the Jacobson technique). The chief topics discussed with the psychologist are current problems such as those of approach and retreat, separation and farewell, tests, dealing with performance demands stress, dealing with pruritus. These concern both the affected patient and his family (Bosse and Hünecke 1987).

The dialogue is necessarily limited in topics and time because of the small number of team psychologists at the hospital and is generally restricted to the duration of inpatient treatment, or perhaps covering also the transfer to supplementary psychological aftertreatment elsewhere. The type of methodologic procedure seems of secondary importance compared with the need for a trustful relationship of patient to psychologist. We prefer to refer children to educational advisers, to be cared for with parental involvement (Bosse et al. 1985).

Our experience with a group of eczematic patients under medical and psychological direction indicates that if possible such a group should not be homogeneous, i. e. should not be composed exclusively of eczematic patients. Sufferers from other skin diseases (e. g., psoriasis) should participate in such a group for the comparative sharing of disease experience, and the healthy (e. g., partners) should also take part. The long take-off phase of the homogeneous group, which is devoted predominantly to rather unconstructive self-pity, may in a mixed group be modified and enriched by the variable nature of the stresses predominant for the different patients (disfigurement and reactive behavior of the psoriatic patients, on the one hand, pruritus and precipitating factors in atopic eczematic patients, on the other). These types of encounter groups under medical psychological direction seem sensible as a supplement to outpatient treatment or treatment after hospitalization. The conceptual goals are principally improved management of the disease and acquisition of social competence.

Forms of cooperation other than those with the psychologist attached to the unit are inferior in our experiece. There is less acceptance by the patient of any form of counselling care from psychosomatic practitioners, psychiatrists, or psychologists. This also applies to the intensity of cooperation with the physicians in charge of treatment, especially the reciprocal information and knowledge of the hospital-related and individual peculiarities of all those involved in treatment. This experience is valid for diagnostic, therapeutic, and scientific problem formulations related to the personal knowledge of the patient. In our experience it is important in all forms of collaboration between psychologists and physicians to avoid conflicting and unfulfillable expectations and to accept existing superiorities in certain areas due to the more critical methodology of the psychologist and the greater clinical experience of the physician.

Current Evaluation of our Integrating Inpatient Treatment of the Atopic Eczema Patient

The development of this extended form of dermatologic treatment of the patient with atopic eczema is still in flux. An objective concluding evaluation is impossible for three reasons. A long-term therapeutic assessment of the effects of incorporing psychosocial development into the disease concept would be possible only in terms of decades of life and development. Because of the spontaneous and usually regressive development of the disease, it remains uncertain how much this development may have been accelerated as compared with the spontaneous course. Finally, it must be considered that the psychosocial circumstances and familial developmental preconditions vary extremely from patient to patient, and that therefore a strict comparison of a treatment and a control group becomes increasingly difficult the longer the follow-up period lasts. However, we may already identify the following series of evident advantages:

- A more intensive physician patient relationship results in better compliance.
- The treatment leads to greater independence and self-responsibility in dealing with himself and with the diseased skin through the development of a new disease concept.
- A lessened steroid dependence is of both subjective and objective importance to the patient.
- There are grounds for postulating an improved midterm prognosis through supplementation of current symptom-oriented, local dermatologic treatment, and the patient acquires a greater social competence through reflection and training during the inpatient stay.
- Insight into the familial dynamics and its relationship the disease provides the prerequisites for improvement.

These important advantages of our integrative, psychosomatically oriented treatment of atopic eczema patients require a quantitatively and qualitatively high expenditure of effort in the following respects:

- Constant collaboration of the psychologist as a member of the hospital team.
- Careful organization of the deployment of colleagues on the ward familiar to the patient. In making leave and other replacements, an effort should be made to avoid the temporary employment of staff unconnected with the ward.
- Appropriate timing of extended medical discussions in addition to the usual visits and physician-patient contacts.
- Daily contact of the head of the department with the physicians working in the ward and with the nursing staff, as well as a patient-oriented arrangement of visits with a generous allotment of time.
- Regular team discussions of the Balint group type among all coworkers (physicians, psychologists, nursing staff, possibly attendants and student nurses).
- Deliberate formation, when needed, of an individual, primary relationship to one team member for specific patients. This relationship exists independently of the other functions of the respective member on the ward. The increased contact take place in additional to the dialogues with the psychologist.
- A communication-intensive atmosphere on the ward. This increases the potential for conflict in assessment of the patient and evaluation of the therapeutic outcome, especially because of overlapping of spheres of responsibility and attention to patients. Team discussion, among other measures, is provided for the working out of this conflict.

References

1. Bosse K (1985) Psychosomatische Gesichtspunkte in der Dermatologie. In: von Uexküll T (ed) Psychosomatische Medizin. Urban und Schwarzenberg, München Baltimore
2. Bosse K, Diepold B, Heigl F, Heigl-Evers A, Streeck U (1985) Familiale Sozialisation, Ich-Entwicklung und psychosomatische Krankheit am Beispiel von Patienten mit endogenem Ekzem. In: Leber A, Trescher HG, Büttner Ch (eds) Die Bedeutung der Gruppe für die Sozialisation Kindheit und Familie. Vandenhoeck and Ruprecht, Göttingen
3. Bosse K, Hünecke P (1987) Endogenes Ekzem – Chance eines aktualgenetischen Ansatzes. In: Bosse K, Gieler U (eds) Seelische Faktoren bei Hautkrankheiten. Beiträge zur psychosomatischen Dermatologie. Huber, Bern
4. Harlow HF, Zimmermann RR (1959) Affectional responses in infant monkey. Science 130: 421
5. Hünecke P, Bosse K, Finckh H (1990) Krankheitsverlauf und psychosoziale Ereignisse während der stationären Behandlung atopischer Ekzematiker – eine Pilotstudie. S. Z Haut Geschlechtskr 65: 428–434
6. Meinhold J (1987) Empirische Untersuchungen über Krankheitskonzepte von Patienten mit dermatologischen Erkrankungen. Thesis, Georg-August-Universität, Göttingen
7. Rowold C, Bosse K, Hünecke P (1990) Kurzbeurlaubung als diagnostische und therapeutische Möglichkeit in der psychosomatisch orientierten Behandlung. Z Haut Geschlechtskr 65: 437–443

Histopathological and Immunohistological Aspects of Atopic Eczema

F. Eckert, M.D.

Pathogenesis and histopathological changes in atopic eczema are still a matter of controversy [9, 24, 26–29, 33]. Basically, an unequivocal diagnosis of atopic eczema, by histological means alone, is hampered for the following reasons:

1. The primary lesion of atopic eczema remains to be defined both clinically and histologically. While some authors see flush, papules, or papulovesicles as the first symptoms [10], others describe "itch" as the primary lesion [20, 21].
2. Scratching and prolonged rubbing of pruritic skin result in a variety of secondary histological changes not specifically related to atopic eczema.
3. The histopathology of atopic eczema shares certain similarities with contact, nummular, and dyshidrotic dermatitis and the so-called id reaction.

Therefore, many authors tend to regard the histological findings of clinical lesions in atopic eczema as nonspecific [1, 13, 16, 18, 33].

Histological Findings

According to the various stages of clinical evolution, histological changes in atopic eczema have been universally classified as acute, subacute, and chronic [1, 15, 19, 33]. However, histological stages are not strictly defined and reports vary markedly concerning the characteristic features of each stage.

Acute Atopic Eczema

As proposed by several authors, itchy follicular papules may represent the first visible eruption of atopic eczema [1, 17]. Early in the course of the disease the principal histological changes are found in the upper portion of hair follicles. Spongiosis is limited to the follicular infundibulum leaving the adjacent epidermis uninvolved. Vesicle formations can be seen in some specimens. The follicular lumen shows hyperkeratosis and parakeratosis. Sometimes, the surface epidermis adjacent to the follicles also shows slight hyperkeratosis with areas of parakeratosis. A predominantly lymphocytic infiltrate within and around the upper external root sheath is seen [1, 17].

In contrast, other studies support the presence of slight epidermal hyperplasia in acute lesions [15, 26, 27]. Spongiosis of interfollicular epidermis was not found consistently [15]. Using plastic-embedded thin sections, Mihm et al. noted epidermal psoriasiform hyperplasia in sites of acute lesions [15]. Intercellular edema with vesiculation was only present in two of four patients studied. The epidermal infiltrate consisted of lymphocytes and monocytes/macrophages.

Prose and Sedlis reported the presence of hyperkeratosis, parakeratosis, irregular epidermal hyperplasia, and spongiosis [19]. According to Russel-Jones and MacDonald acute lesions of all types of eczema are primarily characterized by edema of the superficial venular plexus with subsequent transepidermal elimination of this papillary fluid [24].

In acute lesions, most authors [1, 15, 17, 19] note a marked perivenular and slight intervascular inflammatory infiltrate about the superficial venular plexus consisting of lymphocytes, macrophages, occasional neutrophils, eosinophils, and basophils. However, numerous neutrophils and eosinophils were found in urticarial papules resulting from oral provocation of atopic eczema by spices [28]. Leiferman et al. showed that eosinophils degranulate in skin in atopic eczema [12]. Using immunofluorescent methods they demonstrated deposition of two eosinophil granule proteins, namely major basic protein and eosinophil-derived neurotoxin, in specimens of atopic skin [12]. In other studies, influx of eosinophils into the dermis was observed after patch testing with aeroallergens [7, 11]. Melanophages were found throughout the superficial layers of the dermis [15]. While some authors report an increased number of mast cells, Mihm et al. found normal numbers of mast cells in acute vesicular lesions when compared with skin from normal control individuals [15, 33]. However, mast cells exhibited various degrees of hypogranulation [15].

Vascular changes include endothelial cell swelling of the superficial venules, edema, reduplication, and rarely homogenous thickening of the vascular basement membrane [15, 26, 27]. Compaction of erythrocytes without extravasation was noted in the superficial capillary venule by Soter and Mihm [27].

Subacute Atopic Eczema

This stage of disease is rather ill-defined histologically. Most studies are confined to acute and chronic lesions and do not give any descriptions of subacute atopic eczema. Probably due in part to scratching and rubbing, one finds hyperplasia of the epidermis, less spongiosis than that of acute lesions, and in some instances scale crusts. Interfollicular intercellular edema is rarely seen [1, 18].

Chronic Atopic Eczema

Long-standing lichenified lesions of atopic eczema show a psoriasiform hyperplasia of the epidermis, with little or no intercellular edema evident [1, 15, 19, 33]. In addition, hyperkeratosis, dyskeratosis, and scale crusts may be noted [15, 26, 27]. By quantitative evaluation of epidermal thickening, van Neste et al. [32] found that both differentiated and undifferentiated compartments are increased in chronic lesions. Infiltration of the epidermis by lymphocytes is seen only focally [15]. Dermal changes include papillary fibrosis characterized by coarse collagen bundles arranged perpendicular to the overlying epidermis, a significantly increased number of fully granulated mast cells, and a moderate perivascular and intervascular lymphohistiocytic infiltrate in the upper dermis [15]. Further abnormalities concern the superficial venular plexus and deeper venules. The basement membrane of these vessels is thickened, and endothelial cell swelling and enlarged pericytes may be seen [15, 26, 27]. Demyelinization of cutaneous nerves and perineural sclerosis have been detected by Mihm et al. at all levels of the dermis [15].

Clinically Normal Skin

Histological findings in macroscopically normal skin of atopic eczema patients differ from those found in healthy persons. A variety of moderate but obvious histological changes are observed. Epidermal alterations include hyperkeratosis, slight epidermal hyperplasia, and spongiosis, sometimes also spongiosis of the hair follicle [15, 26, 27]. There is a sparse dermal inflammatory infiltrate consisting primarily of lymphocytes. The venules show endothelial swelling with focal luminal obliteration, prominent nuclei, and sometimes basement membrane thickening. Prominent pericytes are found around almost all affected venules [15, 26, 27]. Occasionally, fibrosis and focal demyelinization of cutaneous sensory nerves are noted [26, 27].

On the basis of their findings Mihm et al. concluded that the histopathological changes of clinically normal skin may reflect either subclinical disease or residual involvement from a previous clinical episode [15]. According to Uehara, biopsy specimens of normal-appearing skin in patients with atopic eczema reveal no pathological findings except for a mild perivascular infiltrate of mononuclear cells in the upper dermis [30].

Dry skin

Histological pictures of mild subacute eczema have also been observed in dry, xerotic skin of patients with atopic eczema. The histological changes include thinning of the granular layer, patchy loss of basket weave pattern of the horny layer, small foci of spongiosis and exocytosis, and a discrete mononuclear cell infiltrate in the upper dermis [15, 30]. Uehara believes that the dry skin in patients with atopic eczema is a mild eczematous lesion of this disease [30].

Immunohistological Findings

Immunohistological studies have been performed to further characterize the mononuclear cell infiltrate in skin lesions of atopic eczema. The phenotype of these cells has been determined by means of monoclonal antibodies reacting specifically with different subsets of lymphocytes, macrophages, and Langerhans cells. While in most studies immunohistological findings in acute lesions have been compared with findings in chronic lichenified specimens, there are only two reports on immunohistological findings in subacute atopic eczema [3, 25]. Some authors did not specify the histological stage of the lesions studied [4, 34].

Acute Atopic Eczema

There is little controversy concerning the composition of the mononuclear cell infiltrate in acute lesions of atopic eczema. T lymphocytes represent an important constituent of the cellular infiltrate. In a quantitative study, Zachary et al. showed that over half of the cells infiltrating the dermis were peripheral T lymphocytes expressing the CD5 antigen [35]. This result is in accordance with findings obtained by other authors [4, 14, 23, 25, 34]. According to most studies the majority of these T cells are CD4-positive helper cells with only a few CD8-positive suppressor cells [4, 14, 25, 29, 35]. The helper/suppressor ratio varies considerably and ranges from 2:1 to 20:1. Rocha et al. found CD4-positive T lymphocytes predominantly around small blood vessels of the deeper dermis, while other authors noted a large number of CD4-positive cells particularly in the epidermis [23]. In contrast, CD8-positive cells were demonstrated in the superficial dermis with some cells infiltrating the basal layer of the epidermis [23]. Leu7 positive natural killer cells were present only occasionally. The same is true for B lymphocytes [35]. When compared to normal skin, atopic skin was shown to contain an increased number of Langerhans cells [23]. CD1-positive Langerhans cells were consistently found both in the dermis and, to a lesser extent, in the epidermis [34, 35]. In the epidermis Langerhans cells are present in a tight network extending from the superficial stratum corneum to the basal epidermal layer [23]. In the dermis they are arranged in grouped foci and within the mononuclear cell infiltrate. The majority of Langerhans cells show coexpression of HLA class II antigens [34]. In addition, IgE molecules were recently demonstrated on epidermal Langerhans cells in atopic eczema [2, 6, 8]. In contrast to these studies, Uno et al. found similar numbers of Langerhans cells in acute lesions of atopic eczema and in nonatopic normal skin [31].

Subacute Atopic Eczema

Findings regarding localization and distribution of T cell subsets in subacute lesions are similar to those in acute lesions of atopic eczema [3, 25]. Exocytic cells of both the CD4 and CD8 phenotype are found in small numbers in the epidermis, especially in spongiotic areas [3, 25]. The number and distribution of CD1-positive Langerhans cells varies. In addition, interdigitating cells are seen in the epidermis and as part of the superficial dermal infiltrate in most patients [3, 25]. Leu7-positive natural killer cells and CD22-positive B cells are found only rarely [25].

Chronic Atopic Eczema

According to Leung et al., the major difference between tissue sections of acute versus chronic lesions is that the chronic lesions demonstrate a lesser number of infiltrating lymphocytes, particularly into the epidermis, the staining pattern being similar to that seen in acute lesions [14]. In contrast, Rocha et al. found the chronic lesion to contain more CD8-than CD4-positive T lymphocytes [23]. The number of Langerhans cells is markedly increased in chronic lesions. They appear as focal aggregations in the epidermis adjacent to subepidermal foci of inflammatory cells [3, 14, 25].

Dry skin

In dry skin the majority of infiltrating lymphocytes in the dermis are CD4-positive T cells. CD8-positive T lymphocytes are rarely found, and B cells are virtually absent. CD1-positive Langerhans cells are increased in number, both in the epidermis and in the inflammatory infiltrate in the upper dermis [30].

In all stages, large numbers of cells expressing HLA class II antigens were found in the dermis. They comprise T lymphocytes, interdigitating cells, and a few macrophages/monocytes [3, 14, 25, 31]. IgG and C3 deposits can be demonstrated at the dermoepidermal junction in lesional and uninvolved skin [22].

Summary

Atopic eczema is an inflammatory skin disease showing stage-dependent histological changes difficult to distinguish from other eczematous skin diseases. The histopathological findings in the acute phase are controversial. While spongiosis limited to the follicular infundibulum has been described as characteristic of acute atopic eczema, other authors found slight epidermal hyperplasia, parakeratosis, and spongiosis not strictly confined to the follicular infundibulum [15, 26]. A superficial perivascular inflammatory infiltrate is a constant finding in acute atopic eczema [1, 13, 15, 16, 18, 27, 33].

Histological examination of subacute atopic eczema and chronic atopic eczema reveals increasing changes corresponding to the clinical impression of lichenification. The changes include psoriasiform hyperplasia of the epidermis, thickening of the papillary dermis with coarsening of collagen and parakeratosis. However, according to most authors these findings are due to scratching and prolonged rubbing of pruritic skin and are not specifically related to atopic eczema [1, 15, 27, 33].

During the course of all histopathological stages the cellular infiltrate consists of a majority of CD4-positive T lymphocytes, which are also found to express class II antigens [4, 14, 23, 25]. In contrast, a smaller number of infiltrating cells are CD8-positive T cells. B cells are virtually absent [14, 35]. An increased number of Langerhans cells both in the epidermis and in the dermis probably reflects increased antigen presentation within the affected skin [3, 35].

Interestingly, both normal-appearing skin and dry skin in patients with atopic eczema show varying histological and immunohistological changes of mild eczema. Basically these include parakeratosis, acanthosis, spongiosis, exocytosis, and a superficial perivascular cell infiltrate similar to that observed in acute atopic eczema. On the basis of these findings the concept that normal-appearing and dry skin represent a primary or subclinical lesion of the disease is favored [15, 30].

Histological and particularly immunohistological findings have prompted a variety of hypotheses as to the pathogenesis of atopic eczema. Most authors have concluded that both type I and type IV hypersensitivity mechanisms may be implicated in the etiology of atopic eczema. Langerhans cells may play a crucial role in local antigen processing and lymphocyte activation through binding of allergen to IgE [2, 3, 6, 8, 14, 25, 29, 34, 35].

References

1. Ackerman AB (1978) Histologic diagnosis of inflammatory skin diseases. Lea and Febiger, Philadelphia
2. Bieber T, Dannenberg B, Prinz JC, Rieber EP, Stolz W, Braun-Falco O, Ring J (1989) Occurrence of IgE-bearing epidermal Langerhans cells in atopic eczema: a study of the time course of the lesions and with regard to the IgE serum level. J Invest Dermatol 92: 215–219
3. Bos JD, van Garderen ID, Krieg SR, Poulter LW (1986) Different in situ distribution patterns of dendritic cells having Langerhans (T6+) and interdigitating (RFD1+) cell immunophenotype in psoriasis, atopic dermatitis, and other inflammatory dermatoses. J Invest Dermatol 87: 358–361
4. Braathen LR, Forre O, Natvig JB, Eeg-Larsen JB (1979) Predominance of T-lymphocytes in the dermal infiltrate of atopic dermatitis. Br J Dermatol 100: 511–519
5. Braun-Falco O, Burg G (1974) Zelluläres Infiltrat und Kapillaren bei Neurodermitis diffusa. Quantitativ enzymzytochemische und histochemische Untersuchungen. Arch Dermatol Forsch 249: 113–124
6. Bruynzeel-Koomen CAFM, van Wichen DF, Toonstra J, Berrens L, Bruynzeel PLB (1986) The presence of IgE molecules on epidermal Langerhans cells in patients with atopic dermatitis. Arch Dermatol Res 278: 199–205
7. Bruynzeel-Koomen CAFM, van Wichen DF, Spry CJF, Venge P, Bruynzeel PLB (1988) Active participation of eosinophils in patch test reactions to inhalant allergens in patients with atopic dermatitis. Br J Dermatol 118: 229–238
8. Bruynzeel-Koomen C, van der Donk EMM, Bruynzeel PLB, Capron M, de Gast GC, Mudde GC (1988) Associated expression of CD1 antigen and FC receptor for IgE on epidermal Langerhans cells from patients with atopic dermatitis. Clin Exp Immunol 74: 137–142
9. Gans O, Steigleder GK (1955) Histologie der Hautkrankheiten. Springer, Berlin Göttingen Heidelberg
10. Hanifin JM (1983) Clinical and basic aspects of atopic dermatitis. Semin Dermatol 2: 5–19
11. Henocq E, Vargaftig BB (1988) Skin eosinophilia in atopic dermatitis. J Allergy Clin Immunol 81: 691–695
12. Leiferman KM (1989) Eosinophils in atopic dermatitis. Allergy [Suppl 9] 44: 20–26
13. Lever W, Schaumburg-Lever G (1990) Histopathology of the skin. Lippincott, Philadelphia
14. Leung DYM, Bhan AK, Schneeberger EE, Geha RS (1983) Characterization of the mononuclear cell infilration in atopic dermatitis using monoclonal antibodies. J Allergy Clin Immunol 71: 47–56
15. Mihm MC, Soter NA, Dvorak HF, Austen KF (1976) The structure of normal skin and the morphology of atopic eczema. J Invest Dermatol 67: 305–312
16. Montgomery H (1967) Dermatopathology. Harper and Row, New York
17. Ofuji S, Uehara M (1973) Follicular eruptions of atopic dermatitis. Arch Dermatol 107: 54–55
18. Pinkus H, Mehregan AH (1981) A guide to dermatopathology. Appleton-Century-Crofts, New York

19. Prose PH, Sedlis E (1960) Morphologic and histochemical studies of atopic eczema in infants and children. J Invest Dermatol 34: 149–165
20. Rajka G (1975) Atopic dermatitis. Saunders, London
21. Ring J, Dorsch W (1985) Altered releasability of vasoactive mediator secreting cells in atopic eczema. Acta Derm Venereol [Suppl] (Stockh) 114: 9–23
22. Ring J, Senter T, Cornell RC, Arroyave CM, Tan EM (1978) Complement and immunoglobulin deposits in the skin of patients with atopic dermatitis. Br J Dermatol 99: 495–501
23. Rocha C, de Maubeuge J, Sarfati M, Song M, Delespesse G (1984) Characterization of cellular infiltrates in skin lesions of atopic eczema by means of monoclonal antibodies. Dermatologica 169: 330–338
24. Russel-Jones R, MacDonald DM (1982) Eczema. Immunopathogenesis and histogenesis. Am J Dermatopathol 4: 335–336
25. Sillevis Smitt JH, Bos JD, Hulsebosch HJ, Krieg SR (1986) In situ immunophenotyping of antigen presenting cells and T-cell subsets in atopic dermatitis. Clin Exp Dermatol 11: 159–168
26. Soter NA (1989) Morphology of atopic eczema. Allergy [Suppl 9] 44: 16–19
27. Soter NA, Mihm MC (1980) Morphology of atopic eczema. Acta Derm Venereol [Suppl] (Stockh) 92: 11–15
28. Sterry W (1990) Histologie des atopischen Ekzems. In: Braun-Falco O, Ring J (eds) Fortschritte der praktischen Dermatologie und Venerologie. Springer, Berlin Heidelberg New York, pp 114–119
29. Thestrup-Pedersen K (1989) Immunology of atopic dermatitis. Acta Derm Venereol [Suppl 151] (Stockh) 69: 77–83
30. Uehara M (1986) Dry skin (sebostasis) and inflammation: heterogeneity of "dry skin" in atopic dermatitis. In: Ring J, Burg G (eds) New trends in allergy II. Springer, Berlin Heidelberg New York, pp 135–144
31. Uno H, Hanifin JM (1980) Langerhans' cells in acute and chronic epidermal lesions of atopic dermatitis, observed by L-Dopa histofluorescence, glycol methacrylate thin section, and electron microscopy. J Invest Dermatol 75: 52–60
32. Van Neste D, Douka M, Rahier J, Staquet MJ (1985) Epidermal changes in atopic dermatitis. Acta Derm Venereol [Suppl] (Stockh) 114: 67–71
33. White CR Jr (1983) Histopathology of atopic dermatitis. Semin Dermatol 2: 34–38
34. Willemze R, de Graff-Reitsma CB, Cnossen J, van Vloten WA, Meijer CVLM (1983) Characterization of T cell subpopulations in skin and peripheral blood of patients with cutaneous T cell lymphomas and benign inflammatory dermatoses. J Invest Dermatol 80: 60–66
35. Zachary CB, Allen MH, MacDonald DM (1985) In situ quantification of T-lymphocyte subsets and Langerhans cells in the inflammatory infiltrate of atopic eczema. Br J Dermatol 112: 149–156

Clinical Aspects of Atopic Eczema: Synopsis

B. Przybilla, J. Ring, T. Ruzicka

Allergic rhinoconjunctivitis, allergic asthma, and atopic eczema constitute the classical triad of atopic diseases. There is no definite marker of atopic eczema, its diagnosis being based on a combination of clinical criteria: chronic or chronically relapsing, intensely pruritic, characteristically distributed, eczematous skin lesions of variable morphology in the presence of an atopic diathesis [15].

Epidemiology

Epidemiologic studies on atopic eczema are hampered particularly by the lack of definite diagnostic criteria, by the fluctuant course of the disease, and by the impact of environmental factors on disease manifestation. Nevertheless, available data at least indicate that atopic eczema is a major health problem.

Atopic eczema is very common, indeed, its prevalence even seems to be rising. The cumulative incidence rate of atopic eczema among Danish twins up to the age of 7, for example, rose from 3% for those born between 1960 and 1964, to 10% for those born between 1970 and 1974 [35]. In contrast to previous opinions, the onset of atopic eczema is not rare during the first 3 months of life, and, as it frequently resolves after adolescence, it is more prevalent among young people than among adults [26]. Both sexes are affected, although during the infantile phase the disease is predominant in males ([27]; Schmied and Saurat, this volume). Although our knowledge of the disease is limited, it evidently occurs worldwide and affects all races ([14, 27]; Schmied and Saurat, this volume), but seems to be more prevalent in cooler climates and urban areas than in rural and tropical regions [8].

Genetics

It has been established that atopic eczema, allergic rhinoconjunctivitis, and allergic asthma are genetically linked (Schultz Larsen, this volume). Furthermore, in individuals with atopic eczema the development of atopic respiratory or cutaneous manifestations is determined genetically ("end-organ sensitivity") ([18, 34, 38]; Schultz Larsen, this volume). The exact genetic mode of inheritance of atopic eczema has not yet been elucidated, but present, a polygenic, multifactorial mechanism seems most probable (Schultz Larsen, this volume). The impossibility of defining atopy or atopic eczema definitely hampers genetic studies profoundly. Furthermore, as atopic eczema may not be a homogeneous entity, but rather comprise several still undefined subgroups, genetic heterogeneity within atopic eczema itself has to be considered (Schultz Larsen, this volume). Despite these difficulties, approximate risk figures for the development of atopic eczema can be derived from the available data and used for patient counseling (see p 18).

Clinical Presentation

Usually, three phases of atopic eczema are discerned [17]: the infantile phase, up to 2 years; the childhood phase, up to 12 years; and the adolescent/young adult phase, between 12 years and young adult life. Manifestation or persistence in older subjects may be called late adult atopic eczema. Itching is an essential and subjectively the most stressful feature in all phases of the disease.

Infantile atopic eczema starts to develop on the face

(cheeks, forehead) and scalp with an erythematous and papulovesicular eruption, frequently developing to oozing and crusted lesions ("cradle cap") ([5, 27]; Merk, this volume). Moreover, lesions may extend to involve other skin areas, particularly the extensor aspects of the limbs and the trunk. The course is chronically persistent or relapsing. Healing occurs in many cases by the end of the 2nd year of life. In the childhood phase, flexural eczema typically develops with involvement of the antecubital and popliteal spaces as well as of the wrists. Other sites of predilection are the face, the neck, the retroauricular areas, and the backs of the hands and feet. The disease may extend to involve the entire skin surface. The skin lesions are less exudative than in the infantile phase. On a conspicuously "dry" skin, there are patchy to diffuse erythema, papules, and excoriated scratch marks. Especially in flexural regions, lichenifications or lichenoid prurigo nodules develop. In the adolescent and adult phases, the predilection sites are virtually the same, lichenified eczema now being the predominating type of lesion. Lymphadenopathy may be present in severe cases.

There are special manifestations of atopic eczema which may be divided into morphological and site-specific variants [22]. Among these are the "minimal forms" of atopic eczema which cause only minor morbidity (Wüthrich, this volume). Variants of atopic eczema may be found associated with classical disease manifestations, or they may occur in isolation, in which case they often pose diagnostic problems. Many of them are not unequivocally related to atopic eczema, demanding exclusion of other causes. Important morphological variants are the following: patchy pityriasiform lichenoid eczema (follicular eczema), papular variant of atopic eczema, nummular atopic eczema, prurigo variant of atopic eczema, dyshidrotic eczema (pompholyx), seborrheic atopic eczema, and pityriasis alba ([5, 16, 22]; Wüthrich, this volume). Recent evidence suggests that infantile seborrheic eczema, which has commonly been regarded as strictly different from atopic eczema, may be at least a closely related entity [24]. Site-specific variants of atopic eczema comprise atopic hand eczema, exfoliative and angular cheilitis, median fissuring of the lower lip, retroauricular intertrigo, infra-auricular or infranasal fissuring, eczema of the lower eyelids, nipple eczema, pulpitis sicca, and vulval eczema ([5, 16, 22]; Wüthrich, this volume) Light-provoked atopic eczema also falls into the category of site-specific manifestations. Although some also regard juvenile plantar dermatosis as an atopic disease ([22]; Wüthrich, this volume), this has been questioned by others [40].

Histopathology

Atopic eczema is not a disease which may be diagnosed histologically, as the findings are non-specific and shared by other forms of dermatitis or eczema ([1, 21]; Eckert, this volume). In acute lesions, some investigators have found spongiosis limited to the follicular infundibulum, whereas others have seen slight epidermal hyperplasia, parakeratosis, and spongiosis of the interfollicular epidermis too (Eckert, this volume). A superficial perivascular inflammatory infiltrate is constantly present. Further disease stages are characterized by parakeratosis, epidermal hyperplasia, and thickening of the papillary dermis with coarsening of collagen. Immunohistologically, CD4-positive T-lymphocytes predominate in the cellular infiltrate at all stages, CD8-positive T-cells being found in smaller numbers [20]. However, a predominance of CD8-positive T-cells in chronic lesions has been found in one study [29]. Interestingly, there is an increased number of epidermal and dermal Langerhans cells, possibly reflecting increased antigen presentation [41].

Stigmata of the Atopic Constitution

There are a host of features which are characteristic of atopy, yet, with the exception of clear-cut overt atopic disease, no specific indicators of it. As there is no definite marker of atopic eczema, the characteristic features are used to support the diagnosis. The features listed by Hanifin and Rajka [15] are those referred to most often. However, the validity of these criteria has never been evaluated systematically. Overall, they appear to be highly sensitive but rather unspecific. When used by non-dermatologists – and they have been suggested particularly for this purpose [16] – overdiagnosis of atopic eczema may ensue.

Information on the "atopy status" can be obtained from history, from physical findings and from skin or laboratory testing (see page 32). True stigmata of atopic constitution must be unrelated to disease manifestations, otherwise they would not provide independent information. Furthermore, they should be easily observable. So, "true" constitutional stigmata of atopy comprise particularly dry skin, hyperlinearity of the palms or soles, infraorbital fold, white dermographism, facial pallor, orbital darkening, Hertoghe's sign, and low hairline (Przybilla, this volume). According to the available data, these features are more prevalent among atopic eczema patients than among controls (Przybilla, this volume). Furthermore, with the exception of dry skin, white dermographism, and Hertoghe's sign, these stigmata were also significantly more frequent in patients with "pure" atopic respiratory disease without indications of atopic eczema than in controls [25]. An atopic state can be presumed if several clear-cut stigmata are present.

Some of these features (dry skin, infraorbital fold, white dermographism, orbital darkening, Hertoghe's sign) have been interpreted as direct manifestations or sequelae of atopic eczema. Apparently, this applies to certain, but not to all cases (Przybilla, this volume). This is illustrated by the difficulties in interpreting the clinical impression of dry skin. Biopsies taken in atopic eczema patients from dry, clinically noninflamed skin have been reported to exhibit the histological picture of mild eczema [37], but this was not confirmed by others [11]. Areas of dry skin may be localized or generalized, and, in patients where dry skin is generalized it may fit a diagnosis of ichthyosis vulgaris combined with atopic eczema (Uehara, this volume). However, this concept has been refuted by others [11]. So, dry skin in atopic eczema may be heterogeneous in nature (Uehara, this volume).

Complications in Atopic Eczema

Skin infections caused by various microorganisms are clinically most important. There is an increased susceptibility to and severity of different viral, mycotic or bacterial infections, which is related to the following features (Vieluf and Ruzicka, this volume): (a) inherent immunological abnormalities (particularly decreased cell mediated immunity); (b) a defective barrier function of the skin; (c) a favorable milieu for microbial growth on eczematous skin; and (d) secondary immunosuppression due to prolonged glucocorticosteroid treatment.

With regard to bacterial infections, there is a high rate of colonization with coagulase-positive *Staphylococcus aureus* in atopic eczema. Clinical impetiginization of large skin areas can rapidly develop, but other forms of bacterial skin disease are infrequent (Vieluf and Ruzicka, this volume). If deeper tissue involvement occurs, one should be alerted to the possibility of a hyperimmunoglobulinemia E (hyper IgE) syndrome (Vieluf and Ruzicka, this volume). Osteomyelitis of distal phalanges in severe atopic eczema seems to be a rare, but possibly sometimes overlooked occurrence [4]. Tinea is not a prominent problem in patients with atopic eczema [5], but increased susceptibility and a risk of persistent mycotic infections has been reported (Vicluf and Ruzicka,this volume). Interest in the yeast *Pityrosporum orbiculare/ovale* has increased in recent years, as it may be involved in the etiopathogenesis of atopic eczema, particularly of so-called head, neck and shoulder (HNS) dermatitis ([30]; Vieluf and Ruzicka, this volume).

Proneness to develop viral infections manifests as an increased frequency of warts and mollusca contagiosa, which may be disfiguring and even disabling when widespread and long-standing. Eczema vaccinatum, nowadays extremely rare, and eczema herpeticum are potentially life-threatening complications. Eczema herpeticum develops especially in younger patients with severe atopic eczema, and, as the vesicles do not exhibit characteristic herpetiform grouping, the diagnosis may be missed easily. It seems that eczema herpeticum is much more common than usually presumed, as milder forms frequently go undiagnosed [2]. Also the incidence and severity of other cutaneous or extracutaneous viral infections or parasitic disorders may be increased in atopic eczema patients (Vieluf and Ruzicka, this volume).

Exfoliative erythroderma in atopic eczema is a potentially life-threatening event, which may occur especially after withdrawal of systemic glucocorticosteroid therapy or may result from widespread superinfections or generalized contact reactions. In children with severe or intractable eczema, growth impairment has been observed (Vieluf and Ruzicka, this volume). Besides severe skin disease, other possible causes of growth failure in these patients are prolonged treatment with topical or systemic glucocorticosteroids, coexisting bronchial asthma, gastrointestinal allergy, or inappropriate dietary restrictions (Vieluf and Ruzicka, this volume).

Long-standing disease may result in cosmetically troublesome hyperpigmentation, particularly on the neck (dirty neck; [6]) and the upper trunk. Also, macular amyloidosis may develop in predisposed individuals (Vieluf and Ruzicka, this volume).

Associated Diseases

Allergic rhinoconjunctivitis and allergic asthma are inherently related to atopic eczema. The frequency of respiratory disease in atopic eczema patients lies around 50% [27, 39]. The onset of respiratory manifestations is usually later than that of eczema. In an individual patient, the course of atopic cutaneous or respiratory disease may be alternating, simultaneous, or independent [27]. Atopy-related hypersensitivity to foods can cause also gastrointestinal symptoms, and patients are not always aware of such an association [33].

In view of the impairment of cellular immunity in atopic eczema, it seems a plausible assumption that allergic contact reactions of the delayed type should be less frequent in patients than in nonaffected individuals. Indeed, several studies have shown that patients with atopic eczema may fail to become sensitized to "obligatory" allergens, and this nonreactivity is related to disease severity (Neumann and Marghescu, this volume). Studies on patch test reactions to common environmental contact allergens have provided contradictory results without definite evidence that the reactivity rate to such allergens is reduced in atopic eczema patents ([9]; Neumann and Marghescu, this volume). Also, there are no consistent results with regard to the frequency of contact sensitivity to individual allergens, e.g., nickel salts, in atopic eczema patients compared with other individuals ([9]; Neumann and Marghescu, this volume). As methodological flaws are common in these studies, further investigations are urgently needed. From a practical point of view, patch testing has to be done in any atopic eczema patient with indication of a coincident allergic contact dermatitis. Immunoglobulin-E (IgE)-mediated immunologic contact urticaria or protein contact dermatitis are obviously linked to atopy [7, 10].

It has not yet been clarified, whether there is an association between drug reactions, particularly of the immediate type, and atopy (Vieluf and Ruzicka, this volume). Similarly, available data do not allow us to draw the conclusion that among patients with hymenoptera venom allergy there would be an increased number of atopic individuals (Vieluf and Ruzicka, this volume).

Other skin disorders related to atopy or atopic eczema comprise anhidrotic congenital ectodermal dysplasia, different forms of photosensitivity, hair anomalies (alopecia areata, "uncombable hair"), Netherton's syndrome, and pityriasis rosea (Vieluf and Ruzicka, this volume). Although there is no association between atopic eczema and psoriasis, the prevalence of atopy in patients with inverted psoriasis is increased [12]. Autosomal-dominant ichthyosis vulgaris has been found in 4% of atopic eczema patients [11].

In up to 40% of atopic eczema patients, there are associated ocular diseases, comprising blepharoconjunctivitis, atopic or vernal keratoconjunctivitis, ocular herpes simplex infections, keratoconus, cataracts, or retinal detachment ([13]; Vieluf and Ruzicka, this volume). In earlier studies, atopic cataract has been reported to occur in up to 33% of atopic eczema patients, but today's knowledge suggests that the prevalence, although not exactly known, is low (Vieluf and Ruzicka, this volume). While anterior subcapsular cataract seems to be specific for atopic eczema, posterior subcapsular cataracts are indistinguishable from those induced by glucocorticosteroid therapy (Vieluf and Ruzicka, this volume).

Besides gastrointestinal symptoms due to classical hypersensitivity reactions, other gastrointestinal disorders, e.g., gluten-sensitive enteropathy, eosinophilic gastroenteritis, ulcerative colitis, or ileitis terminalis, have also been reported to be associated with atopy (Vieluf and Ruzicka, this volume). Furthermore, in widespread skin disease so-called dermatogenic enteropathy may develop (Vieluf and Ruzicka, this volume). The precise relationship between atopy and these inflammatory bowel diseases remains to be established. This also holds true for the supposed association between atopic eczema and cystic fibrosis or steroid-responsive nephrotic syndrome, or between atopic eczema-like lesions and some metabolic disorders such as biotin-responsive multiple carboxylase deficiency, phenylketonuria, or histidinemia (Vieluf and Ruzicka, this volume).

As immunological deviations are a characteristic finding in atopic eczema patients, an association between diseases of the immune system and atopic eczema could be expected. With regard to primary immunodeficiency diseases, such linkage has been established only for the Wiskott-Aldrich syndrome, selective immunoglobulin A (IgA) deficiency and the hyper IgE syndrome (Fritsch and Hintner, this volume). In the secondary immunodeficiency state of human immunodeficiency virus (HIV) infection, atopic eczema has been said to exacerbate in predisposed individuals (Vieluf and Ruzicka, this volume) or to occur with decreased frequency (Fritsch and Hintner, this volume). An association between atopy and cutaneous lymphomas may exist in rare cases, and patients with atypical presentations, e.g., onset at older age, cutaneous lymphoma and Hodgkin's disease have to be excluded ([27]; Vieluf and Ruzicka, this volume).

Atopy or atopic eczema have also been reported to be associated with various other diseases, e.g., congenital perceptive hearing loss, Down's syndrome, sudden infant death syndrome, or endometriosis (Vieluf and Ruzicka, this volume).

Occupational Aspects of Atopic Eczema

Occupational skin disease and atopy are strongly interrelated, and this holds true especially for hand eczema ([36]; Rystedt this volume). The etiology of hand eczema usually is multifactorial: Skin lesions typically occur in atopic individuals who are exposed to irritants and are frequently also sensitized to work-related allergens. Hand eczema is, thus, more prevalent and also more severe in atopics than in nonatopics ([23]; Rystedt, this volume). Patients who work in a wet environment are at special risk, and, in women, domestic work adds significantly to the development of hand eczema (Rystedt, this volume). On the other hand, about a quarter of atopic eczema patients working in risk occupations do not develop hand eczema (Rystedt, this volume). A high risk was found to be associated with atopic eczema involvement of the hands during childhood, persistent eczema on parts of the body other than the hands, persistent dry/itchy skin, severe childhood involvement with atopic eczema, and, to a lesser degree, with female sex, a family history of atopic eczema, and respiratory atopic disease [32]. Individuals without any or with only a few of the weaker risk factors do not seem to develop hand eczema to a greater extent than nonatopics.

For prophylactic reasons, individuals with atopic eczema should avoid wet work, stressful jobs, heavy physical work, working places with high, prolonged low, or greatly varying temperature, warm damp environments, and exposure to irritants (dust, dirt, strongly defatting substances, wool) or contact with potent inhalant allergens ([27]; Rystedt, this volume). With regard to the risk of hand eczema, individual factors have to be considered (see above) since the presence of an atopic state as such is not a valid criterion. By means of a good skin care program, working ability can be maintained or restored in many endangered patients. Work-related eczema does not necessarily disappear after a job change (Rystedt, this volume).

Psychosomatic Aspects

Atopic eczema is a somatic disease which may be strongly influenced by psychological factors. The findings in the field of psychoneuroimmunology provide evidence that there are strong immunoneuroendocrine interactions [3], and these may be of relevance also in the etiopathogenesis of atopic eczema. There is no abnormality inherent to the personality of patients with the disease [27, 28], however, manifest eczema causes significant psychological problems by itching, insomnia, or cosmetic disfigurement. Such secondary psychological disturbances may disappear when the skin lesions improve [27]. On the other hand, psychological stress may also deteriorate the clinical condition, and this may lead to a vicious circle [27]. A dysfunctional parent-child relationship has to be considered as a pathogenetic factor in children with intractable disease [19]. Whenever evaluating or treating patients with atopic eczema, the intimate interrelation between psychological and somatic factors has to be taken into account (Bosse, this volume).

Natural History

Atopic eczema tends to heal with increasing age, however, there is conflicting information on the actual figure of this healing rate, which was reported to be 29%–84% ([27]; Vickers, this volume). These divergencies reflect different methodological approaches, particularly with regard to definition of the disease, inclusion of only severe or also mild cases, retrospective or prospective conductance of the study, and investigation by questionnaire or personal assessment. In a prospective study of 2000 children, 91% of whom could be evaluated at age 20, the overall healing rate was found to be 88.6% (Vickers, this volume).

Prognostic factors indicating a more poor outcome were a delayed onset of the disease after 2 years of age and an inverted pattern with knees and elbows involved (Vickers, this volume). Factors not influencing the prognosis were severity at onset, a family history of severe or persistent disease, the type of infant feeding, the presence of discoid lesions, or proven food allergies (Vickers, this volume). Other studies are at variance with this, as factors indicating an unfavorable prognosis were found to be severe disease in childhood, associated respiratory allergy, early age at onset, and female sex [27, 31]. There is no definite age at which clearance occurs, but merely an increasing incidence of clearance through the years (Vickers, this volume). For patients seeking genetic advice, it is important to know that disease severity cannot be correlated in different generations (Vickers, this volume). And, most important with regard to therapeutic efforts, the prognosis of atopic eczema seems to be positively influenced by an aggressive treatment (Vickers, this volume).

References

1. Ackerman AB (1978) Histologic diagnosis of inflammatory skin diseases. Lea and Febiger, Philadelphia
2. Atherton DJ, Harper JI (1988) Management of eczema herpeticum. J Am Acad Dermatol 18: 757–758
3. Besedovsky HO, Del Rey AE, Sorkin E (1985) Immune-neuro endocrine interactions. J Immunol 135: 750s–754s
4. Boiko S, Kaufman RA, Lucky AW (1988) Osteomyelitis of the distal phalanges in three children with severe atopic dermatitis. Arch Dermatol 124: 418–423
5. Braun-Falco O, Plewig G, Wolff HH, Winkelann RK (1991) Dermatologie. Springer, Berlin Heidelberg New York Lndon Paris Tokyo Hongkong Barcelona
6. Colver B, Mortimer PS, Millard PR, Dawber RPR, Ryan TJ (1987) The "dirty neck" – a reticulate pigmentation in atopics. Clin Exp Dermatol 12: 1–4
7. Cronin E (1987) Dermatitis of the hands in caterers. Contact Dermatitis 17: 265–269
8. Davis RH, Sarkany I (1961) Atopic eczema in european and negro west indian infants in London. Br J Dermatol 73: 410–414
9. Enders F, Przybilla B, Ring J (1991) Atopy and contact allergy. In: Ring J, Przybilla B (eds) New trends in allergy III. Springer, Berlin Heidelberg New York (in press)
10. Fabro L, Mühlethaler K, Wüthrich B (1989) Anaphylaktische Reaktion auf Latex, ein Soforttypallergen von zunehmender Bedeutung. Hautarzt 40: 208–211
11. Fartasch M, Diepgen TL, Hornstein OP (1989) Atopic dermatitis – ichthyosis vulgaris – hyperlinear palms – an ultrastructural study. Dermatologica 178: 202–205
12. Garofolo L, Pisani V, Mazzotta F, Bonifazi E (1989) Psoriasis in atopic children. Acta Derm Venereol [Suppl] (Stockh) 146: 63–65
13. Garrity JA, Liesegang TJ (1984) Ocular complications of atopic dermatitis. Can J Ophthalmol 19: 21–24
14. Hanifin JM (1987) Epidemiology of atopic dermatitis. Monogr Allergy 21: 116–131
15. Hanifin JM, Rajka G (1980) Diagnostic features of atopic dermatitis. Acta Derm Venereol [Suppl] (Stockh) 92: 44–47
16. Herzberg J (1973) Wenig bekannte Formen der Neurodermitis. Hautarzt 24: 47–51
17. Hill LW, Sulzberger MB (1935) Evolution of atopic dermatitis. Arch Dermatol Syph 32: 451–463
18. Kjellman NIM (1977) Atopic disease in seven-year-old children. Acta Paediatr Scand 66: 465–471
19. Koblenzer CS, Koblenzer PJ (1988) Chronic intractable atopic eczema. Its occurrence as a physical sign of impaired parent-child relationships and psychologic developmental arrest: improvement through parent insight and education. Arch Dermatol 124: 1673–1677
20. Leung DYM, Bhan AK, Schneeberger EE, Geha RS (1983) Characterization of the mononuclear cell infiltration in atopic dermatitis using monoclonal antibodies. J Allergy Clin Immunol 71: 47–56
21. Lever W, Schaumburg-Lever G (1990) Histopathology of the skin. Lippincott, Philadelphia
22. Marghescu S (1990) Besondere Manifestationsformen des atopischen Ekzems. In: Braun-Falco O, Ring J (eds) Fortschritte der praktischen Dermatologie und Venerologie, vol XII. Springer, Berlin Heidelberg New York, pp 99–102
23. Nilsson E, Mikaelsson B, Andersson S (1985) Atopy, occupation and domestic work as risk factors for hand eczema in hospital workers. Contact Dermatitis 13: 216–223
24. Podmore P, Burrows D, Eedy DJ, Stanford CF (1986) Seborrhoeic eczema – a disease entity or a clinical variant of atopic eczema? Br J Dermatol 115: 341–350
25. Przybilla B, Ring J, Enders F, Winklmann H (1991) Stigmata of atopic constitution in patients with atopic eczema or atopic respiratory disease. Acta Derm Venereol (Stockh) (in press)
26. Queille-Roussel C, Raynaud F, Saurat JH (1985) A prospective computerized study of 500 cases of atopic dermatitis in childhood. I. Initial analyses of 250 parameters. Acta Derm Venereol [Suppl] (Stockh) 114: 87–92
27. Rajka G (1989) Essential aspects of atopic dermatitis. Springer, Berlin Heidelberg New York
28. Ring J, Palos E, Zimmermann F (1986) Psychosomatische Aspekte der Eltern-Kind-Beziehung bei atopischem Ekzem im Kindesalter I. Psychodiagnostische Testverfahren bei Eltern und Kindern und Vergleich mit somatischen Befunden. Hautarzt 37: 560–567
29. Rocha C, De Maubeuge J, Sarfati M, Song M, Delespesse G (1984) Characterization of cellular infiltrates in skin lesions of atopic eczema by means of monoclonal antibodies. Dermatologica 169: 330–338
30. Rokugo SM, Tagami H, Usaba Y, Tomita Y (1990) Contact sensitivity to pityrosporum ovale in patients with atopic dermatitis. Arch Dermatol 126: 627–732
31. Rystedt I (1985) Prognostic factors in atopic dermatitis. Acta Derm Venereol (Stockh) 65: 206–213
32. Rystedt I (1985) Factors influencing the occurrence of hand eczema in adults with a history of atopic dermatitis in childhood. Contact Dermatitis 12: 185–191
33. Sampson HA, McCaskill CC (1985) Food hypersensitivity and atopic dermatitis: evaluation of 113 patients. J Pediatr 107: 669–675
34. Schnyder UW (1960) Neurodermitis – Asthma – Rhinitis. Eine genetisch-allergologische Studie. Acta Genet Stat Med 10 [Suppl 18]: 1–106
35. Schultz Larsen F, Holm NV, Henningsen K (1986) Atopic dermatitis. A genetic-epidemiologic study in a population based twin sample. J Am Acad Dermatol 15: 487–494
36. Shmunes E, Keil JE (1984) The role of atopy in occupational dermatoses. Contact Dermatitis 11: 174–178
37. Uehara M, Miyauchi H (1984) The morphologic characteristics of dry skin in atopic dermatitis. Arch Dermatol 120: 1186–1190
38. Vogel F, Dorn H (1964) Atopische Hauterkrankungen. Atopische Dermatitis. In: Becker PE (ed) Humangenetik, vol 4. Thieme, Stuttgart, pp 418–428
39. Wüthrich B, Schudel P (1983) Die Neurodermitis atopica

nach dem Kleinkindesalter – Eine katamnestische Untersuchung anhand von 121 Fällen. Z Hautkr 58: 1013–1023
40. Young E (1986) Forefoot eczema – further studies and a review. Clin Exp Dermatol 11: 523–528
41. Zachary CB, Allen MH, MacDonald DM (1985) In situ quantification of T-lymphocyte subsets and Langerhans cells in the inflammatory infiltrate of atopic eczema. Br J Dermatol 112: 149–156

Pathophysiology of Atopic Eczema

Regulation of IgE Synthesis

J. C. Prinz and E. P. Rieber

Introduction

Since 1966 when K. Ishizaka and co-workers [42] first detected cytophilic immunoglobulin E (IgE) as the carrier of reaginic activity in the sera of allergic patients, the production of IgE against common and otherwise innocuous antigens has been recognized as a central feature in the pathogenesis of immediate type hypersensitivity. In order to understand the reasons for this pathological immune response, the regulation of IgE production has become the subject of intensive investigation. Confined as they were to in vitro systems, studies of human IgE synthesis proved to be rather problematic. Until lately, they were restricted to spontaneous IgE secretion by plasma cells which had differentiated in vivo. As opposed to IgG, measurement of the extremely small amounts of IgE secreted into culture supernatants was impeded by the limited specificity and sensitivity of the detection methods. In addition, results were often influenced by cytophilic IgE released from cells bearing Fc receptors for IgE ($Fc_{\varepsilon}R$), such as B lymphocytes, monocytes and basophils. Only the development of monoclonal antibody techniques and the rapid progress in molecular biology have facilitated a deeper understanding of the mechanisms of IgE regulation. Since this insight was obtained in humans as well as in rodent models, in the following chapter the results from the human and the animal systems will be summarized separately from each other. Nevertheless, this juxtaposition will demonstrate that despite some species-specific differences, many of the findings in rodents apply to human IgE synthesis also.

The Humoral Immune Response

When an organism encounters foreign material (viruses, bacteria, fungi and their products, transplants, etc.) which is recognized by the adaptive immune system, a specific immune response is generated. This defence mechanism is dominated either by cell-mediated or by antibody-mediated humoral mechanisms, or consists of a combination of both.

In their structure, immunoglobulin (Ig) molecules are composed of two identical smaller and two identical larger polypeptide chains, the light (L) and heavy (H) chains, respectively (Fig. 1). Each chain consists of a variable (V) region, characterized by high sequence variability, and a constant (C) region. The function of the V regions is to specifically bind antigen. They are generated from germline genes by the random recombination of two (L chain: V and J) or three (H chain: V, D and J) gene segments during early B-cell ontogeny. The C region of the H chains is encoded by one of several constant region genes (C_{μ}, C_{γ}, C_{ε}, etc.), which determine the isotype of the Ig molecules. The two combined C(H)regions represent the Fc part of the Ig molecule. They are thus responsible for the different biological activities of the various Ig classes, which include complement fixation, binding to Fc receptors of immunological effector cells and the ability to cross mucosal and placental barriers. The distinct effector mechanisms reflect the organism's compulsion to cope with a large variety of chemically, physically and biologically different antigens (*anti*body *gen*erators).

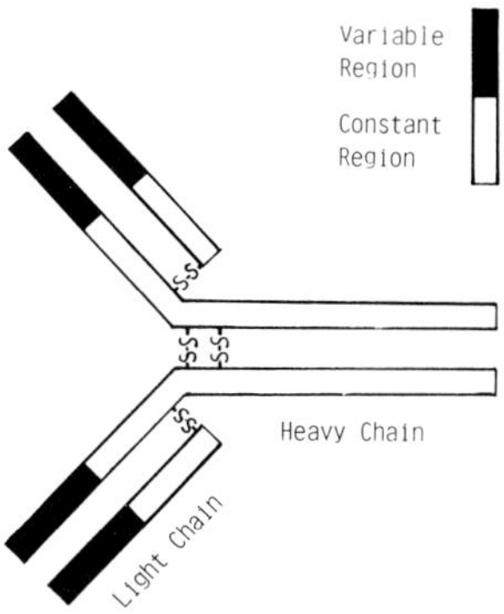

Fig. 1. Basic immunoglobulin (Ig) structure. Each Ig molecule consists of two identical light (L) and two identical heavy (H) chains. Paired variable regions of adjoining L and H chain determine the antigen binding site. The Ig isotype is determined by the constant region of the heavy chain (see text)

It is therefore obvious that the pattern of Ig isotypes secreted in response to a defined antigen crucially affects the course of an immune reaction. Production of inappropriate Ig classes may result not only in incomplete antigen elimination but can also give rise to a pathological immune response harmful to the organism. This is the case in immediate type hypersensitivity: IgE antibodies, phylogenetically evolved to fight parasitic worm infections, are produced against otherwise irrelevant antigens such as pollen, bee venom or chemical haptens. Secondary exposure to these substances will activate IgE-mediated effector mechanisms and thereby trigger the well-known allergic symptoms.

Generation of Functional Antibody Diversity by the Isotype Switch

Each antigen-stimulated proliferating and differentiating B cell gives rise to a clone of Ig-secreting plasma cells, which produce Ig of only one antigen specificity. Functional diversity of these antibodies is generated by the isotype switch: during an antibody response the B cells can change from secretion of IgM to the synthesis of other Ig classes, since the V region gene complex of the heavy chain (VDJ, antigen specificity) can associate with different constant region genes (isotype, Fig. 2). In humans the C_H region genes are aligned downstream of the V_H region genes in the order (5' to 3') VDJ – C_μ-C_δ-$C_{\gamma 3}$-$C_{\gamma 1}$-$C_{\alpha 1}$-$C_{\gamma 2}$-$C_{\gamma 4}$-C_ε-$C_{\alpha 2}$, and in rodents in the order (5' to 3') VDJ–C_μ-C_δ-$C_{\gamma 3}$-$C_{\gamma 1}$-$C_{\gamma 2b}$-$C_{\gamma 2a}$-C_ε-C_α. At the beginning of an antibody response, B lymphocytes first produce IgM because the C_μ gene is closest to the V region gene complex. During an isotype switch this IgM constant region gene is replaced by other C_H region genes further downstream, whereas the V region remains the same. Thus, the V region gene complex in the descendants of a single B cell can be transcribed with different constant region genes, generating different classes of Ig with the same antigen specificity.

The different requirements for coping with a great variety of antigens ask for a well-directed expression of the distinct Ig classes. Although the mechanisms are only partially clarified, isotype switch and isotype secretion have been shown to be regulated by T lymphocytes and their soluble products (reviewed by Teale and Abraham [110]).

Cooperation Between T Cells, B Cells and Accessory Cells

Initiation of antibody secretion to most antigens requires help from activated antigen-specific helper T cells. Therefore, the activation of T cells following recognition of antigen is a key step in the initiation of a humoral immune response. T cells, however, cannot be stimulated by antigen in the soluble state. T-cell receptors only recognize fragments of antigen that are exhibited in association with the individual's own major histocompatibility complex (MHC) molecules on the membrane of antigen-presenting cells (APC, macrophages, Langerhans cells of the skin, follicular dendritic cells, B lymphocytes etc.) This so-called *antigen presentation* requires processing of the antigen by the APCs which includes its uptake, denaturation and proteolytic cleavage. The resulting highly immunogenic peptides are then exhibited on the membrane of the APCs in a complex with MHC molecules. These polymorphic structures were originally detected as transplantation antigens responsible for graft rejection and were named human leucocyte antigens (HLA). Their function as peptide-binding molecules which present fragments of protein antigens to the receptors of immunocompetent T lymphocytes has been proven only recently (Bjorkman et al. [4, 5]). Although additional signals are required, it is the recognition of antigen fragments in association with

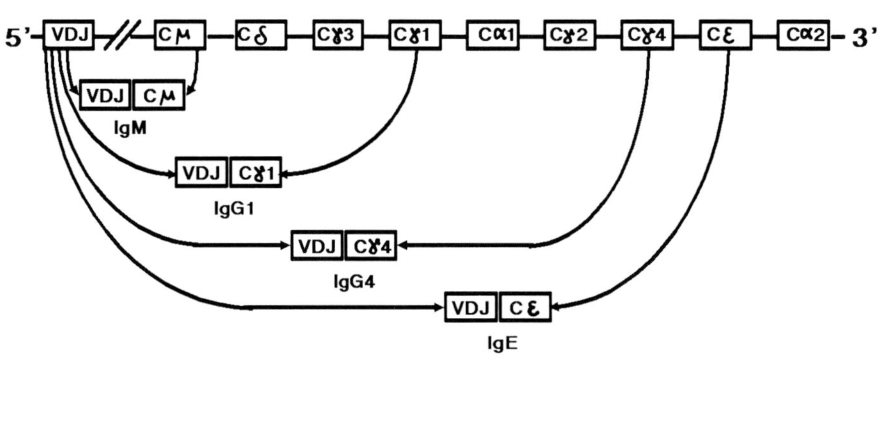

Fig. 2. Generation of functional antibody diversity by the isotype switch in humans. The *C* region genes are located downstream from the rearranged *V* region gene complex (*VDJ*). During antibody production the VDJ segment can be recombined with different C region genes to form antibodies with a single specificity but of different isotypes.

MHC molecules by the T-cell receptor that delivers the main signal for activation of T lymphocytes. The activated T cells then provide help to antigen-stimulated B cells in two ways: by cognate, i.e. MHC-dependent, cell/cell interaction and by secreting soluble mediators which influence B-cell growth and differentiation.

Thus, generation of an antibody response involves several events (reviewed by Grey and Chestnut [32]):

1. Antigen is taken up and processed by APC. The resulting peptide fragments are then presented in a complex with MHC molecules on the membrane of the APC to be recognised by antigen-specific T cells, which are subjected to activation, proliferation and differentiation.
2. Native antigen interacts with Ig receptors on B cells, becomes internalized, processed and expressed on the B-cell surface complexed with MHC molecules. (In the induction of Ig synthesis, this step may replace step 1 as it leads to antigen-specific T-cell activation and simultaneously guarantees direct interaction between T and B cells specific for the same antigen.)
3. The antigen fragments presented on B cells are recognized by the T-cell receptor of the expanded antigen-specific T cells. This cognate interaction with and the secretion of soluble mediators by the activated T cells lead to clonal expansion of the B cells and differentiation into plasma cells, and to the deliberate formation of distinct antibody classes.

Regulation of IgE Production

Since the same basic mechanisms apply for T and B cell activation irrespective of the type of antibodies formed in a humoral immune response, a central question in unraveling the aetiology of allergic diseases has been concerned with the identification of signals that selectively trigger the production of IgE antibodies. For both the rodent and human IgE response three major regulatory components have been delineated: regulatory T cells, IgE binding factors (IgE-BF) and cytokines. These partially overlapping entities obviously operate in concert at different levels of the IgE response to control isotype switch, IgE secretion and provision of effector cells for cytophilic IgE. The overall capacity to mount an IgE response appears to be genetically controlled.

Regulatory T Cells and Genetic Predisposition

Rodent System

In 1967 Ogilvie [73] observed that rats responded to infection with the nematode, *Nippostrongylus brasiliensis* (Nb), with high titres of IgE antibodies which persisted even after termination of infection. Furthermore, these animals showed a rapid secondary IgE response following reinfection with Nb [74]. Immunization of animals of the same strain with protein antigens using *Bordetella pertussis* (Bp) vaccine as an adjuvant, however, initiated only a transient, low level primary and no secondary IgE response (for this reason it is called the low IgE responder strain), although a pronounced secondary IgG response was observed [3]. These findings indiated that IgE synthesis is controlled independently of IgG. The need for regulatory T cells in the production of IgE was first reported by Okumura and Tada [76, 77] who found that neonatal thymectomy completely abolished the ability of rats to mount a primary IgE antibody response. In contrast, when adult animals from a low IgE responder strain were selectively depleted of T cells by thymectomy, by sub-lethal doses of whole body irradiation or by treatment with cyclophosphamide, a prolonged and enhanced IgE antibody response was observed following immunization with protein antigens. This IgE production could be selectively terminated by subsequent T-cell reconstitution with syngeneic thymocytes or spleen cells obtained from normal or antigen-primed rats. Thus, according to these experiments, the generation of an IgE response apparently required helper T cells, whereas the limited and transitory IgE response pattern of low responder strains was due to control by suppressor T cells.

Induction of IgE production was influenced by the experimental conditions chosen. While some antigens were capable of inducing an IgE response when administered in extremely low doses, application of higher antigen amounts elicited only IgG but no, or only little, IgE production. Also, various adjuvants used for immunization of rodents with haptenic conjugates of DNP (dinitrophenyl) coupled to carrier proteins caused a clear dissociation of the DNP-specific IgG and IgE antibody responses [49]. Use of aluminium hydroxide gel (alum) or BP vaccine as adjuvants promoted the production of both DNP-specific IgG and IgE antibodies, whereas inclusion of antigen in complete Freund's adjuvant (CFA) selectively induced IgG antibodies. Preadministration of DNP-coupled *mycobacterium tuberculosis* into mice was found to suppress an anti-DNP IgE response [50]. A differential activation of suppressor T cells was help responsible for these effects: T lymphocytes from animals secreting only DNP-specific IgG antibodies selectively hampered the in vitro IgE production to DNP without affecting IgG synthesis [105], an effect directly proportional to the number of T cells added.

Collectively, rodent IgE production to most antigens appears to be restrained by suppressive mechanisms. Therefore, the ability to initiate an IgE response requires either particular immunization procedures, a perturbation in the regulatory T-cell compartment or as yet undetermined qualities of the antigen. Furthermore, detection of a high IgE responder strain of rats by Jarret and Stewart [44] suggested a genetic predisposition for IgE production. Immune response (Ir) genes for IgE production have also been described in mice. They are linked to the MHC and determine the capacity of animals to respond to defined antigens with high titres of primary and secondary IgE antibody [18, 90].

Human System

In humans, diseases associated with perturbations of the T-cell compartment are often accompanied by distorted IgE production. A marked elevation of serum IgE is found in patients with hyper IgE syndrome [29] and severe atopic diseases [53], both of which display decreased numbers of circulating $CD8^+$ cytotoxic or suppressor cells. Patients with illnesses accompanied by partial T-cell deficiencies, like ataxia teleangiectasia and DiGeorge, Nezelof and Wiskott-Aldrich syndromes, often display elevated serum IgE levels [6]. Similar increases in IgE levels are also found in patients who develop acute graft versus host disease (GVH) after allogeneic bone marrow transplantation [28]. A selective deficiency of $CD8^+$ T cells or an imbalance between $CD4^+$ helper and $CD8^+$ suppressor T cells resulting in decreased suppressor T-cell activity has been accused of causing the elevated IgE levels in these disorders, thereby suggesting that suppressor T lymphocytes may represent a limiting component for the human IgE antibody response, too.

Involvement of genetic factors in the development of allergic disorders was first suggested by Coca and Cooke [10] who defined the inherited predisposition to develop immediate type hypersensitivity as "atopy". Further studies have revealed three genetic parameters which affect IgE antibody production. (1) High IgE levels were shown to be inherited by a recessive gene unrelated to HLA [60]. (2) Linkage between particular HLA haplotypes and an IgE response to defined antigens of allergic patients was first reported by Levine et al. [56] for the allergen Amb a I from ragweed pollen (*Ambrosia artemisifolia*). HLA associations have been found for other allergens as well. They become more obvious with allergens of lower molecular weight and when related to HLA DR/Dw types instead of HLA-A and -B types. An obligatory association with the haplotype DR2/Dw2 was demonstrated for the IgE response to Amb a V, another pollen allergen from ragweed [62]. (3) Certain HLA haplotypes, like A2–B7, A1–B8, Dw2 and Dw3, were found in atopic patients at significantly increased frequencies [61].

For a long time, the reasons of this concomitance remained elusive. The recently described function of MHC molecules in antigen presentation [4, 5], however, offers a clue to a novel understanding of the HLA-association of the IgE response to defined antigens. It suggests that different MHC molecules may have different capabilities for binding and presenting antigens taken up in the lowest quantities (ng/year) or for presenting unique allergenic epitopes of an antigen. Furthermore, presentation of antigen fragments by certain MHC molecules might provide information favouring an IgE response. Thus, the signals delivered during interaction of MHC molecules with antigen receptors on T cells could possibly influence the type of the developing immune reaction.

For a long time, helper activity was associated with $CD4^+$ helper T cells, and, conversely, suppressive activity with $CD8^+$ suppressor T cells. Recently, however, a second concept of immune regulation has evolved, which is based on mutually inhibitory factors secreted by $CD4^+$ T lymphocytes.

Role of Cytokines in the IgE Response

Many of the regulatory signals which control activation, growth and differentiation of B cells, as well as a variety of other cell types, are delivered by T-cell-derived mediators. In 1971, Dutton et al. [19] observed that some functions of activated T lymphocytes could be transferred by their supernatants. These activities were designated T-cell-derived mediators or T-cell-replacing factor (TRF [96]). Further investigations proved that distinct activities could be assigned to different factors, and finally molecular cloning techniques and the production of recombinant cytokines facilitated their biological characterization. Studies on the effect of recombinant factors on the subclass of Ig secreted by B lymphocytes disclosed that the induction of both rodent and human IgE production is dominated by two T-cell-derived lymphokines, interleukin 4 (IL-4) and interferon-gamma (IFN-γ).

Rodent System

Originally, IL-4 was detected by its ability to enhance B-cell proliferation [35] and thus designated as B-cell growth factor (BCGF), later on as B cell stimulatory factor-1 (BSF-1 [71]). It was purified to homogeneity by Ohara and Paul [75] and first cloned and sequenced by Lee et al. [52]. Resting B cells respond to IL-4 by increased expression of class II MHC molecules [91] and of Fc receptors for IgE ($Fc_\varepsilon R$ [36]), by enlarged cell volume and by preparation for transition into S phase in response to stimulation with IgM-specific antibodies [89]. IL-4 also acts as an autocrine growth factor for a subpopulation of helper T cells and for some T-cell lines [20, 57, 65]. Most strikingly, IL-4 enhanced both IgG1 [99] and IgE synthesis [11] in bulk cultures of lipopolysaccharide (LPS)-stimulated B cells. In particular the IgE secretion showed a progressive rise with increasing concentrations of IL-4 whereas the production of IgM, IgG3, IgG2a and IgG2b was markedly reduced [100]. The essential involvement of IL-4 in generating and sustaining an IgE response was also confirmed in vivo since injection of an IL-4-neutralizing monoclonal antibody into mice suppressed the polyclonal IgE response [21, 22]. The mode of action of IL-4 on IgE production has not yet been entirely clarified, results from various experimental systems reported by Lutzker et al. [59], Bergstedt-Lindqvist et al. [1] and by Lebman and Coffman [51], however, suggested that IL-4 directs the isotype switch selectively to the expression of IgG1 and IgE.

Most of the activities of IL-4 are markedly antagonized by IFN-γ. The latter inhibits in vitro IgG1 and IgE production [11] while stimulating the expression of IgG2a [100]. Furthermore, when injected at the time of initiation of an immune response, IFN-γdiminished and neutralising antibodies to IFN-γ enhanced the concentrations of serum IgG1 and IgE in mice [23]. IFN-γ not only antagonized the activities of IL-4 but also inhibited the proliferation of T cells secreting IL-4 [26]. Based on the lymphokine patterns secreted by rodent T cells, two types of helper T-cell clones were defined, both of which promote Ig synthesis but favour the secretion of different isotype patterns [66]. They were designated as T_H1 and T_H2. Both types produce IL-3, but only T_H1 cells secrete IL-2, lymphotoxin and IFN-γ. By these lymphokines they induce synthesis of IgG2a in vitro and are inhibitory for IgG1 and IgE. The T_H1 subset thereby seems to contain the effector cells responsible for delayed type hypersensitivity [9]. In response to the same antigenic stimuli, T_H2 cells secrete IL-4 and IL-5, which drive B cells to the production of IgG1 and IgE. Furthermore, through these lymphokines, T_H2 cells promote the development of two cell types essentially involved in the effector function of cytophilic IgE: IL-4 together with IL-3 enhance the growth of mucosal mast cells in vitro [65], and IL-5 induces growth and differentiation of eosinophils [7].

Although in rodents IL4 does not interfere with the production of IFN-γ by T_H1 clones, T_H2 cells still antagonize T_H1 activities: they secrete a factor that inhibits cytokine production by T_H1 clones [25]. Astonishingly, this cytokine synthesis inhibitory factor (CSIF, IL-10) seems to be of relevance not only for the regulation of immune functions: its protein sequence shows extensive homology to a so far uncharacterized open reading frame, BCRFI, in the Epstein-Barr virus genome, suggesting that a captured gene may enhance virus survival in the host by inhibiting antiviral effector mechanisms [64].

The physiological relevance of the alternative lymphokine patterns becomes most evident in infection of mice with *Leishmania major* or *Schistosoma mansoni*, where the course of disease appears to be strictly related to the lymphokines produced by the parasite-specific T cells. Whereas a predominant activation of T_H2 cells leads to a devastating visceral infection, generation of a T_H1-dominated response is followed by healing of infection and establishment of a long lasting immunity. Furthermore, exogeneous application of IFN-γ or of neutralising antibodies to IL-4 during a predominant recruitment of T_H2 cells resolves infection [33, 97]. The resistance or susceptibility to infection seems to result from different effector mechanisms: whereas IFN-γ is a critical macrophage-activating factor mediating cellular defence against the obligate intracellular pathogens [68, 70], T_H2 cells not only fail to activate monocyte functions [103] but via IL-4 inhibit macrophage activation by IFN-γ, and via IL-5 mediate high eosinophil levels [97, 12].

Collectively, the data indicate that the IgE response is reciprocally controlled by IL-4 and IFN-γ. In rodents, this functional dichotomy is reflected at the cellular level through at least two types of helper T cells that appear to be mutually inhibitory. However, pleiotropic effects of IL-4 beyond regulation of the IgE response are suggested by the wide distribution of IL-4 receptors which are found on many hemopoietic and non-hemopoietic cell types [58].

Human System

Human IL-4 was first identified by screening cDNA libraries prepared from activated human T-cell clones using a cDNA fragment of mouse IL-4 [122]. This was feasible because of the high degree of sequence homology of the two cytokines [124]. Only a region of approximately 40 amino acids in the middle of both proteins lacks such homology. This may explain why both mouse and human IL-4, despite their high structural resemblance, display species-specific activity only [67].

As in rodents, human IL-4 causes a significant increase in the volume of resting B cells and enhances their proliferative response to polyclonal stimulation [14]. B cells cultured in the presence of IL-4 show an increased expression of the low affinity $Fc_\varepsilon R$ ($Fc_\varepsilon R2$/CD23, Defrance et al. 1986) and an augmented release of IgE-BF (soluble CD23, see below). Most important for the generation of allergic diseases, IL-4 plays a key role in the human IgE response by inducing a high rate of in vitro IgE production by polyclonally stimulated human B cells. Although this effect requires the presence of T cells and monocytes, it was specifically inhibited by an IL-4-specific antiserum, thus demonstrating that IL-4 was responsible for the in vitro-induced IgE synthesis [81, 82]. At suboptimal IL-4 concentrations, IgE production was enhanced considerably by addition of IL-5 and was dependent on the presence of IL-6, whereas both factors by themselves failed to induce IgE production [83, 117]. Yet, as in rodents, the role of human IL-4 in the IgE response by far exceeds the induction of IgE secretion. Simultaneously with IgE initiation it provides a differentiation signal for a variety of important immunological effector and regulator cells involved in the IgE response by inducing or enhancing $Fc_\varepsilon R$ expression on monocytes [116], Langerhans cells of the skin [2], B cells [13] and T lymphocytes [87]. A similar functional dominance of a single lymphokine has also been reported for mouse IFN-γ, which induces the production of IgG2a [34] and enhances the expression of Fc receptors for this isotype on macrophages [119].

As for other Ig isotypes, commitment of B cells to IgE secretion occurs in at least two distinct stages: cognate interaction between T and B cells and action of T-cell-derived cytokines on B cells. In all experiments, reported soluble signals alone were insufficient to induce IgE production by activated B lymphocytes, but depended on the presence of T lymphocytes. Additional isotype-specific signals seem to be delivered during MHC-dependent T/B contact: rodent T cells favouring an IgG2a response were insufficient to support IgG1 production by B cells despite the presence of high levels of IL-4 [102], and for the in vivo IgE response in mice, a late acting form of T-cell help other than IL-4 was observed [24]. Similar conditions apply for human IgE secretion. Although IgE synthesis by IL-4 is hampered by monoclonal antibodies against CD2, CD3, CD4, LFA-1 and MHC class II molecules [118], the IgE isotype-specific signals in cellular T/B interaction have not yet been identified.

As in rodents, the functional antagonism between IL-4 and IFN-γ is a feature of the human IgE response, too. IL-4-induced IgE synthesis and $Fc_\varepsilon R2$/CD23 expression on B and T cells are strongly inhibited by IFN-γ as well as by IFN-γ and prostaglandin E_2 [81]. Vice versa, IL-4 suppresses in vitro synthesis of IFN-γ by mononuclear cells and IFN-γ-induced monocyte activation and expression of Fc receptors for IgG [80, 111]. Still the activities of IL-4 and IFN-γ in the IgE response are not entirely exclusive since IFN-γ was found to induce expression of $Fc_\varepsilon R$ on platelets and on Langerhans cells of the skin [2, 79].

In contrast to mice, the antagonistic effects of IL-4 and IFN-γ on IgE secretion are not reflected at the cellular level. In humans, both lymphokines can be secreted by one and the same T cell. The patterns of secreted lymphokines could not be assigned to different types of human helper T cells, and the relative amounts of IL-4 and IFN-γ produced by single T-cell clones in vitro depended on the mode of stimulation. Most of the $CD4^+$ and a proportion of the $CD8^+$ T-cell clones tested simultaneously secreted IL-2, IL4 and IFN-γ, even though at various ratios [78]. Thus, the ability of human T-cell clones to launch IgE synthesis in vitro resulted from the ratio of IL-4 and IFN-γ present in their supernatants. Consequently, IgE production induced by T-cell supernatants could be further enhanced by the addition of an antiserum to IFN-γ and was inhibited by antibodies neutralizing IL-4 [82]. Lately, however, growing experience with cytokine secretion of human T cells indicates that the pattern of lymphokines may be altered by in vitro degeneration of the T-cell clones, since their spectrum often broadens with ongoing T-cell propagation. Careful interpretation is therefore required regarding the exact T-cell function in vivo.

Collectively, IL-4 appears to be the most prominent lymphokine in the initiation of the human IgE antibody response, too. It mediates the secretion of IgE antibodies and simultaneously promotes the differentiation of important effector cells necessary for the biological activities of cytophilic IgE. Yet it should be emphasized that human IL-4 is also a pleiotropic cytokine with effects on various cell types, and that IgE secretion results from many different agonistic and antagonistic signals influencing isotype expression.

Cytokine Production in Allergic Diseases

To determine the role of cytokines in allergic disesases, the lymphokine patterns of T cells from allergic donors have been examined by several investigators. As compared to normal individuals, lectin-stimulated T-cell clones from atopic donors secreted significantly more IL-4 whereas the production of IFN-γ was diminished. T-cell clones obtained from patients with hyper IgE syndrome showed a normal secretion of IL-4, whereas the number of clones producing IFN-γ was strongly reduced

[16]. Furthermore, in allergic patients IL-4 synthesis by allergen-specific T-cell clones was increased and that of IFN-γ reduced as compared to T-cell clones specific for conventional recall antigens such as tetanus toxoid [120, 126]. An imbalance between IL-4 and its antagonistic lymphokines may thus represent a basic feature of diseases characterized by an exaggerated IgE production and offer new therapeutic approaches. As reported by de Vries et al. [17], treatment of a patient suffering from the hyper IgE syndrome with subcutaneous injections of IFN-α improved the clinical symptoms. Although much more experience is needed, these preliminary results indicate that clinical application of cytokines in allergic diseases may become a helpful therapeutic tool.

The Role of $Fc_\varepsilon R2$/CD23 in IgE Regulation

Rodent System

When examining the pronounced IgE response of rodents following helminth infection, Suemura and Ishizaka [104] observed that T cells from mesenteric lymph nodes (MLN) of Nb-infected rats spontaneously released soluble factors, which selectively enhanced the IgE production by antigen-primed lymphocytes in vitro. Further analysis led Ishizaka and co-workers to propose a model of IgE regulation which is dominated by two T-cell-derived factors with selective affinity for IgE. These IgE-BFs act directly on surface IgE^+ B lymphocytes and either enhance or suppress IgE formation (IgE-potentiating or – suppressive factor, IgE-PF or IgE-SF). Both, IgE-PF and IgE-SF are actively secreted by T lymphocytes expressing $Fc_\varepsilon R$ and probably represent their secreted form [38]. They are glycoproteins encoded by one and the same structural gene [63], and their specific activity is determined by post-translational processing: IgE-PF contains N-linked and O-linked oligosaccharides both with a terminal sialic acid residue, whereas IgE-SF has only O-linked oligosaccharides with terminal galactose-*N*-acetylgalactosamine. This glycosylation pattern is reflected by their affinity for different lectins and sensitivity to tunicamycin: IgE-PF binds to concanavalin A (con A) and lentil lectin, and IgE-SF has affinity for peanut agglutinin. When cells producing IgE-PF are treated with tunicamycin, which inhibits the assembly of N-linked oligosaccharides on proteins, the cells form IgE-SF.

Glycosylation of the IgE-BF is regulated by two factors, the glycosylation enhancing and glycosylation inhibiting factors (GEF and GIF). GEF is released from $Fc_\varepsilon R^+$ helper T lymphocytes and enhances N-glycosylation of IgE-BF, whereas GIF is released from suppressor T cells and inhibits their glycosylation (for review see [40]). Recently, Iwata et al. [43] suggested that fractions of both GEF and GIF have specific affinities for the inducing antigen, thereby drawing parallels to the antigen-specific suppressive (TsF) and augmentation (TaF) T cell factors described by Takemori and Tada [109] and Tokuhisa et al. [113].

Human System

Since in 1977 Gonzalez-Molina and Spiegelberg [30] first described the ability of human lymphocytes to bind IgE, the structure, cellular distribution and function of $Fc_\varepsilon R2$/CD23 have puzzled many investigators. Although it was soon recognised that $Fc_\varepsilon R2$/CD23 is not related to the high affinity $Fc_\varepsilon R1$ of basophils and mast cells, its precise role in the IgE response is still controversial.

Two types, $Fc_\varepsilon R2a$ containing 321 amino acids and $Fc_\varepsilon R2b$ containing 320 amino acids, could be distinguished by molecular cloning and RNAse protection assays, which differ only in their N-terminal intracellular amino acid sequence [47, 123]. Whereas $Fc_\varepsilon R2a$ is constitutively expressed on B lymphocytes, $Fc_\varepsilon R2b$ can be induced on several cell types including monocytes [116], B cells [124], T lymphocytes [85], Langerhans cells of the skin [2], eosinophils [8] and platelets [45].

$Fc_\varepsilon R2$/CD23 is a member of the C-type family of animal lectins, and its sequence homology suggests a function in ligand internalization [47]. Kehry and Yamishita [46], and Pirron et al. [84] demonstrated for rodents and humans, respectively, that antigen complexed with IgE is processed and presented by $Fc_\varepsilon R2$/$CD23^+$ B cell lines 10^2 times more efficiently than non-complexed antigen, thus suggesting a role of $Fc_\varepsilon R2$/CD23 in IgE-dependent antigen focussing. This process, however, is very slow and leads to Fc-receptor uptake of only a small proportion of the bound immune complexes (Prinz and Rieber, unpublished data).

On B lymphocytes $Fc_\varepsilon R2$/CD23 expression is confined to IgM^+ and IgD^+ cells and is lost after isotype switching. In non-allergic individuals, it is found on average on 50% of peripheral B lymphocytes [48], whereas atopic patients display significantly increased numbers of circulating $Fc_\varepsilon R2$/CD23 B cells. Gordon et al. [31] have proposed a role of $Fc_\varepsilon R2$/CD23 as a receptor for low molecular weight B-cell growth factor (BCGF). Yet, as shown by Vazquez et al. [115], expression of $Fc_\varepsilon R2$/CD23 is not necessary for BCGF-mediated B-cell proliferation. An essential role of B-cell $Fc_\varepsilon R2$/CD23 and of B-cell-derived IgE-BFs in the IgE response, however, is indicated by the observation that in vitro IgE synthesis by B cells was selectively suppressed in the presence of $Fc_\varepsilon R$-specific mAb [83] or by binding of IgE-immune complexes to the B-cell $Fc_\varepsilon R$ [98]. Furthermore, $Fc_\varepsilon R2$/$CD23^+$ B cells and B cell lines release IgE-binding factors (soluble CD23) with potentiating activity on in vitro IgE production, the effect of which was converted to IgE suppression by treatment of the B cells with tunicamycin [93, 94]. The IgE-potentiating activity was most prominent at suboptimal concentrations of IL-4 [83]. In contrast to rodents IgE-BF released from human B cells are not secreted, but represent breakdown products shedded after proteolytic cleavage of the cell-surface $Fc_{\varepsilon}R$ [69]. In this context it is an interesting correlation that IL-4 as the essential lymphokine for IgE induction strongly enhances $Fc_{\varepsilon}R2$/CD23 expression on B lymphocytes and release of IgE-BF [13, 48, 83], whereas B-cell $Fc_{\varepsilon}R2$/CD23 expression is markedly reduced by IFN-γ [27, 92].

Another function of IgE-BF was suggested by Swendeman and Thorley-Lawson [108] who demonstrated that sCD23 purified from culture supernatants of a human B-cell line could act as autocrine growth factor for anti-IgM stimulated B lymphocytes and some B-cell lines. A genetically engineered recombinant sCD23, however, failed to display this activity [114]. Instead, recombinant sCD23 could inhibit in vitro IgE-mediated reactions by interfering with the binding of IgE to $Fc_{\varepsilon}R1$ and $Fc_{\varepsilon}R2$ [107]. The existence of $Fc_{\varepsilon}R2$/CD23$^+$ T cells has long remained controversial. Several studies have suggested low or lacking $Fc_{\varepsilon}R2$/CD23 expression on T cells [47, 101, 106, 121]. Other investigators have reported on elevated numbers of $Fc_{\varepsilon}R^+$ T cells in the blood of patients with severe atopic disease or hyper IgE syndrome [72, 112, 125]. The difficulties in determining $Fc_{\varepsilon}R2$/CD23$^+$ T lymphocytes, however, seem to result from the fact that on T cells $Fc_{\varepsilon}R2$/CD23 represents an activation antigen the expression of which is too low to be detected on resting but enhanced on activated T lymphocytes. As demonstrated recently, $Fc_{\varepsilon}R2$/CD23 expression is found on a subpopulation of lectin-stimulated peripheral T cells [85]. Also, a high level of expression has been reported on HTLV-1 transformed T cell lines obtained from patients with the hyper IgE syndrome [72]. Above all, however, $Fc_{\varepsilon}R2$/CD23 expression is a selective property of allergen-specific T cell blasts, and its expression is included in the cytokine network regulating IgE secretion: IL-4 enhances and IFN-γ strongly suppresses $Fc_{\varepsilon}R2$/CD23 expression on activated T cells [87]. An important role of $Fc_{\varepsilon}R2$/CD23$^+$T cells in IgE secretion is suggested by the recent finding that T cells pretreated with the $Fc_{\varepsilon}R2$/CD23-specific monoclonal antibody M-L25 were inacapable of supporting IL-4-induced in vitro IgE secretion by polyclonally stimulated B lymphocytes [86, 88].

The mode of action of $Fc_{\varepsilon}R2$/CD23$^+$ T cells in IgE secretion is not yet clear. $Fc_{\varepsilon}R2$/CD23 on T cells could interact with surface-IgE on the membrane of B lymphocytes and thereby deliver the IgE-isotype-specific signal required for IgE induction during cognate T/B interaction. Experiments by Ishizaka and Sandberg [41] demonstrated that T lymphocytes of ragweed-allergic patients produced IgE-Bfs following incubation with specific antigen and IgE. Later on, Saryan et al. [95] identified IgE-PFs when evaluating the selective ability of T-cell supernatants from patients with hyper IgE states to enhance in vitro IgE synthesis, and Huff et al. [37, 39] established a T-cell hybridoma secreting IgE-BF. These factors had affinity for IgE and con A, and their activity was sensitive to the treatment of the T cells with tunicamycin or cycloheximide. In addition, IgE-BFs with IgE-enhancing capacity could be isolated from sera of hyper IgE patients [55] whereas sera of non-atopic donors yielded IgE-SF [54]. Paralleling the influence of *Mycobacterium tuberculosis* used as adjuvant in rodents, T cells from patients with pulmonary tuberculosis that had been stimulated with purified protein derivative from tuberculin (PPD) in the presence of IgE, suppressed in vitro IgE production without affecting the IgG response. This suppressive activity could be absorbed by an IgE column or immobilized mouse antiserum to the human lymphoid $Fc_{\varepsilon}R$ [15].

Conclusions

The previous paragraphs have attempted to summarize the most prominent findings obtained by many different investigators during several decades of IgE research. They can be compiled to suggest a model of IgE regulation which is dominated by T cells and their soluble products in both rodents and humans (Fig. 3).

Antigen is taken up by APCs, processed and presented in the context of MHC class II molecules to T lymphocytes which become activated after antigen recognition. During this step some unknown signal is delivered to the T cells which determines the course of the immune response by deciding the pattern of lymphokines to be secreted or by recruiting a special subset of helper T cells. The predominant secretion of IL-4 as compared with IFN-γ directs the isotype switch to the production of IgE by activated B lymphocytes and simultaneously promotes the generation of important immune effector cells necessary for the biological activity of cytophilic IgE. However, the in vivo concentrations of lymphokines may not reach those used to induce in vitro IgE production. Therefore, much of the in vivo effect of IL-4 may depend on its modification by other lymphokines, such as IL-5.

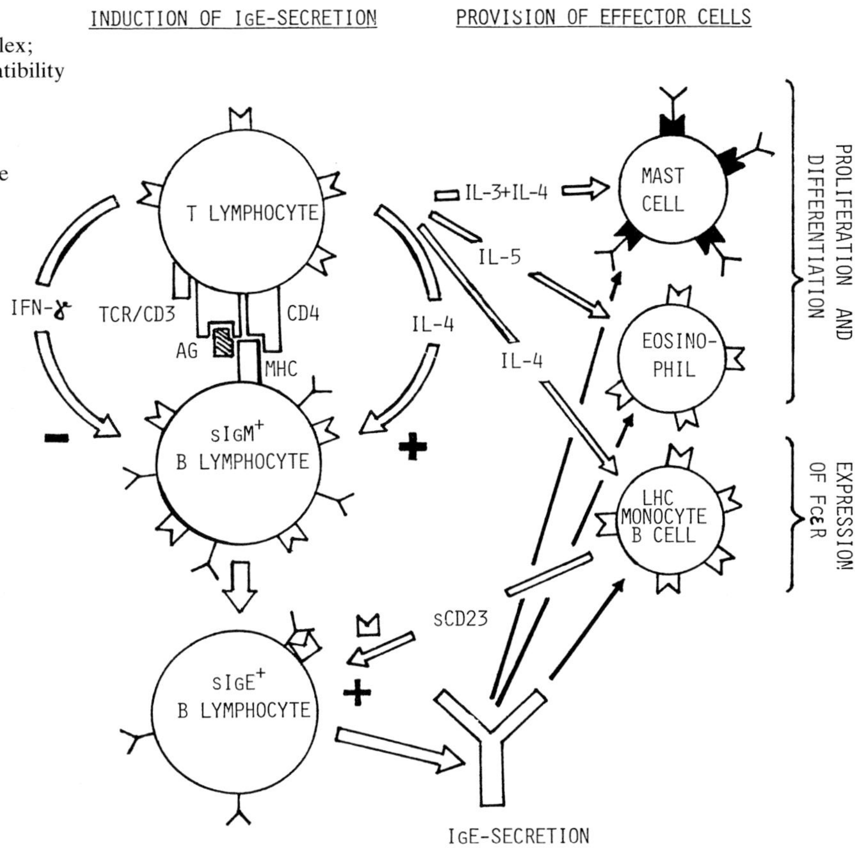

Fig. 3. Synopsis of IgE regulation. *TCR/CD3*, T-cell receptor/CD3 complex; *AG*, antigen; *MHC*, major histocompatibility complex class II molecule; *LHC*, Langerhans cell of the skin; ꟷ, Fc_{ε}R2/CD23; ■, high affinity Fc_{ε}R1; *sCD23*, soluble CD23; for further explanation see text

Once initiated by IL-4, it seems reasonable that IgE secretion is subject to additional control mechanisms. These may be represented by IgE-BF, which may enhance or suppress an ongoing IgE synthesis. IgE secretion thus is the consequence of a multitude of distinct regulatory events the interaction of which by far exceeds the regulatory effects observed for single lymphokines in vitro.

Although there has been much speculation about the nature of the allergic as compared with the physiological IgE immune response, the reasons for the exaggerated IgE production in allergic diseases still remain to be clarified. The inherited nature of atopic diseases has been recognized for a long time. It seems to include the transmission of certain MHC haplotypes whose gene products may specifically present allergenic epitopes to T cells, display a higher efficiency in presenting low amounts of antigen or deliver IgE-inducing signals during antigen presentation.

Also, a partial immunodeficiency, consisting of a selective defect of suppressor T lymphocytes, has been suggested to cause a breakthrough of IgE production to ordinary antigens. The ability to respond to minute quantities of antigen, however, may also be interpreted as a state of increased immune responsiveness.

As demonstrated by the altered lymphokine patterns of patients with atopic diseases or hyper IgE states, an immuneo defect in the form of misregulated cytokine production may be a relevant feature in the pathogenesis of the exaggerated IgE secretion. An enhanced IL-4 production inhibiting the antiviral and other biological activities of IFN-γ would also explain the reduced resistance to infection of atopic individuals.

The obligatory IgE response to parasitic worm infections suggests specific structural or biological properties of antigens that favour IgE production, the definition of which would help to better understand the normal and allergic IgE responses.

In conclusion many questions regarding the regulation of normal and allergic IgE responses remain unanswered. Considering the morbidity of allergic diseases they provide a critical challenge for further allergy research.

References

1. Bergstedt-Lindqvist S, Moon HB, Persson U, Möller G, Heusser C, Severinson E (1988) Interleukin 4 instructs uncommitted B lymphocytes to switch to IgG1 and IgE. Eur J Immunol 18: 1073–1077
2. Bieber T, Rieger A, Neuchrist C, Prinz JC, Rieber EP, Boltz-Nitulescu G, Scheiner O, Kraft D, Ring J, Stingl G (1989) Induction of Fc_{ε}RII/CD23 on human epidermal Langerhans cells by human recombinant interleukin 4 and γ interferon. J Exp Med 170: 309–315
3. Binaghi RA, Benacerraf B (1964) The production of anaphylactic antibody in the rat. J Immunol 92: 920–925
4. Bjorkman PJ, Saper MA, Samraoui B, Bennet WS, Strominger JL, Wiley C (1987a) Structure of the human class I histocompatibility antigen, HLA-A2. Nature 329: 506–512
5. Bjorkman PJ, Saper MA, Samraoui B, Bennet WS, Strominger JL, Wiley C (1987b) The foreign antigen binding site and T cell recognition regions of class T histocompatibility antigens. Nature 329: 512–518
6. Buckley RH, Fiscus SA (1975) Serum IgD and IgE concentrations in immunodeficiency diseases. J Clin Invest 55: 157–165
7. Campbell HD, Tucker WQJ, Hort Y, Martinson ME, Mayo G, Clutterbuck EJ, Sanderson CJ, Young IG (1987) Molecular cloning, nucleotide sequence, and expression of the gene encoding human eosinophil differentiation factor (interleukin 5). Proc Natl Acad Sci USA: 6629–6633
8. Capron M, Kusnierz JP, Prin L, Spiegelberg HL, Ovalque G, Gosset P, Tonnel AB, Capron A (1985) Cytophilic IgE on blood and tissue eosinophils: detection by flow microfluorometry. J Immunol 134: 3013–3018
9. Cher DJ, Mosmann TR (1987) Two types of murine helper T cell clones. II. Delayed type hypersensitivity is mediated by T_H1 Clones. J Immunol 138: 3688–3694
10. Coca AF, Cooke RA (1923) On the classification of the phenomena of hypersensitiveness. J Immunol 8: 163–171
11. Coffman RL, Carty J (1986) A T cell activity that enhances polyclonal IgE production and its inhibition by interferon-gamma. J Immunol 136: 949–954
12. Coffman RL, Seymour BWP, Hudak S, Jackson, Rennik D (1989) Antibody to interleukin 5 inhibits helminth induced eosinophilia in mice. Science 245: 308–310
13. Defrance T, Aubry JP, Rousset F, Vanbervliet B, Bonnefoy Y, Arai N, Takebe Y, Yokota T, Lee F, Arai K, De Vries JE, Banchereau J (1986) Human recombinant interleukin 4 induces $Fc_{\pm}$ receptors (CD23) on normal human B lymphocytes. J Exp Med 165: 1459–1467
14. Defrance T, Vanberfliet B, Aubry JP, Takebe Y, Arai N, Miyajima A, Yokota T, Lee F, Arai K, deVries JE, Banchereau J (1987) B cell growth-promoting activity of recombinant human interleukin 4. J Immunol 139: 1135–1141
15. Deguchi H, Suemura M, Ishizaka A, Ozaki Y, Kishimoto S, Yamamura Y, Kishimoto T (1983) IgE class-specific suppressor T cells and factors in humans. J Immunol 131: 2751–2756
16. Del Prete G, Maggi E, Tiri A, Parronchi P, Macchia D, Ricci M, Romagnani S (1989) In: Proceedings of the 7th international congress of immunology, Berlin, July 30–August 5, 1990, pp 75–8 (Abstract)
17. De Vries JE, Souillet G, Robert J, Rousset F (1989) Administration of interferon-α to an allergic patient resulted in reduction of serum IgE levels and clinical improvement. 7th International congress of Immunology, Berlin, July 30–August 5, 1990, pp. 75–9 (Abstract)
18. Dorf ME, Newburger PE, Hamaoka T, Katz DH, Benacerraf B (1974) Characterization of an immune response gene in mice controlling IgE and IgG antibody responses to ragweed pollen extract and its 2,4-dinitrophenylated derivative. Eur J Immunol 4: 346–353
19. Dutton RW, Falkoff R, Hirst JA, Hoffmann M, Kapler JW, Kettman JR, Lesley JF, Vann D (1971) Is there evidence for a non-antigen specific diffusable chemical mediator from the thymus derived cell in the initiation of the immune response? Prog Immunol 1: 355–364
20. Fernandez-Botran R, Krammer PH, Diamantstein T, Uhr JW, Vitetta ES (1986) B cell stimulatory factor 1 (BSF-1) promotes growth of helper T cell lines. J Exp Med 164: 580–593
21. Finkelman FD, Katona IM, Urban JF, Snapper CM, Ohara J, Paul WE (1986) Suppression of in vivo polyclonal IgE response by monoclonal antibody to the lymphokine B cell stimulatory factor 1. Proc Natl Acad Sci USA 83: 9675–9678
22. Finkelman FD, Katona IM, Urban JF, Holmes J, Ohara J, Tung AS, vG Sample J, Paul WE (1988a) IL-4 is required to generate and sustain in vivo IgE responses. J Immunol 1 41: 2335–2341
23. Finkelman FD, Katona IM, Mosman TR, Coffman RL (1988b) Interferon-γ regulates the isotypes of immunoglobulin secreted during in vivo humoral immune responses. J Immunol 140: 1022–1027
24. Finkelman FD, Holmes J, Urban JF, Paul WE, Katona IM (1989) T help requirements for the generation of an in vivo IgE response: a late acting form of T cell help other than IL-4 is required for IgE but not for IgG1 production. J Immunol 142: 403–408
25. Fiorentino DF, Bond MW, Mosmann TR (1989) Two types of mouse T helper cells. IV. T_H2 clones secrete a factor that inhibits cytokine production by T_H1 clones. J Exp Med 170: 2081–2095
26. Gajewski TF, Fitch FW (1988) Anti-proliferative effect of IFN-γ in murine regulation. I. IFN-γ inhibits the proliferation of T_H2 but not T_H1 murine helper T lymphocyte clones. J Immunol 140: 4245–4252
27. Galizzi JP, Cabrillat H, Rousset F, Menetrier C, DeVries J, Bancherreaus J (1988) IFN-γ and prostaglandin E2 inhibit IL-4 induced expression of Fc_{ε}R2/CD23 on B lymphocytes through different mechanisms without altering binding of IL-4 to its receptor. J Immunol 141: 1982–1988
28. Geha RS, Twarog F, Rappaport J, Parkman R, Rosen FS (1980) Increased serum IgE levels following allogeneic bone marrow transplantation. J Allergy Clin Immunol 66: 78–80
29. Geha RS, Reinherz EL, Leung D, McKee KT, Schlossman SF, Rosen FS (1981) Deficiency of suppressor T cells in the hyperimmunolglobulinemia E syndrome. J Clin Invest 68: 783–791
30. Gonzalez-Molina A, Spiegelberg HL (1977) A subpopulation of normal human B lymphocytes that bind IgE. J Clin Invest 59: 616–624
31. Gordon J, Rowe M, Walker L, Guy G (1986) Ligation of the CD23, p 45 (BLAST-2, EBVCS) antigen triggers the cell-cyle progression of activated B lymphocytes. Eur J Immunol 16: 1075–1080

32. Grey HM, Chestnut R (1985) Antigen processing and presentation to T cells. Immunol Today 6: 101–104
33. Heinzel FP, Sadick MD, Holaday BJ, Coffman RL, Locksley RM (1989) Reciprocal expression of interferon γ or interleukin 4 during the resolution or progression of murine leishmaniasis. Evidence for expansion of distinct helper T cell subsets. J Exp Med 169: 59–72
34. Heusser CH, Anderson CL, Grey HM (1977) Receptors for IgG subclass specificity on different mouse cell types and the definition of two distinct receptors on a macrophage cell line. J Exp Med 145: 1316–1327
35. Howard M, Farrar M, Hilfiker M, Johnson B, Takatsu K, Hamaoka T, Paul WE (1982) Identification of a T cell derived B cell growth factor different from IL-2. J Exp Med 155: 914–923
26. Hudak SA, Gollnick SO, Conrad H, Kehry MR (1987) Murine B-cell stimulatory factor (interleukin 4) increases expression of the Fc receptor for IgE on mouse B cells. Proc Natl Acad Sci USA 84: 4606–4610
37. Huff TH, Ishizaka K (1983) Formation of IgE-binding factors by human T-cell hybridomas. Proc Natl Acad Sci USA 81: 1514–1518
38. Huff TF, Yodoi Y, Uede T, Ishizaka K (1984) Presence of an antigenic determinant common to rat IgE-potentiating factor, IgE-suppressive factor and Fc_εreceptors on T and B lymphocytes. J Immunol 132: 406–412
39. Huff TH, Jardieu P, Ishizaka K (1986) Regulatory effects of human IgE-binding factors on the IgE response of rat lymphocytes. J Immunol 136: 955–962
40. Ishizaka K (1985) Twenty years with IgE: from the identification of IgE to regulatory factors for the IgE response. J Immunol 135: I–X
41. Ishizaka K, Sandberg K (1981) Formation of IgE-binding factors by human T lymphocytes. J Immunol 126: 1692–1696
42. Ishizaka K, Ishizaka T, Hornbrook MM (1966) Physicochemical properties of human reaginic antibody. V. Correlation of reaginic activity with gE globulin antibody. J Immunol 97: 844–851
43. Iwata M, Adachi M, Ishizaka K (1988) Antigen-specific T cells that form IgE-potentiating factor, IgG-potentiating factor, and antigen-specific glycosylation-enhancing factor on antigenic stimulation. J Immunol 140: 2534–2542
44. Jarret EEE, Stewart DC (1972) Potentiation of rat reaginic antibody (IgE) by Helminth infection. Simultaneous potentiation of separate reagins. Immunology 23: 749–756
45. Joseph M, Capron A, Ameisen, Capron M, Vorng H, Pancre V, Kusnierz JP, Auriault C (1986) The receptor for IgE on blood platelets. Eur J Immunol 16: 306–312
46. Kehry MR, Yamishita LC (1989) Fc_ε receptor II (CD23) function on mouse B cells: role in IgE dependent antigen focusing. Proc Natl Acad Sci USA 86: 7560–7566
47. Kikutani H, Inui S, Sato R, Barsumian EL, Owaki H, Yamasaki K, Kaisho T, Uchibayachi N, Hardy RR, Hirano T, Tsunasawa S, Sakiyama F, Suemura M, Kishimoto T (1986a) Molecular structure of human lymphocyte receptor for immunoglobulin E. Cell 47: 657–665
48. Kikutani H, Suemura M, Owaki H, Nakamura H, Sato R, Yamasaki K, Barsumian EL, Hardy RR, Kishimoto T (1986b) Fc_ε receptor, a specific differentiation marker transiently expressed on mature B cells before isotype switching. J Exp Med 164: 1455–1469
49. Kimoto M, Kishimoto T, Noguchi S, Watanabe T, Yamamura Y (1977) Regulation of antibody response in different immunoglobulin classes. II. Induction of in vitro IgE antibody response in murine spleen cells and demonstration of a possible involvement of distinct T helper cells in IgE and IgG antibody response. J Immunol 118: 840–848
50. Kishimoto T, Hirai Y, Suemura M, Yamamura Y (1976) Regulation of antibody response in different immunolobulin classes. I. Selective suppression of anti-DNP IgE response by preadministration of DNP-coupled mycobacterium. J Immunol 117: 396–402
51. Lebman DA, Coffman L (1988) Interleukin 4 causes isotype switching to IgE in T cell-stimulated clonal B cell cultures. J Exp Med 168: 853–862
52. Lee F, Yokota T. Otsuka T, Meyerson P, Villaret D, Coffman R, Mosmann T, Rennick D, Roehm M, Smith C, Zlotnik A, Arai K (1986) Isolation and characterization of a mouse interleukin cDNA clone that expressed B-cell stimulatory factor-1 activities and T-cell and mast-cell stimulating activities. Proc Natl Acad Sci USA 83: 2061–2065
53. Leung DYM, Rhodes AR, Geha RS (1981) Enumeration of T cell subsets in atopic dermatitis using monoclonal antibodies. J Allergy Clin Immunol 67: 450–455
54. Leung DYM, Brozek C, Frankel R, Geha RS (1984) IgE-specific suppressor factors in normal human serum. Clin Immunol Immunopath 32: 339–350
55. Leung DYM, Frankel R, Brozek C, Geha RS (1986) Potentiation of human IgE synthesis by plasma IgE binding factors from patients with the hyper IgE syndrome. J Clin Invest 77: 952–957
56. Levine BB, Stember RH, Fotino M (1972) Ragweed hay fever: genetic control and linkage to HLA-haplotypes. Science 178: 1201–1205
57. Lichtmann H, Kurt-Jones EA, Abbas AK (1987) B cell stimulatory factor-1 and not interleukin 2 is the autocrine growth factor for some helper T lymphocytes. Proc Natl Acad Sci USA 84: 824–827
58. Lowenthal JW, Castle BE, Schreurs J, Rennick D, Arai N, Hoy P, Takebe Y, Howard M (1988) Expression of high affinity receptors for murine interleukin 4 (BSF 1) on hemopoetic and non-hemopoetic cells. J Immunol 140: 456–464
59. Lutzker S, Rothman P, Pollock R, Coffman R, Alt FW (1988) Mitogen- and IL-4-regulated expression of germline IgG2b transcripts: evidence for direct heavy chain class switching. Cell 53: 177–184
60. Marsh DG, Bias WB, Ishizaka K (1974) Genetic control of basal serum immunoglobulin E level and its effect on specific reaginic sensitivity. Proc Natl Acad Sci USA 71: 3588–3593
61. Marsh DG, Meyers DA, Friedhoff LR, Husain R, Hsu SH, Bias WB (1980) Association of HL-A phenotypes A1, B8, Dw3 and A3, B7, Dw2 with allergy. Fed Proc 39: 936–943
62. Marsh DG, Hsu SH, Roebber M, Kautsky E, Friedhoff LR, Meyers DA, Pollard MK, Bias WB (1982) HLA-Dw2: A genetic marker for human immune response to short ragweed pollen allergen Ra5. I. Response resulting primarily from natural antigenic exposure. J Exp Med 155: 1439–1451
63. Martens C, Huff TF, Jardieu P. Trounstine ML, Coffman RL, Ishizaka K, Moore KW (1985) cDNA clones encoding IgE binding factors from a rat-mouse T cell hybridoma. Proc Natl Acad Sci USA 82: 2460–2464

64. Moore KW, Vieira P, Fiorentino DF, Trounstine ML, Khan TA, Mosmann TR (1990) Homology of cytokine synthesis inhibitory factor (IL-10) to the Epstein-Barr Virus Gene BCRFI. Science 248: 1230–1234
65. Mosmann TR, Bond MW, Coffman RL, Ohara J, Paul WE (1986a) T cell and mast cell lines respond to B cell stimulatory factor-1. Proc Natl Acad Sci USA 83: 5654–5658
66. Mosmann TR, Cherwinski H, Bond MW, Giedlin MA, Coffman RL (1986n) Two types of murine helper T cell clones. I. Definition according to profiles of lymphokine activities and secreted proteins. J Immunol 136: 2348–2357
67. Mosmann TR, Yokota T, Kastelein R, Zurawski S, Arai N, Takebe Y (1987) Species-specificity of T cell stimulating activities of IL-2 and BSF-1 (IL-4): comparison of normal and recombinant, mouse and human IL-2 and BSF-1 (IL-4). J Immunol 138: 1813–1816
68. Murray HW, Rubin BY, Rothermel CD (1983) Killing of intracellular Leishmania donovani by lymphokine-stimulated human mononuclear phagocytes. Evidence that interferon-γ is the activating lymphokine. J Clin Invest 72: 1506–1511
69. Nakajima T, Sarfati M, Delespesse G (1987) Relationship between human IgE-binding factors (IgE-BF) and lymphocyte receptors for IgE. J Immunol 139: 848–854
70. Nathan CF, Murray HW, Wiebe ME, Rubin BY (1983) Identification of interferon-γ is the lymphokine that activates human macrophage oxidative metabolism and antimicrobial activity. J Exp Med 158: 670–681
71. Noelle R, Krammer PH, Ohara J, Uhr JW, Vitetta ES (1984) Increased expression of Ia antigens on resting B cells: an additional role for B cell growth factor. Proc Natl Acad Sci USA 81: 6149–6153
72. Nutman TB, Delespesse G, Sarfati M, Volkman DJ (1987) T-cell-derived IgE-binding factors. I. Cloned and transformed T cells producing IgE binding factors. J Immunol 139: 4049–4054
73. Ogilvie BM (1967) Reagin-like antibodies in rats infected with the nematode parasite *Nippostrongylus brasiliensis*. Immunology 12: 13–21
74. Ogilvie BM, Jones VE (1971) *Nippostrongylus brasiliensis*. A review of immunity and the host/parasite relationship in the rat. Exp Parasitol 29: 138–152
75. Ohara J, Paul WE (1985) Production of a monoclonal antibody to and a molecular characterization of B-cell stimulatory factor-1. Nature 315: 333–336
76. Okumura K, Tada T (1971a) Regulation of homocytotropic antibody formation in the rat. III. Effect of thymectomy and splenectomy. J Immunol 106: 1019–1026
77. Okumura K, Tada T (1971b) Regulation of homocytotropic antibody formation in the rat. IV. Inhibitory effect of thymocytes on the homocytotropic antibody response. J Immunol 107: 1682–1695
78. Paliard X, De Waal Malefijt R, Yssel H, Blanchard D, Chretien I, Abrams J, De Vries J, Spits H (1988) Simultaneous production of IL-2, IL-4, and IFN-γ by activated human $CD4^+$ and $CD8^+$ T cell clones. J Immunol 141: 849–855
79. Pancre V, Joseph M, Capron A, Wietzerbin J, Kusnierz JP, Vorng H, Auriault C (1988) Recombinant human interferon-γ induces increased IgE receptor expression on human platelets. Eur J Immunol 18: 829–832
80. Peleman R, Wu J, Fargeas H, Delespesse G (1989) Recombinant interleukin 4 suppresses the production of interferon γ by human mononuclear cells. J Exp Med 179: 1751–1756
81. Pene J, Rousset F, Briere F, Chretien I, Bonnefoy JY, Spits H, Yokota T, Arai N, Arai KI, Bancherau J, De Fries JE (1988a) IgE production by normal human lymphocytes is induced by interleukin 4 and suppressed by interferons γ and α and prostaglandin E_2. Proc Natl Acad Sci USA 85: 6680–6684
82. Pene J, Rousset F, Briere F, Chretien I, Paliard X, Banchereau J, Spits H, De Vries JE (1988b) IgE production by normal human B cells induced by alloreactive T cell clones is mediated by IL-4 and suppressed by IFN-γ. J Immunol 141: 1218–1224
83. Pene J, Rousset F, Briere F, Chretien I, Wideman J, Bonnefoy JY, De Vries JE (1988c) Interleukin 5 enhances interleukin 4-induced IgE production by normal human B cells. The role of soluble CD23 antigen. Eur J Immunol 18: 929–935
84. Pirron U, Schlunck T, Prinz JC, Rieber EP (1990) IgE-dependent antigen focusing by human B lymphocytes is mediated by the low-affinity receptor IgE. Eur J Immunol 20: 1547–1551
85. Prinz JC, Endres N, Rank G, Ring J, Rieber EP (1987a) Expression of Fc_εreceptors on activated human T lymphocytes. Eur J Immunol 17: 757–761
86. Prinz JC, Rieber EP (1987b) Fc-receptors for IgE on human lymphocytes. Detection with a rosetting assay using a recombinant human/mouse IgE antibody and characterization with monoclonal antibodies. Hybridoma 6: 1–16
87. Prinz JC, Baur X, Mazur G, Rieber EP (1990a) Allergen-directed expression of Fc-receptors for IgE (CD23) on human T lymphocytes is modulated by interleukin 4 and interferon γ. Eur J Immunol 20: 1259–1264
88. Prinz JC, Endres N, Rieber EP (1990b) In vitro IL-4-induced IgE secretion requires activated $Fc_\varepsilon R2/CD23^+$ T lymphocytes (abstract) Immunobiology 181: 158
89. Rabin EM, Ohara J, Paul WE (1985) B cell stimulatory factor 1 activates resting B cells. Proc Natl Acad Sci USA 82: 2935–2939
90. Revoltella R, Ovary Z (1969) Reaginic antibody production in different mouse strains. Immunology 17: 45–53
91. Roehm NW, Leibson HJ, Zlotnik A, Kappler JW, Marrack P, Cambier JC (1984) Interleukin-induced increase in Ia expresion by normal mouse B cells. Exp Med 160: 679–694
92. Rousset F, Waal Malefijt R, Slierendregt B, Aubry JP, Bonnefoy JY, Defrance T, Bancherau J, DeVries J (1988) Regulation of Fc receptor for IgE (CD23) and class II MHC antigen expression on Burkitt's lymphoma cell lines by human IL-4 and IFN-γ. J Immunol 140: 2625–2632
93. Sarfati M, Delespesse G (1988) Possible role of human lymphocyte for IgE (CD23) or its soluble fragments in the in vitro synthesis of IgE. J. Immunol. 141: 2195–2199
94. Sarfati M, Rector E, Sehon AH, Delespesse G (1984) In vitro synthesis of IgE by human lymphocytes. IV. Suppression of the spontaneous IgE synthesis by IgE-binding factors secreted by tunicamycin-treated RPMI 8866 cells. Immunology 53: 783–790
95. Saryan JA, Leung DYM, Geha RS (1983) Induction of human IgE synthesis by a factor derived from T cells of patients with hyper IgE states. J Immunol 130: 242–247
96. Schimpl A, Wecker E (1972) Replacement of T cell function by a T cell product. Nature New Biol 237: 15–16

97. Scott P, Pearce E, Cheever AW, Coffman RL, Sher A (1989) Role of cytokines and CD4+ and CD8+ T cell subsets in the regulation of parasite immunity and disease. Immun Rev 112: 161–182
98. Sherr E, Macy E, Kimata H, Gilly M, Saxon A (1989) Binding the low affinity $Fc_\varepsilon R$ on B cells suppress ongoing human IgE synthesis. J Immunol 142: 481–489
99. Sideras PS, Bergstedt-Lindquist S, MacDonald HR, Severinson E (1985) Secretion of IgG1 induction factor by T cell clones and hybridomas. Eur J Immunol 15: 593–598
100. Snapper CM, Paul WE (1987) Interferon-gamma and B cell stimulatory factor-1 reciprocally regulate Ig isotype production. Science 236: 944–947
101. Spiegelberg HL, Thompson LF, McNeil D, Buckley RH (1985) IgE Fc receptor positive T, B and NK cells in patients with the hyper IgE syndrome. Int Arch Allergy Appl Immunol 77: 277–279
102. Stevens TL, Bossie A, Sanders VM, Fernandez-Botran R, Coffman RL, Mosmann TR, Vitetta ES (1988) Regulation of antibody isotype secretion by subsets of antigen-specific helper T cells. Nature 334: 255–258
103. Stout RD, Bottomly K (1989) Antigen-specific activation of effector macrophages by IFN-γ producing (T_H1) T cell clones. Failure of IL-4-producing (T_H2) T cell clones to activate effector function in macrophages. J Immunol 142: 760–765
104. Suemura M, Ishizaka K (1979) Potentiation of IgE response in vitro by T cells from rats infected with Nippostrongylus brasiliensis. J Immunol 142: 760–765
105. Suemura M, Kishimoto T, Hirai Y, Yamamura Y (1977) Regulation of antibody response in different immunoglobulin classes. III. In vitro demonstration of IgE class-specific suppressor functions of DNP-mycobacterium-primed T cells and soluble factor released from these cells. J Immunol 119: 149–155
106. Suemura M, Kikutani H, Barsumian EL, Hattori Y, Kishimoto S, Sato R, Maeda A, Nakamura H, Owaki H, Hardy RR, Kishimoto T (1986) Monoclonal anti-Fc_ε receptor antibodies with different specificities and studies on the expression of $Fc_\varepsilon R$ on human B and T cells. J Immunol 137: 1214–1220
107. Suemura M, Kikutani H, Aitani M, Yamatodani A, Kuritani T, Kishimoto S, Uchibayashi N, Sugiyama K, Barsumian EL, Kishimoto T (1989) Suppression of IgE-mediated allergic reactions with recombinant soluble $Fc_\varepsilon RII$. In: Proceedings of the 7th international congress on immunology, Berlin, July 30–August 5, 1990, pp 19–55 (Abstract)
108. Swendeman S, Thorley-Lawson DA (1987) The activation antigen BLAST-2, when shed, is an autocrine BCGF for normal and transformed B cells. EMBO J 6: 1634–1639
109. Takemori T, Tada T (1975) Properties of antigen-specific suppressive T cell factor in the regulation of antibody response of the mouse. I. In vivo activity and immunochemical characterizations. J Exp Med 142: 1241
110. Teale JM, Abraham KM (1987) The regulation of antibody class expression. Immunol Today 8: 122–126
111. Te Velde AA, Huijbens RJF, De Vries JE, Figdor CG (1990) IL-4 decreases FcγR membrane expression and FcγR-mediated cytotoxic activity of human monocytes. J Immunol 144: 3046–3051
112. Thompson LF, Spiegelberg HL, Buckley RH (1985) IgE Fc receptor positive T and B lymphocytes in patients with the hyper IgE syndrome. Clin Exp Immunol 59: 77–84
113. Tokuhisa T, Taniguchi M, Okumura K, Tada T (1978) An antigen-specific I region gene product that augments the antibody response. J Immunol 120: 414–421
114. Uchibayashi N, Kikutani H, Barsumian EL, Hauptmann R, Schneider FJ, Schwendenwein R, Sommergruber W, Spevack W, Maurer-Fogy I, Suemura M, Kishimoto T (1989) Recombinant soluble Fc_εreceptor II ($Fc_\varepsilon R2$/CD23) has IgE binding activity but no B cell growth promoting activity. J Immunol 142: 3901–3908
115. Vazquez A, Mills S, Sharma S (1988) Expression of CD23 antigen is not necessary for human 12-kDa B cell growth factor-mediated B cell proliferation. Eur J Immunol 18: 1647–1650
116. Vercelli D, Jabara HH, Lee BW, Woodland N, Geha RS, Leung DYM (1988) Human recombinant interleukin 4 induces $Fc_\varepsilon R2$/CD23 on normal human monocytes. J Exp Med 167: 1406–1416
117. Vercelli D, Jabara HH, Arai KI, Yokota T, Geha RS (1989a) Endogeneous interleukin 6 plays an obligatory role in interleukin 4-dependent human Ige synthesis. Eur J Immunol 19: 1419–1424
118. Vercelli D, Jabara HH, Arai KI, Geha RS (1989b) Induction of human IgE synthesis requires interleukin 4 and T/B cell interactions involving the T cell receptor/CD3 complex and MHC class II antigens. J Exp Med 169: 1295–1307
119. Warren MK, Vogel SN (1985) Opposing effects of glucocorticoids on interferonγ-induced murine macrophage Fc-receptor and Ia antigen expression. J Immunol 134: 2462
120. Wierenga EA, Snoek M, De Groot C, Chretien I, De Vries JE, Kapsenberg ML (1989) High allergen-specific IgE levels are associated with an imbalanced interleukin 4 and interferon-γ production by functional allergen-specific Cd4+ helper T lymphocytes. In: Proceedings of the 7th international congress of immunology, Berlin, July 30–August 5, 1990, pp 75–41 (Abstract)
121. Yodoi J, Ishizaka K (1979) Lymphocytes bearing Fc receptors for IgE. Presence of human and rat lymphocytes with Fc_ε receptors. J Immunol 122: 2577–2583
122 Yokota T, Otsuka T, Mosman T, Banchereau J, Defrance T, Blanchard D, De Vries JE, Lee F, Arai K (1986) Isolation and characterization of a human cDNA clone, homologous to mouse B-cell stimulatory factor 1, that expresses B cell- and T cell-stimulatory activities. Proc Natl Acad Sci USA 83: 5894
123. Yokota A, Kikutani H, Tanaka T, Sato R, Barsumian EL, Suemura M, Kishimoto T (1988) Two species of human Fc_ε receptorII ($Fc_\varepsilon RII$/CD23): Tissue specific and IL-4-specific regulation of gene expression. Cell 55: 611–618
124. Yokota T, Arai K, De Vries J, Spits H, Banchereau J, Zlotnik A, Rennick, Howard M, Takebe Y, Miyatake S, Lee F, Arai KI (1988) Molecular biology of interleukin 4 and interleukin 5 genes and biology of their products that stimulate B cells, T cells, and hemopoietic cells. Immunol Rev 102: 137–188
125. Young MC, Leung DYM, Geha RS (1984) Production of IgE-potentiating factor in man by T cell lines bearing Fc receptors for IgE. Eur J Immunol 14: 871–878
126. Yssel H, DeWaal Malefijt R, Spits H, De Vries JE (1989) Quantitative and qualitative differences in lymphokine production by house dust mite specific human T cell clones upon different modes of activation. In: Proceedings of the 7th international congress of immunology, Berlin, July 30–August 5, 1990, pp 75–42 (Abstract)

IgE Receptors on Langerhans Cells: Their Significance in the Pathophysiology of Atopic Eczema

C. Bruijnzeel-Koomen, G. Mudde, P. Bruijnzeel, and T. Bieber

Introduction

Origin and Function of Langerhans Cells

A Langerhans cell (LC) is a dendritic, bone marrow-derived cell belonging to the macrophage-monocyte cell lineage [34, 67]. In the epidermis LCs account for some 3%–8% of the epidermal cell population. It has been suggested that LCs and interdigitating cells may originate from the same stem cell [2, 30], however, the exact phenotype of the LC precursor cell [2] and the homing mechanism of the epidermal LC are still unknown [24]. The LC is MHC (major histocompatibility complex) class II positive [35] and bears the CD1a antigen [42], the CD4 antigen [69] and receptors for the Fc fragment of IgG and C3b [58]. The expression of the CD4 antigen is lower than that of the CD1a antigen. Ultrastructurally, the LC is characterised by the presence of a characteristic cytoplasmic organelle, called the Birbeck granule, whose origin (from the Golgi or from the cell membrane) is still a matter of dispute [31]. The function of these Birbeck granules is still unclear, but they seem to be involved in the intracellular traffic of surface antigens after their endocytosis [31]. The most important and best documented function of the LC is antigen presentation to T lymphocytes in contact allergic reactions [54, 55, 56, 59]. The precise location where antigen presentation to T cells occurs is still unknown. Evidence has been put forward that after antigen binding LC move to the dermis and leave as veiled cells via the lymphatics to present antigen as interdigitating cells to T cells in the paracortical area of the lymph node [55]. The antigen-presenting capacity of the LC is much greater than that of blood-derived antigen-presenting cells [12, 13, 45]. Epidermal LCs produce interleukin-1 (IL-1) [52] and prostaglandin D2 (PGD2) [50], and some evidence exists that these cells are also able to produce interferon-gamma (IFN-γ), at least in the mouse [27].

Taken together, these characteristics suggest that epidermal LCs play an important role in the skin immune system, particularly in antigen handling.

Langerhans Cells in Atopic Eczema

In atopic eczema (AE) the number of epidermal LCs (estimated by L-DOPA staining) is elevated in chronic skin lesions [64]. However, enumeration of epidermal LCs on cryosections by morphometric analysis per mm^2 epidermal section surface does not reveal any differences in the number of LCs between normal skin and AE (acute and chronic lesions) [3, 7]. Occasionally, a focal accumulation of LCs in the epidermis is present adjacent to infiltrating mononuclear cells in the papillary dermis. Infiltrating T lymphocytes in the epidermis are predominantly $CD8^+$ [49].

In acute and chronic AE lesions the dermis shows a lymphohistiocytic infiltrate, mainly consisting of T lymphocytes [17]. An increased ratio of $CD4^+$ T cells to $CD8^+$ cells in the dermis has been observed [36, 38]. This ratio (in acute and chronic skin lesions and in "dry skin") may be even higher than the ratio in peripheral blood and also higher than the ratio observed in contact dermatitis. This suggests a selective homing of $CD4^+$ cells in the dermal infiltrate in AE [38]. Apart from activated (HLA-DR^+) T lymphocytes the dermal infiltrate consists of $CD1a^+$ cells (10%–15%) without Birbeck granules [61], macrophages (10%) and interdigitating reticulum cells (20%) [50, 57, 70, 71]. The in vitro antigen-presenting function of LC in AE seems to be intact, although the autologous mixed skin leucocyte reaction is decreased [46].

In summary, the presence of $CD1^+$ and $RFD1^+$ cells in AE skin may indicate the presence of skin-localized antigen presentation and T-cell activation [16].

Presence of IgE-Bearing Langerhans Cells in Atopic Eczema

In Vivo Binding of IgE by Langerhans Cells

Recently, it was demonstrated that in AE skin, apart from mast cells, CD1a$^+$ dendritic cells in the epidermis also bind IgE molecules [5, 6, 18] (Fig. 1). This phenomenon can be observed not only in acute and chronic skin lesions but also, although to a lesser degree, in clinically "normal" looking skin from AE patients with elevated serum IgE levels. IgE molecules were also present on antigen-presenting cells (CD1a$^+$ cells) in the dermis [4, 37]. The anti-IgE staining of CD1a$^+$ dendritic cells in the epidermis (and dermis) disappeared after removal of cell-bound IgE by acid elution and could be reconstituted by incubation of the skin sections with serum with high IgE levels but not by serum from normal controls [8, 18]. Immunoelectron microscopy studies on epidermal cell suspensions from AE patients revealed that IgE molecules were present on CD1a$^+$ cells containing Birbeck granules, therefore being LC (Fig. 2). Occasionally IgE$^+$/CD1$^+$ cells without Birbeck granules (indeterminate cells) were also observed.

Specificity of Anti-IgE Staining of Epidermal Langerhans Cells for Atopic Eczema

Epidermal LCs from atopic patients without AE do not bear IgE molecules, neither do LCs from patients with schistosomiasis or allergic contact dermatitis. However, in some patients with psoriasis, without history of atopy but with elevated serum IgE levels and without specificity to environmental allergens, epidermal dendritic anti-IgE staining can occasionally be observed (Bruijnzeel-Koomen and Bieber, personal observation).

Furthermore, in patients with actinic reticuloid with elevated serum IgE levels, dendritic anti-IgE staining in the dermis may be seen [62]. However, immuno-double-labelling studies with CD1a-specific antibodies were not performed. Nevertheless, these observations suggest that the presence of IgE-bearing dendritic cells is not entirely specific for AE.

Fig. 1. Immunoperoxidase study with IgE-specific antibody. The anti-IgE$^+$ cells in the epidermis show dendritic processes (*arrows*). x 250

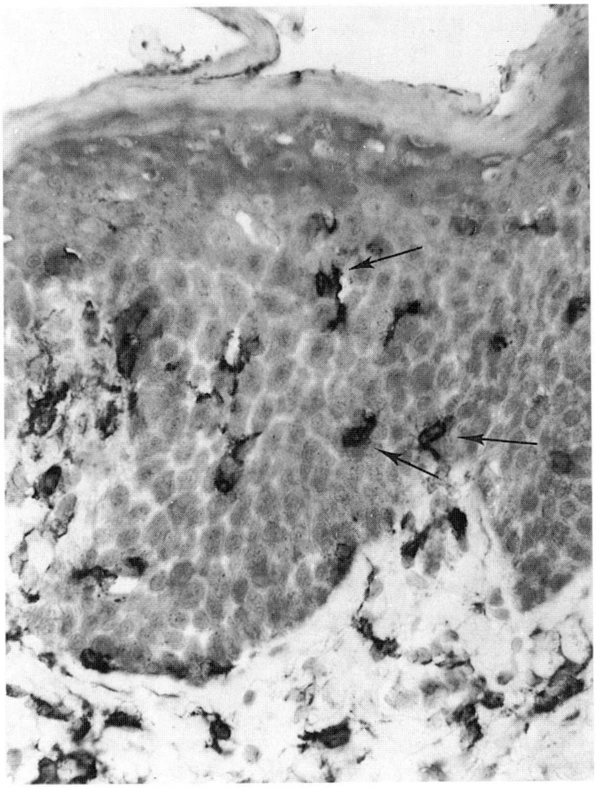

Fig. 2. Immunogold labelling for anti-IgE positivity. Gold particles (*arrows*) are present along the cell membrane of a cell containing Birbeck granules (*Bg*). x 41 700

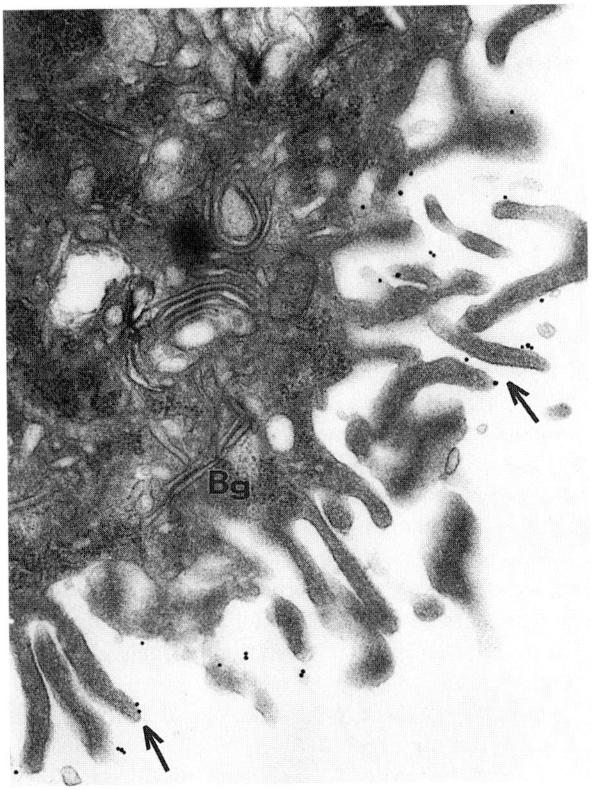

Effect of Topical Treatment with Corticosteroids on the Presence of IgE on Langerhans Cells

The epidermal anti-IgE staining progressively decreases after topical corticosteroid treatment of AE skin over 1 week and completely disappears after 2 weeks. In contrast to the epidermal anti-IgE staining, CD1a$^+$ cells are still present in the epidermis ([9]; Bruijnzeel-Koomen, personal observation).

Presence of $Fc_\varepsilon R$ on Langerhans Cells from Atopic Eczema Patients

Studies on enriched epidermal cell suspensions from AE patients revealed that IgE molecules are bound to LC via their Fc fragments [19]: (a) LC-bound IgE can be eluted and reconstituted by myeloma IgE; (b) pepsin digestion of LC-bound IgE significantly decreased the number of cells staining with light chain-specific antibodies, whereas the number of cells staining with anti-ε heavy chain was not changed ; (c) CD1$^+$ cells form rosettes with sheep red blood cells coated with myeloma IgE.

These experiments demonstrate the presence of a $Fc_\varepsilon R$ on epidermal LCs in AE. LCs from normal non-atopic controls do not show a $Fc_\varepsilon R$. This suggests that either a $Fc_\varepsilon R$ is not present on normal LCs or that its expression per LC or the total number of LCs with a $Fc_\varepsilon R$ is too low to be detected by the above-mentioned rosette assay. Further characteristics of the $Fc_\varepsilon R$ on LCs are: (a) an associated expression with the CD1a antigen; (b) an affinity for IgG, whereas the Fc receptor for IgG on LCs has no affinity for IgE; (c) resistance to trypsinisation [19].

Type of $Fc_\varepsilon R$ on Langerhans Cells in Atopic Eczema Patients

It is still unclear what type of $Fc_\varepsilon R$ is expressed on LCs in AE. Since it is supposed that the LC belongs to the monocyte-macrophage cell lineage, one might expect the presence of the low affinity-type receptor for IgE ($Fc_\varepsilon R_2$/CD23). However, staining with CD23-specific antibodies on AE skin sections was negative (Bruijnzeel-Koomen, personal observation). Furthermore, CD23-specific antibodies could not inhibit the rosette assay with myeloma IgE-coated sheep red blood cells. The rosette assay could, however, be significantly inhibited by BB10, a monoclonal antibody directed against the $Fc_\varepsilon R_2$ on human eosinophils, platelets and macrophages [21]. This antibody also stained in AE skin sections anti-IgE dendritic cells in the upper part of the epidermis. This would suggest that for LCs the same type of $Fc_\varepsilon R$ is involved as on eosinophils. This type of $Fc_\varepsilon R$ may be different from the CD23 type of $Fc_\varepsilon R$ on B cells, T cells and monocytes, since it is still unclear whether or not the BB10 antibody reacts with human CD23$^+$ cells. Other possibilities are that: (a) the $Fc_\varepsilon R$ on LC is CD23, but the epitope for CD23-specific antibodies is hidden by CD1 which is stereometrically associated with the $Fc_\varepsilon R$; (b) the $Fc_\varepsilon R$ on LC is CD23, but its molecular structure and affinity for IgE are changed by local inflammatory mediators like platelet-activating factor, histamine or leukotriene B_4, which have been reported to increase the affinity for IgE on eosinophils [68].

In Vitro Induction of the $Fc_\varepsilon R_2$ on Human Langerhans Cells

It has been stated that normal human LCs neither bind IgE molecules nor react with any anti-$Fc_\varepsilon R$ reagents. This indicates that in AE LCs are induced to express a specific receptor for IgE. Moreover, the fact that in uninvolved skin of patients with AE, anti-IgE-staining is very weak but increases in involved areas suggests a possible role of locally released mediators in the upregulation of the expression of this receptor. Since infiltrating cells are mostly comprised of T cells, T-cell-derived cytokines are presumably involved in this induction process. On the other hand, keratinocyte-derived cytokines may contribute to the regulation of this event.

The putative role of such cytokines in the induction of the $Fc_\varepsilon R_2$ on normal epidermal LC was investigated [10]. To address this issue, LC-enriched human epidermal cells (50%–70% LC) were prepared by negative selection and cultured for 8–36 h in the presence or absence of various concentrations of recombinant human IL-4 (rhIL-4), rhIFN-γ, phorbol myristate acetat (PMA), rhIL-2, recombinant human granulocyte-macrophage colony stimulating factor (rhGM-CSF), rhIL-1, rhIL-3, rhIL-6 and cycloheximide. $Fc_\varepsilon R_2$/CD23 was controlled at various times during culturing by double marker analysis. While LC-enriched epidermal cells either freshly isolated or cultured in media alone did not react with anti-CD23 reagents, rhIL-4 as well as rhIFN-γ led to a gradual, dose-dependent emergence of CD1a/CD23 reactive cells (Fig. 3). A combined use of varying concentrations of rhIL-4 and rhIFN-γ in 24h cultures showed that for each combination chosen, the percentage of CD23-reactive LC was greater than the sum of CD23$^+$

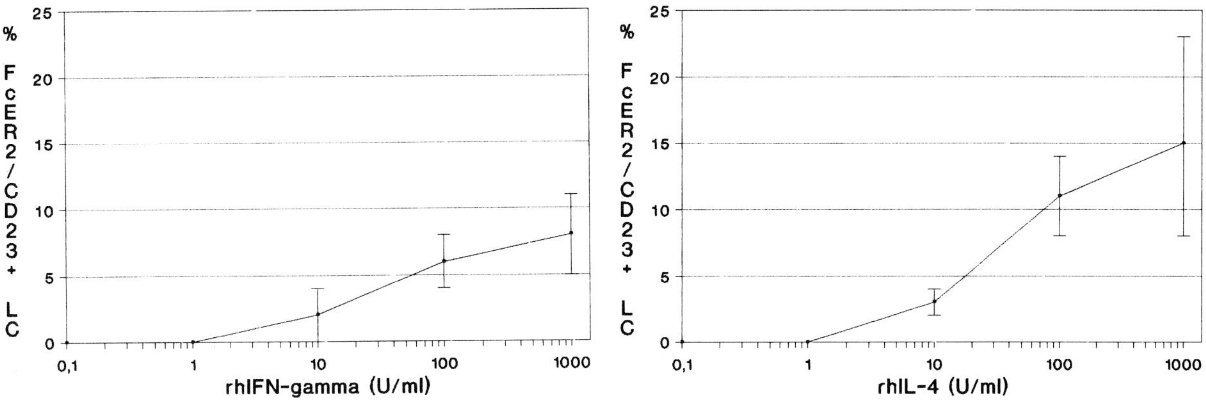

Fig. 3a, b. Recombinant human interleukin-4 (*rhIL-4*) and interferon-γ (*rhIFN-gamma*) induce the expression of $Fc_{\varepsilon}R_2$/CD23 on Langerhans cells (*LC*). LC-enriched (50%) epidermal cell suspensions were stimulated for 24 h with various rhIL-4 (**a**) or rhIFN-gamma (**b**) concentrations and assessed for CD23+ cells (CD23-specific monoclonal antibody-coated ox erythrocytes) and LC (T6/RD1). This figure illustrates the mean ± SE of five experiments

Table 1. Correlation between in vivo and in vitro reactions to house dust allergen (HDA) in atopic patients

In vivo and in vitro responses to HDA in AD patients

pat nr	PRIST kU/l	RAST %	HDA	I.bC. 20 min	PT 24–48 hrs	LPT non-T	IgE on LC	LPT-LC
1	12,000	n.d.		+	n.d.	+	+	−
2	21,000	23%		+	+ −	+	+	+
3	16,000	26%		+	+ +	+	+	+
4	11,000	17%		+	+ +	+	+	+
5	2,550	11%		+	+ +	+	+	−
6	6,800	12%		+	− −	+	+	−
7	3,600	9%		+	+ +	+	+	+
8	9,250	19%		+	n.d.	+	+	+
9	15,000	26%		+	+ +	+	+	+
10	660	6%		+	+ +	+	+	+
11	5,300	9%		+	+ +	+	+	+
12	12,750	21%		+	+ +	+	+	+
13	1,200	5%		+	− −	+	−	−
14	2,100	10%		+	n.d.	+	−	−
15	875	8%		+	+ +	+	−	−
16	1,100	8%		−	− −	+	−	−
17	3,700	11%		+	n.d.	+	−	−
18	2,900	12%		+	− −	−	−	−
19	800	6%		+	+ +	+	−	−
20	16	0%		−	− −	−	−	−

Patient numbers correspond with the experiment numbers in Figs. 4, 7–9. n.d., not done; I.C., intracutaneous test with HDA read after 20 min; PT, patch test with HDA read after 24–48 h; LPT non-T, lymphoproliferation test in the presence of non-T from peripheral blood as antigen-presenting cell (APC); LPT-LC, lymphoproliferation test in the presence of Langerhans cells (LC) as APC.

LPT-LC to HDA was considered negative when the net T-cell response was less than 3000 cpm and when the net T-cell response to HDA in the presence of non-T cells of the same patient was higher.

PRIST, paper-radioimmuno-sorbent text; RAST-radio-allergo-sorbent test

LC after incubation with each cytokine (Table 1) alone, whereas similar studies with U937 cells indicate that these cytokines exert only an additive effect on their CD23 expression. The addition of rhIL-1, rhIL-3 and rhIL-6 decreased the rhIL-4/rhIFN-γ-induced CD23 expression on LCs whereas rhgm-CSF had no effect (Fig. 5). These data show that rhIL-4 and rhIFN-γ induce $Fc_{\varepsilon}R_2$/CD23 expression on normal human LCs and that epidermal cell-derived cytokines may play a regulatory role in this phenomenon.

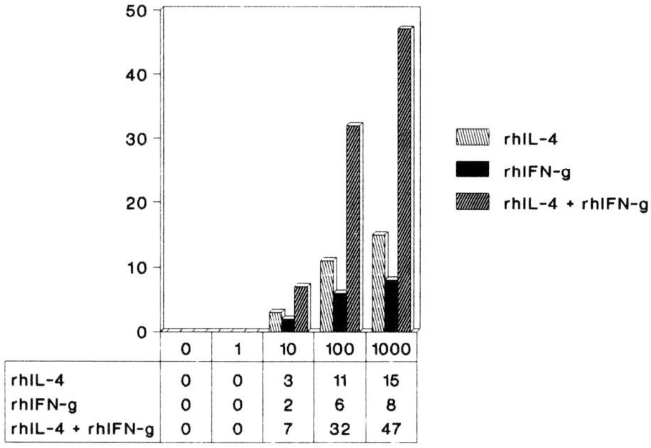

Fig. 4. Recombinant human interleukin-4 (*rhIL-4*) and interferon-γ (*rhIFN-g*) have a synergistic effect on the induction of $Fc_\varepsilon R_2$/CD23 on Langerhans cells (LC) and an additional effect on upregulating the expression of $Fc_\varepsilon R_2$/CD23 on the U937 cell line. LC-enriched (50%) epidermal cell suspensions of U937 were stimulated with various combined concentrations of rhIL-4 and rhIFN-g. After 34 h, the cultures were assessed for CD23+ LC by double marker analysis by (CD23-specific antibody-coated ox erythrocytes) and T6/RD1 (mean ± SE of three experiments)

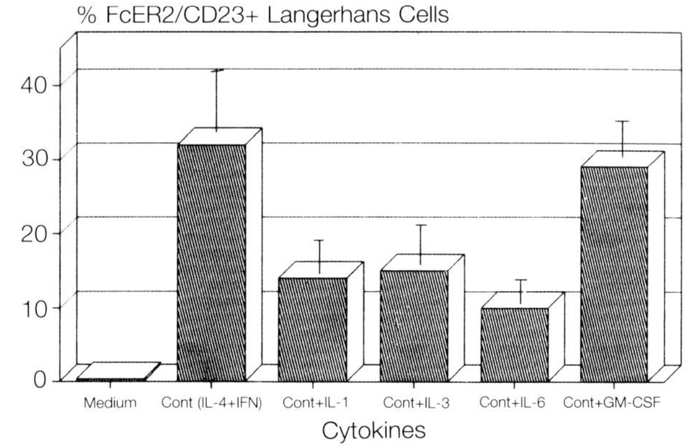

Fig. 5. Modulation of $Fc_E R_2$/CD23 expression on Langerhans cells (LC) by epidermal cell-derived cytokines. LC-enriched epidermal cells were cultured for 24 h with recombinant human interleukin 4 (*IL-4*) and interferon-γ (positive control, *cont*), and in the presence or absence of various epidermal cell-derived cytokines. They were then assessed for CD23+ LC by double staining using CD23-specific monoclonal antibody. This figure illustrates the mean ± SD of five experiments

In summary, it is clear that in the epidermal compartment the LCs are exposed to several cytokines, which exert a complex regulatory network. For example, while in uninvolved skin of atopic patients the effect of IL-4 or IFN-γ on LCs is probably counterbalanced by some epidermal cytokines like IL-6, the presumed locally high amount of IL-4 or IFN-γ produced by infiltrating T cells could be responsible for the increased expression of $Fc_\varepsilon R$ in lesional skin.

These in vitro results support the concept that in atopic disease, under distinct conditions, the expression of $Fc_\varepsilon R$ is induced on LCs which therefore, after binding an aeroallergen, may be able to activate T cells and provoke the eczematous lesions. However, these studies on the rhIL-4/rhIFN-γ-induced CD23 expression on LCs make the question of why the $Fc_\varepsilon R$ on LCs in vivo is CD23 negative even more intriguing.

Function of IgE-Bearing Langerhans Cells in Atopic Eczema

Although the presence of IgE-bearing LCs may not be specific for AE, these cell-bound IgE molecules could play an important role in the pathogenesis of this skin disease, which is associated with atopy. Firstly, it can be hypothesised that like the IgE molecules bound to dermal mast cells, the IgE molecules bound to LCs have specificity for environmental allergens such as house dust, house dust mite, pollen and animal dander (aeroallergens). Secondly, aeroallergens can penetrate the skin of AE patients after epicutaneous contact since they can induce eczematous delayed-type skin reactions which are specific for AE patients [1, 20, 25, 29, 40, 48, 53]. Therefore, it is suggested that aeroallergens bind to allergen-specific IgE molecules on LCs after penetrating the epidermis. Thereafter the following processes may occur.

Activation of Langerhans Cells and Release of Mediators

So far, normal LCs produce IL-1 [52], PGD2 [50] and possibly also IFN-γ [27]. The cytokine spectrum of LC under various pathological conditions is still an unexplored area which needs more attention in the near future. However, in AE, in vivo observations suggest that LCs may release a factor which is chemotactic for eosinophils: in skin biopsies from patch test reactions to aeroallergens, an influx of eosinophils may be observed in the epidermis 24 h after patch testing. Furthermore, some of these eosinophils lie in close contact with IgE-positive LC [20] (Fig. 6).

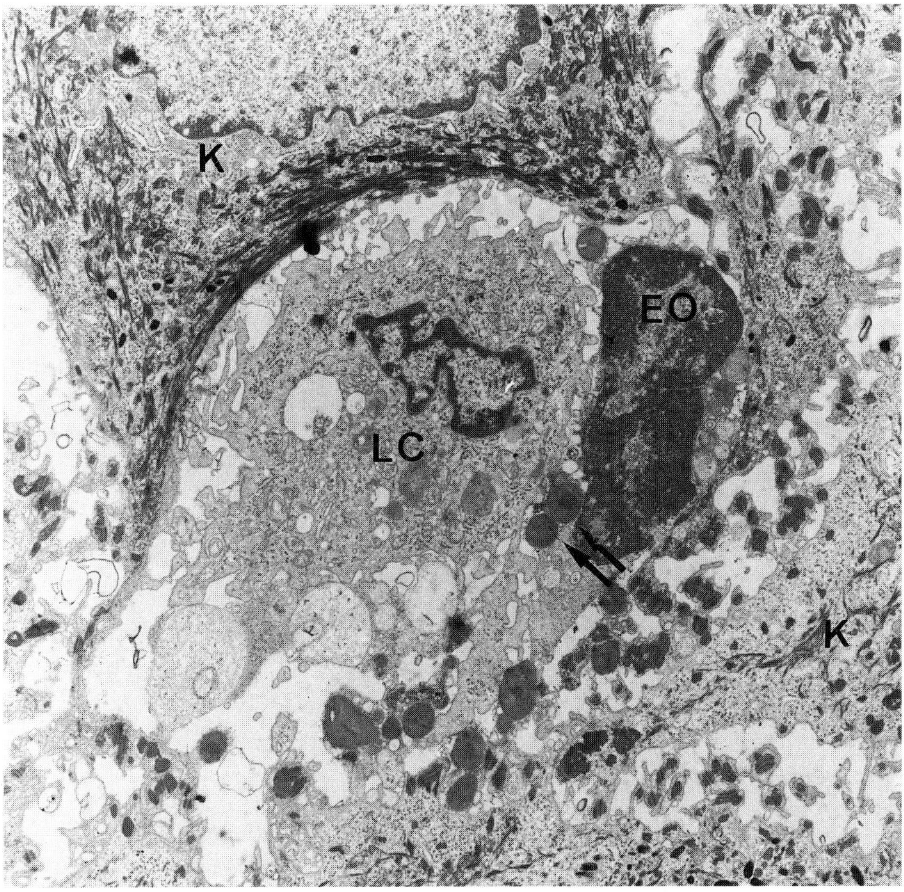

Fig. 6. An epidermal Langerhans cell (*LC*) lying in close contact with an eosinophil (*EO*); *K*, keratinocyte; *double arrows* indicate eosinophil-derived granules. x 9100

Presentation of Aeroallergens by Langerhans Cells to T Cells

As has been documented the best known function of LC is antigen presentation to T cells. To investigate the role of IgE-bearing LC from AE patients in antigen presentation, IgE-positive LC and non-IgE-bearing LC (IgE-negative LC) from AE patients were investigated for their antigen-presenting capacity and compared with antigen-presenting cells from the peripheral blood [41].

Background T-Cell Response in Atopic Eczema

The background T-cell response in the presence of LC in AE patients was increased (Fig. 7). This may be ex-

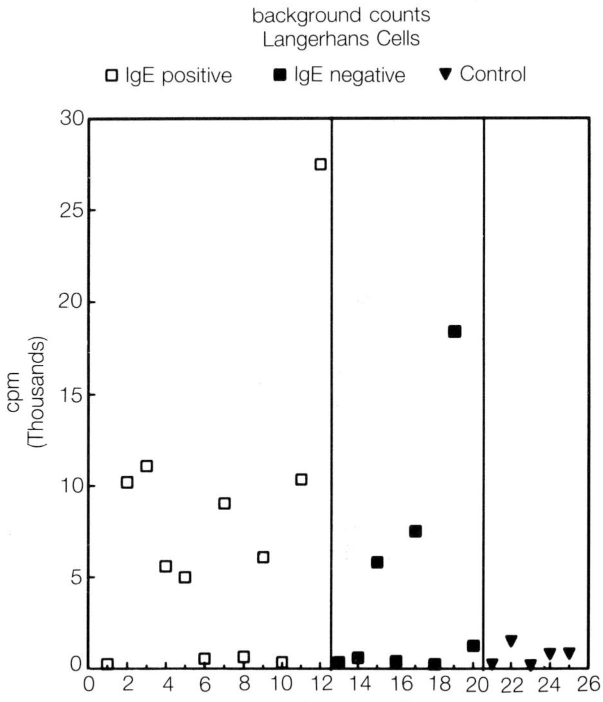

▷

Fig. 7. Background T-cell response in the presence of Langerhans cells (LC). The background in atopic patients was significantly increased compared with normal subjects ($\alpha < 0.05$). There was no significant difference between the background response in the presence of IgE^+ LC (experiment numbers 1–12) compared with IgE-LC (experiment numbers 13–20)

plained in several ways: firstly, as an autologous mixed leukocyte reaction (AMLR) or skin leukocyte reaction (AMSLR); secondly, as an activation of T cells and/or LC from AE patients in vivo; and thirdly, as a reaction to in vivo-bound antigens already present on LC. The first two explanations are not very likely since: (a) the background responses in the presence of non-T cells from AE patients and normal controls are not different; (b) AMLR and AMSLR have been reported to be decreased in AE patients [46]; (c) the T-cell responses to house dust antigens (HDA) in the presence of non-T cells from AE patients and normal controls are not different; (d) the activation of LC by binding of IgE is unlikely, since the background response in the presence of IgE-positive LC or IgE-negative LC is not different.

Moreover, the observation that the T-cell response to *Candida* in the presence of IgE-positive LC or IgE-negative LC is not different also argues against in vivo activation of IgE-positive LC by binding of IgE. Therefore, the third explanation is most likely. This explanation is strengthened by the observation that the background T-cell response can be completely inhibited by HLA-DR-specific antibodies.

Presentation of House Dust Allergen by Langerhans Cells

The T-cell response to *Candida albicans*, using IgE-positive LC from AE patients as APC, was in the same range as with IgE-negative LC. Also, the T-cell response to *Candida* with autologous APC from the peripheral blood did not significantly differ between these groups. In contrast to this finding, the T-cell response to HDA was dependent on the type of APC used. If non-T cells from the peripheral blood were used as APC, both AE and controls responded to HDA. However, when LCs were used as APC, a T-cell response to HDA was only observed in the case of IgE-positive LC. IgE-negative LCs from AE patients or LCs from normal controls were unable to present HDA (Fig. 8).

HLA-DR-specific HLA-DR-specific antibodies inhibited both the HDA and *Candida* presentation by IgE-positive LC and by nonT cells, indicating that the in vitro T-cell proliferation to both HDA and *Candida* is MHC class II dependent.

The T-cell proliferative response to HDA was a consistent finding, which could be reproduced on different occasions in the same patient (at 1-month intervals). The dependence of the T-cell response to HDA on the presence of cell-bound IgE on LC was illustrated by the observation that in one AE patient T cells proliferated to HDA on the first test occasion, when IgE molecules were present on LC, but failed to respond on the second test occasion, when LC did not bear IgE molecules.

Non-T cells can present HDA in the absence of cell-bound IgE as could be demonstrated in normal controls. This could explain why in earlier studies, using antigen-presenting T cells from the peripheral blood, no significant correlation was found between the magnitude of the T-cell response to allergens and the amount of allergen-specific IgE in the serum [14, 23, 26, 33, 47].

Role for IgE in Allergen Presentation by Langerhans Cells

Further evidence that IgE on LC is involved in allergen presentation is provided by the results of inhibition studies with anti-ε heavy chain (a-IgE) or anti-kappa and anti-lambda light chain antibodies (a-k/λ) [41]. I the case of IgE-positive LC, the T-cell response to HDA could be significantly inhibited by both a-IgE and a-k/λ, whereas the response to *Candida* was not affected (Fig. 9).

In case of non-T cells, a-IgE and a-k/λ did not inhibit the T-cell response to HDA significantly. However, inhibition with a-IgE and a-k/λ could be observed in 3 of

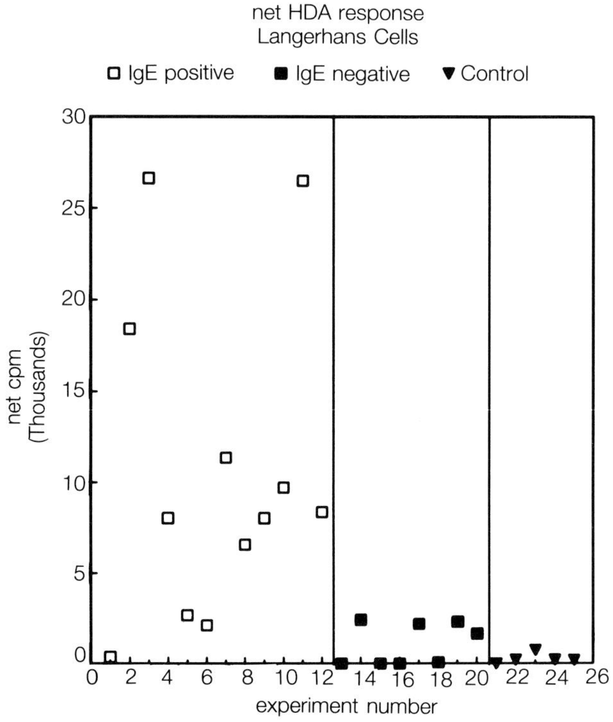

Fig. 8. T-cell response to house dust allergen (*HDA*) using Langerhans cells (LC) as antigen-presenting cells. The results are expressed as net cpm (cpm T-cell response to HDA minus background cpm). There was a significant difference between atopic patients with IgE$^+$LC and IgE-LC ($\alpha<0.005$) and also between IgE$^+$LC and normal controls ($\alpha<0.005$). There was no significant difference between atopic patients with IgE-LC and normal controls

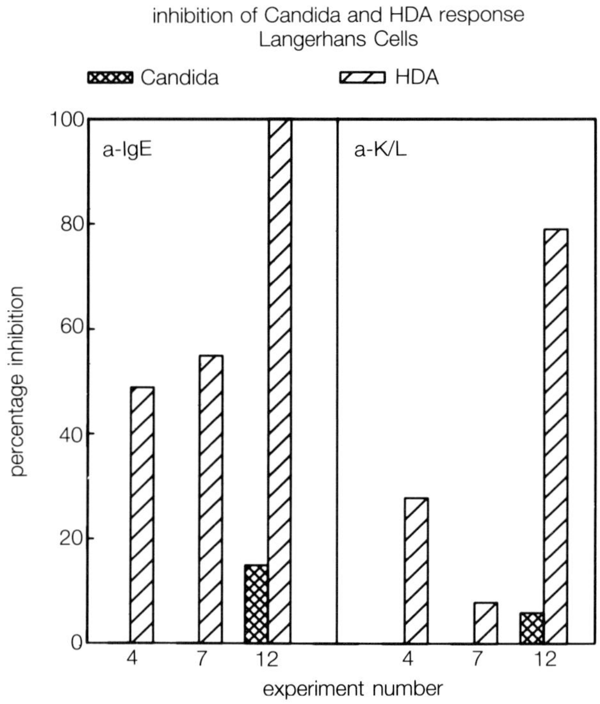

Fig. 9. Comparison of the inhibition by anti-light chain (*a-k/λ*) and anti-IgE antibodies on the T-cell response to *Candida* and house dust allergen (HDA) in the presence of IgE$^+$ LC as antigen-presenting cells ($n = 3$). The inhibition of the T-cell response to *Candida* by both antibodies was not significant compared with the T-cell response to HDA in the same atopic patients

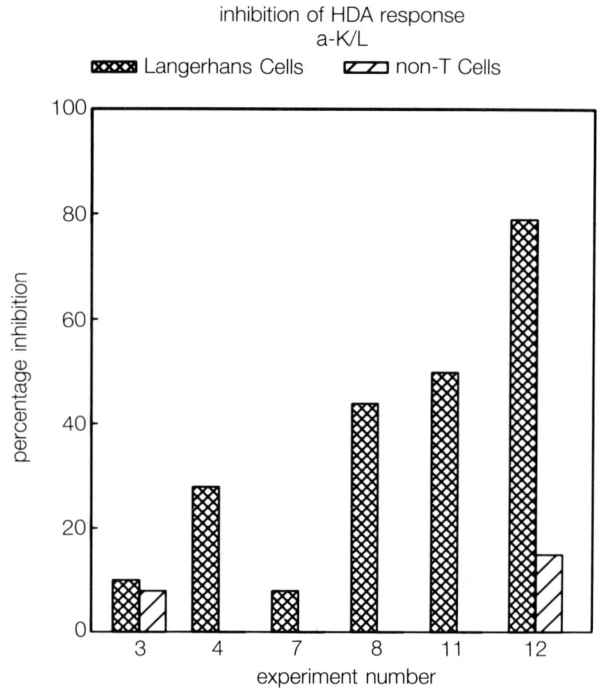

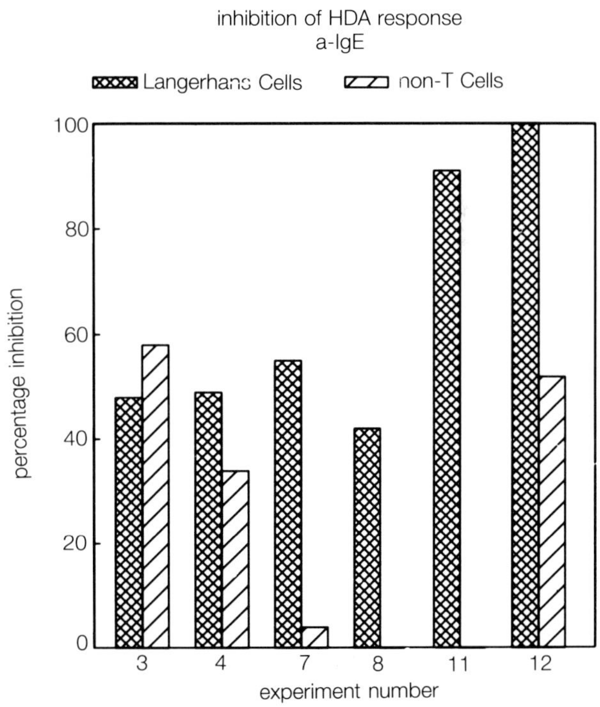

Fig. 10a, b. Inhibition of the T-cell response to house dust allergen (HDA) by anti-light chain (*a-k/λ*) and anti-IgE heavy chain (*a-IgE*) antibodies.
a Inhibition by a-k/λ ($n = 6$). Results are expressed as the percentage inhibition. In the presence of non-T cells no significant inhibition could be observed. **b.** Inhibition by a-IgE ($n = 6$). Results are expressed as percentage inhibition. Although in 3 of 6 patients an inhibition in the presence of non-T cells as antigen-presenting cells could be observed, the mean inhibition by a-IgE was not significant

6 experiments, indicating that even non-T cells from the peripheral blood may use membrane-bound IgE for antigen uptake (Fig. 10). However, these results also imply that at least in part these cells bear IgE on their surface. Indeed, although in contrast to earlier studies from Melewicz [39] – who reported the existence of $Fc_\varepsilon R$ on monocytes in AE patients but did not find IgE on these cells – we found that a substantial proportion of peripheral blood monocytes from patients with IgE-positive LC may bear IgE on their surface. In double-labelling experiments all these IgE cells appeared to be CD_{14}-positive, which indicates that in AE patients with elevated serum IgE levels, IgE-positive monocytes exist. This was also described by Ferreri et al. [28]. The results of this study demonstrate that HDA may be presented to T cells in at least two different ways: IgE dependent (LC) and IgE independent (non-T cells from the peripheral blood).

Correlation Between In Vitro and In Vivo Observations

The above described in vitro observations are supported by the in vivo observation that a higher frequency of positive delayed patch test reactions to HDA is observed in AE patients with IgE-positive LC than in patients with IgE-negative LC (Table 1).

The observations that not all AE patients with IgE-positive LC show a positive patch test reaction to HDA and that in some AE patients with IgE-negative LC the patch test reactions were positive may be explained by local differences in the presence or quantity of LC-bound IgE molecules. Although these studies have to be extended with other and even more purified allergens, the above described in vitro observations may offer an explanation for the reaction mechanism behind the patch test reactions to HDA (and other aeroallergens) in AE patients. The dependence of this T-cell response on LC-bound IgE emphasises the latter's important or even crucial role and explains why the delayed patch test reactions to aeroallergens are specific for patients with AE.

Role of Langerhans Cells in the Regulation of IgE Synthesis

So far, arguments have been put forward which suggest that IgE-positive LCs play a role in the mechanism behind the patch test reaction to aeroallergens. Aeroallergens may bind to allergen-specific IgE on LC, which present the allergen to T cells, inducing an eczematous response. This mechanism may also be involved in the pathogenesis of eczematous skin in AE. However, allergen-specific T cells present in AE skin may not only be involved in the eczematous response but also in the regulation of IgE production by B cells.

Some observations from Carswell [22] and Thompson [60] favour this possibility. Based on differences in serum levels for the specific IgE for allergens derived from house dust mite body and house dust mite faeces in asthmatic children and children with AE, it was hypothesised that sensitisation to allergens from the mite body occurs via penetration of the skin.

Hence, IgE-positive LCs may play a critical role in the regulation of IgE synthesis in at least two different ways: stimulation of IL-4-producing T cells, production of IgE-binding factors or both.

Hauser et al. [32] reported that, in mice, epidermal LC were capable of inducing antigen-specific T cells of the Th-2 subtype, which are able to produce IL-4. IL-4 induces IgE synthesis by B cells [43]. Furthermore, IL-4 is a pluripotent cytokine which (a) induces the expression of a low-affinity Fc receptor for IgE not only on B cells but also on monocytes [66] and LCs [10]; (b) induces normal B cells to produce soluble CD23/IgE-BF [15]; (c) induces the differentiation of monocytes into dendritic cells; (d) increases class II MHC expression of monocytes; (e) inhibits the secretion of IL-1 by monocytes [65].

If we extrapolate this to AE skin, the following pathway is possible after epidermal contact with aeroallergens (Fig. 11): aeroallergens are capable of penetrating the skin, binding to IgE on LC and inducing a T-lymphocytic response. These T cells may be involved in the induction of the eczematous response. However, some

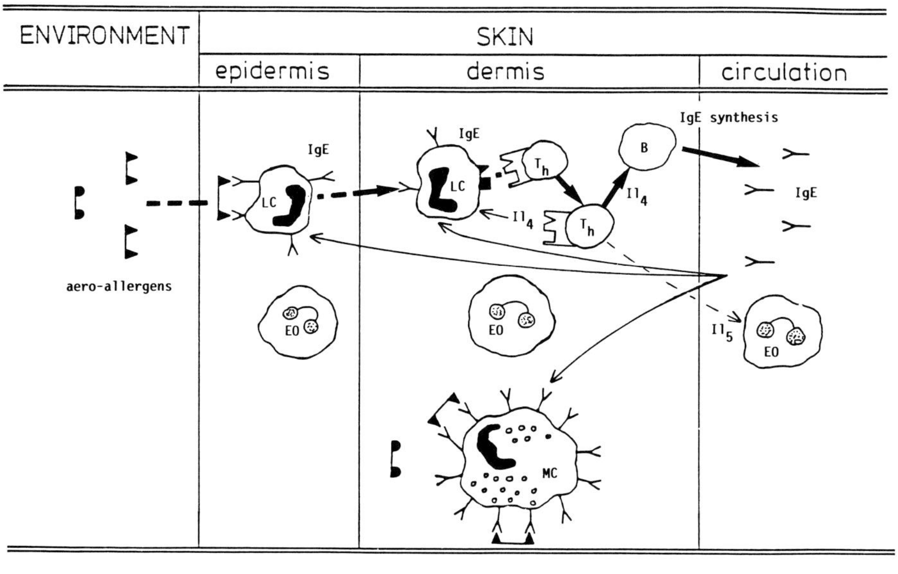

Fig. 11. Allergic reaction mechanism after epicutaneous contact with aeroallergens. *LC*, Langerhans cell: *MC*, mast cell; *EO*, eosinophil; *B*, B cell; T_h, CD4+ cell; Il_4, interleukin-4; Il_5, interleukin-5

T cells may belong to the presumed human equivalent of the Th-2 subtype, which produces IL-4. IL-4 induces IgE production by B cells in afferent lymph nodes. Furthermore, IL-4 may be involved in the induction of $Fc_\varepsilon R$ on monocytes, which further differentiate into dendritic cells, or directly on dendritic cells and LCs in the skin, thereby amplifying the response to allergens. In vitro, IL-4-producing T cells are increasingly present after repeated exposure to antigen, suggesting that they play a particularly important role in the immune response to antigen that persists or is encountered repeatedly [44]. Since contact with aeroallergens occurs via direct skin contact via upholstery, beds and clothes [63], contact occurs frequently or even continuously [11].

Recent work of Bieber et al. (manuscript submitted) argues for the second possibility. It has been reported that IgE-BF are produced by $Fc_\varepsilon R_2/CD_{23}$-positive cells. $Fc_\varepsilon R_2$/CD23 is a 45K glycoprotein which, under some conditions, is cleaved into 25–27K soluble fragments termed IgE-BF because they are still capable of binding to IgE [51]. They exert an inducing or suppressive (depending on their glycosylation) activity on IgE synthesis (see chapter on regulation of IgE synthesis). Since it has been demonstrated that rhIL-4 and rhIFN-γ stimulated LCs become $Fc_\varepsilon R_2/CD_{23}^+$ [10], they are, just like many other $Fc_\varepsilon R_2/CD_{23}^+$ cells, potent producers of IgE-BF. Therefore, the culture supernatants (CSN) of $Fc_\varepsilon R_2/CD23^+$ LCs have been tested for IgE-BF by a radioimmunoassay using a specific non-crossreacting monoclonal antibody reacting with the cleaved moieties of CD23. These investigations have shown that: (a) CSN of unstimulated LCs do not contain IgE-BF; (b) CSN of rhIL-4/rhIFN-γ stimulated, LC-depleted epidermal cells fail to contain IgE-BF; (c) CSN of rhIL-4/rhIFN-γ stimulated, LC-enriched epidermal cells exhibit significant amounts of IgE-BF. These results indicate that rhIL-4 and rhIFN-γ not only induce the expression of $Fc_\varepsilon R_2/CD23^+$ but also the release of IgE-BF by LCs.

However, the question arose as to where IgE-BF-producing LCs exert their regulatory activity. This occurs probably in at least two different areas, namely in the skin and in the afferent lymph nodes. Thus, immunohistochemical investigations of acute inflammatory skin of atopic eczema suggest that IgE-positive LCs may lose their IgE molecules between the keratinocytes by shedding [8]. The immunological significance of this feature remains unclear since as far as we know IgE synthesis has not been demonstrated in the skin. On the other hand, it has been reported that in allergic contact dermatitis LCs may leave the epidermal compartment for the afferent lymph nodes where they probably present the antigen to T cells. Therefore, we may speculate that in AE, $Fc_\varepsilon R_2/CD_{23}^+$ LCs function the same way and participate in the regulation of IgE synthesis in the lymph nodes by producing IgE-BF.

Further studies on the characterisation of the $Fc_\varepsilon R$ on LC in AE are needed to learn us more about its function in IgE-regulation in vivo.

Conclusions

Observations are presented which favour a function for IgE-bearing LC in AE. They are involved not only in the induction of an eczematous response but presumably also in the regulation of IgE synthesis by B cells. By means of this mechanism IgE-bearing LCs form an important link between type I and type IV hypersensitivity reactions in AE. From a practical point of view, the results of this study show that aeroallergens play a more important role in the pathogenesis of AE than has been accepted so far.

References

1. Adinoff A, Tellez P, Clark R (1988) Atopic dermatitis and aeroallergen contact sensitivity. J Allergy Clin Immunol 81: 736–742
2. Agel N (1986) Defining bone marrow progenitor cell for human Langerhans cells and the lack of specific markers. J Pathol 149: 67–68
3. Baier U, Burg G, Kaudewitz P, Bieber T, Ryckmanns F (1987) Correlation of the number of Langerhans cells with epidermal thickness in normal skin and atopic dermatitis. J Invest Dermatol 89: 44
4. Barker J, Alegre V, MacDonald DM (1988) Surface-bound immunoglobulin E on antigen presenting cells in cutaneous tissue of atopic dermatitis. J Invest Dermatol 90: 117–121
5. Bieber T, Baier U, Burg G, Ring J, Rieber P (1987) Quantitative assessment of IgE bearing cells in atopic dermatitis. J Invest Dermatol 89: 499
6. Bieber T, Prinz JC, Rieber P, Ring J (1988) Immunochemical study of IgE bearing cells in atopic eczema. J Invest Dermatol 90: 238
7. Bieber T, Ring J, Braun-Falco O (1988) Comparison of different methods for enumeration of Langerhans cells in vertical cryosections of human skin. Br J Dermatol 118: 385–392
8. Bieber T, Dannenberg B, Ring J, Braun-Falco O (1989) Keratinocytes of lesional skin of atopic eczema bear HLA-DR, CD1a and IgE molecules. Clin Exp Dermatol 14: 35–39
9. Bieber T, Dannenberg B, Prinz JC, Rieber EP, Stolz W,

Braun-Falco O, Ring J (1989) Occurrence of IgE bearing epidermal Langerhans cells in atopic eczema: a study of the time course of the lesions and with regard to the IgE serum level. J Invest Dermatol 92: 215–219
10. Bieber T, Prinz JC, Rieger A, Rieber EP, Boltz-Nitulescu G, Neuchrist C, Kraft D, Stingl G (1989) Induction of FcεR2/CD23 on human epidermal Langerhans cells by human recombinant interleukin-4 and gamma interferon. J Exp Med 170: 309–314
11. Bisschoff E, Kniest F, Liebenberg B (1987) House dust mites in upholstery and clothing: possibilities of involuntarily transporting mites and ways of preventing this. Sixth congress of SEP, Amsterdam
12. Bjerke S, Elgo J, Braathen L, Thorsby E (1984) Enriched epidermal Langerhans cells are potent antigen-presenting cells for T cells. J Invest Dermatol 83: 286–289
13. Bjerke S, Gaudernack G, Braathen L (1985) Enriched Langerhans cells express more HLA-DR determinants than blood derived adherent cells (monocytes and dendritic cells). Scand J Immunol 21: 489–492
14. Black P, Marsh D (1980) Correlation between lymphocyte responses and immediate hypersensitivity to purified allergens. J Allerg Clin Immunol 66: 394–401
15. Bonnefoy J, Defrance T, Peronne C, Menetrier C, Rousset F, Pene, De Vries J, Banchereau (1988) Human recombinant interleukin 4 induces normal B cells to produce soluble CD23/IgE-binding factor analogous to that spontaneously released by lymphoblastoid B cell lines. Eur J Immunol 18: 117–122
16. Bos J, van Garderen I, Krieg S, Poulter L (1986) Different distribution patterns of dendritic cells having Langerhans (T6) and interdigitating (RFD1) cell immunophenotype in psoriasis, atopic dermatitis and other inflammatory dermatoses. J Invest Dermatol 87: 358–361
17. Braathen L, Forr O, Natvig J, Eeg-Larsen T (1979) Predominance of T-lymphocytes in the dermal infiltrate of atopic dermatitis. Br J Dermatol 100: 511–519
181. Bruijnzeel-Koomen C, van Wichen D, Toonstra J, Berrens L, Bruijnzeel P (1986) The presence of IgE molecules on epidermal Langerhans cells from patients with atopic dermatitis. Arch Dermatol Res 278: 199–205
19. Bruijnzeel-Koomen C, van den Donk E, Bruijnzeel P, Capron M, de Gast G, Mudde G (1988) Associated expression of CD1 antigen and the Fc receptor for IgE on epidermal Langerhans cells from patients with atopic dermatitis. Clin Exp Immunol 74: 137–142
20. Bruijnzeel-Koomen C, van Wichen D, Spry C, Venge P, Bruijnzeel P (1988) Active participation of eosinophils in patch test reactions to inhalant allergens in patients with atopic dermatitis. Br J Dermatol 118: 229–238
21. Capron M, Jouault T, Prin L, Joseph M, Ameisen J, Butterworth A, Papin J, Kusnierz J, Capron A (1986) Functional study of a monoclonal antibody to IgE Fc receptor (FcER2) on eosinophils, platelets and macrophages. J Exp Med 164: 72–89
22. Carswell F, Thompson S (1986) Does natural sensitization in eczema occur through the skin? Lancet II: 13–15
23. Cavaillon J, Fitting C, Guinnepain M, Rassemont R, David B (1988) Lymphocyte proliferative responses to purified *Dermatophagoides farinae* major allergen (Der F1) in untreated and hyposensitized atopic patients. Allergy 43: 146–151
24. Choi K, Sauder D (1986) The role of Langerhans cells and keratinocytes in epidermal immunity. J Leukocyte Biol 39: 343–358
25. Desager K, Van Bever H, Stevens W (1987) Contact sensitivity to aeroallergens in children with atopic dermatitis demonstrated by patch test. J Allergy Clin Immunol 79: 236
26. Elliston W, Heise E, Huntley C (1982) Cell-mediated hypersensibility to mite antigens in atopic dermatitis. Arch Dermatol 118: 26–29
27. Enk A, Knop J (1987) Production of interferons by Langerhans cells after stimulation with contact sensitizers. J Invest Dermatol 89: 443
28. Ferreri N, Zeiger R, Spiegelberg H (1988) IgG, IgA, and IgE induced release of leukotriene C4 by monocytes from patients with atopic dermatitis. J Allergy Clin Immunol 82: 556–567
29. Gondo A, Saeki N, Tokuda Y (1986) Challenge reactions in atopic dermatitis after percutaneous entry of mite antigen. Br J Dermatol 115: 485–492
30. Goordyal P, Isaacson P (1985) Immunocytochemical characterization of monocyte colonies of human bone marrow: a clue to the origin of Langerhans cells and interdigitating reticulum cells. J Pathol 146: 189–195
31. Hanau D, Fabre M, Schmitt D, Garaud J-C, Pauly G, Cazenave J-P (1988) Appearance of Birbeck granule like structure in anti-T6 antibody-treated human epidermal Langerhans cells. J Invest Dermatol 90: 298–304
32. Hauser C, Snapper J, O'Harra W, Paul W, Katz S (1988) Cultured Langerhans cells activate type 2 T helper cells which produce IL-4/BSF1. J Invest Dermatol 90: 568
33. Hiratami M. Muto K, Oshida Y, Ito S, Kasei M (1981) Lymphocyte responsiveness to *Dermatophagoides farinae* extract in mite sensitive patients: effect of immunotherapy on cellular proliferative response and specific immunoglobulin E antibody (RAST score). J Allergy Clin Immunol 68: 205–211
34. Katz S, Tamaki K, Sachs D (1979) Epidermal Langerhans cells are derived from cells originating in bone marrow. Nature 282: 324–326
35. Klareskog L, Tjernlund U, Forsum U, Peterson P (1977) Epidermal Langerhans cells express Ia antigens. Nature 268: 248
36. Leung R, Bhan A, Schneeberger E, Geh R (1983) Characterization of the mononuclear cell infiltrate in atopic dermatitis using monoclonal antibodies. J Allergy Clin Immunol 71: 47–56
37. Leung D, Schneeberger E, Siraganian R, Geha R, Bhan AK (1987) The presence of IgE on macrophages and dendritic cells infiltrating into the skin lesions of atopic dermatitis. Clin Immunol Immunopathol 42: 328–337
38. Lever R, Turbitt M, Sanderson A, Mackie R (1987) Immunophenotyping of the cutaneous infiltrate and the mononuclear cells in the peripheral blood of patients with atopic dermatitis. J Invest Dermatol 89: 4–7
39. Melewicz F, Zeiger R, Mellon M, O'Connor R, Spiegelberg H (1981) Increased peripheral blood monocytes with FcER for IgE in patients with severe allergic disorders. J Immunol 126: 1592–1595
40. Mitchell B, Chapman M, Pope F, Crow S, Jouhal S, Platts-Mills T (1982) Basophils in allergen-induced patch test sites in atopic dermatitis. Lancet I: 127–131
41. Mudde G, van Reysen F, Boland G, de Gast G, Bruijnzeel P, Bruijnzeel-Koomen C (1990) Allergen presentation by epidermal Langerhans cells from patients with atopic dermatitis is mediated by IgE. Immunology 69: 335–341
42. Murphy G, Bhan A, Sato S, Mihm M, Harrist T (1981) A new immunologic marker for epidermal Langerhans cells. N Engl J Med 304: 791
43. Pene J, Rousset F, Briere F, Chretien I, Bonnefoy J, Spits H, Yokotu T, Akai N, Akai U, Banchereau J (1988) IgE

production by normal human lymphocytes is induced by interleukin-4 and suppressed by interferons τ and α and prostaglandin E2. Proc Natl Acad Sci USA 85: 6880–6884

44. Powers G, Abbas A, Miller R (1988) Frequencies of IL-2- and IL-4-secreting T cells in naive and antigen-stimulated lymphocyte populations. J Immunol 140: 3352–3357
45. Räsänen L, Lehto M, jansen C, Reunala T, Leinikki P (1986) Human epidermal Langerhans cells and peripheral blood monocytes. Scand J Immunol 24: 503–508
46. Räsänen L, Lehto M, Reunala T, Jansen C, Lehtinen M, Leinikki P (1987) Langerhans cell and T-lymphocyte function in patients with atopic dermatitis with disseminated cutaneous herpes simplex virus infections. J Invest Dermatol 89: 15–18
47. Rawle F, Mitchell E, Platts-Mills T (1984) T-cell responses to the major allergen from the house dust mite *Dermatophagoides pteronyssinus* antigen P1: comparison of patients with asthma, atopic dermatitis and perennial rhinitis. J Immunol 133: 195–201
48. Reitamo S, Visa K, Kahonen K, Stubb S, Salo O (1986) Eczematous reactions in atopic dermatitis patients caused by epicutaneous testing with inhalant allergens. Br J Deratol 114: 303–310
49. Rocha L, de Maubeuge J, Sarfati M, Sing M, Delespesse G (1984) Characterization of cellular infiltrates in skin lesions of atopic dermatitis by means of monoclonal antibodies. Dermatologica 169: 330–338
50. Ruzicka T, Auböck J (1987) Arachidonic acid metabolism in guinea pig Langerhans cells. Studies on cyclooxygenase and lipoxygenase pathways. J Immunol 138: 539–543
51. Sarfati M, Nutman T, Fonteyn C, Delespesse G (1986) Presence of antigenic determinants common to Fc IgE receptors on human macrophage, T and B lymphocytes and IgE-binding factors. Immunology 59: 569–576
52. Sauder D, Dinarello C, Morhenn V (1984) Langerhans cell production of interleukin-1. J Invest Dermatol 82: 605
53. Seifert H, Wollemann G, Seifert B, Borelli B (1987) Neurodermitis. Eine Protein-kontakt Dermatitis? Dtsch Derm 35: 1204–1214
54. Shelley W, Juhlin L (1976) Langerhans cells from an reticuloendothelial trap for external contact allergens. Nature 261: 46
55. Silberberg-Sinakin I, Thorbecke G, Baer R, Rosenthal S, Berezowsky V (1976) Antigen-bearing Langerhans cells in the skin, dermal lymphatics and lymph nodes. Cell Immunol 25: 137–151
55. Silberberg I, Baer R, Rosenthal S (1976) The role of Langerhans cells in allergic contact sensitivity. A review of findings in man and guinea pigs. J Invest Dermatol 66: 210–215
57. Sillevis Smitt J, Bos J, Hulsebosch H, Krieg SR (1986) In situ immunophenotyping of antigen presenting cells and T cell subsets in atopic dermatitis. Clin Exp Dermatol 11: 159–168
58. Stingl G, Wolf-Schreiner E, Pichler W, Gschnait F, Knapp W, Wolff K (1977) Epidermal Langerhans cells bear Fc and C3 receptors. Nature 268: 245
59. Stingl G, Katz S, Clement L, Green I, Shevach E (1978) Immunologic functions of Ia-bearing epidermal Langerhans cells. J Immunol 121: 2005–2013
60. Thompson S, Whitley H, Naysmith J, Carswell F (1988) IgE antibodies to *Dermatophagoides pteronyssinus* in atopic patients. Immunology 64: 311–314
61. Tong A, Mihm M (1986) The pathology of atopic dermatitis. Clin Rev Allergy 4: 27–42
62. Toonstra J, van der Putte S, van Wichen D, van Weelden H, Henquet C, van Vloten W (19899 Actinic reticuloid: immunohistochemical analysis of the cutaneous infiltrate in 13 patients. J Am Acad Dermatol 21: 205–214
63. Tovey E, Chapman M, Wells C, Platts-Mills T (1981) The distribution of dust mite allergen in the house of patients with asthma. Am Rev Respir Dis 124: 630–635
64. Uno H, Hanifin J (1980) Epidermal Langerhans cells and chronic lesions of atopic dermatitis observed by L-dopa. J Invest Dermatol 75: 52–60
65. Te Velde A, Klomp J, Yard B, de Vries J, Figdor C (1988) Modulation of phenotypic and functional properties of human peripheral blood monocytes by IL-4. J Immunol 140: 1548–1554
66. Vercelli D, Jabara HH, Lee B, Woodland N, Geha RS, Leung DYM (1988) Human recombinant interleukin 4 induces FcεR2/CD23 on normal human monocytes. J Exp Med 167: 1406–1416
67. Volc-Platzer B, Stingl G, Wolff K, Hinterberg W, Schneidl W (1984) Cytogenetic identification of allogeneic epidermal Langerhans cells in a bone marrow graft recipient. N Engl J Med 310: 1123
68. Walsh G, Nagakura T, Tikura Y (1988) Flow cytofluorometry analysis of increased IgE uptake by normal eosinophils following activation with PAF-acether and other inflammatory mediators. J Allergy Clin Immunol 81: 209
69. Wood G, Warner N, Warnke R (1983) Anti Leu3/T4 antibodies react with cells of monocyte/macrophage and Langerhans cell lineage. J Immunol 131: 121–216
70. Zachary C, Allen M, MacDonald D (1985) In situ quantification of T-lymphocyte subsets and Langerhans cells in the inflammatory infiltrate in atopic eczema. Br J Dermatol 112: 149–156
71. Zachary C, Poulter L, MacDonald DM (1985) Cell-mediated immune responses in atopic dermatitis: the relevance of antigen presenting cells. Br J Dermatol 113 [Suppl 28]: 10–16

IgG Subclasses in Atopic Eczema

R. C. Aalberse

Atopic Eczema and the Humoral Immune System

Atopic eczema (AE) is often accompanied by abnormalities in the humoral immune system. Most striking in this respect is often a marked increase in IgE production. However, abnormalities are also found regularly in other immunoglobulin isotypes, particularly IgG1 and IgG4. Before I review the data on IgG antibody levels in AE it might be useful to provide some background information on the humoral immune system in general and on the immunoglobulin isotype switch in particular.

Immunoglobulin Isotypes: Classes and Subclasses

Immunoglobulins are produced by plasma cells, which derive from identical B-cell precursors in the bone marrow. The immunoglobulins in the body fluids are highly variable. However, a plasma cell produces only one type of immunoglobulin. It is obvious, therefore, that during the development of B cells diversification and specialisation occur. The resulting cellular phenotypes are largely stable in lineage. This is achieved by a set of modifications in the DNA of the B cell. Two or three pairs of chromosomes are affected by these DNA modifications: either or both of the two pairs of chromosomes that contain the genes of the immunoglobulin light chains (kappa and lambda) and either or both of the chromosomes that contain the genes for the immunoglobulin heavy (H-) chains. For the present discussion only the rearrangement of the latter are of interest.

In the B-cell precursor, this chromosome contains a large number of isolated gene segments. During B-cell differentiation some of these gene segments are excised and lost, while others are joined; the result is a functional gene that can be transcribed into RNA. Two distinct rearrangements of this chromosome occur. The first results in the selection of a particular immunoglobulin variable (antigen-binding) segment, which is coupled to the constant part of the *mu* gene. This rearrangement, which occurs independent of antigen, enables the B cell to produce IgM antibodies, which are bound on the B-cell surface. If this B cell encounters a fitting antigen, further differentiation will occur, during which the DNA rearranges for a second time. Again a part of the DNA is excised and lost. This rearrangement concerns the gene segments that code for the immunoglobulin constant regions, some of which are lost. This process is called the *isotype switch* because the final result is that the B cell now starts to make an antibody with the same antigen-binding specificity but with a different constant part of the heavy chain; instead of producing IgM antibody the cell may now produce IgE antibody, IgG4 antibody or any of the other isotypes. In humans, nine immunoglobulin heavy chain isotypes exist for which the genes are all located in tandem on the same chromosome: mu, delta, gamma 3, gama 1, alpha 1, gamma 2, gamma 4, epsilon and alpha 2 [9]. Early in evolution five isotypes existed, schematically:

M D G E A

In relatively recent times (approximately at the time the mammalian species started to diversify) the number of isotypes increased by gene duplication:

M D *G2* G1 E A

followed by another duplication:

M D G3 G1 Ep A1 *G2 G4 E A2*

The gene coded as Ep (pseudo-epsilon) mutated into a nonfunctional gene.

The reason the nine isotypes are grouped into "classes" and "subclasses" is partially historical: immunoglobulins were grouped into classes when antisera could be produced that reacted with all subclass members of that class. If, for example, an antiserum was produced by immunisation with the heavy chain of IgG1, most antibodies in this antiserum would also react with the three other IgG subclasses; no reaction with immunoglobulins of the other classes would be found.

One important point with respect to the differences between classes and subclasses is that comparisons between species can be made with respect to classes but cannot be made with respect to subclasses. The reason is that subclasses developed after species evolved. Some analogies regarding subclasses between species can occasionally be made, notably with respect to the IgG antibody analogous to human IgG2. It is quite confusing that the corresponding mouse isotype is called IgG3. In some respects a weak analogy is found between human IgG4 and mouse IgG1. It should be stressed, however, that these analogies are far weaker than between e.g. mouse and human IgE.

With respect to function the differences between subclasses are often as marked as between classes. The same holds true with respect to the regulation of the immune response of the subclasses. In this respect, for example, IgG2 is more like IgM than like any of the other IgG subclasses.

For these reasons, it is often advisable to use the "isotype" terminology rather than to use "classes" and "subclasses". One practical advantage of the class/subclass terminology is in the case of tests using class-specific reagents such as anti-IgG or staphylococcal protein A. Good anti-IgG reagents react equally well with all four subclasses; protein A reacts with IgG1, IgG2 and IgG4. It is sometimes assumed that the reactivity of an anti-IgG reagent depends upon the presence of distinct antibodies, some reactive with IgG1, others with IgG2, etc. This is not the case. Almost all antibodies in a polyclonal anti-IgG antisera react with all subclasses because the subclasses have many antigenic determinants in common.

An important point concerning the isotype switch is its T-cell dependence. T cells exert a major regulatory role in determining the frequency and direction of the isotype switch. Some isotypes are markedly T-cell dependent (IgE, IgG4), others less so (IgG2). The precise mechanism of this influence is a very active field of research. The roles of the interleukins 3, 4 and 5 are of interest especially, as is the role of gamma-interferon.

The IgG4 Immune Response

The total serum IgG4 level is approximately ten times lower than the IgG1 level, whereas the half-lives of these two isotypes are indistinguishable. A further difference between IgG1 and IgG4 is the ontogeny of these responses: very little IgG4 is made in the first year of life.

We studied the IgG1 and IgG4 antibody response upon immunisation with various protein antigens: insect venom proteins, ingested foods, inhaled organic dust (employees in animal houses, grain handlers, pig farmers), injected allergen extracts (i.e. immunotherapy) and antigens from some tropical parasites. We invariably found that the early IgG response is predominated by IgG1 antibody; upon continuing immunisation the IgG1 response levels off and may even start to decline, whereas the IgG4 response slowly but steadily increases. We therefore postulated that an elevated IgG4 antibody response indicates chronic antigen stimulation [1]. In the large majority of subjects investigated we did not find any evidence of harmful effects of IgG4 antibodies. On the contrary, we found surprisingly few effects of the often substantial levels of antigen exposure; in particular we found little or no evidence of type III allergic disease.

Properties of IgG4 Antibodies

IgG4 and Type I Allergic Reactions

In many mammalian species IgG antibodies that sensitise mast cells (non-reaginic anaphylactic antibodies) have been described [5]. Also, in humans, a number of researchers have described skin-sensitising, homocytotropic (i.e. specific for primate cells), short-time sensitising IgG antibodies: IgG S-TS [11]. A major problem hampering investigators who attempt to establish the relevance of these antibodies is that the only assay procedure available is the bioassay, which requires suitable primate target cells. Most studies have been performed in monkeys using the passive cutaneous anaphylaxis (PCA) test. Three extensive studies on the prevalence of IgG S-TS were performed. Stanworth [30] investigated 250 asthmatic patients and found a positive PCA with heated sera in only 2%. Nelson and Branch [19] tested 149 patients strongly allergic to inhalant allergens and found no positive PCA after heating the sera. A strikingly high prevalence was found by Brighton [7], who investigated 84 sera from patients suspected of hypersensitivity to food and/or environmental allergens: 26% showed IgG S-TS to cow's milk, 6% to other allergens.

Parish [20] found indirect evidence that IgG4 and IgG S-TS might be related. In attempting to define the subclass of the IgG responsible for the sensitising activity, Stanworth and Smith [31], Malley et al. [16] and Vijay and Perelmutter (38] used myeloma proteins of different subclasses in PCA-inhibition experiments. It must be stressed that in these experiments the inhibition of IgE-mediated PCA reactions was investigated, not the inhibition of PCA reactions induced by IgG S-TS. The results from these and other analogous experiments were not consistent: inhibitory myeloma proteins (IgG4, IgG2) were found, but other myeloma proteins of the same isotype were not inhibitory. Analogous experiments were performed in vitro using human basophils as target cells. Again the results were not consistent, some researchers finding inhibition of IgE-induced sensitisation by IgG4 myeloma protein [38] whereas others failed to find inhibition by various IgG4 myeloma proteins [36, 39]. Stanworth [29] claimed to be able, using a guinea pig antiserum, to distinguish between two sets of IgG4 myelomas, inhibitory and non-inhibitory.

Most investigators would presumably accept the statement that IgG4 does not effectively bind to the IgE receptor on mast cells or basophils. This obviously does not exclude the possibility that IgG4 might be homocytotropic via a separate receptor. There is some evidence that IgG4 could be bound to human basophils which then may be triggered by IgG4 antibody. Most investigators do not find, however, that antigen can trigger basophils incubated with IgG4 antibody. It is important to stress that IgG4 antibodies, e.g. to foods, are found in many asymptomatic individuals [37].

For a detailed discussion on this subject, see [33]

IgG4 and Type III Allergic Reactions

The first investigations on the properties of IgG4 with respect to complement activation were performed with myeloma proteins without known antibody activity. It was found that aggregated IgG4 did not activate complement and therefore differed from the other IgG subclasses. This inability to activate the complement cascade was demonstrated by Ishizaka et al. [14] in experiments with native and chemically aggregated myeloma IgG4. However, Isenmann et al [13] provided evidence that IgG4-Fc fragments were as active in activating C1 as IgG1-Fc fragments were. For this reason, it has been suggested that IgG4 antibodies might be complement-activating after interaction with antigen [15, 32]. We demonstrated, however, that IgG4 antibodies in immune-complex form do not bind C1q and do not cause complement activation [34]. In contrast, we found a pronounced inhibition of activation when IgG4 antibodies were added to IgG1 antibodies. This inability of IgG4 to bind C1q not only results in a lack of complement activation, but it also prevents the formation of large immmune complex aggregates. We found that human IgG1 antibodies in vitro often do not form well-precipitating antigen-antibody complexes unless C1q is present. Heating a serum will destroy C1q activity; this treatment often results in a marked reduction in the amount of immune complex formed. This C1q-induced aggregation of antigen-antibody complexes does not occur with IgG4-containing complexes.

Apart from these C1q-dependent effects, IgG4 antibody differs from IgG1 antibody in the number of antigen molecules that can be bound per molecule antibody. Even in large antigen excess we found that only one antigen molecule per IgG4 antibody molecule was bound, whereas two antigen molecules were bound per IgG1 antibody molecule [35]. This monovalency of IgG4 is possibly due to a steric effect: as soon as a first antigen molecule is bound by either of the two antigen-binding sites of IgG4, the other antigen-binding site is blocked. This effect was found even with relatively small antigens like phospholipase A from honeybee venom (17Kd). It would be of interest to test even smaller antigens like peptides or haptens.

It must be stressed that in *antibody* excess, IgG4 antibodies do form complexes which were found to bind to rheumatoid factors. It is unlikely therefore that the monovalency of IgG4 is responsible for the inability to bind C1q. However, these complexes in antibody excess were still considerably smaller than comparable IgG1-containing immune complexes, even in the absence of C1q.

It is tempting to postulate that the appearance of IgG4 antibodies after prolonged antigenic stimulation is a protective mechanism against complement-induced damage.

IgG and Atopic Eczema: Review of Clinical Data

An extensive review on the IgG subclasses was published recently [25].

In 1977 Shakib et al. [26] reported that in 29 adult or adolescent patients with AE not only was the total IgE level often high (in six patients over 1500 IU/ml) but also the total IgG4 level, which was judged to be elevated in ten patients. As with IgE this increase was more marked in patients with AE than in patients with atopic asthma or rhinitis without eczema. Elevated IgG4 levels were not obviously associated with markedly elevated IgE levels: only three of the patients had high levels of both IgE and IgG4.

Gwynn et al. [12] described elevated IgG4 levels in asymptomatic first-degree relatives of atopic patients. Some 35% of 34 asthmatic children (often with AE) were found to have raised levels of IgG4, and 17% of 104 relatives had raised IgG4, usually without any symptoms. It is not clear from the data presented whether this incidence is significantly higher than expected in a random sample.

Shakib et al. [27, 28] investigated patients with milk intolerance, often accompanied by AE. They concluded that, although IgG4 antibodies to milk and egg are more frequently found in atopic children than in controls, the presence of these antibodies was found to be of no relevance to the child's food sensitivity.

Merret et al. [17] studied 32 adult patients with AE. One of the intake criteria was an IgE level greater than

180 IU/ml; geometric mean total IgG4 level in this group was 0.73 mg/ml. This AE group was compared with 28 patients with atopic asthma and/or rhinitis (total IgG4: 0.35 mg/ml) and with 156 adult healthy controls (total IgG4: 0.38 mg/ml). Allergen-specific IgG4 was measured against three inhalant allergens and seven foods. IgG4 antibodies to the inhalant allergens were almost exclusively found in sera that contained IgE antibodies to that allergen, but not all sera with IgE antibodies to an inhalant allergen had IgG4 antibodies to that allergen. No difference between the AE patients and the asthma/rhinitis patients was found; however, the difference with the control group was highly significant. With respect to IgG4 antibodies to foods, no such correlation with IgE antibodies was found: IgG4 antibodies to many foods, particularly egg white, were found in the majority of the sera investigated. However, AE patients tended to have higher titers than asthma/rhinitis patients, which in turn were usually higher than the controls.

Gondo et al. [10] studied different patient groups: 10 infants with AE (age $<$ 2 years), 10 children with AE (age 3–12 years), 45 adult AE patients (age 18–36 years) and 45 non-atopic healthy controls. Total IgG4 levels were increased in most of the adult AE patients. Ovalbumin-specific IgG4 was increased in the adults; no conclusions can be drawn from the data presented for the infants and children because age-matched controls were not included.

Rowntree et al. [22, 23] investigated 60 patients (35 adult, 25 children; mean age 4 years, range 1–10 years) with AE and 15 adult non-atopic subjects with negative skin prick tests and no history of skin disease. These investigators measured IgG (total), i.e. IgG1 + IgG2 + IgG3 + IgG4, and IgG4 antibodies to two inhalant allergens (a grass pollen allergen and a house dust mite allergen) and three food allergens (ovalbumin, ovomucoid and lactoglobulin). For the three food allergens the difference with the control group was marked for IgG (total) antibody; with respect to IgG4 antibody, the distinction still existed but was less marked. The variation between atopic patients and controls is even more pronounced when IgG (total) antibodies to the inhalant allergens are analysed: IgG antibodies to these two allergens are usually present in the serum of atopic patients with IgE antibodies to the allergen, whereas controls rarely have these IgG antibodies [8]. The contribution of IgG4 to the IgG antibody response is usually lower in the case of inhalant allergens than in the case of food allergens [24].

Nakano et al. [18] investigated 101 children and 19 adults with allergic disease, often with AE. IgG (total) antibodies to egg white and to *D. pteronyssinus* were measured. Increased antibody levels were found relative to age-matched controls.

Barnes et al. [2] investigated 56 adults with AE and 262 blood donors as controls. IgG subclass antibodies to dietary proteins (wheat gliadin, bovine milk and ovalbumin) were measured. Compared with patients with coeliac disease, the AE patients were found to have a more marked IgG4-restricted anti-gliadin response, but this was also found in the controls. Occasional IgA anti-gliadin and anti-milk antibodies were detected in Crohn's disease and dermatitis herpetiformis, but not in AE. These investigators conclude that production of IgG4 isotype antibodies may reflect a normal immune response to dietary protein antigens presented to mucosal surfaces [3, 4].

Reinhold et al. [21] investigated 15 adult patients with severe AE; phytohaemaglutinin-(PHA)-induced production of IFN-γ and the percentage of lymphocytes positive for the CD23 marker were measured. The CD23 marker is a low-affinity receptor molecule present on activated B cells, which is induced among other means by the action of IL-4. This induction by IL-4 is counteracted by IFN-γ. In seven of the patients IFN production was normal; in the other eight IFN production was very low. Regrettably, in only seven were the IgG subclass levels measured and compared with six controls. Three of the seven patients had IgG4 levels higher than 1 mg/ml; IgE levels were 2600, 2200 and 1600 IU/ml. A high correlation between CD23 expression and IgG4 serum concentration was found. Patient 5 in this study is interesting: this patient had a normal IgG4 serum level and a high IgE level (2800 IU/ml) whereas CD23 expression was low.

Discussion

How are the abnormalities in the skin on the one hand and the excessively active humoral immune system related? None of the three possibilities has been ruled out as yet:

1. The abnormal humoral immune system causes the dermatitis, e.g. via a type I allergic reaction induced by foods, other environmental allergens or possibly by endogenous allergens (e.g. "human dander").
2. The abnormalities in the humoral immune system are largely innocent epiphenomena, secondary to some hypothetical primary defect that is responsible both for the dermatitis and for the immunoglobulin abnormalities. Hypothetical example: due to abnormalities in the handling of macromolecules by the gut, increased quantities of insufficiently digested macro-

molecules enter into the circulation; some of these macromolecules stimulate the immune system, others are retained in the skin and cause toxic damage resulting in dermatitis. It should be noted, however, that there does not seem to be a major defect in intestinal permeability in AE [6].

3. The dermatitis is the primary defect causing abnormalities in the humoral immune system, e.g. by the resulting over-activity of the antigen-presenting cells in the skin.

In this paper AE is discussed without further qualification. However, it is unclear whether AE really is a single entity. It might be argued that AE is a symptom which may be induced by various mechanisms. Possibly, one might have to distinguish between AE patients with low total IgE and those with markedly elevated total IgE. Furthermore, juvenile AE might well have to be distinguished from AE in adults. In some papers such distinctions were not made, and it was not always possible to deduce IgE levels and ages of individual patients from the pooled data published.

IgG4 and Atopy

If one assumes that AE is a manifestation of an antibody-mediated allergic reaction (an assumption which is far from established), then several hypothetical possibilities might be considered for the involvement of IgG4 in AE:

1. IgG (4) [IgG (total) with emphasis on IgG4] as protective or blocking antibody in type I allergic reactions. IgE antibodies to foods or inhalant allergens may contribute to AE; the effects of these IgE antibodies might to some degree be blocked by IgG(4) antibodies.
2. IgG4 as protective or blocking antibody in type III allergic reactions. Complement-fixing antibodies to foods might contribute to AE; the effects of these IgG antibodies are to some degree blocked by IgG4 antibodies.
3. IgG4 as anaphylactic antibody in type I reactions. As discussed above it has been claimed that IgG4 antibodies to foods or inhalants have a mast cell-sensitising effect and thus might contribute in some way to the dermatitis.
4. IgG(4) antibodies as "innocent bystanders", indicating some disturbance in the antigen handling capacity of the gut and/or skin and/or in the regulation of the immune system.

Based on the literature presented above the most likely possibility would seem to be hypothesis 4: IgG4 as innocent bystanders.

Does a Relationship Exist Between IgE and IgG4 Antibodies?

Why is the IgG4 response sometimes associated with the IgE response, whereas in other situations no such association is found?

The distinction between atopic patients and controls with respect to the IgE and IgG1/IgG4 antibody levels is clearly found to depend on the antigenic stimulus.

When stimulated by a *weak antigenic stimulus*, e.g. normal levels of exposure to grass pollen allergens or mite allergens, only the most reactive (i.e. atopic) immune system is triggered, which results in the production of IgE and some IgG1.

Upon continuing stimulation by a *moderately potent antigenic stimulus*, e.g. food allergens or animal dander allergens in heavily exposed individuals, everyone will respond by producing IgG antibodies, IgG1 at first and later on IgG4; only atopic individuals will produce IgE antibodies.

A *very strong antigenic stimulus* (e.g. parasitic infections, tetanus immunisation, repeated bee stings in bee keepers) will induce IgE as well as IgG1 antibodies in the majority of exposed individuals, atopic as well as non-atopic; upon continued exposure the IgG4 respone become dominating.

All antigens which are good inducers of IgE antibodies also seem to induce a pronounced IgG4 response, provided the stimulus is chronic. This presumably reflects the marked T-cell dependency of both the IgE response and the IgG4 response.

Conclusions

1. Total IgG4 levels are often increased in AE; the increase is less marked than for IgE; increased IgG4 levels are associated with increased IgE levels.
2. IgG antibodies to foods are often increased in AE; this is true for IgG4, and presumably also for IgG1. The difference with non-atopic controls is quantitative rather than qualitative: IgG4 antibodies to foods are found in many asymptomatic individuals. No close association is seen between IgE antibodies and IgG4 antibodies to the same food.
3. IgG antibodies to inhalant allergens are often increased in AE; this increase is largely *not* IgG4, but presumably IgG1. The difference seems to be qualitative: non-atopic controls do not usually have IgG antibodies to the major allergens of grass pollen or house dust mites. A close association exists between IgE antibodies and IgG antibodies to the same inhalant allergen. No marked differences between atopic patients with or without dermatitis are seen.
4. The diagnostic value of IgG4 assays in AE is very limited.
5. IgG4 antibodies cannot be equated with IgG S-TS; no serologic assay for IgG S-TS is available. It is uncertain whether IgG S-TS plays a significant role in AE.
6. There is no good evidence that IgG4 antibodies are responsible for the dermatitis, neither do these antibodies seem to protect against dermatitis (as blocking antibodies). The increased levels of IgG4 seem to be an epiphenomenon in AE, reflecting chronic antigenic stimulation of an incompletely controlled, or overexposed, humoral immune system [1].

References

1. Aalberse RC, Van der Gaag R, Van Leeuwen J (1983) Serologic aspects of IgG4 antibodies. I. Prolonged immunization results in an IgG4-restricted response. J Immunol 130:722–726
2. Barnes RMR, Harvey MM, Blears J, Finn R, Johnson PM (1986) IgG subclass of human serum antibodies reactive with dietary proteins. Int Arch Allergy Appl Immunol 81:141–147
3. Barnes RMR, Johnson PM, Blears J, Harvey MM, Finn R (1988) Human serum antibodies reactive with dietary proteins. Antigenic specificity. Int Arch Allergy Appl Immunol 87:189–193
4. Barnes RMR, Johnson PM, Harvey MM, Blears J, Finn R (1988) Human serum antibodies reactive with dietary proteins. IgG subclass distribution. Int Arch Allergy Appl Immunol 87:184–188
5. Binaghi RA (1983) Nonreaginic anaphylactic antibodies in animals. In: Halpern GM (ed) Nonreaginic anaphylactic and/or blocking antibodies. Clinical reviews in allergy, vol 1, no 2. Elsevier, New York, pp 237–247
6. Bjarnason I, Goolami SK, Levi AJ, Peters TJ (1985) Intestinal permeability in patients with atopic eczema. Br J Dermatol 12:291
7. Brighton WD (1980) Frequency of occurrence of IgG(S-TS)9. Clin Allergy 10:97–100
8. Chapman MD, Rowntree S, Mitchell EB, Di Prisco de Fuenmajor MC, Platts-Mills TAE (1983) Quantitative assessments of IgG and IgE antibodies to inhalant allergens in patients with atopic dermatitis. J Allergy Clin Immunol 72:27–33
9. Flanagan JG, Rabbitts TH (1982) Arrangement of human immunoglobulin heavy chain constant region genes implies evolutionary duplication of a segment containing gamma, epsilon and alpha genes. Nature 300:709–713
10. Gondo A, Saeki N, Tokuda Y (1987) IgG4 antibodies in patients with atopic dermatitis. Br J Dermatol 117:301–310
11. Goodwin BFJ (1983) Nonreaginic anaphylactic antibodies in man. In: Halpern GM (ed) Clinical reviews in allergy, vol 1. Elsevier, Amsterdam pp 249–258
12. Gwynn CM, Morrison Smith J, Leon Leon G (1979) IgE and IgG4 subclass in atopic families. Clin Allergy 9:119–123
13. Isenman DE, Dorrington KJ, Painter RH (1975) The structure and function of immunoglobulin domains. J Immunol 114:1726–1729
14. Ishizaka T, Ishizaka K, Salmon S, Fudenberg H (1967) Biologic activity of aggregated gamma-globulin. J Immunol 99:82–91
15. Hasemann CA, Capra JD (1989) Immunoglobulins: structure and function. In: Paul WE (ed) Fundamental immunology. 2nd ed. Raven, New York, pp 209–233
16. Malley A, Beacher L, Porter G, Gerding R (1974) Competitive inhibition of reagin-mediated histamine release by human IgG2 myeloma protein. Int Arch Allergy Appl Immunol 47:194–210
17. Merrett J, Barnetson RS, Burr ML, Merrett TG (1984) Total and specific IgG4 antibody levels in atopic eczema. Clin Exp Immunol 56:645–652
18. Nakano H, Hosoi S, Mikawa H (1987) Specific IgG antibodies to *Dermatophagoides pteronyssinus* and egg white – their changes with age. Ann Allergy 59:262–266
19. Nelson HS, Branch LB (1977) Incidence of IgG short-term sensitizing antibodies in an allergic population. J Allergy Clin Immunol 60:266–270
20. Parish WD (1974) Skin sensitizing non-IgE antibodies. Association between human IgG S-TS and IgG4. In: Brent L, Holborow J (eds) Progress in immunology II, part 4. North Holland, Amsterdam, pp 19–28
21. Reinhold U, Pawelec G, Wehrmann W, Herold M, Wernet P, Kreysel HW (1988) Immunoglobulin E and immunoglobulin G subclass distribution in vivo and relationship to in vitro generation of interferon-gamma and neopterin in patients with severe atopic dermatitis. Int Arch Allergy Appl Immunol 870:120–126
22. Rowntree S, Mitchell EB, Platts-Mills TAE (1986)

Assessment of skin reactivity and specific antibody to egg and milk proteins in patients with atopic dermatitis: comparison with responses to the house dust mite antigen. Int Arch Allergy Appl Immunol 79:132–139

23. Rowntree S, Platts-Mills TAE, Cogswell JJ, Mitchell EB (1987) A subclass IgG4-specific antigen-binding radioimmunoassay (RIA): comparison between IgG and IgG4 antibodies to food and inhaled antigens in adult atopic dermatitis after desensitization treatment and during development of antibody responses in children. J Allergy Clin Immunol 80:622–630
24. Sampson HA (1987) Immunologically mediated reactions to foods: IgE in eczema. Ann Allergy 59:71–76
25. Shakib F (1986) Monogr Allergy vol 19, Karger, Basel
26. Shakib F, McLaughlin P, Stanworth DR, Smith E, Fairbairn E (1977) Elevated serum IgE and IgG4 in patients with atopic dermatitis. Br J Dermatol 97:59
27. Shakib F, Brown HM, Stanworth DR (1984) Relevance of milk- and egg-specific IgG4 in atopic eczema. Int Arch Allergy Appl Immunol 75:107–112
28. Shakib F, Brown HM, Redhead R, Phelps A (1985) IgE and IgG4 antibodies to bovine milk fat globule membrane in atopic eczema patients: a study of their occurrence, relevance and antigenic specificity. Clin Allergy 15:265–271
29. Stanworth DR (1983) IgG4 antibodies in atopics and their families. In: Kerr JW, Ganderton MA (eds) Proceedings of the XIth international congress on allergology clinical immunology, London 1982. Macmillan, London, pp 337–340
30. Stanworth DR (1983) Immunochemical aspects of human IgG4. In: Halpern GM (ed) Clinical reviews in allergy, vol 1. Elsevier, New York, pp 183–195
31. Stanworth DR, Smith K (1973) Inhibition of reagin-mediated PCA reactions in baboons by the human IgG4 subclass. Clin Allergy 3:37–41
32. Turner MW (1977) Structure and function of immunoglobulins. In: Glyn LE, Steward MW (eds) Immunochemistry: an advanced textbook. Wiley, Chichester, p 1–57
33. Van der Zee JS, Aalberse RC (1987) The role of IgG in allergy. In: Lessof MH, Lee TH, Kemeny DM (eds) Allergy: an international textbook. Wiley, London, pp 49–67
34. Van der Zee JS, Van Swieten SP, Aalberse RC (1986) Inhibition of complement activation by IgG4 antibodies. Clin Exp Immunol 64:415–422
35. Van der Zee JS, Van Swieten P, Aalberse RC (1986) Serologic aspects of IgG4 antibodies. II. IgG4 antibodies form small, nonprecipitating immune complexes due to functional monovalency. J Immunol 137:3566–3571
36. Van Toorenenbergen AW, Aalberse RC (1981) IgG4 and passive sensitization of basophil leukocytes. Int Arch Allergy Appl Immunol 65:432–440
37. Van Toorenenbergen AW, Aalberse RC (1982) IgG4 and release of histamine from human peripheral blood leukocytes. Int Arch Allergy Appl Immunol 67:117–122
38. Vijay HM, Perelmutter L (1977) Inhibition of reagin-mediated PCA-reactions in monkeys and histamine release from human leucocytes by human IgG4 subclass. Int Arch Allergy Appl Immunol 53:78–87
39. Zhou T, Conroy MC, Spengler H, De Weck AL (1984) Failure of covalently cross-linked human IgG myeloa subclass protein to release histamine from human leukocytes. Int Arch Allergy Appl Immunol 74:108–122

Mast Cells in the Skin

R. C. Benyon and M. K. Church

Morphology and Distribution of Human Skin Mast Cells

The ability of mast cells to be readily stained by basic dyes such as toluidine blue which bind tightly to proteoglycans of the secretory granules [40] has meant that their morphology and anatomical distribution have been well described. Mast cells of human skin are 5–15 μm in diameter and contain a single unsegmented nucleus and relatively few mitochondria [44, 102]. Cytoplasmic microtubules and perinuclear intermediate filaments are frequently seen [24]. In common with mast cells of other human tissues, the plasma membrane of skin mast cells is folded into numerous microvilli. Perhaps the most striking feature of these cells is the presence of a large number of membrane-bound secretory granules. These granules, of which there may be several hundred per cell, are 0.1–0.5 μm in diameter and contain the mast cell pre-formed mediators. Unlike the secretory granules of rat peritoneal mast cells, these granules in common with those of mast cells from human lung, intestine and nasal mucosa are observed under electron microscopy to contain distinct intragranular substructures consisting of whorls, scrolls and lattices [18, 44, 58, 78, 102]. These sub-structure are presumed to reflect the ordered packaging of pre-formed mediators, evidence for this deriving from the observations of Craig et al. [35] that the detailed internal structure of granules depends on the content of neutral proteases.

Mast cells are relatively abundant in human skin, which is in accord with their proposed important role in defence and homeostasis. As it contains a large number of mast cells, skin resembles other tissues such as intestinal mucosa and lung epithelium which form a barrier between the human body cavities and the external environment. Soter et al. [133] counted ~12 mast cells per mm^2 in 1-μm sections of skin whilst Mikhail and Miller-Milinska [95] found ~7 x 10^3 mast cells per mm^3 following staining of sections with toluidine blue. The latter workers found that the density of these cells varied little with gender, age or body region, although other workers [16, 57, 151] have reported decreases in mast cell density with increasing age and a heterogeneous distribution depending on the site examined. A close correlation has been found between the mast cell number and histamine content of human skin [38], this amine being present at a concentration of ~200 ng/mg wet weight of skin in normal individuals [114]. Mast cells are found in the greatest density in the papillary dermis and the superficial dermal zone immediately below the dermal-epidermal junction [34]. They are concentrated particularly around dermal nerve endings and in contact with blood vessels [38, 148] and are therefore ideally situated to play a part in the nervous control of blood flow as discussed below. Skin mast cell numbers increase dramatically in several diseases including urticaria pigmentosa [47] and some forms of chronic urticaria [98], this is associated with increased tissue levels of histamine [74, 106]. Mast cell hyperplasia has also been observed around skin tumours such as basal cell carcinomas [25]. Although histamine has been found in significant amounts in the epidermis [130], mast cells have rarely been observed in this layer in normal individuals. This discrepancy may be due to the presence in the epidermis of mast cell precursors which are not stained by basic dyes or to the uptake of histamine by epidermal phagocytic cells.

Role of IgE in Mast Cell Activation

Mast cells have 10^4–10^5 plasma-membrane receptors for immunoglobulin E (IgE) [32, 33]. The receptors of rat basophil leukaemia (RBL) cells, a tumour hybrid cell line from which large quantities of the receptor may be isolated, are tetrameric structures consisting of one α, one β and two γ subunits. The highly glycosylated α subunit faces the cell exterior and binds the Fc portion of IgE with high affinity ($K=10^9$–10^{12}mol/l) [93]. These receptors have been termed IgE FcR_I to distinguish them from the monomeric IgE receptors (IgE FcR_{II}) recently described on the cell surface of eosinophils, platelets, monocytes and lymphocytes, which have 100- to 1000-fold lower affinity for IgE [21].

Following sensitisation of individuals to an allergen,

allergen-specific IgE is secreted from plasma cells derived from clonal expansion of stimulated B lymphocytes. Even in such individuals, circulating levels of IgE are maintained at low levels due to its rapid adsorption to tissue mast cells and circulating basophils [88]. Due to this property, IgE has been termed cytophilic antibody. The mechanism of mast cell activation by allergens has been the subject of a series of studies by Professors Teruko and Kimishige Ishizaka. They showed that intracutaneous injection of pre-formed allergen-IgE complexes into human skin resulted in a mast cell-dependent wheal and flare reaction only when two or more molecules of IgE were present per molecule of allergen, i.e. the allergen was at least divalent [69]. These observations suggested that mast cell secretion is triggered by the formation of cross-linkages between cell surface IgE receptors, this hypothesis being supported by the findings that both IgE-specific and receptor-specific antibodies (anti-RBL) were effective secretagogues [70]. Although mast cells bear many thousands of IgE receptors, it is likely that only a few percent of them need to be cross-linked for the release of appreciable quantities of mediators [86].

Mast cells undergo a series of morphological changes following IgE-dependent activation [24, 37, 102]. Granules swell due to changes in the flux of anions across the perigranular membrane and at the same time lose their ordered sub-structures as the matrix is solubilised. There is widespread fusion of granules with the formation of large intracellular lacunae which eventually form pores to the cell exterior through which pre-formed mediators escape at various rates depending on their relative affinities for the granule membrane. With stimuli other than antigens, a different secretory mechanism is sometimes observed. For example, compound 48/80, an IgE-independent activator of mast cells, stimulates the rapid expulsion of whole granules from rat peritoneal mast cells [71]. The biochemical changes which follow IgE-dependent activation have been most extensively studied in rat mast cells and RBL cells which are easy to isolate and purify in large numbers. In these cells, IgE-dependent stimuli increase the breakdown of phosphoinositides and polyphosphoinositides, increase Ca^{2+} influx into the cytoplasm, increase cyclic AMP levels, increase protein kinase C activity and cause changes in cytoskeletal elements (reviewed by Ishizaka and Ishizaka [70]; Metzger et al. [93]; Benyon [15]).

Structures and Activities of Mast Cell Mediators

Histamine

Although both histamine and 5-hydroxytryptamine are synthesized by rat mast cells [11], only the former amine has so far been detected in human mast cells. Due to its basic (cationic) nature, histamine is bound tightly to the numerous anionic carboxylic acid and sulphate groups of intragranular proteoglycans [144]. Human dispersed skin mast cells contain 3–6 pg of histamine per cell, similar to the content of mast cells of other human anatomical sites [13]. Following its release from mast cells, histamine slowly dissociates from the granule matrix to exert its large variety of effects by binding to histamine H_1 and H_2 receptor subtypes [17]. A further receptor subtype (H_3) has recently been defined, although this may not be present outside the central nervous system. Binding of histamine to these receptors in various tissues of the body gives rise to the clinical effects of histamine release include pruritus, flushing, hypotension due to widespread vasodilation, palpitation, diarrhoea and headache.

Intradermal injection of picomole quantities of histamine results in the so-called triple response of flushing, flaring and whealing described [81]. Within seconds there is a rapidly developing vasodilation (flushing) at the injection site due to a direct effect of histamine on the microvasculature. Over the next 5–10 min, the vasodilation gradually spreads away from the injection site (flaring) by an axon reflex mechanism involving antidromic impulses in neuropeptide-containing primary afferent nerves which have been activated by both the injected histamine and histamine released locally by dermal mast cells. The final phase of the triple response is the development of oedema (whealing) following the leakage of plasma from blood vessels, generally post-capillary venules, which is mainly due to the direct effect on the blood vessels of peptides released from the primary afferent neurons. Studies with the recently available specific H_1-antihistamines suggest that both the wheal and flare reactions are mediated via this receptor subtype [48]. However, this conclusion is complicated by the findings of Robertson and Greaves [113] which suggest an additional involvement of H_2-receptors. Increased vascular permeability allows high molecular weight serum components such as kininogen, angiotensinogen and C3 to be proteolytically cleaved by mast cell proteases as detailed below with the resulting generation of secondary mediators such as bradykinin, angiotensin and C3a [110, 149].

Apart from its effect on the dermal vasculature,

histamine has other actions relevant to the development of inflammation, being chemotactic for eosinophils and increasing their expression of C3b receptors [3] and ability to neutralise parasites [4]. Histamine-mediated vasodilation and increases in vascular permeability potentiate the ability of the chemotactic factor leukotriene B_4 to cause neutrophil infiltration into the dermis. Down-regulation of the response probably occurs by the rapid degradation of histamine, the major pathway in skin probably being N-methylation [64].

Using the skin chamber technique, various workers have demonstrated directly that allergens activate the release of histamine from skin mast cells in vivo [8, 36, 135]. However, although the early vascular response to allergens and histamine is similar, the former stimulus frequently causes prolonged late vascular and cellular responses at 4–6 h after challenge [129] which are not seen following histamine provocation.

Proteoglycans

These molecules are a common feature of all human mast cells. Proteoglycans have a complex structure consisting of a polypeptide core, largely composed of alternating glycine and serine residues in rat mast cell heparin, to which are linked side chain branches of modified carbohydrate polymers. In the heparin/heparan proteoglycans, the side chains are repeating heterodimers of iduronic acid and *N*-sulphated glucosamine, whilst in the chondroitin sulphates, glucuronic acid and *N*-acetylgalactosamine heterodimers are present. Both types of proteoglycan are highly negatively charged due to the large number of O- and N-sulphates at various positions of the hexosamines and uronic acids.

The proteoglycan content of human mast cells varies according to their anatomical site. Studies of human mastocytosis skin tissue indicate that dermal mast cells contain mainly heparin [92] and our preliminary studies in collaboration with Drs. H. Thompson and D. Metcalfe of the National Institutes of Health, Bethesda, USA, confirm that highly purified preparations of these cells contain heparin as their major proteoglycan together with smaller amounts of chondroitin sulphates. They therefore closely resemble human lung parenchymal mast cells in proteoglycan content [91, 137] and differ from mast cells of human intestine which contain mainly chondroitin sulphate E [39, 49].

Mast cell-derived proteoglycans have several biological activities. Heparin is a potent anti-coagulant [125] and amplifies the alternative pathway of complement fixation whilst suppressing the classic pathway [118]. This proteoglycan also stabilises mast cell tryptase [119] thereby allowing expression of its catalytic activity. In the area of healing skin wounds where mast cell hyperplasia is commonly observed [6, 104], increased release of heparin may assist tissue repair and remodelling by activating fibroblasts [108], increasing neutrophil elastase activity [82] and stimulating capillary endothelial cell migration into the wound area [89].

Neutral Proteases

Human mast cells contain both chymotrypsin-like and trypsin-like neutral proteases, designated chymase and tryptase, respectively. Tryptase of human lung mast cells has been characterised as a tetrametric protein consisting of two 31 500 dalton and two 33 000 Dalton subunits, with each subunit having a single active site [120, 128]. Dissociation of subunits from the tetramer results in the loss of catalytic activity, this being preventable by the binding to tryptase of heparin proteoglycan [119]. Tryptase has several activities relevant to its proposed role as a pro-inflammatory mediator, in particular its ability to cleave the complement protein C3 to generate the anaphylatoxic and vasoactive C3a [121] and inactivate high molecular weight kininogen, thereby preventing the release of bradykinin in response to kallikrein [87, 109]. The observations that tryptase has a long plasma half-life (of ~2 h) relative to histamine (~1 min) and is virtually absent from human basophils [23] suggest that it may be more useful than histamine as a specific marker of mast cell degranulation in vivo. To date, increased concentrations of tryptase have been measured in the plasma of patients with active systemic mastocytosis and during anaphylaxis [124].

Immunoreactive tryptase has been localised to human skin mast cells [66, 123] and is released into skin chamber fluid following epicutaneous challenge with allergen [122]. The amounts of tryptase detected were closely related to the allergen concentration and reached a maximum at 30–60 min after challenge, being released into the chamber fluid more slowly than histamine, which peaked within 30 min. The finding of a close correlation between the amounts of tryptase and histamine in chamber fluid 1 h after challenge supports the hypothesis that tryptase is released from skin mast cell granules. In a study of mediator release into skin chambers during prolonged allergen challenge, Shalit et al. [126] found that the concentrations of both histamine and tryptase peaked within 1 h of challenge. However, whilst histamine levels remained significantly higher than unchallenged controls over the following 8 h, levels of tryptase dropped more rapidly, being greater than control only over the next 4 h. This difference in the time course of release of the two mediators was suggested to be possibly due to the recruitment and activation of basophils which, unlike mast cells, release histamine in the absence of PGD_2.

Mast cells dispersed from adult foreskin contain 35 pg/cell of tryptase, 2–3 times the amount contained in mast cells dispersed from infant foreskin [123]. The histamine content of these cells is similar, however, suggesting that production or storage of tryptase is delayed relative to that of histamine during maturation of skin mast cells.

High salt extracts of human skin contain chymase in addition to tryptase. The major chymase of human skin is a monomeric protein with a molecular weight of 30 000 daltons [115, 116]. It appears to differ structurally from bovine chymotrypsin, human neutrophil cathepsin G and the chymase of rat peritoneal mast cells (rat mast cell protease I) [116, 134, 149]. The observation that the skin of mastocytosis patients contains greater amounts of chymase than normal skin [115] suggests that mast cells are the major repository of chymase in this tissue. The recent in vitro studies of Schwartz et al. [123] demonstrate that mast cells dispersed from adult foreskin contain ~1 pg of chymase per cell, approximately 10 times more than is found in mast cells of infant foreskin. Chymase released from skin mast cells in vivo may play a role in the formation of blisters due to its ability to degrade the connective tissue of the dermal-epidermal junction [19].

The isolation of a monoclonal antibody to tryptase and polyclonal antibodies to chymase has allowed immunohistochemical studies of the distribution of these proteases in the human mast cell population [66, 68, 123]. A mast cell sub-population containing tryptase only predominates in the small and large intestinal mucosa and lung whilst in skin, intestinal submucosa and conjunctiva, mast cells containing both chymase and tryptase predominate. These sub-populations have been designated MC_T and MC_{TC}, respectively. Tryptase appears to be ubiquitously distributed in the human mast cell population, mast cells containing chymase only not having been observed. MC_T and MC_{TC} differ in morphology, the secretory granules of the latter being larger, more uniformly shaped and present in greater numbers per cell [35]. The granules of MC_T also lack lattice and grating sub-structures which are frequently observed in those of MC_{TC}. As well as differing morphologically, the two sub-populations may also vary in their requirement for T-lymphocyte factors for their development. Irani et al. [67] have shown that individuals with AIDS or severe combined immunodeficiency disease and therefore having diminished T-lymphocyte activity have lower numbers of MC_T in various regions of the intestine whilst the numbers of MC_{TC} remain unaffected. In this respect, MC_T resemble intestinal mucosal mast cells of rat and mouse, which require the lymphokine IL-3 for their development [63].

Chemotactic Factors

Cutaneous challenge with allergens often results in biphasic responses consisting of an early phase of mainly vascular changes and a late phase characterised by marked perivascular accumulation of inflammatory leukocytes. Accumulation of neutrophils, monocytes and eosinophils has been observed at sites injected with allergens [129], after cold challenge of skin of patients with cold urticaria [26] and in necrotising venolitis [133]. Accumulation of inflammatory cells is presumably due to the release of leukocyte chemoattractants by cells originally resident within the challenged skin sites. Several chemotactic factors have been associated with human mast cells. Histamine has eosinophil chemotactic activity demonstrable in vitro, but injection of this amine into human skin usually gives vascular changes only. Several groups have reported increased circulating levels of polypeptides chemotactic for neutrophils and eosinophils following challenge of atopic asthmatic patients with relevant allergens [7, 94, 97], but release of such factors in human skin has been less well investigated. Ting et al. [138] reported in vivo release of eosinophil chemotactic activity in human allergic skin reactions, whilst high molecular weight neutrophil chemotactic factors have been detected in the venous effluent of thermally challenged limbs of patients with cold-induced urticaria [132, 147]. Platelet activating factor (PAF), which attracts and activates eosinophils and neutrophils, has been detected in skin chambers placed over allergen-challenged skin sites [145], but its late appearance relative to histamine suggests that it is not a skin mast cell product. Another potent neutrophil chemotactic factor, leukotriene B_4, is not produced by dispersed skin mast cells following IgE-dependent activation (Robinson, Benyon, Holgate and Church, unpublished observations).

Newly Generated Mediators of Skin Mast Cells

A number of in vivo studies indicate that the major eicosanoid products of human skin mast cells are prostaglandin (PG) D_2 and leukotriene (LT) C_4. Firstly, individuals with systemic mastocytosis who have increased numbers of mast cells within their skin have large quantities of PGD_2 and its metabolites in their urine [112]. Secondly, individuals with cold-induced [56, 75] heat-induced [76] and cholinergic [73] urticaria have increased circulating levels of PGD_2 and histamine. Thirdly, epicutaneous challenge of the skin of allergic individuals with allergen results in the release of PGD_2, LTC_4 and histamine into overlying skin chamber fluid [8, 135].

The recent development of techniques for the dispersion of mast cells from human skin has allowed detailed studies of eicosanoid release from these cells. In suspensions of cells dispersed from human foreskin by collagenase and hyaluronidase by the method shown in Fig. 1, mast cells are present at a purity of 4%–8% of total nucleated cells [12, 13]. Percoll density-gradient centrifugation of dispersates results in the separation of cells into fractions which are depleted (< 1%) or enriched (> 90%) in mast cell purity. Gradient-separated human skin cells release both histamine and immunoreactive (i-) PGD_2 following activation with calcium ionophore A23187 [14]. There was a significant correlation between the net release of both mediators in preparations containing mast cells over a wide purity range (0.5%–94%), suggesting that mast cells were the major source of PGD_2. In contrast, the release of i-PGE_2 and thromboxane B_2 did not correlate with that of histamine, suggesting that these eicosanoids were derived from cells other than mast cells. In similar gradient studies in which anti-IgE was used to stimulate mast cells, significant correlations were seen between releases of i-PGD_2 and histamine and i-LTC_4 and histamine, providing strong evidence that both are released from skin mast cells following IgE-dependent stimulation. In preparations of highly purified skin mast cells, anti-IgE released i-PGD_2, i-LTC_4 and histamine in a concentration-dependent manner, maximum release of these mediators being 115.6, 9.1 and 4628 pmol/10^6 mast cells, respectively (Table 1).

Although these in vivo and in vitro studies provide strong evidence that PGD_2 and LTC_4 are produced by skin mast cells, the role of these eicosanoids in the development of allergic and inflammatory responses in the skin is uncertain. PGD_2 has a variety of pro-inflammatory actions, being chemokinetic for leukocytes [50], chemotactic for neutrophils [131] and en-

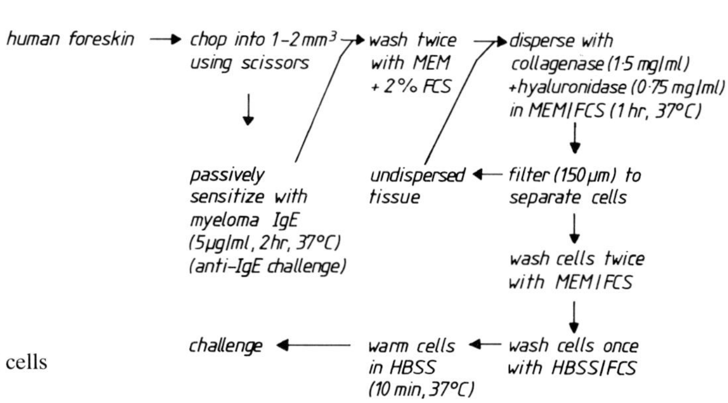

Fig. 1. Technique for the enzymatic dispersion of mast cells from human foreskin

Table 1. Release of histamine and eicosanoids from human purified skin mast cells activated with anti-IgE

Anti-IgE (µg/ml)	Mediator net release (pmol/10^6 mast cells) PGD$_2$	LTC$_4$	Histamine	Histamine release (% of cell total)
0.25	17.6± 4.0	0.2±0.1	361± 72	1.1±0.5
0.83	29.8± 4.9	1.1±0.3	701±181	2.3±0.6
2.5	77.8±12.2	4.5±1.0	1758±401	5.4±1.2
8.3	90.0±12.7	7.8±1.4	3551±869	12.0±3.7
25	115.0±12.1	9.1±1.8	4628±836	16.4±4.3

Results shown are from four experiments in which mast cell purity was 73.2% ± 2.4%.

hancing IgE-dependent release of histamine from basophils [105]. When injected intradermally in subnanomolar quantities, both PGD_2 and LTC_4 induce rapidly developing wheal and flare reactions [20, 131]. Neither eicosanoid produces a late reaction similar to that seen with allergens although neutrophil infiltrates are observed at the sites of injection of PGD_2 [131]. Although, as stated above, increased concentrations of PGD_2 have been measured in the circulation of patients with thermally induced urticaria [56], these concentrations are several hundred-fold lower than those of histamine in the same individuals. Histamine/PGD_2 molar ratios of 133–1532 measured in the plasma of patients with cold urticaria were higher than those measured in skin chambers placed over allergen-challenged dermis [8] or following IgE-dependent activation of skin mast cells in vitro. The small increases in plasma PGD_2 relative to histamine observed in thermal urticarias may be explained by the rapid breakdown of PGD_2 in plasma in vivo or the possible activation of basophils which release histamine but not PGD_2. Alternatively, under these conditions, skin mast cells may be activated by stimuli such as neuropeptides which, as described below, differ from allergens in causing histamine release in the virtual absence of PGD_2.

Characteristics of Skin Mast Cell Activation by IgE-Dependent and Non-immunological Stimuli

Various studies have demonstrated the ability of allergens and other IgE-dependent stimuli such as anti-IgE to release histamine and eicosanoids from human skin mast cells [28, 30, 51, 79, 136]. Recent studies with human dispersed skin mast cells [13, 83] have shown that histamine release by such stimuli is relatively slow, being complete in 5–7 min, requires extracellular concentrations of Ca^{2+} of 1–3 m*M* for optimum secretion and requires an intact cellular mechanism for ATP generation, this last observation suggesting that secretion is not cytotoxic. In responding to IgE-dependent stimuli, skin mast cells thus resemble mast cells of other human anatomical sites such as lung, intestinal mucosa and submucosa, tonsil and adenoids [84]. However, skin mast cells differ from these in being additionally responsive to a number of non-immunological (IgE-independent) stimuli. To date, compound 48/80, poly-*L*-lysine, morphine, dynorphin, substance P, vasoactive intestinal polypeptide (VIP) and somatostatin have all been shown to activate skin mast cells [13, 83]. That skin mast cells are activated by these stimuli in vitro is perhaps not surprising in the light of their ability to induce wheal and flare reactions in human skin in vivo [2, 22, 43, 45, 81]. However, the availability of dispersed cells allows the mechanism of mediator release from skin mast cells activated by non-immunological stimuli to be examined in detail. Such studies have highlighted important differences between the characteristics of histamine release by these stimuli and by anti-IgE [83] (Table 2). Histamine release by non-immunological stimuli is rapid, requiring only 15–20 s for completion and only partially dependent on the presence of extracellular Ca^{2+} ions. This contrasts with histamine release by anti-IgE which is relatively slow (> 5 min to completion) and entirely dependent on extracellular Ca^{2+} ions. However, histamine release by non-immunological stimuli is abrogated by inhibitors of ATP synthesis, suggesting that secretion occurs via a non-cytotoxic mechanism. Anti-IgE and non-immunological stimuli differ further in their ability to activate the release of eicosanoids from skin mast cells. Anti-IgE releases up to 21-fold more PGD_2 and 18-fold more LTC_4 than substance P, VIP, somatostatin and compound 48/80 (Table 3).

Due to the close anastomical association between mast cells and nerve terminals [42, 99, 127, 148], it is likely that neuropeptides represent the major in vivo non-immunological stimulators of these cells. Sensory nerves (primary afferent neurons) containing substance P, VIP and somatostatin are present in human dermis [54, 59, 60, 72]. These primary afferent neurons branch extensively within the dermis, often covering an area of several square millimetres. Some nerve branches terminate at polymodal nociceptors sensitive to physical

Table 2. Characteristics of histamine release from human skin mast cells activated by IgE-dependent and non-immunological stimuli

	IgE-dependent	Non-immunological
Maximum net release	15%–20%	15%–20%
Time course	Complete in 5–6 Min	Complete in <20 s
Requirement for ATP synthesis	+	+
Requirement for extracellular Ca^{2+}	Complete	Partial or no requirement
Inhibition by substance P antagonist	–	+
Stimulation of PGD_2 and LTC_4 release	+	–

stimuli such as heat and deep pressure as well as to chemical stimuli such as 5-HT and histamine. Stimulation of these sensory terminals generates orthodromic impulses which give rise to sensations of pain and itching. Antidromic impulses are also generated which spread to further branches of the same nerve and activate the release of neuropeptides from their terminals. The ability of neuropeptides to activate release of vasodilator histamine from mast cells provides a mechanism for the neurogenic control of blood flow through the microvasculature. The gradual development of flare following intradermal injection of histamine is due to the activation of mast cells increasingly distant from the injection site due to spreading away from this site of antidromic impulses. Support for the neurogenic origin of the spread of flare comes from observations of its blockade following the section of sensory nerves innervating the test area of skin [81], by topical application of local anaesthetics [43] or by topical application of capsaicin, a compound which depletes sensory neurons of their neuropeptide content [2].

Table 3. Histamine, i-PGD_2 and i-LTC_4 release from human purified skin mast cells activated by anti-IgE and non-immunological stimuli

Stimulus	Net mediator release (pmol/10^6 cells)		
	Histamine	PGD_2	LTC_4
Anti-IgE (25 μg/ml)	3576±450	90.9±17.5	7.1± 1.2
Substance P (30 μ*M*)	4432±531.	4.1± 1.0	0.5±0.4
VIP (10 μ*M*)	4261±600	4.9± 1.7	0.5±0.3
Somatostatin (30 μ*M*)	4225±606	1.7± 0.7	0.5±0.4
Compound 48/80 (10 μg/ml)	3950±521	2.9± 1.0	0.1±0.1

Results are from four experiments in which mast cells of purity 76.2% ± 4.2% were incubated with the stimuli shown for 30 min before measurement of release of eicosanoids by radioimmunoassay and histamine by spectrophotofluorometry.

Characterisation of the Skin Mast Cell Receptor for Non-immunological Stimuli

The recent availability of methods for the dispersion of mast cells from human skin has allowed detailed studies of mast cell activation by non-immunological stimuli. Histamine release induced by substance P, somatostatin, VIP, compound 48/80, poly-*L*-lysine and morphine is inhibited by the substance P antagonist [*D*-Pro^4, *D*-Trp^{7,9,10}] substance P fragment 4–11 (SPA), suggesting that each of these compounds binds to skin mast cells by the same receptor [83]. SPA appears to act as a specific inhibitor of mast cell secretion as it does not affect histamine release activated by anti-IgE or calcium ionophore A23187. That the receptor binds such a variety of non-immunological stimuli and that the tachykinins eledoisin, physalaemin, neurokinin A and neurokinin B are poor histamine releasers indicate that it is not one of the NK-1, NK-2 or NK-3 tachykinin receptors identified on smooth muscle cells [80].

Studies with substance P fragments have helped to identify the molecular features of non-immunological stimuli which are required for the activation of skin mast cells. The undecapeptide substance P (Arg^{2+}-Pro-Lys^+-Pro-Gln-Gln-Phe-Phe-Gly-Leu-$MetNH_2$) has basic amino acids near the N-terminal which are positively charged at physiological pH and hydrophobic, aromatic amino acids at positions 7 and 8. Histamine release from human skin mast cells requires that both features be present as both fragment SP_{4-11}, which lacks the basic residues, and fragment SP_{1-4}, which lacks the aromatic residues, have insignificant histamine-releasing activity [83]. These preliminary studies therefore suggest that the substance P receptor of human skin mast cells, which presumably also binds the other non-immunological stimuli mentioned above, resembles that of rat peritoneal mast cells [111].

Pharmacological Modulation of Histamine Release from Skin Mast Cells

Sodium Cromoglycate

Whilst sodium cromoglycate (Intal) inhibits histamine release from mast cells of human dispersed lung [29], bronchoalveolar lavage fluid [41], adenoids [117] and intestine [10], it appears to have little effect on mediator release from skin mast cells. In vivo studies have shown that cromoglycate has little effect on the immediate phase of the wheal and flare reactions induced by histamine, IgE-dependent stimuli or codeine [53, 107, 139, 141]. It does, however, weakly inhibit late reactions induced by allergens [52] or PAF [5], probably due to its effects on eosinophil and neutrophil function [96]. Sodium cromoglycate at concentrations of up to 1 m*M* has no significant effect on IgE-dependent histamine release from human skin slices [30, 103] or on anti-IgE- or substance P-induced histamine release from human dispersed skin mast cells [85], thus supporting the concept that skin mast cells are refractory to this compound. The recently developed successor of cromoglycate, nedocromil sodium, is similarly ineffective on secretion from these cells.

β-Adrenoceptor Agonists

Studies of the in vivo effects of β-adrenoceptor agonists on the response of human skin to allergens have given equivocal results. No inhibition of immediate allergen-induced skin reactions were observed in atopic individuals following oral administration of terbutaline [1, 27, 65], whilst inhibition of such responses has been observed following systemic administration of the mixed α- and β-adrenoceptor agonist adrenaline and the β-adrenoceptor agonist isoprenaline [77, 146]. However, these findings are complicated by the ability of β-agonists to inhibit histamine-induced increases in microvascular permeability by a direct effect on blood vessels [100].

Several studies have addressed the effects of β-agonists on skin mast cells more directly. Ting et al. [140] showed that topical terbutaline reduced both the ultrastructural changes in human skin mast cells and the release of histamine into skin chambers following allergen stimulation. In vitro studies have demonstrated inhibition of IgE-dependent histamine release from human skin slices by adrenaline [150] and salbutamol [30]. Histamine release from dispersed skin mast cells activated by anti-IgE or substance P is inhibited by salbutamol at concentrations between 1 and 10 μM [85]. Histamine release from human skin mast cells is also inhibited by drugs that increase mast cell cyclic AMP levels by mechanisms different to β-adrenoceptor agonists. The cyclic AMP phosphodiesterase inhibitor theophylline decreases histamine release from allergen-challenged skin slices [150], and the related compound 3-isobutyl-1-methylxanthine inhibits histamine release from dispersed mast cells activated with anti-IgE or substance P (Benyon, Lowman and Church, unpublished observations).

Antihistamines

H_1-antihistamines are widely used in the management of allergic disorders and urticaria. H_1-antihistamines such as astemizole, terfenadine and hydroxyzine when given orally inhibit wheal and flare reactions induced by intradermal injection of histamine [48, 61, 62] or allergens [46, 61]. Whilst some component of this inhibitory effect is presumably due to direct antagonism of blood vessel H_1-histamine receptors, these compounds may also act by inhibiting mediator release from skin mast cells. In support of this, Ting et al. [142] have shown that oral hydroxyzine inhibits degranulation of these cells following intradermal injection of allergen as well as blocking the release of histamine into skin chambers placed over the challenged site. More recently, it has been shown that the specific H_1-histamine receptor antagonist terfenadine at a concentration of 10 μM inhibits by $> 50\%$ histamine release from dispersed skin mast cells activated by anti-IgE without significantly affecting secretion induced by substance P (Benyon, Lowman and Church, unpublished observations).

Conclusions

Mast cells and their associated complement of pro-inflammatory mediators have traditionally been associated with the development of allergic responses following activation by an IgE-dependent mechanism. However, recent observations of the ability of skin mast cells to be activated by a wide variety of IgE-independent stimuli, in particular neuropeptides localised to the dermis, might suggest that these cells have further functions. It is becoming increasingly apparent that there are extensive interactions between the peptidergic nervous system and immunocompetent leukocytes such as macrophages, monocytes and lymphocytes [55, 90, 101]. The ability of mast cells to respond to peptides suggests that these cells may now be included amongst those involved in the neuro-immune axis. The rapid release of histamine, presumably in association with other preformed mediators, in the virtual absence of eicosanoid release might allow skin mast cells to be involved in the control of homeostatic activities such as microvascular blood flow, angiogenesis and fibroblast proliferation. Increases in these activities would be required at sites of wound healing, and, indeed, mast cells numbers are often increased in such areas [6, 104]. Activation of skin mast cells by a non-immunological mechanism may also be a feature of skin diseases such as chronic idiopathic urticaria (CIU), cold and heat-induced urticaria and cholinergic urticaria, which are responsive to H_1-anthistamines but in which no causative allergen is apparent. Preliminary studies indicate that defects in the response of skin mast cells to neuropeptides may underlie the pathology of several skin diseases. For example, in individuals with cold- or heat-induced urticaria, areas of skin depleted of neuropeptides by topical application of capsaicin show diminished vascular responses to thermal challenge [143]. In addition, individuals with CIU have enhanced wheal and flare responses to codeine, a non-immunologifcal activator of skin mast cells [31] and show increased histamine release into skin chambers placed over dermis challenged with compound 48/80 [9]. It is therefore apparent that the non-immunological mechanism of skin mast cell activation may have great physiological and pathological relevance.

References

1. Abramowitz PW, Perez MM, Johnson CE, McLean JA (1980) Effect of theophylline, terbutaline, and their combination on the immediate hypersensitivity skin test reaction. J Allergy Clin Immunol 66:123–128
2. Anand P, Bloom SR, McGregor GP (1983) Topical capsaicin pretreatment inhibits axon reflex vasodilation caused by somatostatin and vasoactive polypeptide in human skin. Br J Pharmacol 78:665–669
3. Anwar ARE, Kay AB (1978) Enhancement of human eosinophil complement receptors by pharmacologic mediators. J Immunol 121:1245–1250
4. Anwar ARE, McKean JR, Smithers SR, Kay AB (1980) Human eosinophil and neutrophil-mediated killing of schistosomula of *Schistosoma mansoni in vitro*. I. Enhancement of complement-dependent damage of mast cell-derived mediators and formalmethionyl peptides. J Immunol 124:1122–1129
5. Archer CB, Page CP, Paul W, Morley J, MacDonald DM (1985) Actions of disodium cromoglycate (DSCG) on human skin responses to histamine, codeine and PAF-acether. Agents Actions 16:6–8
6. Atkins FM, Clark RAF (1987) Mast cells and fibrosis. Arch Dermatol 123:191–193
7. Atkins PC, Norman ME, Weiner H, Zwieman B (1977) Release of neutrophil chemotactic activity during immediate hypersensitivity reactions in humans. Ann Intern Med 86:415–418
8. Barr RM, Koro O, Francis DM, Kobza-Black A, Numata T, Greaves MW (1988) The release of prostaglandin D2 from human skin in vivo and in vitro during immediate allergic reactions. Br J Pharmacol 94:773–780
9. Bedard PM, Brunet C, Pelletier G, Hebert J (1986) Increased compound 48/80 induced local histamine release from non-lesional skin from patients with chronic urticaria. J Allergy Clin Immunol 78:1121–1125
10. Befus AD, Dyck N, Goodacre R, Bienenstock J (1987) Mast cells from the human intestinal lamina propria: isolation, histochemical subtypes, and functional characterization. J Immunol 138:2604–2610
11. Benditt EP, Wong RL, Arase M (1955) 5-Hydroxytryptamine in mast cells. Proc Soc Exp Biol Med 90:303–304
12. Benyon RC, Church MK, Clegg LS, Holgate ST (1986) Dispersion and characterization of mast cells from human skin. Int Arch Allergy Appl Immunol 79:332–334
13. Benyon RC, Lowman MA, Church MK (1987) Human skin mast cells: their dispersion, purification and secretory characterization. J Immunol 138:861–867
14. Benyon RC, Robinson C, Holgate ST, Church MK (1987) Prostaglandin D2 release from human skin mast cells in response to ionophore A23187. Br J Pharmacol 92:635–638
15. Benyon RC (1988) Stimulus-secretion coupling in mast cells and basophils. In: Holgate ST (ed) Mast cells, mediators and disease. MTP Press, Lancaster, pp 195–226
16. Binazzi M, Rampichini L (1959) Investigations on the regional distribution of mast cells in human skin. Ital Gen Rev Dermatol 1:17–21
17. Black JW, Duncan WAM, Durant CJ, Ganellin CR, Parsons EM (1972) Definition and antagonism of histamine H2-receptors. Nature 236:385–390
18. Bowyer A (1968) Observations on the granularity of mast cells in human skin. Acta Derm Venereol (Stockh) 48:574–577
19. Briggman RA, Schechter NM, Fraki JE, Lazarus GS (1984) Degradation of the epidermal-dermal junction by a proteolytic enzyme from human skin and human polymophonuclear leukocytes. J Exp Med 160:1027–1042
20. Camp RDR, Coutts AA, Greaves MW, Kay AB, Walport MJ (1983) Responses of human skin to intradermal injection of leukotrienes C4, D4 and B4. Br J Pharmacol 80:497–502
21. Capron A, Dessaint JP, Capron M, Joseph M, Ameisen JC, Tonnel AB (1986) From parasites to allergy: the second receptor for IgE. Immunol Today 7:15–18
22. Casale TB, Bowman S, Kaliner M (1984) Induction of human cutaneous mast cell degranulation by opiates and endogenous opioid peptides: evidence for opiate and nonopiate receptor participation. J Allergy Clin Immunol 73:775–781
23. Castells M, Irani AA, Schwartz LB (1987) Evaluation of human peripheral blood leukocytes for mast cell tryptase. J Immunol 138:2184–2189
24. Caulfield JP, Lewis RA, Hein A, Austen KF (1980) Secretion of dissociated human pulmonary mast cells: evidence for solubilization of granule contents before discharge. J Cell Biol 85:299–311
25. Cawley EP, Hoch-ligeti C (1961) Association of tissue mast cells and skin tumours. Arch Dermatol 83:92–96
26. Center DM, Soter NA, Wasserman SI, Austen KF (1979) Inhibition of neutrophil chemotaxis in assocation with

experimental angioedema in patients with cold urticaria: a model of chemotactic deactivation in vivo. Clin Exp Immunol 35:112–118
27. Chipps BE, Sobotka AK, Sanders JP, Teets KC, Norman PS (1980) Effect of theophylline and terbutaline on immediate skin tests. J Allergy Clin Immunol 65:61–64
28 Church MK, Clegg LS, Holgate ST (1984) Histamine secretion from human skin slices induced by anti-IgE, calcium ionophore A23187, poly-L-lysine and compound 48/80 (abstract). Br J Clin Pharmacol [Suppl] 82:282
29. Church MK, Hiroi J (1987) Inhibition of IgE-dependent histamine release from human dispersed lung mast cells by anti-allergic drugs and salbutamol. Br J Pharmacol 90:421–429
30. Clegg LS, Church MK, Holgate ST (1985) Histamine secretion from human skin slices induced by anti-IgE and artificial secretagogues and the effects of sodium cromoglycate and salbutamol. Clin Allergy 15:321–328
31. Cohen RW, Rosenstreich DL (1986) Discrimination between urticaria-prone and other allergic patients by intradermal skin testing with codeine. J Allergy Clin Immunol 77:802–807
32. Coleman JW, Godfrey RC (1981) The number and affinity of IgE receptors on dispersed human lung mast cells. Immunology 44:859–863
33. Conrad DH, Bazin H, Sehon AH, Froese A (1975) Binding parameters of the interaction between rat IgE and rat mast cell receptors. J Immunol 114:1688–1691
34. Cowen T, Trigg P, Eady RAJ (1979) Distribution of mast cells in human dermis: development of a mapping technique. Br J Dermatol 100:635–640
35. Craig SS, Schechter NM, Schwartz LB (1988) Ultrastructural analysis of human T and TC mast cells identified by immunoelectron microscopy. Lab Invest 58:682–691
36. Dunsky EH, Zweiman B (1978) The direct demonstration of histamine release in allergic reactions in the skin using a skin chamber technique. J Allergy Clin Immunol 62:127–130
37. Dvorak AM, Galli SJ, Schulman ES, Lichtenstein LM, Dvorak HF (1983) Basophil and mast cell degranulation: ultrastructural analysis of mechanisms of mediator release. Fed Proc 42:2510–2515
38. Eady RAJ (1976) The mast cell: distribution and morphology. Clin Exp Dermatol 1:313–329
39. Eliakim R, Gilead L, Ligumsky M, Okon E, Rachmilewitz D, Razin E (1986) Histamine and chondroitin sulfate E proteoglycan released by cultured human colonic mucosa: indication for possible presence of E mast cells. Proc Natl Acad Sci USA 83:461–464
40. Enerbäck L (1966) Mast cells in the gastrointestinal mucosa. II. Dye binding and metachromatic properties. Acta Pathol Microbiol Scand 66:303–312
41. Flint KC, Leung KBP, Pearce FL, Hudspith BN, Brostoff J, Johnson NMcI (1985) Human mast cells recovered from bronchoalveolar lavage: their morphology, histamine release and effects of sodium cromogylcate. Clin Sci 68:427–432
42. Foreman JC, Piotrowski W (1984) Peptides and histamine release. J Allergy Clin Immunol 74:127–131
43. Foreman JC, Jordan CC, Oehme P, Renner H (1983) Structure-activity relationships for some substance P-related peptides that cause wheal and flare reactions in human skin. J Physiol (Lond) 335:449–465
44. Fujita H, Asagami C, Murozumi S, Yamamoto K, Kinoshita K (1969) Electron microscopic studies of mast cells of human fetal skins. J Ultrastruct Res 28:353–370
45. Fuller RW, Conradson TB, Dixon CMS, Crossman DC, Barnes PJ (1987) Sensory neuropeptide effects in human skin. Br J Pharmacol 92:781–788
46. Galant SP, Bulloch J, Wong D, Maibach HI (1973) The inhibitory effect of anti-allergic drugs on allergen and histamine induced wheal and flare response. J Allergy Clin Immunol 51:11–21
47. Garriga MM, Friedman MM, Metcalfe DD (1988) A survey of the number and distribution of mast cells in the skin of patients with mast cells disorders. J Allergy Clin Immunol 82:425–432
48. Gendreau-Reid L, Simons KJ, Simons FER (1986) Comparison of the suppressive effects of astemizole, terfenadine, and hydroxyzine on histamine-induced wheals and flares in humans. J Allergy Clin Immunol 77:335–340
49. Gilead L, Livni N, Eliakim R, Ligumski M, Fich A, Okon E, Rcahmilewitz D, Razin E (1987) Human gastric mucosal mast cells are chondroitin sulfate E-containing mast cells. Immunology 62:23–28
50. Goetzl EJ, Weller PF, Valone FH (1976) Biochemical and functional bases of the regulatory and protective roles of the human eosinophil. Adv Inflamm Res 1:157–167
51. Greaves MW, Yamamoto S, Fairley VM (1972) IgE-mediated hypersensitivity in human skin studied using a new in vitro method. Immunology 23:239–248
52. Gronneberg R, Zetterstrom O (1985) Effect of disodium cromoglycate on anti-IgE-induced early and late responses in man. Clin Allergy 15:167–171
53. Haddad ZH, Gillman SA (1973) Disodium cromoglycate and human reagin (IgE) mediated reactions. Effect on wheal and flare skin reactions and histamine release from rat mast cells in vivo. Int Arch Allergy Appl Immunol 45:439–446
54. Hartschuh W, Weihe E, Reinecke M (1983) Peptidergic (neurotensin, VIP, substance P) nerve fibres in the skin. Immunohistochemical evidence of an involvement of neuropeptides in nociception, pruritis and inflammation. Br J Dermatol 109 [Suppl 25]:14–17
55. Hartung HP, Toyka KV (1983) Activation of macrophages by substance P: induction of oxidative burst and thromboxane release. Eur Pharmacol 89:301–305
56. Heavey DJ, Kobza-Black A, Barrow SE, Chappell CG, Greaves MW, Dollery CT (1986) Prostaglandin D2 and histamine release in cold urticaria. J Allergy Clin Immunol 78:458–461
57. Hellmstrom B, Holmgren H (1950) Numerical distribution of mast cells in human skin and heart. Acta Anat (Basel) 10:81–107
58. Hibbs RG, Burch GE, Phillips JM (1960) Electron microscopic observations on human mast cells. Am Heart J 60:121–127
59. Hokfelt T, Kellerth JO, Nillson G, Pernow B (1975) Experimental immunohistochemical studies on the localization and distribution of substance P in cat primary sensory neurones. Brain Res 100:235–252
60. Hokfelt T, Elde R, Johansson O, Luft R, Nillson G, Arimura A (1976) Immunohistochemical evidence for separate populations of somatostatin-containing and substance P-containing primary afferent neurones in the rat. Neuroscience 1:131–136
61. Howarth PH, Emanuel MB, Holgate ST (1984) Astemizole, a potent histamine H1-receptor antagonist: effects in allergic rhino-conjunctivitis, on antigen and histamine induced skin wheal responses and relationship to serum levels. Br J Clin Pharmacol 18:1–8

62. Huther KJ, Renftle GT, Barraud N, Burke JT, Kock-Wesser J (1977) Inhibitory activity of terfenadine on histamine induced skin wheal in man. Eur J Clin Pharmacol 12:195–199
63. Ihle JN, Keller J, Oroszlan S, Henderson LE, Copeland TD, Fitch F, Prytsowsky MB, Goldwasser E, Schrader JW, Palaszynski E, Dy M, Lebel B (1983) Biological properties of homogeneous interleukin 3: demonstration of WEHI-3 growth factor activity, mast cell growth factor activity, P-cell stimulating factor activity, colony-stimulating activity and histamine producing cell stimulating factor activity. J Immunol 131:282–287
64. Imamura S, Tachibara T, Taniguchi S (1985) Impaired histamine metabolism in human erythematous dermatoses. J Dermatol 12:308–312
65. Imbeau SA, Harruff R, Hirscher M, Reed CE (1978) Terbutalines effect on the allergy skin site. J Allergy Clin Immunol 62:193–196
66. Irani AA, Schechter NM, Craig S, DeBlois G, Schwartz LB (1986) Two types of human mast cells that have distinct neutral protease compositions. Proc Natl Acad Sci USA 83:4464–4468
67. Irani AA, Craig SS, DeBlois G, Elson CO, Schechter NM, Schwartz LB (1987) Deficiency of the tryptase-positive chymase-negative mast cell type in gastrointestinal mucosa of patients with defective T-lymphocyte function. J Immunol 138:4381–4386
68. Irani AA, Butrus S, Schwartz LB (1988) Distribution of T and TC mast cell subsets in vernal conjunctivitis (VC) and giant papillary conjunctivitis (abstract). NER Allergy Proc 9:451
69. Ishizaka K, Ishizaka T (1968) Induction of erythema wheal reactions by soluble antigen-IgE antibody complexes in man. J Immunol 101:68–78
70. Ishizaka T, Ishizaka K (1984) Activation of mast cells for mediator release through IgE receptors. Prog Allergy 34:188–235
71. James MP, Kennedy AR, Eady RAJ (1981) A microscopic study of inflammatory reactions in human skin induced by histamine and compound 48/80. J Invest Dermatol 78: 406–413
72. Johansson O (1986) A detailed account of the NPY immunoreactive nerves and cells of the human skin. Comparison with VIP-, substance P- and PHI-containing structures. Acta Physiol Scand 128:147–153
73. Kaplan AP, Gray L, Shaff RE, Horakova Z, Beaven MA (1975) In vivo studies of mediator release in cold urticaria and cholinergic urticaria. J Allergy Clin Immunol 55:394–402
74. Kaplan AP, Horokova Z, Katz SI (1978) Assessment of tissue fluid histamine levels in patients with urticaria. J Allergy Clin Immunol 61:350–354
75. Kobza-Black A, Ormerod AD, Dawes J, Murdoch RD, Koro O, Barr RM, Greaves MW (1988) Release of histamine and prostaglandin D2 in cold urticaria without evidence of platelet activation. Skin Pharmacol 1:69
76. Koro O, Dover JS, Francis DM, Kobza-Black A, Kelly RW, Barr RM, Greaves MW (1986) Release of prostaglandin D2 and histamine in a case of localized heat urticaria and effects of treatments. Br J Dermatol 115: 721–728
77. Kram JA, Bourne HR, Maibach HI, Melmon KL (1975) Cutaneous immediate hypersensitivity in man: effects of systemically administered adrenergic drugs. J Allergy Clin Immunol 56:387–392
78. Lagunoff D (1972) Contributions of electron microscopy to the study of mast cells. J Invest Dermatol 58:296–311
79. Lawrence ID, Warner JA, Cohan VL, Hubbard WC, Kagey-Sobotka A, Lichtenstein LM (1987) Purification and characterization of human skin mast cells. Evidence for human mast cell heterogeneity. J Immunol 139:3062–3069
80. Lee CH, Campbell NJ, Williams BJ, Iverson LL (1986) Multiple tachykinin binding sites in peripheral tissues and in brain. Eur J Pharmacol 130:209–217
81. Lewis T (1927) The blood vessels of the human skin and their responses. Shaw, London
82. Lonky SA, Marsh J, Wohl H (1978) Stimulation of human granulocyte elastase by platelet factor 4 and heparin. Biochem Biophys Res Commun 85:1113–1118
83. Lowman MA, Benyon RC, Church MK (1988) Characterization of neuropeptide-induced histamine released from human dispersed skin mast cells. Br J Pharmacol 95:121–130
84. Lowman MA, Rees PH, Benyon RC, Church MK (1988) Human mast cell heterogeneity: histamine release from mast cells dispersed from skin, lung, adenoids, tonsils and intestinal mucosa in response to IgE-dependent and nonimmunological stimuli. J Allergy Clin Immunol 81:590–597
85. Lowman MA, Benyon RC, Church MK (1988) Human skin mast cells: effects of salbutamol and sodium cromoglycate on histamine release induced by anti-IgE and substance P. Skin Pharmacol 1:63–64
86. MacGlashan DW, Lichtenstein LM (1983) Studies of antigen binding on human basophils. I. Antigen binding and functional consequences. J Immunol 130:2330–2336
87. Maier M, Spragg J, Schwartz LB (1983) Inactivation of human higher molecular weight kininogen by human mast cell tryptase. J Immunol 130:2352–2356
88. Malveaux FJ, Conroy MC, Adkinson NF, Lichtenstein LM (1978) IgE receptors on human basophils: relationship to serum IgE concentration. J Clin Invest 62:176–181
89. Marks RM, Roche WR, Czerniecki M, Penny R, Nelson DS (1986) Mast cell granules cause proliferation of human microvascular endothelial cells. Lab Invest 55:289–294
90. McGillis JP, Organist ML, Payan DG (1987) Substance P and immunoregulation. Fed Proc 46:196–199
91. Metcalfe DD, Lewis RA, Silbert JE, Rosenberg RD, Wasserman SI, Austen KF (1979) Isolation and characterization of heparin from human lung. J Clin Invest 4:1537–1543
92. Metcalfe DD, Soter NA, Wasserman SI, Austen KF (1980) Identification of sulfated mucopolysaccharides including heparin in the lesional skin of a patient with mastocytosis. J Invest Dermatol 74:210–215
93. Metzger H, Alcarez G, Hohman R, Kinet J-P, Pribluda V, Quarto R (1986) The receptor with high affinity for immunoglobulin E. Annu Rev Immunol 4:419–470
94. Metzger WJ, Richerson HB, Wasserman SI (1986) Generation and partial characterisation of eosinophil chemotactic activity and neutrophil chemotactic activity during early and late-phase asthmatic responses. J Allergy Clin Immunol 78:282–290
95. Mikhail GR, Miller-Milinska A (1964) Mast cell population in human skin. J Invest Dermatol 43:249–254
96. Moqbel R, Walsh GM, Macdonald AJ, Kay AB (1986) Effect of disodium cromoglycate on activation of human eosinophils and neutrophils following reversed (anti-IgE) anaphylaxis. Clin Allergy 16:73–83

97. Nagy L, Lee TH, Kay AB (1982) Neutrophil chemotactic activity in antigen-induced late asthmatic reactions. N Engl J Med 306:497–501
98. Natbony SF, Phillips ME, Elias KM, Godfrey HP, Kaplan AP (1983) Histologic studies of chronic idiopathic urticaria. J Allergy Clin Immunol 71:177–183
99. Newson B, Dahlstrom A, Enerback L, Ahlman H (1983) Suggestive evidence for a direct innervation of mucosal mast cells. Neuroscience 10:565–570
100. O'Donnell SR, Persson CGA (1978) β-adrenoceptor mediated inhibition by terbutaline of histamine effects on vascular permeability. Br J Pharmacol 62:321–314
101. O'Dorisio MS (1987) Biochemical characteristics of receptors for vasoactive intestinal polypeptide in nervous, endocrine and immune systems. Fed Proc 42:192–195
102. Orr TSC (1977) Fine structure of the mast cell with special reference to human cells. Scand J Respir Dis 98:1–7
103. Pearce CA, Greaves MW, Plummer VM, Yamamoto S (1974) Effect of disodium cromoglycate on antigen evoked histamine release in human skin. Clin Exp Immunol 17:437–440
104. Pessinger MA, Lepage P, Simard JP, Parker GH (1983) Mast cell numbers in incisional wounds in rat skin as a function of distance, time and treatment. Br J Dermatol 108:179–187
105. Peters SP, Kagey-Sobotka A, MacGlashan DW, Lichtenstein LM (1984) Effect of prostaglandin D2 in modulating histamine release from human basophils. J Pharmacol Exp Ther 228:400–406
106. Phanuphak P, Schocket AL, Arroyave CM, Kohler PF (1980) Skin histamine in chronic urticaria. J Allergy Clin Immunol 65:371–375
107. Philips MJ, Meyrick T, Moodley I, Davies RJ (1983) A comparison of the in vivo effects of ketotifen, clemastine, chlorpeniramine and sodium cromoglycate on histamine and allergen-induced wheals in human skin. Br J Clin Pharmacol 15:277–286
108. Pillarisetti V, Rao S, Friedman MM, Atkins FM, Metcalfe DD (1983) Phagacytosis of mast cell granules by cultured fibroblasts. J Immunol 130:341–349
109. Proud D, Lichtenstein LM (1984) Human lung mast cell kininogenase: apparent identity to tryptase. Fed Proc 43:1807
110. Proud D, MacGlashan DW, Newball HH, Schulman ES, Lichtenstein LM (1985) IgE-mediated release of a kininogenase from purified human lung mast cells. Am Rev Respir Dis 132:405–408
111. Repke H, Pitrowski W, Bienert M, Foreman JC (1987) Histamine release induced by Arg-Pro-Lys-Pro (CH2) 11CH3 from rat peritoneal mast cells. J Pharmacol Exp Ther 243:317–321
112. Roberts LJ, Sweetman BJ, Lewis RA, Austen KF, Oates JA (1980) Increased production of prostaglandin D2 in patients with systemic mystocytosis. N Engl J Med 303:1400–1404
113. Robertson I, Greaves MW (1978) Responses of human skin blood vessels to synthetic histamine analogous. Br J Clin Pharmacol 5:319–322
114. Ruzicka T, Gluck S (1983) Cutaneous histamine levels and histamine releasability from the skin in atopic dermatitis and hyper-IgE syndrome. Arch Dermatol Res 271:41–44
115. Schechter NM, Fraki JE, Geesin JC, Lazarus GS (1983) Human skin chymotryptic proteinsase: isolation and relation to cathepsin G and rat mast cell protease. J Biol Chem 258:2973–2978
116. Schechter NM, Choi JK, Slavin DA, Deresienski DT, Sayama S, Dong G, Lavaker RM, Proud D, Lazarus GS (1986) Identification of a chymotrypsin-like proteinase from human mast cells. J Immunol 137:962–970
117. Schmutzler W, Delmich K, Eichelberg D, Gluck S, Greven T, Jurgensen H, Riesener KP (1985) The human adenoidal mast cell. Susceptibility to different secretagogues and secretion inhibitors. Int Arch Allergy Appl Immunol 77:177–178
118. Schwartz LB, Austen KF (1984) Structure and function of the chemical mediators of mast cells. Prog Allergy 34:271–321
119. Schwartz LB, Bradford TM (1986) Regulation of tryptase from human lung mast cells by heparin: stabilization of the active tetramer. J Biol Chem 261:7372–7379
120. Schwartz LB, Lewis RA, Seldin D, Austen KF (1981) Acid hydrolases and tryptase from secretory granules of dispersed lung mast cells. J Immunol 126:1290–1294
121. Schwartz LB, Kawahara MS, Hugli TE, Vik D, Fearon DT, Austen KF (1983) Generation of C3a anaphylatoxin from human C3 by human mast cell tryptase. J Immunol 130:1891–1895
122. Schwartz LB, Atkins PC, Bradford TR, Fleekop P, Shalit M, Zweiman B (1987c) Release of tryptase together with histamine during immediate cutaneous response to allergen. J Allergy Clin Immunol 80:850–855
123. Schwartz LB, Irani AM, Roller K, Castells M, Schechter NM (1987b) Quantitation of histamine, tryptase, and chymase in dispersed human T and CT mast cells. J Immunol 138:2611–2615
124. Schwartz LB, Metcalfe DD, Miller JS, Earl H, Sullivan T (1987a) Tryptase levels as an indicator of mast cell activation in systemic anaphylaxis and mastocytosis. N Engl J Med 316:1622–1626
125. Scully MF, Ellis V, Seno N, Kakkar VV (1986) The anticoagulant properties of mast cell product, chondroitin sulphate E. Biochem Biophys Res Comun 137:15–22
126. Shalit M, Schwartz LB, Golzar N, von Allman C, Valenzano M, Fleekop P, Atkins PC, Zweiman B (1988) Release of histamine and tryptase in vivo after prolonged cutaneous challenge with allergen in humans. J Immunol 141:821–826
127. Skotfisch G, Savitt JM, Jacobowitz DM (1985) Suggestive evidence for a functional unit between mast cells and substance P fibres in the rat diaphragm and mesentery. Histochemistry 2:5–8
128. Smith TJ, Hougland MW, Johnson DA (1984) Human lung tryptase, purification and characterization. J Biol Chem 259:11046–11049
129. Solley GO, Gleich GJ, Jordan RE, Schroeter Al (1976) The late phase of the immediate wheal and flare skin reaction: its dependence on IgE antibodies. J Clin Invest 58:408–420
130. Sondergaard J, Zachariae H (1968) Epidermal histamine. Arch Klin Exp Dermatol 233:323–328
131. Soter NA, Lewis RA, Corey EJ, Austen KF (1983) Local effects of synthetic leukotrienes (LTC4, LTD4, LTE4 and LTB4) in human skin. J Invest Dermatol 80:115–119
132. Soter NA, Wasserman SI, Austen KF (1976) Cold urticaria: release into the circulation of histamine and eosinophil chemotactic factor of anaphylaxis during cold challenge. N Engl J Med 294:687–690
133. Soter NA, Mihm MC, Dvorak HF, Austen KF (1978) Cutaneous necrosing venulitis: a sequential analysis of the morphological alterations occurring after mast cell

degranulation in a patient with a unique syndrome. Clin Exp Immunol 32:46–58

134. Starkey PM, Barrett AJ (1985) Human cathepsin G: catalytic and immunologic properties. Biochem J 155: 273–278
135. Talbot SF, Atkins PC, Goetzl EDJ, Zweiman B (1985) Accumulation of leukotriene C4 and histamine in human allergic skin reactions. J Clin Invest 76:650–656
136. Tharp MD, Suvunrungsi RT, Sullivan TJ (1983) IgE-mediated release of histamine from human cutaneous mast cells. J Immunol 130:1896–1901
137. Thompson HL, Schulman ES, Metcalfe DD (1988) Identification of chondroitin sulfate E in human lung mast cells. J Immunol 140:2708–2713
138. Ting S, Zweiman B, Lavker RM, Dunsky EH (1981) In vivo release of eosinophil chemoattractant activity in human allergic skin reactions. J Immunol 127:557–560
139. Ting S, Zweiman B, Lavker RM (1983) Cromolyn does not modulate human allergic skin reactions in vivo. J Allergy Clin Immunol 71:12–17
140. Ting S, Zweiman B, Lavker RM (1983) Terbutaline modulation of human allergic skin reactions. J Allergy Clin Immunol 71:437–441
141. Ting S, Reiman EF, Zweiman B (1984) Effects of cromolyn on codeine-induced histamine release in vivo. Allergy 39:493–497
142. Ting S, Rauls DO, Reiman BEF (1985) Inhibitory effect of hydroxyzine on antigen-induced histamine release in vivo. J Allergy Clin Immunol 75:63–66
143. Toth-Kasa I, Jancso G, Obal F, Husz S, Simon N (1983) Involvement of sensory nerve endings in cold and heat urticaria. J Invest Dermatol 80:34–36
144. Uvnas B, Aborg C-H, Bergendorf A (1970) Storage of histamine in mast cells. Evidence for ionic binding of histamine to protein carboxyls in the granule heparin protein complex. Acta Physiol Scand [Suppl] 336:1–26
145. Valone F, Shalit M, Atkins P, Goertzl E, Zweiman B (1987) Platelet activating factor release in allergic skin site in humans (abstract). J Allergy Clin Immunol 79:248
146. Warren JB, McCusker M, Fuller RW (1988) Systemic adrenaline attenuates skin response to antigen and histamine. Clin Allergy 18:197–199
147. Wasserman SI, Soter NA, Center DM, Austen KF (1977) Cold urticaria: recognition and characterization of a neutrophil chemotactic factor which appears in serum during experimental cold challenge. J Clin Invest 60:189–196
148. Wiesner-Menzel L, Schulz B, Vakilzadeh F, Czarnetzki BM (1981) Electron microscopical evidence for a direct contact between nerve fibres and mast cells. Acta Derm Venereol (Stockh) 61:465–469
149. Wintroub BU, Kempfer CE, Schechter NM, Proud D (1986) Human lung mast cell chymotrypsin-like enzyme: identification and partial characterization. J Clin Invest 77:196–201
150. Yamamoto S, Greaves MW, Fairley VM (1973) Cyclic AMP-induced inhibition of IgE-mediated hypersensitivity in human skin. Immunology 24:77–83
151. Zachariae H (1964) Histamine in human skin. Arch Dermatol Venereol (Stockh) 44:219–222

Role of Eosinophils in Atopic Eczema

B. M. Czarnetzki

Introduction

Recent scientific investigations have made it increasingly apparent that a strict distinction between immediate and delayed type immunological processes cannot be justified. Atopic eczema is a model example for this since pathological alterations of IgE-dependent reactions coexist with lymphocyte-dependent reactions. This mixed involvement of both types of immune processes is also evident when one focuses on the role of eosinophils in this disease. In this chapter, in vivo evidence for a possible involvement of eosinophils in the pathology of atopic eczema will first be examined. On that basis, experimental data that might explain the in vivo observations will be considered. This includes new findings on factors that regulate the generation of these cells in the bone marrow and their infiltration into the skin. Finally, the potential functional significance of eosinophils in atopic eczema will be discussed in view of recent data in the literature.

Clinical and in vivo Experimental Data

Although most dermatohistopathologists would agree that eosinophils are often seen in biopsies from lesional skin of patients with atopic eczema (Fig. 1), systematic studies on the presence of these cells in the skin and peripheral blood of atopic eczema patients are scarce. The most careful examination of the general pathology of involved and normal skin in atopic eczema patients was published more than a decade ago and has been unchallenged since [1] (Table 1). In contrast to rather striking increases in mast cells, only half of the specimens from vesicular and one-fifth from lichenified skin contained scattered dermal eosinophils. In a more recent study, a few eosinophils were noted in the lesional skin of almost all patients with proven allergy to mite or pollen allergens [2] (Table 1).

Fig. 1. Histopathology of chronic lesional skin in a patient with atopic eczema. Note the eosinophils in epidermis (*E*) and in the dermal (*D*) infiltrate (*arrows*).

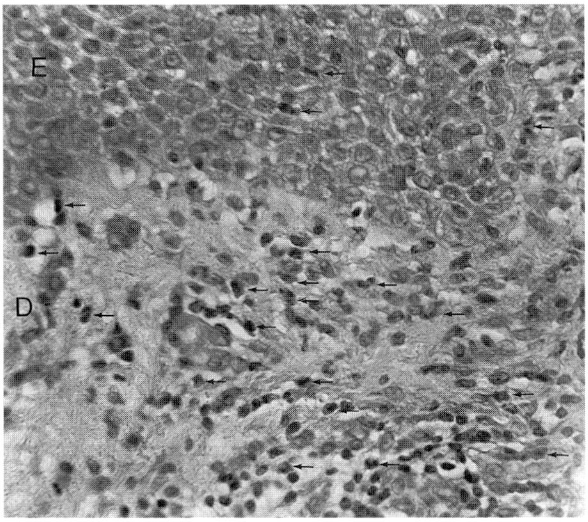

More recently, eosinophil infiltration in atopic skin has been examined in greater detail and in an experimental setting. Patch testing with mite and pollen antigens over stripped skin in sensitized atopic eczema patients yielded localized dermal eosinophil infiltrations in skin patches taken from 11 of 15 patients; the maximum number of cells was observed by 6 h. These dermal eosinophils were partly degranulated and activated, as demonstrated with the EG2 monoclonal antibody. A few non-activated eosinophils were also found in the epidermis in 8 of 11 patients, some of them in close proximity to Langerhans

Table 1. Eosinophil infiltrates in atopic eczema

Vesicular areas [1]	Lichenified skin [1]	Lesional skin [5]
2/4	1/5	9/10

The data are summarized from two different studies [1, 5]. The number of patients with eosinophil infiltrates vs the total number of patients examined is shown. The quantity of eosinophils was said to be few [1]. Nonlesional skin was examined as well and was negative for eosinophils.

cells [2]. In a similar study [3], maximal eosinophil infiltration was noted only at 72 h. Quantification of the infiltrate showed that eosinophils made up only 9% of the inflammatory cells in atopic eczema skin. Atopics without skin involvement had even fewer eosinophils in the dermal infiltrate.

In another study that used the skin window technique [4], 28% ± 2.6% eosinophils were noted on cover slips which had been placed over denuded, antigen exposed skin of atopic patients for 20–24 h.

From clinical observations, it appears that peripheral blood eosinophilia in patients with atopic eczema is of only moderate degree, if present at all. This impression seems to be supported by the scarce amount of data in the literature. In one small study involving 15 patients, blood eosinophils ranged from 200 to 400/mm^3 [5]. In another study, levels were higher, but increases above normal were noted in only 50% of the patients [2] (Table 2). However, this might be an overestimate of the actual figures since the data come from institutions that would select for patients with more severe disease.

Further evidence for the participation of eosinophils in atopic eczema comes from studies with major basic protein (MBP), the major constituent of the eosinophil granule (see below). In one study, peripheral blood MBP levels were elevated in 51% of the patients [2] (Table 2). In tissue sections, fibrillar reaction patterns to MBP antibodies were found along the elastic fibers, and granular staining was observed in the vicinity of the relatively few dermal eosinophils [6]. The source of dermal MBP is unclear in view of the relative paucity of eosinophils in the same sections. MBP depositions could be the persisting document of disintegrated eosinophils. Alternatively, they could come from transudation of plasma proteins or from infiltrating basophils which are known to contain small amounts of this protein. It should also be noted that, in the blood of atopic eczema patients, the quantity of MBP is not strikingly higher than that found in a totally unrelated disease such as psoriasis (Table 2).

Viewed together, these data leave no doubt that eosinophils are present in the blood and involved skin of patients with atopic eczema, albeit to a moderate degree. However, an unambiguous correlation between blood and tissue eosinophils or serum IgE levels could not be established in any of the above studies. The reasons for this discrepancy can partly be found by examining factors that regulate eosinophil production in the bone marrow and the infiltration of these cells into tissues.

Table 2. Blood eosinophil and MBP levels

Disease	Number of patients	Eosinophils cells/mm^3	Eosinophils % patients	MBP ng/ml	MBP % patients
Atopic eczema	16	709 ± 1540 (0–6370)	50	687 ± 299 (312–1360)	51
Psoriasis	10	624 ± 735 (50–2200)	40	572 ± 163 (376–880)	40
Normals	105	115 ± 107 (11–678)	5	454 ± 90 (312–800)	3

The data are excerpted from [3] and show absolute values of eosinophil counts as well as the percentage of patients who had levels raised above normal (eosinophils ⩾ 350/mm^3 MBP ⩾ 600 ng/ml). Note that the data are similar for patients with psoriasis and atopic eczema.

Regulation of Eosinophil Production and Tissue Infiltration

It has long been established that the proliferation and maturation of eosinophils in the marrow depend on genetic factors and on substances produced by mononuclear cells after stimulation with certain types of antigens and adjuvants (e.g. parasitic antigens and aluminum hydroxide or pertussis vaccine). Eosinophilia arises in a great variety of diseases and can be prevented or reversed by treatment with corticosteroids, sympathomimetics, complete Freund's adjuvant, or acute phase mediators (reviewed in [7]).

Recently, the molecular mechanisms underlying these processes have been clarified. Thus, it has been shown that granulocyte-macrophage colony stimulating factor (GM-CSF) and interleukin (IL)-3 induce stem cell differentiation in bone marrow and cord blood to yield mixed colonies containing eosinophils up to the stage of metamyelocytes. IL-5, by contrast, acts only on committed cells, starting with promyelocytes, and induces mature, pure eosinophil colonies [8, 9] (Fig. 2).

GM-CSF and IL-3 are produced by T helper (T_H) cells,

mast cells and squamous cell carcinoma cells [10–12]. In mast cell-deficient mice, eosinopoiesis, as well as recruitment of eosinophils into the tissue, are deficient [13]. This could mean that not only eosinophilotaxis, but also eosinophil maturation and proliferation could potentially be regulated outside the bone marrow in tissues such as the skin.

Additional findings along this line shed light not only on the regulation of eosinopoiesis, but also on that of IgE synthesis and the pathogenesis of atopy in general, as illustrated in Fig. 3. A subtype of T_H cells, the T_{H2} cells, as well as mast cells, produce IL-4, IL-5 and IL-6 [11]. In contrast, T_{H1} cells are induced by Freund's adjuvant, produce IL-2, interferon-γ and lymphotoxin and are viewed as effector cells of classical delayed type hypersensitivity reactions. IL-4 causes increased IgE production and, together with IL-3, enhances mast cell differentiation. IL-4 also inhibits T_{H1} activity. Decreased T_{H1} activity may, for example, explain the deficient handling of cutaneous viral infections seen in patients with atopic eczema. Finally, T suppressor (T_S) cells, which are induced during specific immunization and which bear histamine receptors, are thought to downregulate T_{H2} function and may be deficient in atopic patients (reviewed in [14, 15]). These recent findings shed new light on the pathogenesis of atopic eczema and, at the same time, offer a plausible explanation for the association of increased IgE levels, mast cell proliferation, eosinophil infiltration and partial defects in cellular immune reactions.

Migration of eosinophils into tissue is a complex process that requires receptor expression on the cell surface for detection of chemical signals (chemotactic factors), adherence of cells to endothelial cells, and an intact metabolic and locomotor machinery to enable the cell to migrate towards the highest concentrations of the chemoattractant in the tissue.

So far, only one recent study has demonstrated that a great variety of factors (IL-1, tumor necrosis factor α (TNFα), lipopolysaccharide (LPS), tissue plasminogen activator (TPA), and platelet activating factor (PAF), cause eosinophil adherence to umbilical vein endothelial cells [16]. None of these substances (except PAF) are known eosinophil chemotactic factors (Table 3). IL-5 is the only cytokine that induces both eosinopoiesis and eosinophil migration.

Recently, there has been much controversy about the potency, cell specificity, and relative selectivity of the chemotactic factors listed in Table 3 (reviewed in [7]). This is most likely due to differences in the in vitro test systems employed and, above all, the source of the eosinophils used regarding both species and the specific disease state. There is general agreement that, on a molar basis, complement factor C5a and leukotriene B_4 (LTB_4)

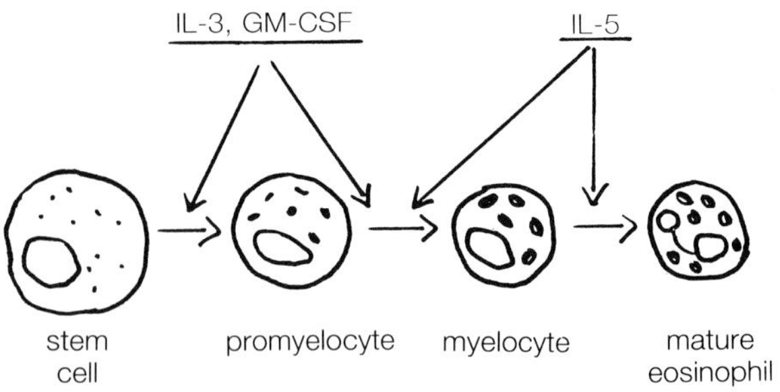

Fig. 2. Influence of cytokines on eosinophil maturation. IL, interleukin; *GM-CSF*, granulocyte/macrophage colony stimulating factor

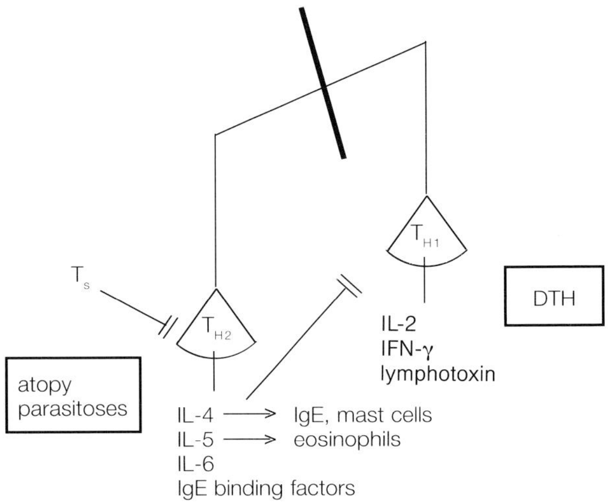

Fig. 3. Production of cytokines by T_{H2} lymphocytes which are overactive in atopy and parasitoses and by T_{H1} lymphocytes which are suppressed by IL-4 and which mediate classical delayed type hypersensitivity (*DTH*) reactions. A lack of antigen-specific, histamine receptor-bearing T suppressor (T_S) lymphocyte activity may explain the overactivity of T_{H2} cells

Table 3. Eosinophil chemotactic factors in atopic eczema

Factor	*Chemical properties*	*Cell specificity*
PAF	ether phospholipid	eos, PMN, monos
LTB_4, 20-OH-LTB_4	eicosanoid	eos, PMN, monos, fibros
mono-HETEs	eicosanoid	PMN, eos
C5a	peptide	PMN, eos, monos, basos, fibros
NFMLP	peptide	PMN, eos, monos
IL-5	protein	eos, ...?
HILDA[a]	protein	eos, ...?
ECF-A	tetrapeptides	–
histamine	amine	–

All of these factors might be operative in eosinophil infiltration into tissues, although their degree of activity is controversial, particularly for the ECF-A tetrapeptides and histamine.
[a]Human interleukin DA, a recently described 41 kDA protein; a potent chemoattractant and activator of eosinophils [23].
eos, eosinophils; PMN, polymorphonuclear neutrophils; monos, monocytes; basos, basophils; fibros, fibrocytes.

Table 4. Differential responsiveness of leukocytes from atopic eczema patients to LTB_4 and PAF

Patient	PAF (10^{-6} *M*)		LTB_4 (10^{-8} *M*)		Control		Peripheral,
	% eos	(PMN)	% eos	(PMN)[a]	% eos	(PMN)	eosinophilia (%)
1	6	(1200)	3	(2000)	0	(801)	11
2	2	(205)	4	(34)	0	(0)	5
3	2	(1350)	6	(500)	0	(250)	10
4	2	(1070)	4	(556)	0	(262)	4
5	74	(464)	71	(104)	79	(88)	4
6	5	(1550)	10	(1250)	5	(750)	6
7	52	(612)	80	(102)	80	(90)	21
8	0	(702)	28	(160)	22	(154)	17
9	1	(819)	35	(476)	33	(247)	7
10	6	(835)	14	(298)	13	(294)	10
11	0	(945)	17	(1690)	4	(140)	6
12	n.d.	(n.d.)	90	(502)	2	(16)	23

[a] Note the lack of correlation between total number of migrating cells through the filter in five high power microscopic fields (PMN), the % eosinophils (% eos) responding to PAF, LTB_4 and buffer control, and the peripheral eosinophilia (n.d. = not done).

are equipotent chemoattractants, but C5a is less active on eosinophils, and 20-OH-LTB_4, the mono-HETEs (hydroxyeicosatetraenoic acids) and PAF need to be used at higher concentrations to yield the same effects as LTB_4. There is disagreement as to whether PAF or LTB_4 are more selective for eosinophils. In our hands, this depends on the patients from whom the eosinophils are obtained (Table 4) [17]. Others have shown that this variation may be due to the density of eosinophils, with hypodense cells being inactive or less responsive [18, 19]. The last two factors listed in Table 3, eosinophil chemotactic factor of anaphylaxis (ECF-A) and histamine, have been found to be inactive by all but a few laboratories. The ECF-A tetrapeptides can, however, modulate some eosinophil functions (reviewed in [20]), and histamine has been found to be a potent inhibitor of eosinophil and neutrophil chemotaxis, both in vitro and in vivo [7, 21].

With the exception of the very recently described cytokines IL-5 and human interleukin DA (HILDA) [22, 23] (Table 3), which so far have not been examined with other cell types, all other known eosinophil chemotactic factors also act on a variety of other cells (Table 3). This would explain the mixed cell infiltrate found in atopic skin. A dissection of the in vivo activity and the relative significance of the different chemotactic factors is, however, difficult, and little data have been published on this topic. The issue is further complicated by the altered responsiveness of pathological, compared to normal, tissue. Thus, PAF and LTB_4 are inactive towards monocytes from normal donors, but elicit a chemotactic response towards cells from patients with atopic eczema and psoriasis [24]. Similarly, PAF has been shown to induce in vivo migration of eosinophils only in atopic and not in normal subjects' skin [5]. In this latter study, PAF alone could not explain the allergen-induced eosinophil influx, and additional factors were postulated. LTB_4 is a likely candidate since it has been shown to be present in atopic skin [25, 26].

In passive cutaneous anaphylaxis (PCA) reactions, low molecular weight eosinophil chemotactic factors (PAF, LTB_4 and possibly mono-HETEs) have been isolated within the first 6 h, C5a after 12 h, and high molecular weight factors (possibly cytokines) after 24 h [27]. The isolation of substances such as LTB_4 in chronic lesions speaks, however, against a strict sequential separation of the activity of the different factors. Their interaction with each other and their activity in the presence of inhibitory factors such as histamine, IgA, and T cell-derived inhibitors [28] will have to be further elucidated.

Eosinophil Function in Atopic Eczema

Most of our knowledge on eosinophil function comes from studies of parasitic infestations. Apart from their cytotoxic effect on parasites, eosinophils are particularly well equipped to participate in IgE- and mast cell-dependent inflammatory reactions. This is evident when one examines the basic properties of these cells (Fig. 4). They can be stimulated by antigens and IgE complexes via their low affinity IgE receptor; they express HLA-DR on exposure to GM-CSF [29]; they produce a plethora of immediate type mediators; and they induce or modulate important inflammatory processes by means of their enzymes and basic proteins. Eosinophil

Fig. 4. Basic properties of eosinophil leukocytes

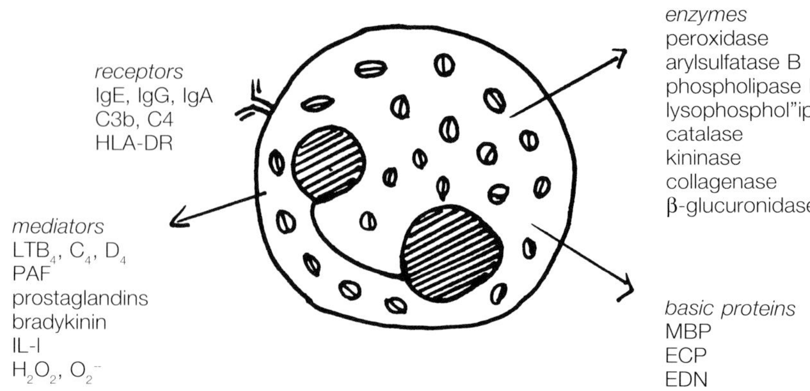

functions that may be important in atopic eczema include:

1. Cytotoxicity against keratinocytes, lymphocytes, fibroblasts, bacteria and nerve cells
2. Histamine release from mast cells and basophils
3. Release of vasoactive and chemotactic lipids
4. Release of enzymes and H_2O_2
5. Increase and inhibition of fibroblast mitogenesis
6. Inhibition of convertases of the complement system

In contrast to neutrophils, eosinophils produce 7–40 times more LTC$_4$ than LTB$_4$ [30]. The peroxidase inactivates leukotrienes and histamine and is cytotoxic for parasites and tumor cells. MBP, which constitutes all the protein in the core of eosinophil granules, is cytotoxic for many cells including keratinocytes and causes basophil and mast cell histamine release [7, 31]. Eosinophil cationic protein (ECP) and neurotoxin (EDN) are ribonucleases with neurotoxic properties. Whether this neurotoxicity is of significance in atopic eczema is as yet unknown. Similarly, the effect of eosinophils on fibroblasts and their modulation of collagen metabolism, lymphocyte proliferation, and complement activation is poorly understood.

The most fascinating insights into eosinophil function in disease have come from the recent differentiation of normodense from hypodense eosinophils. The latter have been found to be increased in diverse pathological states and make up 30%–65% of peripheral blood eosinophils in atopy. The cells have been induced in vitro from normal eosinophils by incubation with TNF, known eosinopoietic factors (Fig. 2), and eosinophil chemotactic factors (PAF, C5a, *N*-formyl-met-leu-phe and ECF-A tetrapeptides) [20, 32]. Hypodense cells are much better equipped to exercise effector functions in allergic disease than normodense cells, due to enhancement of the following functions:

1. Expression of Fc$_\varepsilon$ and complement receptors, IgE binding
2. Respiratory burst
3. Peroxidase activity and release
4. LTC$_4$ and PAF synthesis
5. Activity of lysosomal enzymes
6. Antibody-dependent cytotoxicity
7. Surface charge
8. Conversion of ECP and EDN to their secretory forms
9. Chemotaxis
10. Survival

Summary

This review of recent data on eosinophils in general and their role in atopic eczema specifically leads to the following conclusions:

1. There is evidence for eosinophil presence in atopic eczema.
2. Eosinophil production in atopy is regulated by specific factors that are produced by a subtype of T$_H$ cells.
3. Eosinophil infiltration into tissue is regulated by many factors which have additional cell specificites and functions.
4. Eosinophils in atopy are in an activated hypodense state that enhances their responsiveness in numerous ways.

Despite this knowledge, the fundamental question of whether eosinophils are beneficial to the host in allergic disease, or whether they instead maintain the disease state, has not been answered.

References

1. Mihm MC, Soter NA, Dvorak HF, Austen KF (1976) The structure of normal skin and the morphology of atopic eczema. J Invest Dermatol 67: 305–312
2. Wassom DL, Loegering DA, Solley GO, Moore SB, Schooley RT, Fauce AS, Gleich GJ (1981) Elevated serum levels of the eosinophil granule major basic protein in patients with eosinophilia. J Clin Invest 67: 651–661
3. Mitchell EB, Chapman MD, Pope FM, Crow J, Jouhal SS, Platts-Mills TAE (1982) Basophils in allergen-induced patch test sites in atopic dermatitis. Lancet I:127–130
4. Henocq E, Vargaftig BB (1986) Accumulation of eosinophils in response to intracutaneous PAF-acether and allergens in man. Lancet I:1378–1379
5. Bruynzeel-Koomen CAFM, van Wichen DF, Spry CJF, Venge P, Bruynzeel PLB (1988) Active participation of eosinophils in patch test reactions to inhalant allergens in patients with atopic dermatitis. Br J Dermatol 118:229–2386
6. Leiferman KM, Ackerman SJ, Sampson HA, Haugen HS, Venencie PY, Gleich GJ (1985) Dermal deposition of eosinophil-granule major basic protein in atopic dermatitis. Comparison with onchocerciasis. N Engl J Med 313: 282–285
7. Czarnetzki BM (1987) Les polynucléaires éosinophiles. Ann Dermatol Venereol 114:1147–1156
8 Sonoda Y, Arai N, Ogawa M (1989) Humoral regulation of eosinophilopoiesis in vitro: analysis of the targets of interleukin-3, granulocyte/macrophage colony-stimulating factor (GM-CSF), and interleukin-5. Leukemia 3:14–18
9. Ishizaka T, Saito H, Hatake K, Dvorak AM, Leiferman KM, Arai SN, Ishizaka K (1989) Preferential differentiation of inflammatory cells by recombinant human interleukins. Int Arch Allergy Appl Immunol 88:46–49
10. Wodnar-Filipowicz A, Heusser CH, Moroni C (1989) Production of the haemopoietic growth factors GM-CSF and interleukin-3 by mast cells in response to IgE receptor-mediated activation. Nature 339:150–152
11. Plaut M, Pierce JH, Watson CJ, Hanley-Hyde J, Nordan RP, Paul WE (1989) Mast cell lines produce lymphokines in response to cross-linkage of $Fc_{\varepsilon}RI$ or to calcium ionophore. Nature 339: 64–67
12. Tanno Y, Stadler B, Denburg JA (1987) Human interleukin-3-like activity, basophil and eosinophil growth promoting activities and colony stimulating factor derived from several cell lines. Int Arch Allergy Appl Immunol 83:1–5
13. Nawa Y, Owhashi M, Imai J, Abe T (1987) Eosinophil response in mast cell-deficient w/wv mice. Int Arch Allergy Appl Immunol 83: 6–11
14. O'Garra A (1989) Interleukins and the immune system 2. Lancet I:1003–1005
15. Sustiel A, Rocklin R (1989) T cell responses in allergic rhinitis, asthma and atopic dermatitis. Clin Exp Allergy 19:11–18
16. Lama AM, Mulroney CM, Schleimer RP (1988) Studies on the adhesive interaction between purified human eosinophils and cultured vascular endothelial cells. J Immunol 140: 1500–1505
17. Czarnetzki BM, Scato M (1989) Comparative studies of human eosinophil migration towards PAF and LTB_4. Int Arch Allergy Appl Immunol 88: 191–193
18. Gosset P, Prin L, Capron M, Aurialt C, Tonnel AB, Capron A (1986) Presence of factors chemotactic for granulocytes in hypereosinophilic syndrome sera: relation with alterations in eosinophil migration. Clin Exp Immunol 65: 654–663
19. Sigal CE, Valone FH,Holtzman MJ, Goetzl EJ (1987) Preferential human eosinophil chemotactic activity of the platelet-activating factor (PAF) 1-0- hexadecyl-2-acetyl-sn-glyceryl-3-phosphocholine (AGEPC). J. Clin Immunol 7: 179–184
20. Fukada T, Gleich G (1989) Heterogeneity of human eosinophils. J Allergy Clin Immunol 83: 369–373
21. Ting S, Zweiman B, Lavker R, Dunsky EH (1981) Histamine suprression of in vivo eosinophil accumulation and histamine release in human allergic reactions. J Allergy Clin Immunol 68: 65–71
22. Yamaguchi Y, Hayashi Y, Sugama Y, Kasahara T, Kitamura S, Torisu M, Mita S, Tominaga A, Takatsu K (1988) Highly purified murine interleukin 5 (IL-5) stimulates eosinophil function and prolongs in vitro survival. IL-5 as an eosinophil chemotactic factor. J Exp Med 167: 1737–1742
23. Moreau JF, Bonneville M, Godard A, Gascan H, Gruart V, Moore MA, Soulillou JP (1987) Characterization of a factor produced by human T cell clones exhibiting eosinophil-activating and burst-promoting activities. J Immunol 138: 3844–3849
24. Czarnetzki BM (1983) Increased monocyte chemotaxis towards leukotriene B4 and platelet activating factor in psoriasis and atopic eczema. Clin Exp Immunol 54: 486–492
25. Ruzicka T, Simmet T, Peskar BA, Ring J (1986) Skin levels of arachidonic acid-derived inflammatory mediators and histamine in atopic dermatitis and psoriasis. J Invest Dermatol 86: 105–108
26. Rosenbach T, Grabbe J, Möller A, Schwanitz HJ, Czarnetzki BM (1985) Generation of leukotrienes from normal epidermis and their demonstration in cutaneous disease. Br J Dermatol 113 (Suppl 28): 157–167
27. Hirashima M, Tashiro K, Hirotsu Y, Hayashi H (1983) The mediation of tissue eosinophilia in hypersensitivity reactions. V. Comparative study of tissue eosinophilia in the skin lesions of local and systemic passive cutaneous anaphylactic reactions. Immunology 50: 85–91
28. Tashiro K, Sakata K, Hirashima M, Hayashi H (1985) The regulation of tissue eosinophilia. III. In vitro production of eosinophil-directed chemotactic inhibitory factor by T lymphocytes of complete Freund's adjuvant-treated guinea-pigs. Immunology 55: 115–124
29. Lucey DR, Nicholson-Weller A, Weller PF (1989) Mature human eosinophils have the capacity to express HLA-DR. Proc Natl Acad Sci USA 86: 1348–1351
30. Weller PF, Lee CW, Foster DW, Corey EJ, Austen KF, Lewis RA, Dana CA (1983) Generation and metabolism of 5-lipoxygenase pathway leukotrienes by human eosinophils: predominant production of leukotriene C4. Proc Natl Acad Sci USA 80: 7626–7630
31. Gleich GJ, Ottesen EA, Leiferman KM, Ackerman SJ (1989) Eosinophils and human disease. Int Arch Allergy Appl Immunol 88: 59–62
32. Silberstein DS, Schoof DD, Rodrick ML, Tai PC, Spry CJ, David JR, Eberlein TJ (1989) Activation of eosinophils in cancer patients treated with IL-2 and IL-2-generated lymphokine-activated killer cells. J Immunol 142: 2162–2167

Role of Inhalant Allergens in Atopic Eczema

T. A. E. Platts-Mills, M. D. Chapman, B. Mitchell, P. W. Heymann, and B. Deuell

History

The discovery that many patients with hay fever give immediate wheal and flare skin responses to extracts made from common environmental agents such as pollen, animal dander, of house dust was followed by testing of patients with other diseases [7]. Positive skin tests were found to be common not only in patients with rhinitis and asthma but also in patients with Besnier's prurigo [4, 62]. The term atopic eczema (AE) was introduced by Coca and others, not only because the patients were atopic but also because they felt that these allergens played an important role in the pathogenesis of the disease. Reports were published showing that patients with food allergy and AE improved if they avoided the relevant food [25, 61]. In addition, Rost reported in 1932 [55] that patients with AE who were allergic to house dust improved often dramatically when they stayed in an "allergen-free room". This observation was interpreted as showing that inhalants in the patients' house were an important "cause" of AE. The view that allergen exposure was the major cause of AE was put very forcefully by Louis Tuft in a series of articles in the 1940s. His findings and views can be summarized as follows [64]:

- Positive skin tests to house dust from the patient's house are very common in adults with AE (46 out of 54 cases).
- Children with AE are commonly allergic to foods, but by the age of 7 years they usually become allergic to inhalants, and these are the dominant allergens in adults.
- Adult patients not only improve when they are taken away from their houses but may also improve when their houses are cleaned.
- Finally, Dr. Tuft reported exacerbation of skin rash following nasal challenge with house dust.

During the 1950s several different arguments were advanced against the view that allergens cause AE, and gradually general nihilism developed about the disease not only on the part of dermatologists but also among allergists [16]. Four arguments appear to have been critical:

- The observation that injecting allergen into the skin causes urticaria rather than eczema.
- The patients were usually *not* aware that dust or pollen exposure caused exacerbations of their skin rash.
- The fact that patients with AE often had allergic rhinitis or asthma as well as dermatitis was considered to explain their sensitivity to inhalants.
- Finally, it was generally agreed that specific desensitization therapy did not help these patients. Indeed it was often found that injection therapy made the rash worse.

Although certain aspects of the argument are often quoted, perhaps the most important factor was that the specific diagnosis of allergen sensitivity in patients with AE was not perceived as leading to a useful change in treatment [21, 52]. This was not only because desensitization didn't work but also because the most important allergen identified in adults was house dust. House dust was a problem because its constituents were poorly understood and avoiding it was very difficult. Furthermore, Dr. Hill, who was a major proponent of the role of foods in AE, did not believe that inhalant allergens could give rise to an eczematous skin reaction. By the mid 1960s there was agreement that foods could be a cause of AE in some young children, but few allergists or dermatologists recognized a role for inhalants or foods in adults with AE. During the 1960s the scientific basis of allergy received a major boost with the discovery first of dust mites and second of IgE, both being of great importance for the understanding of AE [27, 65).

The discovery of IgE and two patients with IgE myeloma led to the development of specific anti-IgE reagents and assays for measuring both total serum IgE and specific IgE antibodies. Within 2 years results were published showing that patients with AE had high or very high (i.e., > 5000 IU/ml) levels of total serum IgE. In addition, using the radioallergosorbent technique (RAST) it was clear that many of these patients had high levels of IgE antibodies against several different inhalant allergens. Indeed, from the serum data there was little doubt that patients with AE are "more allergic" than any other patients seen in non-tropical countries [29, 30, 45]. Surprisingly, these findings had very little effect on the analysis of causes of AE, and they were dismissed because: IgE was thought to be not specific; a few patients with apparent AE didn't have raised total IgE; the antibodies could be explained by other allergic diseases.

The discovery that dust mites are an important source of allergens in house dust was not at first seen as relevant to AE, although early reports demonstrated high levels of IgE antibody to dust mites [45]. Initially, there were considerable problems with dust mite extracts, including contamination with horse proteins or human serum proteins contained in the growth media. With better growth conditions, better extracts were produced, and the quantities of mite culture available were sufficient to allow isolation of mite allergens [13]. Purification of a major allergen from *Dermatophagoides pteronyssinus* (Der p I) made possible a variety of immunological experiments. These included not only in vitro studies on isotype-specific antibodies and T cells but also in vivo patch tests designed to study further the way in which eczematous lesions can be produced [14, 41, 53]. A variety of other studies over the last few years have adressed that same question looking at T cells, eosinophils and eosinophil products in the skin of patients with AE [19, 32, 33, 34]. Recent studies can be divided into those on the nature of the immune response to allergens in patients with AE, studies on the immunopathology of either naturally occurring or induced eczematous lesions and finally evidence that particular levels of antigen exposure may be "sufficient" to exacerbate AE.

Specificity of the Immune Response to Inhalant Allergens in Patients with Atopic Eczema

IgE Antibodies

Skin tests in patients with AE pose many problems. Involved skin will often not demonstrate wheal and flare responses, giving false negative results. In addition, local steroids as distinct from systemic steroids have a marked inhibitory effect on skin tests. Multiple skin tests can exacerbate AE and like densensitization may occasionally produce generalized relapses. Finally, in young children with AE, skin tests may be particularly liable to give false negative results. Thus, with different patients it may be best to use skin tests and/or serum assays. Some authorities consider severe AE as one of the indications for using RAST as the primary diagnostic technique. RAST is generally carried out with crude extract (rather than purified allergen) attached to a solid phase immunosorbent which is usually a cellulose disc. The solid phase has two effects: first, relatively low affinity IgE antibodies will bind; and second, the background or nonspecific binding of radiolabelled anti-IgE is directly related to the total serum IgE. For any sera with > 1000 IU/ml the background must be adjusted, and for sera with total IgE > 5000 IU/ml only strongly positive RAST results are relevant. This background binding is easy to understand if one considers that nonspecific binding of IgE is around 0.1% and thus a serum with 5000 IU/ml will bind 5 IU or ~ 12 ng nonspecifically if assayed undiluted; if assayed at 1:10 this binding will fall to ~ 1.2 ng. Clearly, the specific antibody must be at least two fold greater than this and preferably more than that since nonspecific backgrounds are not consistent [2]. Thus, in general only 3+ RAST results or 20 ng of specific IgE per ml should be regarded as definitely positive if the serum has a very high total IgE. Nonetheless, RAST is much the simplest way of measuring IgE antibody to inhalants since most antigens can be bound easily and the procedure is simple.

Using purified antigens IgE antibody can be measured either by RAST or if they can be radiolabelled by radioimmunoprecipitation [49]. Using radiolabelled Der p I

Fig. 1. Serum IgE antibodies to a dust mite allergen in sera from patients with atopic dermatitis. IgE antibodies expressed as IgE binding activity for antigen P_1 (Der p I). *Solid symbols* indicate patients with positive skin tests. Proportion of patients showing detectable serum IgE binding activity is indicated: for patients < 7 years old, those between 7 and 1, and those over 21 years old. Reprinted from Chapman et al. [14].

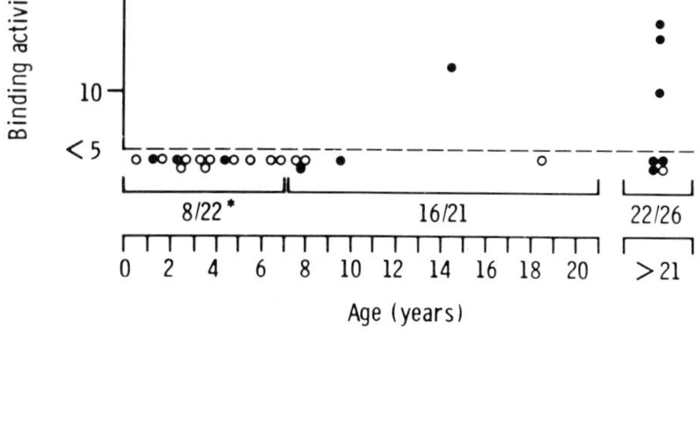

Table 1. Antibodies to antigen P_1 and total serum IgE in patients with perennial rhinitis, asthma, and/or atopic eczema

Patient group	Total IgE[a] (IU/ml)	Incidence of positive skin test to mite	Antibodies to Der p I[b] (U/ml) IgG	IgE
Rhinitis	410	25/26	83	25
$n = 26$	(58–3708)		(10–805)	(8–63)
Asthma	494	22/24	244	96
$n = 24$	(32–5500)		23–1325)	(8–618)
Atopic eczema[c]				
All patients	4008	36/38	263	160
$n = 38$	(125–23000)		(6–2400)	(14–838)
With asthma	5288	20/21	274	165
$n = 21$	(1350–23000)		(20–1575)	(24–768)
No asthma	5159	11/11	268	200
$n = 11$	(2100–17712)		(6–1775)	(14–700)

[a] Values are geometric means and values in parentheses are the range of values observed.
[b] Antibodies to Der p I measured using an antigen binding radioimmuno-precipitation assay. Values in arbitrary units of binding activity.
[c] Patients with atopic eczema were regarded as having asthma if they had been treated for airway obstruction in the past 2 years. Patients with "no asthma" had never been treated for asthma and had no symptoms suggestive of it. Six patients were excluded because their history was equivocal. Results from Chapman et al. [14].

(originally called antigen p I), IgE antibodies can be measured directly in parallel with IgG antibodies, and the results show that a large proportion of adult AE patients and almost all patients with positive skin tests to dust mites have IgE and IgG antibodies to Der p I (see Fig. 1) [14]. Also shown in Fig. 1 is the increasing prevalence of IgE antibody to mites with age. Just as had been described by Dr. Tuft, the prevalence of IgE antibody to inhalants increases with age, and most patients with severe or moderately severe AE who are over the age of 7 years will have high levels of IgE antibody to Der p I. As with most allergens the source material for dust mites includes multiple different proteins which can provoke an IgE antibody response. It is possible to identify IgE antibodies to multiple proteins either by purifying other proteins or by crossed radioimmunoelectrophoresis (CRIE). Preliminary studies have shown that patients with AE have IgE antibodes to mulitple dust mite-derived allergens. Most patients with AE have higher levels of IgE antibody than patients with rhinitis or asthma (Table 1). This high level could represent either responses to a larger number of different proteins or increased quantities of IgE antibody to the same proteins.

It seems likely that both phenomena occur, i.e., that patients with AE produce IgE antibodies to many different dust mite proteins and that they also produce larger quantities of IgE antibody to each protein. To take the argument one step further, it is possible to ask whether IgE antibodies in the serum of patients with AE are directed against the same epitopes on allergenic molecules as IgE antibodies from individuals with asthma. At present there is no clear evidence. However, a serum that could inhibit the binding of multiple different monoclonal antibodies to Der p I was isolated from a patient with AE [15].

Several researchers have observed that patients with AE have IgE antibodies to multiple different inhalant and food allergens, which has led to the suggestion that IgE responses are in some sense nonspecific. In part, this impression can be obtained by over-interpretation of weakly positive RAST results or by using immunoblots which have a great potential for nonspecific binding. However, being aware of these problems, it is still clear that patients can have IgE antibodies to pollen, cat dander, mites and/or a range of inhaled fungi [6, 14, 26, 45]. The question then arises whether these patients have made specific responses to exposure or are responding with nonspecific polyclonal IgE antibody responses. Studies using some less common antigens leave little doubt about the specificity. Thus, in the UK patients who had not been exposed to horses did not have IgE antibody to horse dander; only one of our patients had significant IgE antibody to rat urine; and in the USA IgE antibody to cockroach allergens is not found in sera from patients with AE (or asthma) unless they have lived in a house with heavy cockroach infestation. Many of the patients we studied had received immunization with diphtheria toxoid in alum, an immunization regime that normally only gives rise to IgG antibody. Measuring IgE antibodies with radiolabelled toxin we were unable to demonstrate IgE anti-diphtheria toxin antibodies although patients with AE had normal levels of IgG antitoxin [14]. Further evidence that IgE antibody production occurs in response to specific antigen exposure comes from reports that the total and specific IgE antibody levels can fall if the disease goes into remission [28]. We have observed similar falls in total serum IgE in mite-allergic patients who go into remission after cleaning their houses, e.g., total IgE falling from 35 000 IU to 2000 IU/ml progressively over 2 years (Mitchell and Platts-Mills, unpublished observations). It is well-known that total and specific IgE do not go up and down with relapses over the short term, i.e., weeks; however, this probably reflects the normal life span of IgE-producing plasma cells.

It has long been argued whether or not IgE antibodies to other inhalants such as pollens or danders are etiologically significant in the disease. There are occasional patients who report seasonal exacerbations of eczema and several reports in the literature ([18]; see [10]). Our own view is that any inhalant to which a patient has IgE antibodies can exacerbate the disease given sufficient exposure. However, exposure to many indoor allergens is so chronic that patients often do not appreciate variations caused by exposure to seasonal or occasional allergens. There are some adult patients with AE that appears to be associated with IgE antibodies to foods only. We have seen adult patients with skin sensitivity and very high levels of IgE antibody to egg which was associated with persistent dermatitis and was relieved by a strict avoidance diet. One of the problems in AE is whether food sensitivity can be evaluated satisfactorily in vitro [6, 56, 58]. Indeed, some clinics would consider admitting patients or treating them with a short course of systemic steroids to "calm down" the skin sufficiently in order to obtain reliable skin test results with food extracts.

Patients with AE may produce IgE antibodies to a wide range of inhalants and foods. The evidence at present suggests that these IgE antibody responses are immunologically specific, i.e., they are in general high affinity and specific for the antigen in question. In addition, it appears that these patients do not produce IgE antibodies against allergens to which they have not been exposed. We regard the presence of a strongly positive skin test or serum IgE antibody as good evidence that a patient is exposed or has been exposed in the past to the relevant allergen.

IgG and IgG Subclass Antibodies

Using antigen binding or radioimmunoprecipitation assays, sera from patients with AE contain IgG antibodies to all antigens against which they have IgE antibodies (see Table 1). Our data did not show any striking differences between patients with AE, asthma and rhinitis in the IgG antibody response. However, we have consistently found that as total IgE rises and specific IgE antibody levels rise, the ratio of IgG antibodies to IgE antibodes decreases. Thus, it is not unusual to find sera from patients with AE in which there is an equal quantity of IgE antibodies and IgG antibodies to a specific allergen, e.g., Der p I. We think that this reflects the relative saturation of skin mast cells and other mast cells with IgE [48]. Thus, as the antibody response increases, a larger proportion of the IgE stays in the circulation. Merrett and his colleagues have reported high levels of total serum IgG_4 and of specific IgG_4 antibodies in patients with AE [38]. Using monoclonal anti-IgG_4 in an immunoprecipitation assay, we also found that IgG antibody responses in patients with AE included a large proportion of IgG_4 [57]. Although several researchers have suggested a role for IgG_2 or IgG_4 antibodies in mediator release, this now seems unlikely. However, in allergen-specific IgG antibody responses a progressively larger proportion of IgG_4 develops with prolonged exposure [1]. It is also possible that IgG_4 antibodies alter the properties of immune complexes containing IgG and or IgE antibodies.

However, it is difficult to believe that IgG antibodies play a significant role in AE since although the majority of normal children have IgG antibodies to milk or egg the role of these foods in AE appears to be restricted to those children who develop IgE antibody [59].

T-Cell Responses to Mite Allergens

Experiments in mice have established that IgE antibody responses are T-cell dependent, and it is considered inevitable that human IgE antibody responses are also dependent on T-cell help. Thus, it was not a surprise to find that allergic individuals including those with AE had peripheral blood lymphocytes which would proliferate when stimulated with specific allergens. It has clearly been demonstrated that the cells which proliferate in response to allergens are T cells of the helper phenotype [53]. It is also certain that these responses are dependent on antigen-presenting cells. Using Der p I as the antigen, studies were done using peripheral blood mononuclear cells from mite-allergic patients with asthma, rhinitis or AE [53, 54]. Although mite-allergic patients with AE, particularly children, gave good proliferative responses,

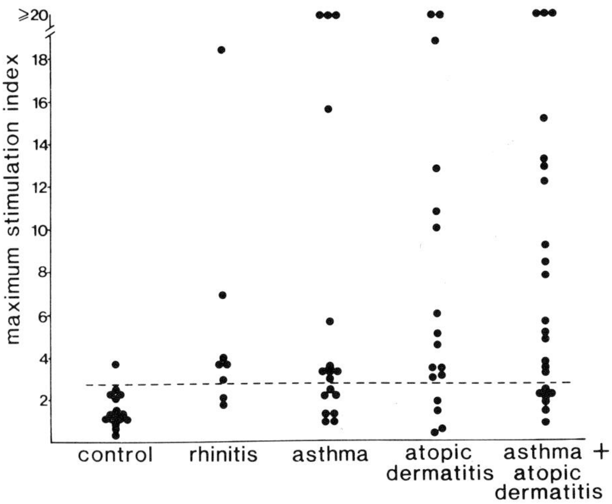

Fig. 2. Maximum stimulation indices with peripheral blood lymphocytes cultured with 10 μg Der p I/ml for 5 or 7 days. Patients who were sensitive to *Dermatophagoides pteronyssinus* are grouped according to symptoms. *Line* (–) shows mean + 2 SD of 14 non-responding controls. Patients groups were all significantly different from controls ($p < 0.01$). Reproduced by permission of the author and *Journal of Immunology* [53].

we could find no evidence that the responses were different among the various diseases. Indeed, comparing mite-allergic patients with asthma, AE or both, it is difficult to identify any immunological difference in their response to mite antigens. They can have similar levels of IgE and IgG antibodies and very similar in vitro T-cell responses (Fig. 2). Perhaps the most important question is what role the T cells play in the local inflammatory lesions and whether T-cell localization is important in the different responses of patients. The normal technique for studying T-cell effector function in vivo is to carry out delayed hypersensitivity skin testing. This is difficult with allergens in allergic individuals because the small quantity of allergen that can safely be injected is diluted by the immediate wheal and flare response, and it appears that this response serves to remove antigen from the local site, so preventing delayed responses [9]. There is an extensive older literature on nonspecific T-cell reactivity in patients with AE (reviewed by Buckley [12]). Those researchers reported difficulty sensitizing patients with AE to such contact sensitizers as DNCB or poison ivy. Other studies showed poor in vitro T-cell responses to nonspecific mitogens. However, it is difficult to assess whether these nonspecific changes are secondary to the inflammatory effects of the disease. Our view is that the antigen-specific responses are more relevant, and it is clear that T cells from patients with AE have excellent proliferative responses to mite allergens in vitro. There are also studies showing that lymphocytes from patients with AE will produce IgE in vitro [12]. However, these studies have not yet reached the point at which they can help us to understand how to reduce IgE production in vivo, which is clearly the long-term objective.

In recent years it has become clear that delayed responses can be either of the classic tuberculin type or of the Jones Mote or cutaneous basophil hypersensitivity type [40]. It could be very important to know whether T cells in patients with AE would produce either of those two types of local responses in vivo. Two approaches to this question are possible: either more detailed studies of the circulating T cells that respond to allergens *or* different techniques for producing delayed reactions on the skin (see next section).

Detailed study of T cells is proceeding with the development of two new techniques, T-cell cloning and the identification of different interleukins produced by T cells. As yet, T-cell cloning with human cells has such a low efficiency that the properties of the cloned T cells probably reflect those cells that can be cloned most easily rather than the dominant cell in that individual. However, clones specific for mite antigens have been produced by several groups, and they include cells which appear to be of the Th_2 type [44]. Production of interleukins by responding T cells from patients with AE has not yet been studied in detail. It is tempting to believe that there might be differences in the relative production of interleukins between patients with asthma and AE; however, it is important to remember that local and systemic eosinophilia is a feature of both diseases and that IL-5 production by T cells may be responsible for eosinophilia in both diseases. Thus, it is possible that detailed analysis of interleukin production in vitro would still leave unresolved the mechanism of localization of inflammation to the skin versus localization to the lung.

Studies on the Immunopathology of Eczema

Use of a Patch Technique to Produce Delayed Eczematous Responses in Patients with Atopic Eczema

The patch technique is a standard way of testing responses to the fat-soluble, low molecular weight chemicals that produce contact sensitivity. In general, this is not considered a useful approach for studying responses to allergens because most allergens are water soluble and of a much higher molecular weight (generally $\geq$ 10 000 daltons). However, it is clear that many mite-allergic patients with AE are chronically exposed to high levels of Der p I in their bedding, and it seems reasonable to ask whether this allergen could produce eczema when applied to the skin. There is a major problem in designing these experiments because inflamed skin gives nonspecific reactions and healthy skin is at least partially "waterproof". The simplest way to obtain consistent eczematous responses is to study patients in remission (i.e., in hospital for 2 weeks) and mildly abrade or "strip" the skin to remove the outer layers of epidermis. This procedure is far less damaging than the scratching the patients apply to their own skin which very commonly causes bleeding. When 5 μg of Der p I is applied in saline on an occluded gauze patch there is an initial swelling of the skin within 30 min followed by an erythematous, papular response with exudation which is usually present by 24 h and by 48 h is macroscopically eczema [41]. The eczematous nature of this response has now been confirmed by at least four groups and completely rebuts the argument that allergens applied to the skin only produce urticaria [3, 11, 20].

In the early studies the main controls have been either saline or an irrelevant allergen applied to the skin of patients with AE *or* Der p I applied to the skin of nonallergic individuals. These controls were negative. Applying Der p I to the skin of mite-allergic individuals who do not have AE was not pursued in the original studies, but more recent results suggest that mite-allergic asthmatic patients show poor patch responses to mite antigen [3]. This suggests that the patch response may actually be a model for studying the differences that lead some individuals to develop AE.

In order to understand the mechanism for induced eczematous responses several groups have studied the cellular infiltrate that occurs both in patch responses and in naturally occurring eczema. There is no question that the response to patch testing includes eosinophils. In our studies and those of Henoque and Gaillard [23] there was no difficulty identifying a basophil infiltrate; however, Bruijnzeel and her colleagues could not identify basophils in their biopsies [10,11]. The issue of whether basophils are present is important because the mechanisms by which basophils are recruited are probably different than those for eosinophils. Basophils are difficult to fix or stain in biopsies from human tissues, and there have also been problems in identifying basophils in nasal secretions from patients with seasonal rhinitis [22]. Our view is that the variations are due to minor technical differences in fixing and staining biopsies and that experimentally induced patches of eczema have both an eosinophil and a basophil dermal infiltrate at 48 h.

Classic experiments in mice have studied the role of T cells by using passive transfer; similar studies for obvious reasons are not possible in humans. However, before the arrival of AIDS it was possible to do passive transfer experiments with serum to try to transfer the eczematous patch test response. Using plasma from patients with AE to provide plasma replacement for patients with severe immunoglobulin deficiency, it was possible to study both immediate skin responses and 48-h patch responses. The patch responses to Der p I following systemic passive transfer were erythematous rather than eczematous and had a significant eosinophil infiltrate but no basophils [42]. Using local transfer of specifically purified IgE and IgG antibodies, we found very similar results. We were inclined to interpret the lack of basophils following passive transfer as evidence that T cells play a role in the recruiment of basophils. However, local transfer of plasma into the skin of nonallergic individuals (e.g. TPM and MDC) and subsequent patch testing produced both eosinophil and basophil infiltration. Thus, there appears to be evidence for a nonantibody serum factor that can contribute to a cellular infiltrate in the skin. Obviously, this factor could be very important in understanding the pathogenesis of eczematous lesions. It is tempting to speculate that T-cell-derived factors similar to those known to control delayed skin responses in guinea pigs are also involved in humans [39, 40]. The only evidence to support this interpretation comes from experiments showing that human T cells can produce a basophil chemotactic factor in vitro [8, 42, 66].

The large numbers of eosinophils present in patch test responses is surprising since routine biopsies of involved skin in patients with AE usually do not show increased eosinophils. However, several pieces of evidence support the view that eosinophil infiltration is a transient feature of the skin response to allergens and is important in AE.

Firstly, Leiferman and her colleagues [32] showed that although skin biopsies from patients with AE contained few eosinophils, they stained very strongly with antibodies against eosinophil major basic protein (MBP). This suggested that eosinophils had been present but had degranulated and so were no longer identifiable.

Table 2. Cellular infiltrate in eczematous response to repeated application of aqueous allergen to patch test

Patch applied	Time of biopsy	Basophils	Mast cells	Eosinophils	Monocytes	Neutrophils	Total
Saline	2 days	2	46	0	303	16	367
Der p I	2 days	26	56	337	795	37	1251
Der p I	6 days	22	77	1249	833	13	2194
Der p I	10 days	21	113	96	932	9	1171

5 μg Der p I was applied to three separate sits and reapplied every 2 days. Cell counts in the dermis of a 4-mm punch biopsy fixed with Karnovsky's fixative, embedded in plastic and stained with Giemsa. Values for a single representative patient from Mitchell et al. [43].

Secondly, when patch tests are maintained with repeated application of allergen over a 10-day period, the number of eosinophils increases up to day 6 and then falls rapidly (Table 2) [43]. Although this experiment did not establish what happens to the eosinophils, in view of the intense MBP staining of AE skin, it seems most likely that the eosinophils are degranulated locally.

Thirdly, a similar discrepancy arises between naturally occurring and experimentally induced contact hypersensitivity. Experimental lesions induced with poison ivy or DNCB include eosinophils and basophils while eosinophils are not obvious in the naturally occurring lesions [17]. It now seems most likely that in both AE and contact hypersensitivity there is an eosinophil infiltrate and that the eosinophils degranulate and are no longer identifiable within a few days. The factors that contribute to eosinophil degranulation are not clear.

The final observation about patch responses is that mast cell numbers in the skin can increase with prolonged antigen exposure. At 48 h we found no significant increase in mast cell numbers compared with control patches. However, by 6 days and more so at 10 days there was a marked increase in mast cells (Table 2). It is not clear whether this increase represents recruitment of cells or differentiation in situ. However, in animal models mast cell recruitment is generally T-cell dependent, which adds more evidence to suggest that T cells are involved in the skin response to persistent allergen exposure.

Further evidence that lymphocytes may play an effector role in the skin comes from direct studies on T cells infiltrating the skin. It has been known for some years that lesions of eczema included mononuclear cells that were presumably lymphocytes. Leung and his colleagues [34] showed that these cells were T cells of the helper phenotype. More recently, it has been confirmed that allergen injection into the skin of atopic patients generally causes an infiltration of CD_4-positive lymphoytes [19]. These results pose the question: is the eosinophil infiltrate in the skin induced by chemotactic products released from mast cells or from T cells? Recent results have shown that PAF is very potent agent in recruiting eosinophils into the skin of atopic patients [24]. However, if the eosinophil infiltrate of patch responses were dependent on the release of PAF, this would not explain why we had no difficulty recruiting eosinophils into the skin of nonatopic individuals after passive transfer of IgE antibody [42]. Another aspect of the skin response is the role of Langerhans cells. It seems very likely that Langerhans cells play a major role in antigen presentation in the skin, particularly to T cells [10, 33]. It has been suggested that IgE plays a role in this antigen presentation; however, that is difficult to fit together with the many known contact sensitivities that do not involve antibodies of any isotype [5, 35].

Natural Exposure to Inhalant Allergens and the Symptoms of Atopic Eczema

The first observation suggesting that the environment was a significant cause of AE was the improvement in hospital. Before the introduction of steroids hospital admission was commonly necessary for patients with AE, and it was well-recognized that the patients improved even without a significant change in their treatment. In 1932 Rost reported that patients with AE would improve if they lived in a climate chamber which was essentially dust free [55]. More recently, during experiments on long-term allergen avoidance and asthma we also admitted mite-allergic patients with AE to "allergen-free" rooms. The results were generally very good, and as with asthma the time taken for improvement was very variable. Some children with extensive, chronically excoriated skin stop scratching their skin within 2 days and show extensive healing within 1 week. It is possible to monitor this improvement by measuring human serum proteins on skin scales in their bedding (see Fig. 3). By

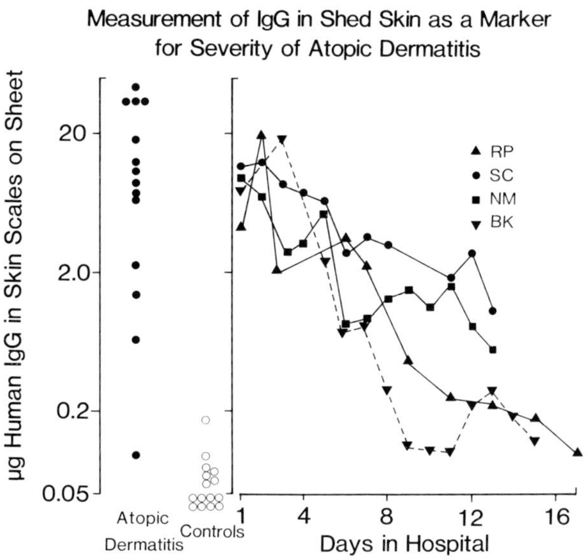

Fig. 3. Radioimmunoassay for IgG in skin scales vacuum cleaned off sheets of patients with atopic dermatitis. Bottom sheet of a hospital bed was cleaned for 2 min with a hand-held vacuum cleaner with a special adaptor to collect scales and dust onto a tissue [63]. The total dust and skin scales were extracted in 15 ml of buffered saline with 0.1% Tween and 0.3% bovine serum albumin. IgG was assayed by double antibody inhibition RIA [47]; values are given as the total IgG extracted. The maximum values are given for 14 patients, and all values are shown for 8 controls who were sampled once or more often. Repeated samples are shown for four patients whose eczema improved progressively in hospital.

contrast, one 20-year-old patient who had used fluorinated steroids on his face and body for years took months before his skin stopped burning. Our impression is that at least 80% of mite-allergic adults with AE experience dramatic improvement in their symptoms when they are admitted to "allergen-free" conditions. These admissions allow some preliminary estimates of the level of mite allergen that can cause or exacerbate AE and also of the decrease necessary to produce improvement. The mean level of Der p I in the hospital was ≤ 0.2 µg/g, while in the patients' houses 15 of 16 studied had > 10 µg Der p I/g in their bedding. We recently studied a group of patients in Virginia and found similar mite allergen levels in the houses of patients with mite allergy and AE (see Table 3). Some of the levels of allergen found in these houses were very high, and they are certainly comparable to those found in the UK.

It has been suggested that the houses of patients with AE are less well kept than average. However, it is clear that *very* high levels, i.e., > 50 µg of mite allergen/g, can be found in dust from carpets or bedding in houses that are apparently well kept.

The big issue from a practical standpoint is whether allergen-specific treatment should be part of the normal management of AE. Our own clinical view is that allergen avoidance pursued aggressively is beneficial for mite-allergic patients. Recent progress in understanding mites has helped to refine the advice that should be given to these patients. In particular, mattresses must be encased (vacuum cleaning mattresses is neither effective for realistic); all bedding including pillows and toys must

Table 3. IgE antibody to house dust mites and exposure to dust mite allergens of patients with atopic eczema in Virginia[a]

Patient		Total serum IgE	IgE anti-mite-antibodies[b] (RAST units/ml) D. pt	D. farinae	Group I[c] mite allergen (µg/g dust)
JB	42/F	8 712	2 250	1 472	3.0
LR	30/F	10 008	2 325	1 150	–
BR	42/M	7 956	7 100	9 366	12.0
GS	29/M	6 28	3 800	4 020	39.6
JL	36/M	1 601	60	48	9.4
VM	44/F	3 150	3 400	2 900	–
VF	15/F	5 760	4 000	10 370	36.7
MT	5/F	1 962	19	43	26.8
PO'M	2/M	11 754	12 200	16 550	43.2
YM	4/M	>20 000	2 800	8 000	38.0
LW	27/F	6 466	970	3 000	304.0
EM	3.5/M	1 254	1 240	740	9.1
Controls		<200	<12	<12	–

[a] Values shown are for 12 patients with moderate to severe atopic dermatitis seen at the University of Virginia who had positive skin tests to dust mite.

[b] IgE antibodies to *Dermatophagoides pteronyssinus* were measured using RAST with a *D. farinae* control curve. The units of IgE antibody equal approximately 0.1 ng IgE (see [51]).

[c] Group I mite allergen is the maximum level found in dust from the patient's house. Values are the sum of Der p I and Der f I/g dust assayed by two-site monocloncal antibody ELISA [37].

be washed at hot temperature (i.e., 57°C) at least every 10 days; and bedroom carpets should be removed if possible. The advantage of this approach is that if done correctly, it requires much less routine work than previous protocols. The next problem comes with carpets and upholstered furniture which cannot be replaced. Decreasing humidity in the house can help to reduce mite growth, but it may be more realistic to recommend some method of killing mites. Several different preparations are currently under trial including pirimiphos methyl or benzyl benzoate which kill mites and tannic acid which can inactivate mite allergens (see Platts-Mills and Chapman [46]). With the availability of acaricides and a better understanding of mites, a successful approach to reducing allergens in houses is now possible. It is clear that a controlled trial of allergen avoidance at home in the treatment of AE is necessary to establish this form of treatment. Such a trial is now realistic for the first time.

The only other form of allergen-specific treatment is desensitization therapy. As discussed previously, the general impression was that injections of allergen often made the disease worse (which makes the case for not using injections but certainly does not argue against these allergens being causally related to the disease!). However, there are allergists in the USA who use desensitization for AE and are convinced that it is beneficial. It is possible that the effectiveness of desensitization depends on the severity of the disease and that only relatively mild cases respond. Alternatively, it may be that as with rhinitis it is a mistake to start desensitization when a patient is exposed to high levels of antigen, which in most cases of AE in older children or adults, includes mite antigen. Thus, it is possible that desensitization therapy should be reevaluated for AE in patients who have already carried out allergen avoidance measures.

Conclusions

It has been known for many years that most adult patients with AE have positive skin tests to house dust extract. In addition, Louis Tuft had argued forcefully that house dust exposure exacerbated the disease, that patients improved in hospital because they were no longer exposed to house dust and that cleaning houses was a useful form of treatment. It is now clear that house dust sensitivity translates into high levels of IgE antibody specific for several different proteins derived from dust mites. In addition, these patients can be highly allergic to other inhalant allergens, i.e., cats, pollens, or fungi. Although some patients with AE have rhinitis and/or asthma, many of them only have AE. It is difficult to take seriously the argument that IgE antibodies are *not* relevant to AE *because* they are explained by other allergic diseases. Applying allergen to the skin of these patients can produce an eczematous response if the allergen is applied for at least 24 h. Thus, it seems likely that the reason why skin tests usually produce only an urticarial reaction must be because injected allergen is "removed" or neutralized by an influx of serum. The delayed nature of the eczematous response to patch testing these patients does much to explain why they do not realize that house dust contributes to their eczema. If a patient responding to something as ubiquitous as house dust, but the response takes between 6 h and 48 h, there is little chance that she or he will connect the two events. Indeed, it appears to be a common misconception that allergic or atopic diseases, because they are associated with immediate skin tests, should show an immediate relationship to exposure. In fact, each of the three diseases associated with exposure to inhalants, i.e. seasonal rhinitis, asthma, and AE, has many features both clinically and pathologically reminiscent of a chronic inflammatory disease. Thus, there is a series of observations that patients with AE are allergic to house dust allergens and are commonly exposed to these allergens and that persistent exposure of their skin can produce eczema.

The view that food allergy is an important cause of AE in young children has recently been strengthened by a series of experiments using double-blind placebo-controlled food challenge. These experiments have established unequivocally that ingested food can exacerbate skin rash in children with AE who have specific IgE antibodies [58, 59]. The results imply that allergen entering the bloodstream can exacerbate the skin rash. This is important for inhalant allergens since it has been proved that allergen inhaled through the nose can enter the circulation and produce an urticarial response in a skin site passively sensitized with IgE antibodies [31]. Thus, it is perfectly possible that allergen inhaled through the nose and absorbed can exacerbate AE. Indeed, anecdotal experiences suggest that this route may be very important in mite- or cat-allergic individuals. One patient who was aware of a rapid (i.e., within 10 min) onset of pruritis and reddening of the rash on his limbs after entering a house with a cat was able to stay in the house for over an hour without symptoms when he wore a mask which filtered the air that he was breathing. The patch test results show that allergen applied to the skin *can* produce a patch of eczema; they do not answer whether this route is important under natural circumstances. The reasons for thinking that direct exposure of the skin may be important are that bedding dust is often found to contain high levels of mite allergen (i.e., > 10 μg Der p I/g) and because in some patients simply cleaning their bedding produces benefit [50]. Also, in thinking about the reasons why these patients develop such high levels of IgE antibodies it seems likely that entry of allergen through the skin is an important stimulus. If the skin is an important route of entry of allergen in patients with AE, it seems possible that IgE production occurs in the lymph nodes draining the skin (which are often enlarged in these patients). At present, it seems likely that both inhaled allergen and direct contact with dust allergens contributes to the dermatitis. Since healthy skin is relatively impermeable to allergens, it is possible that direct contact has an increasing role in skin that is already inflamed. The fact that some sites in the body become involved with eczema repeatedly over many months or years may reflect changes in the local blood vessels and thus be related to the inhaled route more than to direct contact.

The detailed immunological and inflammatory events that lead to the development of an eczematous patch are not clear. However, there is no evidence to suggest that antigens in house dust contribute to either AE or asthma *unless* the individual has an IgE antibody response. Mast cell or basophil triggering via IgE antibodies can lead to the release of prostaglandins and leukotrienes as well as histamine. The arachidonic acid metabolites may either contribute directly or by recruiting cells such as eosinophils. On the other hand, we know that these patients have sensitized T cells and that T cells are part of the infiltrate of AE [34, 53]. T cells could contribute both by local production of inflammatory factors and also by recruiting other cells. T cells are not only capable of recruiting basophils and eosinophils to a local site but are probably a major source of IL-5 which could act to stimulate systemic eosinophilia [36, 60].

There is a large amount of circumstantial evidence that most older children and adults with AE are both allergic to and exposed to inhalant allergens. Most of the observations used to argue against a role for inhalant allergens in AE do not appear convincing. Perhaps most importantly the argument that allergens only produce urticaria on the skin is now seen to be simplistic. To date, the evidence proving that inhaled allergens cause clinical eczema is not available; however, background experiments have been done, and it is now possible to design experiments to prove the point. It is essential that controlled trials of exposure or avoidance be carried out to establish the role of inhalant allergens. In addition, avoidance experiments could prove the usefulness of cleaning houses as a first line treatment for AE.

References

1. Aalberse RC, van de Gaag R, van Leeuven J (1983) Serologic aspects of IgG4 antibodies. 1. Prolonged immunization results in an IgG4-restricted response. J Immunol 130: 722–728
2. Aas K (1978) The diagnosis of hypersensitivity to ingested foods: reliability of skin prick testing and the radioallergosorbent test with different materials. Clin Allergy 8: 39–50
3. Adinoff AD, Tellez P, Clark RAF (1988) Atopic dermatitis and aeroallergen contact sensitivity. J Allergy Clin Immunol 81: 736–742
4. Atherton DJ (1981) Allergy and atopic eczema, I and II. Clin Exp Dermatol 6: 191, 317–326
5. Barker JNWN, Alegre VA, MacDonald DM (1988) Surface-bound immunoglobulin E on antigen-presenting cells in cutaneous tissue of atopic dermatitis. J Invest Dermatol 90: 117–121
6. Barnetson RS, Merrett TG, Ferguson A (1981) Studies on hyperimmunoglobulinaemia E in atopic diseases with particular reference to food allergens. Clin Exp Immunol 46: 54–60
7. Blackley CH (1959) Experimental researches in the causes and nature of catarrhus aestivus (hay fever or hay asthma). Dawson, London, pp 57–58 (reprinted from Bailliere Tindall & Cox 1873)
8. Boetcher DA, Leonard EJ (1973) Basophil chemotaxis: augmentation by a factor from stimulated lymphocyte cultures. Immunol Commun 2: 421–429
9. Brostoff J, Roitt IM (1969) Cell mediated (delayed) hypersensitivity in patients with summer hay fever. Lancet ii: 1269
10. Bruijnzeel-Koomen CAFM (1989) Patch test reactions to aeroallergens: a working model for the pathogenesis of atopic dermatitis. Thesis, Rijksuniversiteit, Utrecht
11. Bruijnzeel-Koomen CAFM, van Wichen DF, Spry CJF, Venge P, Bruijnzeel PLB (1988) Active participation of eosinophils in patch test reactions to inhalant allergens in patients with atopic dermatitis. Br J Dermatol 118: 229–238
12. Buckley RH (1985) Atopic dermatitis. In: Kaplan AP (ed) Allergy. Churchill Livingstone, Edinburgh, pp 417–438
13. Chapman MD, Platts-Mills TAE (1980) Purification and characterization of the major allergen from *Dermatophagoides pteronyssinus*, antigen P_1. J Immunol 125: 587–592
14. Chapman MD, Rowntree S, Mitchell EB, DiPrisco de Fuenmajor MC, Platts-Mills TAE (1983) Quantitative assessments of IgG and IgE antibodies to inhalant allergens in patients with atopic dermatitis. J Allergy Clin Immunol 72: 27–33
15. Chapman MD, Sutherland WM, Platts-Mills TAE (1984) Recognition of two *Dermatophagoides pteronyssinus* specific epitopes on Antigen P_1 using monoclonal antibodies:

binding to each epitope can be inhibited by serum from dust mite allergic patients. J Immunol 133: 2488–2495
16. Chobot R (1951) Pediatric allergy. McGraw Hill, New York p 143
17. Dvorak HF, Mihm MC Jr (1972) Basophilic leukocytes in allergic contact dermatitis. J Exp Med 135:235–254
18. Feinberg SM (1939) Seasonal atopic dermatitis. Arch Dermatol Syphilol 40:200–204
19. Frew AJ, Kay AB (1988) The relationship between infiltrating CD4+ lymphocytes, activated eosinophils, and the magnitude of the allergen-induced late phase cutaneous reaction in man. J Immunol 141:4158–4164
20. Gondo A, Saeki N, Tokuda Y (1986) Challenge reactions in atopic dermatitis after percutaneous entry of mite antigen. Br J Dermatol 115:485–493
21. Hanifin JM (1984) Atopic dermatitis. J Allergy Clin Immunol 73:211–222
22. Hastie R, Heroy JH, Levy DA (1979) Basophil leukocytes and mast cells in human nasal secretions and scrapings studied by light microscopy. Lab Invest 40:554–561
23. Henoque E, Gaillard J (1981) Cutaneous basophil hypersensitivity in atopic dermatitis. Clin Allergy 11: 13–20
24. Henoque E, Vargaftig BB (1988) Skin eosinophilia in atopic patients. J Allergy Clin Immunol 81:691–695
25. Hill IW (1934) Chronic atopic eczema (neurodermatitis) in childhood. JAMA 103:1420–1434
26. Hoffman DR, Yamamoto FY, Sellar B et al. (1975) Specific IgE antibodies in atopic eczema. J Allergy Clin Immunol 55:256–265
27. Ishizaka K, Ishizaka T, Hornbrook MM (1967) Allergen binding activity of γE, γG and γA, antibodies in sera from atopic patients: in vitro measurements of reaginic antibody. J Immunol 98:490–495
28. Johansson SGO, Juhlin L (1970) Immunoglobulin E in "healed" atopic dermatitis and after treatment with corticosteroids and azathioprine. Br J Dermatol 82:10–17
29. Johnson EE, Irons JS, Patterson R, Roberts M (1974) Serum IgE concentration in atopic dermatitis. Relationship to severity of disease and presence of atopic respiratory disease. J Allergy Clin Immunol 54:94–99
30. Juhlin I. Johansson SGO, Bennich H, Hogman C, Thyresson N (1969) Immunoglobulin E in dermatoses. Levels in atopic dermatitis and urticaria. Arch Dermatol 100:12–23
31. Kontou-Karakitsos K, Salvaggio JE, Mathews KP (1975) Comparative nasal absorption of allergens in atopic and non-atopic subjects. J Allergy Clin Immunol 55:241–250
32. Leiferman K, Ackerman S, Sampson M, Haugen M, Venencie P, Gleich G (1985) Dermal deposition of eosinophil granule major basic protein in atopic dermatitis. N Engl J Med 313:282–285
33. Leung D, Geha R (1986) Immunoregulatory abnormalities in atopic dermatitis. Clin Rev Allergy 4:67–86
34. Leung DYM, Bhan AK, Schneeberger EE, Geha RS (1983) Characterization of the mononuclear cell infiltrate in atopic dermatitis using monoclonal antibodies. J Allergy Clin Immunol 71:47–56
35. Leung YM, Schneeberger EE, Siraganian RP, Geha RS, Bhan AK (1987) The presence of IgE on macrophages and dendritic cells infiltrating into the skin lesion of atopic dermatitis. Clin Immunol Immunopathol 42:328–337
36. Lopez AF, Sanderson CJ, Gamble JR, Campbell HD, Young IG, Vadas MA (1988) Recombinant human interleukin-5 is a selective activator of human eosinophil function. J Exp Med 157:219–227
37. Luczynska CM, Arruda LK, Platts-Mills TAE, Miller JD, Lopez M, Chapman MD (1989) A two-site monoclonal antibody ELISA for the quantitation of the major *Dermatophagoides* spp. allergens, Der p I and Der f I. J Immunol Methods 118:227–235
38. Merrett J, Barnetson R, Murr M, Merrett T (1984) Total and specific IgG_4 antibody levels in atopic eczema. Clin Exp Immunol 56:645–662
39. Mitchell EB, Askenase PW (1982) Suppression of T cell mediated cutaneous basophil hypersensitivity by serum from guinea pigs immunized with mycobacterial adjuvant. J Exp Med 156:159–172
40. Mitchell EB, Askenase PW (1983) Basophils in human disease. Clin Rev Allergy 1:427–148
41. Mitchell EB, Crow J, Chapman MD, Jouhal SS, Pope FM, Platts-Mills TAE (1982) Basophils in allergen-induced patch tests sites in atopic dermatitis. Lancet i:127–130
42. Mitchell EB, Crow J, Rowntree S, Webster DB, Platts-Mills TAE (1984) Cutaneous basophil hypersensitivity to inhalant allergens: local tansfer of basophil accumulation with immune serum but not IgE antibody. J Invest Dermatol 83:290–295
43. Mitchell EB, Crow J, Williams G, Platts-Mills TAE (1986) Increase in skin mast cells following chronic house dust mite exposure. Br J Dermatol 114:65–73
44. O'Hehir RE, Eckels DD, Frew AJ, Kay AB, Lamb JR (1988) MHC class II restriction specificity of cloned human T lymphocytes reactive with *Dermatophagoides farinae* (house dust mite). Immunology 64:627–631
45. Ohman S, Johansson SG (1974) Allergen specific IgE in atopic dermatitis. Acta Derm Venereol (Stockh) 54:283–290
46. Platts-Mills TAE, Chapman MD (1987) Dust mites: immunology, allergic disease, and environmental control. J Allergy Clin Immunol 80:755–775
47. Platts-Mills TAE, Ishizaka K (1975) IgG and IgA diphtheria antitoxin responses from human tonsil lymphocytes. J Immunol 114:1058–1064
48. Platts-Mills TAE, Snajdr MJ (1977) Studies of the half life of IgE, IgA and IgG antibodies to pollen antigens. Allergol Immunopathol 5:340–341
49. Platts-Mills TAE, Snajdr MJ, Ishizaka K, Frankland AW (1978) Measurement of IgE antibody by an antigen binding assay: correlation with PK activity and IgG and IgA antibodies to allergens. J Immunol 120:1201–1212
50. Platts-Mills TAE, Mitchell EB, Rowntree S, Chapman MD, Wilkins SR (1983) The role of dust mite allergens in atopic dermatitis. Clin Exp Dermatol 8:233–247
51. Pollart SM, Chapman MD, Fiocco GP, Rose G, Platts-Mills TAE (1989) Epidemiology of acute asthma: IgE antibodies to common inhalant allergens as a risk factor for Emergency Room visits. J Allergy Clin Immunol 83:875–882
52. Rasmussen JE, Provost TT (1978) Atopic dermatitis. In: Middleton E, Reed C, Ellis E (eds) Allergy principles and practice. Mosby, St Louis, pp 1039–1054
53. Rawle FC, Mitchell EB, Platts-Mills TAE (1984) T cell responses to the major allergen from the house dust mite *Dermatophagoides pteronyssinus* antigen P_1: comparison of patients with asthma, atopic dermatitis, and perennial rhinitis. J Immunol 133:195–201
54. Rawle FC, Platts-Mills TAE, Mitchell EB (1985) Quantitative aspects of the T cell proliferation response to Antigen P_1 from *D. pteronyssinus*: suppression by added histamine and limited effects of basophil depletion. Clin Exp Immunol 59:101–109

55. Rost GA (1932) Über Erfahrungen mit der allergenfreien Kammer nach Storm van Leeuwen: insbesondere in der Spätperiode der exsudativen Diathese. Arch Dermatol Syphilol 155:297–308
56. Rowntree S, Cogswell JJ, Platts-Mills TAE, Mitchell EB (1985) The development of IgE and IgG antibodies to food and inhalant allergens in children at risk of allergic disease. Arch Dis Child 60:727–735
57 Rowntree S, Platts-Mills TAE, Cogswell JJ, Mitchell EB (1987) A subclass IgG_4 specific antigen binding radioimmunoassay (RIA): comparison between IgG and IgG_4 antibodies to food and inhaled antigens, in adult atopic dermatitis, after desensitization treatment and during development of antibody responses in children. J Allergy Clin Immunol 80:622–630
58. Sampson HA (1983) Role of immediate food hypersensitivity in the pathogenesis of atopic dermatitis. J Allergy Clin Immunol 71:473–480
59. Sampson HA (1988) The role of food allergy and mediator release in atopic dermatitis. J Allergy Clin Immunol 81: 635–645
60. Sanderson CD, Warren J, Strath M (1985) Identification of a lymphokine that stimulates eosinophil differentiation in vitro. J Exp Med 162:60–68
61. Schloss OM (1915) Allergy to common foods. Arch Pediatr 32:349–355
62. Sulzberger MB, Vaughan WT (1934) Experiments in silk hypersensitivity and inhalation of allergen in atopic dermatitis (neurodermatitis disseminatus). J Allergy 5:544–560
63. Tovey ER, Chapman MD, Wells CW, Platts-Mills TAE (1981) The distribution of dust mite allergens in the houses of patients with asthma. Am Rev Respir Dis 124:630–635
64. Tuft LA (1949) Importance of inhalant allergen in atopic dermatitis. J Invest Dermatol 12:211–219
65. Voorhorst R, Spieksma FThM, Varekamp H, Leupen MJ, Lyklema AW (1967) The house dust mite (*Dermatophagoides pteronyssinus*) and the allergens it produces. Identity with the house dust allergen. J Allergy 39:325–337
66. Ward PA, Dvorak HF, Cohen S, Yoshida T, Data R, Selvaggio SS (1975) Chemotaxis of basophils by lymphocyte-dependent and lymphocyte-independent mechanisms. J Immunol 114:1523–1531

Role of Food Allergy in Atopic Eczema

J. Bernhisel-Broadbent and H. A. Sampson

Introduction

Attempts to identfy the primary pathogenic mechanism(s) in atopic eczema (AE) have been unsuccesful to date. In patients with AE, itching is the dominant symptom and the driving force that leads to the damaging excoriations and skin lichenification characteristic of this disease. Numerous factors triggering flares (itching) have been identified [1]. Patients with AE fulfilling the diagnostic criteria of Hanifin and Rajka [2] are a heterogenous group, but substantial evidence exists that IgE-dependent responses play a pathogenic role in a large number of them. This article will focus on the role of immunologically mediated reactions to food in the pathogenesis of AE. A recent study reported that food allergy is an important trigger factor in the development of AE in approximately one-third of children [3].

Atopic Eczema: Allergic (IgE-Mediated) Etiology

The earliest association of AE with allergy was made in 1892 by Besnier [4], who described a hereditary pruritic skin disorder that occurred commonly with asthma and hay fever and was characterized by its chronic or relapsing course. Wise and Sulzberger [5] coined the term "atopic eczema" in 1933, to emphasize the association of asthma, allergic rhinitis, and eczematous rash, i.e., the "allergic triad". The potential pathogenic role of IgE in this disorder is suggested by the following clinical and laboratory observations: Two-thirds of patients with AE have a positive family history (first-degree relative) for atopic disease [6], and 50%–80% of patients have or will develop allergic rhinitis and/or asthma [7]. Serum IgE concentrations, which correlate roughly with disease severity, are elevated in 80%–90% of patients with AE [8], and most patients have positive prick skin tests or radioallergosorbent tests (RAST), indicating the presence of antigen-specific IgE molecules to various environmental or dietary antigens [9]. Numerous studies correlate eczematous flares with exposure to certain foods and inhalants [10].

The pathogenic role of IgE in AE is further supported by the recent elucidation of the IgE-mediated, cutaneous, late-phase response. Previously, skin biopsies from patients with AE were thought to be inconsistent with an IgE-mediated mechanism because they revealed a non-specific dermatitis characterized by a lymphocytic infiltrate, which appeared indicative of a type IV cell-mediated response. Acute skin lesions of AE are described histologically as having spongiosis, epidermal hyperplasia, and ballooning of the keratinocytes secondary to intracellular edema. Mast cell and basophil numbers are normal, and eosinophils are rare. Chronic skin lesions have moderate to marked hyperplasia of the epidermis with elongation of the rete ridges and prominent hyperkeratosis. Spongiosis is variable, and the number of mast cells and Langerhans cells is significantly increased. Eosinophils are sparse. Demyelination and fibrosis of cutaneous nerves are observed at all levels of the dermis. Capillary numbers are often increased, and their walls may be thickened. Although this pattern is not considered typical of IgE-mediated responses, it is consistent with an end-stage, cutaneous, IgE-dependent, "late-phase" reaction.

IgE-Mediated, Cutaneous, Late-Phase Reaction

The cutaneous, late-phase reaction of IgE-mediated hypersensitivity was first described by Dolovich et al. [11] and by numerous others since [12–14]. These investigators have demonstrated that within minutes of encountering an allergen, mast cells and basophils become activated by antigen-induced bridging of IgE molecules, which are bound to the cell membrane by high-affinity FcE receptors. Mast cell mediators are released and cause an initial flare (vasodilation) and wheal (capillary leakiness) lesion that peaks at 15–30 min and then becomes less distinct. By 90 min the lesion is diffuse, erythematous, and edematous but largely asymptomatic. Clinically, mild pruritus begins by 4 h, moderate pruritus, erythema, tenderness, and warmth of the involved skin develop over 6–12 h, and then symptoms slowly resolve over 24–48 h. The histologic appearance of the late-phase lesion begins with an influx of neutrophils and eosinophils within 2–4 h after the immediate reaction. This influx is promoted by neutrophil and eosinophil chemotactic factors released from mast cells, endothelial cells, and possibly other cell sources. Once present, the neutrophils and eosinophils release other mediators of inflammation (platelet activating factor, leukotrienes, major basic protein, O_2^-, etc.) which perpetuate the response.

Skin biopsies obtained after 6–8 h reveal primarily mononuclear cells and eosinophils, and lesser numbers of neutrophils, basophils, and mast cells. During the ensuing 24–48 h the infiltrating cell population again changes, and later biopsies show primarily a mononuclear cell infiltrate, which is virtually indistinguishable from a type IV cell-mediated response.

Antigen interaction with surface-bound IgE may activate other cell types. Low-affinity FcE receptors have been identified on B cells, T cells, monocytes, macrophages, eosinophils, and platelets [15–17]. Recently, Bruynzeel-Kooman et al. [18] demonstrated the presence of IgE molecules on epidermal Langerhans cells in biopsies of lichenified and acutely eczematous skin in 20 of 23 patients with AE. This finding appears specific for AE; IgE molecules were not found on Langerhans cells in patients with contact dermatitis, sehistosomiasis, or allergic asthma. Langerhans cells are involved in antigen presentation and the synthesis of various mediators of inflammation, especially prostaglandin D_2 [19]. Thus, IgE-antigen-induced activation of a variety of "non-mast cells" could lead to cytokine release and further augmentation of the IgE-mediated late-phase reaction.

Previously, eosinophils were not considered to play a pathogenic role in the skin lesions of AE because they are not abundant in histologic sections of eczematous lesions. However, their participation is suggested by the deposition of eosinophil major basic protein (MBP), the most abundant protein of eosinophilic granules. MBP is a cytolytic protein secreted almost exclusively by eosinophils and is known to damage skin epithelial cells [20] and promote further mast cell degranulation [21]. Leiferman et al. [22] performed skin biopsies on 20 patients with AE. Utilizing an antibody specific for MBP and an indirect fluorescein-staining technique, biopsies of eczematous skin lesions were shown to have extensive extracellular MBP deposition in a fibrillar pattern in the superficial dermis. MBP was not found in biopsy specimens from uninvolved skin sites in these same patients, indicating that this eosinophil product was the result of specific deposition and not due to nonspecific sequestration. Control studies on patients with contact dermatitis revealed no dermal deposition of MBP. This study provided further evidence that the typical mononuclear cell infiltrate in lesions of AE may result from IgE-induced, cutaneous, late-phase reactions, with eosinophil degranulation and dermal deposition of MBP.

Food Hypersensitivity

The role of IgE-mediated food hypersensitivity in AE is controversial because of the lack of well-controlled studies and the frequently variable clinical improvement observed while patients are maintained on food elimination diets. In the 1920s and 1930s, Walzer and his colleagues [23, 24] demonstrated that ingested food antigens rapidly cross the gastrointestinal mucosal barrier and are quickly disseminated to cutaneous mast cells via the circulation. These investigators passively sensitized nonallergic volunteers with an intradermal injection of sera from either egg- or fish-allergic individuals. Then 24 h later these nonallergic volunteers ingested egg or fish, and within several minutes to 2 h, they developed a wheal and flare response at the sensitized site but not at control sites.

Engman's case report in 1935 [25] provided more convincing evidence for a pathogenic role of food hypersensitivity in AE. The report details the course of a wheat-sensitive child with AE who was hospitalized and placed on a wheat-free diet until his skin symptoms cleared. An occlusive dressing was placed on one-half of the child's body prior to instituting an oral wheat challenge. Following the ingestion of wheat, the patient experienced marked generalized pruritus, but eczematous lesions developed only on the part of his body that was exposed and traumatized by scratching.

In order to address further the etiological role of IgE-mediated food hypersensitivity in AE, we utilized double-blind, placebo-controlled, oral food challenges (DBPCFC) in a controlled hospital environment with 210 patients with severe AE refractory to conventional therapy. Sixty percent of this selected referral population was found to have clinically significant allergic reactions to food.

Details of the study protocol have been published previously [26]. Briefly, 7–10 days prior to admission to the hospital Clinical Research Unit (RR-30 or RR-00052), the children entering the study were restricted from all suspected food allergens and antihistamines. The patients were also taken off β-agonists 12 h prior to admission. No patient had received oral corticosteroids for at least 1 month prior to admission. On the day of admission, the patients were tested to a battery of food extracts applied by the prick technique to determine which foods would be administered in the DBPCFC and to standardize skin test results. Commercial glycerinated extracts were used (1:20 weight/volume; Greer Laboratories, Lenior, NC, USA). A wheal reaction 3 mm greater than the negative saline control was considered positive. Based on positive prick skin tests and suggestive history, the patients underwent DBPCFC. Patients with a "convincing" history of anaphylaxis were not challenged. A history of anaphylaxis was accepted as "convincing" only when the allergic reaction occurred immediately after the isolated ingestion of the suspect food, was potentially life threatening (laryngeal edema, severe wheezing, and/or hypotension), and required emergency evaluation and treatment.

Egg, peanut, milk, wheat, soy, and fish accounted for the majority (90%) of the positive skin tests. Foods frequently claimed to exacerbate AE such as strawberry, tomato, corn, citrus fruits, and chocolate rarely elicited a positive skin test. However, these foods may act directly as contact irritants to the skin.

In a previous study, it was concluded that a positive prick skin test is only suggestive of clinically relevant food hypersensitivity [27], necessitating a more definitive study to establish a diagnosis of food hypersensitivity. Conversely, a negative prick skin test was found to be an excellent means of excluding immediate food hypersensitivity in the pathogenesis of a patient's AE. The study also compared the results of RASTs with prick skin tests and determined that the RAST provides no advantage when used alone or in combination with prick skin tests in diagnosing food hypersensitivity. The RAST should be reserved for patients with such severe dermatitis that skin testing is impossible, or for patients who cannot tolerate discontinuation of their antihistamines.

Overall, 647 initial DBPCFC have been conducted in these 210 patients: 412 of the challenges (64%) were negative, and 235 were positive. Some 130 (62%) of the 210 children were determined to be food allergic. DBPCFC were not conducted in 25 instances. All patients had a strongly positive skin test to the food in question. No patient experienced a severe anaphylactic reaction during the DBPCFC, although several required antihistamines and inhaled β-agonists for severe pruritus and wheezing.

The symptoms induced by food challenges may be expressed in one or more target tissues. The basis of the preferential reactivity of one target organ over another in a food-allergic individual is unknown. Perhaps more surprising is the variation in target organ response to different food antigens within the same individual. Symptoms generally developed abruptly within 10–120 min of initiating the oral challenge. Cutaneous reactions occurred in 75% of positive challenges and consisted of a pruritic, erythematous, macular, or morbilliform rash, and commonly involved predilection sites. Gastrointestinal symptoms, characterized by nausea, vomiting, abdominal pain, and diarrhea, occurred in 45% of the challenges. Respiratory symptoms, manifested by wheezing, congestion, sneezing, and stridor, were induced in 53% of the challenges. Patients frequently develop symptoms during DBPCFC that were never suggested by their history. Several factors may account for this: The patient is restricted of the suspected allergen for at least 1 week which may overcome a partial desensitization, oral challenges are performed by giving the antigen on an empty stomach in pure form, the patients are off antihistamines, and the patient's skin is cleared sufficiently on the restriction diet and with intensive topical skin care to allow minor changes or development of a new rash to be more obvious. In the home setting these patients are subject to a variety of trigger factors and are receiving multiple daily ingestions of these allergens. Consequently, the resulting symptoms following ingestion blend into each other.

Some patients experiencing positive DBPCFC develop a slight temperature elevation and fall asleep soon after the reaction begins to subside. Food antigens reacting with IgE bound to cutaneous Langerhans cells or tissue macrophages could induce IL-1 secretion, which may account for these symptoms. Occasionally, patients developed pruritus and a less pronounced erythematous macular rash 4–8 h later, but these late reactions have always followed an initial immediate positive reaction.

It is commonly believed that patients with AE are allergic to a large number of foods. The majority (78%) of the children with food hypersensitivity documented by these DBPCFC is allergic to only one or two foods [28], despite the fact that most patients have positive prick skin tests to 3–6 food antigens out of a standard battery of 20 [29]. Although the Western diet consists of a wide variety of food antigens, six foods (egg, peanut, milk, fish, soy, and wheat) account for about 90% of the positive food challenges. Most identified food antigens are glycoproteins with similar molecular weights (20–60 K), are water soluble, and are resistant to heat, acid, and proteolytic enzymes.

Clinically relevant food hypersensitivity appears very specific despite the frequent skin test and RAST cross-reactivity among members of a botanical family or animal species. Of 69 patients, only 2 had clinical reactivity to more than one member of the legume family (peanut and soy; both patients lost their soy sensitivity within 2 years on a soy restriction diet) [30]. In our patient population, there was only one instance of intraspecies (milk and beef) clinical hypersensitivity. Consequently, the common practice of avoiding all legumes (e.g., soybean, pea, green bean, etc.) when a patient is allergic to peanuts or chicken if the patient is allergic to eggs is unwarranted and nutritionally unsound. Adherence to a food elimination diet is challenging and difficult, and therefore a diet restricting as few foods as possible improves compliance and ease in obtaining a nutritionally complete diet for the child.

The increased cutaneous pruritus and rash with positive oral food challenges was speculated to be the result of food antigen reacting with IgE-bearing cutaneous mast cells and leading to mediator release. This reasoning is supported by a previously published report in which only children experiencing positive DBPCFC developed a rise in plasma histamine level from a mean of 296 ± 80 pg/ml to 1055 ± 356 pg/ml ($P < 0.001$), whereas children having a negative or placebo challenge had no change in plasma histamine level [31]. There was no change in complement levels, basophil number, total basophil histamine content, or unstimulated basophil histamine release at any point prior, during, or after a positive oral food challenge. These results suggest that the rise in plasma histamine level predominantly reflects mast cell histamine release.

Two food-allergic patients whose skin lesions had cleared while they maintained appropriate food allergen-restricted diets were demonstrated to have MBP deposition after positive DBPCFC. Both patients developed a pruritic, morbilliform skin rash within 30–60 min. Skin biopsies from the provoked skin rash taken at 4 and 14 h revealed an infiltration of eosinophils and early MBP deposition. The dermal infiltrate contained more eosinophils and less prominent MBP deposition than was observed with the chronic lesions [22]. The unique presence of FcE receptors on Langerhans cells of patients with AE and the frequent improvement in patients with AE exposed to ultraviolet light (which selectively deactivates Langerhans cells) suggest a central role for Langerhans cells in the pathogenesis and another mechanism by which food antigen could contribute to pathogenic skin changes.

In a recent study, food-allergic patients with AE were found to have high "spontaneous" basophil histamine release in vitro [32]. Once the appropriate food allergen was excluded from the diet for 6–12 months and skin symptoms largely improved, the spontaneous basophil histamine release normalized. This spontaneous basophil releasibility was associated with the "spontaneous" production of histamine releasing factor by peripheral blood mononuclear cells in vitro. It was speculated that the histamine releasing factor could account for the increased basophil releasibility reported in some patients with AE [33] and could lead to a state of cutaneous hyperreactivity similar to that in the airways of patients with IgE-mediated asthma.

The appropriate diagnosis and exclusion of foods eliciting a positive reaction by DBPCFC in these study patients resulted in significant symptomatic improvement compared with children not adhering to their diet or children with no demonstrable food hypersensitivity. This study showed that the diagnosis of food hypersensitivity and the subsequent elimination of foods provoking hypersensitivity responses can favorably affect the course of AE. Therefore, any child with severe AE who is unresponsive to routine therapy (lubricating creams, topical corticosteroids) should be evaluated for food hypersensitivity. This conclusion is further strengthened by the recent findings of Burks et al. [3]. Using a similar DBPCFC protocol, they determined that 35% of children with AE presenting to a university-based dermatology and allergy clinic were food allergic.

Recent evidence by Adinoff et al. [34] established that selected patients with AE might flare after cutaneous contact with various aeroallergens. The parents of our food-sensitive patients often report cutaneous symptoms after their child comes in contact with a food to which he or she is known to be allergic (i.e., a toddler handling "playdough" containing peanut butter). It is reasonable that in addition to ingestion of certain food allergens, topical contact, which can be extensive in a young child at meal time, may trigger an eczematous flare secondary to the pruritus induced.

Diagnosing Food Hypersensitivity in Patients with Atopic Eczema

A DBPCFC provides a scientifically acceptable method of diagnosing food hypersensitivity and is the standard for clinical research investigations. However, in a practice setting, a brief elimination diet may be tried if immediate food hypersensitivity is suspected after obtaining a careful history, physical examination, and skin testing. Any food implicated by the history to have caused a severe anaphylactic reaction should not be tested at home because of the potential of inducing anaphylactic shock [35]. The child may be placed on a diet which strictly eliminates foods suspected by history or prick skin tests for 2–3 weeks. Symptoms are recorded in a diary during the trial period. If unequivocal improvement is documented, foods felt least likely to be responsible are added back to the diet. If a clear deterioration in the patient's AE occurs, the food should be removed from the diet. If cause and effect can be so established, the patient should remain on the restriction diet unless it requires elimination of more than one "major" food (egg, milk, soy, wheat) and/or two or more "minor" foods (all others).

If severe symptoms persist on the elimination diet and food allergy is still in question, a brief trial (1–2 weeks) of a severely restricted diet may be undertaken. The following diets may be used: $<$ 4 months, milk substitute (Nutramigen®, Pregestemil®, or Vivonex®); 4–8 months, milk substitute, rice cereal (cereal labels should be read since many cereals contain milk and/or more than one grain), and pears; 9–24 months, same as 4–8 months plus rice, carrots, squash, and lamb; $>$ 2 years of age, same as 9–24 months plus fresh lettuce, potato, sunflower oil, tea, and sugar. If the elimination diet results are equivocal or several foods are implicated, the patient should be referred for blinded oral food challenges to establish the diagnosis. Widespread dietary restrictions are rarely necessary. Most families with children with severe AE are desperate for a cure, and given the current social and media popularity of food allergy, every effort must be made to make a correct diagnosis [36]. The institution of restriction diets is an enormous task and emotional burden to the patients and families, and unnecessarily restricted diets may lead to feeding disorders, as well as further disease secondary to nutritional deficiency [37].

Once food hypersensitivity is diagnosed, therapy is straightforward. The patient is placed on a diet strictly eliminating the offending food allergen. The assistance of a dietician is helpful in providing a nutritionally balanced diet. Instructing the patient and family to read food labels to find hidden sources of the suspect food (e.g., ovalbumin listed on an ice cream bar wrapper for an egg-sensitive patient) is also very useful. Antihistamines and epinephrine may modify the symptoms of an immediate food hypersensitivity reaction after an accidental ingestion, but they have no prophylactic role in the treatment of food allergy. Prevention of food allergen-induced symptoms with oral cromolyn has been advocated by some investigators. However, in a well-controlled, blinded trial of oral cromolyn in patients with "challenge-proven" food hypersensitivity, no benefit was demonstrated [38]. Other modalities for the diagnosis of food hypersensitivity such as sublingual provocation with drops of antigen extracts, subcutaneous provocation with varying concentrations of food extracts, and measurements of IgE-or IgG_4-specific antibody have never been shown to be useful or effective in controlled studies [39]. Treatment of food hypersensitivity with oral desensitization, immunotherapy, and rotational diets also have not been proven effective in controlled trials. In discussing these controversial procedures for the diagnosis and treatment of food allergy, Bock [40] emphasizes that patients may improve by healing and/or the placebo effect when the physician or provider convincingly suggests that the patient's condition will improve with the performance of expensive tests and treatments.

Natural History of Food Hypersensitivity

Roughly one-third of our patients with food allergy who have been rechallenged have lost their clinical sensitivity over 1–3 years [41]. Several investigators have reported similar findings in other patient populations with food hypersensitivity. Bock [42] reported negative challenges in 19% of children over 3 years of age with previously positive food challenges, and 44% of children less than 3 years of age with previously positive food challenges. Businco et al. [43] concluded that 32% of patients presenting with chronic diarrhea secondary to milk allergy lost their sensitivity over 4 years, and Esteban et al. [44] found that 29% of their food-allergic children developed tolerance to the incriminated food antigen over 3 years. The loss of clinical sensitivity appears to vary among antigens, with fish being more persistent than milk or soybean. Therefore, patients should be rechallenged every 1–2 years to document whether their food sensitivity has been lost, so that their restriction diets may be discontinued. All patients experiencing no reaction to both blinded and open challenge had the challenge food added back into their diets. There have been no recurrences of allergic symptoms or worsening of eczema in these patients. The reason clinically apparent food hypersensitivity is lost remains an enigma.

Role of Diet in the Prevention of Atopic Eczema and Atopic Disease

There is intense interest in the prevention of allergic disease by manipulation of the infant's diet and environment. Since Grulee and Sanford [45] reported a decrease in the incidence of AE in breast-fed infants in the 1930s, there have been numerous conflicting studies about the relative merits of breast feeding infants to prevent or delay the onset of atopic disease [46–48]. Unfortunately, the ideal study has not yet been completed [49] to determine (a) the extent or amount of benefit, if any, of allergy-preventive efforts in compliant families following a strict prophylaxis protocol; (b) the identification of the subgroup of patients in whom this effort would be most likely to benefit (e.g., infant with a highly atopic family history); (c) the preventative measures that are the most important (i.e., breast feeding, avoidance of aeroallergens) and practical in a normal family environment. Despite these shortcomings, the type of infant feeding and manipulation of the maternal diet during lactation are (at present) the only available methods by which patients can postpone/ decrease the development of food allergy and AE.

The choice of breast milk as the ideal nutritional source for the potentially atopic infant appears logical for several reasons. Many protective mechanisms which limit the uptake of intestinal antigens in the newborn are underdeveloped [50], and human breast milk contains cellular and noncellular factors that facilitate the maturation of the intestinal mucosa [51]. This effect has been demonstrated in several studies which report lower serum IgG and IgM in exclusively breast-fed infants compared with formula-fed infants by 9 months of age [52], and lower serum agglutinins to milk and soy in breast-fed infants during the first 3 months of life [53]. In addition, breast milk secretory IgA is postulated by Machtinger and Moss [54] to protect the nursing infant passively by binding foreign antigens and thus lessening the antigenic load presented to the newborn's gastrointestinal surface. These investigators found that of 57 mother-infant pairs entered into their study, the 11 infants with the highest allergy symptom scores all received breast milk with total and cow's milk-specific secretory IgA antibody concentrations below the median value.

Several recent prospective studies that evaluated exclusive breast feeding (no solid food or supplementation) for at least 4 months support this proposed benefit and show that the incidence of AE was significantly decreased in breast-fed infants [55, 56]. For the most part, studies demonstrating no benefit of breast feeding are generally flawed by a short duration of breast feeding and non random assignment to study groups. A recent study by Lindfors and Enocksson [57] has raised new interest in the role of high-dose tolerance. These researchers concluded that initial and early regular feedings with a cow's milk formula followed by a gradual replacement with prolonged breast feeding reduced the development of allergy symptoms in 112 infants in the first 18 months of age to 18%, compared with 33% in the 104 exclusively breast-fed infant group.

The proposed benefit of breast feeding is further clouded by the confirmation that infants can react to food antigens transmitted in their mother's breast milk [58, 59]. Six infants (aged 2.5–6 months) who developed classic infantile AE while being exclusively breast fed were evaluated in our study. These infants all had positive prick skin tests to egg and showed complete clearing of their skin while their mothers maintained a strict egg-free diet. Four of these infants underwent an in-hospital indirect food challenge in which the mothers were fed egg, and each infant developed an eczematoid rash within 4–36 h afterwards. This evidence and findings from recent studies support the recommendation of placing selected mothers on diets that avoid highly allergenic foods during the period of lactation. Hattevig et al. [60] observed the delayed onset of allergic disease, as well as milder disease in infants of mothers who strictly avoided eggs, milk, and fish for the first 3 months of lactation compared with babies of mothers on a regular diet. Falth-Magnusson and Kjellman [61] also studied the effects of manipulating the maternal diet during the last trimester of pregnancy. In this study, four different diets were compared in 400 pregnancies: total avoidance of egg, milk, and fish; avoidance of visible amounts of these foods; normal diet; and a diet consisting of at least one egg and one liter of cow's milk daily. There was no difference in the cord blood IgE concentrations or clinical symptoms of allergy in any infant group during the first 18 months of life. This study concluded unequivocally that antigen-avoidance diets during the third trimester of pregnancy are unwarranted, especially because of the inherent nutritional hazards to the mother and developing fetus.

Conclusion

Current evidence clearly implicates a pathogenic role for food hypersensitivity in a significant portion of children with AE. The continued elucidation of IgE-mediated immediate and late-phase reactions has increased our understanding of the mechanism by which food antigens can behave as trigger factors in these children and lead to increased cutaneous pruritus and resultant skin damage. Contrary to popular belief, the majority of these children are allergic to only 1 or 2 foods, and approximately one-third of these patients outgrow their food allergy within 3 years on antigen restriction diets. Despite conflicting studies on the prevention of AE and food allergy in infants, it seems reasonable to encourage exclusive breast feeding for 6 months in infants from highly atopic families and to restrict lactating mothers' diets from highly allergic foods in select instances.

References

1. Hanifin JM (1988) Atopic dermatitis. In: Middleton E, Reed CE, Ellis EF, Adkinson NF, Yunginger JW (eds) Allergy: principles and practice. Mosby, St Louis, pp 1403–1428
2. Hanifin JM, Rajka G (1980) Diagnostic features of atopic dermatitis. Acta Derm Venereol [Suppl] (Stockh) 92:44–47
3. Burks AW, Mallory SB, Williams LW, Shirrell MA (1988) Atopic dermatitis: clinical relevance of food hypersensitivity reactions. J Pediatr 113:447–451
4. Besnier E (1892) Premiere note et observations preliminaries pour sevir d'introduction a l'etude des pruriqos diathesiques. Ann Dermatol Syphil 23:634
5. Wise F, Sulzberger MD (1933) Yearbook of dermatoloy and syphilogy. Year Book Medial, Chicago, p 59
6. NIAID Task Force Report (1979) Dermatologic allergy: asthma and other allergic diseases. NIH Publication no. 79–387, p 375
7 Stifler WC (1965) A twenty-one year follow-up of infantile eczema. J Pediatr 66:166–167
8. Gurevitch AW, Heiner DC, Reisner R (1973) IgE in atopic dermatitis and other common dermatitises. Arch Dermatol 107:712
9. Hoffman PR, Yamanoto FY, Sellow B, et l. (1975) Diagnosis of IgE-mediated reactions to food antigens by radioimmunoassay. J Allergy Clin Immunol 55:256–267
10. Rajka G (1975) Atopic dermatitis. In: Rook A (ed) problems in dermatology, vol. 3. Saunders, London, pp 46–130
11. Dolovich J, Hargreave FE, Chalmers R, et al. (1973) Late cutaneous allergic responses in isolated IgE-dependent reactions. J Allergy Clin Immunol 52:38
12. Solley GO, Gleich GJ, Jordan RE, Schroeter AL (1976) Late phase of the immediate wheal and flare skin reaction: its dependence on IgE antibodies. J Clin Invest 58:408
13. Atkins PC, Zweiman B (1987) The IgE-mediated late-phase skin response – unraveling the enigma. J Allergy Clin Immunol 79:12
14. Gleich CJ (1982) The late phase of the immunoglobulin E-medicated reactions: a link between anaphylaxis and common allergic disease? J Allergy Clin Immunol 70:160
15. Spiegelberg HL (1984) Structure and function of Fc receptors for IgE on lymphocytes, monocytes and macrophages. Adv Immunol 35:61
16. Joseph M, Capiron A, Ameisen J-C et al (1986) The receptors for IgE on blood platelets. Eur J Immunol 16:306
17. Capiron M, Capiron A, Joseph M (1983) IgE receptors on phagocytic cells and immune response to schistosome infection. Monogr Allergy 18:33
18. Bruynzeel-Kooman C, VanWicker DF, Toonstra J, et al (1986) The presence of IgE molecules on epidermal Langerhans cells in patients with atopic dermatitis. Arch Dermatol Res 297:199
19. Ruzicka T, Aubock J (1987) Arachidonic acid metabolism in guinea pig Langerhans cells: studies on cyclooxygenase and lipoxygenase pathways. J Immunol 138:539
20. Gleich GJ, Frigas E, Loegering DA, et al. (1979) Cytotoxic properties of eosinophilic major basic protein. J Immunol 123:2925–2927
21. O'Donnell MC, Ackerman SJ, Gleich GJ, Thomas LL (1983) Activation of basophil and mast cell histamine release by eosinophil granule major basic protein. J Exp Med 157:1981

22. Leiferman KM, Ackerman SJ, Sampson HA, et al. [1985) Dermal deposition of eosinophil granule major basic protein in atopic dermatitis. Comparison with onchocerciasis. N Engl J Med 313:282–285
23. Brunner M, Walzer M (1928) Absorption of undigested proteins in human beings – the absorption of unaltered fish protein in adults. Arch Intern Med 42:173
24. Wilson SJ, Walzer M (1935) Absorption of unaltered egg protein in infants. Am J Dis Child 50:49
25. Engman WF, Weiss RS, Engman MF (1936) Eczema and environment. Med Clin North Am 10:651–663
26. Leinhas JL, McCaskill C, Sampson HA (1987) Food allergy challenges: guidelines and implications. J Am Diet Assoc 87:604–608
27. Sampson HA, Albergo R (1984) Comparison of results of skin tests, RAST and double-blind placebo controlled food challenges in children with atopic dermatitis. J Allergy Clin Immunol 74:26–33
28. Sampson HA, McCaskill CM (1985) Food hypersensitivity in atopic dermatitis: evaluation of 113 patients. J Pediatr 107:669
29. Atherton DJ (1983) The role of foods in atopic eczema. Clin Exp Dermatol 8:227
30. Bernhisel-Broadbent J, Sampson HA (1989) Cross-allergenicity in the legume botanical family in children with food hypersensitivity. J Allergy Clin Immunol 83:434–440
31. Sampson HA, Jolie PL (1984) Increased plasma histamine concentrations after food challenges in children with atopic dermatitis. N Engl J Med 311:372–376
32. Sampson HA, Broadbent KR, Bernhisel-Broadbent T (1989) Spontaneous release of histamine from basophils and histamine-releasing factor in patients with atopic dermatitis and food hypersensitivity. N Engl J Med 321:228–232
33. Marone G, Giugliano R, Lembo G, Ayala F (1986) Human basophil releasability. II. Changes in basophil releasability in patients with atopic dermatitis. J Invest Dermatol 87:19
34. Adinoff AD, Tellez P, Clark RAF (1988) Atopic dermatitis and aeroallergen contact sensitivity. J Allergy Clin Immunol 87:736
35. David TJ (1984) Anaphylactic shock during elimination diets for severe atopic dermatitis. Arch Dis Child 59:983
36. The shot doctors (1988) Consumer Reports 53:96–100
37. Bierman CW, Shapiro GC, Christle A, et al. (1978) Eczema, rickets and food allergy. J Allergy Clin Immunol 61:119–127
38. Burks AW, Sampson HA (1988) A controlled trial of oral cromolyn in children with atopic dermatitis and documented food hypersensitivity. J Allergy Clin Immunol 77:184
39. Reisman RE (1981) American Academy of Allergy: position statement – controversial techniques. J Allergy Clin Immunol 67:333–338
40. Bock SA (1988) Food allergy: a primer for people. Vantage, New York, pp 54–59
41. Sampson HA (1985) Persistence of food hypersensitivity in children with atopic dermatitis. J Allergy Clin Immunol 75:179
42. Bock SA (1982) The natural history of food sensitivity. J Allergy Clin Immunol 69(2):173–177
43. Businco L, Benincori N, Cantani A, Tacconi L, Picarazzi A (1988) Chronic diarrhea due to cow's milk allergy. A 4 to 10 year follow-up study. Ann Allergy 55:844
44. Esteban MM, Pascual C, Madero R, Diaz Pena JM, Ojeda JA (1985) Natural history of immediate food allergy in children (abstract). The First Latin Food Allergy Workshop, 28–29 June 1985. Rome, Italy.
45. Grulee CG, Sanford HN (1936) The influence of breast and artificial feeding on infantiled eczema. J Pediatr 9:223–225
46. Kramer MS, Moroz B (1981) Do breast-feeding and delayed introduction of solid food protect against subsequent atopic eczema? J Pediatr 98:546–550
47. Chandra RK, Puri S, Cheema PS (1985) Predictive value of cord blood IgE in the development of atopic disease and role of breast-feeding in its prevention. Clin Allergy 15:517–522
48. Van Asperen PP, Kemp AS, Mellis CM (1984) Relationship of diet in the development of atopy in infancy. Clin Allergy 14:525–532
49. Zeiger RS (1988) Development and prevention of allergic disease in childhood. In: Middleton E, Reed CE, Ellis EF, Adkinson NF, Yunginger JW (eds) Allergy: principle and practice. Mosby, St Louis, pp 930–968
50. McNeish AS (1984) Enzymatic maturation of the gastrointestinal tract and its relevance to food allergy and intolerance in infancy. Ann Allergy 53:643
51. Heird WC, Hanse JH (1977) Effect of colostrum on growth of intestinal mucosa. Pediatr Res 11:406A
52. Savilahti E, Salmenpera L, Jainio VM, et al. (1987) Prolonged exclusive breast-feeding results in low serum concentrations of immunoglobulin G, A and M. Acta Paediatr Scand 76:1–6
53. May CD, Fomon SJ, Remigio L (1982) Immunologic consequences of feeding infants with cow milk and soy products. Acta Paediatr Scand 71:43–51
54. Machtinger S, Moss R (1986) Cow's milk allergy in breast-fed infants: the role of allergen and maternal secretory IgA antibody. J Allergy Clin Immunol 77:341–347
55. Kajosaari M, Saarinen U (1983) Prophylaxis of atopic disease by six months total solid food elimination. Acta Paediatr Scand 72:411
56. Fergusson DM, Horwood LJ, Beautrais AL, et al. (1981) Eczema and infant diet. Clin Allergy 11:325–331
57. Lindfors A, Enocksson E (1988) Development of atopic disease after early administration of cow milk formula. Allergy 43:11–16
58. Jakobsson I, Lindberg T, Benediktsson B, et al. (1985) Dietary bovine B-lactoglobulin is transferred to human milk. Acta Pediatr Scand 74:342
59. Sampson HA (1988) The role of food allergy and mediator release in atopic dermatitis. J Allergy Clin Immunol 81:536–645
60. Hattevig G, Kjellman B, Siguns N, et al. (1989) The effect of maternal avoidance of eggs, cow's milk and fish during lactation upon allergic manifestations in infants. Clin Exp Allergy 19:27–32
61. Falth-Magnusson K, Kjellman N-IM (1987) Development of atopic disease in babies whose mothers were on exclusion diet during pregnancy – a randomized study. J Allergy Clin Immunol 80:868–875

Bacteria and Atopic Eczema: Merely Association or Etiologic Factor?

D. Abeck and T. Ruzicka

Introduction

Atopic eczema (AE) is a common dermatological condition that attracts great scientific interest worldwide. Although knowledge concerning the pathogenesis of AE has increased dramatically in recent years, there is no universally accepted pathogenetic concept. Nevertheless, it is generally agreed that AE arises on a genetic background and may be triggered by a variety of nonrelated environmental factors, termed flare factors by Dahl [15]. We discuss here the role of bacterial colonization or infection as one possible flare factor.

Flora of Normal Human Skin

Microbial inhabitants of the skin surface represent a very inhomogeneous group. The mite *Demodex folliculorum* living in the hair follicles and sebaceous glands chiefly on the face is a member of this group, as are fungi or the two lipophilic yeasts *Pityrosporon ovale* and *P. orbiculare*. Also, viruses such as *Herpesvirus hominis*, the cause of "cold sores," must also be regarded as cutaneous residents [47]. Yet the greatest attention has always been paid to the bacterial flora of the skin, particularly the aerobic bacteria, although they are outnumbered by anaerobic ones by a ratio of more than 10:1 [20].

Aerobic Bacterial Flora of Normal Human Skin and Factors Influencing its Ecology and Density

According to Price [51], the "transient" flora which includes a large variety of organisms present at one time or another on the skin surface can be distinguished from the "resident" flora consisting of relatively few types of bacteria which apparently multiply freely in the skin. Although Price's concept must be regarded as an oversimplification [47], it has proven useful. In 1942 Pillsbury et al. [50] divided the resident bacterial skin flora into three major groups: organisms found constantly such as *Staphylococcus albus* (now *Staphylococcus epidermidis*), those found occasionally such as *Staphylococcus aureus*, and those found rarely such as *Streptococcus viridans* or *Sarcina lutea*. According to Noble [47] following genera must be considered as resident bacterial inhabitants: *Staphylococcus, Micrococcus, Peptococcus, Corynebacterium, Brevibacterium, Propionibacterium*, and *Actinobacter.*

Besides identification of the bacteria present in the skin quantitative estimates of their extent are of great importance. Many different methods have been used for sampling the bacterial flora [20, 37, 68], but all have lacked reproducibility. Nowadays most quantitative investigations of cutaneous bacteria are performed using the method of Williamson and Kligman [77], using a buffered nonionic detergent as sampling fluid to assure complete removal of bacteria from the skin so that subsequent colony counts reflect single bacterial cells rather than aggregates.

Differences in numbers of bacteria from one area of the skin to another have been observed [67]. Using the method of Williamson and Kligman [77], Selwyn and Ellis [61] reported a mean of 80 000/cm^2 aerobic bacteria on the axillary skin of 42 adult subjects. Other regions investigated revealed much lower numbers of bacteria, for example the mean aerobic count for forearm skin was 2300/cm^2. The ecology and total number of bacteria on the skin surface is influenced by a large variety of factors, including seasonal variations [11], hydration [19], sex [43], and skin pH [43]. Skin flora maps have proven to be useful in studying the dynamics of cutaneous microbial populations [7].

Bacteria and Eczema: Historical Development of Concepts

The role of cutaneous bacterial flora as a cause of eczematous conditions has been discussed since the beginning of this century. Coinciding with the development of new bacteriologic techniques, Unna postulated "morococci" ("gram-positive cocci") to be the causative organisms of eczema as early as 1899 [65]. Although other researchers found no support for his hypothesis, special attention was drawn to staphylococci and streptococci in the following years. It could be demonstrated that staphylococci brought into close contact with slightly irritated skin for 24 h could produce eczematous lesions in normal skin. The lesions persisted for several days [66]. Whereas staphylococci attracted most interest in German-influenced areas, in France the focus was rather on streptococci as a possible bacterial cause of eczema. Experiments in this field are closely related to the name of Sabouraud. Detection of streptococci in eczematous lesions, intracutaneous reactions with steptococcal vaccines and therapeutic success with the use of parasiticidal ointments led to the classification of different forms of "streptococcide eczematiforme" [56]. In contrast to the extensive research around the turn of the century, only few reports concerning the possible role of bacteria in the expression or exacerbation of eczema have been published in the subsequent years. New impetus and the use of modern scientific methods were brought into this field after World War II by Miescher [40] and Storck [64], investigating the pathogenetic role of bacteria in eczema by challenging patients epicutaneously and intracutaneously with bacterial strains and filtrates gained from their own eczema.

Bacterial Flora in Patients with Atopic Eczema

Gloor and his group [24] compared the resident aerobic bacterial flora in unaffected skin of patients with AE and in healthy controls. They demonstrated a significant increase in colony-forming units (CFU) in patients with AE. For sampling of bacteria the scrub method of Williamson and Kligman [77] was used. With the same method skin flora maps were constructed from a patient with severe AE and from a healthy volunteer with 162 and 175 skin sites sampled, respectively. Striking differences in the density of the aerobic flora were observed between the two subjects, both in affected and in unaffected skin sites [7].

A quantitative study in 70 patients with AE, calculating the total number of aerobes per square unit recovered from various atopic skin manifestations, revealed a mean density of 18 417 000/cm^2 in acute lesions, 593 800/cm^2 in chronic plaques, and 232 307/cm^2 in clinically unaffected skin; these differences were statistically significant [35]. The results were subsequently confirmed by other researchers [3, 28]. Eczematous skin does not only provide favorable conditions for bacterial colonization and multiplication but also shows marked qualitative differences concerning the bacterial ecology compared with skin of healthy subjects. Two studies of Selwyn [58, 59] published in 1963 and 1965 reported a high incidence of *S. aureus* in patients with various types of eczema, but without differentiating them. In the former study 44 of 106 patients without clinical signs of infection carried *S. aureus*, and in the latter, *S. aureus* was found in 56 out of 113 patients, of whom 24 showed clinical evidence of infection.

Table 1 summarizes the detection rates for *S. aureus* in studies undertaken with AE patients.

Carriage of *S. aureus* on normal unaffected skin was detected in up to 76% [3], this figure rising to 100% in exudative lesions [35]. These data are in sharp contrast to the isolation rate of *S. aureus* from skin of healthy subjects. In the study of Gloor [24] the presence of *S.*

Table 1. Isolation rate of *Staphylococcus aureus* in patients with atopic eczema

		Affected skin	
Reference	Normal unaffected skin	Acute, exudative lesions	Chronic, lichenified lesions
Leyden et al. [35]	–	20/20 (100%)	60/66 (91%)
Bibel et al. [8]	22/44 (55%)	–	34/40 (85%)
Aly et al. [3]	30/39 (76%)	–	37/39 (93%)
Gloor et al. [24]	9/14 (64%)	–	–

aureus was demonstrated in only one of 12 healthy subjects. Noble [45] detected *S. aureus* in fewer than 5% of isolates taken from various skin sites of 382 normal children and 378 normal adults. In a study of the microbiological features of the skin of the upper part of the shoulder *S. aureus* could be recovered from only two out of 146 samples [20]. While the nasal carriage of *S. aureus* in the normal population ranges between 10% and 45% [71, 76], there is general agreement that *S. aureus* is not a customary member of the cutaneous microflora except for occasional resident status in the perineum [2]. In addition, normal cutaneous flora may even inhibit the growth of *S. aureus* [38, 62].

Besides a significantly higher carrier rate of *S. aureus* in patients with AE, quantitative assessment of aerobic bacterial flora revealed further remarkable differences when compared with normal subjects. Noble and coworkers [42], looking for the carriage of *S. aureus* in random samples of a normal population, recovered the organism nine times in 201 samples analyzed. More than six colonies could only be detected in one sample [42]. The first quantitative study analyzing *S. aureus* in skin lesions and in unaffected skin of patients with AE was conducted by Leyden and his group [35]; the mean density of *S. aureus* was 14 x 10^6 organisms per square centimeter in exudative lesions, 5 x 10^6 in chronic lichenified plaques, and 1.3 x 10^3 in normal skin. A 100–1000 times higher density of *S. aureus* in different types of lesional skin ompared to normal skin in patients with AE could be confirmed by others in the following years [3, 28]. In addition, a significantly higher frequency of *S. aureus* has been demonstrated in apparently normal skin of AE patients compared to skin of healthy subjects [28].

However, an increased colonization by *S. aureus* is not a specific characteristic in AE. In the series of Selwyn and Chalmers [59] 41 of 114 psoriatic lesions were colonized by *S. aureus* as well. Noble and Savin [44] performed colony counts on lesional and uninvolved skin of psoriatic patients; 9 of 34 patients carried *S. aureus*, with no difference in the number of organisms in involved and uninvolved skin. In the study of Marples and coworkers [39] 42 of 92 (46%) psoriatic lesions were colonized by *S. aureus*. Unaffected skin yielded *S. aureus* in only 14 of 52 sampled sites (27%), which was significantly less than in psoriatic lesions but still much higher than in normal persons. Density of *S. aureus* on psoriatic skin ranged from 20 000 to 300 000/cm^2 with a geometric mean of 928 cm^2, and *S. aureus* counts were higher in lesions compared to uninvolved skin. Thus, there is an increased prevalence of *S. aureus* in psoriatic skin, but the density only rarely reaches the numbers seen in atopic eczematous lesions.

Leyden [35] noticed that eczematous lesions seemed to support preferential growth of *S. aureus*. A density of 10^6 CFU/cm^2 usually resulted in pure cultures of *S. aureus*. He suggested that the organism may be aggravating the underlying dermatosis. In contrast, Bibel [8] reported that the presence of *S. aureus* actually tended to increase the populations of total aerobic flora, a phenomenon that was also noted in sites under occlusion [62].

Although the indigenous flora of AE skin shows a wide range of unrelated qualitative changes [8], the striking ecological aspect of *S. aureus* colonization has led to a concentration of scientific effort on its possible pathogenic role in this disease.

Increased Numbers of S. aureus in Atopic Skin: Harmless Colonization or Primary Cutaneous Infection?

Exacerbation of atopic eczema due to massive secondary bacterial infection is commonly known. Controversial, however, is the question whether there is a primary superficial infection of *S. aureus*. Although the high carriage rate of *S. aureus* in patients with atopic eczema has been confirmed by several groups [3, 29, 46, 74], distinction between colonization and infection is difficult to make.

Leyden [35] demonstrated high-density colonization in lesions of nearly all patients with AE, the highest density, i.e., 10^7/cm^2 or more, being seen in most acute, exudative lesions. He noted, however, that despite the huge numbers of *S. aureus* the lesions did not look infected. Only in the acute form did slight serous exudate and thin crust indicate a possible harmful effect of *S. aureus*. Over a period of 1.5 years Hanifin and Rogge [27] detected superficial staphylococcal pustules associated with a considerable degree of pruritus on the skin of 22 patients with AE. These lesions were commonly found with severe exacerbations of AE. Predominant location of lesions was on the extremities. Although pustules were occasionally found surrounding hairs, the vast majority were not follicular. The relatively frequent palmar localization, however, indicated that hair follicles were not the only site of infection, and even on hairy areas the pustules were distributed randomly with no consistent follicular localization. Furthermore, histopathology of lesions from three patients showed subcorneal, intraepidermal collections primarily of neutrophils with few eosinophils and mononuclear leukocytes. Serial sections failed to show either sweat duct or hair follicle localization. Although in a different study White and Noble [74] found pustulation related mainly to hair follicles a possible explanation for the different findings might be that pustules were already removed by excoriation and could therefore no longer be detected. In summary, there is strong evidence that *S. aureus* is capable of producing actively superficial pustules on the skin of atopic patients, resulting in increased pruritus and in a high number of cases in exacerbation of AE.

S. aureus and Atopic Eczema: General Characteristics of S. aureus

S. aureus is a common pathogen and belongs to a genus which is currently composed of 20 species [34]. It is a nonmotile, non-spore-forming gram-positive, aerobic, and facultatively anaerobic organism [34]. *S. aureus* is relatively resistant to environmental changes, withstanding temperatures as high as 60°C for 30 min or remaining alive for months on the surface of sealed agar plates stored at 4°C. The pH optimum is 7.0–7.5, although the bacteria are able to multiply in a pH range from 4.8 to 9.4. Temperature optimum is between 30°C and 37°C [34]. The cell wall contains peptidoglycan and teichoic acid [18]. Cellular antigens comprise species-specific polysaccharide A (a teichoic acid composed of *N*-acetylglucosamine residues attached in either α- or β-linkage to a polyribitol phosphate "backbone"), protein A, and several capsular antigens [18]. *S. aureus* produces a variety of different entero-(types A through D) and exotoxins (coagulase, staphylokinase, lipase, hyaluronidase, DNAse) [18]. In most laboratories typing of *S. aureus* is performed by bacteriophage typing, a technique for the differentiation of staphylococcal strains on the basis of phage susceptibility. It allows the division into five host-range (lytic) groups consisting of groups I–IV for strains reacting exclusively with phages of one group and group V consisting of isolates reacting with phages of more than one group and with unclassified phages or being untypable [70].

In a recent study the in vitro susceptibility to chemotherapeutic agents of *S. aureus* strains isolated in a department of dermatology was determined using the microdilution test [32]. Table 2 summarizes the results obtained. 35% of the isolates were fully susceptible to penicillin G and 62% to tetracyclin. No resistance was observed to ciprofloxacin, flucloxacillin, or cotrimoxazole. Fewer than 10% of the isolates were resistant to cefotaxim, erythromycin, and gentamycin.

Table 2. Minimum inhibitory concentrations (MICs) of eight antimicrobial agents against 230 strains of *Staphylococcus aureus*. (From [32])

Antimicrobial agent	MIC (mg/L) Range	MIC^{50}	MIC^{90}
Penicillin	0.062–16	1	16
Tetracyclin	2 –16	4	4
Erythromycin	0.25 –16	0.25	2
Cefotaxime	2 –16	4	4
Ciprofloxacin	0.125– 2	0.25	0.5
Flucloxacillin	0.25 – 1	0.25	0.5
Gentamycin	nt	0.25	2
Cotrimoxazol	nt	0.5	16

Characteristics of S. aureus Possibly Associated with Atopic Eczema: S. aureus Phage Typing

Table 3 summarizes the distribution of phage types found in patients with AE. In the study of White and Noble [74] staphylococci from carrier sites and those from lesions were indistinguishable in 30 of the 41 patients who were nasal and/or perineal carriers of *S. aureus*. Whereas Aly and coworkers [3] could not detect any strain belonging to phage group II, these strains were isolated from 5% of patients in the study of White and Noble [74]. Group II staphylococci have been associated with impetigo and toxic epidermal necrolysis [25]. In the studies in which phage typing was performed only a small percentage of strains belonged to phage group I, the majority belonged to group III or were nontypable. A possible explanation for the high number of group III strains is, according to Aly, either the patients' lack of contact with bacteria of phage type I or II (i.e., a chance phenomenon) or ecologic reasons favouring group III strains in atopic patients.

Table 3. Distribution of phage groups in patients with atopic eczema

Reference	I	II	III	IV	V
Aly et al. [3]	13%	0%	38%	0%	40%
White and Noble [74]	11%	5%	11%	0%	73%

Anti-S. aureus Specific IgE in Patients with Atopic Eczema and Their Clinical Significance

Mean serum IgE levels are generally significantly elevated in patients with AE as compared to healthy individuals or subjects with nonatopic dermatoses [13, 26, 63]. The IgE levels show some correlation with the severity of the disease [26]. Extremely elevated serum levels of IgE in combination with chronic eczematous dermatitis and the occurrence of staphylococcal abscesses and chronic mucocutaneous candidiasis characterize the hyperimmunoglobulin E (HIE) syndrome ([21, 52]. Specific IgE antibodies to *S. aureus* (and to *Candida albicans*) could be detected in these patients. Production of these antibodies might contribute to the increased susceptibility of patients with the HIE syndrome to infections with these particular organisms [6, 57].

Due to the clinically almost identical picture of chronic eczematous dermatitis in HIE and AE, the role of IgE-antibodies to *S. aureus* in the pathogenesis of AE has been the subject of interest in recent investigations. The main results of these studies are summarized in Table 4. Whereas Hauser et al. [29] reported a prevalence of 60% of anti-*S. aureus* IgE antibodies in atopic patients, Friedman et al. [23] could detect these antibodies in only 12% of patients with AE and clinical signs of infection. This discrepancy can be explained, at least partly, by the different antigens used as immunosorbent. Whole organisms develop high levels of nonspecific binding [23]. On the other hand, when purified cell walls are used as immunosorbent, detection of specific IgE antibodies to other *S. aureus* cellular proteins is prevented.

Table 4. *Staphylococcus aureus* specific antibodies in atopic eczema

Reference	Year	a.-S.a.-IgE-RAST antigen used as immunosorbent	Main results
Abramson et al. [1]	1982	Whole bacterial pellets	Increased levels of a.-S.a.-IgE in patients with a high serum IgE and no history of furuncles or severe staphylococcal infection.
Henocq et al. [30]	1982	Whole bacterial pellets	Increased levels of a.-S.a.-IgE in patients with *S. aureus* superinfected AE and atopic patients with total IgE levels of more than 1000 U/ml.
Hauser et al. [29]	1985	Purified cell walls (PCW)	a.-S.a.-IgE in 12/21 patients. Elevated PCW-IgE was associated with regional lymphadenopathy but not with impetiginization.
Friedman et al. [22]	1985	Purified cell walls (PCW)	In 4/25 patients with AE and superimposed impetiginization or pustules serum IgE to PCW could be detected. In 1/44 patients with no clinical signs of cutaneous infections but positive cultures for *S. aureus* serum IgE to PCW could be detected.
Motala et al. [41]	1986	Supernatant proteins of sonicated cells	19/64 children and 14/60 adults with AE showed a.-S.a.-IgE antibodies. a.S.a.-positive children had more extensive disease, greater prevalence of cutaneous S.a. infections than those who were negative. a.S.a.-positive adults had more and prolonged disease than those who were negative.
Kapp and Schöpf [31]	1989	Supernatant proteins of sonicated cells	2/52 patients with atopic eczema showed significant levels of specific IgE antibodies (RAST class 2)

a.-S.a.-IgE-RAST = anti-*Staphylococcus aureus*-IgE RAST

These two disadvantages, i.e., the high level of nonspecific binding and the lack of detection of other than cell wall directed antibodies, are avoided by the radioallergosorbent test (RAST) system of Motala et al. using proteins of sonicated cells as immunosorbent [40]. This test system has also been used by Kapp and Schöpf [31] to assess the prevalence of specific IgE antibodies to *S. aureus* in AE. Motala et al. detected positive *S. aureus* results in 14 out of 16 adults [40]. A subdivision into different RAST classes has not been performed. The study of Kapp and Schöpf [31] revealed IgE antibodies to *S. aureus* in only 19 of 52 serum samples with RAST class 2 considered clinically significant in only two. The clinical relevance of specific *S. aureus* IgE antibodies is controversial. Kapp and Schöpf [31] as well Friedman and coworkers [23] conclude that the presence of *S. aureus* is not correlated with disease activity and do not believe that specific anti-staphylococcal IgE represents an important diagnostic feature in AE. On the other hand, Motala et al. [40] discuss the possibility that anti-*S. aureus* IgE antibodies predict a more chronic and less favourable course in patients with AE. Via an IgE-mediated reaction, *S. aureus* might initiate the itch-scratch-excoriation sequence thus resulting in disruption of the epidermis with consequent loss of its barrier function would allow invasion of *S. aureus* followed by further sensitization via IgE receptors on mast cells and macrophages. Further mediator release, cellular recruitment, and chronic inflammation would be the consequences.

Immediate and Delayed Hypersensitivity to Staphylococcal Allergens

The response of patients with AE to staphylococcal allergens has been studied by several investigators in order to support or reject the concept that allergic reactions to *S. aureus*, the inhabitant of virtually all AE lesions, are of pathogenetic importance. Rajka [53, 54] used a "combined staphylovaccine", prepared from heat-killed bacteria of several hospital strains for intradermal testing. In ten children with AE, ranging on age from 6–24 month, there was a weak immediate reactivity in two cases and a delayed reactivity in six [53]. In a further study, performed in patients with AE and a healthy control group, all more than 15 years of age, no difference in the immediate skin reactions to the *S. aureus* extract was seen, but there was a highly significant difference in delayed skin reactions recorded after 48 h which were diminished in the AE group [54].

Analyzing the immediate reactions to staphylococcal antigens, Rudzki and coworkers [55] could show that the percentage of patients with AE who reacted strongly, was higher in the AE group than in the controls. The overall frequency of reactions in atopic patients and controls, however, did not differ. Bode and coworkers [12] studying 15 patients with AE and 15 healthy individuals by intradermal testing with *S. aureus* showed a positive immediate-type reaction in 38% of patients and in 17% of the controls, White and Noble [73] investigated the cutaneous reaction to staphylococcal protein A. From experiments it is known that protein A, a component of the cell wall of *S. aureus*, induces a specific IgE response in humans and the presence of staphylococcal protein A modifies in vitro RAST sensitivity [48]. Furthermore, the reaction to intradermal protein A in humans is dose dependent, and there is individual variation in healthy subjects [49, 72]. By intradermal testing with staphylococcal protein A White and Noble [73] observed an immediate weal and flare response in all groups. Despite marked individual variation patients with AE had less erythema at 15 min and 24 h compared to normal or psoriatic individuals. At 48 h the greatest reaction was observed in psoriatic individuals.

Adherence of S. aureus to Skin of Patients with Atopic Eczema

The adherence of bacterial pathogens to the epithelial cell surfaces of various host tissues is the initial step in the pathogenesis of many infections. The unusual tendency of atopic skin to become colonized by *S. aureus* stimulated investigations of the adherence phenomenon. Adherence of *S. aureus* to corneocytes seems to be both a species-specific and corneocyte-specific phenomenon. *S. aureus* exhibits a statistically much greater degree of adherence ($p = 0.05$; Student's t test) to corneocytes of patients with atopic eczema as compared to corneocytes collected from normal controls or those with psoriatic lesions or other dermatological diseases [14]. Assays performed with three different species of gram-positive bacteria again revealed *S. aureus* as the only bacterial species that was able to adhere avidly to atopic corneocytes [14]. Although there is agreement on the basic finding of increased adherence of *S. aureus* to atopic corneocytes, the question of the adhesin, i.e., the microbial component responsible for adhesion, remains controversial. Cole and Silverberg [14] favor protein A since it inhibits the adherence of *S. aureus* to corneocytes in an in vitro assay system. On the other hand, it has been shown that *S. aureus* binds to fibronectin [33]. Fibronectin is a family of high molecular weight glycoproteins found in blood and body fluids and on many cell surfaces. Bibel et al. [4, 9, 10] identified teichoic acid and not protein A as being responsible for *S. aureus* adhesion to fibronectin. Further work should provide information on the molecular mechanisms of *S. aureus* adhesion to corneocytes of atopic subjects.

Effect of Antimicrobial Therapy on Atopic Eczema

If bacteria or bacterial antigens are indeed involved in the pathogenesis of AE, their elimination by appropiate antibiotic treatment should result in a marked clinical improvement.

In a case described recently by Luber and coworkers [36] elimination of *S. aureus* led to dramatic improvement of the skin condition of a 4-year-old boy diagnosed with AE at 21 months of age. This child with severe AE became colonized with a methicillin-resistant strain of *S. aureus* that resisted eradication by oral and parenteral antibiotic therapy including intravenously administered vancomycin. Sensitivity testing to routine topical antibiotics and to mupirocin ointment revealed mupirocin as the most effective drug. Therefore, in addition to the routine use of 2.5% hydrocortisone ointment and 5% liquor carbonis detergens, applications of mupirocin ointment three times a day was started. Within 7 days *S. aureus* was absent from the boy's skin. Concomitantly there was immediate improvement in his skin condition with resolution of areas of erythema, crusting, and oozing and reduced need for antihistamines. Lichenification, hyperpigmentation, and a few excoriations persisted.

Improvement of AE by antibiotic treatment has been known for a long time. In the mid-1950s, Baer [5] reported an improvement of AE when patients were treated with oral antibiotics [5]. Leyden and his group [35] recommended initial antibiotic therapy of AE, even in the absence of the usual signs of infection. Antibiotics should best be administered for only 1 week, which is sufficient to lower *S. aureus* counts to a harmless level. Usually a clinical improvement was accompanied by a dramatic drop in the quantity of *S. aureus*. In a recent study David and Cambridge [17] also recommended the use of oral antibiotics in any child with troublesome AE. Topical antibiotics were not used because of the possibility of sensitization and the difficulty of application to widespread lesions. An improvement in AE by the use of topical antimicrobial agents has also been reported [69, 75]. However, both oral and topical use of antimicrobial treatment usually achieves only an improvement, not a complete healing of AE. The assessment of an antibiotic treatment effect and resulting conclusions drawn on the pathogenetic role of bacteria are, according to Dahl [16], difficult to make due to the failure of complete eradication of the bacteria from the skin surface. A small number of remaining bacteria may still suffice to provoke dermatitis by immunologic mechanisms. Also, products of dead bacteria left on the skin surface could serve as antigens even in the absence of viable organisms.

Summary and Future Considerations

Within the group of atopic patients there seem to exist subgroups whose disease can be provoked by various flare factors. In analogy to atopic patients in whom food allergies can initiate cutaneous reactions, another subgroup which has not yet been clearly identified may exist in whom eczema is triggered by bacterial factors.

Aerobic bacteria colonize the skin of patients with AE in significantly higher numbers than in healthy individuals. Among the bacteria *S. aureus* seems to play the predominant role. The organism which is not considered a member of the normal resident flora can be isolated in the majority of atopic patients with frequency rates reaching almost 100% in acute exudative lesions. In addition to the colonization, there is clear evidence that a subtle primary cutaneous staphylococcal infection occurs in atopic patients. The reasons for increase carriage of *S. aureus* are still unclear but might be associated with special bacteriophage types and increased adherence to corneocytes derived from patients with AE. Intradermal injection of staphylcococcal antigens led to diminished hypersensitivity reactions in atopic patients, suggesting a defect in cell-mediated immunity. So far, immunologic studies have not been able to establish a pathogenetic significance of IgE antibodies to *S. aureus*. On the other hand, reducing the number of staphylococci by antimicrobial therapy resulted in improvement of AE.

In summary, from the data presented here there is little doubt that bacteria and especially *S. aureus* act as flare factors in AE. The question whether bacteria play a causal role in the disease process cannot conclusively be answered at present. Further experiments using bacteriophage typing should clarify whether AE is associated with specific *S. aureus* types. If such an association is established, it may be due to the presence of specific adhesion molecules. The detection and characterization of possible adhesins responsible for interaction between corneocytes and infecting organisms should be given high priority because it opens the possibility to displace *S. aureus* by pharmacological means.

Besides the question of *why* there is increased colonization of atopic skin with staphylococci, a further question awaiting clarification is the mechanism of *how* bacteria cause eczematous changes. Thus, further investigations into humoral and cellular immunity seem clearly warranted.

References

1. Abramson JS, Dahl MV, Walsh G, Blumenthal MN, Douglas SD, Quie PG (1982) Antistaphylococcal IgE in patients with atopic dermatitis. J Am Acad Dermatol 7:105–110
2. Allen AM, Taplin D, Lawry JA, Twigg L (1972) Skin infections in Vietnam. Military Medicine 137:295–299
3. Aly R, Maibach HJ, Shinefield HR (1977) Microbial flora of atopic dermatitis. Arch Dermatol 113:780–782
4. Aly R, Shinefield HR, Litz C, Maibach HI (1980) Role of teichoic acid in the binding of *Staphylococcus aureus* to nasal epithelial cells. J Infect Dis 141:463–465
5. Baer RL (1955) Atopic dermatitis. New York, New York University Press.
6. Berger M, Kirkpatrick CH, Goldsmith PK, Gallin JK (1980) IgE antibodies to *Staphylococcus aureus* and *Candida albicans* in patients with the syndrome of hyperimmunoglobulin E and recurrent infections. J Immunol 125:2437–2443
7. Bibel DJ, Lovell DJ (1976) Skin flora maps: a tool in the study of cutaneous ecology. J Invest Dermatol 67:265–269
8. Bibel DJ, Greenberg JH, Cook JL (1977) *Staphylococcus aureus* and the microbial ecology of atopic dermatitis. Can J Microbiol 23:1062–1068
9. Bibel DJ, Aly R, Shinefield HR, Maibach HI, Strauss WG (1982) Importance of the keratinized epithelial cells in bacterial adherence. J Invest Dermatol 79:250–253
10. Bibel DJ, Aly R, Shinefield HR, Maibach HI (1983) The *Staphylococcus aureus* receptor for fibronectin. J Invest Dermatol 80:494–496
11. Blank IH, Dawes RK (1965) Survival of bacteria on the skin. In: Skin bacteria and their role in infection. Maibach HI and Hiddick-Smith G (eds) Mc Graw-Hill, New York
12. Bode U, Ring J, Neubert U (1982) Intrakutantestungen und bakteriologische Untersuchungen bei Patienten mit atopischem Ekzem. Allergologie 5:259–261
13. Church JA, Kleban DG, Bellanti JA (1976) Serum immunoglobulin E concentrations and radio-allergosorbent tests in children with atopic dermatitis. Pediatr Res 10:97–99
14. Cole GW, Silverberg NL (1986) The adherence of *Staphylococcus aureus* to human corneocytes. Arch Dermatol 122:166–169
15. Dahl MV (1977) Atopic dermatitis: the concept of "flare factors." South Med J 70:453–455
16. Dahl MV (1983) *Staphylococcus aureus* and atopic dermatitis. Arch Dermatol 119: 840–846
17. David JJ, Cambridge GC (1986) Bacterial infection and atopic eczema. Arch Dis Childhood 61:20–23
18. Davis BD, Dulbecco R, Eisen HN, Ginsberg HS, Wood BW, McCarty M (1973) Microbiology (2nd ed) Harper and Row, Maryland
19. Duncan WC, McBride ME, Knox JM (1969) Bacterial flora. The role of environmental factors. J Invest Dermatol 52:479–484
20. Evans CA, Smith WM, Johnston EA, Giblett ER (1950) Bacterial flora of the normal human skin. J Invest Dermatol 15:305–324
21. Gallin JI, Wright G, Malech HL, Davis JM, Klempner MS, Kirkpatrick CH (1980) Disorders of phagocyte chemotaxis. Ann Intern Med 92:520–538
22. Friedman SJ, Schroeter AL, Homberger HA (1984) Whole organisms and purified cell walls compared as immunosorbents for the detection of IgE antibodies to *Staphylococcus aureus.* J Immunol Methods 66:369
23. Friedman SJ, Schroeter AL, Homburger HA (1985) IgE antibodies to *Staphylococcus aureus.* Arch Dermatol 121:869–872
24. Gloor M, Peters G, Stoika D (1982) On the resident aerobic bacterial skin flora in unaffected skin of patients with atopic dermatitis and in healthy controls. Dermatologica 164:258–265
25. Goerz G, Ruzicka T (1978) Lyell-Syndrom, Grosse Scripta 2, Grosse Verlag, Berlin
26. Gurevitch AW, Heiner DC, Reissner RM (1973) IgE in atopic dermatitis and other common dermatoses. Arch Dermatol 107:712–715
27. Hanifin JM, Rogge JL (1977) Staphylococcal infections in patients with atopic dermatitis. Arch Dermatol 113:1383–1386
28. Hauser C, Wuethrich B, Matter L, Wilhelm JA, Sonnabend W, Schopfer K (1985) *Staphylococcus aureus* skin colonization in atopic dermatitis patients. Dermatologica 170:35–39
29. Hauser C, Wuethrich B, Matter L, Wilhelm JA, Schopfer K (1985) Immune response to *Staphylococcus aureus* in atopic dermatitis. Dermatologica 170:114–120
30. Henocq E, Hewitt B, Guerin B (1982) Staphylococcal and human dander IgE antibodies in superinfected atopic dermatitis. Clin Allergy 12:113–120
31. Kapp A, Schöpf E (1989) Spezifisches IgE gegen *Staphylococcus aureus* bei Patienten mit atopischer Dermatitis. Hautarzt 40:19–22
32. Korting HC, Abeck D, Grimm W, Schiller Y (1990) Heutige in vitro-Empfindlichkeit von Hautbakterien gegenüber unterschiedlichen Chemotherapeutika. Quantitative Ergebnisse des Mikrodilutionstestes. Akt Dermatol 12: 217–220

33. Kuusela P (1978) Fibronectin binds to *Staphylococcus aureus*. Nature (London) 276:718–720
34. Lennette H, Balows A, Hausler WJ, Shadomy HJ (1985) Manual of Clinical Microbiology (4th ed) American Society for Microbiology, Washington
35. Leyden JL, Marples RR, Kligman AM (1974) *Staphylococcus aureus* in the lesions of atopic dermatitis. Br J Derm 90:525–530
36. Luber H, Amornsiripanitch S, Lucky AW (1988) Mupirocin and the eradication of *Staphylococcus aureus* in atopic dermatitis. Arch Dermatol 124:853
37. Marples MJ (1965) The ecology of the human skin. Springfield, Ill.
38. Marples RR, Kligman AM (1969) Pyoderma due to *Staphylococcus aureus* following topical application of neomycin. J Invest Dermatol 53:11–13
39. Marples RR, Heaton CL, Kligman AM (1973) *Staphylococcus aureus* in psoriasis. Arch Dermatol 107:568–570
40. Miescher G (1949) Betrachtungen zur Ekzemfrage. Die Bedeutung der Mikrobenbesiedelung. Arch Derm Syphil 188:36–57
41. Motala C, Potter PC, Weinberg EG, Malherbe D, Hughes J (1986) Anti-*Staphylococcus aureus*-specific IgE in atopic dermatitis. J Allergy Clin Immunol 78:583–589
42. Noble WC, Volkenburg HA, Wolters CHL (1967) Carriage of *Staphylococcus aureus* in random samples of a normal population. J Hyg (Camb) 65:567–573
43. Noble WC (1968) Observations on the surface flora of the skin and on the skin pH. Br J Derm 80:279–281
44. Noble WC, Savin JA (1968) Carriage of Staphylococcus aureus in psoriasis. Br Med J i:417–418
45. Noble WC (1969) Skin carriage of the micrococcaceae. J Clin Path 22:249–252 (1969)
46. Noble WC (1981) Microbiology of human skin. Lloyd-Luke, London
47. Noble WC (1983) Microbiology of skin disease: its epidemiology. In: Philipps IP (ed) Current topics in infection, Edward Arnold (publisher), London
48. Oggel JD, Dockhorn RJ (1983) Staphylococcal protein A and enhancement of disc RAST sensitivity. Ann Allergy 50:178–181
49. Petersson BA, Stalenheim G (1975) Induction of histamine release and desentization in human leukocytes. Effect of anti-IgE or protein A from *Staphylococcus aureus*. Scand J Immunol 4:777–784
50. Pillsbury DM, Shaffer B, Nichols A (1946) Bacterial flora of the normal skin; a study of the effect of sulfathiozole and some ointment bases. J Invest Dermatol 7:365–373
51. Price PB (1938) Bacteriology of normal skin; a new quantitative test applied to the study of bacterial flora and desinfectant action of mechanical cleansing. J Infect Dis 63:301–318
52. Quie PG, Cates KL (1978) Clinical manifestations and disorders of neutrophil chemotaxis. In: Leukocyte chemotaxis. JI Gallin and PG Quie (eds) Raven Press, New York, pp 307–328
53. Rajka G (1967) Delayed dermal and epidermal reactivity in atopic dermatitis (prurigo Besnier). I. Delayed reactivity to bacterial and mold allergens. Acta derm-venereol 47:158–162
54. Rajka G (1982) Studies in hypersensitivity to molds and staphylococci in prurigo Besnier (atopic dermatitis). Acta derm-venereol 13 (suppl 54):1–139
55. Rudzki E, Moskalewska K, Maciejowska E (1965) Bakterienallergie bei Hautkrankheiten. III. Bakterienallergie bei Ekzem, Urticaria and Prurigo. Arch Klin Exp Dermatol 223:245–250
56. Sabourand R (1900) Etude clinique et bacterologique de l'impetigo. Ann Derm (Fr) 62:320–374 and 427–508
57. Schopfer K, Douglas SD, Wilkinson BS (1980) Immunoglobulin E antibodies against *Staphylococcus aureus* cell walls in the sera of patients with hyperimmunoglobulinemia E and recurrent staphylococcal infections. Infect Immun 27:563–568
58. Selwyn S (1963) Bacterial infections in a skin department. Br J Dermatol 75:26–28
59. Selwyn S, Chalmers D (1965) Dispersal of bacteria from skin lesions: a hospital hazard. Br J Dermatol 77:349–356
60. Selwyn S (1965) Mechanisms and preventation of cross infection in dermatology wards. J Hyg 63:59–71
61. Selwyn S, Ellis H (1972) Skin bacteria and skin desinfection reconsidered. Br Med J i:136–140
62. Singh G, Marples RR, Kligman AM (1971) Experimental *Staphylococcus aureus* infections in humans. J Invest Dermatol 75:26–28
63. Stone SP, Muller SA, Gleich GJ (1973) IgE levels in atopic dermatitis. Arch Dermatol 108:806–811
64. Storck H (1948) Experimentelle Untersuchungen zur Frage der Bedeutung von Mikroben in der Ekzemgenese. Dermatologica 96:13–262
65. Unna P (1899) Meine bisherigen Befunde über den Morococcus. Monatsh f prakt Dermat 29:106–113
66. Unna P (1905) Ekzem in: Mracek F (ed), Handbuch der Hautkrankheiten, Hölder, Wien
67. Ulrich JA (1965) Dynamics of bacterial skin populations in skin bacteria and their role in infection. Maibach HI and Hiddick-Smith G (eds) New York: Mc Graw-Hill., p. 219
68. Updegraf DM (1964) A cultural method of quantitatively studying the microorganisms in the skin. J Invest Dermatol 43:129–137
69. Wachs GN, Maibach HI (1976) Co-operative double-blind trial of an antibiotic/corticoid combination in impetiginized atopic dermatitis. Br J Derm 96:323–328
70. Wenthworth BB (1963) Bacteriophage typing of staphylococci. Bacteriol Rev 27:253–272
71. White A, Smith J (1963) Nasal reservoir as the source of extranasal staphylococci. Antimicrob Agents Chemoth 3:679–683
72. White MJ, Noble WC (1980) Skin response to protein A. Proc Royal Soc Edinburgh, 79B, 43–46
73. White MJ, Noble WC (1985) The cutaneous reaction to staphylococcal protein A in normal subjects and patients with atopic dermatitis or psoriasis. Brit J Dermatol 113:179–183
74. White MJ, Noble WC (1986) Consequences of colonization and infection by *Staphylococcus aureus* in atopic dermatitis. Clin Exp Dermatol 11:34–40
75. Wilkinson RD, Collins JP, Raymond GP, Mailhot R, Penas MA, Ricard P (1980) Therapy of infected dermatitis: comparative response to two corticosteroid antimicrobial creams. J Am Acad Dermatol 2:207–211
76. Williamson REO (1963) Healthy carriage of *Staphylococcus aureus:* its prevalence and importance. Bacteriol Rev 27:56–71
77. Williamson P, Kligman AM (1965) A new method for the quantitative investigation of cutaneous bacteria. J Invest Dermatol 45:498–503

Changes in Cell-Mediated Immunity in Atopic Eczema

Ö. Strannegård and I.-L. Strannegård

Introduction

During recent years, an increasing amount of evidence has accumulated suggesting that atopic eczema (AE) should be classified as an immunological disease. The early findings of associations between AE and severe viral infections and cutaneous anergy [1] and the frequent occurrence of raised levels of IgE in AE [2] certainly support this notion. The most convincing evidence, however, stems from observations that the correction of immunological abnormalities by bone marrow transplantation in patients suffering from the Wiskott-Aldrich syndrome also leads to clearing of the dermatitis which almost invariably accompanies it [3]. This dermatitis is indistinguishable from that occurring in classic AE, and the curing effect by bone marrow transplantation is most likely due to the establishment of normal T-lymphocyte function, thereby replacing an abnormal one [4]. Thus T cells, which constitute the major effectors in cell-mediated immunity (CMI), have come into the focus of interest concerning pathogenetic mechanisms in AE. It is the purpose of this chapter to describe the changes of CMI in AE, to review critically the evidence that these changes are of a primary nature and not only secondary consequences of the disease and finally to consider the possible pathological consequences associated with changes in CMI.

Occurrence of Infections Suggesting Defective CMI in AE

Ever since the original description of Kaposi's varicelliform eruption [5], clinicians have been aware of the fact that cutaneous viral infections may run an unusually severe course in patients with AE. It has been found that Kaposi's varicelliform eruption may be caused by herpes simplex, vaccinia, varicella zoster as well as by coxsackie A16 viruses [1, 6, 7]. The reason for the unusual susceptibility to these viruses has been thought to be either cutaneous changes predisposing to infection or defective CMI. The latter possibility is supported by the findings that eczema vaccinatum as well as herpeticum may occur in patients without clinical signs of continuing AE [8, 9]. Similarly, the increased susceptibility to wart virus [10], molluscum contagiosum [11] and the yeast *Pityrosporon orbiculare* [12] as well as the increased incidence of various dermatophytoses [13, 14] are compatible with a defective CMI in AE. In a more recent study, Rystedt et al. [15] found an increased frequency of multiple recurrences of cold sores (presumably caused by herpes simplex virus) and of herpes zoster in adult patients with AE. Although the increased frequencies of these infections were correlated to disease activity, significantly elevated numbers of multiple (> 5 per year) recurrences of cold sores were also found in patients who had had no clinically active disease during the past year. Again, these findlings would be compatible with defective CMI in AE.

Patients with immunodeficiency affecting the cell-mediated rather than the humoral limb of the immune system are particularly prone to developing severe viral and fungal infections. Therefore, if there were a pronounced CMI deficiency in AE, one would expect not only cutaneous but also other viral and fungal infections to run a severe course in this disease. However, there is very little evidence to suggest that this is the case. For instance, there are no reports that common childhood viral infections, like measles and mumps, are particularly severe in atopic children. Although antibody titers to EBV are elevated in AE [16, 17], there is no firm evidence that the clinical outcome of EBV infection is different in atopic as compared with non-atopic individuals. Antibody titers to herpes simplex, varicella zoster, cytomegalovirus, mumps and rubella virus have been found to be similar in atopic and non-atopic individuals [16, 17].

Although there is often heavy colonisation of the skin with *Staphylococcus aureus* and beta-hemolytic streptococci in AE [18–20], there is no indication that this is due to defective CMI; rather, the colonisation is more probably related to the cutaneous alterations associated with the disease [21].

Changes in Delayed Hypersensitivity Reactions

More than 50 years ago Rostenberg and Sulzberger [22] observed that patients with AE had a very low incidence of positive patch tests, used to measure delayed hypersensitivity. Later, Palacios et al. [23] found that atopic patients were less easily sensitised by dinitrochlorobenzene than were normal individuals. Jones et al. [24], who studied contact sensitivity to poison ivy and poison oak, found positive patch tests at a four fold higher frequency in normal than in atopic individuals. Similarly, decreased delayed hypersensitivity responses to various microbial antigens have been observed [25, 26]. Hyporeactivity to PPD (purified protein derivative) has been observed in several studies [25, 27–30].

Both Gudjonsson et al. [28] and Uehara [30] reported that the degree of PPD hyporeactivity correlated with the extent of skin involvement. Thus, there appears to be a correlation between severity of the dermatitis and depression of the delayed hypersensitivity response. Although cutaneous hyporeactivity has been observed during disease-free intervals [8, 9, 31], the studies performed do not allow a firm conclusion that depressed delayed hypersensitivity responses reflect an inherent, dysfunctioning CMI in AE.

Changes in Numbers of T Cells and T-Cell Subpopulations

The relative and absolute number of circulating T cells in AE has been studied in a considerable number of investigations, employing the ability of T cells to bind sheep erythrocytes [32]. The majority of these studies have indicated that T-lymphocyte numbers are indeed decreased in atopic disease. The failure of some investigators to find abnormal T-cell numbers could be explained by an insufficient number of patients studied or by the choice of methods used for enumeration of T cells. In a large investigation Strannegård et al. [33] found significantly depressed numbers of T cells in all types (rhinoconjunctivitis, asthma, AE) of atopic disease. The T-lymphopenia in AE was clearly correlated to the activity of the disease. However, significant T-lymphopenia was observed also in patients with AE that was classified as "mild". As pointed out by Strannegård and Strannegård [32], the fact that T-lymphopenia was clearly demonstrable in most studies measuring high normal relative numbers (65%–70%) of T cells but not in most of those detecting low (about 45%) normal numbers suggests that the T-cell deficiency might be restricted to certain subpopulations of T cells, i.e. those with low avidity for sheep erythrocytes.

Further evidence for a subpopulation-restricted T-cell deficiency has been derived from studies using monoclonal antibodies against various T-cell subsets. As found by several groups, patients with AE display subnormal absolute and relative numbers of T cells of the suppressor/cytotoxic ($CD8^+$) phenotype [34–40]. Most investigators have found normal relative and absolute numbers of $CD4^+$ (helper/inducer) cells and thus a changed balance between $CD4^+$ and $CD8^+$ cells in the circulation.

Additional support for a T-cell defect primarily affecting suppressor T cells has been derived from studies utilising binding of the Fc portions of IgG and IgM as markers for subpopulations of cells. Cells bearing receptors for the Fc portion of IgG (T gamma) and IgM (T mu) have been considered largely to represent suppressor and helper cells, respectively [41]. Schuster et al. [42] and other investigators [37, 43, 44] observed clearly decreased levels of T-gamma cells in AE. In contrast to Schuster et al. [42] who reported that the T-gamma deficit reflected disease activity, others have found the reduction in T-gamma cells to be independent of the extent of the eczematous eruption [43].

Some investigators have failed to find any decrease in circulating T cells of suppressor/cytotoxic phenotypes [45–47]. In view of the rather moderate changes in cell numbers observed by others this is not surprising; an existing slight numerical decrease in a given subpopulation of cells will not be detected in all studies provided they do not include a sufficient number of subjects.

The question of whether the numerical decrease in T-cell numbers is of a primary or secondary nature is unresolved. Several researchers have found the deficiency to be correlated with disease activity, whereas others have claimed that it is independent of this activity. Suggestive evidence for the primary nature of the defect was provided by Juto and Strannegård [48], who found lower numbers of T cells in 1-month-old babies with a genetic predisposition for atopy than in those without a family history of atopy. More recently, Chandra and Baker [49] reported that 1–2-month-old babies who subsequently developed AE had significantly lower numbers of $CD8^+$ cells than babies who did not develop dermatitis. These findings would certainly suggest that the T-cell imbalance in AE is of a primary nature.

In Vitro Studies of CMI in AE

Lymphocyte Response to Mitogens

A vast number of studies on the mitogenic response of lymphocytes from atopic patients have been carried out (reviewed in [1,32]). Taken collectively, these studies indicate that there is a functional defect of cells from patients with AE as evidenced by a decreased response to e.g. phytohaemagglutinin (PHA), concanavalin A_x (ConA), PPD, herpes simplex and *candida* antigens. The defect seems to be moderate, however; some investigators have found subnormal lymphocyte responsiveness only when using suboptimal mitogen concentrations [50, 51]. Others have found the responsiveness to PHA to be more profoundly decreased than that to ConA or phorbol myristate acetate [33]. Hovmark [29] found that hyporeactivity to mitogens was not correlated to activity of disease, treatment or infection and therefore suggested that the functional defect of the T cells in AE was of a primary, intrinsic nature. However, as demonstrated by Elliot and Hanifin [52], an initial subnormal response to PHA may increase to normal levels after culture of the lymphocytes for 4 days. This finding would suggest that the hyporeactivity to mitogens is due to factors associated with disease activity rather than to an intrinsic lymphocyte defect.

Cellular Cytotoxicity

The cytotoxic potential of several types of cells has been found to be decreased in AE. Thus, cytotoxicity evoked by monocytes [53, 54], natural killer (NK) cells [55–57], K cells [58] as well as T cells [59] has been reported to be depressed in patients with active AE. Herlin and Kragballe [54] found depression of antibody-dependent, monocyte-mediated cytotoxicity to be related to the degree of skin involvement. Similarly, Jensen et al. [56] found a relationship between impairment of NK-cell activity and Fc-IgG receptor bearing cells. In agreement with an earlier report by Strannegård and Strannegård [60], Hall et al. and coworkers [57] demonstrated that NK-cell activity in patients with severe AE was significantly more inhibited by histamine than in control subjects. This finding would offer a possible explanation for the depression of NK cell activity in AE.

In apparent conflict with most other studies on NK-cell activity, Leung et al. [61] found cell-mediated cytotoxicity against myeloid target cells (K562) to be normal but cytotoxicity against skin fibroblasts to be increased. This finding raises the interesting possibility that autocytotoxicity against skin cells might play a pathogenic role in AE.

In a study of K-cell-mediated, antibody-dependent cellular cytotoxicity (ADCC), Fritz et al. [58] found that ADCC was reduced in a subset of patients with AE who had a previous history of severe cutaneous infections. This would suggest that defective ADCC in some patients would render them susceptible to such infections.

Since, as described above, patients with AE frequently have reduced numbers of $CD8^+$ cells (suppressor/cytotoxic T cells) it would be logical to assume that T-cell-mediated cytotoxicity is reduced in AE. As shown by Leung et al. [6], this does indeed seem to be the case. These researchers found that cell-mediated lympholysis (CML), but not the proliferative response observed in mixed lymphocyte cultures, was decreased in patients with AE. Also, there was a correlation between CML activity and the percentage of circulating $CD8^+$ cells. The defect in CML was considered to reside not only in the $CD8^+$ but also in the $CD4^+$ (helper/inducer) cell subset.

Taken together, the results of cytotoxicity experiments would be consistent with a very basic immunological disturbance in AE. Since there is direct or indirect interaction between all kinds of cytotoxic cells, a defect in e.g. cells of the macrophage lineage (Langerhans cells, dendritic cells, monocytes, macrophages) manifested as depressed production of IL-1 might account for several of the findings obtained in the experimental systems. As recently described by Räsänen et al. [62], there is indeed suggestive evidence for such a defect (see below).

Chemotaxis

Neutrophils and monocytes from patients with AE have been reported to have generally reduced chemotactic responsiveness [63–69]. This is apparently dependent on the severity of the disease in the various populations studied, however, and widely divergent results ranging from normal to severely depressed chemotaxis have been obtained. It has been suggested that the reason for reduced chemotaxis might be the increased release of histamine associated with AE, since histamine seems to reduce the chemotactic responsiveness of normal neutrophils in vitro [68, 70]. De Shazo and coworkers [69] offered an explanation for depressed monocyte chemotaxis in AE by showing that histamine inhibited the chemotactic responsiveness of monocytes of patients with AE but not those of control subjects. This finding was interpreted to mean that an abnormal sensitivity of monocytes to histamine is an intrinsic feature of AE that may be detectable when the disease is quiescent. Another explanation for impaired chemotaxis might be effects evoked by IgG and IgE immune complexes which can be demonstrated in AE [71, 72] and have been shown to be able to inhibit neutrophil chemotaxis [73].

Taken collectively, results on studies of chemotaxis in AE suggest that the particular defect may be a secondary phenomenon and that it is much less pronounced than that occurring in the hyper IgE syndrome, where it constitutes a hallmark of the disease [74].

Autologous Mixed Lymphocyte Reaction

The autologous mixed lymphocyte reaction (AMLR), which measures the T-cell proliferative response to autologous non-T cells, is considered to represent an inducer circuit for the activation of $CD8^+$ effector cells [75]. Because there is the previously mentioned numerical and functional defect of $CD8^+$ cells in AE, Leung et al. [76] sought an explanation for it by studying AMLR in patients with AE. AMLR in these patients was found to be severely depressed, and the defect was considered to reside at the responder T-cell level rather than at the stimulator non-T-cell level. Furthermore, the defect was associated with a decreased number of circulating T cells bearing the surface marker CD29, which is found on the T-cell subsets that proliferate in AMLR. Impaired AMLR was also observed in patients without evidence of skin disease. These findings suggest that the T-cell defect in AE resides in the $CD29^+$ T-cell subset and that the impaired generation of $CD8^+$ cells is secondary to this defect.

Depression of AMLR in AE has recently been observed by Räsänen et al. [62], who used purified Langerhans cells as stimulators. This depression seems to be a general phenomenon in atopic disease since it has also been described in hay fever and other allergic diseases [77, 78].

Functional Suppressor Cell Assays

The finding that high levels of IgE in atopic patients correlates with low levels of T-gamma cells [44, 79] would suggest that the numerical deficiency of T cells of the suppressor/cytotoxic phenotype reflects a functional defect in these cells. Early studies [32, 80] showed that the generation of Con A-activated suppressor cells, which suppress lymphocyte proliferation, was impaired in atopic individuals. This finding was later verified by other groups [36,43,81]. Some investigators, however, have failed to find any differences between atopic and non atopic individuals regarding ConA-induced suppressor function [82]. This is probably due to a different selection of patients in the different studies; Stingl et al. [43] found a depressed ability to generate ConA-induced suppressor cells in patients with severe generalized AE but not in those with mild disease. This finding was interpreted to suggest that impaired generation of suppressor cells does not represent a primary phenomenon in the pathogenesis of atopic disease.

Since disturbed immunoregulation in AE has been suggested to be responsible for the associated sometimes markedly increased levels of IgE, studies on the suppression of IgE synthesis in vitro are particularly relevant. Results concerning T-suppressor cell function on spontaneous IgE synthesis in vitro have not been consistent and are difficult to interpret [83]. Although suppression of IgE synthesis may be impaired in AE [84], some patients whose B lymphocytes produce excessive amounts of IgE in vitro seem to have normal T-suppressor cell function [85, 86]. Furthermore, Cooper et al. [44] found that T cells from patients with AE generated normal levels of suppression of pokeweed mitogen-driven IgG synthesis.

Presently, there is no firm evidence based on in vitro experiments for a functional defect of suppressor mechanisms in AE which is causally related to hyper IgE production. In fact, the inverse correlation between serum levels of IgE and number of cells of the suppressor/cytotoxic phenotype [44, 79] or ConA-inducible suppressor cell function [81] would constitute more evidence in favour of this assumption than would the results of in vitro experiments of IgE synthesis.

In Vitro Studies of Langerhans Cells

Langerhans cells (LC) are dendritic cells of the monocyte/macrophage lineage [87] which present antigens for T cells [88] and secrete various substances such as the epidermal thymocyte-activating factor (ETAF) [89], which may be identical to IL-1 [90]. LC have been shown to constitute an important part of the cellular infiltrate in AE [91]. In a study by Räsänen and coworkers [62] the antigen-presenting function of purified LC was found to be intact, but their ability to produce ETAF was reduced. Also, autologous mixed cell reactions, using LC as stimulator cells, were impaired. These findings led them to conclude that there may be an abnormality in the generation of effector cells in AE which may be due to diminished production of, or response to, interleukins. As ETAF may be indistinguishable from IL-1, a functional defect of LC, expressed as depressed capacity to produce IL-1, could have consequences regarding the defence against infectious agents and contribute to the pathogenesis of the disease.

It is noteworthy that in other studies monocyte production of IL-1 has been found to be decreased in patients with AE [92]. Strannegård [93] found that glass-adherent mononuclear cells from atopic patients displayed less suppressive activity on the proliferation of autologous T cells than did adherent cells from non-atopic individuals. Thus, it seems possible that the defective function of cells of the monocyte/macrophage lineage may play a central role in the pathogenesis of atopic disease.

Production of Interferon

In view of the recent findings that interferon (IFN) γ and, to a lesser extent, IFN-α has suppressive effects on the synthesis of human IgE [94,95], studies of IFN production in AE are of particular interest. Strannegård and Strannegård [96] found that peripheral blood mononuclear cells from atopic children had a significantly reduced capacity to produce IFN-α upon stimulation with Sendai virus.One patient who had an extremely severe AE was found to lack completely the ability to produce Sendai virus-induced IFN-α. Later, Bengtsson and Strannegård (unpublished data) found that cells from patients with food allergy associated with type I hypersensitivity had an impaired ability to produce IFN-γ after stimulation with the mitogens PHA and phorbol myristate acetate. More recently, Kapp et al. [97] studied the in vitro production of IFN by leukocytes from AE patients in response to a variety of stimuli. Although the lymphoproliferative response to several mitogens was found to be depressed in AE, the production of IFN-α and IFN-γ was not found to be abnormal. In contrast to the findings obtained in patients with AE the production of IFN-γ has been found to be clearly subnormal in patients with the hyper IgE syndrome [98].

The conflicting results on IFN production in atopic disease suggest that abnormalities of IFN production play a minor, if any, role in its pathogenesis. It should be noted, however, that atopic patients, more frequently than non-atopic individuals, have demonstrable levels of IFN in their circulation [99]. This is reminiscent of findings in patients with systemic lupus erythematosus, who display elevated serum levels of IFN concomitantly with a depressed cellular ability to produce IFN upon stimulation with mitogens or viruses [100].

Altered Cellular Reactivity to Physiological Substances

Histamine, which is a potent regulator of various immune responses, generally suppresses the lymphocyte response to T-cell mitogens [101]. Lymphocytes from atopic children appear to be more sensitive to the inhibitory effect of histamine than lymphocytes from non-atopic individuals [102, 103]. Not only the mitogen responsiveness but also NK-cell activity has been claimed to be more easily suppressed in atopic than in non-atopic individuals [57, 60], and similar findings have been reported regarding the chemotactic response of monocytes in patients with AE [69].

Since histamine may act at least partly via increasing intracellular levels of cyclic AMP, effects of other substances promoting cyclic AMP accumulation are of particular interest in AE. Strannegård and Strannegård [104], using cholera toxin and dibutyryl-cAMP as cyclic AMP promoting agents, found an altered sensitivity of lymphocytes to these substances, suggesting an increased sensitivity to the action of cyclic AMP in atopic individuals. Further support for this suggestion was derived from studies of cell viability in lymphocyte cultures, in which it was found that mononuclear cells from atopic children were less viable than cells from non-atopic children, in particular in the presence of dibutyryl-cAMP [105]. In another study the same investigators [106] found that cyclic AMP-elevating substances in low concentrations were able to enhance, but in high concentrations suppressed, in vitro IgE synthesis of cells from AE patients.

The finding of effects of cyclic AMP on IgE synthesis may be linked with results obtained in studies of cyclic nucleotides in atopic disease. β-adrenergic blockade in AE [107] is expressed as a reduced leukocyte response to adenylate cyclase-active agonists [108]. The reduced responsiveness is associated with elevated cyclic AMP-phosphodiesterase (PDE) activity, which is considered to be an intrinsic feature of leukocytes from atopic patients [109–111]. Increased PDE activity may be responsible for the increased leukocyte histamine releasability [112] as well as for the hyper IgE synthesis by AE cells in vitro [106, 113].

Possible Reasons for Defective CMI in AE

Influence of Inflammatory Mediators

About 90% of patients with AE have elevated levels of IgE directed against a variety of allergens [2]. Cells possessing surface receptors for IgE include, among others, mast cells, basophils, monocytes and Langerhans cells [114]. Binding of allergens to cell-bound IgE will result in release of a variety of inflammatory mediators, including histamine and arachidonic acid metabolites such as prostaglandins and leukotrienes. The latter metabolites have been shown to be able to suppress T-cell proliferation in vitro [115, 116].

Histamine, which occurs in elevated concentrations in the skin and plasma of patients with AE [117–119], has a variety of effects on immune responses [101]. Of particular interest in this context are recent results showing that histamine inhibits the production of IFN-γ via suppression of IL-2 synthesis by human T-cells [120, 121]. Also, histamine has been found to suppress the production of IL-1 [122]. These observations are interesting in view of the recent finding that IFN-γ and IL-4, which possibly are produced by different human T-helper cell subsets, have opposing effects on IgE synthesis [94, 95]. Thus, via suppression of IFN-γ production, histamine might enhance IgE synthesis and create a vicious circle.

Through various effects on IL production and the ability to induce cyclic AMP accumulation, histamine might, in conjunction with other mediators, in fact be responsible for most of the abnormalities of CMI in AE referred to above. In addition, these mediators will, if they induce cyclic AMP accumulation, bring about a state of "desensitisation" of cells caused by increased cyclic AMP PDE activity [109]. As mentioned above, elevated PDE levels might enhance IgE synthesis and also stimulate the cellular releasability of histamine, again creating a vicious circle.

Immune Complexes

Several investigators have described the presence of IgG and IgE immune complexes (IC) in atopic diseases [71, 72, 123, 124]. Such IC may consist of allergen and antibody, or of IgE and IgG autoantibodies to IgE [124]. Both IgG and IgE IC have been shown to have the ability to inhibit neutrophil chemotaxis [73] and to cause leukotriene and prostaglandin release by macrophages [125, 126]. Quinti et al. [124] found a significant correlation between serum IgE levels and IgG anti-IgE activity. In view of the often extremely high serum IgE levels observed, IC formation with the ensuing release of inflammatory mediators from macrophages which in turn may lead to changes in CMI should be expected to be a common event in AE.

Evidence for a Primary, Intrinsic, Cellular Defect Associated with Changed CMI

Even if, as described above, the types of changes of CMI seen in AE may well be explained as being secondary phenomena, there are certain studies suggesting that changed CMI is of a primary nature and indeed causally related to the disease. This evidence can be summarised as follows: (a) changes in CMI have not always been found to reflect disease activity but may also occur in disease-free intervals; (b) subnormal numbers of T cells have been observed in newborns with a genetic predisposition for atopy but without clinically evident disease [48]; (c) in a prospective study, babies who later developed AE had low numbers of $CD8^+$ cells [49]; (d) in AE patients with T-cell imbalance who were treated with thymopoietin (TP-5), there was an improvement of the clinical status concomitantly with a tendency towards normalisation of the T-cell abnormality [37, 127].

The evidence cited above is, however, circumstantial; even in the absence of clinically overt disease there may be an abnormal release of inflammatory mediators which cause changes in CMI. Likewise, the observed association between clinical improvement and normalisation of immunological abnormalities does not necessarily imply that the latter is a primary intrinsic feature of the disease.

Hanifin and coworkers [109, 110, 111] have advanced the hypothesis that elevated cAMP PDE activity is an intrinsic, basic abnormality of atopic cells. The hypothesis is based on findings that increased PDE activity has been found in blood leukocytes from newborns with hereditary predisposition to atopy, is present even during remissions of AE and does not fluctuate with disease activity. However, since increased PDE activity may be a consequence of increased intra-cellular cAMP accumulation, it is difficult to exclude the possibility that increased PDE is a secondary phenomenon resulting from increased release of, or stimulation by, cAMP-inducing factors. Thus, the same objections can be raised against the two hypotheses of elevated PDE activity and T-cell imbalances.

Additional evidence for a basic, intrinsic cellular abnormality that is specific for the immune system can be derived from the cure by bone marrow transplantation of Wiskott-Aldrich syndrome [3]. Some data suggest that the blood mononuclear cells of atopic patients are less viable than cells from non-atopic individuals [105], and other data imply that the lipid composition of atopic leukocytes is abnormal [128]. The latter finding would agree with the results of Strannegård et al. [129] showing an abnormality of the serum composition of essential fatty acids in AE and a similar abnormality in umbilical cord sera containing high levels of IgE.

Pathogenic Implications of Changed CMI in AE

Recently obtained evidence suggests that CMI reactions may play a pathogenic role in AE. The cellular infiltrate in the skin of patients with AE is not suggestive of an IgE-mediated immediate hypersensitivity reaction but is rather similar to that seen in contact dermatitis [91, 130]. Patch tests to inhalant allergens may be positive in AE, giving rise to late reactions that are similar to the inflammatory reaction in AE [131, 132]. Furthermore, IgE has been shown to bind to alveolar macrophages [133] as well as to macrophages and Langerhans cells, which constitute part of the cellular infiltrate in AE [134, 114], and to be able to bring about mediator release from macrophages [125, 126]. IgE-mediated release of mediators from mast cells and macrophages may result in immediate as well as delayed-type hypersensitivity reactions, including the attraction of eosinophils and release of toxic factors. One of these, MBP, has been found to be widely deposited in the superficial and deep dermis in AE [135].

From the above it seems reasonable to assume that the pathological picture in AE results from a combination of cell-mediated and humoral immune reactions. Thus, any change in CMI would be presumed to affect the course and clinical manifestations of the disease.

Defective CMI, whether an inherent or a secondary phenomenon in AE, may aggravate the disease by several mechanisms. Firstly, it may increase susceptibility to various cutaneous infections, thereby worsening the dermatitis. Available evidence does not, however, implicate infections as any major exacerbating factors in AE [136]. Secondly, defective CMI might play a pathogenic role in AE by increasing IgE synthesis. Recent results suggest that IgE production is largely regulated by subsets of $CD4^+$ cells producing IFN-γ or IL-4 [94, 95]. Although there seems to be a functional heterogeneity among human $CD4^+$ T-cell clones with regard to the type of lymphokines secreted, so that some clones may secrete both IL-4 and IFN-γ [137, 138], it appears entirely possible that hyper IgE synthesis results from a functional imbalance between IFN-γ and IL-4 secreting $CD4^+$ cells. A functional defect in a subset of $CD4^+$ cells which produces IFN-γ and suppresses IgE synthesis will have a number of secondary consequences. In particular, it should be noted that $CD4^+$ cells are involved in the activation of $CD8^+$ cells, which may have a negative regulatory effect on IgE synthesis.

IgE seems to play a crucial role in AE by its ability to mediate release of inflammatory mediators from mast cells and macrophages. In addition to causing disease symptoms, these mediators, in particular histamine, will have profound effects on CMI and on cyclic nucleotide metabolism, in both cases possibly creating vicious circles. It may be argued that AE can occur without apparent signs of hyper IgE production. The serum levels of IgE may not, however, always reflect the levels of cell-bound IgE. Also, the possibility that the pathogenic events described above may not always be due to increased release of the various mediators, but instead to increased cellular sensitivity to these mediators, should be considered.

Conclusions

A vast number of investigations employing different methodologies have shown that various parameters of CMI are depressed in AE. Most, if not all, of the observed changes in CMI may be secondary phenomena, ascribed to the effects of inflammatory mediators. IgE and histamine seem to be two dominating factors in the pathogenesis of AE. Cytophilic IgE, bound to mast cells and macrophages, may lead to the release of mediators which evoke both immediate and late hypersensitivity reactions. Histamine and other mediators may suppress CMI and affect cyclic nucleotide metabolism, resulting in increased cellular histamine releasability and, possibly, increased IgE synthesis, thus creating vicious circles. A basic abnormality in a subset of $CD4^+$ cells, perhaps aggravated by histamine, appears to be the most likely explanation for the hyperproduction of IgE, with ensuing consequences, in AE.

Finally, the intimate relationship between immunological and pharmacological changes in AE and the present uncertainty regarding the nature of the genetically determined basic abnormality in AE would perhaps make it appropriate to label AE an immunopharmacological rather than an immunological disease.

References

1. Hanifin IM, Lobitz WC (1977) Newer concepts of atopic dermatitis. Arch Dermatol 113:663–670
2. Juhlin L, Johansson SGO, Bennich H, Högman L, Thyresson N (1969) Immunoglobulin E in dermatoses: levels in atopic dermatitis and urticaria. Arch Dermatol 100:12–16
3. Saurat J-H (1985) Eczema in primary immunodeficiencies. Acta Derm Venereol (Stockh.) 114:125–128
4. Parkman R, Rappaport D, Geha R, Belli J, Cassady R, Levey R, Nathan DG, Rosen FS (1978) Complete correction of the Wiskott-Aldrich syndrome by allogeneic bone marrow transplantation. N Engl J Med 298:921–927
5. Kaposi MJ (1987) Pathologie und Therapie der Hautkrankheiten. Urban and Schwarzenberg, Berlin, p 483
6. Marks MJG (1978) Atopic dermatitis, eczema herpeticum, infectious mononucleosis, and depressed cell-mediated immunity. South Med J 71:330–333
7. Verbov J, Hart A (1986) Severe varicella in a child with atopic eczema and ichtyosis. Practitioner 230:15–16
8. Monckton Copeman PW, Wallace HJ (1964) Eczema vaccinatum. Br Med J 2:906–908
9. Verbov JL, Munro DD, Miller A (1972) Recurrent eczema herpeticum associated with ichthyosis vulgaris. Br Med J 86:638–640
10. Currie JM, Wright RC, Miller OG (1971) The frequency of warts in atopic patients. Cutis 8:244–245
11. Dupré A, Christol B, Lassère J (1981) Dermatite atopique et surinfection. Ann Dermatol Venereol 108:829–834
12. Waersted A, Hjort N (1985) Pityrosporum orbiculare – a pathogenic factor in atopic dermatitis of the face, scalp and neck? Acta Derm Venereol (Stockh.) 114:146–148
13. Jones HE, Reinhard JH, Rinaldi MG (1973) A clinical, mycological and immunological survey for dermatophytosis. Arch Dermatol 108:61–65
14. Hanifin JM, Ray LF, Lobitz WC Jr (1974) Immunologic reactivity in dermatophytosis. Br J Dermatol 90:1–8
15. Rystedt I, Strannegård I-L, Strannegård Ö (1986) Recurrent viral infections in patients with past or present atopic dermatitis. Br J Dermatol 114:575–582
16. Strannegård I-L, Strannegård Ö (1981) Epstein-Barr virus antibodies in children with atopic disease. Int Arch Allergy Appl Immunol 64:314–319
17. Rystedt I, Strannegård I-L, Strannegård Ö (1984) Increased serum levels of antibodies to Epstein-Barr virus in adults with a history of atopic dermatitis. Int Arch Allergy Appl Immunol 75:179–183
18. Leyden JJ, Marples RR, Kligman AM (1974) *Staphylococcus aureus* in the lesions of atopic dermatitis. Br J Dermatol 90:525–530
19. Aly R, Maibach HI, Shinefield H (1977) Microbial flora of atopic dermatitis. Arch Dermatol 113:780–782
20. David TJ, Cambridge GC (1986) Bacterial infection and atopic eczema. Archs Dis Child 61:20–23
21. Hanifin JM, Homburger HA (1986) Staphylococcal colonization, infection and atopic dermatitis – association not etiology. J Allergy Clin Immunol 78:563–566
22. Rostenberg A Jr, Sulzberger MB (1937) Some results of patch tests. Arch Dermatol 35:433–454
23. Palacios J, Fuller EW, Blaylock WK (1966) Immunological capabilities of patients with atopic dermatitis. J Invest Dermatol 47:484–490
24. Jones HE, Lewis C, McMarlin SL (1973) Allergic contact sensitivity in atopic dermatitis. Arch Dermatol 107: 217–222
25. Rajka G (1968) Delayed dermal and epidermal reactivity in atopic dermatitis (prurigo Besnier). III. Further studies with bacterial and viral allergens. Acta Derm Venereol (Stockh.) 48:186–191
26. Mc Geady SJ, Buckley RH (1975) Depression of cell-mediated immunity in atopic eczema. J Allergy Clin Immunol 56:393–406
27. Rajka G (1967) Delayed dermal and epidermal reactivity in atopic dermatitis. I. Delayed reactivity to bacterial and mold allergens. Acta Derm Venereol (Stockh.) 47:158–162
28. Gudjonsson H, Lodin A, Modée J (1966) Besnier's prurigo (atopic dermatitis in children). Acta Derm Venereol (Stockh.) 46:159–166
29. Hovmark A (1977) An in vitro and in vivo study of cell-mediated immunity and of T and B lymphocytes in atopic dermatitis. Acta Derm Venereol (Stockh.) 57:237–242
30. Uehara M (1977) Atopic dermatitis and tuberculin reactivity. Arch Dermatol 113:1226–1228
31. Dahl B, Thestrup-Pedersen K, Ellegaard J, Zachariae H (1975) Lymphocyte transformation, IgE and T cells in eczema vaccinatum treated with transfer factor. Acta Derm Venereol (Stockh.) 55:187–190
32. Strannegård Ö, Strannegård I-L (1978) T lymphocyte numbers and function in human IgE-mediated allergy. Immunol Rev 41:149–170
33. Strannegård I-L, Lindholm L, Strannegård Ö (1976) T lymphocytes in atopic children. Int Arch (Allergy) Appl Immunol 50:684–692
34. Leung DYM, Rhodes AR, Geha RS (1981) Enumeration of T cell subsets in atopic dermatitis using monoclonal antibodies. J Allergy Clin Immunol 67:450–455
35. Faure MR, Nicolas JF, Thivolet J, Gaucherand MA, Czerhielewski JM (1982) Studies of T cell subsets in atopic dermatitis. Human T-cell subpopulations defined by specific monoclonal antibodies. Clin Immunol Immunopathol 22:139–146
36. Butler M, Atherton D, Levinsky RJ (1982) Quantitative and functional deficit of suppressor T cells in children with atopic eczema. Clin Exp Immunol 50:92–98
37. Strannegård Ö, Strannegård I-L, Kang K, Cooper KD, Hanifin JM (1982) FcIgG receptor-bearing lymphocytes and monoclonal antibody-defined T cell subsets in atopic dermatitis. Effect of treatment with thymopoietin pentapeptide (TP-5). Int Arch Allergy Appl Immunol 69:238–244
38. Kang K, Cooper KD, Vanderbark A, Strannegård I-L, Strannegård Ö, Hanifin JM (1983) Immunoregulation in atopic dermatitis: T-lymphocyte subsets defined by monoclonal antibodies. Semin Dermatol 2:20–25
39. Zachary CB, McDonald DM (1983) Quantitative analysis of lymphocyte subsets in atopic eczema using monoclonal antibodies and flow cytometry. J Invest Dermatol 108: 411–422
40. Braathen LR (1985) T-cell subsets in patients with mild and severe atopic dermatitis. Acta Derm Venereol [Suppl.] (Stockh.) 114:133–136
41. Moretta L, Webb SR, Grossi CE, Lydyard PM, Cooper MD (1977) Functional analysis of two human T-cell subpopulations: help and suppression of B-cell responses by T-cells bearing receptors for IgM or IgG. J Exp Med 146:184–200
42. Schuster DJ, Bongiovanni BA, Pieron DL, Barbaro JF, Wong DT, Levinson AI (1980) Selective deficiency of a T-

cell subpopulation in active atopic dermatitis. J Immunol 124:1662–1667
43. Stingl G, Gazze L, Czarnecki N, Wolff K (1981) T cell abnormalities in atopic dermatitis patients: imbalances in T cell subpopulations and impaired generation of ConA-induced suppressor cells. J Invest Dermatol 76:468–473
44. Cooper KD, Kazmierowski JA, Wuepper KD, Hanifin JM (1983) Immunoregulation in atopic dermatitis: functional analysis of T-B cell interactions and the enumeration of Fc receptorbearing T cell. J Invest Dermatol 80:139–145
45. Hsieh KH (1982) Study of T-cell subpopulations defined by monoclonal antibodies in asthmatic children with or without atopic eczema and normals. Ann Allergy 48:345–347
46. Miadonna A, Tedeschi A, Leggieri E, Cottini M, Menni S, Froldi M, Zanussi C (1985) Characterization of T-cell subsets in patients with atopic dermatitis using OKT monoclonal antibodies. Ann Allergy 54:321–324
47. Podmore P, Burrowa D, Eedy D (1988) T-cell subset assay. A useful differentiation marker of atopic and seborrhoic eczema in infancy? Arch Dermatol 124:1235–1238
48. Juto P, Strannegård Ö (1979) T lymphocytes and blood eosinophils in early infancy in relation to heredity for allergy and type of feeding. J Allergy Clin Immunol 64:38–46
49. Chandra RK, Baker M (1983) Numerical and functional deficiency of suppressor T cells precedes development of atopic eczema. Lancet ii:1393–1394
50. Rachelefsky GS, Opelz G, Mickey R, Kiuchi M, Terasaki PI, Siegel SC, Stiehm ER (1976) Defective T cell function in atopic dermatitis. J Allergy Clin Immunol 57:569–576
51. Thestrup-Pedersen K, Ellegaard J, Thulin H, Zachariae H (1977) PPD and mitogen responsiveness of lymphocytes from patients with atopic dermatitis. Clin Exp Immunol 27:118–126
52. Elliot ST, Hanifin JM (1979) Lymphocyte response to phytohemagglutinin in atopic dermatitis. Arch Dermatol 115:1424–1426
53. Kragballe K (1979) Antibody-dependent monocyte-mediated cytotoxicity in severe atopic dermatitis. Allergy 34: 35–41
54. Herlin T, Kragballe K (1980) Impaired monocyte cyclic AMP responses and monocyte cytotoxicity in atopic dermatitis. Allergy 35:647–655
55. Kusaimi NT, Trentin JJ (1982) Natural cell-mediated cytotoxic activity in the peripheral blood of patients with atopic dermatitis. Arch Dermatol 118:568–571
56. Jensen JR, Sand TT, Jörgensen AS, Thestrup-Pedersen K (1984) Modulation of natural killer cell activity in patients with atopic dermatitis. J Invest Dermatol 82:30–34
57. Hall TJ, Rycroft R, Brostoff J (1985) Decreased natural killer cell activity in atopic eczema. Immunology 56:337–344
58. Fritz KA, Norris DA, Morris RL (1980) ADCC effector function in patients with atopic dermatitis. J Am Acad Dermatol 3:167–173
59. Leung DYM, Wood N, Dubey D, Rhodes AR, Geha RS (1983) Cellular basis of defective cell-mediated lympholysis in atopic dermatitis. J Immunol 130:1678–1682
60. Strannegård I-L, Strannegård Ö (1980) Regulatory effects of histamine on lymphocyte responsiveness. In Oehling A (ed) Advances in allergology and immunology. Pergamon, p 223–230
61. Leung DYM, Parkman R, Feller J, Wood N, Geha RS (1982) Cell-mediated cytotoxicity against skin fibroblasts in atopic dermatitis. J Immunol 128:1736–1741
62. Räsänen L, Lehto M, Reunala T, Jansén C, Lehtinen M, Leinikki P (1987) Langerhans cell- and T-lymphocyte functions in patients with atopic dermatitis with disseminated cutaneous herpes simplex virus infection. J Invest Dermatol 89:15–18
63. Rogge JL, Hanifin JM (1976) Immunodeficiencies in severe atopic dermatitis. Depressed chemotaxis and lymphocyte transformation. Arch Dermatol 112:1391–1396
64. Snyderman R, Rogers E, Buckley RH (1977) Abnormalities of leukotaxis in atopic dermatitis. J Allergy Clin Immunol 60:121–126
65. Furukawa CT, Altman LC (1978) Defective monocyte and polymorphonuclear leukocyte chemotaxis in atopic disease. J Allergy Clin Immunol 61:288–293
66. Fischer TJ, Gard SE, Rachelefsky GS, Kline RB, Borut TC, Stiehm ER (1980) Monocyte chemotaxis under agarose: defects in atopic disease, aspirin therapy and mucocutaneous candidiasis. Pediatr Res 14:242–246
67. Dahl MV, Cates KL, Quie PG (1978) Neutrophil chemotaxis in patients with atopic dermatitis without infection. Arch Dermatol 114:544–566
68. Radermecker M, Maldague MP (1981) Depression of neutrophil chemotaxis in atopic individuals: an H_2 histamine receptor response. Int Arch Allergy Appl Immunol 65:144–152
69. de Shazo RD, Hase T, Wright DG, Diem JE (1982) Evidence for histamine-mediated inhibition of monocyte chemotaxis in atopic dermatitis. J Allergy Clin Immunol 69:429–434
70. Hill HR, Quie PG (1974) Raised serum IgE levels in defective neutrophil chemotaxis in 3 children with eczema and recurrent infections. Lancet 1:183–187
71. Brostoff J, Johns P, Stanworth DR (1977) Complexed IgE in atopy. Lancet ii:741–42
72. Ferguson AC, Salinas FA (1984) Elevated IgG immune complexes in children with atopic eczema. J Allergy Clin Immunol 74:678–682
73. Setsukoito, Shinomiya K, Mikawa H (1983) Suppressive effect of IgE soluble immune complex on neutrophil chemotaxis. Clin Exp Immunol 51:407–412
74. Leung DYM, Geha RS (1988) Clinical and immunological aspects of the hyperimmunoglobulin E syndrome. Hematol./Oncol. Clin North Am 2:81–100
75. Smolen JS, Chused TM, Novotny EA, Steinberg AD (1982) The human autologous mixed lymphocyte reaction. III. Immune circuits. J Immunol 129:1050–1053
76. Leung DYM, Saryan JA, Frankel R, Lareau M, Geha RS (1983) Impairment of the autologous mixed lymphocyte reaction in atopic dermatitis. J Clin Invest 72:1482–1486
77. Dirienzo W, Bagnasco M, Caria M, Chimini G, Ciprandi G, Ferrini S, Canonica GW (1984) Activation of T lymphocytes and autologous mixed lymphocyte reaction in allergic patients. Ann Allergy 53:272–277
78. Bovbjerg DH, Wang VA, Schwab R, Lebenger KS, Siskind GW, Weksler ME (1985) Lymphocyte transformation induced by autologous cells. XVII. Lower autologous mixed lymphocyte reaction in subjects with a history of hayfever. Int Arch Allergy Appl. Immunol 78:332–334
79. Perelmutter L, Potvin L (1980) Role of T gamma and T mu subset lymphocytes in allergic disease. Ann Allergy 45:18–22

80. Strannegård I-L (1979) Lymphocyte stimulation with phorbol myristate acetate in atopic and non-atopic individuals. Int Arch Allergy Appl. Immunol 58:175–181
81. Rola-Pleszczynski M, Blanchard R (1981) Abnormal suppressor cell function in atopic dermatitis. J Invest Dermatol 76:279–283
82. Martinez JD, Santos JS, Stechschulte MD, Abdou NI (1979) Nonspecific suppressor cell function in atopic subjects. J Allergy Clin Immunol 64:485–491
83. Sampson H, Buckley R (1981) Human IgE synthesis in vitro: a reassessment. J Immunol 127:829–834
84. Hemady Z, Gellis S, Chambers M, Rocklin RE (1985) Abnormal regulation of in vitro IgE synthesis by T cells obtained from patients with atopic dermatitis. Clin Immunol Immunopathol 35:156–168
85. Fiser P, Buckley R (1979) Human IgE biosynthesis in vitro: studies with atopic and normal blood mononuclear cells and subpopulations. J Immunol 123:1788–1794
86. Saxon A, Morrow C, Stevens RH (1980) Subpopulations of circulating B cells and regulatory T cells involved in in vitro IgE production in atopic patients with elevated serum IgE. J Clin Invest 65:1457–1468
87. Tew JG, Thorbecke GJ, Steinman RM (1982) Dendritic cells in the immune response: characteristics and recommended nomenclature. J Reticuloendothel Soc 31:371–380
88. Stingl G, Katz SI, Clement L, Green I, Shewach EM (1978) Immunologic function of Ia-bearing epidermal Langerhans cells. J Immunol 121:2005–2013
89. Sauder DN (1984) Epidermal cytokines: properties of epidermal cell thymocyte-activating factor (ETAF), Lymphokine Res 3:145–151
90. Breathnach SM, Katz SI (1986) Cell-mediated immunity in cutaneous disease. Hum Pathol 17:161–167
91. Leung DYM, Bhan AK, Schneeberger EE, Geha RS (1983) Characterization of the mononuclear cell infiltrate in atopic dermatitis using monoclonal antibodies. J Allergy Clin Immunol 71:47–56
92. Mizoguchi M, Furusawa S, Okitsu S, Yoshino K (1985) Macrophage-derived interleukin 1 activity in atopic dermatitis (abstract). J Invest Dermatol 84:303
93. Strannegård I-L (1981) Adherent suppressor cells in atopic disease. Int Arch Allergy Appl Immunol 64:308–313
94. Del Prete G, Maggi E, Parronchi P, Chrétien I, Tiri A, Macchia D, Ricci M, Banchereau J, de Vries J, Romagnani S (1988) IL-4 is an essential factor for the IgE synthesis induced in vitro by human T cell clones and their supernatants. J Immunol 140:4193–4198
95. Pène J, Rousset F, Brière F, Chrétien I, Bonnefoy J-Y, Spits H, Yokota T, Arai N, Arai K-I, Banchereau J, de Vries J (1988) IgE production by normal human lymphocytes is induced by interleukin 4 and suppressed by interferons gamma and alpha and prostaglandin E_2. Proc Natl Acad Sci USA 85:6880–6884
96. Strannegård I-L, Strannegård Ö (1980) Natural killer cells and interferon production in atopic disease. Acta Derm Venereol (Stockh.) [Suppl] 92:48–51
97. Kapp A, Gillitzer R, Kirchner H, Schöpf E (1987) Production of interferon and lymphoproliferative response in whole blood cultures derived from patients with atopic dermatitis. Arch Dermatol Res 279:55–58
98. Matricardi PM, Capobianchi MR, Paganelli R, Faccini J, Sirianni MC, Seminara R, Dianzani F, Aiuti F (1984) Interferon production in primary immunodeficiencies. J Clin Immunol 4:388–394
99. Skurkowich SV, Eremkina EI (1975) The probable role of interferon in allergy. Ann Allergy 35:356–360
100. Strannegård Ö, Hermodsson S, Westberg G (1982) Interferon and natural killer cells in systemic lupus erythematosus. Clin Exp Immunol 50:246–252
101. Rocklin RE, Beer DJ (1983) Histamine and immune modulation. Adv Intern Med 28:225–251
102. Strannegård I-L, Strannegård Ö (1977) Increased sensitivity of lymphocytes from atopic individuals to histamine-induced suppression. Scand J Immunol 6:1225–1231
103. Brostoff J, Pack S, Lydyard PM (1980) Histamine suppression of lymphocyte activation. Clin Exp Immunol 39:739–745
104. Strannegård I-L, Strannegård Ö (1979) Stimulatory and inhibitory effects of cyclic AMP on lymphocytes from atopic children. Int Arch Allergy Appl Immunol 58:167–174
105. Strannegård Ö, Strannegård I-L (1984) Viability of cultured peripheral blood mononuclear cells from atopic individuals. Int Arch Allergy Appl Immunol 75:289–293
106. Strannegård Ö, Strannegård I-L (1984) Effect of cyclic AMP-elevating agents on human spontaneous IgE synthesis in vitro. Int Arch Allergy Appl Immunol 74: 9–14
107. Szentivanyi A (1968) The beta adrenergic theory of the atopic abnormality in bronchial asthma. J Allergy Clin Immunol 42:203–232
108. Parker CW, Kennedy S, Eisen AZ (1977) Leukocyte and lymphocyte cyclic AMP responses in atopic eczema. J Invest Dermatol 68:302–306
109. Grewe SR, Chan SC, Hanifin JM (1982) Elevated leukocyte cyclic AMP-phosphodiesterase in atopic disease. A possible mechanism for cyclic AMP-agonist hyperresponsiveness. J Allergy Clin Immunol 70:452–457
110. Heskel NS, Chan SC, Thiel ML, Hanifin JM (1984) Elevated umbilical cord blood leukocyte cyclic adenosine monophosphate-phosphodiesterase activity in children with atopic parents. J Am Acad Dermatol 11:422–426
111. Hanifin JM (1988) Atopic dermatitis. Allergy 43 [Suppl 8]:36–38
112. Butler JM, Chan SC, Stevens S, Hanifin JM (1983) Increased leukocyte histamine release with elevated cyclic AMP-phosphodiesterase activity in atopic dermatitis. J Allergy Clin Immunol 71:490–497
113. Cooper KD, Kang K, Chan SC, Hanifin JM (1985) Phosphodiesterase inhibition by R020–1724 reduces hyper-IgE synthesis by atopic dermatitis cells in vitro. J Invest Dermatol 84:477–482
114. Bruynzeel-Koomen C, van Wichen DF, Toonstra J, Berrens L, Bruynzeel PLB (1986) The presence of IgE molecules on epidermal Langerhans cells in patients with atopic dermatitis. Arch Dermatol Res 278:199–205
115. Goodwin JS, Webb DR (1980) Regulation of the immune response by prostaglandins. Clin Immunol Immunopathol 15:106–122
116. Payan DG, Missirian-Bastian A, Goetzl EJ (1984) Human T-lymphocyte subset specificity of the regulatory effects of leukotriene B_4. Proc Natl Acad Sci USA 81:3501–3505
117. Johnson HH, de Oreo GA, Lascheid WP, Mitchell F (1960) Skin histamine levels in chronic atopic dermatitis. J Invest Dermatol 34:237–238
118. Juhlin L (1967) Localization and content of histamine in normal and diseased skin. Acta Derm Venereol (Stockh.) 47:383–391

119. Ring J, Senter T, Cornell RC, Arroyave CM, Tan EM (1979) Plasma complement and histamine changes in atopic dermatitis. Br J Dermatol 100:521–30
120. Carlsson R, Dohlsten M, Sjögren HO (1985) Histamine modulates the production of interferon gamma and interleukin 2 by mitogen-activated human mononuclear blood cells. Cell Immunol 96:104–112
121. Dohlsten M, Sjögren HO, Carlsson R (1986) Histamine inhibits interferon-gamma production via suppression of interleukin 2 synthesis. Cell Immunol 101:493–501
122. Dohlsten M, Kalland T, Sjögren HO, Carlsson R (1988) Histamine inhibits IL-1 production by LPS-stimulated human peripheral blood monocytes. Scand J Immunol 27:527–532
123. Paginelli R, Atherton DJ, Levinsky RJ (1983) Differences between normal and milk-allergic subjects in their immune responses after milk ingestion. Arch Dis Child 58:201–206
124. Quinti I, Brozek C, Wood N, Geha RS, Leung DYM (1986) Circulating IgG autoantibodies to IgE in atopic syndromes. J Allergy Clin Immunol 77:586–594
125. Rankin JA, Hitchcock M, Merill W, Bach MK, Brashler JR, Askenase PW (1982) IgE-dependent release of leukotriene C4 from alveolar macrophages. Nature 297:329–331
126. Rouzer CA, Scott WA, Hamill AL, Liu F-T, Katz DH, Cohn ZA (1982) IgE immune complexes stimulate arachidonic acid release by mouse peritoneal macrophages. Proc Natl Acad Sci USA 79:5656–5660
127. Kang K, Strannegård Ö, Strannegård I-L, Cooper K, Hanifin JM (1983) Suppressor phenotype deficiency and its restoration by thymopoietin pentapeptide in atopic dermatitis. Monogr Allergy 18:181–185
128. Rocklin RE, Thistle L, Gallant L, Manku MS, Horrobin D (1986) Altered arachidonic acid content in polymorphonuclear and mononuclear cells from patients with allergic rhinitis and/or asthma. Lipids 21:17–20
129. Strannegård I-L, Svennerholm L, Strannegård Ö (1987) Essential fatty acids in serum lecithin of children with atopic dermatitis and in umbilical cord serum of infants with high or low IgE levels. Int Arch Allergy Appl Immunol 82:606–607
130. Zachary C, Allen M (1985) In situ quantification of T lymphocyte subsets and Langerhans cells in the inflammatory infiltrate of atopic eczema. Br J Dermatol 112:149–156
131. Mitchell EB, Chapman MD, Pope FM, Crow J, Jouhal SS, Platts-Mills TAE (1982) Basophils in allergen-induced patch test sites in atopic dermatitis. Lancet I:127–130
132. Bruynzeel-Koomen CA, Bruynzeel PL (1988) A role for IgE in patch test reactions to inhalant allergens in patients with atopic dermatitis. Allergy 43 [Suppl] 5:15–21
133. Joseph M, Tonnel A-B, Torpier G, Capron A, Arnoux B, Benveniste J (1983) Involvement of immunoglobulin E in the secretory process of alveolar macrophages from asthmatic patients. J Clin Invest 71:221–230
134. Leung DYM, Schneeberger EE, Siraganian RP, Geha RS, Bhan AK (1987) The presence of IgE on macrophages and dendritic cells infiltrating into the skin lesion of atopic dermatitis. Clin Immunol Immunopathol 42:328–337
135. Leiferman KM, Ackerman SJ, Sampson HA, Haugen H, Venencie PY, Gleich GI (1985) Dermal deposition of eosinophil granulae major basic protein in atopic dermatitis. N Engl J Med 313:282–285
136. Rystedt I, Strannegård I-L, Strannegård Ö (1989) Infections as contributing factors to atopic dermatitis. Int Allergy 44, Suppl 9:79–83
137. Umetsu DT, Jabara HH, De Kruyff RH, Abbas AK, Abrams JS, Geha RS (1988) Functional heterogeneity among human inducer T cell clones. J Immunol 140:4211–4216
138. Paliard X, Malefijt RDW, Yssel H, Blanchard D, Chrétien I, Abrams J, De Vries J, Spits H (1988) Simultaneous production of IL-2, IL-4, and IFN-gamma by activated human $CD4^+$ and $CD8^+$ T cell clones. J Immunol 141:849–855

Role of Cyclic Nucleotide Metabolism in the Pathophysiology of Atopic Eczema

J. M. Hanifin and S. Ch. Chan

A study of the non-allergic, pharmacological mechanisms establishes a separate basic plane of investigation in atopic eczema (AE). Considerable clinical research is focussed at the level of environmental exacerbants while the more fundamental level – the realm of the genetically determined, constitutional predisposition to atopy – is largely ignored. Szentivanyi quoted Rackemann, who recognised this disparity in 1931: "The situation is somewhat analogous to that of a loaded gun. A good deal of knowledge is being obtained about a great variety of triggers (extrinsic and intrinsic causes) which fire the charge; but why is the gun loaded? And, what constitutes the load?" [1, 2]

We continue to focus on the "triggers", e.g. foods, mites, staphylococci, and we have learned a lot in recent years about the "load", e.g. mast cell, basophil and eosinophil inflammatory substances, but we do not know why the gun is "loaded", why the atopic individual is hyperreactive to so many varied stimuli. This is the realm of regulation and control of cellular function. A fundamental regulatory defect in the mast cells or B lymphocytes of an atopic individual could account for the inflammatory lesions and increased serum IgE production that characterise AE. A major dichotomy arises at this point between immunological and pharmacological views of regulation [3]. The immunologist might suggest that early antigen exposure in the genetically programmed individual initiates a central immunological perturbation of T lymphocytes which results in a multifaceted cell activation cascade of cytokine release, receptor expression and cell proliferation. Pharmacophysiological abnormalities would be secondary to this immune activation.

The biochemical/pharmacological view suggests that a basic molecular defect disrupts one or more of the cell regulation systems; e.g. phosphoinositide, calcium or cyclic nucleotide metabolism, causing inappropriate immune and inflammatory responses. Antigen- or irritant-initiated reactions may simply lack a shut-off switch. Ironically, our inability to resolve this dichotomy results from the fact that the basic molecular defect in atopy resides in the cells which mediate immune and inflammatory responses. Knowledge of this fact stems from bone marrow transplantation observations which documented transfer of the atopic defect to non-atopic individuals [4] and resolution of the eczematous condition in Wiskott-Aldrich syndrome [5]. Thus, in AE, we know the molecular defect is in one or, more likely, many cell types derived from the bone marrow lineage. Most of these cells are accessible and demonstrate both immunological and pharmacological abnormalities, so they appear to be worthy of investigation.

Among the different regulatory mechanisms, no information is available pertaining to disturbed calcium metabolism. One preliminary study suggested an irregularity of the phosphoinositide system [6] in atopic leukocytes, but techniques are not yet practical enough given the limited number of blood cells available. In contrast, numerous investigations of cyclic nucleotide metabolism have come forth in the 20 years since Szentivanyi [1] published his β-adrenergic theory of atopic disease causation. He suggested that while histamine and other mast cell factors are responsible for initiating the bronchoconstrictor response in asthma, catecholamines are the principle natural antagonists of that constrictor response. Though studies of cyclic AMP in tracheal smooth muscle had not yet been carried out, he correctly inferred from uterine studies that intracellular cyclic AMP causes bronchial relaxation. He reviewed other functional effects of β-adrenergic agents such as eosinopenia and glycogenolysis and cited studies which showed blunting of these responses in atopic patients. He described the β-adrenergic receptor as an enzyme, adenyl cyclase, though we now know it is only part of a multimolecular complex associated with adenylate cyclase. He suggested that an imbalance of autonomic regulation might account for the pharmacological abnormalities associated with asthma.

Szentivanyi and colleagues stated that a model must imitate not only the immunological but also the pharmacological abnormalities of the asthmatic state. With Fishel and Talmadge [7] numerous studies were carried out with the *Bordetella pertussis* mouse model. Szentivanyi summarised the relevance to asthma of this model:

- Hypersensitivity to histamine, serotonin and bradykinin, and to acetylcholine in one strain.
- Hypersensitivity to non-specific stimuli such as cold and irritants.

- Reduced sensitivity to catecholamines.
- Enhanced formation of reaginic antibodies.
- Marked eosinophilia.
- Loss of normal β-adrenergic inhibition of extrahepatic glucose uptake.

He proposed that this model was characterised by an imbalance between the α- and β-adrenergic systems, possibly due to a reduced functioning of the β-adrenergic receptor or other reactions between receptor activation and adrenergic endresponse. Interestingly, in the past few years a molecular site of action has been found for pertussis toxin. This substance causes ADP-ribosylation of an inhibitory GTP-binding "G-protein" associated with adenylate cyclase [8].

As the principle tenet of the β-adrenergic theory, Szentivanyi regarded asthma not as an immunological disease but as an unique pattern of bronchial hyperreactivity to a broad spectrum of immunological, psychic, chemical and physical stimuli. Thus, a variety of nonspecific exacerbants could function to trigger a central defective homeostatic mechanism, not only in asthma but in other atopic conditions as well.

Szentivanyi detailed many examples in which the β-adrenergic theory accounted for the clinical manifestations of asthma including: (a) bronchial hypersensitivity to histamine and other mediators of the type I immune response; (b) induction of similar hypersensitivity by β-adrenergic blocking agents; (c) increased tolerance to adrenaline; (d) eosinophilia; (e) worsening with onset of respiratory infections; and (f) the therapeutic effect of agents which augment adrenergic activity.

Despite the fact that Szentivanyi's β-adrenergic theory was formulated around asthma, it had perhaps even more impact on research into the causation of AE. The concept of multiple trigger factors coincided especially well with the clinical observations. Also, AE is characterised by aberrant pharmacological and physiological responses, and many investigators found in Szentivanyi's theory some possible explanations for the many pharmacological reactivities that had been observed through the years. Areas of evidence in support of an altered pharmacophysiological reactivity in AE include a variety of systemic abnormalities such as metabolic functions, thyroid and other endocrine associations, psychophysiological abnormalities and defects of sweating and cutaneous physiological and pharmacological responses [9].

Metabolic Abnormalities

A paradoxical defect is that described by Snyderman [10], who observed that children deprived of dietary histidine developed an eczematous skin rash. The paradox is that histidine is the precursor of histamine, which is often considered to be a prime pharmacological mediator of AE. However, whether the rash was truly AE is uncertain.

A condition similar to AE was described in 25% of children with phenylketonuria [11], although other observers who have critically examined such children dispute this claim. Observers have noted altered carbohydrate metabolism and flattened glucose tolerance curves in patients with AE [1, 9, 12–13]. Following a glucose load, blood sugar levels failed to show a normal rise, and conversely no rebound hyperglycaemia was observed. However, the definition of "eczema" was unclear in these reports, and in another study this glucose tolerance abnormality was also seen in patients with miscellaneous forms of eczematous dermatitis [14]. Irregularities were inferred from reports of altered blood glucose responses to adrenaline in patients with asthma [15]. Such observations were considered supportive of Szentivanyi's theory, though different interpretations were also proposed [16].

A number of disturbances of thyroid function have been described in association with AE. Stokes [17] described reduced basal metabolic rates in patients with AE, and he recommended that they be treated with desiccated thyroid. Other investigators suggested a high incidence of thyrotoxicosis or non-toxic goiter in patients with constitutional eczema [18]. In contrast, another study suggested an increased prevalence of hypothyroidism among atopic individuals [19]. Subsequent studies failed to confirm reports of abnormal basal metabolism in patients with AE [20, 21].

Psychophysiological Abnormalities

Most clinicians who have cared for patients with AE have been impressed that they are often characterised by above-average intelligence and certain common personality traits including hyperactivity, compulsive behaviour and emotional lability. A variety of reports through the years described psychoanalytic interpretations [22], personality profiles [23], psychodynamic studies [24] and maternal rejection factors [25]. Later, more critical observers such as Sulzberger [26] and Rostenberg [27] refuted the concept of a psychophysiological basis for AE and suggested instead that the personality variants were the result of the chronic disease burden.

Perhaps because of the focus of psychology on AE, some good psychophysiological studies have resulted. For example, Kalz et al. [28] tested histamine reactions in patients with AE and showed a good correlation between reduced or absent histamine wheal and flare responses and decreased aptitude for open emotional expression. Jordan and Whitlock [29] showed that patients with AE developed conditioned scratch reflexes more rapidly than did normal subjects, and they observed that patients frequently scratched during stressful interviews. Their results confirmed the studies of Graham and Wolf [30], who used measurements of skin temperature and reactive hyperaemia thresholds to demonstrate that patients with flares of AE could be precipitated during experimental stress interviews. These studies also showed quite clearly that erythema precedes the onset of the itch response. While itch had been considered by most investigators since the time of Jacquet [31] to be the primary clinical event in AE, these psychophysiological studies showed that erythema occurs even earlier.

Erythema may well be due to the release of histamine and other factors from skin mast cells. The mechanism for such triggering remains unknown, though recent speculations have suggested that substance P or other neuropeptides from sensory nerves may act upon the mast cells to cause release of vasoactive mediators [32, 33]. Alternatively, neurotransmitters could act directly on cutaneous blood vessels to cause vasodilatation, which is perceived as erythema. The interrelationship between neuropeptides and cyclic nucleotide metabolism remains to be delineated.

Sweating Abnormalities

Dermatologists almost universally agree that sweating leads to itching in patients with AE. Beyond this observation, very little is clear. Physiological and structural studies of sweat disturbances in AE are characterised by controversy and confusion. Sulzberger et al. [26] developed the hypothesis of poral occlusion to explain the deleterious effects of sweating and suggested that this response was similar to that seen in miliaria. They hypothesised that either dermal oedema or swelling of the otherwise dry keratin in patients with AE caused blockage of the sweat pore, creating the miliaria-like lesion. They also proposed that sweat which leaked into the dermis as a result of poral occlusion caused itching and urticaria in some cases and that these effects were even greater when allergens were carried in the sweat [34]. However, much of the genesis of this theory appears to have derived from a single case study [35]. Critical review suggests that the patient had increased sweating in areas of dermatitis such as the elbow and knee flexures but anhidrosis over the uninvolved skin. Subsequent studies provided some support for Sulzberger's concept [36], but, in spite of tedious histological studies, no one has been able to demonstrate a plug in the sweat pores of patients with AE [37]. Perhaps the most contradictory study is that of Rovensky and Saxl [38], who measured exercise-induced sweat output in children with AE. They noted consistently increased sweating over lichenified skin compared with uninvolved areas. Sweating began with low levels of exertion on lichenified areas while the response on unaffected skin required considerably more exertion. The sweat response was suppressed by atropine iontophoresis into the skin.

Possibly as a result of Szentivanyi's theory, studies in the 1970s examined sweat production after cholinergic stimulation. Both Warndorff [39] and Kaliner [40] suggested that cholinergic agents caused increased sweat production in patients with AE. Both authors also stated that their observations were consistent with Szentivanyi's theory and that patients with atopic disease have cholinergic hypersensitivity of the sweat glands, analogous to the hypersensitivity seen when cholinergic agents are inhaled into the bronchial system. Hemels [41] also showed increased cholinergic sweat responses in patients with AE and in normal control subjects whose skin was prepared by local injection of the β-adrenergic antagonist propranolol. He likewise suggested that patients with AE had in intrinsic β-adrenergic blockade which could not be augmented with β-adrenergic antagonists, though such a blockade could be produced in normal individuals. More recent studies by Foster et al. [42]

failed to confirm this. Likewise, other studies by Kiistala [43] and by Murphy et al. 44] have shown no differences in cholinergic sweat responses in atopic skin. Perhaps the main conclusion that can be drawn from all this is that sweating is difficult to evaluate and is subject to too many variables such as the considerable variation in cholinergic and adrenergic responses during autumn versus summer months [45, 46]. Abnormal sweat and itch responses are obviously part of AE but the relationship of sweat abnormalities to the adrenergic and cholinergic system remains to be clarified.

Cutaneous Physiological Responses

A large number of abnormal cutaneous responses have been described through the years:
white dermographism, reduced acral skin temperature, rapid vasoconstriction and rewarming, increased cold-pressor response and increased piloerection.

Perhaps the best known of these is white dermographism, in which the stroking of the skin leads to a paradoxical blanching in patients with AE [47]. This, like many other abnormal reactions described in AE, is probably a result of inflammatory activity in the skin rather than a reflection of basic vascular dysfunction [9, 48].

Abnormal reactions to temperature change appear to be somewhat more characteristic of AE. The basal skin temperature is typically lower in patients with AE, especially over acral areas [49]. Cutaneous blood vessels constrict rapidly in a cold environment and dilate slowly upon rewarming. Patients with AE also show an abnormal cold pressor test [50]. This abnormality is characterised by an excessive elevation of blood pressure when one extremity is immersed in cold water. Observations such as these have suggested to investigators that patients with AE may have a general vasoconstrictor tendency or other autonomic abnormality due to an imbalance of sympathetic and parasympathetic respones.

Pharmacological Abnormalities

A large number of abnormal responses have been documented in patients with AE after injection, epicutaneous application or iontophoresis of a variety of pharmacological agents into the skin:

Delayed blanch response
Increased cholinergic sweat response
Lowered cholinergic bronchoconstrictor threshold
Greater cholinergic pupillary responsiveness
Increased skin acetylcholine level
Lowered blanch threshold to adrenergic agents
Increased vasoconstriction and pupillary responses to phenylephrine
Increased skin adrenaline binding
Increased flush from intramuscular histamine
Reduced flare to intradermal histamine
Increased histamine wheal volume
Nicotinic acid blanching
Increased skin blister leukotriene concentration

Lobitz and Campbell [51] were the first to describe the delayed blanch response which occurs 2–5 min after the injection of cholinergic agents. Initially, a wheal and flare response occurs, but in patients with AE or in other inflammatory conditions blanching soon replaces the erythema. The mechanism of the delayed blanching is controversial, with some evidence for a vasoconstrictor response while other investigations have suggested that it is due to oedema [9, 52]. Laser doppler techniques have demonstrated highly variable responses consistent with vascular lability and defective vasoregulatory mechanisms [53].

Because early studies suggested that the response was due to vasoconstriction, Juhlin [54] reasoned that it occurred as a result of acetycholine-induced release of tissue catecholamines. He noted that iontophoresis of adrenaline predisposed to a delayed blanch response in normal skin. He also noted that the skin of patients with AE required less noradrenaline and adrenaline to cause blanching. He depleted adrenaline stores by pretreatment with guanethidine and thus eliminated the delayed blanch response [55]. Such studies also led to attempts at treating AE with guanethidine to reduce the adrenaline levels and with the oral α-adrenergic blocker, phenoxybenzamine [56]. While the initial studies suggested a beneficial effect, other investigators found only a partial improvement in pruritus in 6 of 13 patients and no change in the delayed blanch response [57]. Their evidence conflicted with Juhlin's concept, as did the finding that cutaneous denervation does not influence the delayed blanching nor does blockade with procaine, though the response is blocked by intradermal injection of atropine [58, 59].

The mechanism of the delayed blanch response reflects abnormal cholinergic responsiveness in AE and provides support to Szentivanyi's theory of autonomic imbalance. The cholinergic abnormality in the inflamed skin may be analogous to the reduced bronchoconstrictor threshold for inhaled methacholine, a widely used diagnostic test for asthma. A recent application of this test to patients with AE but no history of allergic respiratory disease showed airways hyperreactivity in over 50% [60]. Pupillary cholinergic hyperresponsiveness has been reported in atopic patients [61], although contradictory evidence exists [42]. Also, as shown by Clark et al. [62], parenteral methacholine administration produced similar vascular and cardiovascular responses in patients with atopy as in normal control subjects. It is quite difficult to draw any firm conclusions from past studies of cholinergic reactivity in AE. There is a general sense of altered cholinergic reactivity but responses, both in the skin and in bronchial smooth muscle, may be secondary to inflammatory conditions present in these tissues. Evidence for increased skin acetylcholine levels [63] needs confirmation by modern techniques.

Responses of patients with AE to adrenergic agents are likewise highly variable. Clinical observations have suggested a general vasoconstrictor tendency, suggesting increased adrenergic tone [49, 55]. Additionally, the increased piloerection seen in many is an indication of enhanced α-adrenergic tone [64]. Increased pupillary responsiveness as well as cutaneous vasoconstrictor responses to phenylephrine have been demonstrated [65]. The relationship between nocturnal asthma and circadian reductions in plasma adrenaline level has been offered as evidence for a permissive effect upon histamine release from mast cells [66]. It is interesting to speculate also that such a mechanism might help explain the nocturnal pruritus which is so characteristic of AE.

Cutaneous responses to catecholamines have varied in different reports. Intracutaneous adrenergic agonists caused normal responses in two studies [51, 67], while Juhlin [54] reported increased vascular reactivity to such agents. He postulated increased tissue levels of noradrenaline to account for many of the physiological abnormalities in atopic skin. This concept was supported by evidence for increased binding of isotope-labelled noradrenaline in the skin of patients with AE [68].

Cutaneous responses to histamine appear to be abnormal in AE. Patients often show an absent flare response after intradermal histamine administration [28, 50, 69]. A recent preliminary report showed no difference in flare area but significantly greater wheal volume after intradermal histamine injection into uninvolved forearm skin of patients with AE [70]. Williams [71] measured skin temperature responses after intramuscular histamine injections and showed that patients with AE had increased erythema at sites of predilection for lesions, specifically the face and neck and the antecubital and popliteal flexures. He suggested that these patients have a particular vascular sensitivity to histamine, and this is supported by recent evidence of increased skin wheal response to histamine [70]. Such observations may also relate to the increased histamine sensitivity of asthmatic patients to bronchoprovocation, cited by Szentivanyi [1] as evidence for autonomic imbalance in asthma. Increased sensitivity was also demonstrated in laboratory animals injected with pertussis toxin, sometimes known as "histamine sensitizing factor" [7]. The fact that pertussis toxin affects adenylate cyclase may be relevant to the role of cyclic nucleotide abnormalities in the pathogenesis of AE [8].

A role for histamine and other mast cell mediators in AE appears to be reasonably well documented. The flushing over the neck, face and flexural areas during spontaneous flares of AE and after experimental stress interviews [30] or food challenges [72] is similar to the pattern seen by early investigators after intravenous injection of histamine [73, 74]. Several other lines of evidence support the involvement of histamine in the pathogenesis of AE:
erythema and pruritus, increased plasma histamine, flares from food allergy, increased skin histamine and high basophil histamine release.
Mast cell numbers appear to be increased, especially in areas of chronic dermatitis [75], and investigations have shown increased histamine levels in both the uninvolved and involved skin of patients with AE [76]. Sporadic elevations of plasma histamine have demonstrated remarkably high plasma levels in some cases [77,78]. Elevated plasma histamine shortly after double-blind food challenge in food-allergic children coincided with the onset of erythema and itching [72].

Histamine releasability is clearly governed by cyclic nucleotide regulatory influences [79, 80]. While only scant evidence for increased histamine releasability has been uncovered for mast cells, several reports have demonstrated the high releasability in basophils from patients with atopy and AE [81, 82].

In addition to the many studies relating to adrenergic and cholinergic agents and histamine, a variety of other agents have been studied in atopic patients including nicotinic acid blanching, responses to serotonin, tachykinins and skin blister eicosanoids [9]. Little definitive information has arisen from these studies.

Cyclic Nucleotide Abnormalities

While not necessarily based on consistently sound clinical and in vivo observations, Szentivanyi's β-adrenergic theory stimulated a great deal of research in the realm of cyclic nucleotide abnormalities. As a result of Szentivanyi's theory, varied probes of the autonomic and cyclic AMP systems began. At first, these were mainly studies of functional effects of adrenergic stimulation in atopic versus normal humans. Bernstein et al. [83] showed that adrenaline caused a doubling of urinary cyclic AMP excretion in normal but not in asthmatic individuals.

In vitro studies soon followed, demonstrating impaired leukocyte cyclic AMP responses to isoproterenol from patients with asthma [84, 85]. Reed and colleagues then turned their attention to AE. Carr, Busse and Reed [86] studied DNA synthesis in normal epidermis and noted up to 50% inhibition by adrenaline in the range of $10^{-6}M$. In contrast, no inhibition occurred in epidermis from patients with AE. Because of the difficulty of obtaining homogenous tissue specimens from skin, these early investigators began using leukocytes for cyclic nucleotide studies. Similar results were seen in leukocyte preparations from patients with AE as had previously been reported in asthma patients [87–90]. A key question was whether the impaired cyclic AMP response in leukocytes was limited only to the adrenergic receptor. Prostaglandin E_1 (PGE_1) was used as an alternative adenylate cyclase stimulus, and initial results suggested a normal response, supporting a specific β-adrenergic receptor defect [88]. However, Parker et al. [89] were able to discern an impaired response to PGE_1 as well as to isoproterenol in mononuclear leukocytes. Later, Busse and Lantis [90] noted a similarly blunted response to histamine in granulocytes.

These studies were very important because they implied a defect not strictly limited to the β-receptor. Szentivanyi's hypothesis of β-receptor dysfunction in atopic disease also led to a number of studies using radioligands to quantitate receptor numbers and affinities on leukocytes. While reports appeared showing decreased β-adrenergic receptors, numbers or affinities in asthma [91] and AE [92], other assessments tended to show no abnormality [93].

Extrapolating from receptor pharmacology, the concept of desensitisation emerged along with the suspicion that many of the early cyclic AMP and receptor studies in asthma may have been flawed by treatment of patients with β-adrenergic agonists [94, 95]. Such agents cause a down-regulation of receptor function. Greenacre et al. [94] demonstrated that desensitisation could be heterologous, i.e. exposure of leukocytes to PGE_1 caused desensitisation not only for PGE_1 but also for isoproterenol. This information led us to investigate normal mononuclear leukocytes which were desensitised in vitro as a model for cyclic nucleotide abnormalities in AE [96]. We exposed these normal leukocytes to histamine, isoproterenol or PGE_1 at in vitro concentrations ranging from 10^{-7} to $10^{-5}M$ for periods ranging from 15 min to 1 h. We then washed the cells and exposed them to stimulatory concentrations (e.g. $10^{-3}M$) of the same agonists and found heterologous desensitisation; cells desensitised by any one of the adenylate cyclase-active agonists showed blunted cyclic AMP responses to all three agents. Cells in this desensitised state evidenced responses very similar to those observed in mononuclear leukocytes from patients with AE (Fig. 1). These studies

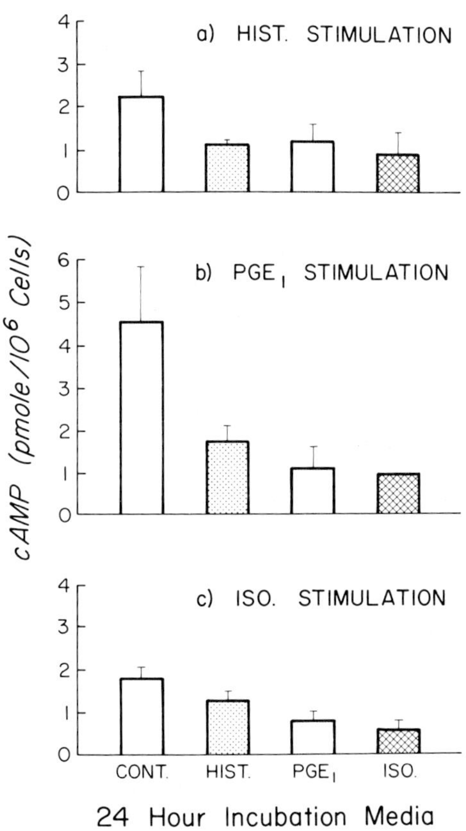

Fig. 1a–c. cAMP levels of mononuclear leukocytes (from four normal volunteers) incubated for 24 h in 20% AB serum/RPMI-1640 (control) or medium containing $10^{-6}M$ histamine, $3 \times 10^{-6}M$ prostaglandin E_1 or $10^{-6}M$ isoproterenol, then washed and stimulated (*cross-hatched bars*) with $10^{-3}M$ histamine (**a**), $10^{-5}M$ prostaglandin E_1 (**b**) or $10^{-3}M$ isoproterenol (**c**). *Open bars,* basal, non-stimulated levels. Responses were significantly reduced below control values for histamine ($P < 0.01$), prostaglandin ($P < 0.01$) and isoproterenol ($P < 0.05$) incubated cells

also confirmed earlier reports that leukocytes from patients with AE have reduced cyclic AMP responses not only to β-adrenergic agonists but to histamine and PGE_1 as well. Thus, the defect in cyclic nucleotide metabolism cannot be limited to the β-adrenergic receptor alone. These studies suggested to us that the defect was likely to be at some site distal to the receptor. Possibilities included a defect in adenylate cyclase generation of cyclic AMP or increased catabolism by cyclic AMP phosphodiesterase.

We elected first to pursue the latter possibility. We showed that desensitisation with either PGE_1, isoproterenol or histamine caused increased cyclic AMP phosphodiesterase activity in normal mononuclear leukocytes, under conditions identical to those in which we had desensitised the cells to agonist stimulation of cyclic AMP [97]. The increase occurred within 15 min and was accompanied by a mirror-image decrease in agonist-stimulated cyclic AMP levels. This phosphodiesterase activity remained elevated for up to 72 h in cultured cells but generally began decreasing within 24 h. As with previous desensitisation studies [96], the optimal phosphodiesterase-stimulatory concentrations for histamine were 1–10 μM, certainly well within the range that might be expected in inflammatory tissues after histamine release had occurred. Thus, our initial hypothesis was that increased phosphodiesterase activity and the resultant, blunted cyclic AMP intracellular levels were secondary to exposure of infiltrating leukocytes, and perhaps circulating leukocytes, to histamine and other inflammatory mediators.

We studied leukocyte phosphodiesterase activity, comparing cells from patients with AE with those of normal control subjects, patients with other atopic conditions such as allergic rhinitis and patients with no personal or family history of atopy but with widespread eczematous dermatitis from allergic contact dermatitis [98]. We were aided in these quantitations by the recently completed basic studies of Thompson et al. [99], who had defined optimal assay conditions and substrate concentrations for the measurement of cyclic AMP phosphodiesterase in mononuclear leukocytes. Using similar conditions, we found very consistent, significant elevations in leukocyte homogenates from patients with AE, even among these whose disease was in remission [98]. Similar, though slightly lower, phosphodiesterase activity levels were detected in patients with allergic rhinitis, while levels were normal in the non-atopic patients with allergic contact dermatitis, providing evidence that the phosphodiesterase defect was not a result of cutaneous inflammation alone. Previous studies in leukocytes by Greenacre et al. [94] as well as in skin homogenates by Holla et al. [100] had failed to detect abnormal phosphodiesterase activity in either desensitised leukocytes or in skin from patients with AE. Inspection of those reports revealed that the substrate concentrations were outside the range of detectable abnormality seen in our studies. It should be noted also that if unusually elevated phosphodiesterase activity is a primary, gene-related defect in leukocytes, the abnormality may not be present in skin cells. The above-mentioned report of bone marrow transfer of atopy suggests that this may well be the case [4].

We next investigated the issue of the biological relevance of abnormally elevated cyclic AMP phosphodiesterase levels in atopic leukocytes. In any study of the mechanisms of allergy, histamine assumes an important role, and a large body of literature has developed around the relationship of the cyclic nucleotide system to tissue histamine release. As early as 1966, Grotti et al. [101] reported that adrenaline could reduce histamine release from guinea pig heart during anaphylactic reactions. Lichtenstein and Margolis [79] then studied histamine release from peripheral blood leukocytes and found inhibition of release by adrenergic agents as well as by phosphodiesterase inhibitors. These principles were extended to lung mast cells, and in a series of excellent studies, Orange et al. [80] demonstrated an inverse relationship between cyclic AMP levels and the release of histamine and slow-reacting substances. Pharmacological agents which increase intracellular cyclic AMP inhibited mediator release, while α-adrenergic stimulation or β-adrenergic blockade increased the level of histamine release. Likewise, cholinergic agents increased histamine release, presumably through the enhancing effects of cyclic GMP [102] (Fig. 2). These elegant studies formed a conceptual framework for the understanding of cyclic nucleotide control of mediator release from mast cells and basophils.

Based on this background, we could predict that the increased phosphodiesterase activity in leukocytes from patients with atopic disease might have a permissive, augmenting effect on mediator release from inflammatory cells. Previous workers including Lebel et al. [81] had shown evidence of increased histamine releasability from basophils among peripheral blood leukocytes isolated from patients with AE. These studies clearly established the fact that basophils from atopic individuals have increased histamine releasability when stimulated with antigen or anti-IgE. Butler [82] in our laboratory utilised concanavalinA (ConA) stimulation of dextran-purified peripheral blood leukocytes from patients with AE and from normal, non-atopic individuals. Approximately 75% of the atopic patients showed increased histamine releasability while normal individuals consistently had histamine release levels below 10% (Fig. 3). We then compared phosphodiesterase activity in those leukocyte preparations and found the same four

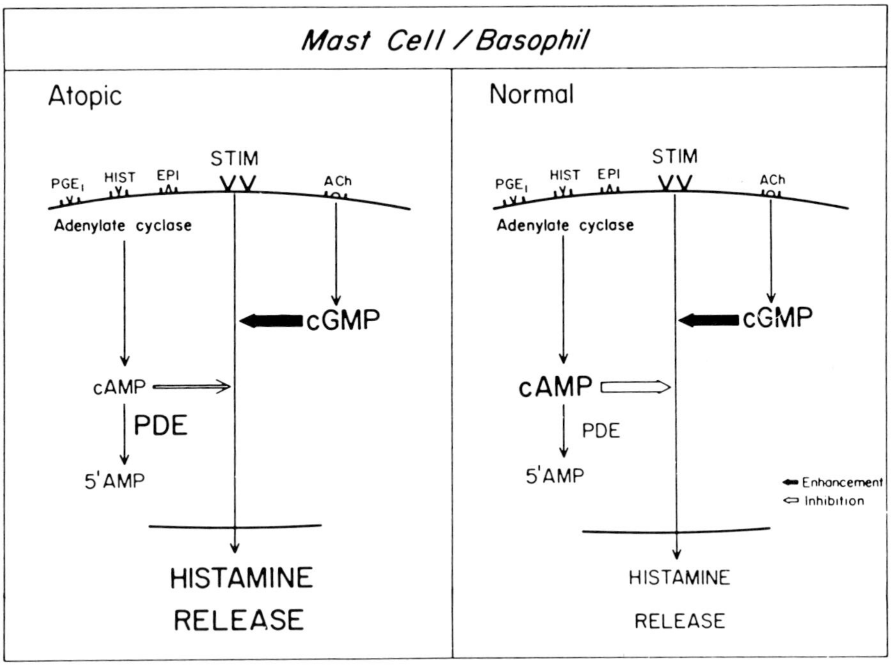

Fig. 2. Cyclic nucleotide regulatory influences on histamine release from normal and atopic mast cells and basophils. Normally, the respective enhancing and inhibiting effects of *cGMP* (cyclic guanosine-3',5'-monophoshate) and *cAMP* (cyclic adenosine-3',5'-monophosphate) are balanced in regulating histamine release. Enhancement may be stimulated by acetylcholine (*ACh*). Activation of adenylate cyclase by prostaglandin E_1 (*PGE_1*), histamine (*HIST*) or epinephrine (*EPI*) would lead to increased cAMP and inhibition of histamine release. In atopic cells, this inhibitory effect is negated by increased phosphodiesterase (*PDE*) hydrolysis of cAMP to 5'-adenosine monophosphate (*5'AMP*), allowing a net enhancement of histamine release

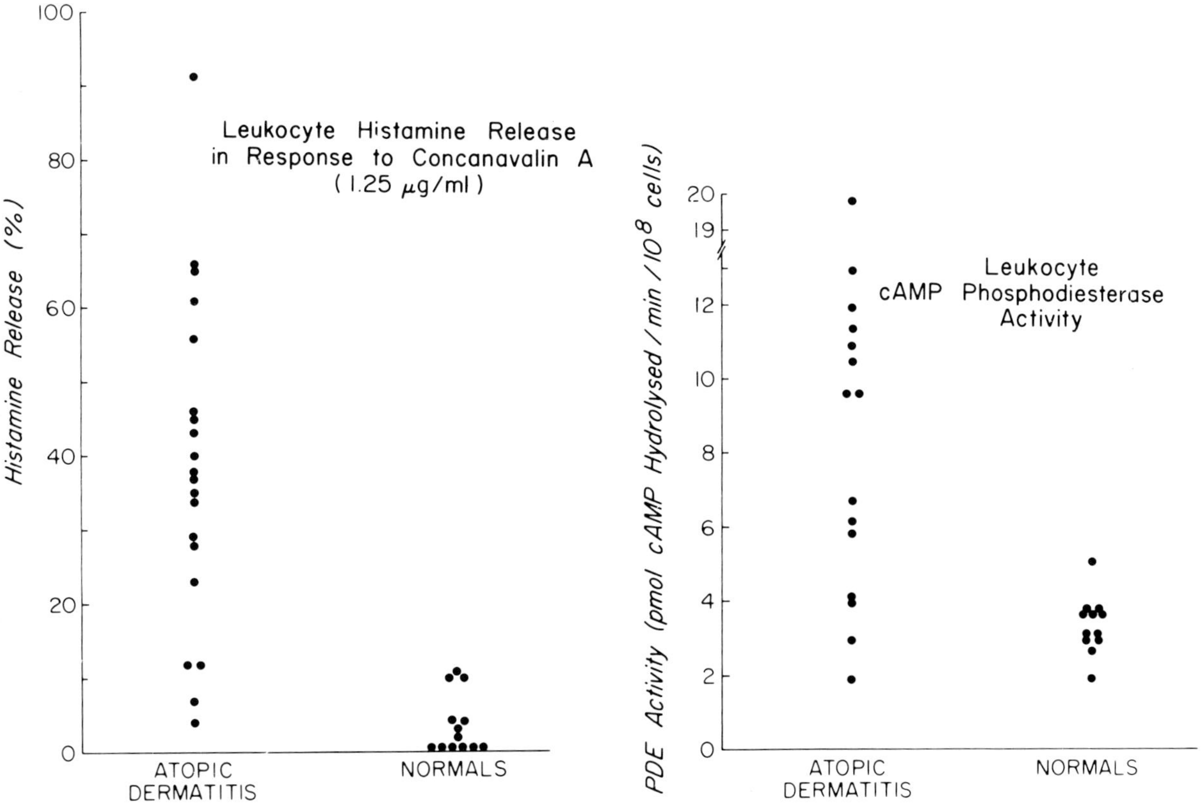

Fig. 3. Leukocyte histamine release (*left*) in response to 1.25 μg/ml concanavalin A and phosphodiesterase (*PDE*) activity (*right*) in leukocytes from the same individual

patients with AE who had low histamine release also had normal levels of phosphodiesterase activity, while the high histamine releasers had consistently elevated enzyme activity. Thus, there was a close correlation between increased histamine releasability and increased phosphodiesterase activity in these atopic individuals. We then exposed leukocytes with high histamine releasability to the phosphodiesterase inhibitor Ro20-1724 which, in every case, reduced histamine releasability to normal levels.

In this study, Butler also demonstrated the effect of the abnormal phosphodiesterase activity on cyclic AMP levels in these leukocyte preparations. As we had shown in a previous study [96] basal cyclic AMP levels in leukocytes from patients with AE were identical with those from normal subjects. Also, within 15 s after stimulation either with isoproterenol or with ConA, cyclic AMP levels increased greatly in both groups. However, after 15 min, during the time when inhibition or modulation of histamine release would be occurring, cyclic AMP levels in the leukocytes from atopic individuals were markedly depressed as a consequence of increased phosphodiesterase hydrolysis. Thus, we demonstrated that in basophils from patients with AE increased histamine releasability relates closely to increased cyclic AMP phosphodiesterase activity and that inhibition of phosphodiesterase restores histamine releasability to normal levels. This information may have considerable relevance to pharmacological intervention in atopic disease, as will be discussed below.

Another irregular functional parameter of AE is the increased spontaneous IgE production by B lymphocytes in culture. We confirmed earlier reports showing consistently increased spontaneous IgE production by mononuclear leukocytes from patients with AE in cultures over 10-day periods [103]. It correlated with elevated serum IgE levels and with increased phosphodiesterase activity in the same mononuclear leukocyte preparations. When these cells were incubated for 60 min with the phosphodiesterase inhibitor Ro20-1724, then washed and continued in culture, a dose-dependent reduction in spontaneous IgE production was demonstrated. Thus, we delineated another relevant abnormal functional parameter in AE that may be a consequence of increased phosphodiesterase activity and decreased intracellular cyclic AMP modulation.

In addition to the functional relationship of elevated phosphodiesterase in AE, we were also interested in its potential as a biochemical marker of the atopic diathesis. We initially considered that the increased enzyme activity was secondary to in vivo histamine desensitisation in patients with AE. An alternative consideration was that this phosphodiesterase abnormality could reflect a basic gene-associated defect. Support for this latter consideration was found by Heskel in our laboratory, who isolated cord blood mononuclear leukocytes from newborn infants with an unilateral or bilateral atopic family history and compared the phosphodiesterase activity with leukocytes from newborns having no family history of atopy [104]. Assays of 120 cord blood preparations revealed significantly elevated mean phosphodiesterase levels in newborns with an atopic history. This association was observed both in newborns with only a paternal atopic history as well as in those with only a maternal family history, thus eliminating the possibility that transplacental passage of histamine or other inflammatory mediators from an atopic mother might be the cause of increased phosphodiesterase. The potential usefulness of phosphodiesterase as a marker for atopy was demonstrated in an 18-month follow-up of a limited number of study infants. Those with elevated cord blood phosphodiesterase activity levels showed a distinctly increased tendency toward atopic symptoms.

Summarising the information to this point, atopic diseases are represented by the triad of conditions (allergic rhinitis or hay fever, asthma and AE) which are familial diseases with an uncertain mode of inheritance. Expression clearly depends upon both genetic and environmental factors, and it seems likely that the primary defect resides in bone marrow-derived cells. Our recent studies have shown several biochemical differences between mononuclear leukocytes of patients with AE as compared with normal individuals. Leukocyte cyclic AMP levels, when stimulated with adenylate cyclase-active agonists, are subnormal in patients with AE, and this observation led to the finding that there is elevated cyclic AMP-specific phosphodiesterase activity in monocytes and lymphocytes of atopic individuals. Paradoxically, however, we found no differences in *basal* cyclic AMP levels between AE and normal mononuclear leukocytes, suggesting that there is increased adenylate cyclase generation of cyclic AMP to offset the increased hydrolysis by phosphodiesterase. Our preliminary turnover studies with intact cells and measurements of adenylate cyclase activity in mononuclear leukocyte homogenates have shown this to be the case. Defective regulation of adenylate cyclase could arise from abnormalities at several sites in the transducer complex which has been characterised in recent years (Fig. 4). Stimulatory (R_s) or inhibitory (R_i) hormone receptors interact with their respective regulatory GTP binding proteins (G proteins) to either stimulate, via G_s, or inhibit, via G_i, the catalytic activity of adenylate cyclase [105]. The G proteins are composed of three subunits: α, β and γ. When the cell receptor binds a stimulatory hormone, α_s binds and hydrolyses GTP, dissociates from the β and γ subunits and interacts with the catalytic unit to increase adenylate cyclase activity. The hydrolysis of

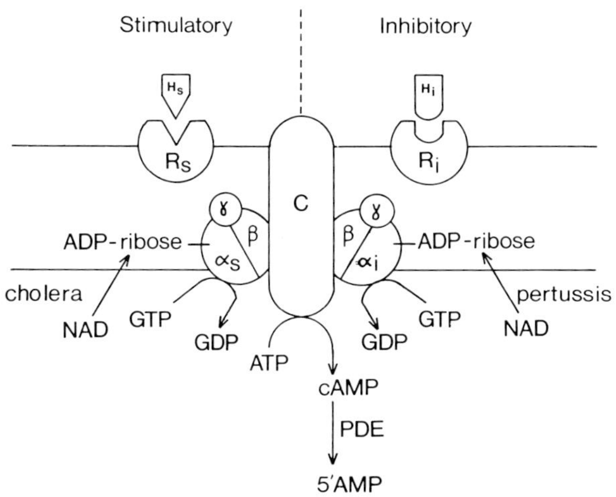

Fig. 4. Model for hormonal signal transduction mediated by guanosine triphosphate (*GTP*)-binding protein regulation of adenylate cyclase. H_s, H_i, hormone stimulatory, hormone inhibitory; R_s, R_i, receptor stimulatory, receptor inhibitory; α, β and γ are subunits of GTP-binding proteins; *cholera, pertussis,* toxins; C, catalytic subunit of adenylate cyclase

GTP to GDP by GTPase terminates G_s protein activation of adenylate cyclase. G_i acts similarly to inhibit adenylate cyclase activation, although it is not yet clear whether inhibition is due to a direct effect of G_i on adenylate cyclase or to an indirect effect.

In recent years the bacterial products cholera toxin (CT) and pertussis toxin (PT) have been used as probes in the study of the regulatory G proteins. CT irreversibly activates G_s by ADP-ribosylation of the α_s subunit, thereby interfering with GTP hydrolysis and eliminating the turn-off mechanism for hormone activation of adenylate cyclase. PT catalyses ADP-ribosylation of G_i. Ribosylation interferes with the ability of α_i to recognise the inhibitory hormone receptor. This uncouples the inhibitory receptor from the catalytic unit of adenylate cyclase, thereby causing a net increase in adenylate cyclase activity.

The idea that the regulatory proteins, in particular G_i, may harbour the site of a defect leading to overactive adenylate cyclase in AE mononuclear leukocytes is suggested by studies which have shown that animals injected with PT develop an atopic-like condition [7]. Additionally, a defect of the transducing proteins in AE would provide a unifying mechanism; otherwise, several hormone receptor defects would have to be invoked to explain the abnormal response of AE leukocytes to isoproterenol, histamine and prostaglandins. If the primary molecular defect does reside in the signal transduction system, we would have to conclude that the increased phosphodiesterase activity is a substrate (i.e. cyclic AMP)-driven enzyme system resulting from exaggerated adenylate cyclase activity.

Much remains to be clarified in relation to the cyclic nucleotide abnormalities in AE. What is the interaction of this system with calcium and phosphoinositide metabolism? Are other tissues such as the epidermis, dermis and endothelium involved? What subsets of lymphocytes and other marrow-derived cells function abnormally as a result of increased phosphodiesterase activity?

While awaiting these basic answers, we clearly can begin to focus on the irregular phosphodiesterase activity as a target for therapeutic intervention. Previous evidence indicates that rapid parenteral theophylline is effective for interrupting pruritus in AE [106]. Our studies question the use of chronic oral theophylline, which appears to cause enzymatic tachyphylaxis, making leukocyte phosphodiesterase more resistant to inhibitors [107]. We also have evidence that topically applied phosphodiesterase inhibitors do significantly reduce clinical parameters in AE. Use of the many new inhibitors being developed may provide a much needed, non-steroidal approach to the management of AE.

References

1. Szentivanyi A (1968) The beta adrenergic theory of the atopic abnormality in bronchial asthma. J Allergy 42:203–232
2. Rackemann FM (1931) Clinical allergy, particularly asthma and hayfever. Mechanism and treatment. Macmillan, New York, p 3
3. Geha RS (1986) Introduction to monograph on atopic dermatitis. Clin Rev Allergy 4:1–2
4. Saarinen UM (1984) Transfer of latent atopy by bone marrow transplantation? A case report. J Allergy Clin Immunol 74:196–200
5. Saurat JH (1985) Eczema in primary immune deficiencies. Clues to the pathogenesis of atopic dermatitis with special reference to the Wiskott-Aldrich syndrome. Acta Derm Venereol [Suppl] (Stockh.) 114:125–128
6. Galey CI, Edelstein RA, Chan SC, Hanifin JM (1986) Altered leukocyte phosphoinositide metabolism in atopic dermatitis. J Invest Dermatol 86:476
7. Fishel CW, Szentivanyi A, Talmadge DW (1964) Adrenergic factors in *Bordetella pertussis*-induced histamine and serotonin hypersensitivity of mice. In: Landy M, Braun W (eds) Bacterial endotoxins. Rutgers University Press, New Brunswick, pp 474–481
8. Kurose H, Katada T, Amano T, Ui M (1983) Specific uncoupling by islet-activating protein, pertussis toxin, of

negative signal transduction via alpha-adrenergic, cholinergic, and opiate receptors in neuroblastoma · glioma hybrid cells. J Biol Chem 258:4870–4875
9. Hanifin JM (1986) Pharmacophysiology of atopic dermatitis. Clin Rev Allergy 4:43–65
10. Snyderman SE (1965) An eczematoid dermatitis in histidine deficiency. J Pediatr 66:212–215
11. Rostenberg A Jr, Solomon LM (1968) Infantile eczema in systemic disease. Arch Dermatol 98:41
12. Rost G, Marchionini A (1932) Asthma-ekzem, Asthma-prurigo and Neurodermitis als allergische Hautkrankheiten. Würzb Abhandl Gesamtgeb Med 27:337–344
13. MacKenna R, Lehmann H (1963) Further observations on the glucose-tolerance test in skin disease. Lancet 1: 1393–1395
14. Hamza SH, El-Mazny HR, Abdallah MA (1978) Glucose tolerance in eczema. Br J Dermatol 98:289–292
15. Lockey S, Glennon J, Reed C (1967) Comparison of some metabolic responses in normal and asthmatic subjects to epinephrine and glucagon. J Allergy 40:349–354
16. Grieco M, Pierson R, Sunyer F (1968) Comparison of the circulatory and metabolic effects of isoproterenol, epinephrine and methoxamine in normal and asthmatic subjects. Am J Med 44:863–872
17. Stokes JH (1930) The eczema problem. Am J Med Sci 179:69–82
18. Readett MD (1955) Constitutional eczema and thyroid disease. J Invest Dermatol 24:126–139
19. Carlson JA (1965) Hypothyroidism in atopics. Ann Allergy 23:331–334
20. Weber R, Roth G, Kierland R (1955) Further contributions to the vascular physiology of atopic dermatitis. J Invest Dermatol 24:19–30
21. Schwartz HJ (1966) The relationship of thyroid disease and the atopic state. Ann Allergy 24:234–237
22. Musaph H (1964) Itching and scratching. Davis, Philadelphia
23. Allerhand M, Gough H, Grais M (1950) Personality factors in neurodermatitis: a preliminary study. Psychosom Med 12:386–390
24. Alexander F (1950) Emotional factors in skin diseases. Norton, New York, pp 164–169
25. Williams D (1951) Management of atopic dermatitis in children: control of the maternal rejection factor. Arch Dermatol and Syphilol 63:545–560
26. Sulzberger MB (1955) Atopic dermatitis: its clinical and historic picture. In: Baer RL (ed) Atopic dermatitis. New York University Press, New York, pp 11–42
27. Rostenberg A (1959) Psychosomatic concepts in atopic dermatitis – a critique. Arch Dermatol 79:692–699
28. Kalz F, Wittkower ED, Vavrusk GW, Telner P, Ferguson S (1957) Studies on vascular skin responses in atopic dermatitis: the influence of psychological factors. J Invest Dermatol 29:67–80
29. Jordan JM, Whitlock FA (1972) Emotions and the skin: the conditioning of scratch responses in cases of atopic dermatitis. Br J Dermatol 86:574–585
30. Graham DT, Wolf S (1953) The relation of Eczema to attitude and to vascular reactions of the human skin. J Lab Clin Med 42:238–254
31. Jacquet L (1904) In: Besnier E, Brocq L, Jacquet L, (eds) La pratique dermatologique, vol 5. Masson, Paris
32. Foreman JC, Piotrowski W (1984) Peptides and histamine release. J Allergy Clin Immunol 74:127–131
33. Ebertz JM, Hirshman CA, Kettelkamp BS, Uno H, Hanifin JM (1987) Substance P-induced histamine release in human cutaneous mast cells. J Invest Dermatol 88:682–685
34. Sulzberger MB, Herrmann F, Borota A, Strauss MB (1953) Studies of sweating. VI. On the urticariogenic properties of human sweat. J Invest Dermatol 21:293–303
35. Sulzberger MB, Herrmann F, Zak FG (1947) Studies of sweating. I. Preliminary report with particular emphasis on a sweat retention syndrome. J Invest Dermatol 9:221–242
36. Davis MJ, Lawler JC (1958) Observations on the delayed blanch phenomenon in atopic subjects. J Invest Dermatol 30:127–132
37. Prose PH (1965) Pathologic changes in eczema. J Pediatr 66:178–199
38. Rovensky J, Saxl O (1964) Differences in the dynamics of sweat secretion in atopic children. J Invest Dermatol 43:171–176
39. Warndorff JA (1970) The response of the sweat gland to acetylcholine in atopic subjects. Br J Dermatol 83:306–311
40. Kaliner M (1976) The cholinergic nervous system and immediate hypersensitivity. I. Eccrine sweat responses in allergic patients. J Allergy Clin Immunol 58:308–315
41. Hemels HGWM (1970) The effect of propranolol on the acetylcholine induced sweat gland response in atopic and non-atopic subjects. Br J Dermatol 83:312–314
42. Foster JG, Haspineall FR, Mollel CL (1971) Effects of propranolol on the response of human eccrine sweat glands to acetylcholine. Br J Dermatol 85:363–367
43. Kiistala R (1982) Stimulated local sweating response in atopic dermatitis. Abstracts, XVI Congressus Internationalis Dermatologiae, Tokyo, p 320
44. Murphy GM, Smith SE, Greaves MW (1984) Autonomic function in cholinergic urticaria and atopic eczema. Br J Dermatol 110:581–586
45. Grosshans E, Woehl M (1982) Troubles vasomoteurs, sudoraux et sebaces de l'eczema constitutionnel. Ann Dermatol Venereol 109:151–162
46. Sato K, Sato F (1983) Individual variations in structure and function of human eccrine sweat gland. Am J Physiol 245:203–208
47. Whitfield A (1938) On the white reaction (white line) in dermatology. Br J Dermatol 50:71–82
48. Uehara M, Ofuji S (1977) Abnormal vascular reactions in atopic dermatitis. Arch Dermatol 113:627–629
49. Champion RH (1961) Abnormal vascular reactions in atopic eczema. Br J Dermatol 81:12–15
50. Eyster WH, Roth GM, Kierland RR (1952) Studies on the peripheral vascular physiology of patients with atopic dermatitis. J Invest Dermatol 18:37–46
51. Lobitz WC Jr, Campbell CF (1953) Physiologic studies in atopic dermatitis (disseminated neurodermatitis). Arch Dermatol Syphilol 67:575–589
52. Ramsay C (1969) Vascular changes accompanying white dermographism and delayed blanch in atopic dermatitis. Br J Dermatol 81:37–42
53. Thune P, Rajka G (1980) Small vessel reactivity in atopic dermatitis. Acta Derm Venereol [Suppl] (Stockh.) 92:30–32
54. Juhlin L (1961) Skin reactions to iontophoretically administered epinephrine and norepinephrine in atopic dermatitis. J Invest Dermatol 37:201–205
55. Juhlin L (1962) Vascular skin reactions in atopic dermatitis. Acta Derm Venereol (Stockh.) 42:218–229
56. Verma BS, Gulati OD, Gokhale SD, Shah KC (1964) Guanethidine and phenoxybenzamine in atopic dermatitis. Arch Dermatol 90:414–417

57. Thomsen K, Osmundsen PE (1965) Guanethidine in the treatment of atopic dermatitis. Arch Dermatol 92:418–421
58. Lobitz WC Jr, Heller M, Dobsen RL (1957) Physiologic studies in atopic dermatitis (disseminated neurodermatitis): the effect of denervation on the "delayed blanch phenomenon." Arch Dermatol 75:228–229
59. Reed WB, Kierland RR (1958) Vascular reactions in chronically inflamed skin. Arch Dermatol 77:181–186
60. Barker AF, Hanifin JM, Hirshman CA, D'Silva R (1985) Airway hyperreaktivity in patients with atopic dermatitis (AD). Am Rev Respir Dis 131:A41
61. Smith LJ, Shelhamer JH, Kaliner M (1980) Cholinergic nervous sysem and immediate hypersensitivity. II. An analysis of pupillary responses. J Allergy Clin Immunol 66:374–378
62. Clark LL, Kierland RR, Roth GM (1960) Methacholine chloride. Arch Dermatol 82:957–964
63. Scott A (1962) Acetylcholine in normal and diseased skin. Br J Dermatol 74:317–322
64. Rajka G (1975) Atopic dermatitis. Saunders, London
65. Henderson WR, Shelhamer JH, Rheingold DB, Smith LJ, Evans R, Kaliner M (1979) Alpha-adrenergic hyperresponsiveness in asthma. N Engl J Med 300:642–647
66. Barnes P, Fitzgerald G, Brown M, Dollery C (1980) Nocturnal asthma and changes in circulating epinephrine, histamine and cortisol. N Engl J Med 303:263–267
67. Soughton RB, DeOreo G, Clendenning W (1960) Effects of intradermal injection of vasopressors in normal and diseased human skin. Arch Dermatol 82:150–157
68. Solomon LM, Wentzel HE, Tulsky E (1964) The physiological disposition of C14-norepinephrine in patients with atopic dermatitis and other dermatoses. J Invest Dermatol 43:193–200
69. Moller H, Rorsman G (1958) Studies on vascular permeability factors with sodium fluorescein, II. The effect of intracutaneously injected histamine and serum in patients with atopic dermatitis. Act Derm Venereol (Stockh.) 38:243–250
70. Coulson IH, Holden CA (1988) Cutaneous reactions to intradermal substance P and histamine in atopic dermatitis. J Invest Dermatol 91:396
71. Williams DH (1938) Skin temperature reaction to histamine in atopic dermatitis (disseminated neurodermatitis). J Invest Dermatol 1:119–129
72. Sampson HA, Jolie PL (1984) Increased plasma histamine concentrations after food challenges in children with atopic dermatitis. N Engl J Med 311:372–376
73. Eppinger H (1913) Quoted by Best CH, McHenry EW (1931) Histamine. Physiol Rev 11:371–477
74. Harmer IM, Harris KE (1926) Observations on the vascular reactions in a man in response to histamine. Heart 13:381–394
75. Mihm MC Jr, Soter NA, Dvorak HF, Austen KF (1976) The structure of normal skin and the morphology of atopic eczema. J Invest Dermatol 67:305–312
76. Johnson HH, DeOreo GA, Lascheid WP, Mitchell F (1960) Skin histamine levels in chronic atopic dermatitis. J Invest Dermatol 34:237–238
77. Hanifin JM (1977) Type I hypersensitivity diseases of the skin: divergent aspects of urticaria and atopic dermatitis. Ann Allergy 39:153–160
78. Ring J, Senter T, Cornell RC, Arroyave CM, Tan EM (1979) Plasma complement and histamine changes in atopic dermatitis. Br J Dermatol 100:512–530
79. Lichtenstein LM, Margolis S (1968) Histamine release in vitro: inhibition by catecholamines and methylxanthines. Science 161:902–904
80. Orange RP, Austen WG, Austen KF (1971) Immunological release of histamine and slow reacting substance of anaphylaxis from human lung. I. Modulation by agents influencing cellular levels of cyclic 3'5'-adenosine monophosphate. J Exp Med [Suppl] 134:136–148
81. Lebel B, Venencie PY, Saurat JH et al. (1980) Anti-IgE induced histamine release from basophils in children with atopic dermatitis. Acta Derm Venereol [Suppl] (Stockh.) 92:57
82. Butler JM, Chan SC, Stevens S, Hanifin JM (1983) Increased leukocyte histamine release with elevated cyclic AMP-phosphodiesterase activity in atopic dermatitis. J Allergy Clin Immunol 71:440
83. Bernstein RA, Linarelli L, Facktor MA et al. (1972) Decreased urinary adenosine 3'5' monophosphate (cyclic AMP) in asthmatics. J Lab Clin Med 80:772–779
84. Parker CW, Smith JW (1973) Alterations in cyclic adenosine monophosphate metabolism in human bronchial asthma. I. Leukocyte responsiveness to beta-adrenergic agents. J Clin Invest 52:48–59
85. Logsdon PJ, Middleton E Jr, Coffey RG (1972) Stimulation of leukocyte adenyl cyclase by hydrocortisone and isoproterenol in asthmatic and nonasthmatic subjects. J Allergy Clin Immunol 50:45–56
86. Carr RH, Busse WW, Reed CE (1973) Failure of catecholamines to inhibit epidermal mitosis in vitro. J Allergy Clin Immunol 55:255–262
87. Reed CE, Busse WW, Lee TP (1976) Adrenergic mechanisms and the adenyl cyclase system in atopic dermatitis. J Invest Dermatol 67:333–338
88. Reed CE (1974) Abnormal autonomic mechanisms in asthma. J Allergy Clin Immunol 53:34–41
89. Parker CW, Kennedy S, Eisen AZ (1977) Leukocyte and lymphocyte cyclic AMP responses in atopic eczema. J Invest Dermatol 68:302–306
90. Busse WW, Lantis SDH (1979) Impaired H2 histamine granulocyte release in active atopic eczema. J Invest Dermatol 73:184–187
91. Sano Y, Watt G, Townley RG (1983) Decreased mononuclear cell beta-adrenergic receptors in bronchial asthma: parallel studies of lymphocyte and granulocyte desensitization. J Allergy Clin Immunol 72:495–503
92. Pochet R, Delespesse G, DeMaubeuge J (1980) Characterization of beta-adrenoreceptors on intact circulating lymphocytes from patients with atopic dermatitis. Acta Derm Venereol [Suppl] (Stockh.) 92:26–29
93. Galant SP, Underwood S, Allred S, Hanifin JM (1979) Beta adrenergic receptor binding on polymorphonuclear leukocytes in atopic dermatitis. J Invest Dermatol 72:330–332
94. Greenacre JK, Schofield P, Connolly ME (1978) Desensitization of the B-adrenoceptor of lymphocytes from normal subjects and asthmatic patients in vitro. Br J Clin Pharmacol 5:199–210
95. Morris HG (1980) Drug-induced desensitization of beta adrenergic receptors. J Allergy Clin Immunol 65:83–86
96. Safko MJ, Chan SC, Cooper KD, Hanifin JM (1981) Heterologous desensitization of leukocytes: a possible mechanism of beta adrenergic blockade in atopic dermatitis. J Allergy Clin Immunol 68:218–225
97. Chan SC, Grewe SR, Hanifin JM (1982) Functional desensitization associated with elevated cAMP phosphodiesterase in human mononuclear leukocytes. J Cyclic Nucleotide Res 8:211–224

98. Grewe SR, Chan SC, Hanifin JM (1982) Elevated leukocyte cyclic AMP-phosphodiesterase in atopic disease: a possible mechanism for cAMP-agonist hyporesponsiveness. J Allergy Clin Immunol 70:452–457
99. Thompson WJ, Ross CP, Pledger WJ, Strada SJ (1976) Cyclic adenosine 3':5'-monophosphate phosphodiesterase: distinct forms in human lymphocytes and monocytes. J Biol Chem 251:4922
100. Holla SWJ, Hollman EP, Mier PD et al. (1972) Adenosine 3'5'-cyclic monophosphate phosphodiesterase in skin. II. Levels in atopic dermatitis. Br J Dermatol 86:147–149
101. Grotti A, Guidotti A, Mannaioni PF, Zilletti L (1966) The influence of adrenotropic drugs and noradrenaline on the histamine release in cardiac anaphylaxis in vitro. J Physiol 184:924
102. Kaliner MA, Orange RP, Austen KF (1972) Immunological release of histamine and slow reacting substance of anaphylaxis from human lung. IV. Enhancement by cholinergic and alpha adrenergic stimulation. J Exp Med 136:556–567
103. Cooper KD, Kang K, Chan SC, Hanifin JM (1985) Phosphodiesterase inhibition by Ro20-1724 reduces hyper-IgE synthesis by atopic dermatitis cell in vitro. J Invest Dermatol 84:477–482
104. Heskel NS, Chan SC, Thiel ML, Stevens SR, Casperson LS, Hanifin JM (1984) Elevated umbilical cord blood leukocyte cyclic adenosine monophosphate-phosphodiesterase activity in children with atopic parents. J Am Acad Dermatol 11:422–426
105. Cassel D, Selinger Z (1977) Mechanism of adenylate cyclase activation by cholera toxin. Inhibition of GTP hydrolysis at the regulatory site. Proc Natl Acad Sci USA 74 (8):3307–3311
106. Epstein E (1946) Theophylline ethylenediamine as an antipruritic agent. Arch Dermatol Syphilol 53:281–284
107. Guistina TA, Chan SC, Thiel MD et al. (1984) Increased leukocyte sensitivity to phosphodiesterase inhibitors in atopic dermatitis: tachyphylaxis after theophylline therapy. J Allergy Clin Immunol 74:252–257

Role of Inflammatory Mediators in Atopic Eczema

T. Ruzicka and J. Ring

Introduction

Inflammatory mediators are molecules which simulate parts of inflammatory reactions by virtue of their effects on microvasculature or inflammatory cells (Fig. 1). They increase vascular permeability and thus may lead to edema. They may cause vasoconstriction or vasodilation by their effects on vascular smooth muscle. In skin, edema and vasodilation may be evident as wheal and erythema, respectively. They may act on nerve endings and produce subjective symptoms such as pain or itch. In addition, inflammatory mediators exert chemotactic and activating effects on leukocytes thus promoting inflammatory infiltration and remodeling of the tissue. Besides these proinflammatory effects, mediators are also involved in immune regulation, frequently exerting a negative immunomodulating action (negative feedback regulation). Finally, inflammatory mediators may act as growth factors and be involved in growth regulation of epithelial tissues.

The best studied inflammatory mediators are histamine, kinins, metabolites of arachidonic acid (collectively termed eicosanoids), and complement-derived peptides. In addition, certain cytokines such as interleukin 1 possess biological properties similar to those of classical mediators of inflammation. Since inflammatory mediators also exert immunoregulatory effects, and the immunoregulatory lymphokines and cytokines exert inflammatory actions, the distinction between these two classes of biologically active molecules becomes obscured and may even disappear.

Although all of the above biological phenomena are believed to be intricately involved in the pathophysiology of atopic eczema, it is surprising how few studies have been devoted to the role of inflammatory mediators in these diseases. This is particularly conspicuous when compared to the host of publications in another common inflammatory dermatosis, psoriasis. Compared to psoriasis, where a variety of effective therapeutic alternatives exist, antiinflammatory treatment of atopic eczema is still very monotonous and largely restricted to glucocorticosteroids. Therefore, increased attention to the role of inflammatory mediators in atopic eczema promises not only a better understanding of the pathophysiology of cutaneous inflammation in this disease, but pharmacologic manipulations of mediator metabolism may lead to the introduction of new pathobiochemically oriented treatment modalities. As already mentioned, only few studies have related to the role of mediators in atopic eczema, most of them dealing with eicosanoids and histamine, which are therefore covered in detail in this chapter.

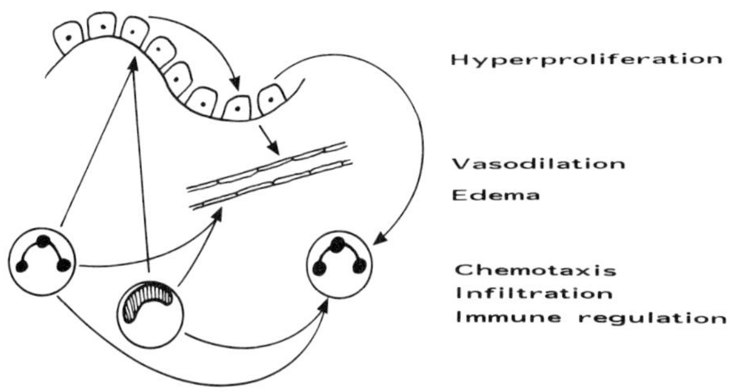

Fig. 1. Effects of inflammatory mediators and cytokines in skin

Eicosanoids

Eicosanoids is the collective term for mediators derived from arachidonic acid (5, 8, 11, 14-eicosatetraenoic acid). The assumption of a pathogenetic role of eicosanoids in inflammatory dermatoses (psoriasis, acne, atopic eczema, etc.) is based upon several lines of evidence: (a) elevated concentrations of eicosanoids in skin; (b) proinflammatory and other biological effects in skin; and (c) inhibition of eicosanoid formation by glucocorticosteroids, the main class of antiinflammatory drugs in dermatology.

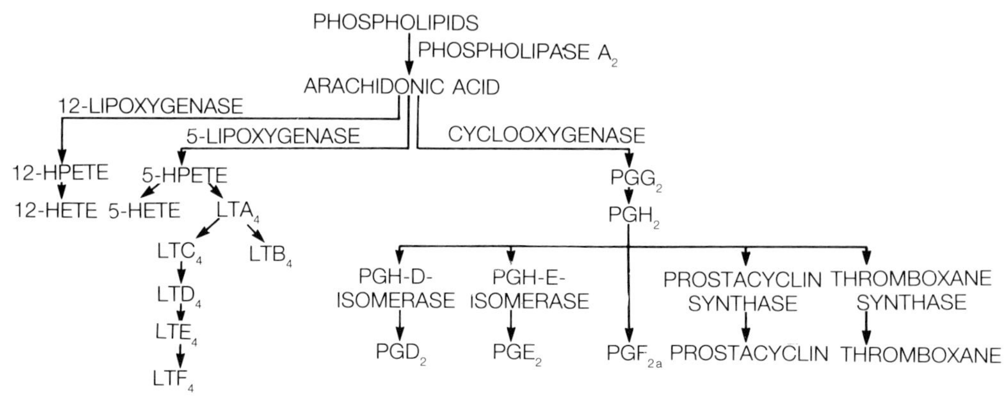

Fig. 2. Metabolism of arachidonic acid

Biochemical Pathways of Arachidonic Acid

Arachidonic acid is esterified in membrane phospholipids of all cells of the organism (Fig. 2). Prior to its metabolic conversions, it must be released from the ester bond by the action of specific phospolipases, particularly phospholipase A_2 (PLA_2) or, in some cases, phospholipase C (PLC).

PLA_2 is of particular interest in dermatology since it is inhibited by glucocorticosteroids [32]. Inhibition of cutaneous PLA_2 by glucocorticosteroids has been demonstrated after topical application of a potent glucocorticosteroid [30]. Inhibition of PLA_2 blocks all subsequent metabolic conversions of arachidonic acid. This relative lack of specificity may offer a therapeutic advantage and at least partly explain the unique therapeutic efficacy of glucocorticosteroids in inflammatory skin diseases which may not be reached by more selective drugs. After release, arachidonic acid becomes the substrate of competing enzymes. The classical pathway of arachidonic acid metabolism is the cyclooxygenase pathway which leads to the formation of prostaglandins (PG) E_2, D_2, and $F\alpha_2$, prostacyclin (PGI_2) and thromboxane (TX) A_2. It is only the cyclooxygenase pathway which is inhibited by nonsteroidal antiinflammatory drugs (NSAIDs) such as aspirin and indomethacin. Since NSAIDs possess very limited therapeutic effects in various skin diseases, but may on the other hand provoke or exacerbate a variety of dermatoses, the pathophysiological significance of cyclooxygenase products in skin seems to be low.

The lipoxygenase pathways deserve greater interest. The 5-lipoxygenase pathway leads to the formation of 5-hydroxyeicosetetraenoic acid (5-HETE) and leukotrienes (LT) A_4, B_4, C_4, D_4, etc.; 12-lipoxygenase forms 12-hydroxyeicosatetraenoic acid (12-HETE). The formation of the lipoxygenase metabolites is nonselectively inhibited by glucocorticosteroids. Selective lipoxygenase and dual lipoxygenase/cyclooxygenase inhibitors are currently being developed by several drug companies.

Metabolism of Arachidonic Acid in Normal Skin

Skin, particularly its epidermal layer, is a site of active metabolic transformations of arachidonic acid. A detailed description of eicosanoid synthesis in normal skin has been provided in recent reviews [71].

Human skin has been shown to possess both PLA_2 and PLC activities. Arachidonic acid released from phospholipid stores by their action can undergo oxygenation by both cyclooxygenase and lipoxygenase pathways. In human epidermis, PGE_2 and PGD_2 are the main cyclooxygenase products formed. In addition, PGD_2 is the predominant eicosanoid of mast cells in various species [68]. With regard to immune regulation, it seems of particular interest that large amounts of PGD_2 are also formed by Langerhans cells [74, 84, 89]. The role of PGD_2 in skin has recently been reviewed in an excellent article by Ikai and Imamura [33].

Besides cyclooxygenase activity, epidermis represents an extraordinarily rich source of 12-lipoxygenase. Its product 12-HETE was identified in skin in 1975 by Hammarström et al. [29]. 12-Lipoxygenase seems to be the major metabolic pathway of arachidonic acid in skin in most species [70]. In contrast to the 12-lipoxygenase activity, epidermis contains only very low 5-lipoxygenase activity, which has been detected by some but not all groups of investigators [77]. Besides eicosanoid-forming enzymes, cutaneous eicosanoid levels may be regulated by catabolic processes. Cytochrome P-450 dependent ω-oxidation of LTB_4 has recently been described in rodent and human keratinocytes [53] . In addition, keratinocytes and melanocytes may catabolize LTC_4 to LTE_4 [51].

Biological Effects of Eicosanoids in Skin

Eicosanoids are pleiotropic mediators affecting a variety of organs. With regard to cutaneous physiology and pathophysiology and the understanding of inflammation and disturbed immunoregulation, the following biological effects are of particular interest:

- Influence on cutaneous microvasculature: edema, erythema
- Leukocyte chemotaxis and activation: inflammatory infiltrate
- Chemotactic effects for fibroblasts and keratinocytes: wound repair (?)
- Growth stimulation: hyperproliferation (indirect)
- Immunoregulatory effects

Influence of Eicosanoids on Cutaneous Microvasculature. The various microcirculatory effects of eicosanoids in skin have recently been reviewed [6, 77]. In brief, intradermal injection of PLA_2, arachidonic acid, PGE_2, PGD_2, and PGI_2 leads to cutaneous vasodilation and prolonged erythema. Prostaglandins may also cause edema and potentiate bradykinin- and histamine-induced plasma exudation in skin. These effects may also be due to oxygen radicals formed in the course of the cyclooxygenase reaction rather than to the terminal prostaglandins. The lipoxygenase-derived HETEs and LTs may also induce plasma exudation and vasoconstriction or -dilation depending on the species and experimental model. Their effects are, in general, rather low and may be enhanced by the concomitant administration of vasodilators such as histamine, bradykinin, and PGE_2.

Leukocyte Chemotaxis and Activation by Eicosanoids. In vitro, mono-HETEs and LTB_4 are potent chemotactic agents for leukocytes. In addition, they may cause activation of their oxidative metabolism and lead to degranulation and enzyme release. Of particular interest to the understanding of inflammatory skin diseases is the preferential migration of eosinophils towards LTB_4 and 12-HETE [16, 17, 25]. The in vitro data are paralleled by in vivo activity. Intradermal injections of HETEs and LTB_4 cause neutrophile adhesion to endothelium, migration through the endothelial layer into the perivascular space, and infiltration of the tissue (reviewed in [77]). Of particular interest to the interpretation of the role of eicosanoids in chronic skin diseases are their chronic effects. LTB_4 applied topically under occlusion to human skin resulted in intraepidermal neutrophil microabscesses and a dermal perivascular infiltrate [14]. Similar effects were obtained with 12-HETE [21]. Repeated intradermal injection of LTB_4 and 12-HETE, which may more closely mimic the in vivo situation than topical application, led to epidermal hyperproliferation and histologic changes suggestive of leukocytoklastic vasculitis in guinea pigs [75]. In addition, a pronounced tissue eosinophilia was observed. Coadministration of PGE_2 and LTB_4 potentiated the vascular aspect of the reaction, with massive vasodilation and edema but completely abrogated the cellular, tissue-destructive changes. From these findings, it has been postulated that PGE_2 may assume a tissue-protective function in skin in analogy to a variety of experimental systems in other organs, particularly the gastrointestinal tract. This may also explain the lack of therapeutic activity of NSAIDs in most dermatoses and their sometimes detrimental effects in skin.

Chemotactic Effects for Fibroblasts in Keratinocytes. Recent data show that lipoxygenase-derived eicosanoids, particularly 5-HETE but also LTB_4 and 12-HETE, are very potent fibroblast chemotactic agents [49, 58]. In addition, these eicosanoids act as chemoattractants for keratinocytes (R. Hein, E. Gross, T. Ruzicka, T. Krieg, manuscript in preparation, and [31]). Thus, release of eicosanoids by epidermal or inflammatory cells may be aimed at restoration of cutaneous integrity after injury. This suggests to us that the physiological role of eicosanoids in skin may in fact be in wound healing.

Growth Stimulation. Hyperproliferative changes are a common characteristic of chronic inflammatory dermatoses, particularly psoriasis, but also chronic lichenified eczema. Therefore, studies showing enhanced epidermal DNA synthesis induced by leukotrienes and 12-HETE in vitro and in vivo [5, 15, 37, 75] are of particular interest. However, despite the unequivocal hyperproliferation observed after topical or intradermal application of LTB and 12-HETE [15, 75], recent studies do not confirm the growth-promoting activity of lipoxygenase-derived eicosanoids on epidermal cells in vitro [26, 55]. Thus, growth-stimulating activity of eicosanoids in skin in vivo may be mediated by infiltrating leukocytes releasing some unidentified growth factors.

Immunoregulatory Effects. Eicosanoids exert a wide spectrum of immunoregulatory effects, thereby modulating the immune response generally in the sense of negative feedback regulation. Prostaglandins show a dualistic action with proinflammatory effects in the early, vascular phase of the inflammatory reaction and antiinflammatory modulation in the chronic, cellular, and proliferative phase [9]. Macrophage-derived PGE_2 may play a role in the down-tuning of an ongoing immune reaction [24]. In skin, an antiinflammatory effect of PGE_2 has been shown by Ruzicka and Burg [75]. In anthralin-induced cutaneous inflammation, topically applied arachidonic acid caused a depression of the late and potentiation of the early inflammatory changes [38].

Lipoxygenase-derived eicosanoids also play a complex role in immune regulation with predominance of inhibitory effects [10].

The immunocompetent cells in epidermis are Langerhans cells, which are characterized by their high capacity to synthesize PGD_2 [74]. This eicosanoid may, similarly to PGE_2, be effective in immune regulation, particularly down-regulation of the immune response [33, 88].

Arachidonic Acid Metabolism in Atopic Eczema

Only very few studies have directly investigated arachidonic acid metabolism in atopic eczema skin. In a study performed by our group [72], suction blisters were raised on involved and uninvolved skin from patients with atopic eczema or psoriasis and at corresponding skin sites of healthy controls. On involved skin, intact blisters sometimes cannot be raised, but the exuding interstitial fluid can be directly collected in the suction bell. The eicosanoid concentrations in the suction blister fluid were analyzed by radioimmunoassay and the identity of LTB_4 confirmed by HPLC. PGE_2 levels showed no significant difference between the various groups. The attempt to measure PGD_2 and its major metabolite by two different antibodies showed levels below the detection limit in all samples. Histamine concentrations were also not elevated in eczematous skin in this study. However, the only mediator found in highly increased concentrations in involved, but not uninvolved, atopic eczema skin was LTB_4. Its concentration in psoriatic lesions was even higher, but the difference between atopic eczema and psoriasis was not striking. Although LTB_4 elevation is not specific to atopic eczema, it is not simply a consequence of cutaneous inflammation, since in UVB erythema, LTB_4 concentrations were within the normal range [73]. No elevation of cutaneous LTB_4 levels was also noted in immediate-type hypersensitivity reactions induced in atopic individuals by ragweed or grass pollen [83], while increaed levels of LTB_4 were measured in suction blister fluid over late cutaneous reactions [20a]. In addition, lack of specificity should not be equated with lack of biological significance. It is likely that in various skin diseases similar inflammatory mechanisms are operative.

In a well-performed study, Fogh et al. [23] recently could show that eicosanoid levels in uninvolved atopic eczema skin do not differ from those in controls. In contrast, lesional and perilesional skin contained elevated concentrations of LTB_4, PGE_2, 12-HETE and 15-HETE. The authors concluded that only PGE_2 and LTB_4 were present in biologically active concentrations, although 12-HETE levels were increased sevenfold in lesional skin and reached a mean concentration of 717 ng/g tissue (!) compared to 5.2 ng/g for LTB_4 and 97.2 ng/g for PGE_2. These conclusions may be questioned since the 12-HETE concentrations were well within the range required for biological effects. Intradermal injection of 100 ng 12-HETE led to pronounced inflammatory changes in guinea pig ears [75]. In addition, the concentrations measured lie within the $K_D$range of epidermal 12-HETE receptors of 0.5 – 2.5 nm [26].

Besides altered eicosanoid concentrations in skin, atopic patients may also show different responsiveness to the effects of eicosanoids. Intradermally injected LTC_4 caused larger wheals in atopics than in controls [28]. Monocytes from patients with atopic eczema and psoriasis showed enhanced chemotaxis towards LTB_4. No such effect was observed in granulocytes [18]. These functional results are corroborated by biochemical findings showing normal affinity and number of LTB_4 receptors on polymorphonuclear leukocytes in patients with atopic eczema and psoriasis [48]. Mononuclear cells from patients with respiratory atopy showed decreased sensitivity to the immunoregulatory effects of PGE_2 and PGD_2 [66]. In particular, these mediators failed to activate suppressor cells from atopic donors.

Eicosanoid Releasability in Atopic Eczema

The concept of enhanced mediator releasability in atopy was tested for eicosanoids by Ruzicka and Ring [76]. We measured the release of PGE_2, LTB_4, and LTC_4 from mixed peripheral blood leukocytes into supernatants by radioimmunoassays in 27 patients with atopic eczema and 22 nonatopic healthy controls. Cells from atopic individuals showed enhanced spontaneous production of LTC_4. Immunological challenge of cells with C5a and anti-IgE resulted in increased production of PGE_2, LTB_4, and LTC_4 in the atopic group, supporting the concept of enhanced generation of vasoactive mediators in atopy. The pharmacologic stimulus calcium ionophore A23127 led to maximal synthesis of all eicosanoids, which was of comparable magnitude in atopics and controls. Similar results were obtained by Ferreri et al. [22] in monocytes from atopic eczema patients after stimulation with the calcium ionophore. IgG-, IgA-, and IgE-induced LTC_4 release was also unaltered in atopics compared to controls.

Several studies have concerned eicosanoid release from blood cells of patients with respiratory atopy.

Monocytes and polymorphonuclear leukocytes (PMNL) from atopic patients showed reduced ability to produce PGE_2 than cells from controls [47, 87]. 5-Lipoxygenase activity was increased in PMNL from asthmatic patients [50].

Therapeutic Implications

Should eicosanoids prove to be indeed of pathophysiological significance in atopic eczema, pharmacologic interventions at various levels of the eicosanoid cascade could have far-reaching therapeutic implications. Potentially useful pharmacologic approaches are shown in Table 1. Since arachidonic acid is the precursor for eicosanoid synthesis, dietary manipulations at the precursor level or topical application of unsaturated fatty acids may be of particular importance (for review, see [13, 34, 91] and Kunz and Ring in this volume). Interest in essential fatty acids (EFAs) dates back to observations showing that EFA-deficient animals and human beings developed inflammatory and hyperkeratotic skin changes which may be corrected by the topical application of linoleic acid. Diet enriched in fish oil containing eicosapentaenoic acid or evening primrose oil (containing linoleic and gammalinolenic acids) may be of some value as adjuvant therapy in atopic eczema [7, 52, 90] although a recent double-blind study demonstrated lack of effect with evening primrose oil in atopic eczema [4], similarly to EPA [37a]. The rationale for supplying gammalinolenic acid is provided by studies of Manku et al. [42, 43] showing normal or increased plasma levels of linoleic acid but decreased levels of gammalinolenic acid and arachidonic acid in patients with atopic eczema, resulting from a postulated defect in the enzyme delta-6-desaturase. Increased linoleic and decreased arachidonic acid levels were also found in neutrophils and monocytes of patients with allergic rhinitis and asthma [67].

Unsaturated fatty acids may also, in addition to compensate for postulated or actual EFA deficiencies, exert direct pharmacologic actions. Of particular interest seem the effects of linoleic acid. In vitro and in vivo, linoleic acid inhibited epidermal cyclooxygenase and 12-lipoxygenase activities, while 5-lipoxygenase and PLA_2 activities in PMNL remained unaffected [78, 79].

Linoleic acid has also been shown to inhibit cyclooxygenase activity in various other cells [54, 56, 81]; furthermore, it has been shown to exert immunosuppressive effects in prolonging skin allograft survival [58a].

Another approach to manipulate arachidonic metabolism at an early stage is inhibition of enzymes releasing arachidonic acid from its phospholipid stores, particularly PLA_2. An example are the glucocorticosteroids, which, however, exert a variety of unrelated effects. More selective inhibition of PLA_2 may be of considerable value in inflammatory skin diseases. Even greater specificity may be obtained by selective inhibitors of 5- and/or 12-lipoxygenase. This specificity, although of great theoretical interest, may prove, however, to be a therapeutic disadvantage, since it seems likely that a variety of mediators formed by different enzymes rather than a single product contribute to cutaneous inflammation. Therefore, dual inhibitors of 5-lipoxygenase and cyclooxygenase are being developed by pharmaceutical companies.

On the other hand, due to the antiinflammatory [9] and tissue-protective effects in skin (discussed in [77]), gastrointestinal tract, and several other organs, the use of stable prostaglandin analogues in cutaneous inflammation may seem an unconventional but rewarding approach, precedented by the use of prostanoids in gastric ulcer disease.

Finally, the identification of 12-HETE receptors on epidermal cells [26] and the presence of LTB_4 receptors on PMNL should lead to the development of receptor antagonists with potential usefulness in inflammatory and hyperproliferative skin diseases.

Table 1: Pharmacologic interventions in eicosanoid metabolism as potential therapeutic approaches in atopic eczema

Unsaturated fatty acids	Linoleic acid Eicosapentaenoic acid (fish oil) Gamma-linoleneic acid (evening primrose seed oil)
Enzyme inhibitors	Phospholipase A_2 5-Lipoxygenase 12-Lipoxygenase Dual inhibitors of 5-lipoxygenase and cyclooxygenase
Prostaglandin analogues	PGE_2 derivatives
Receptor antagonists	12-HETE receptors LTB_4 receptors

Histamine

Histamine is the classical and best characterized mediator of inflammation. Dale and Laidlaw [19] showed as early as 1910 that in vivo effects of this substance resembled the symptoms of anaphylaxis. Besides the discovery of the biological effects of histamine, the major steps in histamine research were the development of antihistamines and the introduction of the H_1 and H_2receptor concept [3,8]. Despite intensive research efforts, knowledge of the physiological role of histamine in health and disease remains incomplete.

Biological Effects of Histamine

Histamine exerts a variety of effects in various organs. It contracts or dilates vascular and extravascular smooth muscles of the bronchi, uterus, gut, etc. It has cardiac, central nervous, and endocrinological effects. Its central effects may be brought about by the recently discovered H_3receptor [1]. Well defined is the role of histamine in the induction of gastric acid secretion, which is mediated by H_2receptors. Of greater relevance to the physiology and pathophysiology of skin is the itch sensation caused by an effect on sensory fibers [20, 27]. Histamine is, in fact, the only inflammatory mediator known so far to cause itch.

With respect to atopic eczema, the pro- and antiinflammatory effects of histamine deserve great interest. The proinflammatory role of histamine as a mediator of immediate-type hypersensitivity reactions caused by allergic or pseudoallergic mechanisms is quite well established. The wheal and flare formation is skin in these reactions is caused predominantly by H_1receptor mediated effects on smooth-muscle cells and endothelium of cutaneous microvasculature (for review, see [63]). The antiinflammatory effects of histamine are brought about by H_2receptors on inflammatory cells which inhibit a variety of immune functions, for example, mediator release by mast cells and basophils [11, 40], neutrophil chemotaxis, phagocytosis and enzyme release [63], lymphocyte proliferation [65], lymphokine production, cytotoxicity and suppressor cell activity [80], and others (Fig. 3).

Histamine Release

Histamine release from its cellular stores in basophils and mast cells can be triggered by a host of chemical and physical stimuli (summarized in [63]) such as IgE and allergen, anti-IgE, anti-ε-receptor, concanavalin A, calcium ionophores, complement peptides, neuropeptides, opioids, enzymes, drugs, cytokines, detergents, heat, cold, pressure, vibration, UV irradiation, etc.

Histamine release from mast cells and basophils is subject to complexe regulatory mechanisms which influence the magnitude and velocity of the release reaction. The main regulatory factor is intracellular cAMP. Adenylate cyclase activation by β-adrenergic agents, histamine via H_2 receptors, PGE_2, and others inhibits the release reaction. Arachidonic acid metabolites modulate histamine release; cyclooxygenase inhibitors enhance, while lipoxygenase inhibitors decrease histamine releasability [57, 62, 85].

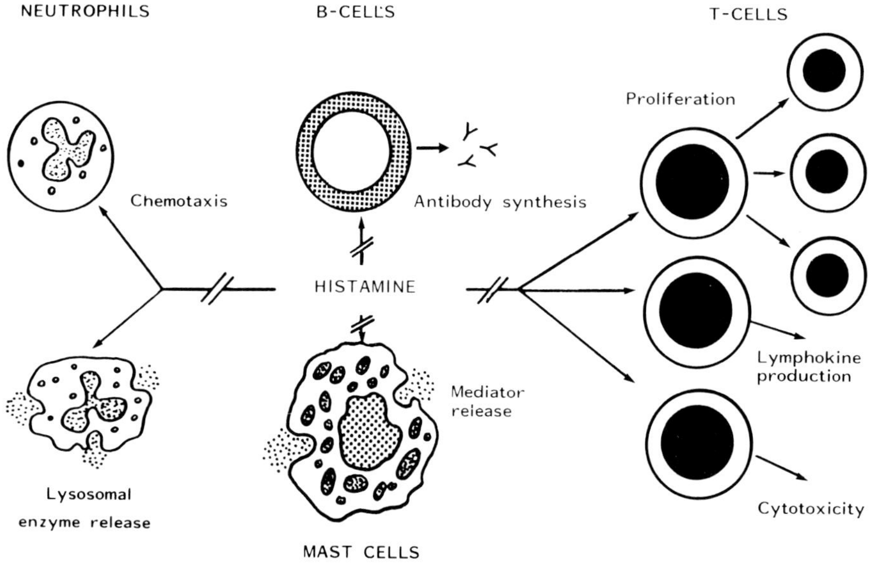

Fig. 3. Immunoregulatory properties of histamine

Histamine Concentrations in Skin and Plasma in Atopic Eczema

In only few studies were histamine concentrations in skin of atopic eczema patients determined. The skin content of histamine in atopic eczema was measured by Johnson et al. [35]. They found increased concentrations in patients, but they concluded that histamine did not seem to be of major importance in the cutaneous alterations of the disease. However, the dinitrofluorobenzene method of histamine determination used in this early study was neither very specific nor sensitive.

Juhlin [36] found increased histamine values in patients with atopic eczema using a combined electrophoretic and fluorometric histamine assay. Interestingly, there was no significant difference between affected and normal-looking skin.

In our study, using a highly sensitive and specific enzymatic double-isotope assay [69], only three of 22 atopic eczema patients showed histamine concentrations in biopsies from lesional skin above the mean ± 2 SD of controls. The difference between controls and patients was not statistically significant. In contrast, a single patient with the hyper-IgE syndrome showed extremely high histamine concentrations in skin, which may contribute to the clinical symptoms of this rare disease. Both in atopic eczema patients and in the hyper-IgE patient, histamine catabolism in skin via methyltransferase was normal. Despite normal steady-state concentrations of histamine in atopic eczema skin, histamine release from skin slices after immunological challenge with anti-IgE was almost twice as high as in controls, supporting the concept of enhanced releasability of vasoactive mediators in atopy (see below). Histamine release induced by the pharmacologic stimulus compound 48/80 was identical in patients and controls, paralleling the findings by Voorhorst et al. [86] in respiratory atopy. No cholinergic histamine release was observed in normal and atopic eczema skin.

Our initial findings of essentially normal histamine concentrations in skin biopsies in atopic eczema patients were confirmed in a subsequent study performed in suction blister fluid. Again, no significant difference between histamine concentrations in lesional and normal atopic eczema skin, psoriasis, and healthy controls was noted [72].

On the other hand, in severe atopic eczema, plasma histamine concentrations may be elevated. In 17 out of 54 patients with atopic eczema, histamine concentrations ranged between 1.2 and 5.2 ng/ml, where in 39 controls the concentration was always below 1 ng/ml. Elevated histamine concentrations were found mostly in patients with severe eczema and high serum IgE levels [60]. Still, from the above studies a key role of histamine as mediator of cutaneous inflammation in atopic eczema cannot be deduced; however, it can be regarded as a marker of mast cell and basophil activation [64a]. This assumption is supported by the lack of antieczematous properties of antihistamines despite their important role as antipruritic agents in this disorder.

Altered Releasability of Vasoactive Mediator-Releasing Cells in Atopic Eczema

Much interest has centered in the past around the concept of altered releasability of vasoactive mediators in atopic eczema [41]. Releasability is defined as the capacity of mediator-secreting cells to release preformed or newly synthesized mediators [63]. The relevant studies dealing with releasability of histamine from basophils in atopic eczema were compiled 1985 by Ring and Dorsch [61].

In most studies basophils released increased amounts of histamine in the atopic population compared to controls, particularly after stimulation with anti-IgE but also other stimuli [2, 12, 39, 44, 45, 62]. In addition, basophils of individuals with atopic eczema showed a faster release kinetics than normals, probably due to a more slowly acting endogenous feedback mechanism by PGE_2 [85].

Altered mediator releasability may be due, among others, to changes in immunopharmacologic or autonomic nervous system control of the release reaction or to genetic factors. Marone et al. [46] were able to show that the capacity of basophils to respond to anti-IgE and calcium ionophore A 23187 is influenced by genetic factors. Only subtle differences between atopics and controls in the immunopharmacologic control of histamine release by the H_2 agonist dimaprit, dibutyryl-cyclic AMP, 5-hydroperoxyeicosatetraenoic acid and indomethacin were noted by Peters et al. [57].

On the other hand, the defective control of mediator release by cyclic nucleotides and the autonomic nervous system in atopy has received great interest by numerous groups of investigators, particularly since the first description of β-adrenergic blockade as a possible explanation for the atopic abnormality in bronchial asthma by Szentivanyi [82]. Studies showing reduced cAMP responses of leukocytes, reduced β-adrenergic reactivity, and dysregulation of the autonomic nervous system in atopic eczema were summarized in recent reviews [61, 63].

Reduced cAMP responses in leukocytes may be due to the enhanced activity of the cAMP-inactivating enzyme phosphodiesterase in atopic patients described by the group of Hanifin [12] (for review, see Hanifin in this volume).

On the basis of the findings of altered releasability of inflammatory mediators and atopy and their immunoregulatory effects, a hypothesis has been proposed by Ring [59] which describes a vicious cycle of vasoactive mediator dysregulation in the pathogenesis of atopic eczema.

Therapeutic Implications

Assuming a role of histamine in the pathophysiology of atopic eczema, pharmacologic interventions are possible at various levels: inhibition of histamine synthesis, blockade of histamine release at different steps of the release reaction, and use of specific receptor antagonist. New developments are taking place particularly in antihistamine therapy with the introduction of nonsedating H_1 antagonists, the combination of H_1 and H_2 antagonists, and the use of H_1 antagonist with mast cell blocking activity. Although many controversies surround the use of H_1 antihistamines in atopic eczema, they have a firm place in the therapeutic armamentarium due to their antipruritic action; the sedating effect of the classical drugs may be desired in in-patients and children but can pose a problem when interfering with normal daily activities. The efficacy of the newer nonsedating antihistamines astemizole and terfenadine in atopic eczema is still subject to some dispute [64a].

Besides pharmacologic therapy, ultraviolet irradiation therapy is gaining increasing importance in the treatment of atopic eczema (see Morrison in this volume). Biochemical basis of ultraviolet efficacy in atopic eczema treatment may be, at least partly, due to the inhibition of histamine release shown recently by our group [64].

Conclusions: Role of Inflammatory Mediators in Atopic Eczema

Intensive biochemical research into the role of vasoactive mediators may provide new information on the pathophysiology of cutaneous inflammation in atopic eczema. In addition, due to the immunoregulatory effects of various mediators, at least part of the immunological disturbances observed in atopic patients may result from their actions.

Based on the evidence of enhanced releasability of vasoactive mediators in atopy, their immunoregulatory effects, the subtle cellular immune deficiency in atopics, and the postulated role of IgE, an integrated concept has been presented by Ring [59] suggesting that atopic eczema is a disease of general vasoactive mediator dysregulation. Experimental data obtained since then support this contention. Based on evidence available today, the following hypothetic scenario of the pathophysiology of atopic eczema is emerging, where altered mediator releasability assumes a central role (Fig. 4). Altered mediator releasability in atopy is caused by genetic factors or defective autonomous and immunopharmacologic control mechanisms. Inflammatory mediators cause, besides inflammatory changes in various target organs, a cellular immune deficiency by virtue of their negative immunoregulatory effects, which in turn may result in reduced suppression of IgE synthesis. Elevated IgE, by leading to enhanced mediator secretion, closes an augmentation loop (vicious cycle).

Better understanding of the inflammatory and immunological aspects of atopic eczema should finally provide new targets for therapeutic-dietary or pharmacologic-manipulations. In particular, inhibition of mediator release or antagonism of mediator action carries the hope of developing new NSAIDs for topical or systemic application, thus enlarging the so far rather limited therapeutic armamentarium in this disease.

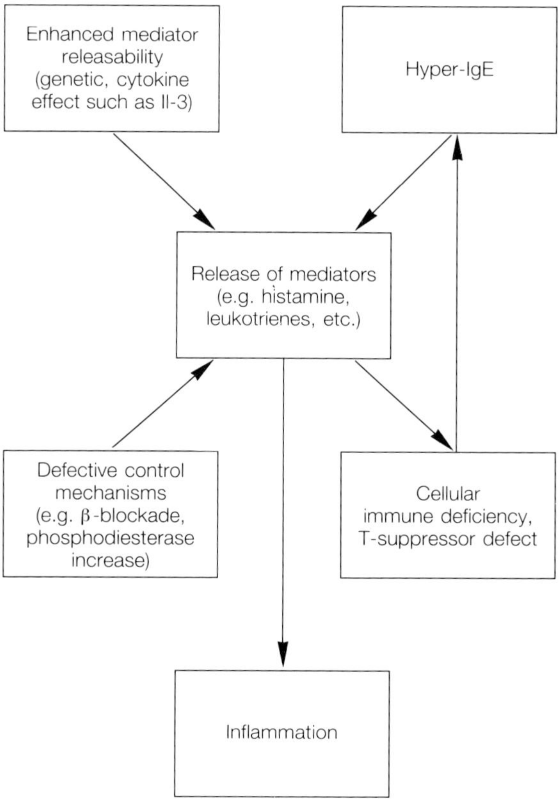

Fig. 4. Integrated concept of the pathophysiology of atopic eczema. (Modified after Ring 1985)

References

1. Arrang J-M, Garbarg M, Lancelot J-C, Lecomte IM, Pollard H, Robba M, Schunack W, Schwartz J-C (1987) Highly potent and selective ligands for histamine H_3-receptors. Nature 327:117–123
2. Assem ESK, Attallah NA (1981) Increased release of histamine by anti-IgE from leukocytes of asthmatic patients and possible heterogenicity. Clin Allergy 11:367–373
3. Ash ASF, Schild HO (1966) Receptors mediating some actions of histamine. Br J Pharmacol 27:427–439
4. Bamford ITM, Gibson RW, Renier CM (1985) Atopic eczema unresponsive to evening primrose oil (linoleic acid and gamma linolenic acids). J Am Acad Dermatol 13:959–966
5. Bauer FW, van de Kerhof PCM, Maassen-de Grood RM (1986) Epidermal hyperproliferation following the induction of microabscesses by leukotriene B_4. Br J Dermatol 124:409–412
6. Bisgaard H (1990) Effects of eicosanoids on microcirculation in the skin. In: Ruzicka T (ed) Eicosanoids and the skin. CRC Press, Boca Raton, pp. 157–170
7. Bjørneboe A, Søyland E, Bjørneboe G-EA, Rajka G, Drevon CA (1987) Effect of dietary supplementation with eicosapentaenoic acid in the treatment of atopic dermatitis. Br J Dermatol 117:463–469
8. Black JW, Duncan WAM, Durant CJ, Ganellin CR, Parsons EM (1972) Definition and antagonism of histamine H2-receptors. Nature 236:385–390
9. Bonta IL, Parnham MJ (1978) Prostaglandins and chronic inflammation. Biochem Pharmacol 27:1611–1623
10. Bray MA (1987) Prostaglandins and leukotrienes: fine tuning the immune response. ISI Atlas of Science Pharmacology 1:101–106
11. Bourne HR, Lichtenstein LM, Melmon KL, Henney CS, Weinstein Y, Shearer GM (1974) Modulation of inflammation and immunity by cyclic AMP. Science 184:19–28
12. Butler JM, Chan SC, Stevens S, Hanifin JM (1983) Increased leukocyte histamine release with elevated cyclic AMP-phosphodiesterase activity in atopic dermatitis. J Allergy Clin Immunol 71:490–497
13. Burton JL (1989) Dietary fatty acids and inflammatory skin disease. Lancet i:27–30
14. Camp R, Russel Jones R, Brain S, Woollard P, Greaves M (1984) Production of microabscesses by topical application of leukotriene B_4. J Invest Dermatol 82:202–204
15. Chan C-C, Duhamel L, Ford-Hutchinson A (1985) Leukotriene B_4 and 12-hydroxyeicosatetraenoic acid stimulate epidermal proliferation in vivo in the guinea pig. J Invest Dermatol 85:333–335
16. Czarnetzki BM, Mertensmeier R (1985) In vitro and in vivo chemotaxis of guinea pig leukocytes toward leukotriene B_4 and its ω-oxidation products. Prostaglandins 30:5–12
17. Czarnetzki BM, Rosenbach T (1986) Chemotaxis of human neutrophils and eosinophils towards leukotriene B_4 and its ω-oxidation products in vitro. Prostaglandins 31:851–859
18. Czarnetzki B (1983) Increased monocyte chemotaxis towards leukotriene B_4 and platelet activating factor in patients with inflammatory dermatoses. Clin Exp Immunol 54:486–492
19. Dale HH, Laidlaw PP (1910) The physiological action of β-imidazolylethylamine. J Physiol 41:318–344
20. Davies MG, Greaves MW (1980) Sensory responses of human skin to synthetic histamine analogues and histamine. Br J Clin Pharmacol 9:461–465

20a Dorsch W, Ring J, Weber PC, Strasser T (1985) Detection of immunoreactive leukotrienes LTC_4/D_4 in skin blister fluid after allergen testing in patients with late cutaneous reactions (LCR). Arch Dermat Res 277:400–401

21. Dowd PM, Black AK, Woollard PM, Camp RDR, Greaves MW (1985) Cutaneous responses to 12-hydroxy-5,8,10,14-eicosatetraenoic acid (12-HETE). J Invest Dermatol 84:537–541
22. Ferreri NR, Zeiger RS, Spiegelberg HL (1988) IgG-, IgA-, and IgE-induced release of leukotriene C_4 by monocytes isolated from patients with atopic dermatitis. J Allergy Clin Immunol 82:556–567
23. Fogh K, Herlin T, Kragballe K (1989) Eicosanoids in skin of patients with atopic dermatitis: prostaglandin E_2 and leukotriene B_4 are present in biologically active concentrations. J Allergy Clin Immunol 83:450–455
24. Gemsa D (1981) Stimulation of prostaglandin E release from macrophages and possible role in the immune response. In: Pick E (ed) Lymphokines. Academic, New York, pp 335–375
25. Goetzl EJ, Gorman RR (1978) Chemotactic and chemokinetic stimulation of human eosinophil and neutrophil polymorphonuclear leukocytes by 12-*L*-hydroxy-5, 8, 10-heptadecatrienoic acid (HHT). J Immunol 120: 520–529
26. Groß EC, Stolz W, von Restorff B, Ruzicka T (1989) High affinity binding and lack of growth promoting activity of 12(S)-hydroxyeicosatetraenoic acid (12(S)-HETE) in a human epidermal cell line. J Invest Dermatol (abstract) 92:437
27. Hägermark Ö, Strandberg K, Grönneberg R (1979) Effects of histamine receptor antagonists on histamine-induced responses in human skin. Acta Derm Venereol 59:297–300
28. Hammarstrom JL (1982) Effects of intradermally injected leukotriene C_4 and histamine in patients with urticaria, psoriasis, and atopic dermatitis. Br J Dermatol [Suppl] 107:106–110
29. Hammarström S, Hamberg S, Samuelsson B, Duell E, Stawiski M, Voorhees JJ (1975) Increased concentrations of nonesterified arachidonic acid, 12-*L*-hydroxy-5, 8, 10, 14-eicosatetraenoic acid, prostaglandin E_2 and prostaglandin $F\alpha_2$ in epidermis of psoriasis. Proc Natl Acad Sci USA 72:5130–5134
30. Hammarström S, Lindgreen JA, Marcello C, Duell EA, Anderson TE, Voorhees JJ (1979) Arachidonic acid transformations in normal and psoriatic skin. J Invest Dermatol 73:180–183
31. Hein R, Groß E, Ruzicka T, Krieg T (1990) Chemotactic effects of eicosanoids for fibroblasts and keratinocytes. In: Ruzicka T (ed) Eicosanoids and the skin. CRC Press Boca Raton
32. Hong LS, Levine L (1976) Inhibition of arachidonic acid release from cells as the biochemical action of anti-inflammatory corticosteroids. Proc Natl Acad Sci 73: 1730–1734
33. Ikai K, Imamura S (1988) Prostaglandin D_2 in the skin. Intern J Dermatol 27:141–159
34. Isseroff RR (1988) Fish again for dinner! The role of fish and other dietary oils in the therapy of skin disease. J Amer Acad Dermatol 19:1073–1080
35. Johnson HH, de Oreo G, Lascheid WP, Mitchell F (1960)

Skin histamine levels in chronic atopic dermatitis. J Invest Dermatol 34:237–238
36. Juhlin L (1967) Localisation and content of histamine in normal and diseased skin. Acta Derm Venereol 47:383–391
37. Kragballe K, Desjarlais L, Voorhees JJ (1985) Leukotrienes B_4, C_4 and D_4 stimulate DNA synthesis in cultured human epidermal keratinocytes. Br J Dermatol 113:43–52
37a Kunz B, Ring J, Braun-Falco O (1989) Eicosapentaenoic acid (EPA) treatment in atopic eczema (AE): a prospective double-blind trial. J Allergy Clin Immunol (abstract) 83:196
38. Lawrence CM, Shuster S (1987) Effect of arachidonic acid on anthralin inflammation. Br J Clin Pharmacol 24:125–131
39. Lebel B, Venencie PY, Saurat JH, Soubrane C, Paupe J (1980) Anti-IgE induced histamine release from basophils in children with atopic dermatitis. Acta Derm Venereol, [Suppl] 92:57–59
40. Lichtenstein LM, Gillespie E (1973) Inhibition of histamine release by histamine is controlled by an H2 receptor. Nature 244:287
41. Lichtenstein LM, Conroy MC (1977) The "releasability" of mediators from human basophils and granulocytes. In: Mathov E, Sindo T, Naranjo P (eds) Allergy and clinical immunology. Excerpta Medica, Amsterdam, pp 109–115
42. Manku MS, Horrobin DF, Morse N, Wright S, Burton DL (1982) Reduced levels of prostaglandin precursors in the blood of atopic patients: defective delta-6-desaturase function as a biochemical basis for atopy. Prostaglandins Leukotrienes Med 9:615–628
43. Manku MS, Horrobin DF, Morse NL, Wright S, Burton JL (1984) Essential fatty acids in the plasma phospholipids of patients with atopic eczema. Brit J Dermatol 110:643–648
44. Marone G, Poto S, Giugliano R, Bonini S (1985) Studies on human basophil releasability. Int Archs Allergy Appl Immunol 77:103–106
45. Marone G, Poto S, Giugliano R, Lembo G, Ayala F (1986) Human basophil releasability. II. Changes in basophil releasability in patients with atopic dermatitis. J Invest Dermatol 87:19–23
46. Marone G, Poto S, Celestino D, Bonini S (1986) Human basophil releasability. III. Genetic control of human basophil releasability. J Immunol 137:3580–3590
47. Matloff SM, Kiselis IK, Rocklin RE (1983) Reduced production of histamine-induced suppressive factor (HSF) by atopic mononuclear cells and decreased prostaglandin E_2 output by HSF-stimulated atopic monocytes. J Allergy Clin Immunol 72:350–364
48. Meier F, Gross E, Klotz K-N, Ruzicka T (1989) Leukotriene B_4 receptors on neutrophils in patients with psoriasis and atopic eczema. Skin Pharmacol 2:61–67
49. Mensing H, Czarnetzki BM (1984) Leukotriene B_4 induces in vitro fibroblast chemotaxis. J Invest Dermatol 82:9–13
50. Mita H, Yui Y, Taniguch N, Yasueda H, Shida T (1985) Increased activity of 5-lipoxygenase in polymorphonuclear leukocytes from asthmatic patients. Life Sci 37: 907–914
51. Morelli JG, Norris DA, Lyons MB, Murphy RC (1988) Metabolism of exogenous leukotrienes by cultured human keratinocytes and melanocytes. J Invest Dermatol (abstract) 90:590
52. Morse PF, Horrobin DF, Manku MS et al. (1989) Meta-analysis of placebo-controlled studies of the efficacy of Epogam in the treatment of atopic eczema. Relationship between plasma essential fatty acid changes and clinical response. Br J Dermatol 121:75–90
53. Mukhtar H, Bik DP, Ruzicka T, Merk H, Bickers DR (1989) Cytochrome P-450-dependent omega-oxidation of leukotriene B_4 in rodent and human epidermis. J Invest Dermatol 93:231–235
54. Needleman SW, Spector AA, Hoak JC (1982) Enrichment of human platelet phospholipids with linoleic acid diminishes thromboxane release. Prostaglandins 24:607–622
55. Otto WR, Barr RM, Dowd PM, Wright NA, Greaves MW (1987) 12-hydroxyeicosatetraenoic acid (12-HETE) does not promote growth of human keratinocytes in vitro. J Invest Dermatol (abstract) 89:339
56. Pace-Asciak C, Wolfe LS (1968) Inhibition of prostaglandin synthesis by oleic, linoleic and linolenic acids. Biochim Biophys Acta 152:784–777
57. Peters SP, Tung RS, Chatham M, Bleecker ER, Lichtenstein LM (1985) Inhibitability and enhanceability of basophil histamine release in asthmatic and normal subjects. Int Archs Allergy Appl Immunol 76:344–349
58. Rieger G, Hein R, Ruzicka T, Wach F, Adelmann-Grill B, Krieg T (1987) Biologic activities of eicosanoids on fibroblasts in culture. Regulation of chemotactic activity and collagen synthesis. J Invest Dermatol (abstract) 89: 339
58a Ring J, Seifert J, Merten J, Brendel W (1974) Prolongation of skin allograft survival in rats by treatment with linoleic acid. Lancet ii:1331
59. Ring J (1979) Atopic dermatitis: a disease of general vasoactive mediator dysregulation. Int Archs Allergy Appl Immunol 59:233–239
60. Ring J (1983) Plasma histamine concentrations in atopic eczema. Clin Allergy 13:545–552
61. Ring J, Dorsch W (1985) Altered releasability of vasoactive mediator secreting cells in atopic eczema. Acta Derm Venereol (Stockh.) [Suppl] 114:9–23
62. Ring J, Walz U (1985) Indomethacin enhances in vitro histamine release induced by anti-IgE and Ca-ionophore but inhibits C5a-induced release reactions from basophils of atopics and normals. Int Arch Allergy Appl. Immunol 77:225–227
63. Ring J, Sedlmeier F, von der Helm D, Mayr T, Walz U, Ibel H, Riepel H, Przybilla B, Reimann H-I, Dorsch W (1986) Histamine and allergic diseases. In: Ring J, Burg G (eds) New Trends in Allergy II. Springer, Berlin·Heidelberg·New York·Tokyo, pp 44–77
63a Ring J (1988) Angewandte Allergologie, 2nd edn. MMV-Vieweg, Munich
64. Ring J, Przybilla B, Eberlein B (1989) Ultraviolet A inhibits histamine release from human peripheral leukocytes. Int Arch Allergy Appl. Immunol 88:136–138
64a Ring J, Thomas P (1989) Histamine and atopic eczema. Acta Derm Venereol (Stockh.) [Suppl] 144:70–77
65. Rocklin RE (1976) Modulation of cellular immune response in vivo and in vitro by histamine receptor-bearing lymphocytes. J Clin Invest 57:1051–1058
66. Rocklin RE, Thistle L, Andera C (1985) Decreased sensitivity of atopic mononuclear cells to prostaglandin E_2 (PGE_2) and prostaglandin D_2 (PGD_2). J Immunol 135: 2033–2039
67. Rocklin RE, Thistle L, Gallant L, Manku MS, Horrobin D (1986) Altered arachidonic acid content in polymorphonuclear and mononuclear cells from patients with allergic rhinitis and/or asthma. Lipids 21:17–20

68. Ruzicka T, Wasserman SI, Soter NA, Printz MP (1983) Inhibition of rat mast cell arachidonic acid cyclooxygenase by dapsone. J Allergy Clin Immunol 72:365–370
69. Ruzicka T, Glück S (1983) Gutaneous histamine levels and histamine releasability from the skin in atopic dermatitis and hyper-IgE-syndrome. Arch Dermatol Res 275:41–44
70. Ruzicka T, Vitto A, Printz MP (1983) Epidermal arachidonate lipoxygenase. Biochim Biophys Acta 751:359–374
71. Ruzicka T, Printz MP (1984) Arachidonic acid metabolism in skin: a review. Rev Physiol Biochem Pharmacol 100: 121–160
72. Ruzicka T, Simmet T, Peskar BA, Ring J (1986) Skin levels of arachidonic acid-derived inflammatory mediators and histamine in atopic dermatitis and psoriasis. J Invest Dermatol 86:105–108
73. Ruzicka T, Przybilla B (1986) Eicosanoids in skin UV-inflammation – lack of leukotriene B_4 elevation in UVB-induced dermatitis. Photodermatology 2:306–307
74. Ruzicka T, Auböck J (1987) Arachidonic acid metabolism in guinea pig Langerhans cells: studies on cyclooxygenase and lipoxygenase pathways. J Immunol 138:539–543
75. Ruzicka T, Burg G (1987) Effects of chronic intracutaneous administration of arachidonic acid and its metabolites. Induction of leukocytoclastic vasculitis by leukotriene B_4 and 12-hydroxyeicosatetraenoic acid and its prevention by prostaglandin E_2. J Invest Dermatol 88:120–123
76. Ruzicka T, Ring J (1987) Enhanced releasability of prostaglandin E_2 and leukotrienes B_4 and C_4 from leukocytes of patients with atopic eczema. Acta Derm Venereol (Stockh.) 67:469–475
77. Ruzicka T (1988) The physiology and pathophysiology of eicosanoids in the skin. Eicosanoids 1:59–72
78. Ruzicka T, Groß E (1989) In vivo and in vitro pharmacologic activities of linoleic acid in skin and polymorphonuclear leukocytes. Arch Dermatol Res (abstract) 281: 163
79. Ruzicka T, Groß E (1989) Pharmacologic effects of linoleic acid (LA) in skin and polymorphonuclear leukocytes. J Invest Dermatol (abstract) 92:510
80. Schwartz A, Sutton SL, Askenase PW, Gershon RK (1981) Histamine inhibition of concanavalin A-induced suppressor T-cell activation. Cell Immunol 60:425–439
81. Spector AA, Hoak IC, Fry GL (1980) Effect of fatty acid modification on prostacyclin production by cultured human endothelial cells. J Clin Invest 65:1003–1012
82. Szentivanyi A (1968) The beta-adrenergic theory of the atopic abnormality in bronchial asthma. J Allergy 42:203–232
83. Talbot SF, Atkins PC, Goetzl EJ, Zweiman B (1985) Accumulation of leukotriene C_4 and histamine in human allergic skin reactions. J Clin Invest 75:650–656
84. Ujihara M, Horiguchi Y, Ikai K, Urade Y (1988) Characterization and distribution of prostaglandin D synthetase in rat skin. J Invest Dermatol 90:440–451
85. Von der Helm D, Ring J, Dorsch W (1987) Comparison of histamine release and prostaglandin E_2 production of human basophils in atopic and normal individuals. Arch Dermatol Res 279:536–542
86. Voorhorst R, van den Hooft van Asbeck MC (1979) Atopic skin test re-evaluated. VI. Skin reactions to compound 48/80 and histamine in patients with atopic and non-atopic chronic respiratory complaints and in normal volunteers. Ann Allergy 42:185–186
87. Wang SR, Yang CM, Wang SSM, Han SH, Chiang BN (1986) Enhancement of A 23187-induced production of the slow-reacting substance on peripheral leukocytes from subjects with asthma. J Allergy Clin Immunol 77:465–471
88. Wasserman J, Hammarström S, Petrini B (1987) Effects of some prostaglandins and leukotrienes on lymphocytes, monocytes and their activity in vitro. Int Archs Allergy Appl Immunol 83:39–43
89. Wong G, Duncan MR, Ziboh VA, Berman B (1987) Purified human Langerhans cells and not epidermal cells generate prostaglandin D_2 (PGD_2) and 15-hydroxy-eicosatetraenoic acid (15-HETE) from arachidonic acid. J Invest Dermatol (abstract) 88:524
90. Wright S, Burton IL (1982) Oral evening-primrose-seed oil improves atopic eczema. Lancet ii:1120–1122
91. Ziboh VA (1989) Implications of dietary oil and polyunsaturated fatty acids in the management of cutaneous disorders. Arch Dermatol 125:241–245

Cytokines in Atopic Eczema

A. Kapp

Immunologic Alterations in Atopic Eczema – Role of Cytokines?

Although atopic eczema (AE) represents an inflammatory skin disorder which has been well-known since the beginning of the century, its pathogenesis is as yet not clearly understood. Many trigger mechanisms have been identified which aggravate the clinical course of AE, but several findings support the concept of a genetic background to the disease [25, 26]. Monozygotic twin pairs are more often concordant for AE than dizygotic twin pairs [78]. Moreover, atopy could be transferred by bone marrow transplantation, pointing to an alteration of immunocompetent stem cells [74, 75].

Accordingly, there exists a variety of studies describing dysregulation of humoral as well as cellular immune functions in AE. Specifically, serum immunoglobulin E (IgE) levels are elevated [29, 59], in particular specific IgE directed to a variety of environmental allergens [37, 41]. In addition, IgE-containing immune complexes have been detected [4, 35], possibly involved in the activation of the complement system [43, 66].

On the other hand, AE is characterized by a number of cellular dysfunctions of nonimmune cells [24, 40, 68] and, particularly, in the T cell compartment. Numerical and functional defects have been described for natural killer (NK) cells [28, 48, 82] and cytotoxic and suppressor T cells [10, 11, 47, 70, 80]. There is increasing evidence that these alterations may be due to imbalances within the cytokine network (Table 1).

Table 1: Cytokine production by MNC in vitro and serum receptor levels in atopic eczema and psoriasis

Cytokine production (stimulus)	Atopic eczema	Psoriasis	Reference
IL-1 (LPS	↓ [a]	N.D. [b]	[36,62]
IL-1 (spontaneous)	unchanged	N.D.	[36,62]
IL-6 (PHA, LPS)	unchanged	unchanged	[56]
IL-6 (spontaneous)	unchanged	↑	[56]
TNF α (PHA, LPS)	↓	unchanged	[42]
IFN α (*C. parvum*, poly I-polyC, HSV)	unchanged	↓	[33,34]
IL-2 (PHA)	↓	unchanged	[36,38]
IL-4 (in serum) [c]	unchanged	N.D.	
TNF β (PHA)	unchanged	unchanged	[42]
IFN γ (PHA, ConA, PWM, PPD, tetanus antigen)	unchanged	↓	[33,34]
Receptors (serum)			
IL-2 receptor	↑	↑	[38,39]
CD4 [c]	unchanged	unchanged	
CD8	unchanged	↑	[30]

a) ↑, increased, ↓, decreased;
b) N.D., not determined
c) W. Czech, A. Kapp (unpublished observation)

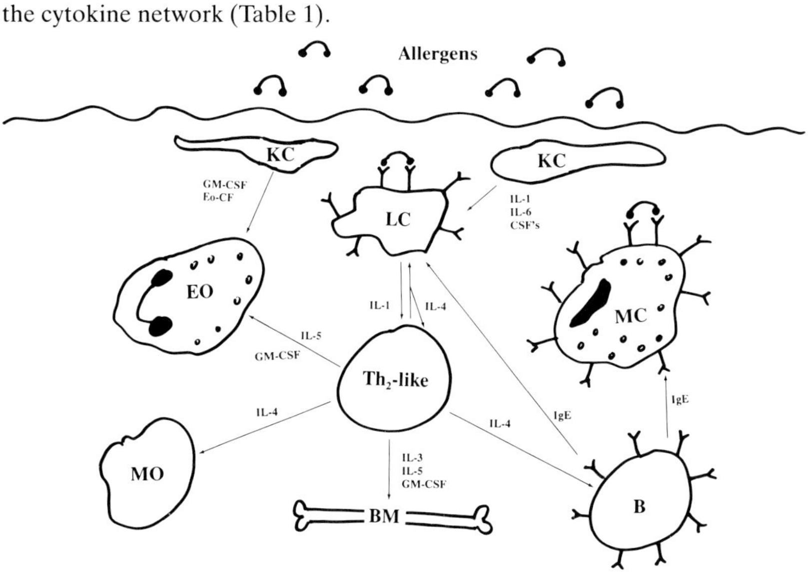

Fig. 1. Possible cytokine interactions and their pathopysiological role in the pathogenesis of atopic eczema. *B*, B-lymphocyte; *EO*, eosinophilic granulocyte; *BM*, bone marrow; *KC*, keratinocyte; *LC*, Langerhans cell, *MO*, monocyte; *MC*, mast cell

Interferons

A predominant feature of AE is the enhanced susceptibility to viral infections [63, 73]. Since first reported by Kaposi, it is well known that Herpes simplex and vaccinia virus infections may cause syndromes of eczema vaccinatum and eczema herpeticum in patients with AE [13, 63]. Furthermore, an increased incidence of warts and molluscum contagiosum has also been reported in AE [14, 63]. Although the cause of this phenomenon has not yet been elucidated, it has been speculated that there is a defect in the capacity to produce interferons in response to viral antigens [82].

The interferon system represents an integral part of the defense system against viral infections [45]. Furthermore, interferon modulates the activity of different effector cells, such as macrophages or NK cells. Surprisingly, it could be shown that there was no significant difference between AE patients (showing moderate to severe disease activity) and controls in the capability of leukocytes to release interferon activity upon stimulation with a variety of interferon-α and interferon-γ inducers in vitro [33]. Since eczema herpeticum often represents a severe complication in AE, Herpes simplex virus was also included as a representative stimulus [33], Moreover, interferon responses were tested upon stimulation with *Corynebacterium parvum*, which is also known to be an inducer of interferon-α in human leukocyte cultures. Nevertheless, no significant differences were observed. Recently, a diminished production of interferon-γ upon stimulation with PHA was observed exclusively in patients with *severe* atopic eczema showing markedly increased serum IgE levels. Therefore, it appears very likely that these findings may be related to the disease activity of AE or a subgroup of the patients [64]. Similarly, there is a report demonstrating that children with AE released significantly less interferon upon stimulation with Sendai virus [82]. However, the investigators used Sendai virus as the only stimulus to test the reactivity of leukocytes. Furthermore, Sendai virus does not seem to be involved in infections observed in AE patients. Therefore, it is suggested that the enhanced susceptibility to viral infections in AE is not due to a primary defect of patients' leukocytes in releasing interferons upon appropriate stimulation. The increase in cutaneous viral infections may be mediated by diminished NK cell activity [28, 48] or decreased cytotoxic T cell function, which may be the result of a dysregulation of suppressor T cell activity reported in AE [10, 11, 47, 70, 80].

Interleukin-1 and Interleukin-2

Activation of T cells is dependent on the release of immunomodulating cytokines: Following binding of the T cell to the antigen-presenting cell, the T cell stimulates the antigen-presenting cell to produce interleukin-1 (IL-1) by a mechanism which is not completely clarified at present [19]. IL-1 in association with antigen stimulation induces interleukin-2 (IL-2) receptors on the T cells and stimulates T cells to release IL-2; this drives antigen-activated cells into proliferation [69]. Therefore, functional alterations of T cells such as decreased lymphoproliferative responses [33, 47, 76] could be the result of a diminished capacity of mononuclear cells to release IL-1 and IL-2 upon appropriate stimulation.

As shown previously, mononuclear cells from AE patients released significantly less IL-1 and IL-2 following stimulation whereas the basal IL-1 production was unchanged [36]. The results are in agreement with a previous report of Räsanen et al. [62], who showed that purified monocytes of AE patients produced clearly less IL-1 in response to stimulation than monocytes from healthy controls. Therefore, the decreased production of IL-1 is apparently not due to suppressive factors derived from T lymphocytes. These data support the hypothesis that monocyte functions are impaired in AE.

Mononuclear cells of AE patients release significantly less IL-2 in the supernatants following stimulation with the T cell mitogen PHA in comparison with healthy controls [36, 38]. Moreover, there was an inverse correlation between IL-2 concentrations and body surface involvement [38]. Therefore, depressed lymphoproliferative responses upon stimulation with T cell mitogens may be caused by diminished production of IL-2 upon stimulation.

Interleukin-6

Interleukin-6 (IL-6) has recently been identified as a multifunctional mediator which regulates various aspects of local and systemic inflammation [51]. IL-6 previously was described as interferon-β_2, hybridoma growth factor, hepatocyte-stimulating factor, or B-cell stimulatory factor 2, and is produced by monocytes, fibroblasts, and epidermal cells. There is a clear parallel between the effects of IL-6 and IL-1 on hematopoietic cells. Many of the biological effects of IL-1 and IL-6 overlap and IL-1 is a potent inducer of IL-6 in many cell types. In contrast to the finding of a decreased release of IL-1 there was no significant difference between AE patients and controls when supernatants of unstimulated or stimulated mononuclear cells were tested for IL-6 activity [56]. In addition, sera of AE patients did not contain increased levels of IL-6.

Tumor Necrosis Factor and Lymphotoxin

Tumor necrosis factor/cachectin/TNF-α (TNF) and lymphotoxin/TNF-β (LT) [23, 61], initially characterized by their cytotoxic properties, are suggested to play an essential role as mediators of inflammatory reactions. TNF was shown to mediate a broad range of regulatory and inhibitory effects on various cell types [1, 19, 44, 53, 60]. Specifically, TNF was shown to be a relevant signal for IL-1 production in vitro and in vivo [20, 54]. In AE patients TNF production by mononuclear cells in vitro was shown to be significantly decreased upon stimulation with PHA and LPS as compared with healthy controls [42]. There was no sign of a continuous in vivo activation in AE patients since no significant spontaneous production of TNF or LT could be detected in vitro. There was no correlation of TNF levels and IgE concentrations or body surface involvement, suggesting that the decreased production of TNF does not directly reflect the inflammatory process in the skin of AE patients. However, it was reported recently that stimulation of polymorphonuclear neutrophils (PMN) in vitro deactivated the cells for subsequent stimulation with the same cytokine [44]. Therefore, it may be possible that excessive stimulation in vivo could be the cause of a decreased TNF production by monocytes in vitro. Alternatively, the decreased production could be a sign of "exhaustion" due to preceding activation of monocytes in vivo. The potential role of monocytes in the pathogenesis of AE is also emphasized by the finding that release of the nonmonocyte product LT did not show any significant changes in AE. Although TNF and LT have similar biological activities, share a common receptor, and are encoded by genes which are structurally related [1, 60], LT is exclusively produced by lymphocytes [15, 81]. In contrast, TNF can be produced by both lymphocytes and monocytes [15, 81].

T Cell Activation In Vivo – Serum Interleukin-2 Receptor

Inflammatory processes are regulated by a network of immunomodulating cytokines including cytotoxins, interferons, colony-stimulating factors, and interleukins. Based on the data presented, AE in particular is characterized by a significantly decreased capacity of monocytes to release immunomodulating cytokines. However, these findings do not reflect an overall decreased capacity of monocytes in AE patients to release immunomodulating cytokines since the production of IL-6 [56] and interferon-α [33] appeared to be unaffected. Furthermore a possible "defect" would probably involve more than one regulating step since TNF and IL-1 production appear to be differentially modulated [9]. Moreover, sera of AE patients contained significantly increased levels of the IL-2 receptor, as compared with healthy controls [39]. In addition, IL-2 receptor levels in AE patients showed a significant correlation with IgE levels and body surface involvement [38]. As mentioned above, IL-2 plays an essential role in triggering proliferation of activated T cells. The response is mediated by binding of the cytokine to a high-affinity membrane receptor [67]. Synthesis and expression of this receptor which was shown to be released from T cells and a subpopulation of B cells upon activation represent a very early sign of T cell activation [71, 72, 83]. Increased levels of IL-2 receptor in serum have been detected in different diseases accompanied by T cell activation, e.g., rheumatoid arthritis, lupus erythematosus, T cell leukemia, and allograft rejection [12, 52, 55, 79]. With respect to increased IL-2 receptor levels, no hyperproliferation of peripheral blood lymphocytes could be observed in AE in vitro, and lymphoproliferative responses upon stimulation were usually normal or even decreased [33, 47, 76]. Therefore, a supposed T cell defect which could be shown by functional assays in the peripheral blood is in direct contrast to signs of hyperactivation, probably in the skin of the patients. In addition, concentrations of cell-free CD8 antigen, which is reported to be released by activated suppressor/cytotoxic T cells [5, 21], were not decreased in the sera of AE patients [30].

Possible Immunoregulatory Mechanisms in AE

Usually investigations on immunologic parameters of AE were done with peripheral blood leukocytes. Since in AE the inflammatory process is focused on the skin, measurement of immune functions and immunomodulating mediators in the peripheral blood only "reflects" immunoregulatory mechanisms at the site of inflammation. It appears very unlikely that the reported alterations of the immune system in AE are the result of a basic defect of patients' monocytes to produce immunomodulating cytokines upon stimulation. It is tempting to speculate that the decreased production of cytokines by blood mononuclear cells is due to downregulation of the immune response in the peripheral blood induced by cytokines released from hyperactivated immune cells in the inflamed skin. Alternatively, the hyporesponsiveness of mononuclear cells in vitro could be a sign of "exhaustion" following excessive stimulation in vivo. These suggestions are supported by the finding that alterations of distinct T-cell functions normalized with clinical remissions [47, 48, 68, 84]. Whereas most of these studies focus on the situation in the peripheral blood, relatively little is known about the inflammatory process in atopic skin. The human skin itself is the source of a variety of inflammatory cytokines, e.g., IL-1, IL-6, TNF, GM-CSF [51]. In addition, these mediators can be released by nonspecific mechanisms: irradiation with ultraviolet light or mechanical irritation (scratching). Moreover, distinct mediators may be rapidly released since they are contained in the epidermal cells as preformed material [27, 32].

Recent reports indicate that contact of skin with inhalant allergens may induce exacerbation of AE [6, 22, 57, 65]. This may be due to an allergen-specific process, which may be mediated by Langerhans cells expressing Fc receptors for specific IgE [3, 8] (Fig. 1). Activation of Langerhans cells, associated with release of IL-1, results in activation of an atopy-specific T-helper lymphocyte subset, which in turn release IL-4, IL-5, or other growth factors. IL-5 is capable of stimulating eosinophil proliferation and function in man [50]. Eosinophils were reported to be important effector cells for propagation of the local inflammatory response in AE [7, 31, 46]. IL-4 mediates various immunologic effects, two of which may be of major importance for the pathogenesis of AE: IL-4 is able to induce the low-affinity receptor for IgE on Langerhans cells (CD23) and regulates IgE synthesis, particularly influencing the switch of IgM to IgE/IgG_1 [2, 16, 58]. Therefore, induction of a local immune response, associated with the release of immunomodulating cytokines, may result in systemic activation of their target cells in the bone marrow [17, 18]. Moreover, during chronification of the disease it is completely possible that an antigen-specific immune response in AE will change to an antigen-independent and selfperpetuating inflammatory process which is triggered by a number of different factors, but also by sympathetic neural mechanisms [49].

However, the data presented are preliminary findings and possibly other immunologic alterations within the skin immune system may also contribute to the pathogenesis of AE.

References

1. Beutler BB, Cerami A (1986) Cachectin and tumour necrosis factor as two sides of the same biological coin. Nature 320:584–588
2. Bieber T, Rieger A, Neuchrist C, Prinz JC, Rieber EP, Boltz-Nitulescu G, Scheiner O, Kraft D, Ring J, Stingl G (1989) Induction of FcεR2/CD23 on human epidermal Langerhans cells by human recombinant interleukin 4 and gamma interferon. J Exp Med 170:309–314
3. Bieber T, Ring J, Braun-Falco O (1989) IgE-tragende dendritische Zellen der Haut. Ein Hinweis auf die pathophysiologische Bedeutung von Langerhans-Zellen beim atopischen Ekzem. Dtsch Med Wochenschr 114:150–153
4. Brostoff J, Johns P, Stanworth DR (1977) Complexed IgE in atopy. Lancet II (8041):741–742
5. Brown M, Carrabis S, Ip S, Kung P (1987) Enzyme immunoassay for the quantitation of cell free human T cell CD8 like molecule. Fed Proc 46:467
6. Bruynzeel-Koomen CA, Bruynzeel PL (1988) A role for IgE in patch test reactions to inhalant allergens in patients with atopic dermatitis. Allergy 43 [Suppl 5]: 15–21

7. Bruynzeel-Koomen CA, van Wichen DF, Spry CJ, Venge P, Bruynzeel PL (1988) Active participation of eosinophils in patch test reactions to inhalant allergens in patients with atopic dermatitis. Br J Dermatol 118:229–238
8. Bruynzeel-Koomen C, van Wichen DF, Toonstra J, Berrens L, Bruynzeel PL (1986) The presence of IgE molecules on epidermal Langerhans cells in patients with atopic dermatitis. Arch Dermatol Res 278:199–205
9. Burchett SK, Weaver WM, Westall JA, Larsen A, Kronheim S, Wilson CB (1988) Regulation of tumor necrosis factor/cachectin and IL-1 secretion in human mononuclear phagocytes. J Immunol 140:3473–3481
10. Butler M, Atherton D, Levinsky RJ (1982) Quantitative and functional deficit of suppressor T cells in children with atopic eczema. Clin Exp Immunol 50:92–98, 1982
11. Chandra RK, Baker M (1983) Numerical and functional deficiency of suppressor T cells precedes development of atopic eczema. Lancet II:1393–1394
12. Colvin RB, Fuller TC, MacKeen L, Kung PC, Ip SH, Cosimi AB (1987) Plasma interleukin 2 receptor levels in renal allograft recipients. Clin Immunol Immunopathol 43:273–276
13. Copeman PW, Wallace HS (1964) Eczema vaccinatum. Br Med J 2:906–914
14. Currie JM, Wright RC, Miller OW (1971) The frequency of warts in atopic dermatitis. Cutis 8:244–254
15. Cuturi MC, Murphy M, Costa-Giomi MP, Weinmann R, Perussia B, Trinchieri G (1987) Independent regulation of tumor necrosis factor and lymphotoxin production by human peripheral blood lymphocytes. J Exp Med 165: 1581–1594
16. Delespesse G, Sarfatti M, Peleman R (1989) Influence of recombinant IL-4, IFN-alpha, and IFN-gamma on the production of human IgE-binding factor (soluble CD23). J Immunol 142:134–138
17. Denburg JA, Telizyn S, Belda A, Dolovich J, Bienenstock J (1985) Increased numbers of circulating basophil progenitors in atopic dermatitis. J Allergy Clin Immunol 76: 466–472
18. Denburg JA, Otsuka H, Ohnisi M, Ruhno J, Bienenstock J, Dolovich J (1987) Contribution of basophil/mast cell and eosinophil growth and differentiation to the allergic tissue inflammatory response. Int Arch Allergy Appl Immunol 83:321–326
19. Dinarello CA (1986) Interleukin-1: amino acid sequences, multiple biological activities and comparison with tumor necrosis factor (Cachectin). Year Immunol 2: 68–89
20. Dinarello CA, Cannon JG, Wolff SM, Bernheim HA, Beutler B, Cerami A, Figari IS, Palladino MA, O'Connor JV (1986) Tumor necrosis factor (cachectin) is an endogenous pyrogen and induces production of interleukin 1. J Exp Med 163:1433–1450
21. Fujimoto J, Levy S, Levy R (1983) Spontaneous release of the Leu-2 (T8) molecule from human T cells. J Exp Med 159:752–766
22. Gondo A, Saeki N, Tokuda Y (1986) Challenge reactions in atopic dermatitis after percutaneous entry of mite antigen. Br J Dermatol 115:485–493
23. Gray PW, Aggarwal BB, Benton CV, Bringman TS, Henzel WJ, Jarrett JA, Leung DW, Moffat B, Ng P, Svedersky LP, Palladino MA, Nedwin GE (1984) Cloning and expression of cDNA for human lymphotoxin, a lymphokine with tumour necrosis activity. Nature 312: 721–724
24. Hanifin JM, Rogge JL, Bauman RH (1980) Chemotaxis inhibition by plasma from patients with atopic dermatitis. Acta Derm Venereol (Stockh.) [Suppl] 92:52–56
25. Hanifin JM, Rajka G (1980) Diagnostic features of atopic dermatitis. Acta Derm Venereol (Stockh.) [Suppl] 92: 44–47
26. Hanifin JM (1987) Epidemiology of atopic dermatitis. Monogr Allergy 21:116–131
27. Hauser C, Saurat JH, Schmitt A, Jaunin F, Dayer JM (1986) Interleukin 1 is present in normal human epidermis. J Immunol 136:3317–3323
28. Jensen JR, Sand TT, Jorgensen AS, Thestrup-Petersen K (1984) Modulation of natutal killer cell activity in patients with atopic dermatitis. J Invest Dermatol 82:30–34
29. Juhlin L, Johansson SGO, Bennich H, Högman C, Thyresson N: Immunoglobulin E in dermatoses (1969) Levels in atopic dermatitis and urticaria. Arch Dermatol 100:12–16
30. Kapp A (1990) Elevated levels of soluble CD8 antigen in sera of patients with psoriasis – a possible sign of suppressor/cytotoxic T cell activation. Arch Dermatol Res 282:6–7
31. Kapp A, Czech W, Krutmann J, Schöpf E (1991) Eosinophil cationic protein (ECP) in serum of patients with atopic dermatitis. J Am Acad Dermatol 24: 555–558)
32. Kapp A, Danner M, Luger TA, Hauser C, Schöpf E (1987) Granulocyte-activating mediators (GRAM): II. Generation by human epidermal cells. Arch Dermatol Res 279:470–477
33. Kapp A, Gillitzer R, Kirchner H, Schöpf E (1987) Production of interferon and lymphoproliferative responses in whole blood cultures derived from patients with atopic dermatitis. Arch Dermatol Res 279:S55–S58
34. Kapp A, Gillitzer R, Kirchner H, Schöpf E (1988) Decreased production of interferon in whole blood cultures derived from patients with psoriasis. J Invest Dermatol 90:511–514
35. Kapp A, Kemper A, Schöpf E, Deicher H (1986) Detection of circulating immune complexes in patients with atopic dermatitis and psoriasis. Acta Derm Venereol (Stockh.) 66:121–126
36. Kapp A, Kirnbauer R, Luger TA, Schöpf E (1987) Altered production of immunomodulating cytokines in patients with atopic dermatitis. Acta Derm Venereol (Stockh.) [Suppl] 144:97–99
37. Kapp A, Löbig K-P, Schöpf E (1989) Allergie gegen Vorratsmilben bei Patienten mit atopischer Dermatitis – Eine RAST Studie. Allergologie 12:315–317
38. Kapp A, Neuner P, Krutmann J, Luger TA, Schöpf E (1991) Production of interleukin-2 by mononuclear cells in vitro in patients with atopic dermatitis and psoriasis – comparison with serum interleukin-2 receptor levels. Acta Derm Venereol (in press)
39. Kapp A, Piskorski A, Schöpf E (1988) Elevated levels of interleukin-2 receptor in sera of patients with atopic dermatitis and psoriasis. Br J Dermatol 119:707–710
40. Kapp A, Schöpf E (1986) Cellular reactivity of polymorphonuclear leukocytes in Psoriasis and Atopic Dermatitis. Acta Derm Venereol 66:285–289
41. Kapp A, Schöpf E (1989) Spezifisches IgE gegen Staphylokokkus aureus bei Patienten mit Atopischer Dermatitis. Hautarzt 40:19–22
42. Kapp A, Textor A, Krutmann J, Möller A (1990) Immunomodulating cytokines in atopic dermatitis and psoriasis – production of tumor necrosis factor/cachectin and lymphotoxin by mononuclear cells in vitro. Br J Dermatol 122:587–592

43. Kapp A, Wokalek H, Schöpf E (1985) Involvement of complement in psoriasis and atopic dermatitis – measurement of C3a and C5a, C3, C4 and C1 inactivator. Arch Derm Res 277:359–361
44. Kapp A, Zeck-Kapp G, Blohm D (1989) Human tumor necrosis factor is a potent activator of the oxidative metabolism in human polymorphonuclear neutrophilic granulocytes (PMN)-comparison with human lymphotoxin. J Invest Dermatol 92:348–354
45. Kirchner H (1986) The interferon system as an integral part of the defense system against infections. Antiviral Res 6:1–17
46. Leiferman KM (1989) Eosinophils in atopic dermatitis. Allergy 44 [Suppl 9]:20–26
47. Leung DY, Geha RS (1986) Immunoregulatory abnormalities in atopic dermatitis. Clin Rev Allergy 4:67–86
48. Lever RS, Lesko MJ, MacKie RM, Parrott DM (1985) Natural killer cell activity in atopic dermatitis: a sequential study. Clin Allergy 15:479–486
49. Livnat S, Madden KS, Felten DL, Felten SY (1987) Regulation of the immune system by sympathetic neural mechanisms. Prog Neuropsychopharmacol Biol Psychiatry 11:145–152
50. Lopez AF, Sanderson CJ, Gamble JR, Campbell HD, Young IG, Vadas MA (1988) Recombinant human interleukin 5 is a selective activator of human eosinophil function. J Exp Med 167:219–224
51. Luger TA, Schwarz T (1989) Epidermal cell derived cytokines. In: (ed.) JD Bos, Skin immune system. CRC Press, Boca Raton, pp 257–291
52. MacKeen L, Brown M, Ip SH, Kung PC, Yasuda N, Harrington D, Hinuma Y, Weisenburger D, Lai P, Purtilo D (1986) Serum interleukin 2 receptor as a marker for active T cell malignancies. Fed Proc 45:454
53. Munker R, Koeffler HPh (1987) Tumor necrosis factor: Recent advances. Klin Wochenschr 65:345–352
54. Nawroth PP, Bank I, Handley D, Cassimeris J, Chess L, Stern D (1986) Tumor necrosis factor/cachectin interacts with endothelial cell receptors to induce release of interleukin 1. J Exp Med 163:1363–1375
55. Nelson DL (1986) Soluble interleukin 2 receptors: analysis in normal individuals and in certain disease states. Fed Proc 45:377
56. Neuner P, Kapp A, Kirnbauer R, Schwarz T, Krutmann J, Luger TA (1989) Monocytes derived from patients with psoriasis synthesize and release increased levels of interleukin 6. J Invest Dermatol 92:490
57. Norris PG, Schofield O, Camp RD (1988) A study of house dust mite in atopic dermatitis. Br J Dermatol 118: 435–440
58. O'Garra A, Warren DJ, Holman M, Popham AM, Sanderson CJ, Klaus GGB (1986) Interleukin 4 (B-cell growth factor II/eosinophil differentiation factor) is a mitogen and differentiation factor for preactivated murine B lymphocytes. Proc Natl Acad Sci USA 83:5228–5232
59. Ogawa M. Berger PA, McIntyre OR, Clendenning WE, Ishizaka K (1971) IgE in atopic dermatitis. Arch Dermatol 103:575–580
60. Old LJ (1987) Tumour necrosis factor: Polypeptide mediator network. Nature 326:330–331
61. Pennica D, Nedwin GE, Hayflick JS, Seeburg PH, Derynck R, Palladino MA, Kohr WJ, Aggarwal BB, Goeddel D (1984) Human tumour necrosis factor: precursor structure, expression and homology to lymphotoxin. Nature 312:724–729
62. Räsanen L, Lehto M, Reunala T, Jansen C, Leinikki P (1987) Decreased monocyte production of interleukin-1 and impaired lymphocyte proliferation in atopic dermatitis. Arch Dermatol Res 279:215–218
63. Rajka G (1986) Natural history and clinical manifestations of atopic dermatitis. Clin Rev Allergy 4:3–26
64. Reinhold U, Wehrmann W, Kukel S, Kreysel HW (1990) Evidence that defective interferon-gamma production in atopic dermatitis patients is due to intrinsic abnormalities. Clin Exp Immunol 79:374–379
65. Reitamo S, Visa K, Kähönen K, Käyhkö K, Stubb S, Salo OP (1986) Eczematous reactions in atopic dermatitis caused by epicutaneous testing with inhalant allergens. Br J Dermatol 114:303–309
66. Ring J, Senter T, Cornell RC, Arroyave CM, Tan EM (1979) Plasma complement and histamine changes in atopic dermatitis. Br J Dermatol 100:521–530
67. Robb RJ (1984) Interleukin 2:the molecule and its function. Immunol Today 5:203–209
68. Rogge JL, Hanifin JM (1976) Immunodeficiencies in severe atopic dermatitis. Arch Dermatol 112:1391–1396
69. Roitt IM, Brostoff J, Male DK (1985) Immunology. Gower, London
70. Rola-Pleszczynski M, Blanchard R (1981) Abnormal suppressor cell function in atopic dermatitis. J Invest Dermatol 76:279–283
71. Rubin LA, Jay G, Nelson DL (1986) The released interleukin 2 receptor binds interleukin 2 efficiently. J Immunol 137:3841–3844
72. Rubin LA, Kurman CC, Fritz ME, Biddison WE, Boutin B, Yarchoan R, Nelson DL (1985) Soluble interleukin 2 receptors are released from activated human lymphoid cells in vitro. J Immunol 135:3172–3177
73. Rystedt I, Strannegård IL, Strannegård Ö (1986) Recurrent viral infections in patients with past or present atopic dermatitis. Br J Dermatol 114:575–582
74. Saarinen UM (1984) Transfer of latent atopy by bone marrow transplantation? A case report. J Allergy Clin Immunol 74:196–200
75. Saurat JH (1985) Eczema in primary immunedeficiencies. Clues to the pathogenesis of atopic dermatitis with special reference to the Wiskott-Aldrich syndrome. Acta Derm Venereol (Stockh.) 114:125–128
76. Schöpf E, Kapp A, Kim CW (1978) T-cell function in atopic dermatitis – controlled examination of concanavalin A dose-response relations in cultured lymphocytes. Arch Derm Res 262:37–44
77. Schultz-Larsen F, Grunnet (1985) Lymphocyte transformation tests and subpopulations of lymphocytes in a population-based material of atopic dermatitis in twins. Scand J Immunol 21:375–381
78. Schultz-Larsen FS, Holm NV, Henningsen (1986) Atopic dermatitis. A geneticepidemiologic study in a population-based twin sample. J Am Acad Dermatol 15:487–494
79. Sethi KK, Näher H (1986) Elevated titers of cell-free interleukin-2 receptor in serum and cerebrospinal fluid specimens of patients with acquired immunodeficiency syndrome. Immunol Lett 13:179–184
80. Stingl G, Gazze LA, Czarnecki N, Wolff K (1981) T cell abnormalities in atopic dermatitis patients: imbalances in T cell subpopulations and impaired generation of ConA-induced suppressor cells. J Invest Dermatol 76:468–473
81. Stone-Wolff DS, Yip YK, Kelker HK, Le J, Henriksen-Destefano D, Rubin BY, Rinderknecht E, Aggarwal BB, Vilcek J (1984) Interrelationships of human interferon-

gamma with lymphotoxin and monocyte cytotoxin. J Exp Med 159:828–843

82. Strannegård IL, Strannegård Ö (1980) Natural killer cells and interferon production in atopic dermatitis. Acta Derm Venereol (Stockh.) [Suppl] 92:48–51
83. Uchiyama T, Broder S, Waldmann TA (1981) A monoclonal antibody (anti-Tac) reactive with activated and functionally mature human T cells. J Immunol 126: 1393–1397
84. Zachary CB, Mac Donald DM (1983) Quantitative analysis of T-lymphocyte subsets in atopic eczema, using monoclonal antibodies and flow cytometry. Br J Dermatol 108:411–422

Vascular Reactivity in Atopic Eczema

T. J. Ryan

The term "atopy" describes the altered reactivity characteristic of asthma, hayfever and eczema. These are common problems tending to run in families, and especially affecting children. The principal manifestations involving the lung, nose or skin have attracted an enormous volume of literature. That the blood vessels play some part in the mechanisms underlying the disorder is clear, especially in the congested and oedematous nasal mucosa of hayfever and the urticarial response and vasodilation in eczema, but less obviously so in asthma. Infact, urticaria was a prominant feature in 11% of children in one large French study [78]. The contribution of a raised surface temperature to itch is also important in the skin.

In this review of vascular reactivity in atopic eczema, the relevant inflammatory processes, which are believed to be active or disordered in the atopic state, will be discussed and relevant chapters elsewhere in this volume will be referred to. Much of this book concerns the biochemical and pharmacological mechanisms influencing vasoactivity and thus impinges on this section, which will deal with flushing, pallor and thermoregulation, together with the vascular contribution to itching.

Disorders of the Inflammatory Response in Atopic Eczema

In a recent review, Cooper [20] wrote of the multiplicity of immunobiochemical abnormalities in atopic eczema. Hanifin's observations [35] on cyclic nucleotide changes in leucocytes and on elevated activity of cyclic adenosine monophosphate (cAMP) phosphodiesterase (in adults but less so in some children [22], are believed to explain increased IgE production. They may also explain the increased histamine release from basophils or mast cells and the therapeutic role of papaverine in the control of itching [6]. These biochemical changes are believed to be triggered by stress via sympathetic tone, or by histamine release and/or prostaglandin E production from monocytes and macrophages which infiltrate the tissues of atopic eczema [76]. Cooper also referred to the role of thymic-like hormones or interleukins which emanate from the epidermis and are believed to modulate T-cell differentiation by cAMP-mediated mechanisms. The β-adrenergic theory of the atopic abnormality in bronchial asthma, described by Szentivanyi [99], has been an important influence on our thinking during the past two decades since it has pointed to a disturbance in cAMP regulation.

Neutrophil and monocyte function is sensitive to cAMP effects and hence chemotactic migration and cytotoxicity are also found to be defective in atopic eczema. Recently, Ring [83] suggested that the essential defect in these cells is an altered pattern of release of vasoactive mediators such that excess histamine is a consequence of a decreased response to adrenergic stimuli and an increased response to cholinergic stimuli. Increased eisosanoids also play a role in atopic eczema. Finally, as Ring has repeatedly emphasised, one cannot ignore the role of stress and the influence of the psyche on the manifestations of atopic eczema.

In considering vasoreactivity in atopic eczema, the main response appears to be an increase in the permeability of the vessels so that there is a continual flushing out of the interstitium by excess transudate. Altered control of vasoconstriction and vasodilatation is a significant determinant of this response.

It is useful to compare atopic eczema to psoriasis, a disease which has collected an even greater volume of literature. Ryan [86] has reviewed the role of the microcirculation in that disorder. Many of the more obvious changes that are present in psoriasis are not a major feature of atopic eczema and the simultaneous occurrence of psoriasis and atopic eczema is much less common than might be expected of two such common diseases [19]. The abnormal vascular patterns of psoriasis, with cotton ball coiling of the vasculature, suggestive of angiogenesis, is rarely seen in atopic eczema. In psoriasis, one may conceive that the increase in blood supply plays some part in the high turnover of the epidermis; in turn, injury to the epidermis may be a stimulus to the blood supply. However, such a concept seems not to apply to atopic eczema, in spite of obvious repetitive injury both to the epidermis as a consequence of scratching and a clear increase in some aspects of microcirculatory response. In his review of psoriasis, Ryan emphasised, in general terms, the importance of the lymphatic system in disease processes. The lymphatic system in atopic eczema has not been studied, in spite of the fact that massive lymphadenopathy is a feature of the infant with atopic eczema. At least one explanation of this lymphadenopathy may be an increased traffic through the lymphatics. The lymphatic literature, especially of venous disease of the lower leg, emphasises that excess traffic may lead to exhaustion of the lymphatics and ultimately to lymphoedema. This is not a feature of atopic eczema, though it is sometimes described in contact dermatitis and chronic lichen simplex of non-atopic aetiology. Recurrent episodes of infection are believed to play a part in lymphoedema and these are present in atopic eczema but seem to have different consequences with no long-term ill effects. This too suggests that the lymphatics are functioning surprisingly well. If this is so, then one has to draw attention to possible changes in T cell reactivity that are determined by the efficiency of the lymphatic pathways.

Another feature of atopic eczema is its association with ichthyosis vulgaris which, in comparison with psoriasis, is a slight atrophy of the skin. Ichthyosis does not give rise to telangiectasia in the manner of some other atrophies such as poikiloderma, in which the upper dermis is characteristically thin with loss of papillary vasculature and increased visibility and dilation of the horizontal venous plexus. If telangiectasia is seen at all, then it is mostly as a response to the use of steroids in the atopic patient. Some atopics have a persistent facial pallor with episodes of flushing and repeated inflammatory episodes due to scratching and infection, but this is not followed by permanent redness of the cheeks unless steroids have been abused. In atopic skin there is preservation of the papillary vasculature but without the exaggeration of the undulations of the epidermal-dermal junction to the extent seen in psoriasis.

Histopathology

In atopic eczema there are distinctive histopathological changes in the skin vasculature. Sedlis and Prose [96] recorded oedema and perivascular mononuclear cell infiltration and reported an apparent increased number of mast cells. Mihm et al. [67] also noted increased numbers of mast cells in lichenified skin with degranulation of some cells. Endothelial cell hypertrophy was noted in venules of most microscopic sections but, unlike allergic contact dermatitis, there was little interstitial fibrin deposition. Leung et al. [56] using monoclonal antibody techniques, identified T helper cells in excess, whereas suppressor cytotoxic cells were significantly reduced. There is, of course, an association between endothelial hypertrophy of the high endothelial type and T helper cell activity. Similar findings have also been made in contact dermatitis; in one study of patch testing with known allergens [82], the dermal infiltrates consisted mainly of T lymphocytes ($T_4 : T_8 = 2.6 : 1$) and, to a lesser degree, Langerhans and indeterminate T_6 cells. Between 50% and 90% of the cells were Ia positive; the number of mast cells and basophils did not exceed 10%–15%. In a study of juvenile plantar dermatosis (possibly also an atopic condition), an apparent predilection for the dermal infiltrate to surround sweat ducts was thought to reflect the distribution of blood vessels rather than that of sweat glands themselves [5].

Functions of the Vasculature

The functions of blood vessels include:

1. Permeability, leakiness and barrier control
2. Maintenance of blood flow
3. Contractility and lumen size control
4. Oxygen supply and control
5. Coagulation and fibrinolysis, platelet interaction adherence and slipperiness of surface
6. Pharmacological production and detoxication
7. Recognition and removal of macromolecules and cells

The cell which characterises blood vessels and lymphatics is the endothelial cell (recently the subject of a four-volume review by Ryan [90]. It can no longer be regarded simply as an interface between the blood and the extravascular compartment, but it is also the source of activation and inhibition of many vasoactive agents. Since the endothelium of the blood vessel is situated in the presence of platelets and fibrin-related material, it must be involved in controlling aggregation and maintains a thin film of fibrin and fibrinolytic materials (believed to be responsible for the slipperiness of the luminal cell surface). This is done while maintaining tight adhesion to the surrounding connective tissue to protect itself from the shearing forces of blood flow.

The functions of vascular endothelium which are most likely to be important in atopic eczema are the maintenance of a selective permeability barrier and the regulation of vascular tone. The maintenance of haemostasis and the regulation of angiogenesis are perhaps not as important as in psoriasis, but in both disorders the regulation of immune and inflammatory responses is an important function of the endothelium. The role of antigen presentation and cell adhesion factors is discussed elsewhere in this volume. A further characteristic of skin vasculature which is relevant to the atopic skin is that it has to be responsive both to temperature changes and to external mechanical stresses or injury.

Histamine

The pharmacological responses of blood vessels to histamine are well known and the ready release of this agent when the skin is scratched has been studied for some 70 years. Histamine, given intramuscularly to atopic patients, causes flushing of face, neck and cubital fossae. It is not certain whether this is due to heightened receptor activity or merely greater delivery because of a richer blood supply to these areas in such patients. As with the greater sensitivity of bronchial smooth muscle in asthmatics, the atopic response to histamine is probably not simply a question of blood supply. Increased plasma histamine levels have been reported in atopic eczema [91]; Mallet et al. [61] measuring urinary histamine and its metabolites in severe adult atopic eczema, found that levels were higher in remission than during active disease. They proposed that, during active phases, steroid therapy may suppress these levels. In another study, basophils from 21 young atopic patients released significantly more histamine in response to a number of pharmacological challenges than did the controls [62]. High plasma levels of histamine impair macrophage functions and could thus contribute to high rates of skin infection [41]. How histamine acts in the atopic state is not clear. In spite of the belief that altered β-adrenergic responses may determine the release of histamine, infusion of histamine in the standing position produces no greater rise in plasma adrenaline, cAMP or noradrenaline than in normal controls [3]. Psoralens and ultraviolet A (PUVA) therapy for atopic eczema is often effective and it could be relevant that photoactivation of rat peritoneal mast cells suppresses histamine release [112].

Acetylcholine

Acetylcholine increases cyclic guanosine monophosphate (cGMP) in mast cells and may augment histamine release. This effect is greater in mast cells stimulated by IgE. Inhaled methacholine causes bronchoconstriction and this has been used as a diagnostic test of respiratory atopy [63]. Scott [95] found elevated levels of acetylcholine in the skin of patients with atopic eczema, and, as discussed below, there is a well recognised delayed blanching response to inoculation of acetylcholine and its analogues into the skin. The development of this white reaction is prevented by prior treatment with atropine. Scott [94] also observed that it was prevented by sympathectomy. The red flare induced by the inoculation of acetylcholine in normal subjects is accompanied by the release of acetylcholine esterase; such release is not seen in the atopic [94]. The role of acetylcholine as a transmitter in the autonomic nervous system is discussed below.

Endothelium-Derived Relaxing Factor

A number of studies of the effect of acetylcholine on arteries resulted eventually in the identification of an endothelial-derived relaxing factor which is nitric oxide. The release of nitric oxide by acetylcholine acting on muscarinic receptors has led to an understanding of how many agents, such as vasopressin, serotonin, noradrenaline and substance P, produce relaxation of arteries in certain circumstances (Fig. 1). Essentially, the smooth muscle of arteries is made to relax as a result of the release of nitric acid from endothelial cells which line the arteries. The nitric acid acts through a protein kinase and stimulates the cGMP system [71, 75]. There is also an endothelium-derived contracting factor which causes prolonged vasoconstriction. Interaction of these systems provides constant blood flow when perfusion pressure varies [2].

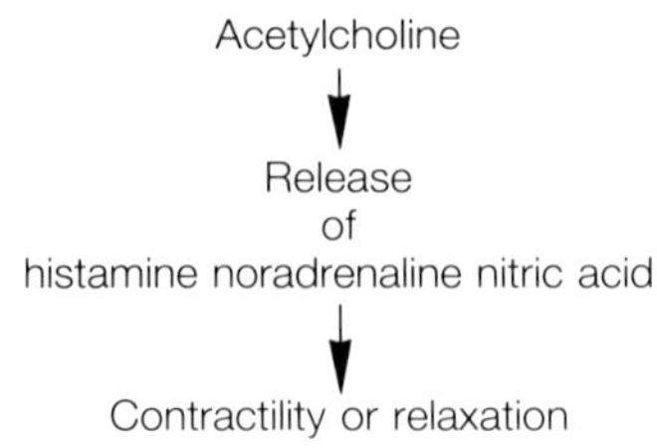

Fig. 1. Actions of acetylcholine

Arachidonic Acid Metabolism

Early studies of agents later termed prostaglandins showed that they caused smooth muscle contraction and lowered blood pressure. Much is written elsewhere in this book about the role of arachidonic acid-derived material in inflammation. The importance of prostaglandin endoperoxides in inducing platelet aggregation and of unstable vasoconstrictor agents such as thromboxane A_2 have excited great interest amongst pharmacologists and microvascular experts. When Moncada et al. [69] and Needleman et al. [72] found that endoperoxides were metabolised by rabbit aorta and thence produced a labile substance able to relax distal arterial vessels, the interest in vasoactivity erupted. PGI_2 (prostacyclin) remains one of the most fascinating of the vasoactive agents. It is quite clear that endothelial cells are the most active producers of PGI_2 and that they can do this in response to a number of chemical and physical stimuli. An example of its relevance in dermatology has been the recent interest in primrose oil and linoleic acid as a treatment for atopic eczema. Linoleic acid metabolism influence the production of eicosanoids [98]. Howbeit, levels of PGE_2 are low in the skin of atopics [28]. Lovell et al. [59] proposed primrose oil containing linoleic acid for the management of atopic eczema after observing that PGE enhanced the itching produced by histamine applied to the base of blisters. It is of interest that prolonged release of PGI_2 from human endothelial cells in vitro can be induced by histamine via occupancy of H_1 receptors [13]. As described elsewhere, the major source of arachidonic acid is within the cell membrane in the form of phosphatidylinositol, phosphatidylcholine and phosphatidylethanolamine. It is at this point that phospholipases A_2 and C are involved [43] since these enzymes liberate arachidonic acid from the precursor. Furthermore, both 1-2-diacylglycerol and calcium are active. At one time it was thought that cAMP and calmodulin played a part in such activity because PGI_2 release could be inhibited by both intracellular calcium and calmodulin or by increased cAMP levels [10, 36, 97, 108]. However, Brotherton et al. [11] have shown that PGI_2 production is not inhibited by increased cAMP levels induced by other agents such as forskolin.

There is some evidence that intact endothelial cells can synthesise PGI_2 from exogenous endoperoxide PGH_2 [92]. Such endoperoxides could be obtained from platelet activation. The relevance of platelet aggregation or the provision of platelets as a source of PGI_2 in atopic eczema becomes apparent when one considers the inhibition by aspirin of the white dermatographic response in the Trafuril (tetrahydrofurfyl nicotinic acid ester) reaction ([110] and see below). If endothelial cells are treated with aspirin and then exposed to thrombin and platelets, increased platelet adherence and reduced PGI_2 release occurs. Recovery from this effect of aspirin is prevented by cycloheximide [23] which inhibits the synthesis of PGI_2 required to prevent the adherence of platelets. Stimulation of PGI_2 release by histamine or shear stress are of interest; such studies have investigated endothelial cell culture systems but we lack knowledge of activity in vivo. Frangos et al. [29] and Grabowski et al. [31] found that the shearing forces produced by pulsatile blood flow increased the production of PGI_2. If one examines Lewis's manouevre [57] in which the skin is subjected to shearing stresses by stretching it, white dermatographism is induced, especially in the atopic state. In this respect, the only studies of the effects of shear stress on endothelial cells have used cells from neonatal skin or adipose tissue. These suggested that skin endothelial cells produce equal amounts of PGE_2 and $PGF_{2\alpha}$ but considerably less 6-keto-$PGF_{1\alpha}$ [18], than other cell types. From studies of skin in scleroderma, many aspects of endothelial cell behaviour suggest that arachidonic acid metabolism in the skin has some relevance to vasoconstrictor versus vasodilator responses.

In Raynaud's phenomenon, it has been suggested hat there is an imbalance between the vasoconstrictor and the vasodilator properties of thromboxane and PGI_2. Neri Serneri et al. [73] found that cooling of the skin caused platelet aggregation, with raised plasma levels of β-thromboglobulin and thromboxane B_2, which was not influenced by the administration of aspirin. Gresele et al. [34] were unable to confirm this finding. Thus, the effects of cooling on the metabolism of endothelium need further study and cannot be entirely explained by changes in blood flow.

Although agents such as PGD_2 cause dose-related increases in blood flow and erythema but not weals, they do not potentiate the erythema and blood flow effects of histamine and their exact role in skin disease is uncertain [64]. Studies of basophils suggest that in atopics histamine release is more rapidly and that this may be an effect of endogenous PGE_2 [105]. However, it would be difficult to rule out the chronic or repetitive effects of scratching as an influence in this respect.

Coagulation and Thrombosis

There is very little evidence of a defect in coagulation or thrombosis in atopic eczema but fibrinolysis has been implicated. The interaction of both coagulation and fibrinolysis with other biochemical factors controlling biological functions of the tissues is such that they cannot be ignored by dermatologists. One only has to examine the way in which the plasmin system interacts with the kinin or complement system or the way in which coagulation and heparin interact with other glycosaminoglycans to see how complex this area may be. Alterations in protease activity induced by oestrogens are also relevant when one considers that atopic eczema is worse 1 week before menstruation and improves 1 week after menstruation [53]. There is evidence that histamine increases tissue plasminogen activator production but not the production of plasminogen activator inhibitor, whereas endotoxin causes the reverse [36]. Interleukin-1 (IL-1), by contrast, is believed to inhibit tissue plasminogen activator production while stimulating that of the inhibitor of plasminogen activator. Some 25 years ago, Japanese workers reported an anti-pruritic effect of certain inhibitors of fibrinolysis and a local anti-fibrinolytic activity in several skin disorders [37]. Haustein [38] also reported low fibrinolytic activity in the affected skin of atopic eczema. Turner et al. [102] reported that abraded normal skin showed impairment of fibrinolysis 24 h later, while Ryan et al. [89] studying mediators such as histamine, suggested that they caused an early release and subsequent exhaustion of fibrinolytic enzymes (Fig. 2). Moulin and Manuel [79] observed increased fibrinolytic activity in the blisters of dyshidrotic eczema. Such increased local activity is a relatively common characteristic of spongiosis [38, 89]. Acute anaphylaxis and urticaria can be prevented by inhibitors of fibrinolysis [7] depending on whether they are given early or late and on the type of mediator responsible [85]. Yamamoto [111] reported decreased blood fibrinolytic activity in atopic eczema subjects.

Fibrin is not usually deposited in atopic eczema. Studies of the histopathology of the skin affected by delayed cellular hypersensitivity are worth noting since, under these circumstances, fibrin is usually deposited. One of the best known functions of endothelium is the production of factor VIII, which is a complex of factor VIII c synthesised in the liver, with von Willebrand's factor, synthesised by endothelial cells. The polymers are stored in Weibel-Palade bodies and serve as a means of identifying vascular endothelium on microscopy. The von Willebrand's factor is an adhesive material an absence of which causes endothelial disruption and more frequent bleeding. It is needed if the endothelium is to be protected from shearing forces tending to detach it from the vessel wall.

Finally, with respect to coagulation factors, one must refer to platelet activating factor which is released by platelets when they aggregate and which can contract visceral smooth muscle but relaxes vascular smooth muscle. It stimulates aggregation and chemotaxis and plays a part in vascular permeability. Archer et al. [4] observed that inoculation of platelet activating factor intradermally caused an eosinophilic response in atopics compared to a neutrophilic response in normal non-atopic skin.

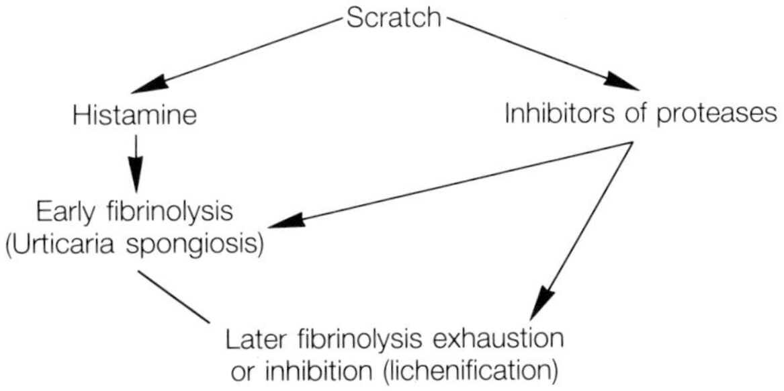

Fig. 2. Relationship between scratching and protease activity

Neutrophil-Endothelial Interaction

Unlike psoriasis, neutrophil adherence does not seem to play a major role in atopic eczema. Nevertheless, the failure of control of bacterial infection in many patients with atopic eczema merits attention to defects in neutrophil adherence.

Endothelial cells produce a glycoprotein CD18 within the venule lumen in response to complement factor C5 [106]. Hoover et al. [44, 45] have shown that adherence of neutrophils to endothelium occurs as a result of the administration of C5a or leukotriene B4. Human monocyte derived IL-1 can also be shown to stimulate neutrophil adherence. A newly described soluble leucocyte adhesion inhibitor [107] which is stimulated by IL-1 could be of interest in this respect. Lymphocyte adherence is increased by IL-1 [16] and interferon-γ [113] and by certain lipopolysaccharides [114]. One of the many factors inducing IL-1 from keratinocytes is the neuropeptide substance P which might link the clinical picture of atopic eczema to the nervous system [12].

Neuropeptides

No discussion of the effects of acetylcholine or noradrenaline on the microvascular system would be complete without reference to the advances in our understanding of such neuropeptides. The complex innervation of the capillary bed includes: (a) a vasoconstriction system of noradrenaline and neuropeptide Y, (b) a vasodilatory system of acetylcholine, vasoactive intestinal peptide and peptide histidine isoleucine and (c) an afferent system which includes substance P (SP) neurokinin A (NKA) and calcitonin gene-related peptide (CGRP).

The vasoconstrictor fibres originating in sympathetic ganglia can directly cause vasoconstriction, potentiate noradrenaline or, paradoxically, inhibit the release of noradrenaline. The parasympathetic system causes vasodilation, employing acetylcholine, which affects smooth muscle relaxation only if the endothelium is intact. Vasoactive intestinal peptide and peptide histidine isoleucine act directly on smooth muscle and do not need the endothelium as an intermediary. These various agents necessarily act on different receptors. SP and NKA are also dependent on endothelium but CGRP is not. The latter is a strong activator of adenylate cyclase and induces a prolonged erythema with an increase in blood flow without weal formation [9]. SP also induces keratinocyte-derived inflammatory mediators such as IL-1 [12] (Fig. 3).

In normal subjects, neuropeptides produce local erythema and an axon flare when inoculated into the skin. SP is the most potent in this respect. Most such flare responses last up to 2 h, but CGRP acts for 12 h. Antihistamines inhibit the response to NKA and the flare response, but not the local erythema of CGRP. Aspirin blocks the axon reflex induced by SP, NKA and CGRP, but not that caused by neurokinin B (NKB) or histamine. There is thus some dependency on histamine and cyclooxygenase products for the effects of some neuropeptides [30], and histamine release might be an important mechanism in atopic eczema.

The use of capsaicin to inhibit neuropeptides while examining the leakage of dyes, such as Evan's blue, after inoculation of histamine, serotonin, the histamine liberator 48/80, bradykinin or SP into the skin has shown that all these mediators are blocked when neuropeptides are suppressed in rats [49]. Bull et al. [13] have compared this response to that of neuropeptides in vitro using large vessel endothelial cells and dermal endothelial cells from neonatal foreskin. They found that the latter are less responsive in most respects, including the generation of cAMP and vasoactive prostaglandins. This could be relevant to the relative nonresponsiveness of the neonate which subsequently develops atopic eczema to a number of phenomena compared to non atopic infants. Neonatal cells cannot sustain production of urokinase inhibitor [46]. Consequent protease activity may be advantageous for remoulding in the embryonic or neonatal period [87]. CGRP, which activates adenylate cyclase, is protease sensitive, and its action is transient in the presence of mast cell proteases [8], which are more plentiful in neonatal tissue. While the itch response to neuropeptides is not different in atopics compared to controls [31], a reduced weal and flare is observed in adults; however, as discussed below, such tachyphylaxis could be secondary to the tissue stiffness induced by scratching.

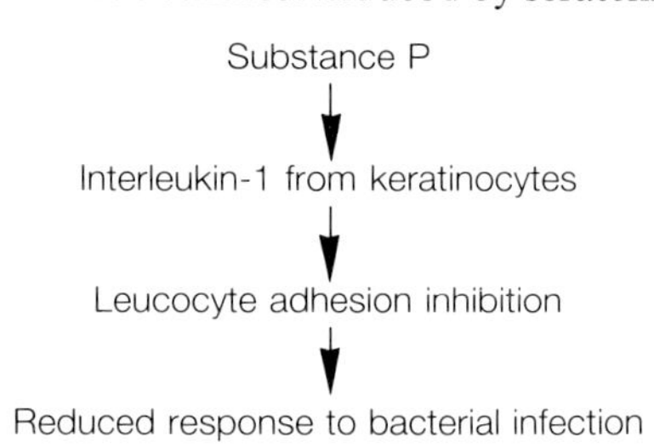

Fig. 3. Actions of substance P

Cutaneous Vascular Reactions in Atopic Eczema

For several decades it has been noticed that, whereas normal skin when rubbed becomes red, atopic skin tends after a few seconds to become white (Fig. 4). Lewis [57] showed that stretch could produce the same effect. Schonberger et al. [93] in an attempt to quantify the reaction, observed that white dermatographism took significantly longer to develop than red dermatographism in controls. Using capillary microscopy, Ryan [84] observed the response and noted reversal of flow in papillary vessels. This may have been a myogenic stretch reflex on precapillary myosins, but a reversal of flow carrying pharmacological agents was also possible. This abnormal response is characteristic, but probably not specific, since it can occur in other diseases. Of equal interest was the observation by Lobitz and Campbell [58] that, when one injects acetylcholine intradermally into patients with atopic eczema, the flare develops as in normal skin but is slowly replaced by pallor which may be quite intense and lasts 15–30 min.

The debate that has developed concerning the mechanism underlying these results sometimes fails to take into account what it is exactly that is being observed. In other words, what is a white skin? Essentially, it depends on the amount of blood visible in the vessels at the surface. Such visibility depends not only on the vessel capacity but also on whether there is any veil of tissue fluid (not withstanding pigment) between the vessel and the observer. Pallor can quite definitely occur due to vasoconstriction and consequent emptying of the vessel but it can also be due to oedema, as can be easily

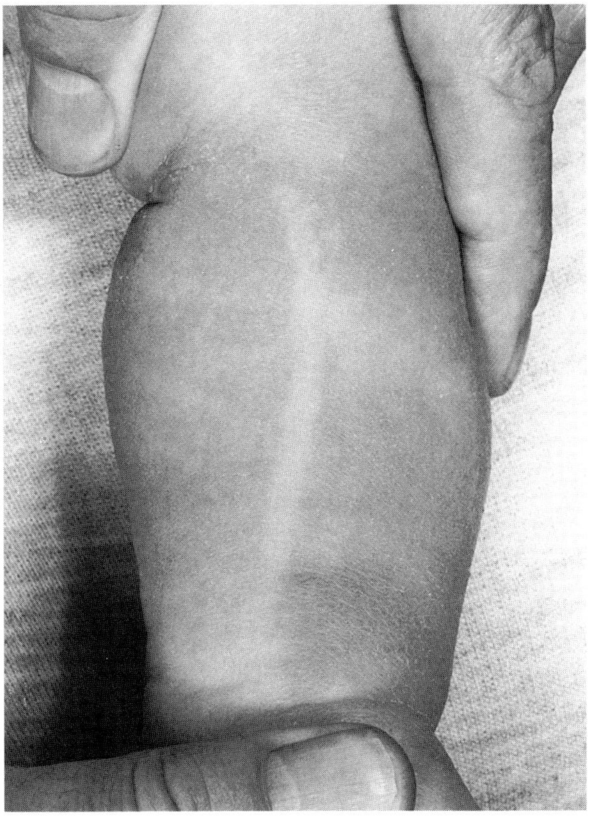

a

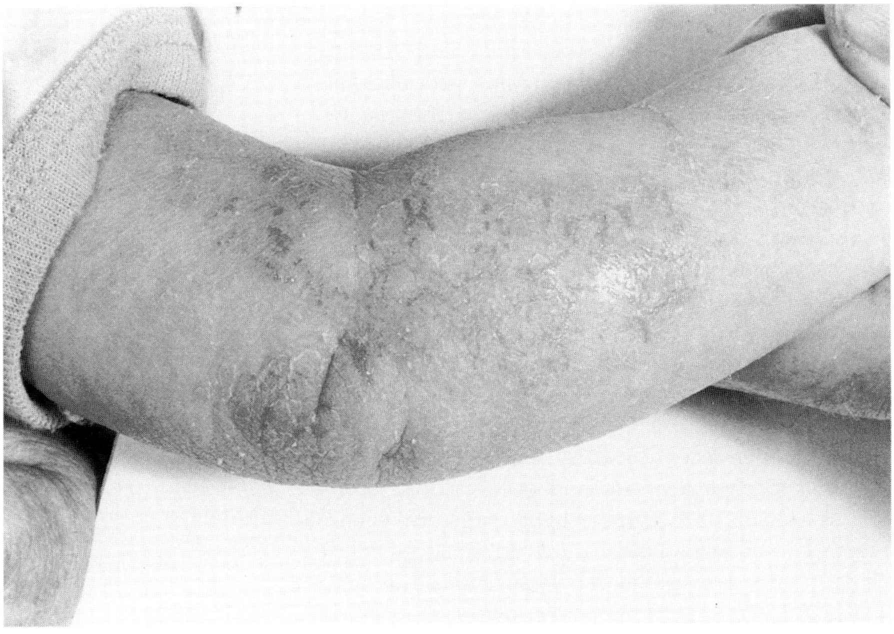

b

Fig. 4a–c. a White dermatographism 15 s after a gentle scratch on the leg of an atopic infant occurring as soon as the infant was able to scratch and had developed **b** eczema, and **c** Morgan's fold of the lower eyelid

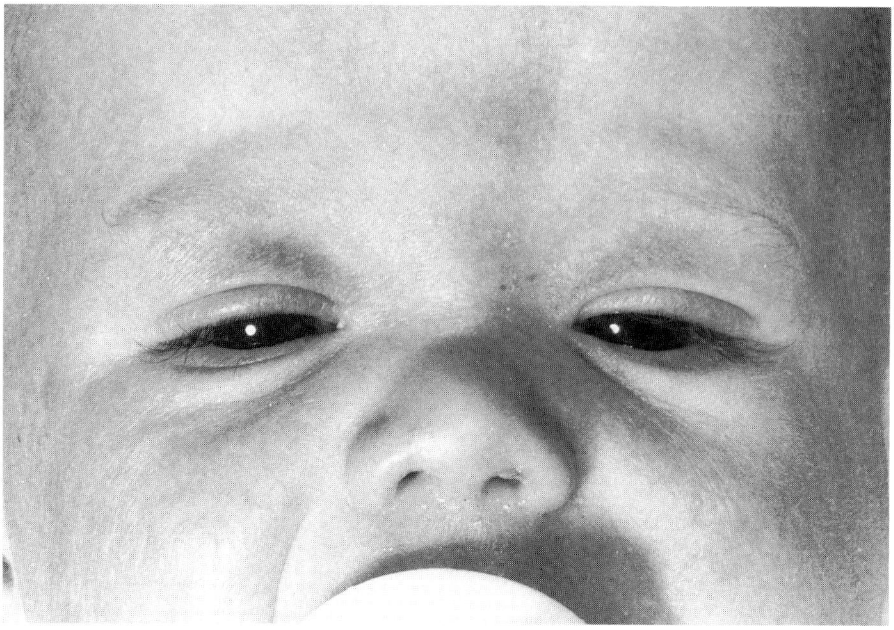

Fig. 4c

observed in urticaria or the pallor of nephrosis. If one takes a blunt instrument and indents the skin, tissue fluid can be pushed to one side and the mark of indentation appears red, whereas in the adjacent area where the tissue fluid has accumulated, the tissue looks whiter. Provided there is enough tissue fluid to obscure the vessels, it matters not at all whether they are filled and pulsatile since, under there circumstances, an increase in blood flow will not necessarily be observed as redness.

The difficulty in atopic eczema is to decide whether the pallor is due to oedema or vasoconstriction. White dermatographism is macular but oedema does not necessarily result in clinical swelling either. Ramsey [79] observed white dermatographism in seven or eight atopics when the skin was rubbed, and, with photoplethysmography, demonstrated vasoconstriction in two patients with severe disease (Figs. 5–7). In the other patients, pallor was incomplete and the recording showed either no change or a slight increase in pulsation. In the case of a definite delayed blanch reaction from acetylcholinelike drugs, even when the area was completely pale, the photoelectric pulse meter showed an increase in the height of pulsations, indicating vasodilatation. One of the difficulties of this type of technique is that the photoelectric plethysmograph detects not only the most superficial vessels, but also picks up some deeper, possibly shunting, vessels [60]. When upper dermal vessels contain less blood, there is less absorption of the probes light; as a consequence, readings from deeper vasculature are enhanced [79]. It could be argued that vasoconstriction or the obscuring of superficial vessels by oedema can occur while deeper

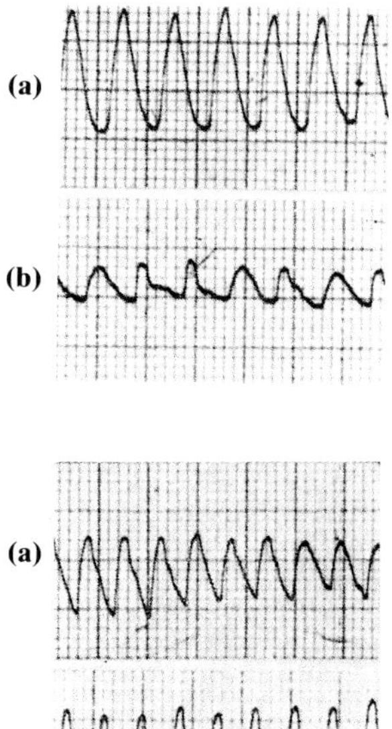

Fig. 5a,b. Photoplethysmographic reading from a patient with atopic eczema. White dermatographism **a** before and **b** after a light scratch. This degree of reduction in blood volume was observed in only two out of eight atopics; in the other subjects, there was either no change or a slight increase in pulsation. (From Ramsey 1969, with permission)

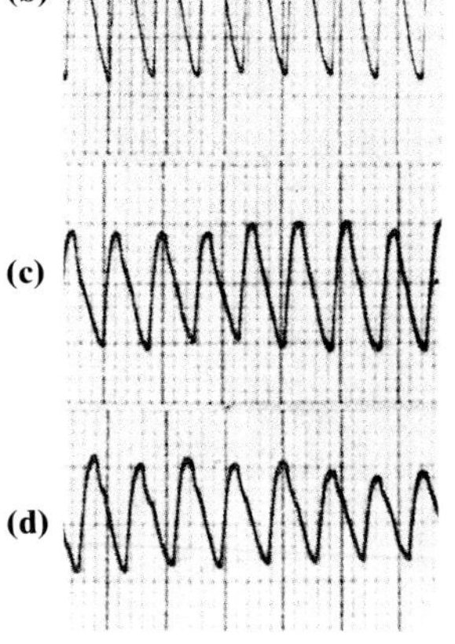

Fig. 6a–d. Photoplethysmographic reading from a patient with atopic eczema. Effect of intradermal acetyl β methacholine **a** before injection, **b, c** and **d** 10, 20 and 40 min, respectively, after injection. The area was completely pale at the time of the 10 and 20 minute records. (From Ramsey 1969, with permission)

vessels picked up by the photoelectric sensor are open and free-flowing. Using capillary microscopy, one can at least observe the most superficial vessels. Lobitz and Campbell [58] Reed and Kierland [80] and Davis and Lawler [24] observed dilated blood vessels, even in the presence of blanching. Again, it has to be understood that papillary vessels even when dilated, usually do not contribute greatly to skin colour. It is the subpapillary venous plexus which accounts for pinkness of the skin. Only when the papillary vessels are extremely coiled and dilated, as in psoriasis, do they significantly contribute to the colour observed microscopically.

Earlier experiments using a scratch or the inoculation of acetylcholine were shown to produce nonspecific and variable results. Juhlin [50] found that a delayed blanch could be produced by both methacholine and the histamine liberator 48/80 in about half of the atopic patients tested. He avoided the effect of scratching by employing iontophoresis. In a subsequent examination of some 50 patients, methacholine induced blanching in 44% of the patients, redness in 24%, and an intermediate colour in the remaining 32%. By injecting intravenous sodium fluorescein (4 mg/kg), Juhlin observed that white areas induced by methacholine did not turn yellow, but white areas induced by 48/80 did so, provided a weal was induced. Blanched areas without wealing showed no fluorescence. It was assumed that vasoconstriction was the explanation. Using Coomassie blue, Kalz and Fekete [52] were unable to demonstrate oedema in the region of the delayed blanch. Moller and Rorsman [68] also failed to show capillary leakage in the delayed blanch of atopic eczema using the same technique. However, Scott [94] was able to produce a red flare with acetylcholine in skin pretreated with hyaluronidase and in such cases acetylcholine esterase was detected. It was suggested that oedema was dispersed in this treatment. Current theory would indicate that oedema dispersion lowers interstitial pressure acutely and that this encourages vasodilatation, a mechanical explanation which makes pharmacological events more difficult to interpret.

Juhlin [50] posed the question of why drugs such as methacholine and 48/80, which normally cause vasodilatation, should produce vasoconstriction in atopic eczema? Using iontophoresis, it was shown that the doses of adrenaline or noradrenaline required to produce vasoconstriction (i.e. blanching) were rather less in patients with atopic eczema than in controls. For this reason, guanethidine (which was believed to effectively block normal metabolism of the transmitter substance at nerve terminals) was employed, knowing that it augments the response of the effector organ to injected noradrenaline [65]. After guanethidine pretreatment of the skin in normal subjects and patients with atopic eczema, blanching previously caused by methacholine

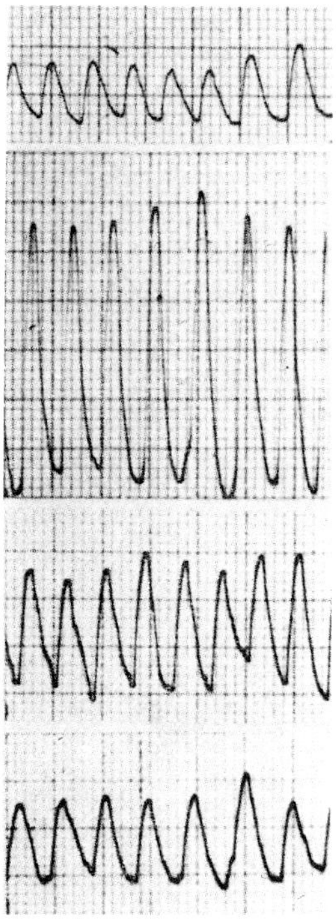

Fig. 7a–d. Photoplethysmographic reading from a patient with atopic eczema. Effect of intradermal normal saline **a** before injection, **b, c** and **d** 10, 20 and 40 min, respectively, after injection. (From Ramsey 1969, with permission)

and 48/80 was replaced by normal reddening in the pretreated areas. It was suggested therefore that the increased blanching in atopic eczema was due to the increased release of noradrenaline caused by methacholine and 48/80. This might be due to increased sensitivity to acetylcholine and nicotine, as described by Kottegoda [55] and Burn [14]. Kottegoda had found that, in the rabbit ear, the acetylcholine-induced vasoconstriction converted to vasodilatation when a sympathicolytic agent was added. Burn [15] showed that in the cat and rabbit, acetylcholine and nicotine probably acted by liberating noradrenaline and adrenaline from chromaffin cells. Burn [14], in a classic review, proposed that all sympathetic post-ganglionic fibres release acetylcholine, which in turn releases noradrenaline. Juhlin's experiments using iontophoresis simply increased the amount of adrenaline available for release by methacholine and 48/80 and hence produced blanching. In those patients who responded by a red reaction to methacholine, presumably with no release of adrenaline, the guanethidine had no effect. The authors also blockaded α-adrenergic receptors by injecting phenoxybenzamine hydrochloride intravenously and β-receptors by injecting isopropyl, both of which had no clear effect. Studies on lymphocytes and neutrophils isolated from patients with atopic eczema showed a decreased rise in intracellular levels of cAMP after incubation of β-agonists [81]. Hornqvist et al. [47], using iontophoresis, came to the conclusion that the sympathetic adrenoreceptor-mediated response of blanching was mediated by α-adrenoreceptors, whereas erythema was induced by β_2-adrenoreceptors. They used phenylephrine (10 ug/ml) as an α-agonist and isoproterenol (100 ug/ml) as a non-selective β-agonist. The α-agonist caused increased blanching response; the non-specific β-agonist produced blanching in up to 60% of the atopic patients. They concluded that an increased sensitivity towards phenylephrine and blanching in response to isoproterenol in atopic eczema confirmed the existence of an altered adrenoreceptor reactivity (increased α-adrenoreceptor and/or decreased β-adrenoreceptor). In Champion's studies of the use of methacholine (Table 1), both oedema and vasoconstriction could be induced but this depended on the dilutions used. A true delayed blanch occurs with increasing dilutions from 10^{-4} to 10^{-6} and the dose response curve becomes flatter so that on further dilution the blanching may be the same. Oedema may occur if dilutions are only 10^{-2} or 10^{-3}.

Table 1. Delayed blanch with Mecholyl [17]

	Number of cases	*Delayed blanch positive*
Atopic eczema – typical adult	50	36
Atopic eczema – infantile	7	1
Eczema in atopic person		
• Discoid eczema	5	1
• Pompholyx	6	0
• Contact dermatitis	1	1
Atopic asthma or hay-fever	15	0
Atopic carrier	5	0
Controls		
• Normal	30	0
• Miscellaneous dermatoses	2	0
• Lichen simplex	9	0
• Rheumatic fever	1	0

Champion [17] found that the blanching was less likely to occur in infants; others have also studied the capacity of the neonate to react to pharmacological agents. Because the skin of the neonate is already oedematous, the vessels are maximally permeable and wealing and erythema much more difficult to interpret. Aizawa and Tagami [1] observed that white dermatographism occurred in only 11% of atopic babies aged 1–2 months, but this increased to 88% in those older than 7 months. They referred to Ryan's observations on the anatomical immaturity of the skin with respect to a well-defined papillary system taking time to develop [77]. Of 50 children who showed the delayed blanch phenomenon at birth, 78% still showed the reaction 5 years later but this was unrelated to allergy [74].

Uehara and Ofuji [104] demonstrated blanching in response to Trafuril applied as an ointment. English et al. [27] observed that within 2 h of application, normal subjects showed non-allergic leucocytoclastic vascular damage; this reaction was reduced in five out of six atopic subjects. The effect of this ointment on fibrinolysis and the blockade of the reaction by prostaglandin inhibitors led Ryan and his colleagues to suggest that the main effect of this agent was on prostaglandin release [101]. Wilkin et al. [109] later produced firm evidence of this effect. The role of prostaglandins in atopic eczema was also studied by Juhlin and Michaelsson [51]. Intradermal injection of PGE_1 into human skin in doses of 1–5 μg resulted in prolonged erythema, however, in 15 adult atopics, the erythematous area produced by PGE_1 was significantly smaller at 20 min than in controls.

Copeman and Winkelmann [21] used Evan's blue injected intravenously prior to intradermal methacholine and concluded that blanching was due to release of oedema fluid. In the case of Trafuril, they concluded that some other mechanism was involved since the skin remained white. Thune and Rajka [100] also used Trafuril ointment and in three out of six patients a clear decrease in photoplethysmographic pulsations occurred, but in three other patients the pulse amplitudes were either unchanged or alternatingly decreased and increased. Such variability made interpretation difficult. They suggested that regional variations and the degree of previous inflammation may play some part. They pointed out the difficulty of distinguishing between superficial and deeper vessels and that urticarial weals can either be blue, red or white, even though deeper vasodilation is clearly evident.

Disturbance of Thermoregulation following Warm and Cold Exposure

Recent studies by Hornqvist et al. [48] of the iontophoresis of the α-agonist phenylephrine showed that subjects exhibited decreased reactivity in the winter (Fig. 8). The β-agonist isoproterenol also produced blanching in fewer patients in the winter compared to the summer. A number of possibilities, such as raised IgE levels and histamine release during hayfever season, should be taken into account in such studies. It was suggested that the patients were more vasoconstricted in the winter and therefore could not be subjected to much further blanching. However, studies by Di Palma [25] showed quite clear differences in the reactivity of the skin in summer and winter, which Ryan has interpreted as due to more interstitial fluid or cold-induced stiffness of the interstitium in the winter. This again raises the unresolved argument of oedema versus vasoconstriction. It is generally believed that patients with atopic eczema show greater vasoconstriction in response to thermoregulatory reflexes. Weber suggested that the cubital fossae flushed more readily in atopic persons and hence, by warming the skin, the itch threshold decreased. Heyer et al. [40] studied the temperature changes that occurred in one forearm while the other forearm was subjected to cooling or warmth. It was found that in most atopic patients, during exposure of one forearm to warmth, skin temperature of the contralateral forearm remained unchanged or decreased slightly, whereas exposure to cold induced either a slight rise in skin temperature or an almost indiscernible decrease. In contrast to the normal temperature reaction observed in control subjects, the response of atopic patients to warmth exposure seemed less reactive or even paradoxical.

Ryan has argued that the cubital and popliteal fossae are protected from cooling in neonates who normally, unless overheated, are in a flexed position. The development of thermoregulatory reflexes in response to cooling are thus impaired in these flexures and they remain warm and thus itchy when other areas of skin are vasoconstricted.

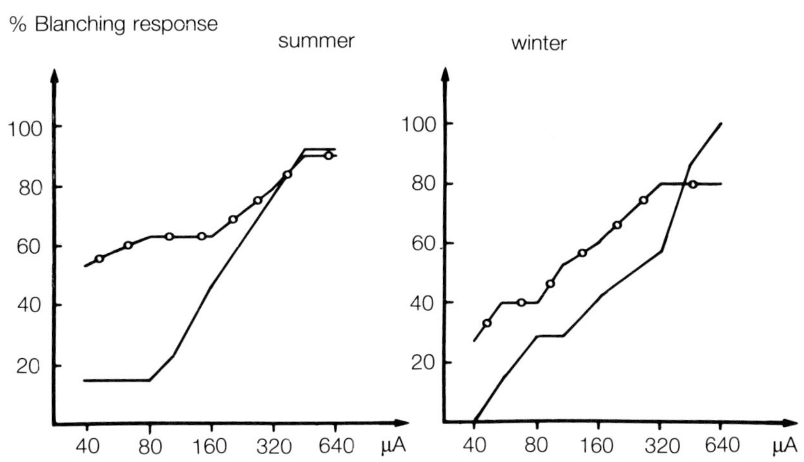

Fig. 8a,b. Dose response curves for phenylephrine, 10 µl/ml, after 5 min, in atopic eczema patients and controls for **a** summer and **b** winter. Percentage blanching response is plotted against iontophoresis current; the dose is directly proportional to the current. Summer, atopic eczema (•; n = 19) and healthy controls (—; n = 13); winter, atopic eczema (•; n = 15) and healthy controls (—; n = 7). The atopics respond to lower doses, especially in the summer. (From Hornquist et al 1988, with permission)

Reactivity of the Skin during Experimental Stress

Whereas most clinicians accept that psychological stress plays some part in atopic eczema, investigation of the vascular mediators of stress has not advanced further than the classic observations of Graham and Wolf [33]. They recorded that discussion of stressful experiences caused flushing with a rise in skin temperature of at least 0.3°C followed by increased itching. Scratching with a pin felt more itchy when the skin was flushed. If anxiety was succeeded by feelings of frustration, then exacerbation of eczema resulted. Their investigation included measurement of the skin temperature on the volar aspects of the forearm while discussing life events. They also measured the resistance of the skin to vasodilatation by applying a weight to the skin long enough to produce an increase in skin colour after it is removed. The resulting zone of erythema is due to minute vessel dilation. Emotional stress caused dilatation which was greater in atopic subjects. Kepecs et al. [54] made a study of the rate of exudation into blisters when discussing life events and observed that flushing was associated with increased exudation. The role of neuropeptides, discussed above, is clearly relevant as is the histamine release in those who are neurotic or where mast cells are sensitized by IgE.

Conclusions

There are many difficulties in the measurement of the responses discussed above. One is the variation in the thickness of the skin due to lichenification. Habitually scratched skin is anatomically and physiologically different (Fig. 9) thus the findings discussed in this review could be explained by chronic scratching. In one study by Uehara [103] lichenified skin consistently showed a reduced erythema or no erythema at all after intracutaneous injection of histamine. A disinclination to show redness is halfway towards a tendency to whiten. On normal skin in the same patients a normal erythematous response was usually produced. Uehara believes that it is difficult to identify uninvolved skin. Even normal looking skin may appear eczematous on histology. Michaelsson [66] reported that patients with healed atopic eczema showed normal reactivity. Thus, atopic eczema is reactive only in the stage of repetitive scratching — an explanation of why all tests are less significant in neonates, who are as yet unable to scratch. Uehara [103] and Englehart [26] refer to reactions similar to that of atopic eczema in contact dermatitis; therefore, it is dermatitis, not atopy, which needs explanation. One such explanation is that there may be a kind of spontaneous tachyphylaxis due to continuous release of histamine in eczematous skin. The release of SP and the effect of mechanical stretching on cell membranes [87] are other factors which must be taken into account. Finally, scratched skin, especially chronically inflamed dermis which is rich in mast cells, is a pharmacological bath for cells traversing it. Such cells retain the effect of the bath while circulating through the blood stream and when examined in vitro. The interstitium is overhydrated because of high interstitial pressure and vessels more easily collapse when intravascular pressure falls. The delayed onset of the white blanch suggests that a nervous or autonomic explanation is less likely than a myogenic reflex. Slight shape change, imperceptibly narrowing the endothelial lumen 12–15 s after a scratch, is sufficient to lower intracapillary pressure below interstitial pressure. A slight pharmacological imbalance tipping the vasoreactivity towards vasoconstriction would do the same. Conversely, when vasodilation is induced, the white reaction should be abolished by raising intracapillary pressure above interstial pressure. A physiological explanation of the vascular behaviour of the dermis in atopic eczema is as valid as an immunological or pharmacological one. Nonetheless, no explanation of the vascular behaviour in atopic eczema is valid unless it has been tested in skin which has been free of scratching for several days. Thus again, all the phenomena described above could be due to the mechanical consequences of scratching. However, the pathophysiology of itch and ichthyosis and their association with asthma remains a mystery which is unlikely to be explained by a fuller understanding of the microvascular system of the skin.

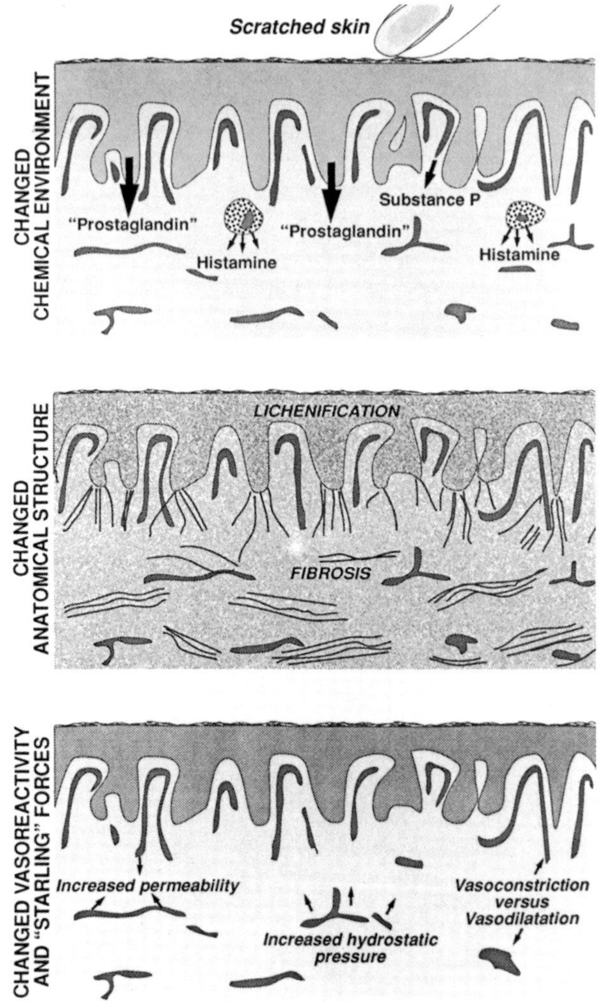

Fig. 9. Some consequences of scratching important for understanding the biochemistry and vasoreactivity of atopic skin and likely to be present at an early age, as illustrated in Fig. 4a, b, c.

References

1. Aizawa H, Tagami H (1989) Inhability to produce white dermographism in the early stage of infantile eczema. Pediatr Dermatol 6:6–9
2. Anonymous (1988) Editorial. Lancet 2:19–20
3. Archer CB, Dalton N, Turner C, Mac Donald DM (1987) Investigation of adrenomedullary function in atopic dermatitis. Br J Dermatol 116;793–800
4. Archer CB, Markey AC, Barker JNWN, Lee TH, MacDonald DM (1989) Effects of the platelet activating factor (PAF) antagonist BN5 2063 on the clinical and histological responses to PAF in atopic skin. J Invest Dermatol 92:397
5. Ashton RE, Russell Jones R, Griffiths A (1985) Juvenile plantar dermatosis: a clinicophathologic study. Arch Dermatol 121:225–8
6. Baer RL (1985) Papaverine therapy in atopic dermatitis. J Am Acad Dermatol 13:806–808
7. Bertelli A (1968) Proteases and anti-proteasic substances in the inflammatory response. Biochem Pharmacol [Suppl] 229
8. Brain SD, Williams TJ (1988) Substance P regulates vasodilator activity of calcitonin gene related peptide. Nature 335:73–75
9. Brain SD, Tippins JR, Morris HR, McIntyre I, Williams TJ (1986) Potent vasodilator activity of calcitonin gene-related peptide in human skin. J Invest Dermatol 87:533–536
10. Brotherton AFA, Hoak JC (1982) Role of Ca2+ and cyclic AMP in the regulation of the production of prostacyclin by the vascular endothelium. Proc Natl Acad Sci USA 79:495–499
11. Brotherton AFA, MacFarlane DE, Hoak JC (1982) Prostacyclin biosynthesis is not inhibited by cyclic AMP. Studies with 3-isobutyl-1-methylxanthine and forskolin. Thromb Res 28:637–647
12. Brown J, Perry P, Ansel J (1989) Substance P induction of keratinocyte cytokines. J Invest Dermatol 92:407
13. Bull HA, Rustin MHA, Dowd PM (1989) Release of prostacyclin from cultured human endothelial cells following prolonged exposure to histamine. Br J Dermatol 120:757–765
14. Burn JH (1961) A new view of adrenergic nerve fibres, explaining the action of reserpine, bretylium and guanethidine. Br Med J 1:1623–628
15. Burn JH, Rand MJ (1960) The relation of circulating noradrenaline to the effect of sympathetic stimulation. J Physiol 150:295–305
16. Cavender DE, Haskard DO, Joseph B, Ziff M (1986) Interleukin 1 increases the binding of human B and T lymphocytes to endothelial cell monolayers. J Immunol 136:203–207
17. Champion RH (1963) Vascular reactions in atopic eczema. Br J Dermatol 75:12–15
18. Charo IF, Karasek MA, Davison PM, Goldstein IM (1984) Prostaglandin I2 is not a major metabolite of arachidonic acid in cultured endothelial cells from human foreskin microvessels. J Clin Invest 74:914–919
19. Christophers E, Henseler T (1987) Contrasting disease patterns in psoriasis and atopic dermatitis. Arch Dermatol Res 48 [Suppl 5]:551
20. Cooper KD (1988) Atopic eczema. In. Orfanos CE, Stadler R, Gollnick H (eds) Dermatology in five continents. Springer, Berlin, Heidelberg, New York, p 280
21. Copeman PWM, Winkelman RK (1969) Vascular changes accompanying white dermographism and delayed blanch in atopic dermatitis. Br J Dermatol 81:944–945
22. Coulson IH, Duncan SN, Holden CA (1989) Peripheral blood mononuclear leukocyte cyclic AMP specific phosphodiesterase activity in childhood atopic dermatitis. Br J Dermatol 120:607–612
23. Czervionke RL, Smith JB, Fry GL, Hoak JC, Haycraft DL (1979) Inhibition of prostacyclin by treatment of endothelium with aspirin. J Clin Invest 63:1089–1092
24. David MJ, Lawler JC (1958) Observations on delayed blanch phenomenon in atopic subjects. J Invest Dermatol 30:127
25. Di Palma JR, Reynolds SRM, Foster FI (1942) Quantitative measurement of reactive hyperemia in human skin. Individual and seasonal variation. Am Heart J 23:377–389
26. Englehardt A (1965) Gefäßreaktionen bei verschiedenen Formen des mikrobiell-seborrhoischen Ekzems als nosologischen Ordnungsprinzips. Arch Klin Exp Dermatol 223:16
27. English JS, Winkelmann RK, Louback et al. (1987) The cellular inflammatory response in nicotinate skin reaction. Br J Dermatol 116:341–349
28. Fogh, K, Herlin T and Kragballe K (1989) Eicosanoids in skin of patients with atopic dermatitis; prostaglandin E_2 and leukotriene B_4 are present in biologically active concentration. J Allergy & Clin Immunol 83: 450–455
29. Frangos JA, Eskin SG, McIntyre LV, Ives CI (1985) Flow effects on prostacyclin production by cultured human endothelial cells. Science 227:1477–1479
30. Fuller RW, Conradson TB, Dixon CMS (1987) Sensory neuropeptide effects on human skin. Br J Dermatol 92:781
31. Giannetti A, Girolomoni G (1989) Skin reactivity to neuropeptides in atopic dermatitis. Br J Dermatol 121: 681–688
32. Grabowski EF, Jaffe EA, Weksler BB (1985) Prostacyclin production by cultured endothelial cell monolayers exposed to step increases in shear stress. J Lab Clin Med 105:36–43
33. Graham DT, Wolf S (1953) The relation of eczema to attitude and vascular reactions of the human skin. J Lab Clin Med 42:238
34. Gresele P, Bounameaux H, Arnout J, Perez-Requejo JL, Deckmyn H, Vermylen J (1985) Thromboxane A2 and prostacyclin do not modulate the systemic haemodynamic response to cold in humans. J Lab Clin Med 106:534–541
35. Grewe SR, Chan SC, Hanifan JM (1982) Elevated leukocyte cyclic AMP phosphodiesterase in atopic disease: a possible mechanism for cyclic AMP agonist hypo-responsiveness. J Allergy Clin Immunol 70:452–457
36. Hanss M, Collen D (1987) Secretion of tissue-type plasminogen activator and plasminogen activator inhibitor by cultured human endothelial cells: modulation by thrombin, endotoxon, and histamine. J Lab Clin Med 109:97–104
37. Hatano H, Yamamoto K, Kono N (1962) Studies on fibrinolytic enzyme system in dermatology: local anti-fibrinolytic activity in several skin diseases. Keio J Med 11:167
38. Haustein UF (1968) Quantitative Bestimmung des Gewebsaktivators der Fibrinolyse in gesunder und kranker Haut. Arch Klin Exp Dermatol 232:245
39. Haustein UF (1969) Die Lokalisation des Gewebsaktivators der Fibrinolyse bei Dermatosen. Arch Klin Exp Dermatol 234:182

40. Heyer G, Schonberger A, Hornstein OP (1988) Disturbances of thermoregulation following warm and cold exposure in patients with atopic eczema. Hautarzt 39:18–22
41. Hill HR, Quie PG (1974) Raised serum IgE levels and defective neutrophil chemotaxis in three children with eczema and recurrent bacterial infections. Lancet 1:183
42. Hirschberg H, Bergh OJ, Thorsby E (1980) Antigen-presenting properties of human vascular endothelium. J Exp Med 152:249s–255s
43. Hong SL, Deykin D (1982) Activation of phospholipases A2 and C in pig aortic endothelial cells synthesizing prosacyclin. J Biol Chem 257:7151–7154
44. Hoover RL, Folger R, Haering WA, Ware BR, Karnovsky MJ (1980) Adhesion of leucocytes to endothelium: roles of divalent cations, surface charge, chemotactic agents and substrate. J Cell Sci 45:73–86
45. Hoover RL, Karnovsky MJ, Ausren KF, Corey EJ, Lewis RA (1984) Leukotriene B4 action on endothelium mediates augmented neutrophil endothelial adhesion. Proc Natl Acad Sci USA 81:2191–2193
46. Horiuchi Y, Ryan TJ (1987) Phorbol ester stimulates urokinase inhibitor synthesis by cultured human fibroblasts. Br J Dermatol 116:419–420
47. Hornqvist R, Bäck O, Henriksson R (1984) Adrenoceptor-mediated responses in human skin studied by iontophoresis. Br J Dermatol 111:561–566
48. Hörnqvist R, Henriksson R, Bäck O (1988) Iontophoretic study of skin vessel reactivity in atopic dermatitis and its correlation to serum IgE levels. J Am Acad Dermatol 18:269–274
49. Jancso G, Obal F, Tothkasa I, Katona M, Husz S (1985) The modulation of cutaneous inflammatory reactions by peptide containing sensory nerves. Int J Tissure React 7:449–457
50. Juhlin L (1962) Vascular skin reactions in atopic dermatitis. Acta Derm Venereol (Stockh.) 42:218–229
51. Juhlin L, Michaelsson G (1969) Cutaneous vascular reactions to prostaglandins in healthy subjects and in patients with urticaria and atopic dermatitis. Acta Derm Venereol (Stockh.) 49:251–261
52. Kaltz F, Fekete Z (1960) Studies on the mechanism of the white response and of the delayed blanch phenomenon in atopic subjects by means of coomassie blue. J Invest Dermatol 35:251
53. Kemmett D (1989) Premenstrual exacerbation of atopic dermatitis. Br J Dermatol 120:715–718
54. Kepecs JG, Robin M, Brunner MJ (1951) Relationship between certain emotional states with exudation into the skin. Psychosom Med 13:10
55. Kottegoda SR (1953) The action of nicotine and acetylcholine on the vessels of the rabbit's ear. Br J Dermatol 8:156–161
56. Leung DYM, Bhaw AK, Schneeberger EE et al. (1983) Characterization of the mononuclear cell infiltrate in atopic dermatitis using monoclonal antibodies. J Allergy Clin Immunol 71:47
57. Lewis T (1927) The blood vessels of the human skin and their responses. Shaw and Sons, London
58. Lobitz WC, Campbell CJ (1953) Physiologic studies in atopic dermatitis (disseminated neurodermatitis) I. The local cutaneous response to intradermally injected acetylcholine and epinephrine. Arch Dermatol Syphilol 67:575
59. Lovell CR, Burton JL, Horrobin DF (1981) Treatment of atopic eczema with evening primrose oil. Lancet 2:1120
60. MacMillan A (1969) Delayed blanch and opacity pulse. Br J Dermatol 81:631
61. Mallet AI, Camp RDR, Rendell NB, Ross JS, Mitchell M, Greaves MW (1989) Measurement of levels of histamine and its major metabolite in the urine of atopic dermatitis patients. J Invest Dermatol 92:475
62. Marone G, Giugliano R, Lembo G, Ayala F (1986) Human basophil releasability. II. Changes in basophil releasability in patients with atopic dermatitis. J Invest Dermatol 87:19–23
63. Masuda T, Naito A, Kinoshita M et al. (1967) Acetylcholine inhalation test in atopic dermatitis. J Allergy 40:193
64. Maurice PDL, Barr RM, Koro O, Greaves MW (1987) The effect of prostaglandin D2 on the response of human skin to histamine. J Invest Dermatol 89:245–248
65. Maxwell RA, Plummer AJ, Schneider F, Povalski H, Daniel AJ (1960) Pharmacology of 2-(octahydro-I-azocinyl)-ethyl-guanidine sulfate (SU-5864). J Pharmacol Exp Ther 128:22–29
66. Michaelsson G (1970) Decreased cutaneous reactions to kallikrein in patients with atopic dermatitis and psoriasis. Acta Derm Venereol (Stockh.) 50:37–41
67. Mihm M, Soter NA, Dvorak HF et al. (1976) The structure of normal skin and the morphology of atopic eczema. J Invest Dermatol 67:305
68. Möller H, Rorsman H (1958) Studies on vascular permeability factors with sodium fluorescein. II. The effect of intracutaneously injected histamine and serum in patients with atopic dermatitis. Acta Derm Venereol (Stockh.) 38:243
69. Moncada S, Gryglewski RJ, Bunting S, Vane JR (1976) An enzyme isolated from arteries transforms prostaglandin endoperoxides to an unstable substance that inhibits platelet aggregation. Nature 263:663–665
70. Moulin G, Manuel Y (1964) Étude immuno-électrophorétique comparative des protéines du sérum et du liquide des bulles dans les dermatoses bulleuses (60 observations). Ann Dermatol Syphilig. 91:505–11
71. Murad F (1986) Cyclic guanosine monophosphate as a mediator of vasodilation. J Clin Invest 78:1–5
72. Needleman P, Bronson SD, Wyche A, Sivakoff M, Nicoloau KC (1978) Cardiac and renal prostaglandin 12.J Clin Invest 839:849
73. Neri Serneri GG, Abbate R, Gensini GF, Galanti G, Paoli G, Laureano R (1982) Platelet aggregation and thromboxane A2 production after adrenergic stimulation in young healthy humans. Haemostasis 11:40–48
74. Olive JT, Connell JO, Winkelmann RK, Logan GB (1970) Delayed blanch phenomenon in children: re-evaluation of 5-year old children originally tested as newborn. J Invest Dermatol 54:256
75. Palmer RMJ, Ferrige AG, Moncada S (1987) Release of nitric oxide accounts for the biological activity of endothelium-derived relaxing factor. Nature 327:524–526
76. Parker CW, Kennedy S, Eisen AZ (1977) Leukocyte and lymphocyte cyclic AMP responses in atopic eczema. J Invest Dermatol 68:302–306
77. Perera P, Kurban AK, Ryan TJ (1970) The development of the cutaneous microvascular system in the newborn. Br J Dermatol 82 [Suppl 5]:86–91
78. Queille-Roussel C, Raynaud F, Saurat JH (1985) A prospective computerized study of 500 cases of atopic dermatitis in childhood. 1. Initial analysis of 250 parameters. Acta Derm Venereol (Stockh.) 114 [Suppl]
79. Ramsey C (1969) Vascular changes accompanying white

dermographism and delayed blanch in atopic dermatitis. Br J Dermatol 81:37

80. Reed WB, Kierland RR (1958) Vascular reactions in chronically inflamed skin. II. Action of epinephrine and phentolamine (Regitine): action of acetylcholine and methacholine (Mecholyl), and the "delayed blanch". A, M, A, Arch Derm 77:181–186
81. Reed CE, Busse WW, Ping Lee T (1976) Adrenergic mechanisms and the adenyl cyclase system in atopic dermatitis. J Invest Dermatol 67:333–338
82. Reitamo S, Visa K, Kahonen K (1986) Eczematous reactions in atopic patients caused by epicutaneous testing with inhalant allergens. Br J Dermatol 114:303–309
83. Ring J (1988) In: Orfanos CE, Stadler R, Gollnick H (eds) Dermatology in five continents. Springer, Berlin, Heidelberg, New York, p 281
84. Ryan TJ (1967) A new technique for studying the microcirculation of the skin In: Bourne GH (ed) In Vivo. Techniques in histology. Williams and Wilkins, Baltimore, pp 192–202
85. Ryan TJ (1977) Urticaria and fibrinolysis. Clin Exp Dermatol 2:177–182
86. Ryan TJ (1984) Microcirculation in psoriasis: blood vessels, lymphatics and tissue fluid. Section 110. In: Baden HP (ed) The chemotherapy of psoriasis. Pergamon, Oxford, pp 145–184
87. Ryan TJ (1989) Biochemical consequences of mechanical forces generated by distension and distortion. J Am Acad Dermatol 21:115–130
88. Ryan TJ (1989) The cutaneous adipose tissue in. Clin Dermatol 7:1–164
89. Ryan TJ, Nishioka K, Dawber RPR (1971) Epithelial-endothelial interaction in the control of inflammation through fibrinolysis. Br J Dermatol 84:501
90. Ryan US (1988) Endothelial cells I. CRC, Boca Raton
91. Sampson HA, Jolie PL (1984) Increased plasma histamine concentrations after food challenge in children with atopic dermatitis. New Engl J Med 311:372–376
92. Schafer AI, Crawford DD, Gimbrone MA (1984) Unidirectional transfer of prostaglandin endoperoxides between platelets and endothelial cells. J Clin Invest 73:1105–1112
93. Schonberger A, Langestein B, Heyer G, Hornstein OP (1988) A method of quantifying dermatographism in atopic eczema. Hautarzt 39:72–76
94. Scott A (1960) Acetyl cholinesterase responses in physiological and pathological vasomotor reactions. In: Rook A (ed) Progress in biological sciences in relation to dermatology. Cambridge University Press, Cambridge
95. Scott A (1962) Acetylcholine in normal and diseased skin. Br J Dermatol 74:317
96. Sedlis E, Prose P (1959) Infantile eczema with special reference to the pathologic lesion. Pediatrics 23:802
97. Seid JM, Macneil S, Tomlinson S (1983) Calcium, calmodulin and the production of prostacyclin by cultured vascular endothelial cells. Biosci Rep 3:1007–1015
98. Spector AA, Hoak JC, Denning GM, Stoll LL (1980) Effect of fatty acid modification on prostacyclin production by cultured human endothelial cells. J Clin Invest 65:1003–1012
99. Sventivanyi A (1968) The beta adrenergic theory of the atopic abnormality in bronchial asthma. J Allergy 42:203
100. Thune P, Rajka G (1980) Small vessel reactivity in atopic dermatitis. Acta Derm Venereol 30 [Suppl 92]:30–32
101. Thune P, Ryan TJ, Powell SM, Ellis JR (1976) The cutaneous reactions to kallikrein, prostaglandin and thurfyl nicotinate in chronic urticaria and the effect of polyphloretin phosphate. Acta Derm Venereol 56:217–221
102. Turner R, Kurban AK, Ryan TJ (1969) Fibrinolytic activity in human skin following epidermal injury. J Invest Dermatol 53 (6)
103. Uehara M (1982) Reduced histamine reaction in atopic dermatitis. Arch Dermatol 118:244–245
104. Uehara M, Ofuji S (1977) Abnormal vascular reactions in atopic dermatitis. Arch Dermatol 113:627
105. Von der Helm, Ring J, Dorsch WE (1987) Comparison of histamine release and prostaglandin E2 production of human basophils in atopic and normal individuals. Arch Dermatol Res 279:536–542
106. Wallis WJ, Hickstein DD, Schwartz BR, June CH, Ochs HD, Beatty PG, Klebanoff SJ et al. (1986) Monoclonal antibody defined functional epitopes on the adhesion-promoting glycoprotein complex (CDw18) of human neutrophils. Blood 67:1007–1013
107. Wheeler ME, Bevilaqua MP, Luscinskas FW, Brock AF, Gimbrone MA (1986) Interleukin-1 treated endothelial cells produce an inhibitor of leukocyte-endothelial adhesion. Fed Proc 45:450
108. Whorton AR, Willis CE, Kent RS, Young SL (1984) The role of calcium in the regulation of prostacyclin synthesis by porcine aortic endothelial cells. Lipids 19:17–24
109. Wilkin JK, Fortner G, Reinhardt LA, Flowers OV, Kilpatrick SJ (1985) Prostaglandins and nicotinate – provoked increase in cutaneous blood flow. Clin Pharmacol Ther 38:273–277
110. Winkelmann RK, Wilhelmj CM, Horner FA (1965) Experimental studies on dermographism. Arch Dermatol 92:436
111. Yamamoto K (1967) The fibrinolysis system (plasmin system) in atopic dermatitis. Speculation of kinin formation. J Clin Dermatol 21:1257–1263
112. Yen A, Barrett KE, Gigli I (1989) Photoactivation of rat peritoneal mast cells suppresses histamine release induced by compound 48/80 and calcium ionphore A23187. J Invest Dermatol 92:546 (abstract)
113. Yu CL, Haskard DO, Cavender D, Johnson AR, Ziff M (1985) Human gamma interferon increases the binding of T lymphocytes to endothelial cells. Clin Exp Immunol 62:554–560
114. Yu CL, Haskard DO, Cavender D, Ziff M (1986) Effects of lipolysaccharide on the binding of lymphocytes to endothelial cell monolayers. J Immunol 136:569–573

The Pathophysiology of Itch

Ö. Hägermark

Introduction

To fulfill its function as an organ of protection, the skin is endowed with a network of sensory receptors and nerves able to discriminate between touch, pressure, heat, cold, pain and itch. The two latter modalities are unpleasant phenomena evoked by noxious stimuli and therefore designated "nociceptive", and they induce opposite defence reflexes. Thus, pain elicits a withdrawal from a possible damaging stimulus, whereas itch provokes an urge to scratch. The obvious purpose of scratching is to remove harmful agents from the skin, such as sharp hairs, destructive chemicals or stinging insects. Here the itch-scratch reflex is rational and may explain why this sensory quality has survived in evolution. On the other hand, the pathological itching occurring in many skin diseases and internal disorders seems meaningless. Here the scratching leads to further irritation of the skin, producing more itching, thus initiating a vicious itch-scratch cycle. A typical example of this is atopic eczema (AE), where scratching plays an important part in the formation of the skin lesions. People who have not suffered from itch may not realise that persistent, generalised itching can be more disabling than severe pain – it has even driven patients to suicide.

Most itching dermatoses are of an immunological/inflammatory nature, such as urticaria, contact dermatitis, AE, lichen planus, dermatitis herpetiformis and bullous pemphigoid. Pruritus may also appear in virtually normal skin in such diverse diseases as uraemia, cholestasis, hyperthyreosis and polycythemia vera. However, our knowledge of the pathophysiology of itch in all these conditions is very incomplete. Clinical research in this field is hampered by difficulties in defining and measuring itch, and there are no suitable animal models because the subjective and descriptive nature of the sensation means that investigations have to be performed with humans; animals have no direct means of communicating sensory experiences. Also, there is still no systemic anti-pruritic drug available. Thus, itch is indeed a challenge both to the basic scientist and the clinician.

Neuroanatomy and Neurophysiology

The progress of sensory physiology in the past few decades has led to considerable gains in our knowledge of the sensory qualities of the skin. Cutaneous receptor populations have been discovered that can be correlated with the perception of warmth, cold, touch and pain, whereas the mechanism by which pruritus is encoded by the peripheral nervous system is less well understood. Pain and itch are related, and much of our knowledge of the pathophysiology of pruritus has actually been inferred from pain studies. Historically, itch has been considered to be sub-threshold pain, since strong noxious stimuli are likely to induce pain and weak ones may cause itch [1]. Supporting this view is the observation that both types of sensation are transmitted in the same type of peripheral nerve, the non-myelinated, slowly conducting C-fibres, and in the same central neurons, the lateral spinothalamic tract. Spinal lesions eliminating pain also eliminate itch perception [2, 3]. The close relation between pain and itch is further illustrated by patients with congenital insensitivity to pain, in whom the itch sensation is also absent [4, 5].

However, there seems to be more reason to regard pain and itch as two separate qualities. For example, itch and pain originating from the same area of the skin can be experienced over a full range of intensities simultaneously and can be separately recognised. Itch is a sensation limited to the superficial layers of the skin, while pain originates from different layers and from several other tissues. Heating of the skin eliminates itch but increases pain. Removal of the epidermis also eliminates itch and enhances pain. Pain and itch initiate different reflexes: withdrawal and scratching. Pain is relieved by analgesics, whereas itch is not – morphine derivatives may in fact intensify itching [6].

Itch Receptors and Neurons

Previously it was thought that itch and pain were transmitted by one type of neuron with the ability to generate different patterns of activity for the two sensations [7]. New evidence obtained by intraneuronal stimulation and recording has changed this traditional view. By inserting microelectrodes percutaneously into the peripheral C-fibres of conscious volunteers it has been convincingly shown that different subsets of receptors and fibres subserve pain and itch. Torebjörk and Ochoa [8] found that intraneuronal microstimulation of a subpopulation of C-fibres evoked a sensation of pruritus, while activation of other C-neurons induced pain. When the frequency of stimulation of the "itch fibre" was increased, only the magnitude of itch was changed but not the quality of sensation; in other words, itch was not changed to pain. Tuckett [9] induced itching by stimulating the skin electrically and showed that the intensity of itch increased with the frequency of stimulation with no change in the quality of the sensation from itch to pain. Handwerker et al. [10] confirmed this by inducing itch with histamine introduced into the skin by iontophoresis. Increasing the dosage led to increased itching but never to pain. Microneurograph recordings from C-fibres showed that only a small population of fibres responded to histamine stimulation, and the researchers concluded that only a small subgroup of C-fibres seems to mediate itch. Most probably these "itch fibres" have their receptors in the most superficial layers of the skin, since iontophoresis introduces histamine only very superficially into the skin.

That the "itch receptors" are located very superficially was determined by Shelley and Arthur as early as the 1950s [11]. In their experiments they used cowhage spicules of "itching powder". They showed that the spicules, obtained from the tropical plant *Mucuna prurnies,* contained a pruritogenic proteolytic enzyme which they named mucunain. Inserting one of these spicules into the skin produced violent itching provided the spicule was located close to the dermo-epidermal junction. When the spicule was inserted deeply into the dermis or very superficially into the epidermis, no itch occurred. Therefore the receptor structures transmitting itch are located in a very limited layer near the dermo-epidermal junction. As yet, no anatomical structure specific for itch receptors has been identified morphologically, but the receptors are assumed to be linked to the free "penicillinate" [12] nerve endings situated at the dermo-epidermal junction [13]. Most C-fibres appear to end near the junction, but some seem to penetrate into the epidermis [14]. Cauna [15] found interesting ultrastructural changes occurring in the free endings close to the dermo-epidermal junction at the site of urticarial reactions. These changes included accumulation of extracytoplasmic glycogen located between the axolemma, Schwann cell membrane and nerve basement membrane. Other types of nerve endings showed a normal morphology. Cauna suggested that these nerve endings may be associated with itch.

Anti-pruritic State

The term anti-pruritic state was introduced by Bickford [2] in the 1930s to describe the observation that experimental, histamine-induced itch could not be elicited in an area made hyperalgesic by a previous noxious stimulus. The phenomenon was further studied by Graham et al. [16], who found that a fairly mild stimulus, e.g. a few pinpricks, could relieve histamine-induced itching for several minutes. The inhibition appeared even if the pinpricks were performed at a distance, as long as they were confined to the same dermatome as the primary stimulus. Other stimuli such as touch, cold, heat and vibration may also cause itch to fade transiently. The gate-control theory proposed by Melzack and Wall [17] in 1965 to explain reduction of pain by mechanical stimulation can probably also be applied to itching and may explain why scratching gives transient relief. According to this theory, signals in the C-fibres reaching the spinal cord are modulated or inhibited by other afferent impulses arriving via large A-fibres transmitting touch or temperature stimuli. In other words, large-fibre inputs would close the "gate" for pain and itch stimuli arriving in thin C-fibres. It could be speculated that the increased itching experienced by many patients with itching diseases after undressing at bedtime is due to decreased stimulation of the skin with fewer impulses in the A-fibres.

Itchy Skin

In contrast to the anti-pruritic state the phenomenon of itchy skin or itch hyperexcitability is due to lowering of the itch threshold [2]. In this state, itching does not occur spontaneously but may be elicited by all kinds of normally inadequate stimuli such as light touch or slight temperature change. Itchy skin is a common finding in many dermatoses and is also observed in experimental itch induced by cowhage or intradermal injections of histamine. Cormia [18] noted that light stroking in the area of the histamine flare frequently produced pruritus or caused its return after the initial pruritus had subsided. Itchy skin has also been observed in partially anaesthetised areas [19]. The neurophysiological mechanisms involved in the phenomenon of itchy skin are unknown, but it may be that in this condition the "gates" for itch are, in some way, opened up.

Peripheral Mediators of Itch

Itch can be produced by chemical, mechanical, thermal or electrical stimuli. Spots on the skin sensitive to itch can be demonstrated by mechanical pressure of a fine probe [11]. Little is known about the biochemical events that elicit stimulation of the itch receptors in the various itching diseases, but since most of them are inflammatory, it has been assumed that the itch impulses are initiated by inflammatory mediators acting upon the itch receptors. However, pathological itch may occur without any sign of inflammation, e.g. in uraemia and cholestasis, and many inflammatory dermatoses, e.g. acne or lupus erythematosus, do not itch. A number of inflammatory mediators have been suggested as causative agents of acute and chronic itching although a scientific basis for this assumption is incomplete, except for the role of histamine in urticaria.

Histamine and Antihistamines

Histamine is the classic itch mediator. Ever since Lewis [20] more than 60 years ago showed that intradermal injection of histamine causes a vascular "triple response" (redness, wheal and flare) and itching, it has been debated whether or not histamine is the ultimate mediator always released in pathological pruritus. It is beyond doubt that histamine contributes to the itching in urticaria, since the administration of antihistamines in this disease usually diminishes or removes the itch. However, some patients with urticaria respond poorly to the antihistaminic drugs, indicating that other mediators may be involved as well.

The role of histamine in other pruritic skin disorders remains to be defined. Experimental itching induced by the intradermal injection of histamine is always associated with a visible vascular response and is easily blocked by H_1-receptor antagonists but not by H_2-inhibitors [21]. Conversely, pathological itching in disease often occurs without whealing and erythema, and antihistamines usually have a poor anti-pruritic effect in many itching disorders. Thus, other mediators than histamine seem to be involved in many itching states. Any relieving effect of antihistamines in itching diseases might be explained by the central, sedative actions of these drugs [22].

In recent experiments the phenomenon of tachyphylaxis for itch and erythema was confirmed after repeated intradermal injections of histamine [23]. When histamine was injected at intervals of 90 min, the cutaneous reactions had almost disappeared by the fifth injection. A similar decrease in histamine reactivity occurred when the interval between injections was extended to 24 h. These observations indicate that histamine cannot be a mediator of the persistent itching lasting for hours in many pruritic diseases. In urticaria in which histamine is the main mediator, the itching of the individual lesions lasts only for a comparatively short time.

Endopeptidases and Kinins

As mentioned above, Shelley and Arthur [11] found an endopeptidase (mucunain) to be the active principle of cowhage. As they subsequently discovered that other endopeptidases such as trypsin, chymotrypsin and papain were also pruritogens when introduced intradermally, they considered endopeptidases to be the naturally occurring mediators of itching, due to their ability to produce itch without visible skin changes and their ubiquitous presence in tissues [11]. However, more recent studies indicate that even though some peptidases such as kallikrein and papain can produce itching without visible skin changes and are not inhibited by antihistamines, other pruritogenic endopeptidases such as trypsin and chymase usually evoke a triple response and are indeed inhibited by antihistamines [24]. The pruritogenic effect of the two latter enzymes, at least, thus seems to be due to histamine release from the dermal mast cells.

The itch evoked by kallikrein and papain was not inhibited by antihistamines, and it had a pricking, not purely itching character [25]. Similar observations have been made with cowhage, which may evoke burning, stinging or pricking as well as itch [26]. It has been speculated that different subpopulations of nociceptive neurons mediate the four sensory qualities of itching, burning, stinging and pricking; histamine might selectively activate the subpopulation serving itch, and cowhage might activate all subtypes (Tuckett, personal communication, cited in [26]).

Bradykinin is a small peptide formed in blood and tissue fluids by the action of kallikrein on the large protein kininogen. Bradykinin is among the most potent pain-producing agents in animals and humans, but when injected intradermally it is only a weak pruritogen and elicits a small triple response which can be inhibited by antihistamines [25]. Therefore, the experimental itching evoked by bradykinin is probably due to the release of histamine [25].

Eicosanoids (Arachidonic Acid Derivatives)

The substances synthesised from arachidonic acid are collectively referred to as eicosanoids. Inflamed skin shows raised levels of these pro-inflammatory derivatives, which include prostaglandins, hydroxyeicosatetraenoic acids (HETEs) and leukotrienes [27]. Prostaglandins E_1, E_2 and the cyclic endoperoxide PGH_2 have no or only a weak pruritogenic effect when injected intradermally but lower the itch threshold for histamine, papain and serotonin [28–30]. Thus, the prostaglandins enhance experimentally induced itching, possibly by sensitising the itch receptors. This is similar to pain responses, which are also enhanced by prostaglandins [31]. However, there is one serious objection to the theory that prostaglandins have a role in clinical pruritus. Aspirin, the analgesic effect of which is due to inhibition of prostaglandin synthesis, seems to have little or no effect in relieving clinical itch.

PGD_2, which is formed in association with mast cell degranulation and histamine release, does not lower the itch threshold [32].

The other pro-inflammatory eicosanoids, i.e. HETEs and leukotrienes, are not pruritogenic when introduced into human skin [33]. Neither do they seem to sensitise the itch receptors (Hägermark, unpublished work).

Serotonin

Serotonin is a weak pruritogen. In a study of 12 volunteers, intradermally injected serotonin evoked itch only in 8, but when injected together with PGE_2 it produced a marked sensation of itch in all subjects [30]. A hypothesis was proposed that the characteristic pruritus of polycythemia vera, appearing after hot baths, may be due to serotonin and prostaglandins released simultaneously from aggregating platelets [30].

Neuropeptides

During the past 20 years an increasing number of peptides have been identified in the central and peripheral nerves. Such neuropeptides have now been found in almost every tissue of the body. Among those so far identified in human skin are substance P, vasoactive intestinal polypeptide (VIP), neurotensin A, γ-melanocyte-stimulating hormone (γ-MSH), somatostatin, neurokinin A, neuropeptide Y (NPY) and opioid peptides [34]. They are found in both sensory and autonomic neurons of the skin. Although much is known about their distribution in the nervous system, much less has been uncovered concerning their physiological role. Because of their localisation within the nerves, releasability and potent biological activities, they are considered to be neurotransmitters or locally acting modulators [35].

One of the most extensively studied peptides is substance P which is regarded as a transmitter for primary nociceptor effects. As early as 1953 Lembeck [36] proposed it as a candidate for transmitting nociceptive impulses of primary sensory neurons to the central nervous system. In recent years Hökfeld et al. [35] have shown, with immunohistochemistry, that substance P is abundant in the C-fibres and formed in the cell bodies of the nerves. It is then transported in two directions: towards the central end of the C-fibres in the spinal cord, where it has a putative transmitter function as predicted by Lembeck [36], and towards the peripheral terminals of these neurons. It is interesting that its rate of transport from the cell body is much greater towards the peripheral terminals than towards the central endings. In the peripheral terminals it can be released by antidromic impulse transmission, leading to vasodilation and inflammation.

In a search for possible itch-mediating agents, substance P and other neurogenic peptides with putative neurotransmitter functions were injected intradermally in humans [37, 38]. The itching evoked by these compounds was accompanied by a wheal and flare reaction, i.e. the same response as after injection of histamine. Moreover, the itching and vascular responses were inhibited by antihistamines and by pretreatment with the histamine liberator compound 48/80, which depletes local histamine stores. Thus, it was concluded that the itching induced by neurogenic peptides was due to the release of histamine from the dermal mast cells (Fig. 1). In fact, substance P and VIP were found to be among the most potent histamine-liberating agents in humans. However, whether neurogenic peptides are responsible for the pruritus associated with clinical diseases remains to be determined.

Opioid Peptides

Research on opiates has made great advances since the discovery in 1975 of the endorphins or enkephalins, i.e. endogenous peptides with morphine-like antinociceptive activity [40]. These neurogenic peptides are believed to be involved in the endogenous control of pain and are recovered both in central and peripheral nerves [41]. Hartschuh et al. [42] have shown that opioid peptides may be present in the Merkel cells of the skin and may also co-localise with substance P in sensory nerves.

It has long been known that morphine is a histamine liberator and induces a triple response at the injection

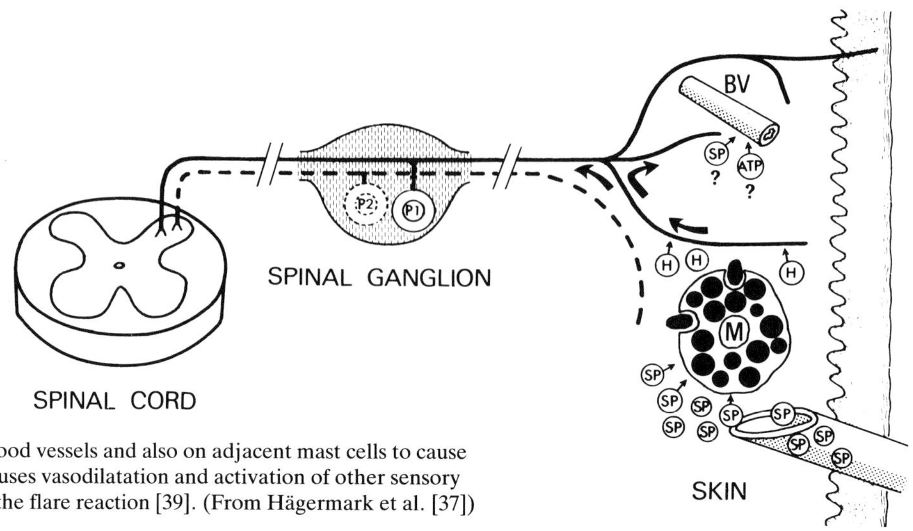

Fig. 1. Hypothetical scheme of events induced by intradermal injection of substance P (*SP*) leading to a wheal and flare response and itching. SP activates dermal mast cells (*M*) to release histamine (*H*), which stimulates two separate populations of "pain" (*P1*) and "itch" (*P2*) nerves. By antidromic stimulation, dilatation of blood vessels (*BV*), i.e. the flare response, is produced via release of SP and possibly other peptides. SP released from the nerve terminals acts directly on the blood vessels and also on adjacent mast cells to cause secretion of H, which in turn causes vasodilatation and activation of other sensory nerves, leading to extension of the flare reaction [39]. (From Hägermark et al. [37])

site when given intradermally [43]. Morphine may also produce histamine release after subcutaneous and intravenous injection. Its pruritogenic effect has therefore been ascribed to its histamine-releasing capacity. However, we found that opioids can cause a potentiation of the itch response similar to that produced by prostaglandins [44]. Subthreshold doses of morphine and the opioid peptides β-endorphin and a stable met-enkephalin analogue, which did not produce any histamine release and itching when injected alone, caused a marked enhancement of histamine-induced itch when injected in a mixture with histamine. This potentiation was influenced by neither local pretreatment with compound 48/80 to deplete the local stores of mast cell-bound histamine nor oral pretreatment with indomethacin to inhibit prostaglandin formation in the skin. Thus, the enhancement did not seem to be due to histamine release or prostaglandin generation.

Surprisingly, the morphine antagonist naloxone failed to inhibit the opioid-induced potentiation, indicating that opioid receptors might not be involved in this peripheral stimulating effect [44, 45]. However, similar findings concerning pain have recently been reported, as it was found that opiates may induce hyperalgesia outside the blood-brain barrier and analgesia within the barrier [46]. The peripheral hyperalgesia appears to be mediated by some mechanism other than opiate receptors since it is not antagonised by specific opiate antagonists [47].

The central pruritic effects of opiates will be discussed below.

In contrast to the opioids, subthreshold (not histamine releasing) doses of substance P and VIP did not cause any enhancement of the histamine-induced responses when injected together with histamine [38].

Lymphokines

Lymphokines (cytokines, interleukins) are soluble proteins generated by lymphocytes and other cells when stimulated with antigens or mitogens. At first, lymphokines were named on the basis of their activity. For example, migration inhibitory factor, or MIF, was generated in cultures of antigen-activated lymphocytes and, when added to macrophages, inhibited their migration from the capillary tubes. Later, it became clear that various biological activities were actually different effects of the same substance. Several hundred activities have been described – among them histamine-releasing factors (HRF) – and the actual number of lymphokines is unknown [48].

In many of the itching dermatoses, e.g. in eczematous skin or in lichen planus, there are accumulations of lymphocytes in the epidermis or upper dermis, i.e. near the itch receptors. The possibility must therefore be considered that pruritogenic lymphokines are secreted by lymphocytes when stimulated. Theoretically, these lymphokines could act directly on the itch receptors or indirectly by inducing mediator release. In preliminiary experiments, it was investigated whether culture supernatants of stimulated lymphocytes obtained from blood samples of healthy volunteers could provoke itching when injected intradermally. Autologous lymphocytes were used and stimulated with the mitogen ConA. Although these in vitro experiments were negative (Wahlgren and Hägermark, unpublished data) this does not exclude the possibility that under in vivo conditions lymphocytes may produce pruritogenic lymphokines in itching skin lesions. This is supported by some clinical reports in which it was observed that cyclosporin — an inhibitor of lymphokine secretion – could inhibit itch in

AE [49, 50, 51] and Sézary syndrome [52]. However, the hypothesis of pruritic lymphokines needs further investigation.

Dry Skin

Dehydration of the stratum corneum, xerosis, is a common cause of pruritus. Cornified epithelium becomes hard and brittle if the water content is less than 10%. Why this condition is associated with pruritus is not known, but it has been assumed that the impaired barrier function of the dry stratum corneum permits the entrance of external agents, leading to a mild but itching dermatitis.

Conclusion

Until now it has not been possible to isolate a universal final mediator to explain all the various kinds of pathological pruritus. Histamine is the classic mediator which induces a "true" itch when injected intradermally and is considered to play an essential role in the pathogenesis of those cases of urticaria that are effectively treated with antihistamines. In all other pruritic states almost nothing is known as to what mediators or other pathogenic mechanisms are involved. The data presented here indicate that mediators can act directly on the itch receptor or indirectly as histamine liberators or enhancing agents.

Central Mediators of Itch

It has long been known that intraventricular injection of morphine and other substances into the brains of laboratory animals can produce a violent scratch syndrome [53, 54, 55], and it has been concluded that an itch center might be located in the lower part of the medulla oblongata [54]. This observation, when related to the recent discovery of opiate receptors and endorphins in the brain, makes it conceivable that these endogenous morphine-like peptides are involved as central transmitters of the itch sensation.

Intraspinal injection of opiates is a very effective way of obtaining segmental pain relief and is frequently used by anaesthesiologists [56]. However, one of its most common side effects is pruritus, which sometimes can be very disabling [57]. The itching may be generalised, but more often it is localised to the segment of injection and sometimes spreads rostrally to the face [57]. There is no redness or whealing in the affected areas that would indicate histamine release. It is not known why this pruritus is so often confined to the face, particularly the nostrils, but it has been speculated that an itch center in the medulla oblongata might be activated [58]. This facial itching from spinal opioids is effectively inhibited by the opioid antagonist naloxone.

Since naloxone effectively inhibits pruritus induced by spinal anaesthesia, it seems natural to investigate its effect in various pruritic diseases. An inhibitory effect on pathological itch would be a strong argument that endogenous opioids are essential transmitters of the itch stimulus. In 1979 there was a report on intractable pruritus due to cholestasis in one patient, who was relieved by naloxone [59]. In a placebo-controlled study of 20 patients with pruritus due to cholestatic liver disease, the itch decreased after naloxone in the 9 placebo non-responders, whereas those who improved after placebo (placebo responders) reported that the itching became worse on naloxone [60]. However, this study has not been confirmed, and my own impression is that naloxone has no obvious itch-relieving effect in pruritic diseases. Thus, whether or not endogenous opioids are involved as mediators or transmitters of pathological pruritus is still an open question.

Pathophysiology of Itch in Atopic Eczema

Although itching is the cardinal symptom of AE and the patient's scratching is responsible for a major part of the skin manifestations, its pathogenesis remains to be explained. Whether any of the mechanisms mentioned previously in this review are involved will be discussed briefly.

Itchy Skin

The clinical experience that atopic patients have itchy skin responding with itch to minor irritants was experimentally confirmed by Rajka [61], who found a lowered itch threshold to histamine and trypsin given intradermally. The biochemical basis for this is unknown, but judging from the previous sections in this chapter it would be interesting to investigate whether enhancing modulators such as prostaglandins or opioid peptides are involved. Well-controlled studies evaluating the effect of prostaglandin inhibitors and opioid antagonists might help in answering this question.

Dry Skin

The skin of the atopic patient gives a dry impression clinically, and recently it was reported that the water content of the stratum corneum in these patients is low [62]. To what extent dry skin contributes to the pruritus is very difficult to assess, however, as the itching of dry skin might be due to a mild dermatitis inseparably linked to AE itself.

Histamine

Much evidence seems to indicate that histamine plays a role in the pathogenesis of AE. Histamine levels are incresed in both involved and uninvolved skin [63, 64]. Ring [65] showed increased plasma histamine in some, but not all, cases of AE. There are more mast cells in the lichenified plaques than in uninvolved skin [66]. There is an increased or faster releasability of histamine from blood basophils of patients with AE [67, 68].

However, the new type of non-sedative H_1-receptor inhibitors does not alleviate the itching of AE [69, 72]. This supports the view that histamine is not of great importance in the pathogenesis of pruritus in AE.

Psychogenic Factors

All kinds of itching, regardless of its aetiology, become worse under emotional stress. This is well-known to all patients with AE. The pathophysiological background for this is unknown. The simplest explanation would be that the nervous patient tends to scratch more, which leads to skin irritation and itch. However, it could be that there is a primary stimulation of the peripheral itch receptors due to release of neurogenic, inflammatory peptides from the cutaneous nerve endings.

Lymphokines

Atopic skin lesions contain an inflammatory infiltrate including lymphocytes and monocytes. The infiltrating T cells are predominantly of the helper/inducer phenotype, which are known to be activated in response to antigen stimulation [70]. It is known that soluble factors (lymphokines) secreted by such activated cells can induce proliferation and collagen biosynthesis by fibroblasts and induce basophil degranulation and mediator release [71]. That lymphokines are involved in the pathogenesis of AE is supported by the observation that cyclosporin, which is known to inhibit lymphokine generation, alleviates itching in some patients with severe AE [49, 50, 51]. We are at present exploring the effect of cyclosporin on itching in AE.

References

1. Zotterman Y (1939) Touch, pain and tickling: an electrophysiological investigation on cutaneous sensory nerves. J Physiol (Lond) 95:1–28
2. Bickford RG (1937–38) Experiments relating to the itch sensation, its peripheral mechanism and central pathways. Clin Sci 3:377–386
3. Arieff AJ, Pyzik SW, Tigay EL (1957) Itch sensation and recovery of sensation in spinal cord injuries. Arch Neurol Psychiatry 77:156–158
4. Kunkle EC, Chapman WP (1943) Insensitivity to pain in man. Ass Rev Nerv Ment Dis Proc 23:100–109
5. McMurray GA (1950) Experimental study of a case of insensitivity to pain. Arch neurol Psychiatry 64:650–659
6. Herndon JH Jr (1975) Itching: the pathophysiology of pruritus. Int J Dermatol 14:465–468
7. Wall PD, Cronly-Dillon JR (1960) Pain, itch and vibration. Arch Neurol 2:365–375
8. Torebjörk HE, Ochoa JL (1981) Pain and itch from C-fiber stimulation. Soc Neurosci Abstr 7:228
9. Tuckett RP (1982) Pruritus evoked by electrical stimulation of the skin. J Invest Dermatol 79:368–373
10. Handwerker HO, Magerl W, Klemm F, Lang E, Westerman RA (1987) Quantitative evaluation of itch sensation. In: Schmidt RF, Schaible H-G, Vahle-Hinz C (eds) Fine afferent nerve fibers and pain. VCH, Weinheim, pp 463–473
11. Shelley WB, Arthur RP (1957) The neurohistology and neurophysiology of the itch sensation in man. Arch Dermatol 76:296–323
12. Cauna N (1973) The free penicillate nerve endings of the human hairy skin. J Anat 115:277–288
13. Bishop GH (1946) The skin as an organ of senses with special reference to the itching sensation. J Invest Dermatol 11:143–154

14. Arthur RP, Shelley WB (1959) The innervation of the human epidermis. J Invest Dermatol 32:397–411
15. Cauna N (1977) Fine morphological changes in the penicillate nerve endings of human hairy skin during prolonged itching. Anat Rec 188:1–11
16. Graham DT, Goodell H, Wolff HG (1951) Neural mechanisms involved in itch, "itchy skin", and tickle sensations. J Clin Invest 30:37–49
17. Melzack R, Wall PD (1965) Pain mechanisms: a new theory. Science 150:971–979
18. Cormia FE (1952) Experimental histamine pruritus, I. Influence of physical and psychological factors on threshold reactivity. J Invest Dermatol 19:21–34
19. Cormia FE, Kuykendall V (1953) Experimental histamine pruritus. II. Nature: physical and environmental factors influencing development and severity. J Invest Dermatol 20: 429–446
20. Lewis T (1927) The blood vessels of the human skin and their responses. Shaw, London
21. Hägermark Ö, Strandberg K, Grönneberg R (1979) Effects of histamine receptor antagonists on histamine-induced responses in human skin. Acta Derm Venereol (Stockh.) 59:297–300
22. Savin JA (1980) Do systemic antipruritic agents work? Br J Dermatol 102:113–118
23. Bäckdahl M, Hägermark Ö, Lins L-E (1988) The sensitivity of uremic and normal human skin to histamine. Acta Derm Venereol (Stockh.) 68:230–235
24. Hägermark Ö, Rajka G, Bergqvist U (1972) Experimental itch in human skin elicited by rat mast cell chymase. Acta Derm Venereol (Stockh.) 52:125–128
25. Hägermark Ö (1974) Studies on experimental itch induced by kallikrein and bradykinin. Acta Derm Venereol (Stockh.) 54:397–400
26. Simone DA, Ngeow JYF, Whitehouse J, Becerra-Cabal L, Putterman GJ, LaMotte RH (1987) The magnitude and duration of itch produced by intracutaneous injections of histamine. Somatosens Res 5:81–92
27. Voorhees JJ (1983) Leukotrienes and other lipoxygenase products in the pathogenesis and therapy of psoriasis and other dermatoses (editorial). Arch Dermatol 119:541–547
28. Greaves MW, McDonald-Gibson W (1973) Itch: role of prostaglandins. Br Med J 111:608–609
29. Hägermark Ö, Strandberg K, Hamberg M (1977) Potentiation of itch and flare responses in human skin by prostaglandins E_2 and H_2 and a prostaglandin endoperoxide analog. J Invest Dermatol 69:527–530
30. Fjellner B, Hägermark Ö (1979) Pruritus in polycythemia vera: treatment with aspirin and possibility of platelet involvement. Acta Derm Venereol (Stockh.) 59:505–512
31. Ferreira SH (1972) Prostaglandins, aspirin-like drugs and analgesia. Nature (New Biol) 240:200–203
32. Maurice PDL, Barr RM, Koro O, Greaves MW (1987) The effect of prostaglandin D_2 on the response of human skin to histamine. J Invest Dermatol 89:245–248
33. Camp RDR et al. (1983) Responses of human skin to intradermal injections of leukotrienes C_4, D_4 and B_4. Br J Pharmacol 80:497–500
34. Johansson O (1987) Pain, motility, neuropeptides and the human skin: immunohistochemical observations. In: Tiengo M et al. (eds) Advances in pain research and therapy, vol 10. Raven, New York, pp 31–44
35. Hökfelt T, Johansson O, Ljungdahl Å, Lundberg JM, Schultzberg M (180) Peptidergic neurons. Nature 284:515–521
36. Lembeck F (1953) Zur Frage der zentralen Übertragung afferenter Impulse. III. Mitteilung. Das Vorkommen und die Bedeutung der Substanz P in den dorsalen Wurzeln des Rückenmarks. Naunyn Schmiedebergs Arch Pharmacol 219:197–213
37. Hägermark Ö, Hökfelt T, Pernow B (1978) Flare and itch induced by substance P in human skin. J Invest Dermatol 71:233–235
38. Fjellner B, Hägermark Ö (1981) Studies on pruritogenic and histamine-releasing effects of some putative peptide neurotransmitters. Acta Derm Venereol (Stockh.) 61:245–250
39. Lembeck F, Gamse R (1982) Substance P in peripheral sensory processes. In: Porter R, O'Connor M (eds). Ciba Symposium 91, Substance P in the nervous system. Pitman, London, pp 35–54
40. Hughes J, Smith TW, Kosterlitz H, Fothergill LA, Morgan BA, Morris HR (1975) Identification of two related pentapeptides from the brain with potent opiate agonist activity. Nature 258:577–579
41. Beaumont A, Hughes J (1979) Biology of opioid peptides. Ann Rev Pharmacol Toxicol 19:245–267
42. Hartschuh W, Weihe E, Büchler M, Helmstaedtler V, Feurle GE, Forssmann WG (1979) Met-enkephalin-like immunoreactivity in Merkel cells. Cell Tissue Res 201:343–348
43. Feldberg W, Paton WDM (1951) Release of histamine from skin and muscle in the cat by opium alkaloids and other histamine liberators. J Physiol (Lond) 114:490–509
44. Fjellner B, Hägermark Ö (1982) Potentiation of histamine-induced itch and flare responses in human skin by the enkephalin analogue FK 33–824, β-endorphin and morphine. Arch Dermatol Res 274:29–37
45. Fjellner B, Hägermark Ö (1984) The influence of the opiate antagonist naloxone on experimental pruritus. Acta Derm Venereol (Stockh.) 64:775
46. Van der Kooy D, Nagy JL (1985) Hyperalgesia mediated by peripheral opiate receptors in the rat. Behav Brain Res 17: 203–211
47. Yaksh TL, Harty GJ, Onofrio BM (1986) High doses of spinal morphine produce a nonopiate receptor-mediated hyperesthesia; clinical and theoretic implications. Anesthesiology 64:590–597
48. Hamblin AS (1988) Lymphokines. IRL Press, Oxford
49. van Joost T, Stolz E, Heule F (1987) Efficacy of low-dose cyclosporin in severe atopic skin disease (letter to the editor). Arch Dermatol 123:166–167
50. Logan RA, Camp RDR (1988) Severe atopic eczema: response to oral cyclosporin A. J R Soc Med 81:417–418
51. de Prost Y, Bodemer C (1988) Double-blind, randomised placebocontrolled trial of local cyclosporin in atopic dermatitis. Abstract, Immunointervention in Autoimmune Diseases, Paris, 15–17 June
52. Tötterman TH, Scheynius A, Killander A, Danersund A, Alm GV (1985) Treatment of therapy-resistant Sézary syndrome with cyclosporin-A: suppression of pruritus, leukaemic T cell activation markers and tumour mass. Scand J Haematol 34:196–203
53. Méhes J (1938) Experimentelle Untersuchungen über den Juckreflex am Tier. Arch Exp Pathol Pharmacol 188:650–656
54. Koenigstein H (1948) Experimental study of itch stimuli in animals. Arch Dermatol 57:828–849
55. Feldberg W, Sherwood SL (1954) Injections of drugs into the lateral ventricle of the cat. J Physiol (Lond) 123:148–167
56. Wang JK, Nauss LA, Thomas JE (1979) Pain relief by intrathecally applied morphine in man. Anesthesiology 50:149–151

57. Bromage PR (1981) The price of intraspinal narcotic analgesia: basic constraints (editorial). Anesth Analg 60: 46–463
58. Scott PV, Fischer HBJ (1982) Spinal opiate analgesia and facial pruritus: a neural theory. Postgrad Med J 58:531–535
59. Bernstein JE, Swift R (1979) Relief of intractable pruritus with naloxone. Arch Dermatol 115:1366–1367
60. Summerfield JA (1980) Naloxone modulates the perception of itch in man. Br J Clin Pharmacol 10:180–183
61. Rajka G (1968) Itch duration in the uninvolved skin of atopic dermatitis (prurigo Besnier). Acta Derm Venereol (Stockh.) 48:320–321
62. Werner Y (1986) The water content of the stratum corneum in patients with atopic dermatitis. Measurement with the corneometer CM 420. Acta Derm Venereol (Stockh.) 66: 281–284
63. Johnson HH, De Oreo GA, Lascheid WP, Mitchell F (1960) Skin histamine levels in chronic atopic dermatitis. J Invest Dermatol 34:237–243
64. Juhlin L (1967) Localisation and content of histamine in normal and diseased skin. Acta Derm Venereol (Stockh.) 42:218–226
65. Ring J (1983) Plasma histamine concentrations in atopic eczema. Clin Allergy 13:545–552
66. Mihm MC, Soter NA, Dvorak HF, Austen KF (1976) The structure of normal skin and the morphology of atopic eczema. J Invest Dermatol 67:305–312
67. Ring J (1981) Increased vasoactive mediator releasability: a possible pathogenetic factor of atopic dermatitis. Int Arch Allergy Appl Immunol 66 [Suppl 1]:156–158
68. von der Helm D, Ring J, Dorsch W (1987) Comparison of histamine release and prostaglandin E_2 production of human basophils in atopic and normal individuals. Arch Dermatol Res 279:536–542
69. Savin JA, Dow R, Harlow BJ, Massey H, Yee KF (1986) The effect of a new non-sedative H_1-receptor antagonist (LN 2974) on the itching and scratching of patients with atopic eczema. Clin Exp Dermatol 11:600–602
70. Willemze R, de Graaff-Reitsma CB, Cnossen J, van Vloten W, Meijer CJLM (1983) Characterization of T cell subpopulations in skin and peripheral blood of patients with cutaneous T cell lymphomas and benign inflammatory dermatoses. J Invest Dermatol 80:60–66
71. Thueson DO, Speck LS, Lett-Brown MA, Grant JA (1979) Histamine-releasing activity (HRA). I. Production by mitogen or antigen stimulated human mononuclear cells. J Immunol 123:626–632
72. Wahlgren CF, Hägermark Ö, Bergström R (1990) The antipruritic effect of a sedative and a non-sedative antihistamine in atopic dermatitis. Br J Dermatol 122: 545–551

Sebaceous Gland Activity in Atopic Eczema

M. Gloor

In the skin of a patient with atopic eczema, a multitude of non-immunological factors are alterated compared with the skin of a healthy person [9, 15, 31]. The secretion activity of the sebaceous glands is one of these factors. This may further be of practical importance, as the therapy for atopic eczema partly consists in supplying the skin with lipids. The acknowledged facts on sebaceous gland secretion in the patient with atopic eczema are described herein.

Sebaceous Gland Lipids and Their Significance

Anatomy, Arrangement and Control of Sebaceous Glands

The sebaceous gland shows holocrine secretion. The more cell divisions that take place in the gland, the larger the gland as a rule, and the greater amount of sebaceous cell lipids secreted. When, however, the migration time is greatly prolonged, an exceptional situation may occur: the sebaceous cell secretion is diminished, and the number of cell divisions may be reduced, although the gland itself appears enlarged. An example of this is senile hyperplasia of the sebaceous glands [21].

Plewig et al. [24, 25] have made a distinction between differentiated and undifferentiated cells in the sebaceous gland. Only the differentiated cells display lipid synthesis. After marking with [^{3}H] thymidine, the marked cells take 7 days to appear inside the sebaceous gland. The time from the beginning of synthesis to the release of lipids in the gland is estimated at about 2 weeks.

The sebaceous gland secretion varies considerably in different parts of the body. On the scalp, it is the greatest by far. Other parts with ample secretion are the chest, back and face. Secretion is very low on the limbs and abdomen. The palmae and plantae have no sebaceous glands. The dimension of sebaceous gland secretion is correlated to the histologically found amount and size of the cells.

Sebaceous gland secretion is governed to a high degree by genetic influences. Gloor and Schnyder [8] examined uniovular and binovular twins. They were able to demonstrate that the difference between twins was significantly smaller for uniovular than for binovular twins (Fig. 1).

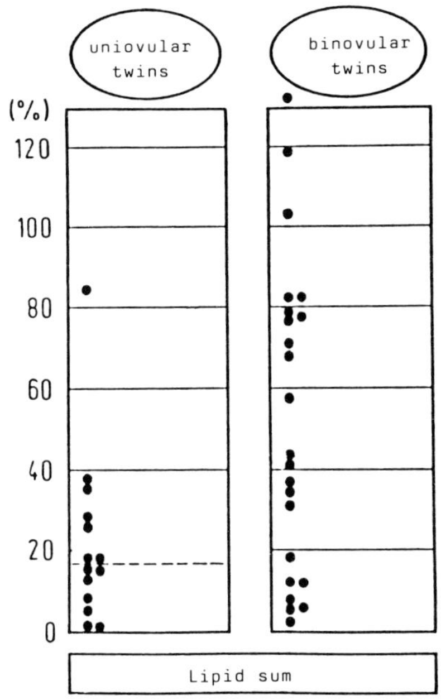

Fig. 1. Differences of the sum of skin surface lipids in 15 uniovular and 26 binovular pairs of twins. Differences were significantly smaller in the uniovular twins than in the binovular twins (taken from Gloor and Schnyder [8]

Sebaceous gland secretion furthermore depends on sex and age. Figure 2 shows results by Cunliffe and Shuster [3], which refer to the determination of sebaceous gland secretion per unit of time after removal of skin lipids. They demonstrate very considerable differ-

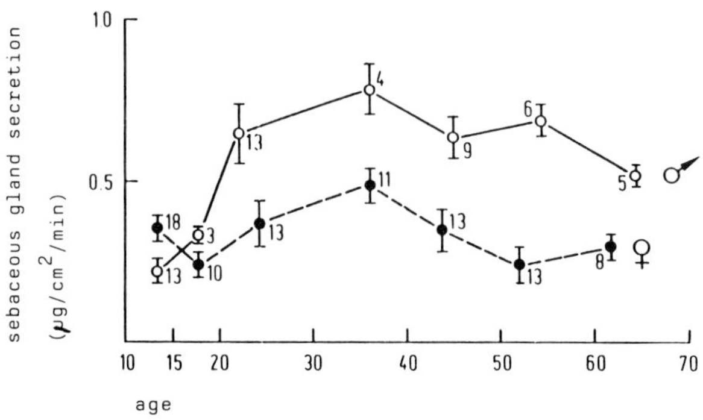

Fig. 2. Replacement sum of the skin surface lipids according to sex and age of the persons examined (taken from Cotterill et al. [2]

Table 1. Sum of skin surface lipids (casual level) according to age and sex (taken from Gloor et al. [12])

	Age (years)	Sum of skin surface lipids (mg/ cm^2)
Male	8–12	0.40
	18–80	1.50
Female	8–12	0.96
	18–80	1.57

ences between the sexes. Results by Gloor et al. [12], however, which apply to the determination of lipid amounts on untreated skin, may be set against this (Table 1). In these surveys, the lipid amount for males and females was nearly identical. It can be asssumed that sebaceous gland secretion after lipid removal sets in faster in males, whereas the secretion lasts longer in females, so that in the end similiar lipid amounts are reached. The results of both teams named above are clearly in agreement about the fact that in children before puberty the secretion of the sebaceous glands is far lower than in adults. After 40 years of age, secretion is gradually reduced. In old age, secretion becomes so low in parts that this, together with other factors, leads to the clinical picture of dry, scaling, senile skin. Histologically, the sebaceous glands become smaller in old age, but they can still be stimulated by hormones to a high degree [32].

The increase of sebaceous gland secretion is chiefly caused by sex hormones. In early adult age, secretion appears to be maximally stimulated by androgens, so that the administration of androgens causes no further increase in secretion [40]. In old age, however, stimulation of sebaceous glands by androgens becomes possible [34]. In the castrated men, secretion is reduced and can be increased by androgens [26]. Administration of androgens raises secretion in women also [40]. Stimulation of sebaceous gland secretion as by androgens may also be achieved by gestagens. On the other hand, so-called antiandrogens lead to a reduction of secretion by blocking the androgen influence. Some gestagens have an antiandrogenic effect as well, for example, estrogens inhibit sebaceous gland secretion.

Seasonal and climatic influences also appear to be important. It is commonly held that secretion rate rises with temperature, and therefore, it is higher in summer than in winter. This is presumably so because high temperature and air humidity cause the excretory ducts to dilate [39]. Because low doses of UV light also stimulate sebaceous gland secretion, this too, may explain a higher secretion rate in summer.

Composition of Sebaceous Gland Lipids

The composition of sebaceous gland lipids is not easy to discuss, because the skin produces a mixture of sebaceous gland lipids and epidermal lipids. Yet it may be assumed that in areas with many sebaceous glands, such as the scalp, back and presternal region, sebaceous gland lipids dominate so greatly over epidermal lipids that the larger part of the lipids analysed is of seborrhoeic origin. On the palmae and plantae, however, only epidermal lipids are detected.

In the sebaceous gland itself only a small amount of free fatty acids compared with the amount of triglycerides is found. Data from the literature agree that the proportions of glycerides and free fatty acids together make up at least half of the sebaceous gland lipids [6]. The triglycerides are composed of extremely varying fatty acids, especially myristic acid, palmitic acid, stearic acid and oleic acid. Free fatty acids are formed in the sebaceous gland infundibula by the hydrolysis of triglycerides. Nearly one third of the triglycerides are split before they reach the surface of the skin. On the scalp, hydrolysis continues outside the infundibula. One day after shampooing, the ratio between triglycerides and free fatty acids is 2:1. Ten days after shampooing, this ratio has reversed to 1:2 [7].

In the sebaceous gland acini no esterases are found [35]. Therefore, lipolysis takes place within the infundibula and microbial esterases in particular become effective. Here, propionibacteria play the main part. They are found in the depths of the sebaceous gland infundibula. *Propionibacterium acnes* is discovered much more frequently than *P. granulosum*. In the upper parts of the infundibula, lipases probably derive to some extent from coagulase-negative staphylococci. For lipolysis on the scalp, other microorganisms are also important. Lipolysis seems to depend on the substrate. Particular strains of propionibacteria split off certain fatty acids more easily than others [17]. On the other hand, some fatty acids, chiefly saturated fatty acids with chain lengths under C16, inhibit the bacteria. Oleic acid, however, enhances bacterial growth [28].

Next to glycerides and free fatty acids, wax esters make up the largest part of sebaceous gland lipids. They amount to about 25% of the total [6]. Mainly seen are chain lengths between C 26 and C 42. Wax esters are hardly present in epidermal lipids. They cannot be split by microbial enzymes and therefore do not form a source of fatty acids.

Among the other components of sebaceous gland secretion, squalene, an intermediate in the synthesis of cholesterol, dominates with about 12%–14%. In the sebaceous glands, cholesterol synthesis nearly always comes to a stop with squalene, so that hardly any cholesterol and only a very small amount of cholesterol ester appear in the secretory product. Because squalene is hardly to be found among the epidermal lipids, it is considered as the characteristic component of sebaceous gland lipids, next to the wax esters. The free cholesterol in epidermal lipids may be esterified with sebogenous free fatty acids on the surface of the skin [29]. The amount of phospholipids in the sebaceous gland is minimal. Paraffins are not secreted in the sebaceous gland but reach the skin through environmental pollution.

Significance of Sebaceous Gland Lipids

The significance of these skin surface lipids for skin and stratum corneum function is disputed. Kligman [18] has denied any effect. Just like many other authors, I hold the opinion that skin surface lipids have a softening and smoothing effect on the stratum corneum. In older literature, occlusive moistening of the skin by sebaceous gland lipids was assumed. Personal surveys, however, have brought forth that the sebaceous gland lipids form no covering film on the skin but are predominantly grouped around the follicles [11]. Schneider and Schuleit [33] demonstrated that the skin of a seborrhoeic patient is moistened more easily than that of a sebostatic patient. This was confirmed later by Gloor et al. [11]. Skin surface lipids thus seem to enhance the capacity for the absorption of water in the stratum corneum. Yet it is questionable whether they take part in the moisturisation of the stratum corneum this way. Findings by Gloor et al. [13] make this assumption seem quite unlikely, because there is no demonstrable correlation between the degree of moisture in the stratum corneum and the amount of lipids.

Sebaceous cell lipids may be of distinct importance for microbial colonisation of the skin. Horaček and Pospišil [16] demonstrated that cleansing of the skin improves the living conditions for staphylococci in seborrhoeic patients, whereas these conditions become worse after regeneration of the lipid film. This result might be explained as an antimicrobial effect chiefly of fatty acids with medium chain length.

Incidence of Acne in Patients with Atopic Eczema

Many researchers have confirmed unanimously that in patients with acne vulgaris, sebaceous gland secretion is increased. Table 2 shows my results which, corresponding with other data in the literature, make it clear that sebaceous gland secretion in the patient with acne, is usually heavier the more severe the acne is. For further data, see the monograph by Gloor [5].

Table 2. Mean values of casual level and replacement sum of skin surface lipids in patients suffering from acne vulgaris and in healthy controls (taken from Gloor et al. [10]
Group A, healthy controls; group B1, acne patients, lightly affected; group B2, acne patients, averagely affected; group B3, acne patients, seriously affected

	n	Casual level ($mg/16 cm^2$)	Replacement sum ($mg/16 cm^2$) over 2h
Group A	18	1.228	0.627
Group B (total)	51	1.883	0.986
Group B1	25	1.658	0.754
Group B2	14	1.971	1.133
Group B3	12	2.251	1.300

The primary efflorescence in acne is the comedo (black head). It originates through keratosis within the inside of the infundibula. The comedo may (but need not) be transformed into an inflamed acne lesion. Lysis of the follicular walls takes place before inflammatory infiltrates in these areas develop. Clinical findings in juvenile, 13–14-year-old patients with acne are mainly comedones, whereas in older patients the inflammatory efflorescences dominate. Inclination towards the formation of inflammatory acne efflorescences can be so pronounced that fully developed comedones are hardly to be seen, as even microcomedones are transformed into inflammatory efflorescences before turning into ripe comedones.

The effect of seborrhoea on the pathogenesis of acne is not perfectly clear. There are no hints to the fact that seborrhoea might be important for inflammatory reactions surrounding the comedo. Yet it is probable that seborrhoea stimulates follicular hyperkeratosis. The large sebaceous glands of the patient with acne secrete increased amounts of squalene [36]. In accordance with this, diffferent teams found increased amounts of squalene in the secretory product of the sebaceous glands [2, 10, 37]. Because squalene enhances the formation of comedones in experimental trials [19], it has been assumed that seborrhoea stimulates follicular hyperkeratosis through squalene. In more recent times, another hypothesis has been discussed. Epidermal lipids are said to have a suppressing effect on follicular hyperkeratosis. The relative decrease of their presence among the skin surface lipids is supposed to promote follicular hyperkeratosis by reducing the suppressor effect of the complete lipid mixture [22].

Many dermatologists suspect a reduced incidence of acne in patients with atopic eczema. Baer [1] reports findings by his collaborator Green, which demonstrate the tendency towards this reduced incidence. It was not possible, however, to confirm these findings by statistical means. Liddel [20] presented studies on a large group of patients with acne. Table 3 compares them with healthy controls of about the same age and sex. It is shown that the number of patients with atopic eczema among those suffering from acne is far lower than in the control group and this difference is highly significant.

Table 4 shows the incidence of atopic eczema in the parents of patients with acne and controls. A highly significant difference was found here also. Parents of patients with acne suffered from atopic eczema to a far lesser extent than the parents of controls. Table 5 demonstrates that the same also applies to the siblings of patients with acne and controls.

It has often been observed that not only the incidence of acne differs between patients with atopic eczema and healthy persons but also the clinical picture of the acne itself. In the most cases, acne in the patient with atopic eczema displays only a few comedones. Inflammatory efflorescences dominate by far, and it is presumed that the age of acne manifestation is higher in patients with atopic eczema.

Table 3. Incidence of atopic eczema in control subjects and subjects with acne (taken from Liddell [20])

	Atopic eczema	Total	Percentage
Acne subjects	4	127	3.2
Non-acne subjects	22	116	19.0

Table 4. Incidence of atopic eczema in the parents of control subjects with acne (taken from Liddell [20])

	Atopic eczema	Total	Percentage
Parents of acne subjects	6	243	2.5
Parents of non-acne subjects	23	220	10.5

Table 5. Incidence of atopic eczema in the siblings of subjects with acne and control subjects (taken from Liddell [20])

	Atopic eczema	Total	Percentage
Siblings of acne subjects	10	236	4.2
Siblings of non-acne subjects	27	202	13.4

All observations mentioned speak for the idea that seborrhoea, which as stated above is an important component in the origin of follicular hyperkeratosis, does not occur in the patient with atopic eczema to the same extent as in other people.

Histological Studies in Patients with Atopic Eczema

Prose [27] has reported extensive histological studies on children suffering from infantile eczema. In these studies, he has, among other topics, focussed his attention on the sebaceous glands. He found remarkable differences in children with infantile eczema, compared with healthy children. Instead of normal, plump, lipid-filled sebaceous glands, only atrophied gland structures were seen. These were composed of small, basaloid cells and contained no lipids. The glands looked as if they had evacuated their lipids into the infundibulum a short time ago, yet the infundibula contained no lipids either.

The same researcher gives an account of histochemical surveys. Contrary to previous studies by others, he found no two layers of lipids in frozen sections, but a regular distribution of lipids through the whole stratum corneum. The types of lipids in children with infantile eczema appeared to differ from those in healthy children. In both groups, phospholipids were detectable. Staining for wax esters and neutral fat, however, showed far lower amounts of these in children with eczema than in healthy children. In individual cases, neither wax esters nor neutral fat were found at all.

The relatively low number of sebaceous glands and their smaller size in the patient with atopic eczema is not unknown to the dermatohistologist. Wirth et al. [41], assessed these conditions according to quantity. The studies were made with 18 patients suffering from atopic eczema and 18 healthy controls. The medium age for both groups was 27. In either group, half of the test persons were male, half female. The biopsies examined were taken from the front hairline of the forehead, an area comparatively rich in sebaceous glands. In each case, biopsy specimens of 1 cm length were studied, so that statistically relevant interpretations were possible.

The studies produced impressive differences between the two groups. The number of glands per unit area and the portion of sebaceous gland surface were determined by histology. Figure 3 shows the results. It may be gathered that the size of the glands was significantly smaller in patients with atopic eczema. The differences were so great that no overlapping of results from both groups occurred at all. The patient with atopic eczema and the largest gland surface still had less than half the surface of the control person with the smallest gland surface. The number of glands was also significantly lower in patients with atopic eczema than in controls. Here, too, no overlapping occurred, but the differences were not as great as those relating to the gland surface.

These data make it clear that the number and surface of glands are much smaller in patients with atopic eczema. The surprising thing about these results is the extent of the difference. Sebostatis in the patient with atopic eczema can therefore not be considered as a norm variation but must be looked upon as definitely pathological. It might even be possible to make the diagnosis of atopic eczema solely on grounds of such quantitatively evaluated histological findings.

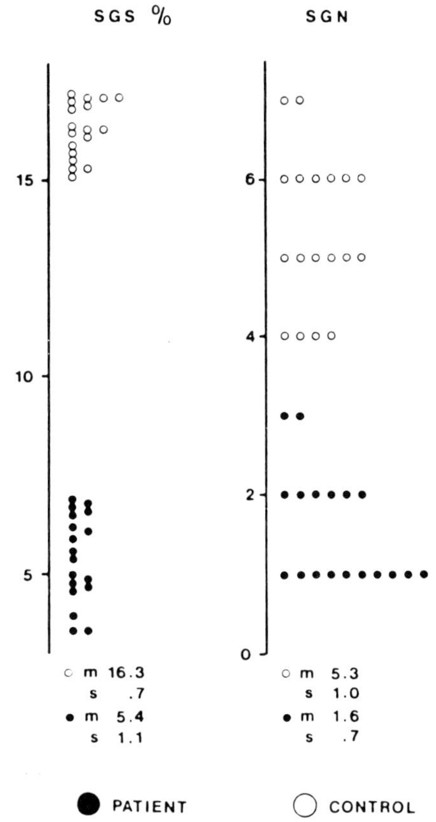

Fig. 3. Number (*SGN*) and size (*SGS%*) of the sebaceous glands in the uninvolved skin of patients suffering from atopic eczema compared with healthy non-atopic control persons; means (*n*) and SE (*s*) are given underneath (taken from Wirth et al. [41]

Studies on Cellular Kinetics in the Sebaceous Glands of Patients with Atopic Eczema

Wirth et al. [41] reported autoradiographic in vitro studies on the same specimens used for the histological surveys mentioned above. The studies thus concern 18 patients with atopic eczema and 18 controls, half of each group male and half female. The medium age for both groups was 27 years. Biopsy specimens 1 cm in length were taken from the hairline on the forehead.

The in vitro incubation with isotopes took place immediately after collecting the specimen.To avoid errors by circadian variations, the specimens were all collected at the same time of day. Conditions for incubation were a P O_2 of 2.2 atm and temperature of 37°C. Total incubation time was 2 h. During the 1st h, 1μCi [^{14}C] thymidine and during the 2nd h 10μCi [^{3}H] thymidine were added to the incubation medium (autologous plasma). After the end of each hour, the specimens were washed carefully with the incubation medium. This method makes it easy to distinguish between ^{3}H- and ^{14}C-labelled specimens. [^{3}H] Thymidine generates short-range radiation, so that a punctiform marking is seen on a thick layer of photoemulsion. The radiation of [^{14}C] thymidine is of much longer range, so that long traces become visible on the photoemulsion layer, when the microscope adjustor is moved. In practice, it is hardly possible to distinguish between cells marked solely by ^{14}C and double-labelled cells.

The number of cells labelled only by ^3H is equivalent to the number of cells entering the S-phase. This number is a unit for cell proliferation. The number of cells labelled only by ^{14}C and the number of double-labelled cells together is equivalent to the number of cells that stay in the S-phase over 2 h. If the number of cells marked only by ^{14}C plus the double-labelled cells is divided by the number of cells marked solely by ^3H, the duration of the S-phase results. For methodological details, see the monography by Gloor [5].

Figure 4 shows the results of these studies. As in the histological surveys, highly significant differences between the groups were found. The differences were so great that no overlapping occurred. As in the histological surveys, the results must therefore be considered as definitely pathological and not as norm variations. In particular, the number of cells marked solely by ^3H was significantly reduced in the patients with atopic eczema. Therefore, the cell proliferation within the sebaceous glands was reduced. The total number of marked cells was also definitely lower. On the other hand, the duration of the S-phase was significantly prolonged in patients with atopic eczema. According to these surveys, it may be assumed that the generation time of the cell cycle is also very much prolonged.

If a comparison is made between the histological surveys and the autoradiographic findings, a uniform picture emerges. Both studies allow the assumption that the secretion of the sebaceous glands is obviously lower in the patient with atopic eczema.

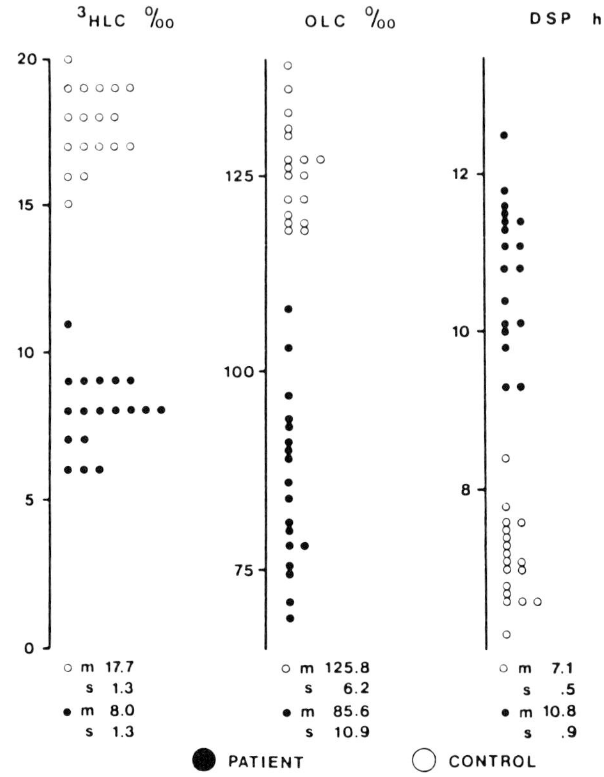

Fig. 4. Single ^3H-labelled cells (*^{3}HLC*), ^{14}C-labelled cells (single ^{14}C- and double-labelled cells, *OLC*) and duration of S-phase (*DSP*) in uninvolved skin of patients suffering from atopic eczema compared with healthy non-atopic control persons; mean (*n*) and SE (*s*) are given underneath (taken from Wirth et al. [41]

Analyses of Skin Surface Lipids

The oldest lipid analyses of patients with atopic eczema known to me are those by Wheatley [38]. The researcher states that the skin surface lipids of the patient with atopic eczema contain essentially more cholesterol and less squalene than those of healthy people. Because cholesterol – as specified above – is the characteristic constituent of skin surface lipids, these studies confirm a relative decrease in the proportion of sebaceous gland lipids among the total. Unfortunately, these publications give no details of test conditions and number of subjects.

Studies by Mustakallio et al. [23] give only limited information on sebaceous gland secretion. They analysed lipids extracted from the total lipid mixture. These lipids were gained by the experimental formation of vesicles. Qualitative analysis was done by thin-layer chromatography. In experimentally formed vesicles a large proportion of epidermal lipids is also found, so that statements on sebaceous gland lipids can only be made to a limited extent. It was demonstrated, however, that the total amount of epidermal lipids is reduced in the patient with atopic eczema. The proportion of cholesterol is clearly increased; these findings might be interpreted as a reduction in the proportion of sebaceous gland lipids among the total lipid mixture, due to decreased sebaceous gland secretion. Noteworthy about these results is the fact that more free fatty acids and fewer glycerides are found in patients with atopic eczema than in healthy persons. The investigators assumed increased lipolytic activity.

Rajka [30] reported extensive surveys with 35 patients with atopic eczema and 21 healthy controls. He used the paper absorption method and subsequent gravimetrical lipid determination. Qualitative lipid analysis was done by thin-layer paper chromatography. The back of the hand was used as the test area. Table 6 shows the results of the quantitative lipid analysis. It can be seen that the amount of lipids in patients with atopic eczema was less than half as large as in healthy controls. Table 7 shows the

Table 6. Surface lipid values on the back of the hands in patients suffering from atopic eczema and in healthy controls (taken from Rajka [30])

	n	Surface lipid values (mg/9 cm^2/3h)
Controls, male	9	0.339
Controls, female	12	0.283
Atopic eczema, male	15	0.152
Atopic eczema, female	20	0.136

Table 7. Composition of the skin surface lipids on the back of the hands in patients suffering from atopic eczema and in healthy controls (taken from Rajka [30]

	Atopic eczema (%)	Controls (%)
Triglycerides	19.7	24.6
Diglycerides	14.6	14.6
Free fatty acids	25.1	21.7
Cholesterol	8.9	3.7
Wax esters	22.2	25.6
Squalene	7.1	9.8

results of the qualitative analysis. It becomes evident that more cholesterol, less squalene and fewer wax esters are found in patients with atopic eczema than in healthy persons. This speaks for an increase in the relative proportion of epidermal lipids at the cost of sebaceous gland lipids among the total lipid mixture. This is in good agreement with the results of Wheatley [38] and Mustakallio [23].

Table 7 shows further that free fatty acids are increased and glycerides reduced in the patient with atopic eczema. Increased microbial lipolysis within the infundibula of the sebaceous glands may be assumed. This observation coincides with the results by Mustakallio et al. [23] referred to previously. Increased microbial lipolysis in the patient with atopic eczema must be assumed. In my own studies, I found a significant increase in *Staphylococcus aureus* and in coagulase-negative staphylococci for the patient with atopic eczema [14]. These findings coincide with other communications. Coagulase-negative staphylococci play an important part in lipolysis. It is unknown to me whether or not propionibacteria are to be seen to a greater extent in the patient with atopic eczema.

Results nearly identical to those of Rajka [30, 31] were found by Ead et al. [4]. Tested area was the forehead. 16 patients suffering from atopic eczema and 27 healthy controls of about the same age and sex were tested. Additionally, 13 patients with acne were included for comparison. The amount of sebaceous gland secretion per unit time was determined by gravimetrical methods. Figure 5 shows the results of the quantitative assessment. Secretion was lower in patients with atopic eczema than in healthy controls, whereas the patients with acne displayed higher values. The difference between patients with atopic eczema and controls, however, was not significant.

The researchers analysed the lipids detected by thin-layer chromatography (Table 8). In agreement with Rajka [30], they found an increase in free cholesterol in patients with atopic eczema. This is caused by the relative increase in the portion of epidermal lipids among the total lipid mixture. The cholesterol value, which was lower than in Rajka's findings [30], is explained by the fact that Rajka examined an area low in sebaceous glands, whereas the area examined by Ead et al. [4] was rich in sebaceous glands. The increased microbial lipolysis in patients with atopic eczema was stated by Ead et al. [4], corresponding with Rajka [30]. Free fatty acids were increased and triglycerides reduced in comparison with the control group.

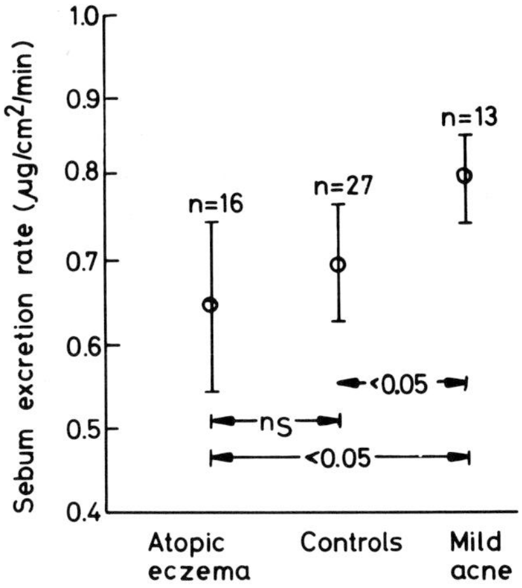

Fig. 5. Sebum excretion rate in control subjects and patients with mild acne and atopic eczema (taken from Ead et al. [4])

Table 8. Composition of the skin surface lipids on the forehead in patients suffering from atopic eczema and in healthy controls (taken from Ead et al. [4]

	Atopic eczema (%)	Controls (%)
Squalene	16.1	12.6
Wax esters	24.4	24.9
Triglycerides	41.1	47.7
Free fatty acids	15.9	14.2
Cholesterol	2.2	0.5

Summary

On account of these results, the following statements can be regarded as certain:

1. Fewer patients with atopic eczema suffer from acne vulgaris than healthy controls.
2. The sebaceous gland secretion in patients with atopic eczema is reduced compared with healthy persons.
3. Microbial lipolysis of glycerides in the secretion product is increased in patients with atopic eczema compared with healthy persons.

References

1. Baer (1965) Contribution to discussion. J Pediatr 66:189
2. Cotterill JA, Cunliffe WJ, Williamson B, Bulusu L (1972) Further observations on the pathogenesis of acne. Br Med J 3:444–446
3. Cunliffe WJ, Shuster S (1969) The rate of sebum excretion in man. Br J Dermatol 81:697–704
4. Ead RD, Fairbank RA, Cunliffe WJ (1977) Sebum excretion rate, surface lipid composition and constitutional eczema. Clin Exp Dermatol 2:361–364
5. Gloor M (1982) Pharmakologie dermatologischer Externa. Springer, Berlin, Heidelberg, New York
6. Gloor M, Horáček J (1979) Über die Hautoberflächenlipide. In: Schwarz E, Spier HW, Stüttgen G (eds) Normale und pathologische Physiologie der Haut II. Springer, Berlin, Heidelberg, New York, pp 263–348 (Handbuch der Haut- und Geschlechtskrankheiten, vol 1, pt 4a)
7. Gloor M, Kohler H (1977) On the physiology and biochemistry of scalp and hair lipids. Arch Dermatol Forsch 257:273–279
8. Gloor M, Schnyder UW (1977) Vererbung funktioneller Eigenschaften der Haut. Hautarzt 28:231–234
9. Gloor, M, Wagner L (1985) Nichtimmunologische Funktionsstörungen der Haut beim Neurodermitiker. Zentralbl. Haut Geschl. Kr 150:505–509
10. Gloor M, Graumann U, Wiegand I, Friederich HC (1972) Über den Einfluß der Tetracyclintherapie bei Acne vulgaris auf Menge und Zusammensetzung der Hautoberflächenlipide bei verschiedener Dosierung. 1. Mitteilung. Arch Dermatol Forsch 242:309–315
11. Gloor M, Franz P, Friederich HC (1973) Untersuchungen über die Physiologie der Talgdrüsen und über den Einfluß der Hautoberflächenlipide auf die Benetzbarkeit der Haut. Arch Dermatol Forsch 248:79–88
12. Gloor M, Kionke M, Friederich HC (1975) Biochemical and physiological parameters on the skin surface of healthy test persons. A contribution towards the interpretation of the results obtained by a screening program. Arch Dermatol Forsch 252:317–330
13. Gloor M, Willebrandt U, Thomer G, Kupferfschmid W (1980) Water content of horny layer and skin surface lipids. Arch Dermatol Res 268:221–223
14. Gloor M, Peters G, Stoika D (1982) On the resident aerobic bacterial skin flora in unaffected skin of patients with atopic dermatitis and in healthy controls. Dermatologica 164:258–265
15. Grosshans E, Woehl M (1982) Troubles vasomoteurs, sudoraux et sébacés de l'eczéma constitutionnel. Ann Dermatol Venereol 109:151–162
16. Horáček J, Pospisil LS (1965) The lipases of the skin surface staphylococci. Bratisl Lék Listy 45:193–197
17. Kellum RE, Toshitani S, Strangfeld K (1973) Humans sebaceous gland lipids: in vitro incubations with 14 C labelled compounds. J Invest Dermatol 60:53–57
18. Kligman AM (1963) The uses of Sebum. Br J Dermatol 75:307–319
19. Kligman AM, Wheatley VR, Mills OH (1970) Comedogenicity of human sebum. Arch Dermatol 102:267–278
20. Liddell K (1976) A familial study of acne and eczema. Br J Dermatol 94:633–637
21. Luderschmidt C, Plewig G (1977) Circumscribed senile sebaceous gland hyperplasia (CSSGH): cellular kinetics and biometrical data. J Invest Dermatol 68:248
22. Melnik B (1988) Epidermale Lipide: Ein neues Konzept für die Pathogenese der Akne. Z Haut Geschlechtskr 154:570–571
23. Mustakallio KK, Kiistala U, Piha HI, Nieminen E (1967) Epidermal Lipids in Besnier's Prurigo (atopic eczema). Ann Med Exp Fenn 45:323–325
24. Plewig G, Christophers E, Braun-Falco O (1971) Cell transition in human sebaceous glands. Acta Derm Venereol (Stockh.) 51:423–428
25. Plewig G, Christophers E, Braun-Falco O (1971) Proliferative cells in human sebaceous glands. Acta Derm Venereol (Stockh.) 51:413–422
26. Pochi PE, Strauss JS (1963) Sebaceous gland function before and after bilateral orchiectomy. Arch Dermatol 88: 729–731
27. Prose PH (1965) Pathologic changes in eczema. J Pediatr 66:178–199
28. Puhvel SM, Reisner RM (1970) Effect of fatty acids on the growth of corynebacterium acnes in vitro. J Invest Dermatol 54:49–52
29. Puhvel SM, Reisner RM, Sakamoto K (1975) Analysis of sebum composition of isolated human sebaceous gland homogenisates after incubation with cutaneous bactera-thin layer chromatography. J Invest Dermatol 64:406–411
30. Rajka G (1974) Surface lipid estimation on the back of the hands in atopic dermatitis. Arch Dermatol Res 251:43–48
31. Rajka G (1975) Atopic dermatitis. Saunders, Philadelphia
32. Rapaport M (1973) The aging skin. J Am Geriatr Soc 21:206–207
33. Schneider W, Schuleit H (1951) Der Fettmantel der Haut und seine Bedeutung für die Benetzung. Arch Dermatol Syph 193:434–459
34. Smith JG, Brunot FR (1961) Hormonal effects on aged human sebaceous glands. Acta Derm Venereol (Stockh.) 41:61–65
35. Steigleder GK (1957) Die Histochemie der Epidermis und ihrer Anhangsgebilde. Arch Klin Exp Dermatol 206:276–317
36. Summerly R, Yardley HJ, Raymond M, Tabiowo A, Ilderton E (1976) The lipid composition of sebaceous

glands as a reflection of gland size. Br J Dermatol 94:45–53

37. Tronnier H, Brunn G (1972) Vergleichsuntersuchungen des Hautoberflächenfettes Hautgesunder und Aknekranker. Berufsdermatosen 20:79–88
38. Wheatley VR (1965) Secretions of the skin in eczema. J Pediatr 66:200–202
39. Williams M, Cunliffe WJ, Gould D (1974) Pilosebacous duct physiology. I. Effect of hydration on pilosebaceous duct orifice. Br J Dermatol 90:631–635
40. Winkler K (1972) Talgdrüsenaktivität im Spiegel endokriner Vorgänge. Z Haut Geschlechtskr 47:925–930
41. Wirth H, Gloor M, Stoika D (1981) Sebaceous glands in uninvolved skin of patients suffering from atopic dermatitis. Arch Dermatol Res 270:167–169

Disturbances of Epidermal Lipid Metabolism and Barrier Function in Atopic Eczema

B. C. Melnik

Introduction

The presence of generalised dry skin is a characteristic feature of atopic eczema (AE) which fluctuates with disease activity. Besides xerosis, ichthyosis vulgaris has been reported in 2%–6% of patients with AE. Intolerance of lipid solvents is another common feature of atopic dry skin [28]. These symptoms correlate with disturbances of the water permeability barrier and diminished hydration [63–65].

The stratum corneum of all terrestrial vertebrates contains a highly specialised permeability barrier which protects the organism from extensive transepidermal water loss. The ultrastructural and biochemical characteristics of this barrier have been clarified recently [11, 40, 68]. It waterproofs the skin and is found within the lowest cell layers of the stratum corneum, just above the living stratum granulosum. Its functional integrity depends predominantly on intercorneocyte sheets of lipids. These keratinocyte-derived, stratum corneum barrier lipids act as a kind of "mortar" around the lipid-depleted corneocytes in the stratum corneum [12, 18]. Recent physical, ultrastructural and biochemical findings support the view that disturbances of epidermal lipid metabolism account for the defect in barrier function in atopic dry skin.

Biochemistry of Epidermal Lipids

The keratinocyte-derived epidermal lipids constitute approximately 10%–14% of the dry weight of mammalian epidermis. During epidermal differentiation, the composition and quantities of epidermal lipids change dramatically from the basal to the granular layer with further striking modulations occurring within the stratum corneum. These compositional changes of epidermal lipids are closely linked to the functional requirements of the differentiating epithelium. The important role of the epidermal lipids in barrier function and desquamation has been recognised in the past few years [10, 25, 44, 74, 77, 81, 82]. On the basis of light microscopy, transmission electron microscopy and freeze-fracture studies, cell fractionation and histochemical analyses, a two-compartment model ("brick-and-mortar" model) of the stratum corneum consisting of protein-enriched corneocytes ("bricks") embedded in lipid-enriched intercellular material ("mortar") has been established [11, 12, 18] (Fig. 1).

With regard to the biochemical process of epidermal differentiation the keratin matrix constituents of corneocytes have been the subject of interest for several decades. However, until recently, the intercellular, lipid-rich compartment of the stratum corneum which accounts for 10%–30% of the volume of the horny layer [15] has received only little attention. Now evidence is growing fast that the intercellular stratum corneum lipids are the biochemical equivalent of the epidermal permeability barrier [14, 40, 43, 68].

The chemical structures of most important stratum corneum lipids are presented in Fig. 2 and 3. The epidermal lipid composition markedly changes in the successive layers of epidermal cells. It had already been recognised in 1932 that phospholipids, present in the viable epidermal layers, were strikingly diminished in the stratum corneum [35].

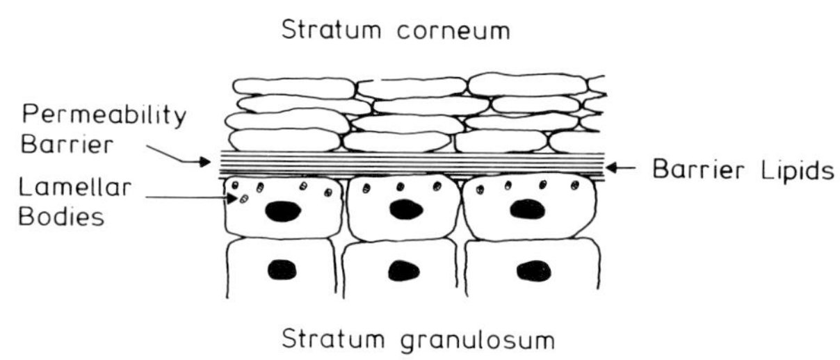

Fig. 1. The epidermal permeability barrier and the two-compartment model of the stratum corneum

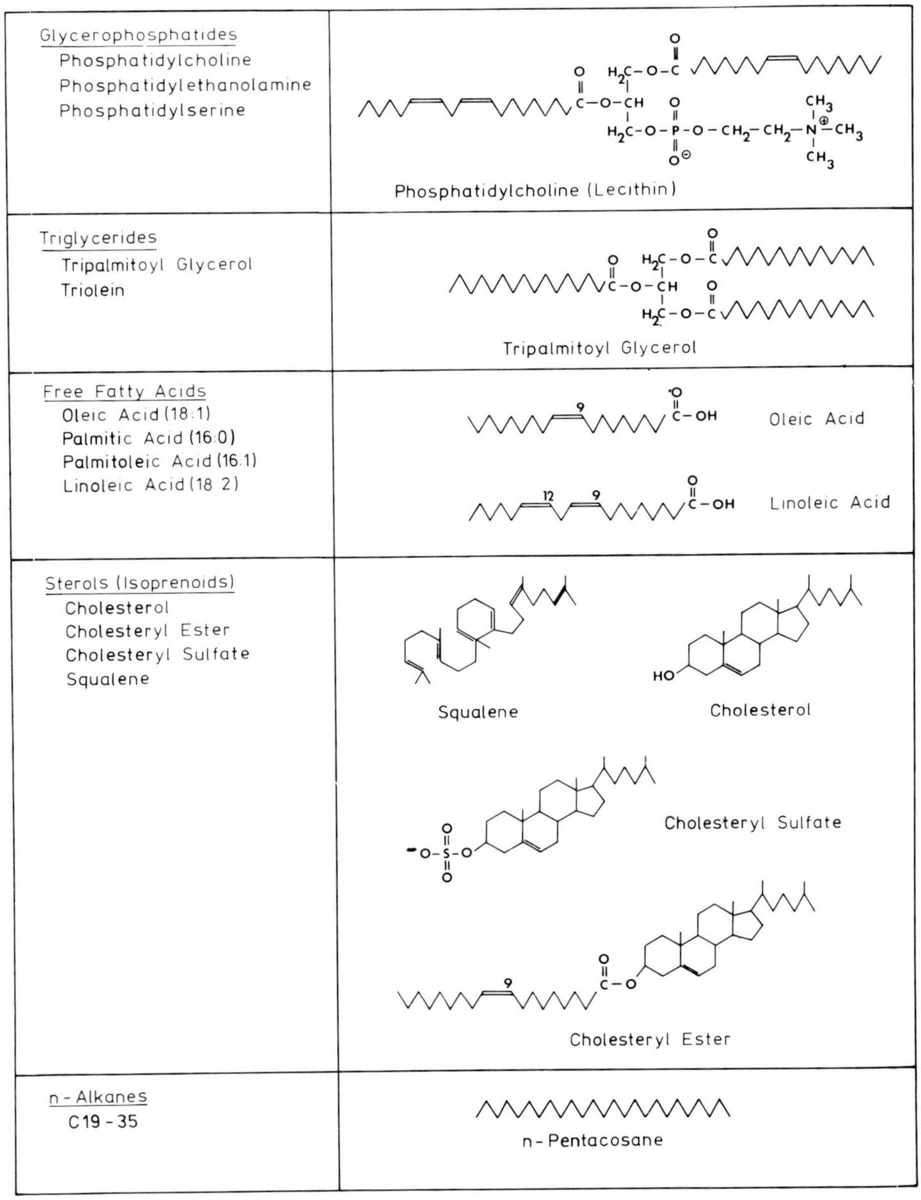

Fig. 2. Chemical structures of important epidermal non-sphingolipids. With permission of Melnik [44]

Phospholipids, which are essential for the maintenance of most cellular membrane bilayers, predominate in the lower layers of the epidermis as in other epithelia [82]. In human stratum corneum, however, phospholipids account for less than 5% of the total [37]. The biotransformation of the stratum granulosum into the stratum corneum is accompanied not only by a remarkable depletion in phospholipids but also by an increase in the levels of neutral lipids as well as by a large increase in the concentration of sphingolipids, especially ceramides [37] (Table 1). The relative amount of shingolipids increases in human epidermis from 7.3% in the basal layers (stratum basale and spinosum) to 18.1% in the whole stratum corneum, reaching 26.6% in the outer stratum corneum [37].

Table 1. Changes of the lipid composition of the epidermal layers during epidermal differentiation. Data according to Lampe et al. [37]

Lipid fraction (Weight %)	Stratum basale and spinosum	Stratum granulosum	Stratum corneum
Phospholipids	44.5 ± 3.4	25.3 ± 2.6	4.9 ± 1.6
Cholesterol sulphate	2.4 ± 0.5	5.5 ± 1.3	1.5 ± 0.2
Clucosylceramides	3.5 ± 0.3	5.8 ± 0.3	Trace
Ceramides	3.8 ± 0.2	8.8 ± 0.3	18.1 ± 0.4
Free sterols	11.2 ± 1.7	11.5 ± 1.1	14.0 ± 1.1
Free fatty acids	7.0 ± 2.1	9.2 ± 1.5	19.3 ± 3.7
Triglycerides	12.4 ± 2.9	24.7 ± 4.0	25.2 ± 4.6
Sterol and wax esters	5.3 ± 1.3	4.7 ± 0.7	5.4 ± 0.9
Squalene	4.9 ± 1.1	4.6 ± 1.0	4.8 ± 2.0
n-Alkanes	3.9 ± 0.3	3.8 ± 0.8	6.1 ± 2.6

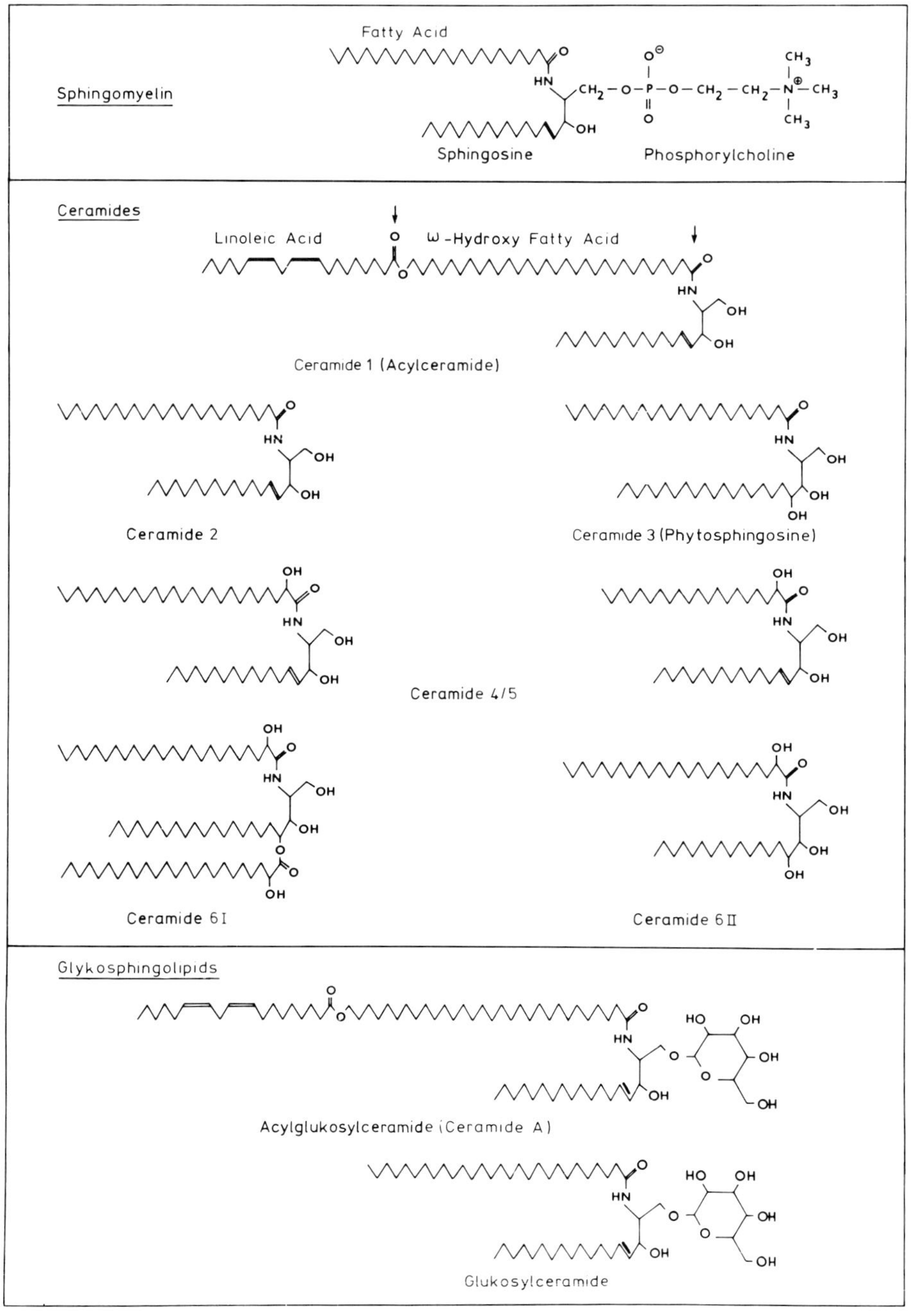

Fig. 3. Chemical structures of important epidermal sphingolipids. With permission of Melnik [44]

The ceramides represent a unique heterogenous class of barrier lipids [25]. In human stratum corneum six structurally distinct series of ceramides were identified [42, 71] (Fig. 3). They are composed of the long-chain aminoalcohols sphingosine or phytosphingosine with amide-linked, non-hydroxy and α-hydroxy fatty acids. The most unusual of the epidermal ceramides, designated ceramide 1, consists of a spingosine base with an amide-linked, long-chain, Ω-hydroxy fatty acid and an ester-linked, non-hydroxy acid, 41% of which proved to be linoleic acid. Evidence has accumulated that this ceramide ester serves as a molecular rivet locking together the multiple intercellular lipid membranes within the stratum corneum [67, 68]. In human keratinocytes cultivated at an air-medium interface, it could be demonstrated that keratinocytes have the ability to incorporate exogenous fatty acids preferentially into complex lipids [56]. Triacylglycerols provide a pool of fatty acids for phospholipid synthesis, whereas palmitate and de novo-synthesised fatty acids are preferentially utilised for sphingolipid synthesis [56]. From time course studies of lipid biosynthesis in pig epidermis after intradermal injection of [^{14}C]acetate, it became apparent that virtually all of the radioactivity in the aliphatic chains was incorporated first into phospholipids and then transferred to glucosylceramides and subsequently into ceramides [31].

The pathway of ceramide esterification with linoleic acid is not completely understood at present. Preliminary data indicate that the essential linoleic acid is transported by a specific cytosolic fatty acid binding protein [57]. It is remarkable that rat, guinea pig and normal human epidermis lack the capacity to transform linoleic acid into arachidonic acid due to an absence of epidermal δ-6- and δ-5-desaturase activities [6, 7]. Therefore, it is most likely that this inability to biosynthesise arachidonic acid from epidermal linoleic acid represents an evolutionary protective mechanism to ensure that plasma-derived linoleic acid is not consumed by eicosanoid biosynthesis but remains available to permeability barrier requirements, i.e. biosynthesis of linoleate-containing acylceramides. Thus, the mode of transport of essential fatty acids to the epidermal cells, the role of epidermal fatty acid binding proteins and cellular fatty acid carrier systems remain to be elucidated.

Glucosylceramides are glucosylated versions of the ceramides in which the β-*D*-glucopyranosyl moiety is glycosidically linked to the 1-hydroxyl group of the long-chain base. Most intriguing among the epidermal glycosphingolipids is a compound called glucosylceramide A, an acylglucosylceramide which accounts for nearly 50% of the total glycolipids [1] (Fig. 3). The Ω-hydroxyl group of the hydroxy acid bears the ester-linked linoleic acid moiety. Acylglucosylceramides are enriched in lamellar bodies (Odland bodies) [70] as will be discussed later. In the keratinising epidermis the ceramides increase proportionately in the stratum corneum while glucosylceramides decrease. Under physiological conditions glucosylceramides are found only in the viable epidermis and not in the stratum corneum [82], whereas in disorders of differentiation glycolipids are detectable in the stratum corneum [82]. Yet, it is not clear to what extent ceramides are synthesised de novo or are derived from hydrolysis of glucosylceramides and sphingomyelin. Interestingly, in human fetal epidermis, after 110 days of estimated gestational age, ceramides and glycosphingolipids become increasingly prominent. These changes in epidermal lipid composition correspond morphologically to the progressive emergence of both folliculocentric epidermal cornification and sebaceous gland development [78].

Sterols, together with ceramides and free fatty acids, account for nearly all the keratinocyte-derived lipids of the stratum corneum. In human epidermis most sterols are present as cholesterol. In human stratum corneum the fraction of free sterols accounts for 14% of total lipids [36]. Sterol esters are more prominent in the stratum corneum than in the Malpighian layers. Both free and esterified cholesterol increase slightly during epidermal differentiation [37].

Cholesterol sulphate, a minor polar lipid of the stratum corneum comprising about 1.5% of the total deserves special mention. It is one of the few remaining polar amphipathic lipids in the stratum corneum and probably is of critical importance in maintaining the intercorneocyte lipid bilayers [74, 77]. Cholesterol sulphate reaches its highest level in the stratum granulosum, diminishing in the stratum corneum and nearly disappearing from the outer stratum corneum [37, 42]. The lower layers of the epidermis actively synthesise cholesterol for their own growth and membrane requirements. In the stratum basale and spinosum a minor cholesterol moiety is sulphated by the action of the enzyme cholesterol sulphotransferase, which transfers a sulphate group from an active sulphate, e.g. 3'-phosphoadenosine-5'-phosphosulphate, to cholesterol [20]. It could be shown that an increase in cholesterol sulphate and cholesterol sulphotransferase activity is related to the multistep process of differentiation in human epidermal keratinocytes [34]. The cholesterol sulphate accumulation as well as the increase in cholesterol sulphotransferase and transglutaminase activities were inhibited by retinoids [34]. These findings indicate that human epidermis accumulates cholesterol sulphate when undergoing squamous differentiation and might explain its increased vulnerability and transepidermal water loss, especially in the epidermis of atopic patients, during retinoid treatment.

Steroid sulphatase (sterol sulphate sulphohydrolase, EC 3.1.6.2) hydrolyses sulphate esters of 3-β-hydroxysterols, including cholesterol sulphate [58]. Steroid sulphatase activity leaves its microsomal location in the stratum granulosum to accumulate in the outer membrane region of corneocytes [19]. Continual and controlled hydrolysis of cholesterol sulphate by steroid sulphatase appears to be a critical factor for the destabilisation of the intercorneocyte lipid lamellae, promoting corneocyte desquamation [74, 77]. This concept is supported by the fourfold decrease of cholesterol sulphate from cohesive versus desquamated stratum corneum [42] and in X-linked recessive ichthyosis by the association with steroid sulphatase deficiency and accumulation of cholesterol sulphate in the stratum corneum [19, 58, 75].

The triglyceride and free fatty acid levels also increase as the epidermis differentiates. In the whole stratum corneum, triglycerides account for 25% and free fatty acids for 19% of total lipids, respectively [36]. Whether the increasing amounts of free fatty acids are derived from hydrolysis of phospholipids and acylglucosylceramides or predominantly from de novo synthesis is not known.

Squalene and *n*-alkanes can be demonstrated in human epidermis under physiological as well as pathological conditions [74, 77]. It is thought that the former represents contamination by sebaceous lipids and the latter, contamination from the environment or topical treatment. However, both hydrocarbons have been detected in plantar stratum corneum [36], where sebaceous glands are absent, as well as in isolated populations of human epidermal cells [37]. The straightchain, fully saturated *n*-alkanes form a homologous series with a bellshaped distribution from C19 to C35 revealing a peak at C25/26 with an equal representation of both odd and even chains [76]. In a series of time-course experiments in which pig epidermal lipids were labelled by intradermal injection of [^{14}C]acetate, biosynthesis of *n*-alkanes was not observed [30]. On the other hand, the biosynthesis of *n*-alkanes by mammalian cells seems possible as there is evidence of alkane synthesis by the sciatic nerve of the rabbit [5].

Furthermore, it has been recognised that mammals are able to catabolise hydrocarbons, and this enzymatic activity most likely resides in the cytochrome P-450 system [2].

The composition of stratum corneum lipids displays remarkable regional intra-individual variations, reflecting differences in stratum corneum thickness as well as skin permeability [36].

The Lipid Concept of the Epidermal Permeability Barrier

The important lipid biochemical events for the formation of the permeability barrier occur at the interface of the stratum granulosum and stratum corneum. At this interface between viable and non-viable epidermal layers, the majority of the intracellular lipids of the granular cells are extruded into the intercorneocyte space. In the granular cells as well as in the intercellular space of the stratum corneum, the lipid molecules are highly ordered and arranged into multilamellar bilayer structures [39, 40, 60].

In the granular layer most of the lipid destined for the intercorneocyte space is packed and transported in unique, 0.2 –0.3 μm diameter, ovoid, secretory organelles, the lamellar bodies (Odland bodies). These contain stacks of lipid-rich discs exhibiting alternately electron-lucent and electron-dense ultrastructure [39]. The organelles are produced primarily in the spinous cells and seem to originate from the Golgi apparatus [38]. After being displaced to the apex of the granular cells, they fuse with the plasma membrane, thereby secreting their contents into the intercellular space of the stratum corneum [11, 29, 80]. Recent lipid biochemical characterisation of the content of lamellar bodies confirmed the electron microscopical observation that the intercellular lipids of the stratum corneum are derived from exocytosis of these organelles [39, 40]. Lamellar body-enriched subcellular fractions contain lipids nearly identical to those found in the stratum corneum [23, 26, 70]. Thus, the process of intercellular lipid sequestration imparts to the stratum corneum the unique two-compartment configuration of lipid-depleted cells embedded in multilamellar lipid sheets.

It has been suggested that the acylglucosylceramides serve in the assembly of the stacks of membranous discs seen within the lamellar bodies [69]. The Ω-hydroxyacyl chain of an acylglucosylceramide could extend through one bilayer of a flattened discoid liposome, while the linoleyl group would extend into an adjacent flattened liposome, thus locking the two together. A similar flattening effect of liposomes is expected from ceramide 1 [67]. This hypothesis is supported by the experimental formation of flattened discoid liposomes by adding 5% of an acylglucosylceramide to spherical phosphatidylcholine:cholesterol liposomes [41]. Further evidence comes from the observation that in essential fatty acid deficiency (EFAD), lamellar bodies lack lamellae [13], most likely due to the absence of linoleic acid from acylglucosylceramides [69].

Upon extrusion into the intercorneocyte space, the tightly packed discs of lamellar bodies are reorganised and coalesce into broad bilayer sheets [16], forming the epidermal barrier to water diffusion. The unstacking of the discs and formation of the sheets involve edge-to-edge fusion of the discs and glycolipid catabolism [39, 67].

The epidermal permeability barrier not only depends on the presence of ceramides but also on the homeostasis of epidermal sterol metabolism. Evidence for this comes from the observation of a two- to threefold stimulation of epidermal sterologenesis after solvent or detergent disruption of the epidermal barrier function [47]. This indicates that the water content of the stratum corneum plays a role in the regulation of epidermal cholesterol biosynthesis. In mice deficient in essential fatty acids and with disrupted epidermal barrier function, the greater transepidermal water loss was accompanied by a twofold increase in epidermal cholesterol synthesis [21]. Taken together, these data indicate that epidermal sterologenesis responds to water barrier requirements [27].

Disturbed Epidermal Permeability Barrier in Essential Fatty Acid Deficiency

The epidermal permeability barrier is a very important functional product of epidermal differentiation, protecting the organism from the loss of essential body fluids and restricting the penetration of chemicals, allergens, water and microorganisms. The principal structural element providing the barrier function is the intercorneocyte lipid lamellae. Further clarification is derived from studies on essential fatty acid-deficient animals, in which oleic acid replaces the essential linoleic acid in the O-acylated sphingolipids [68]. Under these conditions, lamellar bodies reveal an amorphous appearance rather than discrete stacks of lamellae, and the intercellular membranes of the stratum corneum are markedly disturbed, a condition which leads to excessive transepidermal water loss [13].

Recently, it has been discovered that besides the presence of intercorneocyte lipid lamellae each corneocyte appears to possess a lipid envelope consisting of a monomolecular layer of *N*-(Ω-hydroxyacyl)-sphingosines that are ester-linked to proteins of the outer corneocyte membrane [59]. This corneocyte lipid envelope may also play a role in the barrier function and in corneocyte cohesion.

The structural lipids of the intercorneocyte lamellae are not only involved in the regulation of epidermal permeability but are also critical for the water-holding properties of the stratum corneum, providing a reservoir function for stratum corneum hydration [32, 33]. Solvent challenge experiments of human stratum corneum indicate that the water-holding properties of the horny layer depend predominantly on the presence of ceramides [32, 33]. Disturbances of the relative composition of various ceramide fractions in surfactant-induced, dry, scaling human skin without affecting the total lipid content of the stratum corneum support this also [24]. From these observations it can be expected that deficiencies in epidermal ceramide or acylceramide biosynthesis might impair epidermal barrier function, leading to dry, scaling skin.

The essential fatty acid linoleic acid is intimately involved in barrier lipid synthesis and the maintenance of epidermal integrity [4, 45, 83]. The clinical similarities between the skin changes in EFAD and AE might reflect common pathological mechanisms.

The symptoms of EFAD in mammals were first described in 1929 [3]. Experimental EFAD produces an ichthyosiform dermatitis characterised by scaling and impaired barrier function with increased transepidermal water loss [13, 51, 52]. After surgical or dietary intervention, especially prolonged parenteral nutrition or alcoholism, the clinical syndrome of EFAD develops in humans [49, 51, 61].

The essential fatty acids are long-chain, unsaturated lipids, so named because they are essential to the diet of mammals as they cannot be synthesised de novo. Mammalian cells are unable to desaturate fatty acids at the Ω-6 position. There are two major essential fatty acids, both of the Ω-6 configuration (denoting the position of the first methylene-interrupted double bond, numbered from the methyl end of the chains): linoleic acid (18:2n6), the most common essential fatty acid, and arachidonic acid (20:4n6), its chain elongation product and precursor for eicosanoid synthesis [55].

Excessively increased transepidermal water loss is a characteristic feature of EFAD; as the water barrier is known to reside in the multiple intercellular lipid sheets of the stratum corneum, it is conceivable that a deficiency in essential fatty acids affects the structure and function of the lipid bilayers [27]. Arachidonic acid given intraperitoneally will heal the skin scaliness rapidly without repairing the disturbed barrier function. Conversely, topically applied or intraperitoneally administered linoleate has been reported to restore the barrier function of EFAD rats, independent of its role in prostaglandin metabolism [17, 52, 53]. These findings suggest that linoleate or molecules containing linoleate are involved in the maintenance of the epidermal water barrier. These functionally extremely important molecules are the linoleate-rich *O*-acylsphingolipids [25, 67–69, 72]. It was demonstrated that *O*-acylsphingolipids are unique constituents of all keratinising epithelia and reflect the presence of lamellar bodies [67]. The linoleate-rich acylglucosylceramides are the driving force behind the formation and integrity of the lamellar bodies [68]. In EFAD, linoleate is replaced by oleate in *O*-acylspingolipids [69]. Due to this substitution the physical properties of these particular sphingolipids are markedly altered, resulting in the failure to form lamellar bodies and leading to severe disturbances of the intercorneocyte lipid sheets, where only occasional fragments of lipid lamellae are detectable [13]. Consequently, the water barrier breaks down.

At present, there is only scarce information about epidermal biosynthesis of linoleate-containing sphingolipids. Recently, a cytosolic fatty acid binding protein was identified in murine epidermis and human keratinocytes [57]. This 60 K protein, which preferentially binds linoleic acid, probably delivers linoleic acid to ceramide acyltransferase for the synthesis of *O*-linoleyl-ceramides required for the structural and functional integrity of the multilamellar lipid sheets of the stratum corneum.

Disturbed Barrier Function in Atopic Dry Skin

AE is a chronic, intermittent, inflammatory skin condition characterised by erythema, dryness and severe pruritus. Patients with seemingly complete remissions retain a tendency toward dry, easily irritated skin, hand dermatitis and recurrence of disease activity after occupational and emotional stress [8]. Many patients have dry-looking skin in non-predilection areas such as the back and lower legs. A high incidence of viral and bacterial infections of the skin and of non-allergic hand eczema are clinical evidence indicating defective barrier function.

Furthermore, the physical properties of the stratum corneum are altered in dry non-eczematous skin of patients with AE. In dry skin in AE as well as in clinically normal-appearing skin on predilection sites of AE, for instance the hands and forearms, increased transepidermal water loss has been determined [64]. The elevated transepidermal water loss in eczematous and clinically non-eczematous atopic skin indicates a defective epidermal permeability barrier. A low water content of the stratum corneum in atopic dry skin [63] and a reduced water-binding capacity [65] are physical evidence for disturbed barrier function.

It is not known whether atopic dry skin results from subclinical dermatitis, i.e. inflammation-induced alterations of epidermal differentiation leading to defective barrier function [22, 62], or whether atopic xerosis might result from primary barrier defects, predisposing to AE [4].

In comparison with normal skin a relative increase in the volume of lamellar bodies in the transition zone between the stratum granulosum and the stratum corneum has been demonstrated in non-eczematous dry skin of patients with AE [66]. This ultrastructural finding points to disturbances in the maturation or biochemical differentiation of lamellar body contents, which might reflect abnormalities of their lipid compounds. Alterations of lamellar body-derived lipids might result in a leaky barrier which could explain the disturbed barrier properties of atopic dry skin. Indeed, biochemical analyses of epidermal lipids of patients with AE support the hypothesis that defective barrier function of atopic dry skin results from disturbances of epidermal lipid metabolism [4, 45, 48].

Alterations of Epidermal Lipids in Atopic Eczema

In 1967, Mustakallio et al. [48] analysed the composition of epidermal lipids from the volar sites of the forearm of 12 patients with AE after isolation of epidermis by the suction blister technique. They found a decrease of total epidermal lipids content, i.e. 12.4% ± 0.8% in eczematous epidermis compared with 15.4% ± 1.2% in normal epidermis of non-atopic subjects. In eczematous epidermis levels of phosphatidylethanolamine, mono-, di- and triglycerides as well as sterol esters were diminished. In contrast, levels of free fatty acids and sterols were elevated. It should be remembered that increased sterologenesis has been shown to be a response to increased transepidermal water loss or perturbations of barrier function [21, 27, 47]. Some patients with AE exhibit remarkable elevations of *n*-alkanes. Interestingly, cerebrosides and an unidentified fraction "X_2" were decreased compared with normal epidermis. Retrospectively, these diminished fractions most likely represent epidermal ceramides or acylceramides, which was not known at that time.

In order to confirm this proposal, Melnik et al. [45] analysed stratum corneum lipids of untreated, non-inflamed, plantar skin of 10 patients with AE and 10 healthy, age-matched controls by sequential high-performance thin-layer chromatography [46]. A significant decrease in total ceramides, expressed as percentage of total stratum corneum lipids, was determined in patients with AE (29.0% ± 3.6%, mean ± SEM) compared with the controls (35.0% ± 3.2%) [45]. Although statistically not significant, an increase of free sterols in the stratum corneum of patients with AE corresponded to the findings of Mustakallio et al. [48].

These observations point to an impaired ceramide biosynthesis and probably increased compensatory sterologenesis in patients with AE, resulting in xerosis with increased transepidermal water loss and diminished water-holding capacity of "atopic" stratum corneum.

On the other hand, the dry skin of patients with AE has also been explained by impaired sebaceous gland activity. In infantile AE, sebaceous glands with lipid-depleted basal cells were observed histologically [50]. In AE the sebaceous gland size, number of glands per skin area and their proliferative activity were significantly reduced while the S-phase of the sebocytes was prolonged compared with that of normal subjects [79]. Levels of skin surface lipids, which are a mixture of sebaceous and epidermal lipids, were decreased on the back of the hand of patients with AE [54]. Although other investigators found no differences in the sebum secretion rate and sebum composition between atopic and non-atopic subjects, the sebum secretion rate in the former was lower than that of a comparable group with acne [9]. Nevertheless, there appears to be sufficient evidence for diminished sebaceous gland activity in atopic skin [73], but the disturbances of keratinocyte-derived stratum corneum lipids, i.e. the barrier lipids, seem to be of greater relevance for defective barrier function and the dry appearance. Furthermore, impaired sebaceous gland activity appears not to play a major role in the development of atopic xerosis and abnormal transepidermal water loss as clinical experience indicates that there are no quantitative differences in dry scaling skin in prepubertal versus postpubertal atopic individuals. Finally, it should be emphasised that sebaceous glands do not synthesise ceramides and acylceramides, which are the functionally important lipids for the integrity of the permeability barrier.

Perspectives for Improvement of Disturbed Barrier Function in Atopic Dry Skin

The ceramides and acylceramides are very unique mammalian lipids which are predominantly found in two locations, the central nervous system and the epidermis, where they play a crucial role in the integrity of barrier systems.

The chemical isolation and preparation of ceramides from natural sources, for instance from pig epidermis or bovine brain, for topical treatment is very expensive. Chemical ceramide synthesis is uneconomical as well, because the aminoalcohols sphingosine and phytosphingosine are not available on a large scale basis. Thus, the synthesis of ceramide or acylceramide analogues, i.e. chemically synthesised pseudo-ceramide derivatives, might overcome these difficulties. It is remarkable that the influence of this functionally important class of sphingolipids (comprising about 15%–35% of total stratum corneum barrier lipids) was not recognised until some years ago. Subsequently, this class of lipids was not used for topical treatment and restoration of disturbed barrier function in various skin conditions with defective permeability barrier function like AE.

At present, several pharmaceutical companies are focussing their efforts on the identification of efficient ceramide analogues and vehicle conditions in order to provide improved topical steroid-sparing treatment modalities for atopic dry skin. The restoration of the disturbed transepidermal water flux and water-binding capacity of atopic dry skin by pseudo-ceramides is a promising new therapeutic approach, especially in dermatitis-free intervals, which might diminish recurrences of AE as barrier-defective dry skin is known to predispose to exacerbations of inflammatory episodes. Thus, the stabilisation and restoration of disturbed barrier function in atopic skin are of great relevance in occupational dermatology and preventive medicine [43].

References

1. Abraham W, Wertz PW, Downing DT (1985) Linoleate-rich polar lipids of epidermis: structure determination by proton magnetic resonance. Clin Res 33:621 A
2. Bickers DR (1983) Drug, carcinogen, and steroid hormone metabolism in the skin. In: Goldsmith LA (ed) Biochemistry and physiology of the skin, vol 2, 1. Oxford University Press, New York, pp 1169–1186
3. Burr GO, Burr MM (1929) A new deficiency disease produced by the rigid exclusion of fat from the diet. J Biol Chem 82:345–367
4. Burton JL (1989) Dietary fatty acids and inflammatory skin disease. Lancet i:27–31
5. Cassagne C, Carriet D (1977) Evidence of alkane synthesis by the sciatic nerve of the rabbit. FEBS Lett 82:51–54
6. Chapkin RS, Ziboh VA (1984) Inability of skin enzyme preparations to biosynthesize arachidonic acid from linoleic acid. Biochem Biophys Res Commun 124:784–792
7. Chapkin RS, Ziboh VA, Marcelo CL, Vorhees JJ (1986) Metabolism of essential fatty acids by human epidermal enzyme preparations. evidence of chain elongation. J Lipid Res 27:945–954
8. Cheng DS, Hanifin JM (1986) Atopic dermatitis. In: Thiers BH, Dobson RL (eds) Pathogenesis of skin disease. Churchill Livingstone, New York, pp 13–23
9. Ead RD, Fairbank RA, Cunliffe WJ (1977) Sebum excretion rate, surface lipid composition and constitutional eczema. Clin Exp Dermatol 2:361–364
10. Elias PM (1981) Epidermal lipids, membranes, and keratinization. Int J Dermatol 20:1–19
11. Elias PM (1987) Epidermal lipids, barrier function and desquamation. J Invest Dermatol 80:44s–49s
12. Elias PM (1987) Plastic wrap revisited. The stratum corneum two-compartment model and its clinical implications. Arch Dermatol 123:1405–1406
13. Elias PM, Brown BE (1978) The mammalian cutaneous permeability barrier. Defective barrier function in essential

fatty acid deficiency correlates with abnormal intercellular lipid deposition. Lab Invest 39:574–583
14. Elias PM, Friend DS (1975) The permeability barrier in mammalian epidermis. J Cell Biol 65:180–191
15. Elias PM, Leventhal ME (1979) Intercellular volume changes and cell surface expansion during cornification. Clin Res 27:525
16. Elias PM, Goerke J, Friend DS (1977) Mammalian epidermal barrier layer lipids: composition and influence on structure. J Invest Dermatol 69:535–546
17. Elias PM, Brown BE, Ziboh VA (1980) Permeability barrier in essential fatty acid deficiency: Evidence for a direct role for linoleic acid in epidermal barrier function. J Invest Dermatol 74:230–233
18. Elias PM, Grayson S, Lampe MA, Williams ML, Brown BE (1983) The intercorneocyte space. In: Marks R, Plewig G (eds) Stratum corneum. Springer, Berlin, Heidelberg, New York, pp 53–67
19. Elias PM, Williams ML, Maloney ME, Bonifas JA, Brown BE, Grayson S, Epstein EH Jr (1984) Stratum corneum lipids in disorders of cornification: steroid sulfatase and cholesterol sulfate in normal desquamation and the pathogenesis of recessive X-linked ichthyosis. J Clin Invest 74:1414–1421
20. Epstein EH Jr, Bonifas JM, Barber TC, Haynes M (1984) Cholesterol sulfotransferase of newborn mouse epidermis. J Invest Dermatol 83:332–335
21. Feingold KR, Brown BE, Lear SR, Moser AH, Elias PM (1986) Effect of essential fatty acid deficiency on cutaneous sterol synthesis. J Invest Dermatol 87:588–591
22. Finlay AY, Nicholls S, King CS, Marks R (1980) The "dry" non-eczematous skin associated with atopic eczema. Br J Dermatol 102:249–255
23. Freinkel RK, Traczyk TN (1985) Lipid composition and acid hydrolase content of lamellar granules of fetal rat epidermis. J Invest Dermatol 85:295–298
24. Fulmer AW, Kramer GJ (1986) Stratum corneum lipid abnormalities in surfactant-induced dry scaling skin. J Invest Dermatol 86:598–602
25. Gray GM, White RJ (1978) Glycosphingolipids and ceramides in human and pig epidermis. J Invest Dermatol 70: 336–341
26. Grayson S, Johnson-Winegar AG, Wintroub BV, Isseroff RR, Epstein EH Jr, Elias PM (1985) Lamellar body-enriched fractions from neonatal mice: preparative techniques and partial characterization. J Invest Dermatol 85: 289–294
27. Grubauer G, Feingold KR, Elias PM (1987) Relationship of epidermal lipogenesis to cutaneous barrier function. J Lipid Res 28:746–752
28. Hanifin JM, Rajka G (1980) Diagnostic features of atopic dermatitis. Acta Derm Venereol [Suppl] (Stockh.) 92:44–47
29. Hashimoto K (1971) Cementosomes, a new interpretation of the membrane-coating granule. Arch Dermatol Forsch 240: 349–364
30. Hedberg CL, Wertz PW, Downing DT (1988) The nonpolar lipids of pig epidermis. J Invest Dermatol 90:225–229
31. Hedberg CL, Wertz PW, Downing DT (1988) The time course of lipid biosynthesis in pig epidermis. J Invest Dermatol 91:169–174
32. Imokawa G, Hattori M (1985) A possible function of structural lipids in the water-holding properties of the stratum corneum. J Invest Dermatol 84:282–284
33. Imokawa G, Akasaki S, Hattori M, Yoshizuka N (1986) Selective recovery of deranged water-holding properties by stratum corneum lipids. J Invest Dermatol 87:758–761
34. Jetten AM, George MA, Nervi C, Boone LR, Rearick JI (1989) Increased cholesterol sulfate and cholesterol sulfotransferase activity in relation to the multi-step process of differentiation in human epidermal keratinocytes. J Invest Dermatol 92:203–209
35. Kooyman DJ (1932) Lipids of the skin. Some changes in the lipids of the epidermis during the process of keratinization. Arch Dermatol Syph 25:444–450
36. Lampe MA, Burlingame AL, Whitney J, Williams ML, Brown BE, Roitman E, Elias PM (1983) Human stratum corneum lipids: characterization and regional variations. J Lipid Res 24:120–130
37. Lampe MA, Williams ML, Elias PM (1983) Human epidermal lipids: characterization and modulations during differentiation. J Lipid Res 24:131–140
38. Landmann L (1980) Lamellar granules in mammalian, avian and reptilian epidermis. J Ultrastruct Res 72:245–263
39. Landmann L (1986) Epidermal permeability barrier: transformation of lamellar granule-disks into intercellular sheets by a membrane fusion process, a freeze-fracture study. J Invest Dermatol 87:202–209
40. Landmann L (1988) The epidermal permeability barrier. Anat Embryol (Berl) 178:1–13
41. Landmann L, Wertz PW, Downing DT (1984) Acylglucosylceramide causes flattening and stacking of liposomes. An analogy for assembly of the epidermal permeability barrier. Biochim Biophys Acta 778:412–418
42. Long SA, Wertz PW, Strauss JS, Downing DT (1985) Human stratum corneum polar lipids and desquamation. Arch Dermatol Res 277:284–287
43. Melnik B (1989) Epidermale Lipide. In: Macher E, Knop J, Bröcker EB (eds) Jahrbuch der Dermatologie 1988. Regensberg and Biermann, Münster, pp 121–139
44. Melnik B (1989) Epidermal lipids and the biochemistry of keratinization. In: Traupe H (ed) The ichthyoses. Springer, Berlin, Heidelberg, New York, pp 15–42
45. Melnik B, Hollmann J, Plewig G (1988) Decreased stratum corneum ceramides in atopic individuals – a pathobiochemical factor for xerosis? Br J Dermatol 119:547–549
46. Melnik B, Hollmann J, Erler E, Verhoeven B, Plewig G (1989) Microanalytical thin-layer chromatography of all major stratum corneum lipids. J Invest Dermatol 92:231–234
47. Menon GK, Feingold KR, Moser AH, Brown BE, Elias PM (1985) De novo sterologenesis in the skin. II. Regulation by cutaneous barrier requirements. J Lipid Res 26:418–427
48. Mustakallio KK, Kiistala U, Piha HJ, Nieminen E (1967) Epidermal lipids in Besnier's prurigo (atopic eczema). Ann Med Exp Biol Fenn 45:323–325
49. Paulsrud JR, Pensler L, Whitten CF, Stewart S, Holman RT (1972) Essential fatty acid deficiency in infants induced by fat-free intravenous feeding. Am J Clin Nutr 25:897–904
50. Prose PH (1965) Pathologic changes in eczema. J Pediatr 66:178–199
51. Prottey C (1976) Essential fatty acids and the skin. Br J Dermatol 94:579–587
52. Prottey C (1977) Investigation of functions of essential fatty acids in the skin. Br J Dermatol 97:29–38
53. Prottey C, Hartop PJ, Black JG, Mc Cormack JI (1976) The repair of impaired epidermal barrier function in rats by cutaneous application of linoleic acid. Br J Dermatol 94: 13–21
54. Rajka G (1974) Surface lipid estimation on the back of the hand in atopic dermatitis. Arch Dermatol Forsch 251:167–169

55. Ruzicka T (1988) The physiology and pathophysiology of eicosanoids in the skin. Eicosanoids 1:59–72
56. Schürer NY, Monger DJ, Hincenbergs M, Williams ML (1989) Fatty acid metabolism in human keratinocytes cultivated at an air-medium interface. J Invest Dermatol 92:196–202
57. Schürer NY, Bass NM, Pillai S, Williams ML (1989) Murine epidermis and human keratinocytes contain high-affinity cytosolic fatty acid (FA) binding activity (BA). J Invest Dermatol (abstr) 92:515
58. Shapiro LJ (1983) Steroid sulfatase deficiency and X-linked ichthyosis. In: Stanbury JB, Wyngaarden JB, Frederickson DS, Goldstein JL, Brown MS (eds) The metabolic basis of inherited disease. McGraw-Hill, New York, pp 1027–1039
59. Swartzendruber DC, Wertz PW, Madison KC, Downing DT (1987) Evidence that the corneocyte has a chemically bound lipid envelope. J Invest Dermatol 88:709–713
60. Swartzendruber DC, Wertz PW, Kitko DJ, Madison KC, Downing DT (1989) Molecular models of the intercellular lipid lamellae in mammalian stratum corneum. J Invest Dermatol 92:251–257
61. Truchetet E, Brändle I, Grosshans E (1988) Hautveränderungen, Pathophysiologie und Therapie bei Mangel an essentiellen Fettsäuren. Z Hautkr 63:290–301
62. Uehara M, Miyauchi H (1984) The morphologic characteristics of dry skin in atopic dermatitis. Arch Dermatol 120:1186–1190
63. Werner Y (1986) The water content of the stratum corneum in patients with atopic dermatitis. Measurement with the corneometer CM 420. Acta Derm Venereol (Stockh.) 66: 281–284
64. Werner Y, Lindberg M (1985) Transepidermal water loss in dry and clinically normal skin in patients with atopic dermatitis. Acta Derm Venereol (Stockh.) 65:102–105
65. Werner Y, Lindberg M, Forslind B (1982) The water-binding capacity of stratum corneum in dry non-ecxzematous skin of atopic eczema. Acta Derm Venereol (Stockh.) 62:334–337
66. Werner Y, Lindberg M, Forslind B (1987) Membrane-coating granules in "dry" non-eczematous skin of patients with atopic dermatitis. Acta Derm Venereol (Stockh.) 67: 385–390
67. Wertz PW (1986) Lipids of keratinizing tissues. In: Bereiter-Hahn J, Matoltsy AG, Richards KS (eds) Vertebrates. Springer, Berlin, Heidelberg, New York, pp 815–823 (Biology of the integument, vol 2)
68. Wertz PW, Downing DT (1982) Glycolipids in mammalian epidermis: structure and function in the water barrier. Science 217:1261–1262
69. Wertz PW, Cho ES, Downing DT (1983) Effect of essential fatty acid deficiency on the epidermal sphingolipids of the rat. Biochim Biophys Acta 753:350–355
70. Wertz PW, Downing DT, Freinkel RK, Traczyk TN (1984) Sphingolipids of the stratum corneum and lamellar granules of fetal rat epidermis. J Invest Dermatol 83:193–195
71. Wertz PW, Miethke MC, Long SA, Strauss JS, Downing DT (1985) The composition of the ceramides from human stratum corneum and from comedones. J Invest Dermatol 84:410–412
72. Wertz PW, Swartzendruber DC, Abraham W, Madison KC, Downing DT (1987) Essential fatty acids and epidermal integrity. Arch Dermatol 123:1381–1384
73. Wheatley VR (1986) Diseases with apparent or truly altered sebaceous gland activity. In: Jarrett A (ed) The physiology and pathophysiology of the skin, vol 9. Academic, London, pp 2934–2941
74. Williams ML (1983) The ichthyoses – pathogenesis and prenatal diagnosis: a review of recent advances. Pediatr Dermatol 1:1–24
75. Williams ML, Elias PM (1981) Increased cholesterol sulfate content of stratum corneum in recessive X-linked ichthyosis. J Clin Invest 68:1404–1410
76. Williams ML, Elias PM (1982) n-Alkanes in normal and pathological human scale. Biochem Biophys Res Commun 107:322–328
77. Williams ML, Elias PM (1986) The ichthyoses. In: Thiers BH, Dobson RL (eds) Pathogenesis of skin disease. Churchill Livingstone, New York, pp 519–551
78. Williams ML, Hincenbergs M, Holbrook KA (1988) Skin lipid content during early fetal development. J Invest Dermatol 91:263–268
79. Wirth H, Gloor M, Stoika D (1981) Sebaceous glands in uninvolved skin of patients suffering with atopic dermatitis. Arch Dermatol Res 270:167–169
80. Wolff-Schreiner E (1977) Ultrastructural cytochemistry of the epidermis. Int J Dermatol 16:77–102
81. Yardley HJ (1983) Epidermal lipids. In: Goldsmith LA (ed) Biochemistry and physiology of the skin. Oxford University Press, New York, pp 363–381
82. Yardley HJ, Summerly R (1981) Lipid composition and metabolism in normal and diseased epidermis. Pharmacol Ther 13:357–383
83. Ziboh VA, Chapkin RS (1987) Biologic significance of polyunsaturated fatty acids in the skin. Arch Dermatol 123: 1686a–1690

The Phenomenon of Irritable Skin in Atopic Eczema

R. Gollhausen

Introduction

An essential problem of dermatological research and practice is the lack of techniques to measure the overall function of the skin. Every other medical discipline has more instruments to evaluate the organ of interest, e.g., pulmonology uses the plethysmograph, X-ray, spirography, and other techniques. The most valuable tools of the dermatologist, i.e, his eyes and fingertips, are subjective and difficult to standardize. This dermatological poverty inevitably leads to the problem of conceiving subjective symptoms like irritable or sensitive skin or even of defining skin diseases like atopic eczema (AE).

Problems Regarding Definition of Irritable Skin

Irritable skin can be defined as a lowered irritation threshold to very diverse nonallergic stimuli [60]. Among others, it can stand for pure subjective sensations like increased itchiness or some sort of stinging and burning sensation [62, 105], for undefinable variants of dermatopsychological uneasiness [117], for the tendency to develop nonimmunologic contact urticaria [73, 102], or to develop a dermatitis with histologic signs of perivascular infiltrate and spongiosis [107]. Often it is understood as dry itchy skin. However, the term dry skin is itself not yet defined and can be interpreted as a lack of lipids or water, some sort of roughness or a combination of these attributes [43, 99, 131]. Subjects with other skin types such as a seborrhoeic constitution may also have special skin problems like seborrhoeic dermatitis, acne, intertrigo, folliculitis, or pityriasis versicolor. Fair-skinned individuals are easily sunburned, but do not necessarily have irritable skin [60, 64, 78]. Patients with polymorphic light eruptions, which can be seen as another kind of irritable skin with uncertain pathogenesis, do not necessarily have fair skin or another destined skin type [19, 59, 63, 118].

Therefore, we have to define the term irritable skin in this discussion. In the following, irritable skin stands for the tendency to develop an eczematous reaction after contact with nonallergic stimuli or irritants. Irritants vary so much in character that, knowing the strength of reaction to one irritant it is hardly possible to predict the reaction to another. In his extensive study of irritants in hand eczema, Björnberg found no significant correlation between 11 irritants used, i.e., cantharidin, sapo kalinus, sodium lauryl sulfate (SLS), hydrochloric acid, benzalkonium chloride, croton oil, mercury bichloride, potassium hydroxide, sodium hydroxide, phenol and trichloroacetic acid [19]. This lack of correlation was confirmed by Wahlberg et al., who used only tensides, i.e., SLS, nonanoic acid, and benzalkonium chloride [173], and by Czerwinska-Dihm and Rudzki [42]. They mostly used irritants in chamber tests. The mode of action of irritants is wide; many irritants can even provoke an airborne dermatitis [49].

Many factors influence the degree of irritability such as age, ethnic origin, hardening, sun tan, season, pressure, etc. [38, 54, 71, 72, 78, 107, 111, 112, 121]. The reasons for these effects are not always understood. A wide variation in individual susceptibility to skin damage after contact with irritants is known. Besides the wide interindividual variability, a considerable intraindividual variation exists, which is much higher for irritant than for allergic reactions [4, 44] (own unpublished results).

Problems Regarding the Definition of AE

The diagnostic criteria for AE comprise a whole array of symptoms which are hardly adapted for objective assessment and are often differently weighted, depending on the view of the examining dermatologist [10, 13, 34, 47, 80, 82, 141]. The value of skin testing type I allergens as a marker of AE is still a matter of discussion [10, 11, 41, p. 82f). The positive prick test may hint at a relevant cause in the diagnosis of asthma or allergic rhinitis, but it is of little use in the diagnosis of irritable and/or atopic skin. In hand dermatitis, clinical relevance may be evident, since sensitization to type I allergens is often found in patients with atopic hand dermatitis [41], and avoidance of these allergens may be helpful. Some forms of AE exhibit clear correlation to type I allergens, such as AE which gets worse during pollen season, or after contact with cats or house dust mites [3, 15, 16, 32, 33, 182], but often no such correlation can be found. A wheal and flare reaction does not necessarily mean an allergic pathomechanism [83, 102, 107]. Therefore, a positive skin test on its own may be a nonspecific sign of irritable skin in AE rather than a sign of allergy.

Although the term irritable or sensitive skin, which lacks a clear cut definition by itself, is usually not included in the array of diagnostic criteria [113, 118], there are always some paraphrases of irritable skin in the description of AE.

Paraphrases of Irritable Skin in the Description of AE

Pruritus is a basic feature in the list of diagnostic criteria of AE according to Hanifin and Rajka [82]; itch when sweating and intolerance to wool and lipid solvents are minor features. Rajka [141, p. 63] maintained that a well-done exposure experiment in AE should provoke pruritus, but not necessarily clinical signs of dermatitis. Itch when sweating and intolerance to wool are among the highest graded symptoms for AE in a study on the diagnostic features of AE by Diepgen et al. [48]. It is accepted clinical knowledge that patients with AE have a more sensitive skin, especially to soap and lipid solvents. With regard to other irritants the sensitivity is hardly ever defined.

Pruritus and the Intrinsic Type of AE

Many authors see a lowered itch threshold to stimuli as the hallmark of AE, just as increased bronchial reactivity is characteristic of bronchial asthma. One can speculatively subdivide AE into extrinsic and intrinsic categories analogous to bronchial asthma. In the extrinsic type, one or more specific allergens, harmless to nonsensitized persons, elicit a response. In the intrinsic category, nonspecific substances, which can irritate any person depending upon the intensity of contact cause in sensitive patients an exaggerated response to small amounts, which are well tolerated by nonsensitive persons (Fig. 1). This intrinsic type has not been studied in detail up to now [113, 183].

According to Rajka [136–138], who found the itch to last for a longer time period in un- and involved skin of patients with AE compared to patients with nonatopic eczema or psoriasis, there is a much greater difference in itch duration than in itch threshold. Harnack [84] also emphasized the longer itch duration in patients with AE, although there was a considerable overlap between the tested groups.

Using epicutaneous histamine iontophoresis, Heyer et al. [89] found a reduced itch threshold with low stimuli, but weaker ability to discriminate stronger stimuli in patients with AE in comparison to controls. They attributed this finding, together with a reduced vascular reaction, to desensitisation of cutaneous unmyelinated afferent nerve fibers by histamine.

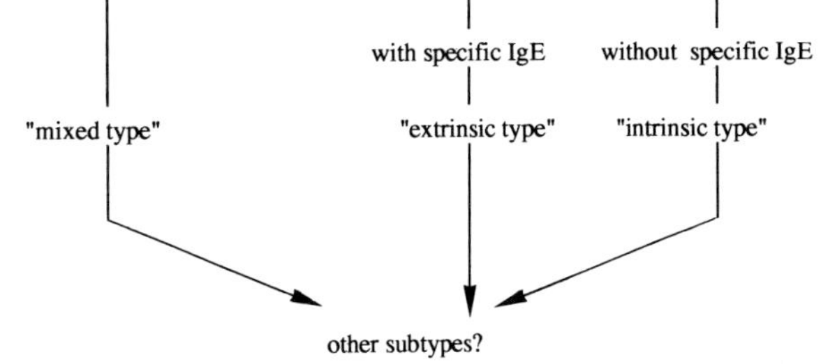

Fig. 1. Classification of atopic eczema. (Modified after Wüthrich [183])

The findings of abnormal pattern of thermoregulation [88], lowered excitation threshold of sudomotor nerves in affected skin [147], altered itch perception, and impaired vasoregulation may indicate a complex regulation disorder of the central and peripheral autonomous nervous system as one pathogenetic factor in AE. Nontheless, satisfying explanations as to why dry, old, or atopic skin itches are lacking.

Pruritus only evokes AE in conjunction with scratching, as demonstrated by Engman et al. [55]. He challenged a 2-year-old atopic child with a known wheat allergen; eczema developed only in skin areas which were not protected from scratching by bandage.

Itch is not only a characteristic sign of AE, but also of many other dermatological disorders, e.g. lichen ruber, nodular prurigo, allergic contact dermatitis, etc. However, response to the itch varies dramatically. In lichen ruber, the patients usually do not so much scratch as rub their skin. In nodular prurigo, they pierce and excoriate the itching papule with their finger nails in order to destroy it. In allergic contact dermatitis, the scratching and rubbing is quite defined to the contact area of the allergen, whereas in AE the region of itching and the response to it are quite diffuse. To date, no reliable method of detecting specific itch responses in AE exists [9, 56, 152].

Itch When Sweating

The nature of itch-inducing stimuli is diverse. No clear data exist about the difference in sweating between patients with AE and controls [141]. There is still some debate about the allergic or irritant nature of sweat-induced itching [2].

Intolerance to Wool

The pruritus of wool intolerance may be induced by the innumerable tiny harpoons of wool fiber endings. It occurs more often in atopic patients, especially those with AE, than in controls or patients with other forms of eczema [17, 79, 86].

Stinging

Another subjective feeling of uneasiness, i.e., burning, or stinging, does not apparently correlate with AE, perhaps due to its short duration. Nonetheless, the clinician should note the AE patients; complaints of stinging sensation after the application of various topical preparations [60, 62, 73, 102, 105, 117].

Intolerance to Lipid Solvents

Intensive use of soap and water is deleterious to atopic skin, although moderate use is harmless [23, 168, 180]. However, the same statement holds true for ichthyotic, dry, or old skin, and any kind of eczema. Since lipids are essential in the "brick and mortar" barrier of the stratum corneum, lipid solvents can break down this first line of defence especially in sebostatic skin conditions [53].

Xerosis

Since dry rough skin can be induced experimentally by irritation, it might be in itself a sign of irritation [61, 129].

Clinical Evidence of Irritable Skin in AE

Recognition and avoidance of irritating factors are considered essential in the management of AE. Large studies involving hand eczema clearly confirm the clinical impression that patients with a personal or family history of atopy are prone to develop hand eczema [14, 36, 40, 41, 103, 109, 130, 150, 151], and patients with atopic hand eczema have a low cure rate [109].

However, Rystedt [149] reported that endogenous factors like the history of hand eczema in childhood, persistent AE, or dry/itchy skin are more important for the development of hand eczema than exogenous factors such as chemicals, water, soil, and wear. In the case of a patient with a history of AE and acute or chronic hand eczema it is nearly impossible to decide whether the nature of the hand eczema is atopic, irritant, or both. This difference is important not only from an academic point of view, but also in the many occupational compensation cases of hand eczema. Why do some atopics and nonatopics develop hand eczema, which predisposes to further skin problems much more than a history of atopy alone [130], and others do not? Children have the highest prevalence of atopic eczema, but not of hand eczema; it is unsettled whether infant skin is more irritable than aged skin. De Boer et al. state that dyshidrotic eczema in metalworkers is a predominantly irritant dermatitis, mainly induced by exposure to soluble oils, and unrelated to atopy [45]. In some studies regarding hand eczema in occupations with exposure to water, atopics are relatively rare. This might be due to the fact that atopics withhold from skin-irritating work [65].

There is much less clinical evidence that atopic patients without AE have more irritable skin than the average population. In spite of this, one should advise atopic patients without present skin symptoms to avoid irritants and to care for their skin, since we know of the easy switch from one atopic symptom to another.

Since neither the diagnosis of irritant dermatitis nor that of AE can be proven by objective tests, the interrelation of reactivity to irritants and AE should be addressed in experimental studies.

Experimental Evidence of Irritable Skin in AE

Irritable skin in AE relates to uninvolved skin beyond the eczematous areas. The problem is how to determine the end of diseased skin and the beginning of normal skin. Dry skin in atopic patients is considered by Uehara [168], and Finlay et al. [57], to be a sign of slight inflammation. However, what is dry skin? Is it skin with a low water or lipid content, or rough skin [131]? Kligman et al. state that it is not definable but represents a family of disorders [99]. If tiny scales are visible [178], the skin is already altered by some kind of damage; a visibly weakened stratum corneum is produced at a greatly accelerated epidermal turnover. A comparison of squamous to normal skin appears senseless, because the skin damage is already visible. In patients with AE, Rajka [141] prefers the term symptomfree skin for the macroscopically normal-looking skin to normal or uninvolved skin, since he believes the total integument of a patient with AE is altered, even if the eczema is only circumscribed. To determine whether the integument of patients with AE is irritable, we have to consider normal-looking skin. Since no definition of what should be regarded as normal-looking and dry skin exists, only a subjective answer can be given.

There are relatively few visually evaluated studies on the effect of irritants in AE. We will not include the reports of altered vascular reactivity which are discussed in a separate chapter (Ryan, this volume).

In an extensive study of sensitive skin by Frosch [60] it was possible to differentiate probands according to their skin sensitivity by a group of tests, i.e., the DMSO test, the ammonium hydroxide minimal blistering time (MBT), the minimal erythema dose (MED) and the chamber test with kerosene, hyamine and croton oil. However, patients with AE and controls were not compared.

Some studies using irritants did not show an increased reactivity in AE. With 1% pentadecylcatechol, similar reactions were induced in probands with and without AE [157]. With dithranol [87] and chrysarobin [141 p.124], even weaker reactions were seen in patients with AE compared to controls. The difficulties of irritant testing are illuminated by a study of Wahlberg et al. [173]: they tested the skin irritancy from various substances in 100 hospitalized patients with different skin diseases and found the highest ID_{50} concentration of SLS and benzalkonium chloride in 16 patients with AE, even though these patients are supposed to be especially sensitive to tensides.

Due to the acid pH of the skin (between 5.4 and 5.9 [24, 153]) the alkali resistance test was considered a valuable test of skin sensitivity [30, 115]. Although alkali resistance can be lowered in the case of status eczematicus, it is of little clinical help in the estimation of skin condition [19]. Burckhardt and Dorta [31] observed a higher incidence of a pathologic alkali resistance test in AE and, comparing the results of several studies, Schnyder et al. [154] came to the same conclusion. However the value of this test is uncertain; other studies could not confirm a lowered alkali resistance in symptomfree skin of patients with AE [66, 70]. The importance of pH of the tenside solution used for washing the skin is often emphasized, but most studies on irritants, especially tensides, show a negligible effect of pH [8, 68, 85, 100, 126, 134, 161, 171]. According to some authors [51, 59, 85, 170, 171], alkaline soaps are better tolerated than syndets.

Rajka [141], Allison and Bettley [6], and Allison and Williamson [7] reported larger cantharidin blisters in AE. Gehse et al. [66] found increased irritability to eight irritant substances, regularly used by nurses and hairdressers, in patients with AE compared to controls, which was significant with two irritants. Gloor et al. [70] tested seven tensides; all of them provoked stronger reactions in patients with AE, although a significant difference was seen with only two tensides. Quite a number of authors have shown the increased aggressiveness of tensides in AE by using noninvasive techniques [74, 164, 170]. Al-Jaberi and Marks [5] found a significantly lowered ammonium hydroxide MBT together with a reduction in the mean corneocyte area in patients with atopic eczema compared to controls.

We looked at the skin sensitivity to UV light, measuring the cutaneous blood flow slope (CBFS) by laser-doppler-flowmetry (Fig. 2). The individual MED to polychromatic UVB (Philips TL/12) was determined on the lower back of eight patients with AE and ten controls.

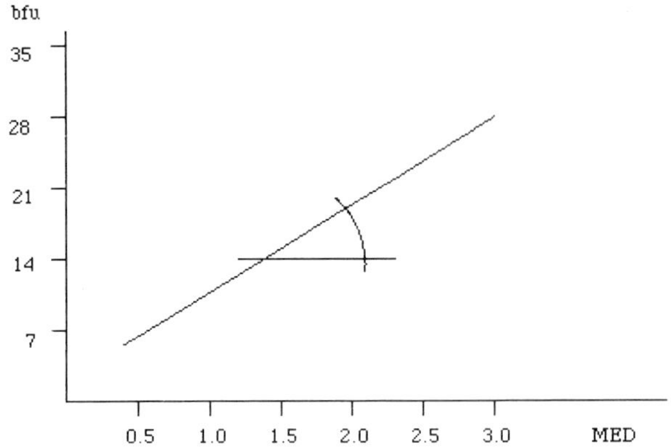

Fig. 2. Determination of the cutaneous blood flow slope (*CBFS*)

Table 1. Minimal erythema dose (MED) and cutaneous blood flow slope (CBFS) in patients with AE and controls

	MED (mJ/cm^2) $x \pm SD$	CBFS (bfu/MED) $x \pm SD$
Patients with AE (8)	66 ± 30	13.8 ± 8.1
Controls (10)	63 ± 25	6.5 ± 4.5
P Value	n.s.	0.027

(x, mean; SD, standard deviation)

Then six fractions of the individual MED, from 0.5–3.0 MED rising in steps of 0.5, were applied. The cutaneous blood flow of each irradiated spot was measured using a laser-doppler flowmeter the following day. The slope of the dose-response curve (increase of cutaneous flood flow per various fractions of the individual minimal erythema), which is approximately linear in the given range, was calculated in each patient. By this method it was possible to differentiate patients with AE and controls, although there was no difference of the MED. Patients with AE had a steeper CBFS, i.e., a higher vascular response to UVB than controls (Table 1) [75, 76].

Stratum Corneum as the Most Important Skin Barrier

The barrier function of the skin is mainly located in the stratum corneum [20, 53]. Although a thinner stratum corneum together with an increased epidermal thickness was reported to occur in AE by some authors [5, 58, 181], this has not generally been described [123] and is not proof of higher irritability. Hamami and Marks [18] found a trend to positive correlation between stratum corneum thickness and irritability in healthy volunteers.

A higher irritability to irritants in dermatitis can be correlated with smaller corneocytes. Al-Jaberi and Marks [5] discussed a link between abnormal small corneocytes and a diminished skin barrier, which was indicated by a lowered ammonium hydroxide MBT. They regarded the higher irritability in uninvolved skin of patients with AE as indicative of an "angry back syndrome" rather than specific for AE. Hölzle and Plewig [91] reported the presence of abnormally small corneocytes in various forms of dermatitis. Studying epidermal structural determinants of the reactions to dithranol and ammonium hydroxide in normal healthy volunteers, Hamami and Marks [78] found a positive correlation between the minimal irritancy dose of dithranol and the mean corneocyte area.

Epidermal lipids are essential for the stratum corneum as the most important skin barrier [50, 53]. Elias [53] developed the two-compartment-model of the stratum corneum where the lipids represent the "mortar" between the "bricks" of cornified cells.

Dry skin is supposed to have too few lipids. Using the absorbent paper technique and chromatography, Rajka [139] measured the skin surface lipids on the back of symptom-free hands of patients with AE and found a decrease in lipids from sebaceous glands such as wax esters, triglycerides, and squalene, and a corresponding increase in epidermal lipids. According to Wirth et al. [181] the sebaceous glands of patients with AE are reduced in size. Jakobza et al. [96] measured an increase of fatty acids with chain length of C14 and C16 and a decrease of branched C18 fatty acids in patients with AE. Abe et al. [1] found significantly lowered sebaceous lipids in uninvolved skin of children with AE compared to controls and a tendency to lower total surface lipids. Mustakallio et al. [127] found a reduction of total epidermal lipids in eczematous skin of atopics. Melnik et al. [122] observed a significant reduction of the ceramides in the stratum corneum of symptom-free plantar skin of patients with AE (see Melnik, this volume). All these studies point to an altered lipid composition in the skin of patients with AE.

There is good correlation between disturbed lipid metabolism of the stratum corneum and transepidermal water loss measured by an evaporimeter, or hydration of the stratum corneum measured by electrical inductivity. Imokawa and Hattori [93] showed a marked decrease in the water-holding capacity of the stratum corneum together with a considerable loss of intercellular lipids such as cholesterol, cholesterol esters and phospholipids. Blanken et al. [21] failed to reduce the elevated

Table 2. Transepidermal water loss (g/m^{2}h) of uninvolved skin in patients with atopic eczema (AE) and controls

Author	Method	Testarea	Controls (C) $x \pm SD$	n	Patients with AE (AE) $x \pm SD$	n	P Value	AE/C quotient
Abe et al. [1]	electrohygrometry	forearm	2.3 ± 0.3	40	3.0 ± 0.6	18	0.001	1.31
Baker and Kligman [12]	electrohygrometry	forearm	2.8 ± 0.3	132	2.9 ± 0.9	22	n.s.	1.04
Finlay et al. [57]	evaporimetry	upperarm	2.9 ± 1.8	11	11.6 ± 5.0	3	0.005	4.04
Gollhausen et al. (unpublished data)	evaporimetry	forearm	9.1 ± 4.2	10	15.3 ± 11.4	8	n.s.	1.68
Rajka [140]	electrohygrometry	back of hand	12.6 ± 1.3	14	16.1 ± 1.5	14	0.025	1.28
Thune [160]	evaporimetry	upperarm	4.8 ± 2.0	17	20.0 ± 7.8	13	not given	4.17
Tupker [164]	evaporimetry	forearm	5.6 ± 1.0	18	7.6 ± 1.5	20	0.05	1.36
Valk v.d. et al. [170]	evaporimetry	forearm	6.5 ± 1.5	19	8.7 ± 2.0	10	0.004	1.34
Werner and Lindberg [176]	evaporimetry	back of hand	9.8 ± 2.2	16	14.6 ± 3.9	16	0.05	1.50
		forearm	4.7 ± 1.9	16	7.6 ± 2.8	16	0.05	1.61
		back	6.6 ± 3.0	16	7.4 ± 2.2	16	n.s.	1.12

x, mean; SD, standard deviation; n.s., not significant

transepidermal water loss (TEWL), caused by SLS, by application of 38% linoleic acid. Perhaps the highly concentrated unsaturated fatty acid caused skin irritation itself. On the other hand Imokawa et al. [94] improved SLS-induced dehydration of the stratum corneum by application of stratum corneum lipids, especially cholesterol ester and sphingolipid fractions, but not by free fatty acids and cholesterol fractions.

An increased baseline TEWL indicating a decreased epidermal barrier, has been shown in so-called symptom-free skin of patients with AE by several authors [1, 58, 92, 140, 160, 164, 170, 176], but also in dry skin unrelated to AE [114, 158, 161]. Only Baker and Kligman [12] did not find an increased TEWL in patients with AE (Table 2). Our own studies revealed an increased baseline TEWL in AE, although the difference between patients with AE and controls was not significant [74]. The difference was statistically significant when considering the TEWL of skin irritated with 1% SLS in a Finn chamber for 24 h (Table 3). There was no difference in TEWL comparing normal-appearing skin of patients with atopic rhinitis and controls [48]. The increased TEWL can be mostly attributed to reduced function of the stratum corneum. The good correlation between epidermal lipids and TEWL has been mentioned above. The TEWL can be greatly enhanced by tape-stripping of the stratum corneum [12, 58, 90]. In a prospective study, Coenraads and Pinnagoda [37] reported a higher baseline TEWL in metal workers who developed some workrelated dermatitis than in their colleagues without skin problems. Tupker et al. [165] reported the value of the baseline TEWL as predictive of susceptibility to SLS-induced irritation. They tested healthy volunteers and observed no influence of history of atopy, history of sensitivity to soap, and/or dry skin. In another study they measured a higher baseline TEWL in patients with healed AE than in patients with healed contact dermatitis and controls [164]. Shahidullah et al. [155] observed higher TEWL in normal appearing skin of patients with various types of eczema, so that the higher baseline TEWL may be a sign of status eczematicus rather than AE.

Table 3. Transepidermal water loss of uninvolved and irritated skin (1% SLS for 24 h) in patients with AE and controls

	Baseline TEWL $x \pm SD$	TEWL after irritation $x \pm SD$
Patients with AE (8)	15.3 ± 11.4	35.4 ± 20.6
Controls (10)	9.1 ± 4.2	16.9 ± 6.6
P Value	0.17	0.01

(x, mean; SD, standard deviation)

A pathologic stratum corneum is believed to have a low hygroscopicity due to smaller capacity for secondary bound water, in addition to increased TEWL [158, 159]. There are conflicting studies about the hydration of the stratum corneum in AE. Measuring electrical impedance Lawler et al. [110], Finlay et al. [57], and Keilhauer et al. [98] reported increased hydration of the stratum corneum at uninvolved sites. According to den Arend et al. [47], who used the same method, there was an increased hydration even in normal-appearing skin of patients with atopic rhinitis. Using infrared spectroscopic determination, Gloor et al. [69] confirmed an increased water content in patients with AE. Using the corneometer, which depends upon the high dielectric constant of water, Werner [175] found decreased hydration of the stratum corneum in dry-looking skin of patients with AE, although there was no statistical difference between normal-looking skin of patients with AE and controls. In vitro they also found a lower water-binding capacity in dry, noneczematous skin of AE [177]. Studying the dry skin in elderly, nonatopic patients with the same methods as Werner, Thune et al. [161] suggested that high TEWL correlated with low hydration of the stratum corneum, but they noticed a high interindividual variability. Using the corneometer, Thune [160] found low hydration values in patients with AE (29.2 ± 21.3) in comparison to controls (79.8 ± 16.9), although old patients with dry skin had even higher hydration values (86.5 ± 16.2). Al-Jaberi and Marks [5] did not detect a difference between normal-looking skin of patients with AE and controls, measuring electrical conductance. Perhaps the differences of the studies can be explained by the different methods applied [163]. With no method is it guaranteed that the measured value really represents stratum corneum hydration. Noninvasive techniques have been developed for better and more objective distinction of delicate differences in skin sensitivity. At the moment they cannot be recommended for daily clinical use due to technical drawbacks [46]. In our experience measurement of baseline TEWL, or parameters defined by noninvasive techniques, is influenced by too many factors to be a reliable indicator of irritable skin in any individual. The influencing factors include the instrument itself, the patient, the examiner and environmental conditions. To exclude some of these factors we prefer to use each proband as his own control, i.e., to measure the reaction of the skin to a small stimulus. Duplicate or even triplicate measurements should be performed if possible in order to calculate the difference between baseline and provocation values. Pinnegoda et al. [132] reported that a high baseline TEWL might be a better indicator of hyperirritability than a high TEWL value after a single 24-h SLS patch test. Tupker [164] found a significant difference in baseline TEWL between patients with AE, or contact dermatitis and controls. Perhaps they used very constant test conditions [133]. In our opinion further studies and improvements of the noninvasive techniques are necessary for wide clinical use.

Gloor et al [70] found increased irritability of the AE skin by tensides in the scarification test, which is independent of stratum corneum function. Perhaps an increased release of inflammatory mediators in the atopic group is responsible for this phenomenon. At the moment no specific mediator can be blamed, although increased release of many mediators has been reported in patients with AE. Likewise down-regulation of other mediators has also been found [25, 39, 81, 97, 101, 143–145, 148] (see Ruzicka and Ring, this volume).

Status Eczematicus and AE

Most of the above mentioned studies clearly indicate that the symptom-free skin of patients with AE is more sensitive to irritation than normal skin. However, the results of these studies are very similar to those of other studies addressing nonatopic eczema.

In his extensive study on irritants in hand eczema, Björnberg excluded patients with AE, but reported an observation which is pertinent to the problem of irritable skin. During the active state of hand dermatitis he found increased reactivity of the skin to SLS, hydrochloric acid, and benzalkonium chloride at a test site far away from the inflamed skin, namely the thigh. This difference was not demonstrable three months after healing of the hand dermatitis [19].

Wilson [180] found the same phenomenon when patch testing patients with allergic contact dermatitis, discoid eczema, AE and controls, each group consisting of 50 members. The threshold of skin reactivity was lowered during the eczema phase and apparently up to 3 months later. He also found a high percentage of false positive reactions to nickel sulfate. However, an increased frequency of contact allergy to nickel together with reduced general contact allergy rate is considered typical of AE [47, 141 p.133]. Positive patch testing with type I allergens in patients with AE has been performed by a number of authors [3, 27–29, 77, 108, 124, 142]. In patients with immediate contact dermatitis on their hands, only predamaged skin, which might look normal, reacts to foods [162]. A valid estimation of possibly lowered skin threshold to patch tests is hard to assess, especially in the comparison of atopic and contact allergic patients. Therefore, the possibility of truly irritant rather than allergic reactions has to be borne in mind during patch testing. Quite a number of further studies show increased reactions to various irritants, including cantharidin, in patients with nonatopic eczema [18, 67, 156, 157, 174].

Al-Jaberi and Marks [5] studied the clinically uninvolved skin of 22 patients with AE, 32 patients with other forms of "constitutional dermatitis", 30 patients with contact dermatitis, and 45 controls. They found a significantly lowered threshold to ammonium hydroxide MBT together with a reduction in the mean corneocyte area in both patients with AE and contact dermatitis compared to controls. The mean corneocyte area was significantly lowered in patients with constitutional dermatitis.

Raffle and Shahidullah [135] observed increased TEWL after standardized skin irritation by a tenside in patients with clinically resolved or normal-looking skin for a time period of 2–3 months after remission of the dermatitis. The baseline TEWL did not show a significant increase. Shahidullah et al. measured a higher TEWL in normal-looking skin during the highly active phase of circumscribed dermatitis than during a more quiescent phase [155].

In studies addressing nonatopic eczema, increased reactivity is regarded as a sign of the status eczematicus described by Jadassohn [95] and Bloch [22]. This term is ill-defined and means a general increase of skin sensitivity due to an eczematous reaction in a circumscribed area that stays for some time I^2 even after healing of the eczema. It occurs in any kind of dermatitis, including AE [5, 18, 19, 135, 180]. There is some overlap, if not identity of this term with other descriptions like "angry back syndrome" or "excited skin syndrome" [26, 116, 125] but its nature is uncertain. One could speculate that it is evoked and maintained by some systemic mediators, which are produced by eczematous skin in accordance with area, duration, and intensity of the eczema. These undefined mediators could disturb epidermal metabolism leading to an altered skin barrier with small corneocytes and altered lipids. Only after disappearance of these mediators could the epidermis rebuild a functioning stratum corneum. Although the phenomenon is closely related to skin reactivity, it has not been studied in detail in AE in the last few years.

Most of the studies finding an increased sensitivity of symptom-free skin in patients with AE cannot exclude the possibility that this hyperirritability is only a secondary phenomenon. Thus, one could speculate that irritable skin in AE is nothing more than status eczematicus. After complete healing of AE, the irritable skin becomes normal. Nonspecific hyperreactivity is also known in other targets of atopic disease, like the nasal, bronchial, and intestinal mucous membranes [128]. Nonetheless, clinicians discern an intrinsic or extrinsic form of asthma bronchiale or vasomotor rhinitis versus allergic rhinitis. Differentiation of skin reactions due to status eczematicus or intrinsic form of AE [113, 183] is extremely difficult. At the moment a lower resistance to irritants in AE remains only a putative primary event in the pathomechanisms of AE, supported mainly by clinical experience.

Outlook

Clinically, it is agreed that patients with AE have more irritable skin in symptom-free areas. Therapeutically one of the most important consequences is the avoidance of irritants. However, it is very difficult to prove this suspected hyperirritability in an experimental design. There are few studies about the problem of irritable skin, not only in AE, but also in any sensitive skin condition, in spite of its vast relevance to the patient's daily life. This might be due to the fact that most of the irritant tests are too short-termed and too simple; they hardly imitate the day to day strain on skin by a variety of physical, chemical and psychic irritants.

It is quite easy to detect acute damage of the skin and to perform correct provocation tests. However, in everyday life it is the repeated action of various microtraumata that finally results not only in a broken skin barrier, but also in hyperirritable skin. Apart from the detrimental effects of irritants on it, the skin has defense mechanisms like skin hardening which have not yet been thoroughly studied [104, 106, 119, 120, 164, 166, 167]. The cumulative-iterative damage of daily life is hard to copy in an experimental study.

At least in short-term tests, a great interindividual variation of skin reactivity exists in normal individuals without skin problems. This variability is much wider in patients with AE, dependent on the mode of patient selection, severity of disease [35], and methods used for determining skin reactivity. Noninvasive techniques cannot decisively diminish the considerable overlap between the two groups. An overlap also exists for the clinical features indicative of irritable skin in AE: dry skin, hand eczema, pruritus, sensitivity to soap, intolerance to wool, and so on [172].

Thus, for a given individual it often remains impossible to predict susceptibility to develop skin damage in, for instance, his future profession. Nonetheless, it has been possible to show, statistically, an increased irritability of symptom-free skin in AE patients. The question still remains whether this increased irritability is a primary phenomenon of AE or a sign of status eczematicus. Therefore studies addressing this problem should always include groups with other forms of chronic eczema besides patients with AE and healthy normal controls.

References

1. Abe T, Ohkido M, Yamamoto K (1978) Studies on skin surface barrier functions – skin surface lipids and transepidermal water loss in atopic skin during childhood. J Dermatol (Tokyo) 5:223–229
2. Adachi K, Aoki T (1989) IgE antibody to sweat in atopic dermatitis. Acta Derm Venereol [Suppl] (Stockh.) 144:83–87
3. Adinoff AD, Tellez P, Clark RAF (1988) Atopic dermatitis and aeroallergen contact sensitivity. J Allergy Clin Immunol 81:736–742
4. Agner T, Serup J (1990) Individual and instrumental variations in irritant patch-test reactions – clinical evaluation and quantification by bioengineering methods. Clin Exp Dermatol 15:29–33
5. Al-Jaberi H, Marks R (1984) Studies of the uninvolved skin in patients with dermatitis. Br J Dermatol 111:437–443
6. Allison JH, Bettley FR (1958) Investigations into cantharidin blisters raised on apparently normal skin in normal and abnormal subjects. Br J Dermatol 70:331
7. Allison JH, Williamson DH (1960) The abnormal cantharidin blister in atopy: an explanation on its production. Br J Dermatol 72:383
8. Antoine JL, Contreras JL, van Neste D (1989) pH influence of surfactant-induced skin irritation. A non-invasive, multiparametric study with sodium lauryl-sulfate. Dermatosen 37:96–100
9. Aoki T, Kushimoto H, Kobayashi E, Ogushi Y (1980) Computer analysis of nocturnal scratch in atopic dermatitis. Acta Derm Venereol [Suppl] (Stockh.) 92: 33
10. Archer CB (1986) Atopic dermatitis – an obvious diagnosis? Clin Dermatol 11:560–563
11. Atherton DJ (1981) Review article. Allergy and atopic eczema II. Clin Dermatol 6:317–325
12. Baker H, Kligman AM (1967) Measurement of transepidermal water loss by electrical hygrometry. Arch Dermatol 96:441–452
13. Bauerdorf R, Borelli S (1989) Neurodermitis. In: Stüttgen G (ed) Standort und Ausblick der deutschsprachigen Dermatologie. Grosse, Berlin, pp 82–97
14. Bäurle G (1986) Handekzeme. Studie zum Einfluß von konstitutionellen und Umweltfaktoren auf die Genese. Schattauer, Stuttgart
15. Beck HI, Korsgaard J (1989) Atopic dermatitis and house-dust mites. Acta Derm Venereol [Suppl] (Stockh.) 144: 125–126
16. Beck HI, Bjerring P, Harving H (1989) Atopic dermatitis and the indoor climate. Acta Derm Venereol (Stockh.) 69:162–165
17. Bendsöe N, Björnberg A, Åsnes H (1987) Itching from wool fibres in atopic dermatitis. Contact Dermatitis 17: 21–22
18. Bettley FR (1964) Non-specific irritant reactions in eczematous subjects. Br J Dermatol 76:116–119
19. Björnberg A (1968) Skin reactions to primary irritants in patients with hand eczema. Isacsons, Göteborg
20. Blank IH (1987) The skin as an organ of protection. In: Fitzpatrick TB, Eisen AZ, Wolff K, Freedberg IM, Austen KF (eds) Dermatology in general medicine, 3rd edn. McGraw-Hill, New York, pp 337–342
21. Blanken R, van Vilsteren MJT, Tupker RA, Coenraads PJ (1989) Effect of mineral oil and linoleic-acid-containing emulsions on the skin vapour loss of sodium lauryl-sulphate induced irritant skin reactions. Contact Dermatitis 20:3–97
22. Bloch B (1924) Pathogenese des Ekzems. Arch Dermatol Syph 145:34–182
23. Braun-Falco O (1988) Hautreinigung bei atopischen Ekzem (Neurodermitis diffusa, endogenes Ekzem). Ärztl Kosmetol 18:276–278
24. Braun-Falco O, Korting HC (1986) Der normale pH der menschlichen Haut. Hautarzt 37:126–129
25. Brown KA, Ellis BA, Dumonde DC (1989) Cytokines in relation to inflammatory skin disease. In: Greaves MW, Shuster S (eds) Pharmacology of skin systems autocoids in normal and inflamed skin. Springer, Berlin Heidelberg New York, Pharmacology of the skin I
26. Bruynzeel DP (1983) Angry back or excited skin syndrome. Kripps, Amsterdam
27. Bruynzeel-Koomen C, van Wichen DF, Toonstra J, Berrens L, Bruynzeel PLB (1986) The presence of IgE molecules on epidermal Langerhans cells in patients with atopic dermatitis. Arch Dermatol Res 278:199–205
28. Bruynzeel-Koomen C, van Wichen DF, Spry C, Venge P, Bruynzeel PLB (1988) Active participation of eosinophils in patch test reactions to inhalant allergens in patients with atopic dermatitis. Br J Dermatol 118:229–238
29. Bruynzeel-Koomen C, Mudde GC, Bruynzeel PLB (1989) New aspects in the pathogenesis of atopic dermatitis. Acta Derm Venereol [Suppl] (Stockh.) 144: 58–63
30. Burckhardt W (1947) Neuere Untersuchungen über die Alkaliempfindlichkeit der Haut. Dermatologica 94:73–96
31. Burckhardt W, Dorta T (1957) Die Alkaliresistenz bei Ekzemen verschiedener Genese und bei Neurodermitis. Dermatologica 114:252–257
32. Burges GE, Lang PG (1987) Atopic dermatitis exacerbated by inhalant allergens. Arch Dermatol 123:1437–1438
33. Carswell F, Thompson S (1986) Does natural sensitization in eczema occur through the skin? Lancet vi:13–15
34. Champion RH, Parish WE (1986) Atopic dermatitis. In Rook A, Wilkinson DS, Ebling FJG, Champion RH, Burton JL (eds) Textbook of dermatology, 4th edin. Blackwell, Oxford pp 419–434
35. Clark RAF (1989) Cell-mediated and IgE-mediated immune responses in atopic dermatitis. Arch Dermatol 125:413–416
36. Coenraads JP (1983) Prevalence of hand eczema. Association with occupational exposure especially in construction workers. Thesis, State University of Groningen
37. Coenraads PJ, Pinnagoda J (1985) Dermatitis and water vapour loss in metal workers. Contact Dermatitis 13:347–348
38. Coenraads PJ, Bleumink E, Nater JP (1975) Susceptibility to primary irritants. Age dependence and relation to contact allergic reactions. Contact Dermatitis 1:377–381
39. Cooper KD (1989) Mechanisms of atopic dermatitis. In: Norris DA (ed) Immune mechanisms in cutaneous disease. Dekker, New York, pp 247–276
40. Cronin E (1985) Clinical patterns of hand eczema in women. Contact Dermatitis 13:153–161
41. Cronin E (1987) Dermatitis of the hands in caterers. Contact Dermatitis 17:265–269
42. Czerwinska-Dihm I, Rudzki E (1976) Skin reactions to primary irritants. Contact Dermatitis 2:314–324
43. Dahl MV (1986) Editorial reflex. Research on atopic dermatitis. Arch Dermatol 122:265

44. Dahl MV, Pass F, Trancik RJ (1984) Sodium lauryl sulfate irritant patch test. II. Variations of test responses among subjects and comparison to variation of allergic responses elicited by toxicodendron extract. J Am Acad Dermatol 11:474–477
45. De Boer EM, Bruynzeel DP, van Ketel WG (1988) Dyshidrotic eczema as an occupational dermatitis in metal workers. Contact Dermatitis 19:184–188
46. De Jongh GJ (1981) Porosity of human skin in vivo assessed via water loss, carbon dioxide loss and electrical impedance for healthy volunteers, atopic and psoriatic patients. Curr Probl Dermatol 9:83–101
47. Den Arend JAC, de Haan AFJ, Malten KE (1988) Seasonal transepidermal water loss and impedance of forearm skin in atopics and non-atopics. Contact Dermatitis 19:376–390
48. Diepgen TL, Fartasch M, Hornstein OP (1989) Evaluation and relevance of atopic basic and minor features in patients with atopic dermatitis and in the general population. Acta Derm Venereol [Suppl] (Stockh.) 144:50–54
49. Dooms-Goossens AE, Debusschere KM, Gevers DM, et al. (1986) Contact dermatitis caused by airborne agents. J Am Acad Dermatol 15:1–10
50. Downing DT, Stewart ME, Wertz PW, Colton SW, Abraham W, Strauss JS (1987) Skin lipids: an update. J Invest Dermatol [Suppl] 88:2s
51. Dyer DW, Hassapis T (1983) Comparison of detergent based versus soap based liquid soaps. Soap Cosmet Chem Spec 59:36–40
52. Elias PM (1983) Epidermal lipids, barrier function and desquamation. J Invest Dermatol [Suppl] 80:44s
53. Elias PM (1987) The special role of the stratum corneum. In: Fitzpatrick TB, Eisen AZ, Wolff K, Freedberg IM, Austen KF (eds) Dermatology in general medicine, 3rd edn. McGraw-Hill, New York, pp 342–346
54. Enders F, Gollhausen R, Kligman AM, Przybilla B (1988) Jahreszeitliche Einflüsse auf die Hautreaktivität (Abstr) Zentralbl Haut 154:631
55. Engman MF, Weiss RS, Engman MF Jr (1936) Eczema and environment. Med Clin North Am 20:651–663
56. Felix R, Shuster S (1975) A new method for the measurement of itch and response to treatment. Br J Dermatol 93:303–312
57. Finlay AY, Nicholls S, King CS, Marks R (1980) The "dry" non-eczematous skin associated with atopic eczema. Br J Dermatol 102:249–256
58. Frödin T, Skogh M (1984) Measurement of transepidermal waterloss using an evaporimeter to follow the restitution of the barrier layer of human epidermis after stripping the stratum corneum. Acta Derm Venereol (Stockh.) 64:537–540
59. Frosch PJ (1982) Irritancy of soaps and detergent bars. In: Frost P, Horwitz SN (eds) Principles of cosmetics for the dermatologist. Mosby, St Louis, pp 5–12
60. Frosch PJ (1985) Hautirritation und empfindliche Haut. Grosse, Berlin (Grosse Scripta 7)
61. Frosch PJ (1989) Irritant contact dermatitis. In: Frosch PJ, Dooms-Goossens A, Lachapelle JM, Rycroft RJG, Scheper RJ (eds) Current topics in contact dermatitis. Springer, Berlin Heidelberg New York, pp 385–398
62. Frosch PJ, Kligman AM (1977) A method for appraising the stinging capacity of topically applied substances. J Soc Cosmet Chem 28:197–209
63. Frosch PJ, Kligman AM (1982) Recognition of chemically vulnerable and delicate skin. In: Frost P, Horwitz SN (eds) Principles of cosmetics for the dermatologist. Mosby, St Louis
64. Frosch PJ, Wissing CH (1982) Cutaneous sensitivity to ultraviolet light and chemical irritants. Arch Dermatol Res 272:269–278
65. Gawkrodger DJ, Lloyd MH, Hunter JAA (1986) Occupational skin disease in hospital cleaning and kitchen workers. Contact Dermatitis 15:132–135
66. Gehese M, Kändler-Stümer P, Gloor M (1987) Über die Bedeutung der Irritabilität der Haut für die Entstehung des berufsbedingten allergischen Kontaktekzems. Dermatol Monatsschr 173:400–404
67. Geiger R (1929) Unspezifische Desensibilisierungsversuche an Ekzematikern mit Terpentinöl auf percutanem Wege. Arch Dermatol Syph 158:76–87
68. Gloor M, Scheer T (1989) In-vivo-Regulation der Hornschichtfeuchtigkeit. Ärztl. Kosmetol 19:31–40
69. Gloor M, Heymann B, Stuhlert T (1981) Infrared spectroscopic determination of the water content of the horny layer in healthy subjects and in patients suffering from atopic dermatitis. Arch Dermatol Res 271:429–436
70. Gloor M, Völlm P, Gehse M, Ringelmann R (1985) Irritationseffekt von Tensiden bei Patienten mit Gewerbeekzemen im Friseur- und Krankenpflegeberuf. Vergleichsuntersuchungen mit Gesunden und Neurodermitikern. Dermatosen 33:86–89
71. Gollhausen R (1990) Implikationen von Irritans-Tests mit Syndetbestandteilen. In: Braun-Falco, Korting HC (eds) Griesbach-Konferenz: Hautreinigungsmittel auf Syndet-Basis – Zusammensetzung, Grundlagen ihrer Anwendung, Effekte, Nebenwirkungspotential. Springer, Berlin Heidelberg New York
72. Gollhausen R, Kligman AM (1985) Effects of pressure on contact dermatitis. Am J Ind Med 8:323–328
73. Gollhausen R, Kligman AM (1985) Human assay for identifying substances which induce non-allergic contact urticaria: the NICU-test. Contact Dermatitis 13:98–106
74. Gollhausen R, Göttsberger K, Winter H, Przybilla B, Ring J (1987) Skin sensitivity in atopic eczema before and after UVA phototherapy – evaluation by visual assessment, evaporimeter and laser doppler flowmeter (Abstr) J Invest Dermatol 89:319
75. Gollhausen R, Göttsberger K, Winter H, Przybilla B, Ring J (1988) The cutaneous blood flow as a new marker of skin sensitivity to UV-B. Evaluation in patients with atopic eczema and in controls (Abstr) J Invest Dermatol 91:385
76. Gollhausen R, Klutke U, Przybilla B, Ring J (1989) The cutaneous blood flow slope (CBFS) as a marker of skin sensitivity to UV-light (Abstr) J Invest Dermatol 92:435
77. Gondo A, Saeki N, Tokuca Y (1986) Challenge reactions in atopic dermatitis after percutaneous entry of mite antigen. Br J Dermatol 115:485–492
78. Hamami I, Marks R (1988) Structural determinants of the response of the skin to chemical irritants. Contact Dermatitis 18:71–75
79. Hambly EM, Levia L, Wilkinson DS (1978) Wool intolerance in atopic subjects. Contact Dermatitis 4:240–241
80. Hanifin M (1984) Atopic dermatitis. J Allergy Clin Immunol 73:211–222
81. Hanifin JM (1989) Pharmacological abnormalities in atopic dermatitis. Allergy [Suppl] 9:41–46
82. Hanifin JM, Rajka G (1980) Diagnostic features of atopic dermatitis. Acta Derm Venereol [Suppl] (Stockh.) 92:44–47

83. Hannuksela M (1980) Atopic contact dermatitis. Contact Dermatitis 6: 30–32
84. Harnack K (1986) Experimental itch as a diagnostic method. Acta Derm Venereol [Suppl] (Stockh.) 92:40–41
85. Hassing JH, Nater JP, Bleumink E (1982) Irritancy of low concentrations of soap and synthetic detergents as measured by skin water loss. Dermatol 164:314–321
86. Hatch KL, Maibach HI (1985) Textile fiber dermatitis. Contact Dermatitis 12:1–11
87. Heite HJ, Kleinhans D (1961) Über die Cignolin-Erythemschwelle bei einigen Dermatosen. Arch Klin Exp Dermatol 212:431
88. Heyer G, Schönberger A, Hornstein OP (1988) Störungen der Thermoregulation auf externe Kälte- und Wärmereize bei Patienten mit atopischem Ekzem. Hautarzt 39:18–22
89. Heyer G, Hornstein OP, Handwerker HO (1989) Skin reactions and itch sensation induced by epicutaneous histamine application in atopic dermatitis and controls. J Invest Dermatol 93:492–496
90. Hofmann H, Maibach HI (1976) Transepidermal water loss in adhesive tape induced dermatitis. Contact Dermatitis 2:171–177
91. Hölzle E, Plewig G (1977) Effects of dermatitis, stripping and steroids on the morphology of corneocytes. A new bioassay. J Invest Dermatol 68:350–356
92. Holzmann H, Korting GW, Oehmichen C (1961) Vergleichende Messungen der Feuchtigkeitsabgabe von Herdbezirk und unveränderter Haut bei verschiedener Hautkrankheiten. Arch Klin Exp Dermatol 212:312–318
93. Imokawa G, Hattori M (1985) A possible function of structural lipids in the waterholding properties of the stratum corneum. J Invest Dermatol 84:282–284
94. Imokawa G, Akasaki S, Minematsu Y, Kawai M (1989) Importance of intercellular lipids in water-retention properties of the stratum corneum: induction and recovery study of surfactant dry skin. Arch Dermatol Res 281:45–51
95. Jadassohn J (1895) Zur Kenntnis der medikamentösen Dermatosen. 5th Congress of the German Academy of Dermatology, Graz, pp 103–129
96. Jakobza D, Reichmann G, Langnick W, Langnick A, Schulze P (1981) Gaschromatographische Untersuchungen des Hautfettes bei endogenen Ekzematikern. Dermatol Monatsschr 167:26–29
97. Kapp A, Kirnbauer R, Luger T, Schöpf E (1989) Altered production of immuno-modulation cytokines in patients with atopic dermatitis. Acta Derm Venereol [Suppl] (Stockh.) 144:97–99
98. Keilhauer A, Wienert V, Pürschel W (1982) Die Hautfeuchtigkeit bei Neurodermitikern in maritimer Klimazone. Z Hautkr 57:1477–1486
99. Kligman AM, Lavker RM, Grove GL, Studemayer TJ (1982) Some aspects of dry skin and its treatment. In: Kligman AM, Leyden JJ (eds) Safety and efficacy of topical drugs and cosmetics. Grune and Stratton, New York, pp 221–238
100. Korting HC, Kober M, Müller M, Braun-Falco O (1987) Influence of repeated washings with soap and synthetic detergents on pH and resident flora of the skin of forehead and forearm. Acta Derm Venereol (Stockh.) 67:41–47
101. Kupper TS (1989) Mechanisms of cutaneous inflammation (Editorial). Arch Dermatol 125:1409–1412
102. Lahti A, Maibach HI (1987) Immediate contact reactions: contact urticaria syndrome. Semin Dermatol 6:313–320
103. Lammintausta K, Kalimo K (1981) Atopy and hand dermatitis in hospital wet work. Contact Dermatitis 7: 301–308
104. Lammintausta K, Maibach HI, Wilson D (1987) Human cutaneous irritation: induced hyporeactivity. Contact Dermatitis 17:193–198
105. Lammintausta K, Maibach HI, Wilson D (1988) Mechanisms of subjective (sensory) irritation. Propensity to non-immunologic contact urticaria and objective irritation in stingers. Dermatosen 36:45–49
106. Lammintausta K, Maibach HI, Wilson D (1988) Susceptibility to cumulative and acute irritant dermatitis. An experimental approach in human volunteers. Contact Dermatitis 19:84–90
107. Lammintausta K, Maibach HI (1988) Exogenous and endogenous factors in skin irritation. Int J Dermatol 27:213–222
108. Langeland T, Braathen LB, Borch M (1989) Studies of atopic patch tests. Acta Derm Venereol [Suppl] (Stockh.) 144:105–109
109. Lantinga H, Nater JP, Coenraads PJ (1984) Prevalence, incidence and course of eczema on the hands and forearms in a sample of the general population. Contact Dermatitis 10:135–139
110. Lawler JC, Davis MJ, Griffith EC (1960) Electrical characteristics of the skin. J Invest Dermatol 34:11
111. Lehmann P, Helbig S, Hölzle E, Plewig G (1988) Bestrahlung mit UV-A oder UV-B wirkt protektiv gegenüber Irritantien. Zentralbl Haut 154:686–692
112. Lejman E, Stoudemayer T, Grove G, Kligman AM (1984) Age differences in poison ivy dermatitis. Contact Dermatitis 11:163–167
113. Leung DYM, Rhodes AR, Geha RS (1987) Atopic dermatitis. In: Fitzpatrick TB, Eisen AZ, Wolff K, Freedberg IM, Austen KF (eds) Dermatology in general medicine, 3rd edn. McGraw-Hill, New York, pp 1385–1408
114. Leveque JL, Garson JC, de Rigal J (1979) Transepidermal water loss from dry and normal skin. J Soc Chem 30:333–343
115. Locher G (1962) Permeabilitätsprüfung der Haut Ekzemkranker und Hautgesunder für den neuen Indikator Nitrazingelb “Geigy”, Modifizierung der Alkaliresistenzprobe, pH-Verlauf in der Tiefe des Stratum corneums. Dermatol 124:159
116. Maibach HI (1981) The E.S.S. – excited skin syndrome (alias the “angry back”). In: Ring J, Burg G (eds) New trends in allergy. Springer, Berlin Heidelberg New York, pp 208–221
117. Maibach HI, Engasser PG (1986) Cosmetic intolerance syndrome. Semin Dermatol 5:273–276
118. Maibach HI, Lammintausta K, Berardesca E, Freeman S (1989) Tendency to irritation: sensitive skin. J Am Acad Dermatol 21:833–835
119. Malten KE, den Arend JACJ (1985) Irritant contact dermatitis. Traumiterative and cumulative impairment by cosmetics, climate and other daily loads. Dermatosen 33:125–132
120. Malten KE, Thiele FAJ (1973) Some theoretical aspects of “orthoergic” (=irritant) dermatitis. Arch Belg Dermatol 28:9–21
121. Mathias CGT (1986) Clinical and experimental aspects of cutaneous irritation. In: Marzulli FN, Maibach HI (eds) Dermatoxicology. Hemisphere, Washington, pp 173–189
122. Melnik B, Hollmann J, Plewig G (1988) Decreased stratum corneum ceramides in atopic individuals – a pathobiochemical factor for xerosis? Br J Dermatol 119:547–549

123. Mihm MC, Nicholas A, Soter MD, Harold F, Dvorak MD, Austen KF (1976) The structure of normal skin and the morphology of atopic eczema. J Invest Dermatol 67:305–312
124. Mitchell B, Chapman M, Pope F, Crow S, Jouhal S, Platts-Mills T (1982) Basophils in allergen-induced pathc test sites in atopic dermatitis. Lancet 1:127–131
125. Mitchell JC (1975) The angry back syndrome: eczema creates eczema. Contact Dermatitis 1:193–194
126. Murahata RI, Toton-Quinn R, Finkey MB (1988) Effect of pH on the production of irritation in a chamber irritation test. J Am Acad Dermatol 18:62–66
127. Mustakallio KK, Kiistala U, Piha HJ, Nieminen E (1967) Epidermal lipids in Besnier's prurigo (atopic exzema). Ann Med Exp Biol Fenn 45:323–325
128. Naclerio RM (1988) The pathophysiology of allergic rhinitis: impact of therapeutic intervention. J Allergy Clin Immunol 82:927–934
129. Neste D, van Mahmoud G, Masmoudi M (1987) Experimental induction of rough dermatitis skin in humans. Contact Dermatitis 16:27–33
130. Nilsson E, Bäck O (1986) The importance of anamnestic information of atopy, metal dermatitis and earlier hand exzema for the development of hand dermatitis in women in wet hospital work. Acta Derm Venereol (Stockh.) 66: 45–50
131. Pierard GE (1987) What does "dry skin" mean? Int Dermatol 26:167–168
132. Pinnegoda J, Tupker RA, Coenraads PJ, Nater JP (1989) Prediction of susceptibility to an irritant response by transepidermal water loss, Contact Dermatitis 20:341–346
133. Pinnegoda J, Tupker RA, Agner T, Serup J (1990) Guidelines for transepidermal water loss (TEWL) measurement. Contact Dermatitis 22:164–178
134. Raab W (1987) Zur Reinigung gesunder und kranker Haut. Ärztl. Kosmetol 17:354–359
135. Raffle EJ, Shahidullah M (1970) The effect of a standardized "skin insult" on transepidermal water loss. Dermatologica 141:208–214
136. Rajka G (1967) Itch duration in the involved skin of atopic dermatitis (prurigo Besnier). Acta Derm Venereol (Stockh.) 47:154–157
137. Rajka G (1968) Evaluation of drug influence on the itch duration in the skin of patients with atopic dermatitis, various eczemas and psoriasis. Acta Derm Venereol (Stockh.) 48:93–97
138. Rajka G (1968) Itch duration in the uninvolved skin of atopic dermatitis (prurigo Besnier). Acta Derm Venereol (Stockh.) 48:320–321
139. Rajka G (1974) Surface lipid estimation on the back of the hands in atopic dermatitis. Arch Dermatol Res 251:111–115
140. Rajka G (1974) Transepidermal water loss on the hands in atopic dermatitis. Arch Dermatol Forsch 251:111–115
141. Rajka G (1989) Essential aspects of atopic dermatitis. Springer, Berlin Heidelberg New York
142. Reitamo S, Visa K, Kahonen K, Stubb S, Salo O (1986) Eczematous reactions in atopic dermatitis patients caused by epicutaneous testing with inhalant allergens. Br J Dermatol 114:303–310
143. Ring J (1988) Entzündungsmediatoren bei atopischem Ekzem. Allergologie 11:60–62
144. Ring J, Dorsch W (1985) Altered releasability of vasoactive mediators secreting cell in atopic eczema. Acta Derm Venereol [Suppl] (Stockh.) 114:9–23
145. Ring J, Thomas P (1989) Histamine and atopic eczema. Acta Derm Venereol [Suppl] (Stockh.) 144:70–77
146. Roper SS, Jones HE (1982) A new look at conditioned hyperirritability. J Am Acad Dermatol 7:643–650
147. Rovensky J, Saxl O (1964) Differences in the dynamics of sweat secretion in atopic children. J Invest Dermatol 43:171–176
148. Ruzicka T (1989) Leukotrienes in atopic eczema. Acta Derm Venereol [Suppl] (Stockh.) 144:48–49
149. Rysted I (1985) Factors influencing the occurence of hand eczema in adults with a history of atopic dermatitis in childhood. Contact Dermatitis 12:185–191
150. Rysted I (1985) Hand eczema and long-term prognosis in atopic dermatitis. Acta Derm Venereol [Suppl] (Stockh.) 117
151. Rysted I (1986) Atopy, hand eczema, and contact dermatitis: summary of recent large scale studies. Semin Dermatol 5:290–300
152. Savin JA, Paterson WD, Oswald I, Adam K (1975) Further studies in scratching during sleep. Br J Dermatol 93:297
153. Schade H, Marchionini A (1928) Der Säurekettenmantel der Haut (nach Gaskettenmessungen). Klin Wochenschr 7:12–14
154. Schnyder KW, Gloor M, Taugner M (1977) Über die sozialmedizinische Bedeutung von Alkaliresistenz, Alkalineutralisation und Hautoberflächenlipidmenge bei Neurodermitis atopica und Ichthyosis vulgaris. Berufsdermatosen 25:101–107
155. Shahidullah M, Raffle EJ, Rimmer AR, Frain-Bell W (1969) Transepidermal water loss in patients with dermatitis. Br J Dermatol 81:722–730
156. Sigel H (1959) Threshold stimulation of the skin and house-wives eczema of the hands. Arch Dermatol 80:461–465
157. Skog E (1960) Primary irritant and allergic eczematous reactions induced in patients with different dermatoses. Acta Derm Venereol (Stockh.) 40:307–316
158. Tagami H, Yoshikuni K (1985) Interrelationship between water-barrier and reservoir functions of pathologic stratum corneum. Arch Dermatol 121:642–645
159. Takenouchi M, Suzuki H, Tagami H (1986) Hydration characteristics of pathologic stratum corneum – evaluation of bound water. J Invest Dermatol 87:574–576
160. Thune P (1989) Evaluation of the hydration and the water-holding capacity in atopic skin and so-called dry skin. Acta Derm Venereol [Suppl] (Stockh.) 144:133–135
161. Thune P, Nilsen T, Hanstad K, Gustavsen T, Lövig Dahl H (1988) The water barrier function of the skin in relation to the water content of stratum corneum, pH and skin lipids. The effect of alkaline soap and syndet on dry skin in elderly, non-atopic patients. Acta Derm Venereol (Stockh.) 68:277–283
162. Tosti A, Fanti PA, Guerra L, Piancastelli E, Poggi S, Pileri S (1990) Morphological and immunohistochemical study of immediate contact dermatitis of the hands due to foods. Contact Dermatitis 22:81–85
163. Triebskorn A, Gloor M, Greiner F (1983) Comparative investigations on the water content of the stratum corneum using different methods of measurement. Dermatol 167:64–69
164. Tupker RA (1990) The influence of detergents on the human skin. A study on factors determining the individual susceptibility assessed by transepidermal water loss. Thesis, State University Groningen
165. Tupker RA, Coenraads PJ, Pinnegoda J, Nater JP (1989)

Baseline transepidermal water loss (TEWL) as a prediction of susceptibility to sodium lauryl sulfate. Contact Dermatitis 20:265–269

166. Tupker RA, Pinnagoda J, Coenraads PJ, Nater JP (1989) The influence of repeated exposure to surfactants on the human skin as determined by transepidermal water loss and visual scoring. Contact Dermatitis 20:108–114
167. Tupker RA, Pinnagoda J, Nater JP (1990) The transient and cumulative effect of sodium lauryl sulphate on the epidermal barrier assessed by transepidermal water loss: inter-individual variaton. Acta Derm Venereol (Stockh.) 70:1–5
168. Uehara M (1986) Dry skin (sebostasis) and inflammation: heterogeneity of "dry skin" in atopic dermatitis. In: Ring J (ed) New trends in allergy II. Springer, Berlin Heidelberg New York, pp 135–144
169. Uehara M, Takada K (1985) Use of soap in the management of atopic dermatitis. Clin Exp Dermatol 10:419
170. Van der Valk PGM, Nater JP, Bleumink E (1985) Vulnerability of the skin to surfactants in different groups of eczema patients and controls as measured by water vapour loss. Clin Exp Dermatol 10:185–193
171. Van Ketel WG, Bruynzeel DP, Bezemer PD, Stamhuis HI (1984) Toxicity of handcleaners. Dermatol 168:94–99
172. Visscher MO, Hanifin JM, Bowman WJ, Reed BR (1989) Atopic dermatitis and atopy in non-clinical populations. Acta Derm Venereol [Suppl] (Stockh.) 144:34–40
173. Wahlberg JE, Wrangsjö K, Hietasalo A (1985) Skin irritancy from nonanoic acid. Contact Dermatitis 13:266–269
174. Wedroff NA, Dogloff AP (1935) Ein Beitrag zur Frage der Reaktionsfähigkeit der Haut bei "chemischen" Ekzemen, auf Grund von Untersuchungen bei ekzemkranken und gesunden Personen mittels der obligaten chemischen Reizmittel. Arch Dermatol Syph 171:641–646
175. Werner Y (1986) The water content of the stratum corneum in patients with atopic dermatitis. Measurement with the Corneometer CM 420. Acta Derm Venereol 66: 281–284
176. Werner Y, Lindberg M (1985) Transepidermal water loss in dry and clinically normal skin in patients with atopic dermatitis. Acta Derm Venereol (Stockh.) 65:102–105
177. Werner Y, Lindberg M, Forslind B (1982) The water-binding capacity of stratum corneum in dry non-eczematous skin of atopic eczema. Acta Derm Venereol (Stockh.) 62:334–336
178. Werner Linde Y (1989) "Dry" skin in atopic dermatitis. I. A clinical study. Acta Derm Venereol (Stockh.) 69:311–314
179. White MI, Mcewan Jenkinson D, Lloyd DH (1987) The effect of washing on the thickness of the stratum corneum in normal and atopic individuals. Br J Dermatol 116:525–530
180. Wilson HTH (1955) Standard patch tests in eczema and dermatitis. Br J Dermatol 67:291–298
181. Wirth H, Gloor M, Stoika D (1981) Sebaceous glands in uninvolved skin of patients suffering from atopic dermatitis. Arch Dermatol Res 270:167–169
182. Wüthrich B (1989) Atopic dermatitis flare provoked by inhalant allergens. Dermatol 178:51–53
183. Wüthrich B (1989) Neurodermatitis atopica. Wien Med Wochenschr 139:156–165

Environmental Pollution and Atopy

F. Riedel

In recent decades an increasing prevalence rate of atopic diseases has been observed [1], and reports of the World Health Organization [2] show these to constitute an important and expensive health problem throughout the world. As is known from many genetic studies, the disposition to react in an allergic manner is inherited [3], however the manifestation of allergic disease may be influenced by extrinsic factors. Environmental pollution must be considered as one such important external factor, for the increasing prevalence of atopy has been reported mainly for allergic respiratory tract disorders and asthma [4–6].

Environmental factors associated with industrialization have thus been implicated in asthma. In developing countries the prevalence of asthma differs among persons with similar genetic background but exposed to different environmental conditions. Van Niekerk et al. [7] studied the occurrence of bronchial asthma in 1375 black South African children from the Xhosa tribe, 694 of whom were from Guguleto, an urban area of Capetown, while 671 lived in the sparsely populated grassland region of Transkei. Twenty-three children showed bronchial hyperresponsiveness (defined by exercise-induced bronchial obstruction), and only one of these came from the rural "homeland." Researchers suggested that the substantial difference in occurrence of asthma between urban and rural communities (3.27% and 0.14%, respectively) may have been due in part to families switching from a tribal life-style to a Westernized industrial habitat in which pollution is common.

In Japan seasonal allergic rhinitis was extremely rare before 1950, but since then a dramatic increase in the prevalence rate (up to 9%) has been observed, together with a similar increase in the number of diesel-powered cars. Among children in polluted districts the prevalence rate for seasonal allergic rhinitis has risen to 33% [8]. In another very recent study the incidence of seasonal allergic rhinitis was significantly lower in rural areas than in Tokyo (8.5% versus 15.7%) [9].

Also from Japan has come experimental support for the view that environmental pollution is a factor in the development of allergic disease; Miyamoto and coworkers [10] showed that diesel exhaust particles have an adjuvant effect on the production of specific IgE in mice. They immunized mice with ovalbumin by intranasal inoculation and studied subsequent specific anti-ovalbumin IgE responses in the serum with and without the antigen being mixed with diesel exhaust particles. The IgE response was found to be clearly higher in mice inoculated with ovalbumin together with diesel exhaust particles than with ovalbumin alone.

Several recent epidemiological studies conducted mainly in children report an association between air pollution and allergic airway disease. Andrae et al. [11] compared the prevalence of allergic disorders in children from areas in southern Sweden having high pollution caused by sulfur dioxide with children from areas having clean air. Questionnaires from the parents of 4990 children were evaluated. Children living near paper pulp plants showed symptoms more frequently that suggested allergic asthma (relative risk 1.3) and especially birch pollen asthma (relative risk 1.8) than children from less industrialized rural areas. Similar results have been published by Goren and Hellman from Israel [12]. They studied school children living in two communities with different levels of air pollution, again using questionnaires. The prevalence of bronchial asthma was found to be higher among children living in the polluted area than among those living in the area with clear air, with a relative risk of 2.66. Children under 6 years of age in North Rhine-Westphalia (FRG) were screened for serum IgE levels in two areas with different air pollution levels, and IgE was found to be higher in the industrial area of Dortmund compared to the rural area of Duelmen. This difference persisted after controlling for smoking and for ethnic and social differences [13]. Similar findings were also reported from a study in Denmark, in which serum IgE levels were determined in 363 nonatopic children under 12 years of age. Again, the mean value of serum IgE increased with the degree of air pollution in the area [14].

A new field of research, allergotoxicology, is thus emerging which examines the interaction between air pollution and natural allergens such as pollen and moulds. Recent experimental studies in allergotoxicology have focused on the hypothesis that inhalation of irritant gases increases the likelihood of allergic sensitization throughout the respiratory tract. Matsumara

[15] first reported this phenominon in the series of articles published in 1970, describing the effects of high concentrations of ozone, nitrogen dioxide, and sulfur dioxide on ovalbumin sensitization measured by antibody assays (hemagglutination technique and radioimmune electrophoresis) and on systemic anaphylactic reaction in inhalative antigen challenge. However, in these studies brief exposures to high concentrations of the irritant gas were used, and enhanced sensitization to ovalbumin occurred only after exposure to concentrations of O_3 over 5 ppm, NO_2 over 70 ppm, and SO_2 over 330 ppm. These concentrations are substantially in excess of those commonly encountered in air pollution.

More recently, experiments with lower concentrations of irritant gas have been performed. Osebold et al. [16] observed increased sensitization to inhaled ovalbumin after 5–6 weeks of intermittent exposure to 0.5–0.8 ppm O_3. In guinea pigs exposed concurrently to inhalative ovalbumin 85%, developed an anaphylactic reaction to intravenous application of ovalbumin compared to only 25% of the control group not exposed to O_3. Biagini et al. [17] exposed monkeys to 1 ppm O_3 for 12 weeks concurrently with inhalation of platinum salt. Two weeks after the exposure period, the animals were examined for platinum hypersensitivity by specific skin test and specific bronchial provocation testing. The combination of O_3 and platinum exposure significantly increased platinum hypersensitivity compared to platinum exposure alone, as shown by the incidence of positive skin tests and positive bronchial provocation results with platinum salt. An experiment in Cuba examined kerosene, commonly used in developing countries for cooking and heating. An increased specific antibody response and tracheal inflammation were found in the serum of guinea pigs exposed to kerosene when inhaled concurrently with ovalbumin [18].

In our laboratory we have developed an animal model to study the effect of damage to bronchial mucosa by inhalation of irritant gases, including SO_2, NO_2, and O_3, on local sensitization to inhaled antigens [19]. Guinea pigs were exposed to mixture of the pollutant and synthetic air in an inhalation chamber on 5 consecutive days for 8 h per day. On days 3, 4, and 5, the animals were sensitized by inhalation of ovalbumin as antigen after the exposure to the irritant gases. After 1 week of rest, bronchial provocation tests with inhaled ovalbumin were performed using a two-chamber body plethysmograph for guinea pigs. Airway obstruction was expressed in measurements of trapped air and significant bronchial obstruction; positive bronchial provocation tests were present when trapped air was greater than 0.08 ml. Pre-exposure to 3.5 ppm SO_2 over 5 days significantly enhanced sensitization to inhaled ovalbumin (Fig. 1). We increased the SO_2 concentration until a maximum of bronchial sensitization was reached beyond which further increases did not result in a higher degree of sensitization.

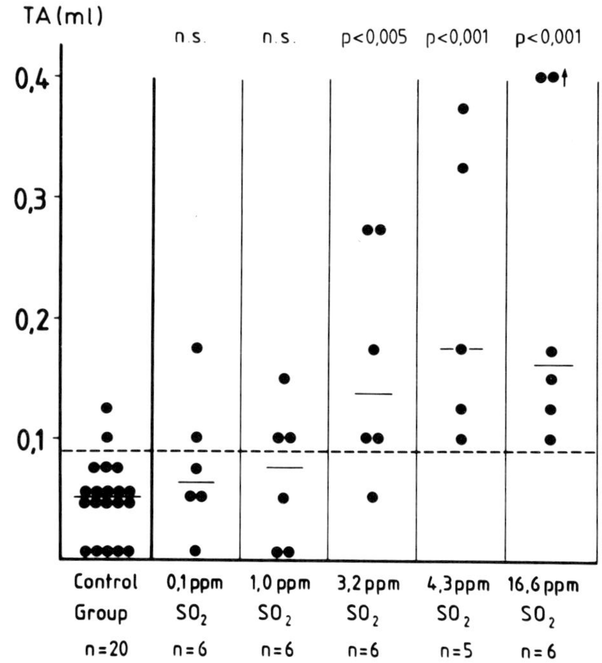

Fig. 1. Bronchial obstruction (*TA*) on specific bronchial provocation after exposure to different SO_2 concentrations

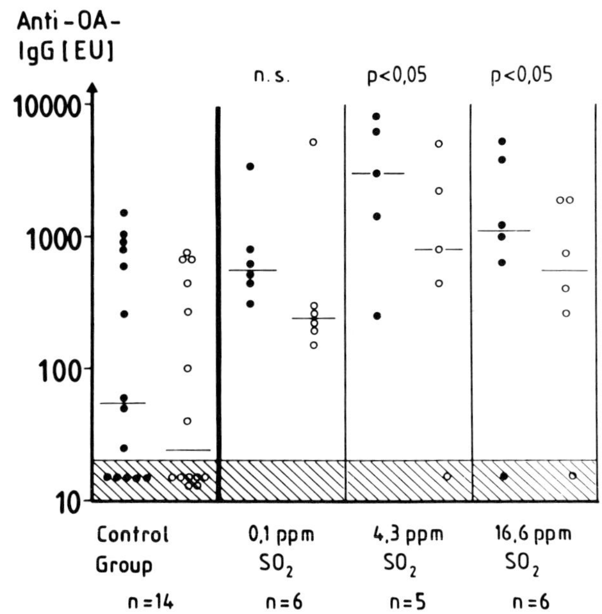

Fig. 2. Specific antiovalbumin antibody (*anti-OA*) concentrations in ELISA units (•, total IgG; ○, IgG_1) after exposure to different SO_2 concentrations

Furthermore, antiovalbumin antibodies of IgG and the IgG subclass IgG_1, the major reagenic antibody in the guinea pig, were measured in serum and bronchoalveolar fluid at the end of the experiment using a direct

ELISA technique (for details see [19]). The results for SO_2 exposures in different concentrations (Fig. 2) also demonstrate clearly that preexposure to the irritant gas increases the sensitization in terms of specific antibody response. Similar results were obtained with other pollutants in this model, the limit of effectiveness being 1 ppm for NO_2 and O_2 [20]. Figure 3 presents the frequency of positive bronchial reactions on specific bronchial provocation testing after exposure to different concentrations of the tested irritant gases. As can be seen from this figure, the combination of 1 ppm SO_2 and 0.5 ppm O_3 has a potentiating and more than an additive effect on the bronchial sensitization in our experiment.

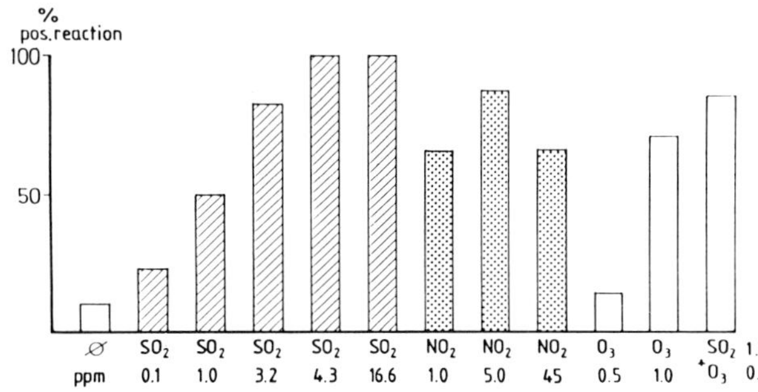

Fig. 3. Positive reactions in percent on specific bronchial provocation testing after exposure to different concentrations (ppm) of irritant gases followed by inhalative sensitization

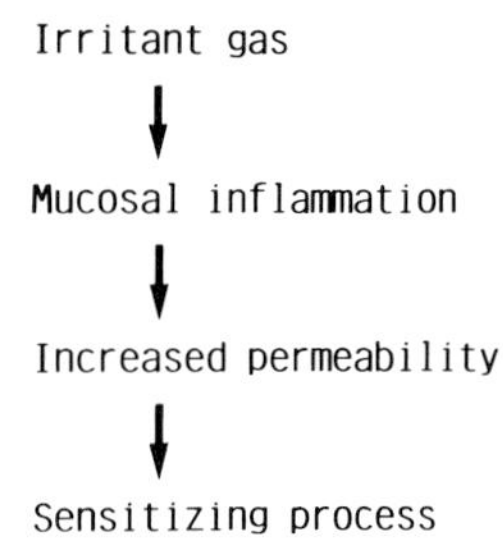

Fig. 4. Hypothesis for the influence of exposure to irritant gas on sensitizing process

Most studies in this field suggest the following hypothesis for pathogenesis of enhancement of allergic sensitization by air pollution (Fig. 4): irritant gas exposure causes inflammation of airway mucosa, leading to increased permeability of the barrier to inhaled antigens which then gain easy access to the submucosal lymphatic tissue and initiate the process of sensitization [21]. All steps in this cascade have been confirmed in experiments. For example, SO_2 inhalation induces airway inflammation and transient bronchial hyperactivity in sheep [22], in humans [23], and in our own model [20]. Inflammation due to SO_2 inhalation causes increased permeability for macromolecules in rats [24], as has been shown for O_3 and NO_2 in other animal species. Furthermore, mucociliary clearance is generally reduced after expose to irritant gas [25]. Matsumura has observed that O_3 exposure causes retention of inhaled radioactively labeled ovalbumin [15]. This may cause longer contact time between antigen and mucosa, further facilitating the sensitizing process.

The most important indoor pollutant is tobacco smoke. An association between active smoking and atopic disposition has been discussed for some time. Increased incidence of positive skin tests to common inhalation allergens as described by Welty et al. [26], and higher prevalence of specific IgE against an occupational allergen in active smokers [27] are indices of this association. Several authors have also reported eosinophilia [28] and increased serum IgE levels [29], although this was not supported by others [30]. Passive smoking seems to be associated with increased incidence of asthma in children according to epidemiological studies carried out in several communities of the United States by Gortmaker et al. [31] and McConnochie and Roghmann [32]. The same applies to recurrent obstructive bronchitis, the early childhood form of asthma [33, 34]. Kjellman measured serum IgE levels in children aged between 0 and 3 years and found higher levels in smoking families at 9 and 36 months of age compared to nonsmoking families [35]. The experimental background was added by Zetterström et al. [36] who found IgE levels in rats exposed to cigarette smoke for 8 weeks to be significantly higher than those in nonexposed animals. Furthermore, rats exposed concurrently to cigarette smoke and ovalbumin aerosol had increased anti-ovalbumin antibodies of the IgG and IgE classes, while subcutaneous immunization with ovalbumin had no effect on the antibody titer [36]. Thus, the importance of the local effect of tobacco smoke on the bronchial mucosa could be emphasized.

In our guinea pig model described above, we exposed animals to tobacco smoke over 8 h on 5 consecutive days, the mean nicotine serum levels at the end of the exposure period being 87 ng/ml [37]. After inhalation of sensitizing ovalbumin all animals showed enhanced sensitization on consecutive bronchial provocation testing compared to the control group, stressing the influence on tobacco smoke in this experimental setting.

In conclusion, there is enough epidemiological and experimental evidence to support the theory that outdoor pollution, i.e., air pollution and irritant gases, as well as indoor pollution, and in this respect mainly tobacco smoke, are associated with an increased prevalence of allergic disorders concerning mainly the airways as the main contact surface between air and tissues. This could partly explain the rising incidence of allergic disease in the second half of this century and could promote measures for reduction of indoor and outdoor pollution.

References

1. Massicot JG, Cohen SG (1986) Epidemiologic and socioeconomic aspect of allergic diseases. J Allergy Clin Immunol 87:954–958
2. World Health Organization (1980) 7th WHO report of a meeting on allergic disease. Geneva, 24–28 July 1978. Clin Allergy 10:1–20
3. Marsh DG, Meyers DA, Bias WB (1981) The epidemiology and genetics of atopic allergy. N Engl J Med 305:1551–1559
4. Morrison-Smith J, Harding JK, Cumming C (1971) The changing prevalence of asthma in school children. Clin Allergy 1:57–61
5. Kjellman B, Petterson R, Hensjö B (1982) Allergy among school children in a Swedish county. Allergy 37 [Suppl 1]: 5–6
6. Daneault S, Infante-Rivard C (1988) Hypotheses sur les changements dans la frequence de l'asthme. (Hypothesis of the changes in the frequency of asthma) Can Med Assoc J 139 (4):297–304
7. Van Niekerk CH, Weinberg EG, Shore SC et al. (1979) Prevalence of asthma: a comparative study of urban and rural Xhosa children. Clin Allergy 9:319–424
8. Kaneko S, Shimada K, Horikuchi H et al. (1980) Nasal allergy and air pollution. Oto-Rhino-Laryngology (Tokyo) 23 [Suppl 4]:270–274
9. Osaka F, Kasuga H, Sugita M et al. (1985) Relationship between housing environment and allergic symptoms of children using ATS-DLD-questionnaires. Tokai J Exp Clin Med 10:51–60
10. Takafuji S, Suzuki S, Koizumi K et al. (1987) Diesel-exhaust particulates inoculated by the intranasal route have an adjuvant activity for IgE production in mice. J Allergy Clin Immunol 79:639–645
11. Andrae S, Acelson O, Björksten B, Fredrikson M, Kjellman N (1988) Symptoms of bronchial hyperreactivity and asthma in relation to environmental factors. Arch Dis Child 63:473–478
12. Goren AI, Hellmann S (1988) Prevalence of respiratory symptoms and diseases in schoolchildren living in a polluted and in a low polluted area in Israel. Environ Res 45:28–37
13. Gleichmann E (1988) Modulation of the immune system by chemical and environmental compounds. XIIIth International Congress of Allergology and Clinical Immunology, Montreux, 16–21 Oct 1988
14. Berciano FA, Crespo M, Gao CG, Alvarez FV (1987) Serum levels of total IgE in non-allergic children. Influence of genetic and environmental factors. Allergy 42(4):276–283
15. Matsumara Y (1970) The effects of ozone, nitrogen dioxide, and sulfur dioxide on the experimentally induced allergic respiratory disorder in guinea pigs. Am Rev Respir Dis 102:420–447
16. Osebold JW, Chung Zee Y, Gershwin LJ (1988) Enhancement of allergic lung sensitization in mice by ozone inhalation. Proc Soc Exp Biol Med 188:259–264
17. Biagini RE, Moorman WG, Lewis TR, Bernstein IL (1986) Ozone enhancement of platinum asthma in a primate model. Am Rev Respir Dis 134:719–725
18. Casacao, Carvajal D, Noa M et al. (1985) Effects of kerosene on airway sensitization to egg albumin in guinea pig. Allergol Immunopathol 13:235–239
19. Riedel F, Kramer M, Scheibenbogen C, Rieger CHL (1988) Effects of SO_2-exposure on allergic sensitization in the guinea pig. J Allergy Clin Immunol 82:527–534
20. Riedel F, Sade U, Rüschhoff G et al. (1991) Initant gases (SO_2, NO_2, O_5) as unspecific triggers for allergic sensitization in the guinea pig. Clinical and Experimental Allergy, in press
21. Hogg JC (1982) Bronchial mucosal permeability and its relationship to airway hyperreactivity. Eur J Respir Dis [Suppl] 122:17–22
22. Abraham WM, Oliver W, Welker MJ et al. (1980) Sulfur dioxide-induced airway hyperreactivity in allergic sheep. Am J Ind Med I:383–390
23. Islam MS, Vastag E, Ulmer WT (1972) Sulphur dioxide-induced bronchial hyperreactivity against acetylcholine. Int Arch Arbeitsmed 29:221–232
24. Vai F, Fournier F, Lafuma JC, Touaty E, Pariente R (1980) SO_2 induced bronchopathy in the rat: abnormal permeability of the bronchial epithelium in vivo and vitro after anatomic recovery. Am Rev Respir Dis 121:851–858
25. Dalhamm T (1956) Mucuous flour and ciliary activity in trachea. Acta Physiol Scand [Suppl] 36:76–87
26. Welty C, Weiss ST, Tager IB et al. (1984) The relationship of airways responsiveness to cold air, cigarette smoking, and atopy to respiratory symptoms and pulmonary function in adults. Am Rev Respir Dis 130:198–203
27. Venables KM, Topping MD, Howe W et al. (1985) Interaction of smoking and atopy in producing specific IgE antibody against a hapten protein conjugate. Br Med J 290:201–204
28. Taylor RG, Gross E, Joyce H et al. (1985) Smoking, allergy, and the differential white blood cell count. Thorax 40:17–22
29. Burrows B, Halonen M, Barbee RA, Lebowitz MD (1981) The relationship of serum immunoglobulin E to cigarette smoking. Am Rev Respir Dis 124:523–525
30. Gerrard JW, Heiner DC, Mink J, Meyers A, Dosmann JA (1980) Immunoglobulin levels in smokers and non-smokers. Ann Allergy 44:261–262
31. Gortmaker SL, Klein Walter D, Jacobs FH, Ruch-Ross H (1982) Parental smoking and the risk of childhood asthma. Am J Public Health 72:574–579
32. McConnochie KN, Roghmann KJ (1986) Parental smoking, presence of older siblings, and family history of asthma increase risk of bronchiolitis. Am J Dis Child 140:806–812
33. Weiss ST, Tager IB, Speizer FE, Rosner B (1980) Persistent wheeze, its relation to respiratory illness, cigarette smoking, and level of pulmonary function in a population sample of children. Am Rev Respir Dis 122:697–707
34. Cogswill JJ, Mitchell EB, Alexander J (1987) Parental smoking, breast feeding, and respiratory infection in development of allergic diseases. Arch Dis Child 62:338–344
35. Kjellman NIM (1981) Effect of parental smoking on IgE levels in children. Lancet I:993–994
36. Zetterström O, Nordwall SL, Björkstein B, Ahlstedt S, Stelander M (1985) Increased IgE antibody responses in rats exposed to tobacco smoke. J Allergy Clin Immunol 75:595–598
37. Riedel F, Nüßlein T, Rieger CHL (1990) Tobacco smoke enhances allergic bronchial sensitization in the guinea pig. Pediatr Allergy Immunol 1: 26–33

Animal Models of Atopic Eczema

T. Willemse

Introduction

Other than humans, the dog is the only animal in which spontaneously occurring atopic disease has been documented and studied. As early as 1941, Wittich [61] described a dog with hay fever-like symptoms, and he was able to transfer immediate skin test reactivity passively to recipient dogs. According to the literature [38, 43, 48, 58], atopic eczema (AE) is the major feature in canine atopy. However, in contrast to findings in humans, other symptoms like rhinitis, sneezing, asthma and conjunctivitis are rare [39, 48, 58]. Therefore, it is the purpose of the present review to focus on the similarities and the comparative aspects between this disease in humans and dogs.

Immunopathogenesis

Immunoglobulin E

As in humans, immunoglobulin E (IgE) in the dog is a homocytotropic antibody, has a sedimentation coefficient of 8–9 *S*, is inactivated by heating at 56°C for 2–4 h and is mercaptoethanol sensitive [44, 46]. Conclusive evidence for antigenic similarities between canine and human IgE were found by Patterson et al. [40] and by Halliwell et al. [15]. However, investigations in experimentally induced respiratory hypersensitivity to *Artemisia gnopheles* in dogs [9] suggested an incomplete antigenic relationship between canine and human IgE.

Canine reagin found in a pollen-allergic dog was found to be non-precipitating, heat labile and incapable of inducing a passive cutaneous anaphylaxis (PCA) reaction in guinea pigs [39], but able to elicit Prausnitz-Küstner (P-K) reactions and active cutaneous anaphylaxis in dogs [37]. Reagins were also found in dogs sensitised to *Ascaris suum* antigen [2], which is in accordance with the presence of elevated IgE concentrations in people with endoparasitic infections [22]. These observations were confirmed by Halliwell [12] in dogs with internal and external parasites and spontaneous hypersensitivity. In addition, a latency period of 24 h was found to be necessary for optimum expression of the P-K test. Receptor sites in canine skin could be saturated and made nonreceptive for P-K testing by injection of a serum selected as likely to be high in reaginic antibody.

In healthy dogs, serum IgE levels were found to be 23–420 μg/ml [13, 51]. No correlation was found between serum IgE concentrations and the presence of IgE in the skin, as demonstrated by immunofluorescence [13]. The above-mentioned discrepancies between IgE levels and clinical observations were not solved when the determination of allergen-specific IgE antibodies was introduced. According to Halliwell and Kunkle [14], the agreement between positive radioallergosorbent test (RAST) scores and skin test results in atopic dogs ranged from 82% for ragweed to 42% for *Dermatophagoides farinae* and only 12% for dandelion. RAST tests using whole house dust extract as antigen were invariably negative, despite the fact that sera of the dogs gave positive P-K tests with the same extract. At that time it was uncertain whether these variable findings were due to the presence of antibodies of other immunoglobulin classes interfering with the binding of IgE antibodies to solid-phase antigens in RAST. Support for this hypothesis was given by the work of Schwartzman et al. [47]. They tried to establish a colony of atopic dogs, by inbreeding dogs with a seasonal AE. Progeny were studied during their first 2 years of life. However, neither the results of testing by passive cutaneous anaphylaxis nor RAST procedures correlated with positive clinical findings. None of the 70 dogs tested had elevated allergen-specific IgE antibodies as determined by RAST.

Non-IgE Anaphylactic Antibodies

The first indication of the presence of non-IgE anaphylactic antibodies in dogs was obtained in the studies of Willemse et al. [59]. They immunised dogs with eggs of *Toxocara canis* or *o*-dinitrocarboxyphenol-bovine serum albumin (*o*-DNCP-BSA), as these antigens were reported to be able to induce considerable amounts of IgE production in dogs [12] and horses [49].

In all dogs, immediate skin test reactivity preceded or accompanied serum P-K and PCA reactivity (Table 1). P-K and PCA reactivity was only observed after 4 h of sensitisation of recipient skin. In addition, heating of the sera at 56°C for 2 h or reduction with 2-mercaphoethanol did not influence the P-K and PCA results. Such properties are not known for IgE [15]. These non-IgE anaphylactic antibodies are most likely IgGd, a subclass of immunoglobulin G. The reference values of serum IgGd in healthy dogs range between 1.6 and 17.8 mg/ml. In one study, allergen-specific IgGd antibodies were determined in dogs with AE by means of an enzyme-linked immunosorbent assay (ELISA) [60]. Of dogs with clinical manifestations of AE together with the presence of immediate skin test reactivity, 89% had allergen-specific IgGd antibodies against one or more allergens. Antibodies were most frequently found against house dust, human dandruff, grass pollens and spring tree pollens. In addition, 55% of the dogs which had atopic signs without immediate skin test reactivity also exhibited elevated IgGd titers. Comparable with the findings of allergen-specific IgE antibodies in relation to skin test reactivity, a partial agreement was found between the two tests also for allergen-specific IgGd. Support for a significant role of IgGd was found by Prelaud [42], who found a high correlation between the occurrence of immediate skin test reactivity to *Dermatophagoides farinae, Dermatophagoides pteronyssinus*, cat dander, *Artemisia vulgaris*, and grass pollen, and the basophil granulation test using an iodonitrotetrazolium stain for canine basophils.

In humans, the immunoglobulin having these properties is IgG S-TS (short-term sensitising) [33, 34]. IgG S-TS probably mediates anaphylactic reactions in patients with little or no detectable IgE against the offending antigen [35], which is in accordance with the findings of Willemse et al. [60] in dogs.

Although it is uncertain whether IgG4 and IgG S-TS are identical or merely share similar properties, comparable evidence has been reported by Gwynn et al. [11], who found significantly elevated levels of IgG4 in patients with asthma and AE.

Table 1. Data of dogs immunised with *o*-DNCP-BSA or *Toxocara canis*

Week no.	Highest antigen dilution causing ISR[a]		Serum dilution causing: 4-h P-K reactivity		4-h PCA reactivity	
	B	C	B	C	B	C
6	1:8	1:1	–	–	–	–
8	1:8	1:16	–	undil	–	–
10	1:8	1:100	–	1:2	–	–
12	1:8	1:100	undil	1:2	–	–
	D	E	D	E	D	E
1	1:2	1:2	–	1:10	–	–
3	1:16	1:4	–	1:20	–	–
5	1:256	1:4	1:80	1:40	1:80	–
7		1:8		1:320		1:60
8		1:32		1:640		1:640

[a] Immediate skin test reactivity.
B,C, data of dogs immunised with 10 μg and 100 μg of *o*-DNCP-BSA, respectively. D,E, data of dogs immunised with embryonated eggs of *Toxocara canis*.

T-Cell Disorders in Relation to Atopy

The relevance of changes in lymphocyte activity as a fundamental feature of atopy is little understood. In humans it is evident that atopy, and in particular AE, is a manifestation of reduced immunocompetence with a selective deficiency of T-cell suppressor activity, which in turn may be a manifestation of impaired endogenous mediator synthesis, thymus hormones and interleukins [36]. The pathogenesis of IgE-mediated allergic disorders has been explained by Katz [23] by means of the "allergic breakthrough" and an imbalance in normal "damping" of IgE. It is postulated that the normal damping is regulated by antigen-specific helper and suppressor T cells and also by non-specific suppressor factors of allergy. If the threshold of the damping mechanism is lowered (e.g. experimentally by administration of anti-lymphocyte serum or cyclophosphamide or by irradiation) to a level insufficient to control the magnitude of IgE antibody synthesis, and exposure to an allergen then occurs, an "allergic breakthrough" might result. Once a given response has entered into the allergic zone, it will remain there until the damping mechanism returns, leading to a return of the IgE antibody response to the non-allergic zone. At that point the normal balance between the threshold activity of the damping mechanism and IgE antibody synthesis will be restored. Evidence for a comparable phenomenon in dogs has been provided by the experiments of Frick and Brooks [10], who suggested that attenuated live virus vaccines may selectively deplete suppressor T lymphocytes, thereby leading to a naturally occurring allergic breakthrough.

Recently an altered *in vitro* cell-mediated immune function was found in atopic dogs, as it is in atopic people [31]. Peripheral blood mononuclear cells (pbmc) of atopic dogs that had been preincubated for 24 h failed to show the enhancement of Con A mitogenesis that the normal canine cells did. Histamine added simultaneously with the Con A also failed to enhance the mitogenesis of atopic dog pbmc, although normal canine pbmc did respond.

A comparable suppressive effect of histamine was observed on the *in vitro* T cell blastogenic responses of canine pbmc to phytohemagglutinin-P [8].

Cellular Mechanisms and Mediator Release

It is commonly accepted that atopy in dogs is a manifestation of an immediate type hypersensitivity reaction. That means that like in humans in its simplest form the sequence of events is as follows. In animals with a hereditary basis for atopic disease, contact with inhalant allergens initiates the formation of the immunoglobulin E or IgGd isotype. Subsequently, these homocytotropic antibodies are fixed to the surfaces of basophil granulocytes and mast cells. Upon re-exposure to the allergen, vasoactive mediators are released from these cells and result in the clinical manifestation of atopic disease [29, 54]. Mast cells release preformed granule-associated mediators, including histamine, neutral proteases, exoglycosidases and eosinophilic chemotactic factor of anaphylaxis (ECF-A), and membrane-derived mediators such as prostaglandins, thromboxanes and leukotrienes. Histamine, proteolytic enzymes and leukotrienes are most important in dogs [1, 51, 62].

Cutaneous histamine concentrations were found to be significantly higher in dogs with AE compared to values of healthy dogs [32]. There was no correlation between serum IgE concentrations and those of plasma histamine, but a very good correlation ($r = 0.84$) was found between mast cell numbers and cutaneous histamine concentrations.

Histamine

An enhanced releasability of histamine has been seen in dogs upon immunological challenge with anti-IgE [5]. This phenomenon has been found to be caused by elevated leucocyte cAMP phosphodiesterase activity [21].

With respect to the role of histamine, the study of Helton Rhodes et al. [19] is of interest. Dogs were challenged with an aerosolised, skin-test-positive antigen by nasal inhalation, and serum histamine concentrations were determined using a radioenzyme and thin-layer chromatography technique. Another group of dogs were exposed to the same regimen, except that they were challenged with a skin-test-negative antigen. The study indicated that environmental allergens identified as skin-test-positive in AE appear to cause an increase in serum histamine higher than that caused by a skin-test-negative allergen. In addition, the increase in serum histamine correlated with the mild increase in clinical signs. Whether these differences were statistically significant or not could not be calculated due to limited data. A priming effect of subsequent challenge with skin-test-negative and skin-test-positive allergens might have contributed to the increase of serum histamine.

Willemse [55] found in only 3 of 45 dogs with clinical manifestations of atopy a significant increase in nasal airway resistance after challenge with grasses and summer weeds ($P < 0.001$). It was only in these animals that in addition a seasonal occurrence of clinical signs and sneezing and bilateral conjunctivitis had been observed, together with the presence of positive P-K tests to the respective allergens. In the same study exposure of the nasal mucosa to histamine (0.5 mg/ml) caused a significant, similar increase in nasal airway resistance in healthy dogs and in atopic animals. In humans, however, no increase may be observed in healthy individuals after histamine exposure in concentrations up to 32 mg/ml [7].

Arachidonic Acid and its Metabolites

Eicosanoids are products of the oxygenation of 20-carbon polyunsaturated fatty acids, in particular arachidonic acid (5, 8, 11, 14-eicosatetraenoic acid). The prostanoids – prostaglandins and thromboxanes – are derived from arachidonate by the action of a cyclo-oxygenase enzyme system, whereas the leukotrienes and hydroxy-acids are synthesised following lipo-oxygenase enzyme activity [20].

Arachidonic acid is the principal substrate for eicosanoid systhesis in animal tissues and is an essential fatty acid derived from the diet either directly or following synthesis from dietary linoleic acid. In dogs with AE, the oral administration of essential fatty acids and eicosatetraenoic acid seems to contribute to the improvement of the dermatitis [27], most likely due to a negative feedback on the release of preformed, granule-associated mediators via prostaglandin formation and intracellular cAMP.

There are only a few reports on the regulatory role of eicosanoids in dogs in relation to atopy. A pruritic dermatitis and increased airway resistance have been described in basenji-greyhound dogs by Butler et al. [5]. In response to antigen challenge, a blunted cAMP response to β-adrenergic agents and in vivo release of histamine and SRS-A (slow reactive substance of anaphylaxis, nowadays believed to be comprised of a mixture of leukotrienes: LTB_4, LTC_4, LTD_4 and LTE_4) were observed. This observation is in accordance with the β-adrenergic blocking theory of the atopic abnormality in bronchial asthma in humans [50]. It was suggested, however, that the airway response of sensitised basenji-greyhound dogs to ascaris antigen was more dependent on factors affecting mediator release frompulmonary sources than on circulating, specific reagenic antibody [41].

Langerhans Cells

In addition to their antigen-presenting function, Langerhans cells have been regarded as interacting with helper T lymphocytes or as specific targets for destruction by cytotoxic T cells [3]. Langerhans cells have been well characterised in rodents and humans. They are epidermal, dendritic macrophages which express abundant Ia antigens and possess a characteristic ultrastructural cytoplasmic organelle, the Birbeck's granule. Dendritic Langerhans-like cells have also been observed in healthy dogs [28]. These cells were identified by their electronlucent, finely granular cytoplasm, irregularly folded nuclear membrane and marginated chromatin. The cytoplasmic compartments of the Langerhans cell characteristically contain multivesicular bodies, phagosomes, coated and smooth vesicles, dispersed microfilaments, rare profiles of granular endoplasmic reticulum and free ribosomes, and sparse mitochondria. However, Birbeck's granules were not observed.

Langerhans cells have been observed in dogs with AE (Willemse 1987, unpublished work). The recent finding in humans that IgE is present on epidermal Langerhans cells of patients with AE but not on those of healthy persons may partly explain the high frequency of positive patch tests to inhalant allergens in AE and may provide a link between immediate and delayed-type hypersensitivity reactions [4]. Although it is very likely that similar phenomena will play a role in the pathogenesis of canine AE, so far no other evidence has been uncovered.

Histopathology

Histopathological examination of lesional skin from atopic dogs reveals varying degrees of chronic non-suppurative dermatitis. Although not diagnostic of canine atopy, the observed changes are consistent and supportive. Angiocentric accumulations of inflammatory cells are confined to the superficial dermal blood vessels. Mononuclear cells and neutrophils, in varying proportions, are the predominant inflammatory cells seen. Eosinophils are observed in only 15% and then only in very small numbers. Mast cell numbers are increased in 35% of atopic dogs [48]. In AE in humans and dogs, the epidermal and dermal changes vary with the severity of clinical signs. The histopathological alterations in clinically normal skin may reflect either subclinical disease or residual involvement from a previous clinical episode. The findings in dogs are comparable with the histopathological features of human patients with AE [26].

Diagnostic Criteria of Atopic Eczema

In an attempt to provide consistency in the diagnosis of AE in humans, Hanifin and Lobitz [17] and Hanifin and Rajka [18] introduced the concept of major and minor diagnostic features. According to their criteria at least three of the following major features must be present: pruritus, a typical morphology and distribution including flexural lichenification in adults and facial and extensor involvement in infants and children, a tendency towards chronic or chronically relapsing dermatitis, and a personal or family history of atopy (asthma, allergic rhinitis, AE). In addition, three or more of the following minor features must be present: early age of onset, immediate skin test reactivity, elevated serum IgE, xerosis, a tendency towards cutaneous infections, impaired cell-mediated immunity, recurrent conjunctivitis, cheilitis, a tendency towards non-specific hand or foot dermatitis, facial pallor, facial erythema, and orbital darkening, food intolerance or intolerance to wool and lipid solvents, itch when sweating, course influenced by environmental or emotional factors, and white dermographism and delayed blanch.

In dogs pruritus has been considered a hallmark of AE, if emphasised by feet licking and nose or head rubbing [48]. Since the occurrence of primary cutaneous lesions has never been firmly established in dogs or in humans [18], it may be that all the cutaneous changes are secondary to itch-induced scratching. This hypothesis is supported by the finding of Willemse and van den Brom [58] that although all of the dogs had signs of face rubbing and feet licking, only two-thirds had cutaneous lesions in the facial and pedal areas.

As far as the distribution is concerned, in dogs the most commonly affected areas are the muzzle and the periocular area (60%), the feet (70%) and to a lesser extent the axillae (35%), the extensor side of the carpal joint (40%) and the flexural side of the tarsal joint (30%) [58]. Obviously, involvement of the extensor and flexural surfaces was only observed in those dogs in which the atopic symptoms were associated with immediate skin test reactivity.

The most frequently observed skin morphology includes erythema, papular reactions, crusts and lichenification. Although lichenified skin is seen in over 80% of the animals with AE, it does not appear to be related to the presence of immediate skin test reactivity.

In addition, there is no apparent age-related difference in distribution or morphology, which is in contrast to the findings in humans [18]. As in humans, AE in dogs tends to be a chronic or chronically relapsing dermatitis as well [29, 58]. The latter study showed the disease to be present for more than 1 year in approximately 80% of the animals, whereas one-third of the dogs had been affected for more than 3 years. Seasonal exacerbations are reported for 30%–40% of the dogs with atopy and tend to progress from seasonal to non-seasonal in 15% during the course of the disease [30, 48].

A personal or family history of atopy may, also in dogs, contribute to the diagnosis. Support for this hypothesis is given by the study of Schwartzman [45]. Of the progeny resulting from brother-to-sister matings of atopic dogs, 30 of 56 animals developed immediate skin test reactivity to inhalant allergens, and 13 showed clinical evidence of atopic disease. Interesting, however, was the development of skin test reactivity prior to the presence of clinical signs. The latter did not occur before the age of 13 months.

With respect to the clinical manifestations which may indicate atopy in relatives in additon to AE, conjunctivitis, reverse sneezing, rhinitis and asthma-like symptoms have to be included [39, 48, 58]. Although the familial nature of the disease is well known, the mode of inheritance is unclear in both humans and dogs [16, 53]. The latter found no relationship between serologically recognised dog leucocyte antigen (DL-A)groups (the major histocompatibility genetic region in dogs) and atopy. Although it was hypothesised that the DL-A haplotype 9,4 might offer protection against the disease while haplotype 3,R15 might be associated with a greater susceptibility, this statement has never been confirmed since. It is generally observed that in dogs with AE the age of onset is low. In 75% the dogs the first symptoms are seen before the age of 3 years [48, 58]. Approximately 80% of dogs with AE exhibits immediate skin test reactivity (after 20 min) to inhalant allergens [30, 48, 58]. Late-phase IgE/IgGd-like reactions at 2–8 h after the intradermal reaction are occasionally seen (Willemse 1988, unpublished work), but delayed reactions at 24 h are not known. Multisensitivity occurs in approximately 60% of animals, with house dust (40%–70%), human dandruff (20%–40%), dog dandruff (25%), cat dandruff (30%), grass pollen and weed extracts (20%–70%) being most commonly reported. The study of Willemse and van den Brom [58] showed a lower number of positive skin test reactions to multiple allergens in dogs older than 6 years ($P < 0.001$), which is in agreement with the findings in middle-aged humans [6].

The significance of elevated IgE/IgGd concentrations has been discussed earlier. However, it is noteworthy that Willemse [55] could demonstrate P-K reactivity at 24 h in only 3 of 46 atopic dogs, despite the presence of characteristic symptoms, immediate skin test reactivity and the fact that a latent period of 24 h was found to be necessary for optimum expression of the P-K test [12]. This suggests that IgE may only occasionally be involved in the pathogenesis of canine AE. Support for this interpretation is found by the inability to demonstrate IgE activity in dogs with AE [47,59]. Xerosis or generalised dryness of the skin is a common feature of animals with AE and has been seen in association with the presence of staphylococcal skin infections [48, 58]. In addition it was noticed that the incidence of a superficial pyoderma was significantly higher in dogs with atopic symptoms together with immediate skin test reactivity than in dogs with clinical manifestations but without a positive skin test. Although the presence of a pyoderma in conjunction with AE in humans is sometimes thought to be related to a decreased cell-mediated immunity with impaired chemotaxis [15], this has not been found in dogs [24, 25].

Recurrent conjunctivitis has often been seen in atopic dogs [30, 48]. Whether this reflects the presence of hay fever-like phenomena is uncertain. However, the improvement of many animals upon the topical application of cromoglycate may emphasise this possibility. Cheilitis, facial erythema and orbital darkening are clinical manifestations which are noticed occasionally but may also be present in a series of other diseases. The concomitant occurrence of a food allergy or a contact allergy in dogs with AE is an uncommon observation. However, it cannot be excluded that a food allergy or food intolerance is part of the atopy complex and must be considered as part of its preliminary stages. An argument in favour of this hypothesis may be the fact that food allergies in the majority of cases are seen below the age of 1 year, and AE after that period of life. In addition, it is of interest that in a considerable percentage of dogs with atopy, immediate skin reactivity has been found to storage mite extracts [52].

It is a clinical impression that stress and sweating contribute considerably to the total amount of itch, as present in atopic dogs. An increased sweating ability has been observed in about 10% of the dogs [48, 58]. Whether this sweating is the result of emotional stress or is an isolated phenomenon has not been investigated. As the remaining minor diagnostic features of AE in humans have not been reported or investigated in dogs, their significance is unclear. It is apparent, however, that most of the diagnostic criteria suggested by Hanifin and Rajka [18] for humans may be used in dogs. Upon this basis a modification of these criteria has been proposed for the definite diagnosis of canine AE [56, 57].

Basic features include:
- Pruritus
- Facial and/or digital involvement
- Lichenification of the flexor surface of the tarsal joint and/or the extensor surface of the carpal joint
- Chronic or chronically relapsing dermatitis
- Individual or family history of atopy
- Breed predisposition

and minor features:

- Onset of symptoms before the age of 3 years
- Immediate skin test reactivity to inhalant allergens
- Elevated allergen-specific IgGd
- Elevated allergen-specific IgE
- Xerosis
- Superficial staphylococcal pyoderma
- Bilateral recurrent conjunctivitis
- Facial erythema and cheilitis
- Sweating

Summary

Many similarities exist between AE in humans and in dogs, not only in the clinical manifestations of the disease but also in the histopathological features and the background mechanisms with regard to the immunopathogenesis. Although in comparison with humans not all aspects of the disease have been investigated in dogs so far, there is substantial evidence that the dog may be a good model for further research of AE humans.

References

1. Becker AB, Chung KF, McDonald DM, Frick OL, Gold WM (1988) Cutaneous allergic response in atopic dogs: relationship of cellular and histamine reponses. J Allergy Clin Immunol 81:441–448
2. Booth BH, Patterson R, Talbot CH (1970) Immediate type hypersensitivity in dogs: cutaneous, anaphylactic and respiratory responses to *Ascaris*. J Lab Clin Med 76:181–189
3. Breathnach SM (1988) The Langerhans cell. Br J Dermatol 119:463–469
4. Bruynzeel-Koomen C, van Wichen DF, Toonstra J (1986) The presence of IgE molecules on epidermal Langerhans cells in patients with atopic dermatitis. Arch Dermatol Res 278:199–205
5. Butler JM, Peters JE, Hirshman CA, White CR, Margolin LB, Hanifin JM (1983) Pruritic dermatitis in asthmatic basenji-greyhound dogs: a model for human atopic dermatitis. J Am Acad Dermatol 8:33–38
6. Champion RH, Parish WE (1979) Textbook of dermatology, 3rd edn. Blackwell, Oxford, pp 349–361
7. Clement PAR, Van Dishoeck A, Van de Wal J (1981) Nasal provocation and passive anterior rhinomanometry (PAR). Clin Allergy 11:293–301
8. Daniel SL, Ogilvie GK, Felsburg PJ (1990) Modulation of Canine lymphocyte blastogenesis via histamine. Vet Immunol Immunopathol 24: 69–77
9. Faith RE, Hessler JR, Small PA (1977) Respiratory allergy in the dog: induction by the respiratory route and the effect of passive antibody. Int Arch Allergy Appl Immunol 53: 530–544
10. Frick OL, Brooks DL (1983) Immunoglobulin E antibodies to pollens augmented in dogs by virus vaccins. Am J Vet Res 44:440–445
11. Gwynn CM, Almosawi T, Stanworth DR (1982) Clinical associations with serum allergen-specific IgG4 antibodies. Clin Allergy 12:459–464
12. Halliwell REW (1973) Studies on canine IgE. Thesis, University of Cambridge
13. Halliwell REW (1973) The localization of IgE in canine skin: an immunofluorescent study. J Immunol 110:422–430
14. Halliwell REW, Kunkle GA (1978) The radioallergosorbent test in the diagnosis of canine atopic disease. J Allergy Clin Immunol 62:236–242
15. Halliwell REW, Schwartzman RM, Rockey JH (1972) Antigenic relationship between human IgE and canine IgE. Clin Exp Immunol 10:399–407
16. Hanifin JM (1982) Atopic dermatitis. J Am Acad Dermatol 6:1–13
17. Hanifin JM, Lobitz WC (1977) Newer concepts of atopic dermatitis. Arch Dermatol 113:663–670
18. Hanifin JM, Rajka G (1980) Diagnostic features of atopic dermatitis. Acta Derm Venereol (Stockh.) 92:44–47
19. Helton Rhodes K, Kerdel F, Soter NA, Chinnici R (1987) Investigation into the immunopathogenesis of canine atopy. Semin Vet Med Surg (Small Anim) 2:199–201
20. Higgins AJ (1985) Eicosanoids in health and in disease: an appraisal. Vet Quart 7:44–59
21. Hirshman CA, Leu DB, Austin DR, Chan SC, Veith L, Hanifin JM (1987) Elevated mononuclear leukocyte phosphodiesterase in allergic dogs with and without airway hyperresponsiveness. J Allergy Clin Immunol 79:46–53
22. Johansson SGO, Mellbin T, Vahlquist B (1968) Immunoglobulin levels in Ethiopean preschool children with special reference to high concentrations of immunoglobulin E (IgND). Lancet i:1118–1121
23. Katz DH (1978) The allergic phenotype: manifestation of allergic breakthrough and imbalance in normal damping of IgE antibody productin. Immunol Rev 41:77–108
24. Kroese FGM, Willemse A, Slappendel RJ (1981) Granulocyte function tests in canine infectious diseases. Vet Immunol Immunopathol 2:455–466
25. Latimer KS, Prasse KW, Mahaffey EA, Dawe DL, Lorenz MD, Duncan FR (1983) Neutrophil movement in selected canine skin diseases. Am J Vet Res 44:601–605
26. Leung DYM, Rhodes AR, Geha RS (1987) Atopic dermatitis. In: Fitzpatrick TB, Eisen AZ, Wolff K, Freedberg IM, Austen KF (eds) Dermatology in general medicine, 3rd edn. McGraw Hill, New York, pp 1385–1409
27. Lloyd HD (1989) Essential fatty acids and skin diseases. J Small Anim Pract 30:207–212
28. Moore PF, Mariassy AT (1986) Dendritic (Langerhans) cells in canine epidermis: ultrastructure and distribution. Anat Histol Embryol 15:178–179
29. Muller GH, Kirk RW, Scott DW (1989) Small Animal Dermatology, 4th edition. Saunders, Philadelphia, pp 427–574
30. Nesbitt GH (1978) Canine allergic inhalant dermatitis: a review of 230 cases. J Am Vet Med Assoc 172:55–60
31. Nimmo Wilkie JS (1990) Cell-mediated immune function in dogs with atopic dermatitis. In: Advances in Veterinary Dermatology. Baillière Tindall, London, vol I, pp 145–154
32. Nimmo Wilkie JS, Yager JA, Eyre P, Parker WM (1990) Morphometric analysis of the skin of dogs with atopic dermatitis and correlations with cutaneous and plasma histamine and total serum IgE. Vet Pathol 27: 179–186

33. Parish WE (1970) Short-term anaphylactic IgG antibodies in human sera. Lancet ii:591–592
34. Parish WE (1974) Skin sensitizing non-IgE antibodies. Association between human IgG S-TS and IgG4. Prog Immunol 4:19–28
35. Parish WE (1981) The clinical relevance of heat-stable, short-term sensitizing anaphylactic IgG antibodies (IgG S-TS) and of related activities of IgG4 and IgG2. Br J Dermatol 105:223–231
36. Parish WE (1988) Atopy: one hundred years of antibodies, mast cells and lymphocytes. Br J Dermatol 119:437–443
37. Patterson R (1960) Investigations of spontaneous hypersensitivity of the dog. J Allergy 31:351–363
38. Patterson R (1969) Laboratory models of reagenic allergy. Prog Allergy 13:332–407
39. Patterson R, Pruzansky JJ, Chang WWY (1963) Spontaneous hypersensitivity to ragweed. Characterization of the serum factor transferring skin, bronchial and anaphylactic sensitivity. J Immunol 90:35–42
40. Patterson R, Roberts M, Pruzansky JJ (1969) Comparisons of reagenic antibodies from three species. J Immunol 102: 466–475
41. Peters JE, Hirshman CA, Malley A (1982) The Basenji-Greyhound dog model of asthma: leukocyte histamine release, serum IgE, and airway response to inhaled antigen. J Immunol 129:1245–1249
42. Prelaud L (1990) Basophil degranulation test in the diagnosis of canine allergic skin diseases. In: Advances in Veterinary Dermatoloy. Baillière Tindall, London, vol I, pp 117–125
43. Reedy LM (1980) The diagnosis of canine atopic disease. In: Kirk RW (ed) Current veterinary therapy. Saunders, Philadelphia, pp 450–453
44. Rockey JH, Schwartzman RM (1967) Skin sensitizing antibodies: a comparative study of canine and human PK and PCA antibodies and a canine myeloma protein. J Immunol 98:1143–1151
45. Schwartzman RM (1984) Immunologic studies of progeny of atopic dogs. Am J Vet Res 45:375–378
46. Schwartzman RM, Rockey JH, Halliwell REW (1971) Canine reaginic antibody. Characterization of the spontaneous anti-ragweed and induced anti-dinitrophenyl reaginic antibodies of the atopic dog. Clin Exp Immunol 9:549–569
47. Schwartzman RM, Massicot JG, Sogn DD, Cohen SG (1983) The atopic dog model: report of an attempt to establish a colony. Int Arch Allergy Appl Immunol 72:97–101
48. Scott DW (1981) Observations on canine atopy. J Am Anim Hosp Assoc 17:91–100
49. Suter M, Fey H (1981) Isolation and characterization of equine IgE. Zentralbl Veterinarmed [B]28:414–418
50. Szentivanyi A (1968) The beta adrenergic theory of the atopic abnormality in bronchial asthma. J Allergy 42:203–233
51. Tizard I (1987) Veterinary immunology, 2nd edn. Saunders, Philadelphia
52. Vollsett I (1986) Immediate type hypersensivity in dogs induced by storage mites. Res Vet Sci 40:123–127
53. Vriesendorp HM, Smid-Mercx BMJ, VisserTP, Halliwell REW, Schwartzman RM (1975) Serological DL-A typing of normal and atopic dogs. Transplant Proc 7:375–377
54. Willemse A (1984) Investigations on canine atopic dermatitis. Thesis, Utrecht University, Utrecht
55. Willemse A (1984) Canine atopic disease: investigations of eosinophils and the nasal mucosa. Am J Vet Res 45:1867–1869
56. Willemse A (1986) Atopic skin disease: a review and a reconsideration of diagnostic criteria. J Small Anim Pract 27: 771–778
57. Willemse A (1987) Atopic dermatitis. In: Nesbitt GH (ed) Dermatology. Churchill Livingstone, New York, pp 57–77 (Contemporary issues in small animal practice, vol 8)
58. Willemse A, Van den Brom WE (1983) Investigations of the symptomatology and the significance of immediate skin test reactivity in canine atopic dermatitis. Res Vet Sci 34:261–265
59. Willemse A, Noordzij A, Rutten VPMG, Bernadina WE (1985) Induction of non-IgE anaphylactic antibodies in dogs. Clin Exp Immunol 59:351–358
60. Willemse A, Noordzij A, Van den Brom WE, Rutten VPMG (1985) Allergen-specific IgGd antibodies in dogs with atopic dermatitis. Clin Exp Immunol 59:359–363
61. Wittich FW (1941) Spontaneous allergy (atopy) in the lower animal. J Allergy 12:247–251
62. Zimmerman I, Ulmer WT (1981) Effect of intravenous histamine, allergen (Ascaris suum extract) and compound 48/80 and inhaled allergen-aerosol on bronchoconstriction and histamine release. Respiration 42:30–42

The Pathophysiology of Atopic Eczema: Synopsis

J. Ring, T. Ruzicka, and B. Przybilla

Introduction

While the pathomechanisms of allergic respiratory diseases such as hay fever or extrinsic bronchial asthma are rather well established, the role of allergic reactions in the pathophysiology of atopic eczema is still controversial. Two main currents can be detected in the history of the literature that try to explain the disease: specifically altered immune reactivity (i.e., allergy), on the one hand, and nonspecifically altered reactivity on the other [5, 18, 31, 36, 47, 52].

The confusion becomes visible in the various names for this skin disease, all emphasizing a certain aspect of a suspected pathophysiology, such as "prurigo diathésique", "neurodermitis constitutionalis" or "neurodermitis diffusa", "endogenous eczema", "asthma eczema", "atopic eczema" or "eczema". We think the term "atopic eczema" is the most honest one since it simply describes the eczema occurring in atopics without inferring other mechanisms or abnormalities (e.g., neurological) or routes of elicitation (e.g., from the inside or the outside).

However, to be fair, we have to first define "atopy", a term with an equally long history [10]. Many think that atopy equals increased IgE production, an assumption which clearly is incorrect when we think of many other diseases like parasitoses, graft-versus-host disease, T cell malignancies, and other conditions with elevated IgE production. It also seems too simple to define atopy as a "condition associated with but not necessarily caused by IgE antibodies" [27]. We have seen that although IgE is more than atopy, atopy is also more than IgE since it describes an altered reactivity towards a variety of nonspecific stimuli too. Nevertheless, atopic diseases can be grouped immunologically among IgE mediated reactions, with the addition of their familial occurrence and the phenomenon of altered reactivity. We define atopy as: "familial hypersensitivity of skin and mucous membranes against environmental agents, associated with increased IgE production and/or altered reactivity" [35].

Like every biological process, atopy is not an all or nothing response. There are marginal manifestations which are difficult to classify. One is tempted to speak of "latent atopy" or of degrees of atopicness. One might think of a Gaussian distribution of atopic diseases, in which the criteria IgE production and altered reactivity are illustrated (see the chapter "Atopy" by J. Ring, this volume). Let us now consider the most frequently discussed etiopathophysiological concepts of atopic eczema. These are:

1. Genetic influences
2. Dry skin
3. Immunological dysfunction (cellular immunodeficiency)
4. Increased IgE production
5. Psychosomatic interaction
6. Autonomous nervous system imbalance

Genetic Influence and Atopic Eczema

There is no doubt that a genetic component favors the manifestation of atopic eczema. Together with allergic rhinoconjunctivitis and allergic asthma this disease is intrinsically connected within families [25, 41, 44]. Twin studies show clearly that the concordance in homozygous twins is around 75% but in heterozygous twins only 30% [44, 52]. Not only the immunological abnormality of atopy but also the organ manifestation seems to be influenced by genetic factors. When both parents suffer from the same organ manifestation of atopy (e.g., father and mother have eczema) the child has a risk of around 70% to also develop atopic eczema. If, however, the two parents suffer from different atopic diseases (e.g., father asthma, mother eczema) the incidence of atopic diseases in the children is only 30% [3].

This clear-cut genetic influence sometimes gives rise to the misleading concept of an inborn, hereditary disease which therefore is incurable. This is not only theoretically and empirically wrong, but also very frustrating for the patient when doctors pronounce this verdict. The patient does not suffer from chromosomal patterns leading to increased IgE production, but from itching skin lesions.

The chromosomes cannot be changed at the moment; however, the itchy skin lesions can be treated very well! Nobody would say that streptococcal angina is incurable only because it may occur again.

Genetic Factors and Dry Skin

The well-known alteration of the skin surface most commonly described as "dry skin" (also known as "xerosis", "asteatosis", "sebostasis", "ichthyosis", "xeroderma") represents a complex mixture of various factors. At least three quite different dimensions have to be considered when talking about dry skin, namely:

"rough" vs "smooth"
"lipid-rich" vs "lipid-poor"
"moist" vs "low in water content" [29].

The role of sebaceous gland function is controversial ([29, 50] and see the chapters by Melnik and Gloor, this volume). Some authors concentrate on the epidermal lipid components, postulating a defect in the enzyme delta-6-desaturase that converts linoleic acid into other essential polyunsaturated fatty acids, mostly arachidonic acid, a major component of the cell membrane [51] (Melnik, this volume). This concept is especially attractive because of the similarity to a scaling dermatosis observed in rats deprived of essential fatty acids. However, the efficacy of therapeutic substitution or application of essential unsaturated fatty acids is still a matter of controversy (Ring and Kunz, this volume).

In atopic eczema the skin is not really dry in the sense of low water content; its dry appearance is mainly due to an increased transepidermal water loss (see the chapter by Gollhausen, this volume).

While many authors regard "dry skin" as a genetic feature of atopic eczema, others point correctly to the variable nature of this dryness, changing rapidly in many patients during exacerbation and remission. It is an attractive hypothesis that the dryness of the skin reflects only the sequelae of an otherwise invisible inflammation (see the chapter by Uehara, this volume).

There is an intimate relation between dry skin and itch, well-known in exsiccation conditions leading to pruritus, scratching, and eczematous skin lesions. Dry skin also is more irritable than normal skin. Some people talk of "sensitive skin" without being able to define it or measure it quantitatively. The possibility to quantitate the irritability of atopic skin with modern techniques, e.g. laser Doppler flowmetry (see the chapter by Gollhausen, this volume), can be regarded as a major advance.

Autonomic Dysregulation in Atopic Eczema

Many of the stigmata of atopic eczema and the phenomenon of dry skin are explained by some authors as a dysregulation in the autonomic nervous system, best described as β-adrenergic blockade [47] together with α-adrenergic and cholinergic hyperreactivity [13]. This autonomic nervous system transmitter imbalance could explain the increased releasability of vasoactive mediators (e.g. histamine or leukotrienes) in atopic eczema and the well-known psychosomatic interactions operating in this condition [5, 36, 39]. The mechanism of this altered autonomic reactivity is not yet clear. The most attractive hypothesis is an increased phosphodiesterase level in leukocytes, already measurable in cord blood which influences both IgE production and vasoactive mediator secretion [13].

The vasoactive mediators which seem to be more easily released, such as histamine or prostaglandins, not only have proinflammatory activities, but also anti-inflammatory effects via receptors on the leukocyte surface. It may be speculated that an increased level of these mediators in tissues may contribute to the well-known minimal immunodeficiency of cellular immune reactions in these patients [36].

Minimal Cellular Immunodeficiency

Decreased resistance to infections especially of the skin is a well-known characteristic of atopic eczema, noted first by Kaposi and since confirmed by a variety of clinical and experimental investigations. Furthermore, a decreased tendency to develop allergic contact dermatitis after dinitrochlorbenzene (DNCB) sensitization has been reported. This has led to a continuous debate on the relation of contact allergy to atopic eczema [24]. While some authors claim there is a decreased frequency of allergic contact sensitization in atopic eczema, others argue that, due to the defective skin barrier, the tendency to develop contact allergy may be increased in atopic eczema. A critical analysis of the literature reveals that most of the studies regarding the prevalence of contact allergy in atopic eczema are retrospective in nature and without adequate controls (see the chapter by Neumann and Marghescu, this volume). In our own experience the prevalence of allergic patch test reactions in patients with atopic eczema is almost equal to that of patients with allergic contact dermatitis. However, with regard to single contact allergens, there were significantly elevated rates of contact sensitization against nickel, cobalt, dichromate, and thiuram in atopics, while other contact reactions, e.g., to lanolin, cainemix, etc., were significantly less frequent in atopics than in nonatopics [12]. A simple explanation for the divergent results may be that these differences simply reflect the different age distributions of patients with atopic eczema and allergic contact dermatitis.

Among the various in vitro abnormalities of cellular immune functions, defects in supressor T cell activities have been reported which might explain the increased IgE production in this disease [42, 46].

Increased IgE Production in Atopic Eczema

Few diseases are characterized by such an elevated production of IgE as is atopic eczema. Not only are total IgE levels increased, but specific antibodies can be measured against common environmental allergens [1, 28]. Many authors interpret this specific IgE production as a mere epiphenomenon, which only gains clinical relevance for concomitant respiratory atopic diseases. The major argument in this debate was stated by Marchionini in 1960 [23], who said that the classic IgE mediated skin reaction is urticaria but not eczema, which is characterized by a lymphocytic inflammatory infiltrate.

Recent studies have, however, put forward a variety of working hypotheses assigning IgE antibodies a role in eliciting eczematous skin lesions (Table 1). The role of IgG antibodies, especially IgG_4, is still unclear (see the chapter by Aalberse, this volume).

The vasoactive mediator substances released from mast cells or basophils after allergen stimulation (such as histamine, eicosanoids, platelet activating factor, et.) induce itch, contact urticaria, or a late-phase reaction which finally, together with a scratch reflex, induce the eczematous skin changes [36]. A very attractive hypothesis focuses on the role of epidermal Langerhans cells bearing a receptor for IgE with low affinity (Fc_{ε} RII) similar to the one found on lymphocytes, macrophages, eosinophils, and platelets [2, 8, 11, 45]. IgE antibodies bound to Langerhans cells might function as receptors for protein antigens after they have passed the stratum corneum barrier and thus mediate antigen presentation to lymphocytes. On the other hand, Langerhans cells may well only exert a regulatory influence. Certain cytokines, such as interleukin-4, are able to enhance expression of this IgE receptor on Langerhans cells; interferon-γ has a synergistic effect in this model, in contrast to its inhibitory effect on peripheral lymphocytes [2].

Nonetheless, lymphocytes might well act directly via certain cytokines, such as histamine releasing factors (HRF), in a proinflammatory way.

Furthermore, eosinophils which were formerly regarded as antiinflammatory effector cells, might release protein mediators of a proinflammatory nature, such as major basic protein (MBP), eosinophil peroxidase (EPO), eosinophil cationic protein (ECP), and others [21]. In patients with severe atopic eczema increased levels of ECP in plasma have been observed [17].

Table 1. Atopic eczema: different hypotheses to explain the elicitation of eczematous skin lesions via IgE-dependent mechanisms

Cells	Mediators/Functions	Consequences
Mast cells/ basophils	Histamine, eicosanoids, PAF, etc.	Itch, "invisible" urticaria, contact urticaria, late phase reaction
Langerhans cells	Antigen presentation, cytokines	Delayed type hypersensitivity, regulation?
Lymphocytes	Cytokines (e.g., HRF, IL-4, etc.)	Mediator secrection, IgE production
Eosinophils	MBP, ECP, etc.	Inflammation

Many patients with atopic eczema show strong sensitization in the skin prick test against aeroallergens and foods; however, the relevance of these test reactions is unclear. Application of these protein allergens, most commonly known as elicitors of IgE antibodies, in a classical patch test to the skin surface (atopy patch test) led to a remarkable rate of positive epidermal test reactions in about 30% of the patients [8, 28, 37]. The most frequent allergen causing positive epidermal reactions was housedust mite.

It cannot be overlooked that the atopy patch test is still an experimental procedure not yet suitable for clinical routine. Many questions remain regarding the nature of allergens (concentration, vehicle, test site, test area, test conditions, etc.). According to our experience it seems to be important to perform an "atopy patch test" only in a phase of remission, when the skin is clear and there is no systemic or topical glucocorticoid treatment.

Apart from aeroallergens, microbial antigens (e.g., *Staphylococcus, Pityrosporum, Trichophyton,* etc. [4, 43, 49] or autologous epidermal proteins (human dander) might play a role in this context.

The role of food allergy in atopic eczema was a matter of debate [30, 31, 52] until well-controlled clinical trials, including double-blind placebo-controlled food challenges [1, 40], showed that in a high proportion of patients with atopic eczema, skin lesions flared after specific oral provocation with certain foods.

Even more controversial is the role of food additives in this condition. Our own data lead us to believe that some cases of severe atopic eczema may be triggered by a hypersensitivity against food additives [48], the mechanism of which is by no means clear. The role of other known elicitors of pseudoallergic reactions, such as acetylsalicylic acid, radiographic contrast media, or local anesthetics, in atopic eczema is not a matter of urgent interest.

Nevertheless, the question regarding the general role of allergy in the pathophysiology of atopic eczema is crucial. Only after a careful allergological diagnosis, including skin test, in vitro diagnostics, and possibly provocation tests can the necessary environmental control measures (e.g., dietary approaches, housedust mite programs, etc.) be successful. In the interpretation of the test results one always has to be very critical and differentiate between the coincidence and the relevance of a given sensitization (Table 2).

Table 2. Allergy and pseudo-allergy in atopic eczema

Type of reaction	Coincidence	Relevance
I	+ + +	+ to + +
II	0	0
III	±	?
IV	− + +	?
V	0	0
VI	± (auto-anti-IgE?)	?
Pseudo-allergy		
Acetylsalicylic acid	±	±
Additives	+	+?
Radiographic contrast media	0	0
Local anesthetics	0	0
UV light hypersensitivity	+	+?

Genetics and Environment in the Pathophysiology of Atopic Eczema

Nearly all the above mentioned abnormalities described in atopic eczema can either be seen as genetically determined defects or as environmental influences, depending upon the view of the observer.

The strategy in the management of patients with atopic eczema will have to be much more diagnosis-oriented than it has been up to now. It will become easier to treat the itchy skin lesions, but more difficult to identify the relevant eliciting factors. Only then, however, will specific avoidance programs be possible, finally making symptomatic antiinflammatory therapy unnecessary. The secret of successful patient management in atopic eczema is: Do not only treat the symptoms but try to find the causal factors which are specific to each patient!

References

1. Atherton DJ (1981) Allergy and atopic eczema. I and II. Clin Exp Dermatol 6:191,317
2. Bieber T, Rieger A, Neuchrist C, Prinz JC, Rieber EP, Boltz-Nitulescu G, Scheiner O, Kraft D, Ring J (1989) Induction of Fc_ε R2/CD23 on human epidermal Langerhans cells by human recombinant Interleukin 4 and γ Interferon. J Exp Med 170:309–314
3. Björkstén B, Kjellman NIM (1987) Perinatal factors influencing the development in allergy. Clin Rev Allergy 5: 339
4. Bode U, Ring J, Neubert U (1982) Intrakutantestungen und bakteriologische Untersuchungen bei Patienten mit atopischem Ekzem. Allergologie 5:259–261
5. Borelli S, Schnyder UW (1962) Neurodermitis constitutionalis sive atopica. II. Ätiologie, Pathophysiologie, Pathogenese, Therapie. In: Miescher G, Storck H (eds) Entzündliche Dermatosen I. Springer, Berlin Göttingen Heidelberg pp 254–319 (Handbuch der Haut- und Geschlechtskrankheiten) vol 1/1
6. Braun-Falco O, Ring J (1984) Zur Therapie des atopischen Ekzems. Hautarzt 35:447–454
7. Brostoff J, Carini C, Wraith DG, Johns P (1979) Production of IgE complexes by allergen challenge in atopic patients and the effect of sodium cromoglycate. Lancet 1:1268–1270
8. Bruijnzeel-Koomen C, van Wichen L, Toonstra J, Berrens Bruijnzeel P (1986) The presence of IgE molecules on epidermal Langerhans cells from patients with atopic dermatitis. Arch Dermatol Res 278:199–205
9. Capron M, Jouault T, Prin L, Joseph M, Ameisen J, Butterworth A, Papin J, Kusnierz J, Capron A (1986) Functional study of a monoclonal antibody to IgE Fc receptor (FcER2) on eosinophils, platelets and macrophages. J Exp Med 164: 72–89
10. Coca AF, Cooke RA (1923) On the classification of the phenomena of hypersensitiveness. J Immunol 8:163–182
11. Dahl MV (1983) Staphylococcus aureus and atopic dermatitis. Arch Dermatol 119:840–846
12. Enders F, Przybilla B, Ring J, Burg G, Braun-Falco O (1988) Epikutantestung mit einer Standardreihe. Ergebnisse bei 12026 Patienten. Hautarzt 39:779–786
13. Hanifin J (1983) Atopic dermatitis and other endogenous eczemas. Semin Dermatol 2:1–44
14. Hjorth N, Roed-Petersen J (1976) Occupational protein contact dermatitis in foodhandlers. Contact Dermatitis 2:28–42
15. Hornstein OP, Bäurle G, Kienlein-Kletschka B (1985) Prospektivstudie zur Bedeutung konstitutioneller Parameter für die Ekzemgenese im Friseur- and Baugewerbe. Dermatosen 33:43–49
16. Ishizaka K (1989) Regulation of immunoglobulin E biosynthesis. Adv Immunol 47:1–44
17. Jakob T, Hermann KJ, Ring J (1991) Eosinophil cationic protein in atopic eczema. Arch. Dermatol. Res. 283: 5–6
18. Korting GW (1954) Zur Pathogenese des endogenen Ekzems. Thieme, Stuttgart
19. Kunz B, Vieluf D, Ring J (1988) Efficacy of oral disodium cromoglycate (DSCG) in atopic eczema. New Engl Reg Allergy Proc 9:411
20. Kunz B, Ring J, Überla K (1989) Frequency of atopic diseases and allergic sensitization in preschool children in different parts of Bavaria. Allergologie [Suppl] 12: 144
21. Leiferman KM, Ackerman SJ, Sampson HA, Haugen HS, Venencie PY, Gleich GJ (1985) Dermal deposition of eosinophil-granule major basic protein in atopic dermatitis. Comparison with onchocerciasis. N Engl J Med 313:282–285
22. Leyden JJ, Marples RR, Kligman AM (1974) Staphylococcus aureus in the lesions of atopic dermatitis. Br J Dermatol 90:525–530
23. Marchionini A (1960) Neuere Untersuchungen über die Neurodermitis constitutionalis. In: Marchionini A (ed) Fortschritte der praktischen Dermatologie und Venerologie, vol 3. Springer, Berlin Göttingen Heidelberg, pp 42–62
24. Marghescu S (1985) Patch test reactions in atopic patients. Acta Derm Venereol (Stockh.) 114:113–116
25. Marsh DG, Hsu SH, Hussam R, Meyer DA, Freidhoff LR, Bias WB (1980) Genetics of human immune response to allergens. J Allergy Clin Immunol 65:322–330
26. Merrett J, Barnetson R, Burr M, Merrett T (1984) Total and specific IgG_4 antibody levels in atopic eczema. Clin Exp Immunol 56:645–662
27. Middleton EC, Ellis B, Reed E (eds) (1978) Allergy: principles and practice. Mosby, St Louis
28. Platts-Mills TAE, Mitchell EB, Rowntree S, Chapman MD, Wilkins SR (1983) The role of dust mite allergens in atopic dermatitis. Clin Exp Dermatol 233–247
29. Pierard GE (1987) What does "dry skin" mean? Int J Dermatol 26:167–168
30. Przybilla B, Ruzicka T, Ring J (1988) Die Bedeutung von Nahrungsmittelallergien bei atopischem Ekzem. Allergologie 2:63–67
31. Rajka G (1989) Essential aspects of atopic dermatitis. Springer, Berlin
32. Reitamo S, Visa K, Kahonen K, Stubb S, Salo O (1986) Eczematous reactions in atopic dermatitis patients caused by epicutaneous testing with inhalant allergens. Br J Dermatol 114:303–310
33. Ring J (1981) Atopic dermatitis: a disease of immuno-vegetative (autonomic) dysregulation. In: Ring J, Burg G (eds) New trends of allergy. Springer, Berlin Heidelberg New York, pp 237–249
34. Ring J (1984) Nahrungsmittelallergie und atopisches Ekzem. Allergologie 7:300–306
35. Ring J (1988) Angewandte Allergologie, 2nd edn., MMV-Vieweg, Munich
36. Ring J, Dorsch W (1985) Altered releasability of vasoactive mediator secreting cells in atopic eczema. Acta Derm Venereol (Stockh.) 114:9–23
37. Ring J, Kunz B, Bieber T, Vieluf D, Przybilla B (1989) The "Atopy Patch Test" with aeroallergens in atopic eczema. J Allergy Clin Immunol 82:195
38. Ruzicka T, Ring J (1987) Enhanced releasability of prostaglandin E_2 and leukotrienes B_4 and C_4 from leukocytes of patients with atopic eczema. Acta Derm Venereol (Stockh.) 67:469–475
39. Ruzicka T, Simmet T, Peskar BA, Braun-Falco O (1984) Leukotrienes in skin of atopic dermatitis. Lancet 1:222–223
40. Sampson HA, MacCaskill CC (1985) Food hypersensitivity and atopic dermatitis: evaluation of 113 patients. J Pediatr 107:669–675
41. Schnyder UW (1960) Neurodermitis–Asthma–Rhinitis. Eine genetisch-allergologische Studie. Int Arch Allergy Appl Immunol [Suppl] 17:1–106
42. Schöpf E (1974) Störung zellvermittelter Immunreaktionen bei Neurodermitis atopica. Verminderte Spontanrosettenbildung von T-Lymphozyten. Dermatologica 149:210
43. Schopfer K, Baerlocher K, Price P, Krech U, Quie PG, Douglas SD (1979) Staphylococcal IgE antibodies, hyper-

immunoglobulinemia E and Staphylococcus aureus infections. N Engl J Med 300:835–838
44. Schultz-Larsen F, Holm NV, Hennigsen K (1986) Atopic dermatitis. A genetic-epidemiologic study in a population-based twin sample. J Am Acad Dermatol 15:487–494
45. Spiegelberg HL, Boltz-Nitulescu G, Plummer JM, Melewiez FM (1983) Characterization of the IgE Fe receptors on monocytes and macrophages. Fed Proc 42:124–128
46. Stingl G, Gazze L, Czarnecki N, Wolff K (1981) T-cell abnormalities in atopic dermatitis patients. Imbalance in T-cell subpopulation and impaired generation of con-A-induced suppressor cells. J Invest Dermatol 76:468–473
47. Szentivanyi A (1968) The beta adrenergic theory of the atopic abnormality in asthma. J Allergy 42:203
48. Vieluf D, Przybilla B, Traenckner I, Ring J (1990) Oral provocation with food additives in atopic eczema. J Allergy Clin Immunol 85: 206
49. Waersted A, Hjorth N (1985) Pityrosporum orbiculare: a pathogenetic factor in atopic dermatitis of the face, scalp and neck. Acta Derm Venereol [Suppl] (Stockh.) 114:146–148
50. Wright S, Burton JL (1982) Oral evening-primrose-seed-oil improves atopic eczema. Lancet 2:1120–1122
51. Wüthrich B (1975) Zur Immunpathologie der Neurodermatitis constitutionalis. Huber, Bern
52. Wüthrich B (1983) Neurodermitis atopica sive constitutionalis. Ein pathogenetisches Modell aus der Sicht des Allergologen. Aktuel Dermatol 9:1–7

Therapy of Atopic Eczema

Atopic Prophylaxis

B. Björkstén

Introduction

Allergic diseases have become a major health problem in industrialised societies, particularly in children and young adults. This may partly be explained by an increased awareness of such conditions, as general health has improved, and infections and malnutrition have become less threatening. But there also appears to be an increased prevalence of atopic diseases, and this is generally ascribed to environmental influences. As a consequence, there has been an increasing interest in the possibility of preventing allergy by various prophylactic measures. In this chapter, the value of such prophylactic measures will be discussed, with emphasis on the possibility of primary prevention, i.e. avoiding sensitisation in healthy infants and children. Secondary and tertiary prevention will only briefly be mentioned. Since available evidence indicates that environmental influences affect the rate of appearance of atopic diseases, mainly in those individuals who have a genetically determined propensity to develop allergy, it is also important to discuss how such risk individuals can be identified.

Environmental Influences on Allergy Development

An individual must be exposed to an allergen in order to become sensitised and to develop an allergy against it. This sensitisation is influenced by the amount and duration of exposure, the sensitising capacity of the allergen, patient's age at exposure and genetic propensity, and environmental triggers. Experience from the development of occupational allergies in adults shows that both high concentrations of allergens and prolonged exposures to them increase the risk. The relationship between exposure and sensitization is, however, not a simple one. There appears to be a threshold concentration above which the risk increases rapidly. This concentration may vary depending on the sensitising potency of the allergen. For very potent allergens, like ragweed, a total exposure of a few micrograms over several weeks may suffice to sensitise an atopic individual.

There seems to be a period in early life during which the individual is more easily sensitised than later in life. As an example, the season of birth seems to play a role. This was indicated by the observation that Scandinavian children born in the spring have a significantly increased risk of subsequent development of allergy to birch and grass pollen as compared with those born in the autumn [4]. Later it was shown that this risk was influenced not only by the month of birth but also by the intensity of the first pollen season [4]. Similar results have been reported for grass allergy in the UK [20] and for ragweed allergy in North America [21]. Recently, it was reported that the relation between season of birth and allergy development was limited to children with a congenital propensity for allergy, as indicated by elevated IgE levels in the cord blood [6].

Similar to the apparent effects of early exposure to pollen, early contact with animal epithelia and house dust mites as well as early feeding with foreign proteins appear to influence the incidence of allergy [2]. This has been indicated by the observation that adolescents with various allergies who had been exposed to cats for at least 3 months during the first year of life more often had positive skin reactions to cat epithelium than those who were not exposed to cats early in life [22]. Analogously, British studies have shown that birth during the period May–October was associated with a significantly increased risk of asthma to house dust mite [20]. These observations in pollen-, dander- and mite-sensitive individuals indicate that early exposure to an allergen increases the risk for allergy later in life. Reasons for this, however, remain unknown.

Intensive exposure to an allergen may increase the risk of sensitisation. Thus, reduction of exposure, i.e. by effective air cleaning devices in industries, appears to reduce the risk for occupational allergy. It is reasonable to assume that a similar reduction of the amount of allergens present in day care centres and schools would reduce sensitisation in susceptible children.

In addition to direct allergenic exposure, there are a number of environmental factors that facilitate sensitisation to almost any allergen to which the individual is exposed:

- Exposure to air pollution, particularly tobacco smoke
- Tight, poorly ventilated houses
- Presence of infections
- Various stress factors
- Sensitisation (of infant) via mother

Air pollution

Tobacco smoke is the most important indoor air pollutant. In fact, the concentration of smoke in a room when someone is smoking by far exceeds that caused by any emission from a polluting industry. There is now a confirmed clear relationship between exposure to tobacco smoke and allergy.

In children with parents who smoke at home, there is significantly earlier onset and higher incidence of allergy and wheezy bronchitis as compared with children of non-smoking parents [17]. In a recent epidemiological survey of 5300 children in Sweden, it was found that bronchial hyperreactivity and pollen allergy were both more common in children of parents who smoked at home [1]. This was particularly obvious in children living in an area near a moderately air-polluting paper factory as compared with children in a forested area with no polluting industry (Fig. 1). This indicates that various sources of air pollution could act synergistically for sensitisation.

The effect of tobacco smoke on sensitisation to allergens may be explained by a local effect on airways rather than by a direct effect on the immune system. This is supported by the finding that smoking rats exposed to aerosolised antigen developed higher IgE antibody responses than subcutaneously immunised animals and non-smoking, aerosol-immunised controls [25]. Other pollutants like ozone, SO_2 and NO_2 may increase serum IgE levels, at least in experimental animals [10].

Housing

Modern housing may be one of the factors influencing the development of allergy. Well-insulated buildings with poor ventilation may thus represent a risk factor for allergic sensitisation. "Sick buildings" characterised by damage due to dampness and indoor mould growth have become increasingly common as a consequence of improved insulation and various other energy-saving procedures.

In an epidemiological survey of 5300 children, comprising all individuals below 16 years of age in six defined areas, it was found that children living in homes with damage due to dampness had a higher incidence of atopic disease and/or bronchial hyperreactivity [1], compared

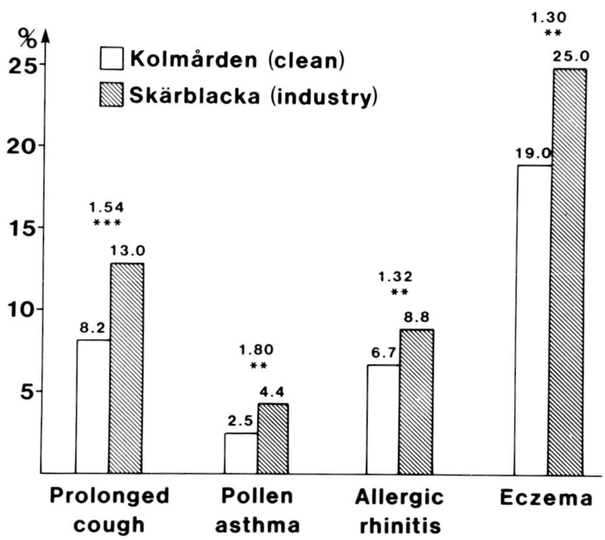

Fig. 1. Prevalence of bronchial hyperreactivity and allergic disease children living in a forested, farming area with no local pollution and in an area near a polluting paper pulp plant. The *asterisked numbers* indicate the relative risk of symptoms in children living near the plant and level of statistical significance (*** γ 0.001; ** γ < 0.01)

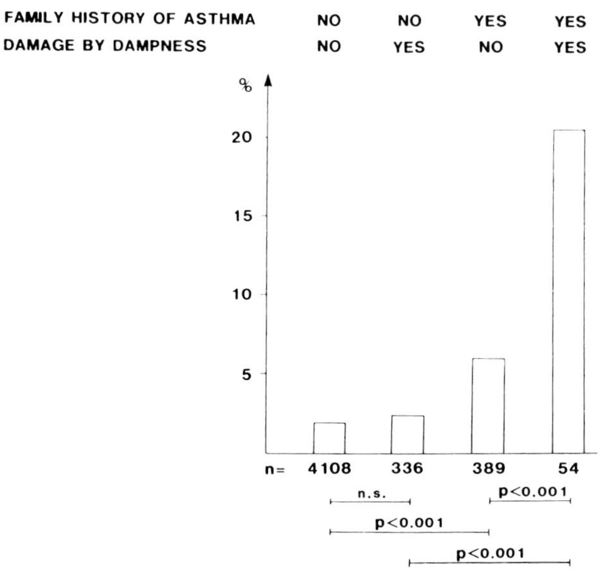

Fig. 2. Presence of asthma in children living in houses with or without damage by dampness (probably indicating poor ventilation) in relation to family history of asthma

with children living in undamaged homes. For children living in houses with damage by dampness whose parents smoked at home, there was a marked increase in allergic asthma and bronchial hyperreactivity as compared with children exposed to only one of the factors. It seems reasonable to explain the synergistic effects of exposure to tobacco smoke and damage by dampness by the fact that these houses are poorly ventilated and thus allow increased concentrations of air pollutants as well as allergens. The effect of these environmental conditions were most marked for children with a family history of asthma (Fig. 2), supporting the notion that environmental influences only play an important role in individuals with a genetic susceptibility for allergic disease.

Infections

There are now several studies suggesting an association between upper respiratory tract infections and appearance of allergic disease [8, 23]. Possible explanations include that infectious agents may facilitate sensitisation to environmental allergens, alter immune defence, act as adjuvants and act as allergens. It is well-known from animal studies that pertussis bacteria are adjuvants for the induction of IgE antibody formation against various antigens. There are also indications that this can be true in humans, suggesting the possibility that whooping cough may trigger allergy. This notion is further supported by the fact that whooping cough often is associated with a prolonged period of bronchial hyperreactivity.

Recently, it was found that IgE antibodies against pertussis toxin are encountered in children and adults during whooping cough and in response to pertussis immunisation [16]. The IgE antibody response was particularly pronounced after immunisation with a vaccine containing $Al(OH)_3$ as adjuvant, supporting animal experiments in which alum was shown to be an excellent adjuvant for IgE antibody formation.

Psychological Factors

Less is known regarding the possible impact of psychological factors for the development of allergy in childhood. Animal studies and recent clinical observations indicate that stress may alter the immune response [13]. Swedish studies have shown that families with a severely affected asthmatic child often demonstrate a rigid or chaotic interaction pattern as compared with families with children that suffer from diabetes and control families with healthy children [12]. Family therapy for such families reduced the severity of the asthma [11]. It is not known whether the particular interaction patterns commonly found in families of asthmatic children are a consequence of the disease or whether they represent a primary factor that may increase the risk for asthma in an atopic individual born into the family. Prospective studies to assess this are presently in progress.

Pre- and Perinatal Influences

Stress during the natal period, e.g. prematurity, complicated delivery and general anaesthesia in early infancy, have all been suggested to be associated with the later development of respiratory tract allergy [16a, 20a]. I have, however, not been able so far to confirm these observations. Since both studies were retrospective and did not control for a number of possible confounding factors, they should be confirmed by prospective studies before any definite conclusions can be drawn.

The possibility that drugs given to infants or their mothers during pregnancy can influence the risk for allergic disease has been little studied. There are, however, indications that drugs administrated to women during pregnancy may have some immune regulatory properties. As an example, progesterone has been suggested to elevate significantly cord blood IgE levels, but it does not seem to increase the risk for allergic disorders later in infancy and childhood [19]. In a double-blind, placebo-controlled study of the β-adrenergic receptor blocking agent metoprolol in pregnant women, it was found that children exposed in utero to the drug more often had elevated IgE levels in the cord blood and/or developed clinical allergy during the first 4 years of life than the children of placebo-treated control mothers [3]. Until confirmed by other studies, these observations should be interpreted with caution. They do, however, add to the list of possible environmental triggers of sensitisation.

Prophylaxis

A logical conclusion from the previous discussion would be to avoid all the various factors in the environment that may influence sensitisation and subsequent development of allergic disease. For a number of them, however, the individual can do very little. The cost-benefit ratio of various allergen avoidance procedures must also be carefully assessed. Some prophylactic measures could radically affect the life of the family, yet the beneficial effect would be only marginal. There are, however, certain prophylactic measures that seem reasonable. They are summarised in Table 1.

Table 1. Preventive measures in individuals at risk for allergic disease

Before birth:
Stop smoking
Consider possible effects of medication
In risk individuals:
Avoid exposure to tobacco smoke
Reduce exposure to strong allergens, e.g. household pets, house dust mites and occupational allergen exposure
Ensure proper ventilation in dwellings, day care centres, schools and workplaces
For infants add:
Exclusive breast feeding for at least 3 months
Total avoidance of other foods
Consider reduction of allergens in diet of breast-feeding mothers. This should be adequately supervised and supported

Avoidance of tobacco smoking is probably the single most important allergy-preventive measure. This is true in adults to avoid occupational allergy and to reduce allergy in their offspring.

Similarly, reduction of industrial emissions would be expected to reduce the risk for sensitisation. The effect of outdoor air pollution is, however, probably limited, since it has not been clearly shown that the incidence of allergic disease is lower in unpolluted rural areas that in industrialised urban zones.

Even if genetic factors play a major role in the development of allergic conditions, the atopic diseases definitely do not belong to those diseases for which genetic counselling is warranted. Although the season of birth has been shown to affect the risk for allergy to pollen in temperate zones, this is not sufficient for any recommendations. It is also true that birth during the autumn or winter is associated with an increased risk for allergy to house dust mites and furred pets. It is, however, reasonable to discourage families with a history of allergy to keep any pets at home, and the exposure to house dust mites should be reduced if possible, i.e. by avoiding wall to wall carpets and by reducing humidity indoors. Regular weekly vacuum cleaning of the house is to be expected, but meticulous cleaning beyond normal efforts does not reduce the mite counts significantly.

From the previous discussion it follows that smoking should be discouraged during pregnancy as well as after the birth of the baby. It is also reasonable to consider the possibility that medication during pregnancy could affect the risk for allergy in the baby. Available evidence of such effects is, however, scarce. Therefore, an awareness of a possible allergy-promoting effect of drugs should not prevent the adequate treatment of diseases during pregnancy.

Although manipulation of the maternal diet during pregnancy has been suggested [5], this practice is questionable. Studies indicating an effect of such manipulation have not been limited to pregnancy but also include the first months of lactation [5, 24]. Two prospective studies that were limited to studying the effects of dietary manipulation during pregnancy both failed to reveal any effect [7, 18]. Furthermore, there are definite hazards involved with dietary manipulation. Thus, it was observed that the mothers on a diet totally avoiding milk, fish and eggs gained less weight during pregnancy than mothers on a unrestricted diet. Their babies also had a tendency to a lower birth weight. The difference in birth weight between babies of mothers on a restricted and an unrestricted diet was statistically significant for the subgroup of infants of smoking mothers.

These effects were obvious despite the fact that all the mothers in the study had repeated individual and group counselling sessions, in which nutritional compensation for milk, fish and egg were discussed by an experienced dietician.

In early infancy all forms of artificial foods should be avoided for the first months, and breast feeding should be strongly encouraged. Human milk is the normal and optimal food for babies, and it provides the infant with immune defense and immune regulatory components. It is, however, undoubtedly true that minute amounts of foreign proteins that may be present in the maternal milk could sensitise the breast-fed baby [9, 14]. As a consequence, the maternal diet during the period of lactation has been discussed. In a recent study [15], the effects of avoidance of cow's milk, fish and egg during the first 3 months of lactation were studied in 115 newborn infants with a high risk for allergy development. All the babies had a strong history of allergy in at least two members of the immediate family and/or one affected family member and an elevated cord blood IgE (above 0.5 kU/l). All the babies were subject to general allergy preventive measures, i.e. breast-feeding was encouraged for at least 3 months, and no smoking or furred pets were allowed in the house. If the babies were not fully breast fed, then they received a protein hydrolysate as supplement.

The diet group comprised 65 mothers who totally avoid all cow's milk-, egg- and fish-containing products, and the control group comprised 50 mothers on a regular, unrestricted diet. The rate of atopic eczema was significantly lower in the diet group at 6 months (11% vs 28%). At 12 and 18 months the comparable figures were 23% vs 38% and 26% vs 40%. These differences were not statistically significant, possibly due to the low numbers in each group. There was, however, a significant reduction in severity of disease up to 9 months of age in the diet group.

These results suggest that dietary manipulation during the lactation period could be considered in an effort to delay the onset of allergy. It should, however, be remembered that total avoidance of all egg- and milk-containing products is not an easy task since they may be hidden in small amounts in various processed foods.

Very recently, various acaracides have appeared on the market. They undoubtedly have the capacity to reduce mite counts. The long-term consequences of regularly spraying the homes, particularly for infants, should, however, be carefully assessed before they are recommended for use.

Conclusions

Several factors play a role in the apparent increase in the incidence of atopic diseases in industrialised countries. The diseases are a consequence of an interplay between a genetic propensity of allergy, time and amount of exposure to sensitising allergens, and exposure to a number of non-specific triggers that facilitate sensitisation. But even if all known and hypothetical environmental influences are taken into account, this would not fully explain why allergic diseases are becoming more common. Since the genetic set-up of humans has not changed appreciably over the past few centuries, unknown environmental triggers must be looked for, including lifestyle patterns, housing conditions, food and environmental pollution.

There seems to be a period in early infancy during which the individual is particularly vulnerable to sensitisation. It is important to identify individuals with an increased risk for allergic disease since they seem to be the ones who suffer from the various environmental influences. Such individuals may act as "biological indicators" of risk factors in the environment. Although much remains to be learned about the development of allergy, several preventive measures can be taken now, including reduction of allergen exposure and avoidance of smoking and exposure to tobacco smoke.

References

1. Andrae S, Axelson O, Björkstén B, Fredriksson M, Kjellman N-I M (1988) Symptoms of bronchial hyperreactivity and asthma in relation to environmental factors. Arch Dis Child 63:473–478
2. Björkstén B, Kjellman N-I M (1987) Perinatal factors influencing the development of allergy. Clin Rev Allergy 5: 339–347
3. Björkstén B, Finnström O, Wichman K (1988) Intrauterine exposure to beta-adrenergic receptor blocking agent metoprolol and allergy. Int Arch Allergy Clin Immunol 87: 59–62
4. Björkstén F, Suoniemi I, Koski V (1980) Neonatal birch pollen contact and subsequent to birch pollen. Clin Allergy 10:581–591
5. Chandra RK, Puri S, Suraiya C, Cheema PS (1986) Influence of maternal food antigen avoidance during pregnancy and lactation on incidence of atopic eczema in infants. Clin Allergy 16:563–569
6. Croner S, Kjellman N-I M (1986) Predictors of atopic disease: cord blood IgE and month of birth. Allergy 41:68–70
7. Fälth-Magnusson K, Kjellman N-I M (1987) Development of atopic disease in babies whose mothers were receiving exclusion diet during pregnancy – a randomized study. J Allergen Clin Immunol 80:868–875
8. Frick OL, German DF, Mills J (1979) Development of allergy in children. Association with virus infections. J Allergy Clin Immunol 63:228–241
9. Gerrard JW (1979) Allergy in breast-fed babies to ingredients in breast-milk. Ann Allergy 42:69–71
10. Gershwin J, Osebold JE, Zee YC (1985) Immunoglobulin E-containing cells in mouse lungs following allergen inhalation and ozone exposure. Int Arch Appl Immunol 65:266–277
11. Gustafsson PA, Kjellman N-I M, Cederblad M (1986) Family therapy in the treatment of severe childhood asthma. J Psychosom Res 30:369–374
12. Gustafsson PA, Kjellman N-I M, Ludvigsson J, Cederblad M (1987) Asthma and family interaction. Arch Dis Child 62:258–263
13. Haggerty RJ (1986) Stress and illness in children. Bull NY Acad Med 62:707–711

14. Hattevig G, Kjellman B, Johansson SGO, Björkstén B (1984) Clinical symptoms and IgE responses to common food proteins in atopic and healthy children. Clin Allergy 14:551–559
15. Hattevig G, Sigurs N, Kjellman B, Kjellman N-I M, Björkstén B (1989) The effect of maternal avoidance of eggs, cow's milk and fish during lactation upon manifestations in infants. Clin Exp Allergy 19:27–32
16. Hedenskog S, Björkstén B, Blennow M, Granström G, Granström M (1989) Immunoglobulin E response to pertussis toxin in whooping cough after immunization with a whole cell and an acellular pertussis vaccine. Int Arch Allergy Appl Immunol 89:156–161
16a. Johnstone DE, Roghwann KJ, Pless IB (1975) Factors associated with the development of asthma and hay fever n children: the possible risks of hospitalization, surgery and anaesthesia. Pediatrics 56:398–403
17. Liard R, Perdrizet S, Retner P (1982) Wheezy bronchitis in infants and parents' smoking habit. Lancet I:332–335
18. Lilja G, Dannaeus A, Fälth-Magnusson K, Graff-Lonnevig V, Johansson SGO, Kjellman N-I M, Öman H (1988) Immune response of the atopic woman and foetus: effects of high- and low-dose food allergen intake during late pregnancy. Clin Allergy 18:131–142
19. Michel J, Bousquet J, Coulomb Y, Robinet-Lévy M (1981) Prediction of the high-allergic-risk newborn. In: Johansson SGO (ed) Diagnosis and treatment of IgE-mediated diseases. Excerp Medica, Amsterdam, p 35–42
20. Morrison-Smith J, Springett VH (17979) Atopic disease and month of birth. Clin Allergy 9:157
20a. Salk L, Grellong BA (1974) Perinatal complications in the history of asthmatic children. Am J Dis Child 127:30–33
21. Settipane RJ, Hagy GW (1979) Effect of athmospheric pollen on the newborn. R I Med J 62:477–482
22. Suoniemi I, Björkstén B, Haahtela T (1981) Dependence of immediate hypersensitivity in the adolescent period on factors encountered in infancy. Allergy 36:263–268
23. Welliver RC, Ogra L (1983) The role of IgE in pathogenesis of mucosal viral infections. Ann NY Acad Sci 165:321–332
24. Zeiger RS, Heller S, Mellon M, O'Connor R, Hamburger R (1986) Effectiveness of dietary manipulations in the prevention of food allergy in infants. J Allergy Clin Immunol 78:224–232
25. Zetterström O, Nordvall SL, Björkstén B, Ahlstedt S, Stelander M (1985) Increased IgE antibody responses in rats exposed to tobacco smoke. J Allergy Clin Immunol 75:594–598

Guidelines for Topical Treatment in Atopic Eczema

O. P. Hornstein

Atopic eczema is the most common cutaneous dermal manifestation of a polygenetic and multifactorial systemic disease that is characterized principally by a preponderance of IgE-dependent type I allergic reactions occurring on the skin and rhinoconjunctival and aerodigestive mucous membranes [8, 22, 31, 61] and by generalized xerosis, pruritic attacks, pallor, and disturbances of both microcirculation and thermoregulation of the skin. The multiple facets of this syndrome, which also include abnormal cutaneous irritability and immunological, neurovegetative, and psychic factors, must be considered when taking the different aspects of topical therapy into account.

Compliance as a Precondition of Good Management

Treatment of atopic eczema (AE) is usually a challenge to the physician's therapeutic skill and patience. To bring about stable compliance it is important to gain the confidence and cooperation of the patient and, in the case of children, their parents. It is advisable to inform the patient or his/her parents about the planned therapy and to explain all the necessary therapeutic steps as precisely as possible. Before giving detailed instructions one should listen carefully to the patient's complaints and enable him to put questions or express concernes without hesitation. In the hospital we offer, moreover, a special atopy treatment service to the patients or their parents in order to train the performance of practical therapeutic skills (e.g., technique of bandages, proper application of ointments, reasonable cleansing procedures of skin) under the supervision of a nurse. The establishment of a stable therapeutic alliance between patient and physician may be the crucial point for achieving lasting success in the cutaneous management of patients suffering from AE.

General Therapeutic Measures

Further prerequisites for therapeutic success include an initial "calming down" of both the excited skin and perturbed general condition by suspending daily work, repeated use of tepid tub water baths, stage-adapted skin treatment with mild emollients, keeping bed rest alternating with slight physical activities. For many sufferers from atopic eczema short walks or moderate bodily exercise (e.g., short ergometer training) are valuable tools to reduce psychic restlessness or "inner tension." Some patients feel relief even after such general measures as intermittent purgation of the bowel or a short-term sodium-poor and potassium-rich dietetic regimen (e.g., by two rice-fruit-days per week). Such simple arrangements may comfort the patient's feeling, particularly when he/she is adhering to diets or similar health care regimens. Such offers may encourage the patient's confidence in being able to overcome his/her eczema with personal cooperation. Relative air humidity in rooms should be kept at 50%–60% to prevent additional skin drying. The basic prerequisites for treating atopic eczema are the following:

- At severe exacerbations of AE complete suspension of professional work with change of environment (e.g., hospitalization)
- Balneotherapeutic regimen (tepid tub water baths emulgated with oil, cool shower against nocturnal itching) followed by application of emollients
- Painstaking avoidance of skin irritation (no rubbing of the skin after bath, wearing loose underwear, no skin contact with either wool or full synthetic textiles)
- Application of well-fitting bandages and/or cotton gloves in phases of widespread or oozing eczema
- Avoidance of exaggerated and skin-irritating cleansing procedures
- Short-term wearing of protective gloves at work and/or disposable plastic gloves (e.g., in the bathroom)

Principles of Topical Therapy in Atopic Eczema

Patients with AE suffer from a vicious circle of severe itching, exacerbation of cutaneous inflammation, and superimposed infection of skin. It is very important to manage these three main pathogenetic components of AE effectively by not only systemic but also appropriate topical treatment (Fig. 1). Consequently the antipruritic, antieczematous, and antiinfective effects of proper topical management should converge in a synergistic manner (Figs. 2 and 3). This means a therapy which is adequately adapted to the varying eczematous phases, so inhibiting both the inflammatory rash and pruritus as well as secondary infections.

The efficacy of topical treatment depends not only on the pharmacological agent itself (e.g., corticosteroid) but also on the type of therapeutic vehicle, which must be adapted to the undulating course of eczematous inflammation. Some principles of a stage-adjusted external therapy of eczema are delineated in Table 1.

In some cases a one-sided trial may be helpful. One applies two different topical agents (e.g., unguentum leniens versus unguentum alcoholum lanae; German Pharmacopoeia, 9th edition) on contralateral skin areas for a few hours and favors then the preparation offering more comfort to the patient. In recalcitrant eczemas, setting a small topical mark of the stronger agent on the lesional skin may be appropriate for testing its individual acceptability before it is applied more extensively.

Since management of AE must as a rule be continued over years, it must be practicable, reasonable, as effective as possible, not hazardous, and economic. Long-

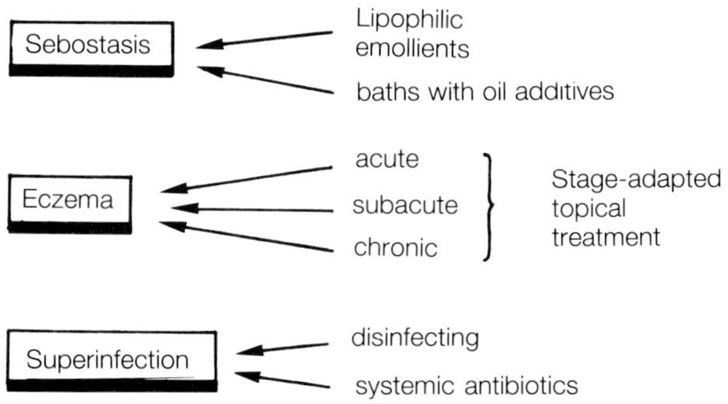

Fig. 2. Principles for external treatment of atopic eczema

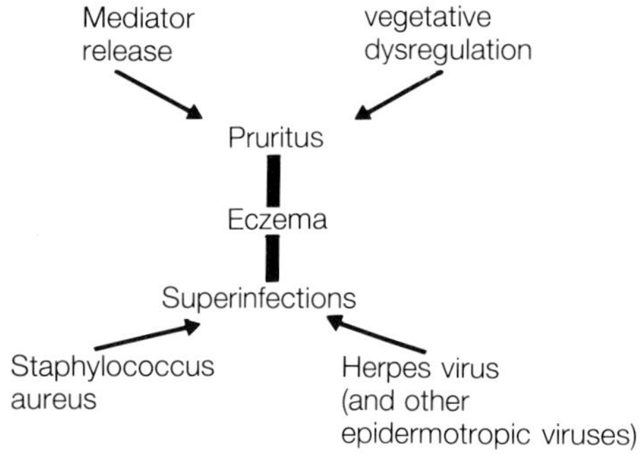

Fig. 1. Targets for therapy of atopic eczema

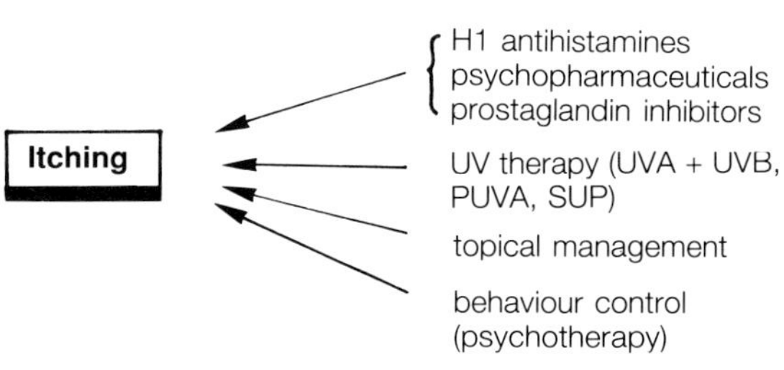

Fig. 3. Therapeutic measures against pruritus

Table 1. Stages of eczema and rules of local therapy

Stage of eczema	*Management*
Acute (vesicles, weeping, crusts, erosions)	Exsiccating (wet on wet), indifferent bases (hydrophilic creams = oil/water emulsions)
Subacute (erythema, edema, seropapules, oozing scales)	Mild exsiccating and antiphlogistic creams or soft pastes, use of mild ingredients
Chronic (dry desquamation, crusts, lichenification, infiltrated papules)	Hydro- to lipophilic ointments (type water/oil), increasingly also stronger ingredients (e.g., distilled tar)
Hyperkeratoses/rhagades (mostly palmoplantar areas)	Keratolytic and rehydrating ointments (containing salicylic acid, urea, sodium chloride), up to 4–12 h under local plastic foil occlusion
Oozing, macerating lesions	Drying (by application of compresses soaked with watery/alcoholic solutions, thin covering by soft zinc pastes or zinc oil)
At all stages	Tub water baths (containing minute proportions of bran or emulgating oils but no surfactants); intermittent use of corticosteroids alternating with the corresponding corticoid-free basic vehicle

lasting application of topical steroids should be avoided in AE because of the danger of unwanted side effects and the enhancement of bacterial and viral superinfections on the eczematous lesions. Early change from dermatosteroids of high or moderate to low potency and discontinuous short-term application of the steroid alternating with the steroid-free vehicle (called either tandem therapy or interval therapy) are important concepts to prevent major side effects and cut the costs remarkably [26, 40].

Warnings in the Management of Atopic Eczema

Atopic subjects usually suffer increased skin irritability and may respond very sensitively even to minor discomfort of topical treatment. Due to their xerotic skin condition atopics usually tolerate lipophilic ointments (water- in-oil emulsion) better than hydrophilic creams (oil-in-water emulsion). Creams and lotions may be irritating due to the drying effects of water evaporation and/ or to chemical ingredients added as preservatives, fragrances, or solubilizers. Preparations containing propylene glycol may be particularly irritating to atopic skin. However, greasy agents should be avoided during periods of excessive heat and air humidity to prevent palmoplantar dyshidrosis or other occlusive effects on sweating. There are also regional differences in the degree of xerosis and grease compatibility in the atopic skin. For instance, the skin on trunk and limbs usually tolerates and needs more greasy ointments than that on head and neck. Children react to discomforting topicals less by crying than by enforced scratching.

Emulsifying ointment should be used in place of soap for cleansing the skin or eliminating the irritative and drying effects of soap. In severe AE, therapy should include frequent tepid tub water baths for the débridement of extensive crusting and weeping as well as for soothing of the excited skin. Placement of wet compresses on the skin without underlying cream or ointment is to be avoided since an increased drying effect may occur by water loss of the skin surface. The same holds true for infants and young children who may easily suffer from a significant heat loss (chilling) effect.

Supporting Psychotherapeutic Influence

It is well known that a wide variety of allergens, reduced air humidity, excessive sweating, and many irritants (wool, acrylic, soaps, detergents, creams, lotions) may precipitate itching and scratching in most patients. Not rarely, children with AE more or less unconsciously use scratching to manipulate their parents and siblings. Even habitual scratching without itch sensation may develop in some patients, particularly in situations of distress or psychic discomfort. In such cases a psychological behavior therapy may be used by teaching the adolescent or adult patients a better situation awareness, so enabling them to control scratching consciously, as reported in a Swedish study [36]. In this study, the patients were motivated to discuss unpleasant aspects of scratching and were taught, in a "competing response practice" procedure, to control the urge to scratch in several psychotherapeutic sessions. As described by Melin et al [36], the patients were stepwise instructed how to avoid direct scratching or to convert the impulse to scratch by grasping an object, then to practice competing responses while pretending to be in distressing situations, and finally how to cope better with everyday situations conflicting them personally. Psychotherapeutic measures such as this may be helpful in highly motivated and comprehensive patients yet cannot be considered a substitute for appropriate topical therapy.

Topical Corticosteroids

Local application of corticosteroids in suitable carrier substances (aqueous, alcoholic, or lipid-containing lotions, creams, pastes, ointments) is a nonspecific but very effective pharmacodynamic therapy, with topical doses suppressing inflammatory local reactions but exceeding physiological amounts needed for systemic supply of the healthy skin via blood (Table 2). All the glucocorticoids, including the topically effective derivatives, apparently have in common the subcellular pharmacokinetic basic mechanisms, namely binding of the steroid molecule to a cytoplasmic receptor, transport of the steroid-receptor complex into the nucleus with

Table 2. Therapeutic effects and side-effects of topical corticosteroids

Effects	*Possible side-effects*
Vasoconstriction	Reversal effect ("tachyphylaxis") generating persistent erythema along with continuous steroid application
Antiinflammation through inhibition of – Eicosanoid synthesis – Cell infiltrate (inhibited expression of receptors on Langerhans cells, lymphocytes, monocytes, macrophages, mast cells)	Enforcement of microbial (bacterial, viral, mycotic) superinfections; acneiform folliculitis, rosaceiform dermatitis
Antiproliferation through inhibition of DNA-synthesis (epidermis, lymphocytes, fibroblasts)	Atrophy (potentially reversible) of epidermis and dermis with teleangiectasis, rubeosis faciei (cf. "tachyphylaxis"), xerosis; increased sensitivity to sunlight
Enhancement of catecholamine-induced cAMP-accumulation ("permissive catecholamine effect") with restored cellular capacity for differentiation	Comedones and ostiofollicular keratotic plucking
Stimulation of vellus hair genesis (in females) and sebaceous gland secretion (by enzyme inhibition)	Hypertrichosis lanuginosa, so-called steroid acne
Inhibition of fibroblast functions – synthesis of hyaluronic acid ↓ – receptor density ↓ – prolin → hydroxyprolin	Atrophy, loss of cutaneous elasticity, propensity for dermal edema, striae distensae

binding to DNA strands, and induction of mRNA matrix enabling neosynthesis of a protein which influences the cell metabolism, including cAMP/cGMP balance, growth rate, and functional activity. Such self-mediated down-regulation of cell action can produce both beneficial and detrimental effects depending on the duration and modalities of topical application even when performed in accordance with the approved rules for treatment with corticosteroids [22, 25–28, 31, 43–45, 57].

The higher the lipid solubility of the applied hormone, the better the molecules permeate into the lower stratum corneum, where they accumulate as in a reservoir and exhibit pharmacological effects in both the inflamed epidermis and papillary dermis. High-potency topical steroids are either more lipid soluble by esterification of the steroid molecule or possess enhanced antiinflammatory and antiproliferative action by double bonding and/or halogenation at distinct sites of the molecule. Differences in the rate of transepidermal absorption may be due to some partitioning of the steroid molecules into the lipid structures and intercellular spaces of the epidermis as well as to the degree of physicochemical adaptation of the carrier substance to the stratum corneum [9, 25, 27, 51].

In exudative eczematous areas the transepidermal route and absorption of topical steroids may be remarkably enhanced. While only little steroid penetrates through healthy skin (1%–5% depending on the anatomical site), absorption may rise up to 25% depending on the degree of the inflammatory epidermal damage. However, major systemic hormonal side effects such as suppression of the endogenous plasma cortisol level need not be feared, except when substantially extended application of high-potency steroid preparations or prolonged covering by large occlusive bandages is executed over several days or weeks [9, 24–26, 39, 42, 45, 52].

For short periods of time, topical steroids are quite effective and relatively safe when the therapy is critically supervised by the physician. For mild inflammation, particularly on neck, face and intertriginous areas, use of a low-potency preparation is preferred, for example, hydrocortisone 17-butyrate 0.5%–1% in ointment or cream. Especially in children, it is best to prescribe as mild a steroid as possible, but hydrocortisone may be too weak for severe exacerbations and only prolong discomfort and frustration.

Within the scope of this chapter only a few corticosteroids developed in the past decade and of interest to the dermatologist are mentioned briefly. Esterifying of the hydrocortisone molecule, for example, by valeranic acid, generates a dermatocorticoid of higher potency [51, 53]. The same has been shown for hydrocortisone 17-butyrate through double-blind studies revealing some superiority of this derivative to the parent compound [56]. Such hydrocortisone derivatives may be safer, in particular less atrophogenic, than fluorinated steroids. Of course, the potency of local steroids must be considered when using steroids on areas with thin skin such as eyelids and scrotum or on intertriginous areas over 1–2 weeks or longer. In the past decade, ointments with amcinonide 0.1% or betametasone dipropionate 0.05%, creams with halcinonide 0.1% or fluocinonide 0.05% have ranked among the most potent steroids used in dermatology. However, the vehicle of the drug is also extremely important in producing efficacy. Betametasone dipropionate and similar high-potency steroids demand prescription restrictions, particularly that no more than 50 g preparation per week be applied to an infant, no usage under occlusion, and limited treatment time of at most 2 weeks [11, 33]. Clobetasol propionate should also be administered cautiously as to the duration and the amount applied per week [45].

The cutaneous blanching effect of topical, but not systemic, steroids can be explained by catecholamine-induced vasoconstriction of the metarterioles, swelling of collagen fiber bundles, and increased hydratation of the intercellular matrix substance. Moreover, some inhibition of prostaglandin synthesis (by formation of lipomodulin acting as phospholipase A2 inhibitor) and increased intracellular calcium influx play an additional role. However, with continuous application of most dermatocorticoids the vasoconstrictive effect decreases quickly (so-called tachyphylactic phenomenon). This weakening of the local blanching effect typical of dermatocorticoids can be measured by the change in cutaneous photoreflection after repeated application of such preparations (Fig. 4).

Due to the antiproliferative effect of topical steroids, also in approved therapeutic doses, the maturation and differentiation of damaged keratinocytes are improved (parakeratosis, orthokeratosis), whereas healthy or lesional epidermis grows more slowly and so becomes thinner.

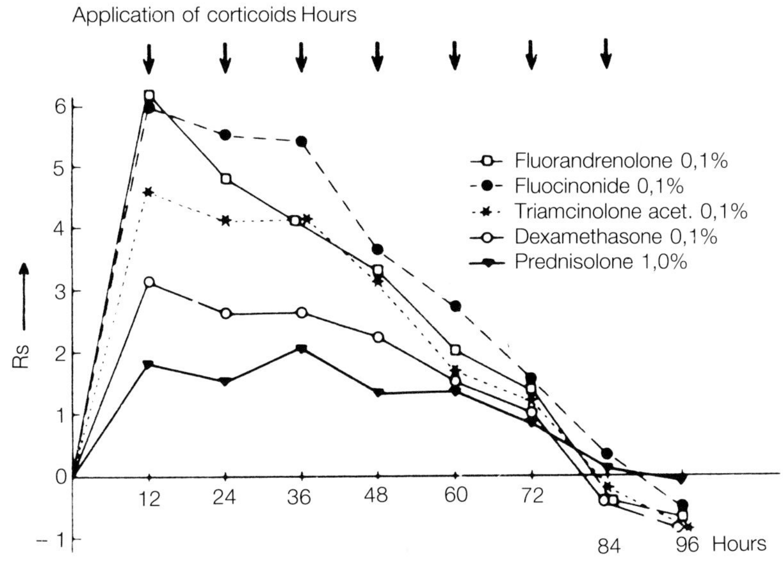

Fig. 4. Reflexphotometrical measurements of local skin blanching after topical application of different corticosteroids on healthy back skin. Note the fall of light reflection (= decrease in vasoconstriction) beginning at 48 h, after the third corticoid application. *Rs*, steroid-induced change in reflection. (From [2])

Alternating Therapy with Dermatocorticoids and Basic Vehicles

In order to prevent topical side effects by prolonged steroid application in AE (and other corticoid-responsive dermatoses) the alternating use of steroid-containing and steroid-free preparations is highly recommended [25, 26, 40, 45, 50, 54]. This rotating of topical preparations with or without steroid can be done either in a diurnal day/night rhythm (tandem therapy) or every one or two days (interval therapy; Fig. 5). Comparative therapeutic studies have yielded evidence that application of the steroid only once or at most twice a day provides about equal success within the same time as the continuous day and night application of the steroid [25, 50, 54]. Moreover, diminution of vasoconstriction and other topical side effects can largely be avoided by such alternating therapy [40].

For all these reasons the discontinuous tandem therapy (or interval therapy) with topical steroids has considerable benefits in comparison to the drawbacks of continuous application of the same drugs. This concept of rotating therapy is in my experience superior also to the well-known step-down therapy using continuous yet rapidly changing application from high to lower potency steroids over one to several weeks.

For tandem therapy, it is reasonable to use the same carrier base (hydrophilic ointment, paste, lipophilic ointment) as for the topical steroid. Prescription of tandem therapy has been facilitated by combining the steroid-containing and the steroid-free preparations in the same package for the majority of newer dermatocorticoids.

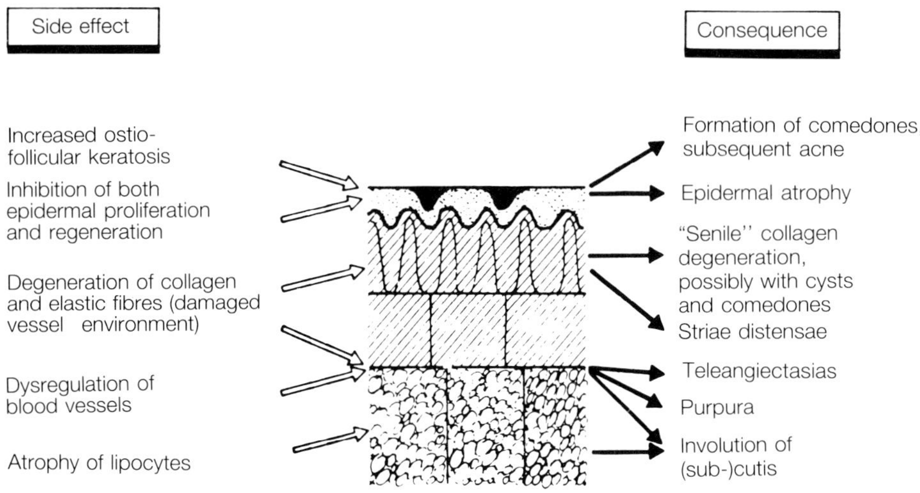

Fig. 6. Major side effects and consequences of prolonged application of topical corticosteroids on epidermis, dermis, and hypodermis [28]

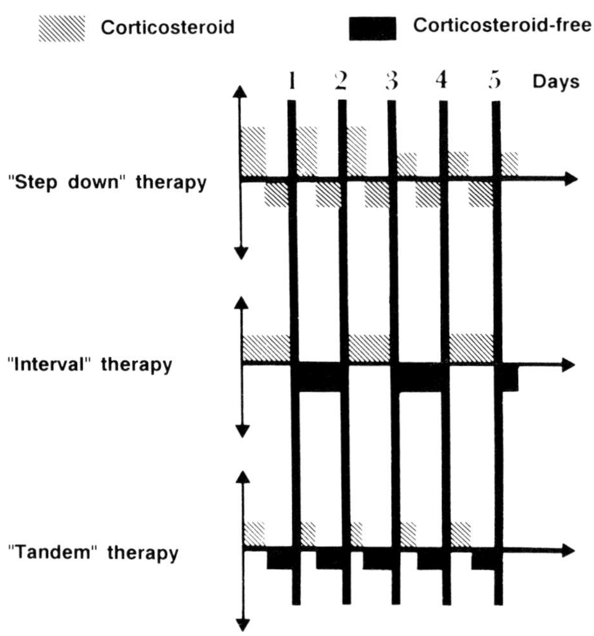

Fig. 5. Time schedule of different therapeutic regimens applying topical corticosteroids on the skin. Note the alternating use of topical agents (same carrier bases) with and without corticoids on interval (day by day) and tandem (diurnal) application

Topical side effects of dermatocorticoids include:

Most frequent

- Skin atrophy
- Teleangiectasias
- Dyspigmentation
- So-called steroid acne
- Increased sunlight sensitivity
- Striae distensae
- Rubeosis faciei
- Rebound phenomenon (after abrupt withdrawal of the steroid)

Less frequent

- Granuloma gluteale infantum
- Hypertrichosis lanuginosa
- So-called colloid milium
- Purpura or ecchymoses
- Camouflage or aggravation of cutaneous infections (drug-induced pathomorphosis)
- Contact allergy to the corticosteroid itself or carrier constituents

Recommended therapeutic measures for sparing dermato-corticoids are the following:

- Reduction of daily steroid application by alternating use of the same but corticoid-free excipient (initially tandem therapy, later interval therapy)
- "Step down" therapy (changing from high- to low-potency dermatocorticoids)
- Preference of intermediate – or low-potency dermatosteroids
- Daily rotating treatment of different skin regions (maximum 20% skin area at each day)
- Combination of short-term systemic and topical corticosteroid therapy (the latter often exceeding the period of systemic treatment) when generalized AE (> 20% skin involvement) is to be managed

General rules for rational use of topical corticosteroids are as follows:

- Avoidance of continuous long-term application.
- *Tandem therapy* (1 or 2 applications at morning and/or noon, then alternating with corticoid-free basic ointment). The reverse sequence (the vehicle by day, the steroid preparation at night) can also be employed in outpatients.
- No simultaneous topical treatment of generalized eczematous lesions (proposed limit of topical corticoid application: 20% skin involved).

- Daily change of the steroid-treated lesional areas. This regimen can avoid both loss in efficacy and expansion of costs.
- On impetiginized areas: firstly topical antimicrobial monotherapy (e.g., topical agents containing povidone-iodine, chlortetracyclin, quinolines), later dermatocorticoid (*sequential monotherapy*).
- When impetiginization is subsiding: so-called sandwich therapy (e.g., antiseptic dye solution covered by a dermatocorticoid and alternately by its vehicle).
- Combined drug preparations, e.g., containing antiseptics and corticoids in the same ointment, can be recommended less than sequential monotherapy (successive application of different topicals) or sandwich therapy (stratified application of different topicals, e.g., antiseptic dye solution covered by soft time paste). Monotherapy enables best control of the therapeutic efficacy of each drug used. Unfortunately, preparations with combined agents, though widely prescribed by general practitioners, are often given more or less empirically as a substitute for either poor diagnostic accuracy and/or therapeutic incompetence.

Nonsteroid Topicals

In many cases sufficient therapeutic success can obviously be achieved merely by applying corticoid-free basic preparations, if these are adequately adapted to the stage of the inflammatory skin condition. Relief of pruritus, discomforting skin tension, weeping, and crusting can often be reached after repeated soothing of the inflamed skin by bland emollients also supported by tepid tub water baths. It should be emphasized that every external therapy must be managed continuously, i.e., applied several times daily overnight and/or under suitable dressings. Exfoliative (sub-)erythroderma will usually require frequent tub water baths, rotating application of topical steroids (alternately replaced by nonsteroid topical agents) and antibacterial chemotherapy against staphylococcus superinfection if present. Tub water baths should be kept at tepid temperature and contain a little emulsifying oil in order to prevent skin exsiccation after emerging from bath. Hydrophobic, nonirritating agents should be applied after bathing and any excess residues gently removed with a cotton towel. Only well-fitting dressings are helpful; bad fitting ones produce additional irritation to the eczematous skin.

Nonsteroidal topical antiphlogistic/antimicrobial preparations include:

Tar preparations
- Pix lithanthracis (5%–10%)
- Liquor carbonis detergens (2%–20%)
- Bituminosulfonate (= ichthammol 2%–10%)
- Arning's solution (without benzoic acid)

Bufexamac (5% in cream or ointment)
Urea (5%–20%)
Sodium chloride (2%–5%, e.g., on hyperkeratotic palmoplantar lesions)
Salicylic acid (5%–10% keratolytic, <3% keratinizing)

Antiseptics
- Triphenylmethane dyes
- Halogenated quinoline derivatives

Antibiotics
- Aminoglycosides (neomycin; gentamycin, bacitracin)
- Macrolides (erythromycin, clindamycin)
- Chlortetracycline (2%–5%)
- Fucidinic acid

For topical treatment of (mainly staphylococcal) superinfection of AE antibiotics or antiseptics in suitable carrier substances are required [9, 25, 26, 31]. Ointments or solutions containing chlortetracycline or iodine-polyvinylpyrrolidone complex are generally effective when applied to impetiginized eczematous areas. Excess colonization by *Candida* species (intertriginous areas) can better be treated by antimycotics of the nystatine or the imidazole type than by antibiotic ointments. Topical application of antibiotics to such areas may even aggravate the AE [12].

Waersted and Hjorth [59] showed that *Pityrosporum orbitale* may be an additional pathogenetic factor in AE when occurring on scalp, neck, and face; these authors used ketoconazole in standard doses to treat patchy *Pityrosporum* colonization and reported good results.

Iodine-polyvinylpyrrolidone complex in ointment or solution has an excellent antiseptic, broad-spectrum efficacy on the superinfected skin. Even extended local application does not produce systemic toxicity except in cases with concomitant hyperthyroidism. Short-term topical treatment with halogenated quinoline derivatives is also well tolerated but may sometimes lead to type IV contact allergy after prolonged administration.

Nowadays, superinfection of AE by herpesvirus makes a systemic therapy with high doses of aciclovir indispensible. This potentially life-saving management can be supported but not replaced by topical aciclovir preparations (5% in hydrophilic base). In cases of eczema herpeticatum hospitalization is mandatory. Topical steroids should not be used or must be withdrawn if a herpetic skin infection is suspected.

In cases of recalcitrant fissures at palms and soles on local painting by coagulating silver nitrate solution (0.01%–0.1%) subsequently covered by soft zinc paste is a helpful measure. For treatment of areas with patchy or confluent weeping and crusting typical of bacterial superinfection in AE, one can rely, instead of antibiotic ointments, on the drying effect of soft zinc pastes (with or without halogenated quinoline derivatives or tannic acid as pharmacological agent). A simple household remedy is the repeated use of compresses soaked with black tea and applied wet for several minutes, also employed as sandwich therapy (e.g., hydrophilic cream covered by black tea compresses). Such remedies make use of the mild adstringent effect of tea infusion.

Tannic acid (1%–20%) produces drying, adstringent and antiinflammatory effects. It is incompatible with iron (no application on deep excoriations or erosions!) and other heavy metal salts (e.g., bismuth, mercury) [25].

In chronic phases of AE tar-containing topical agents are rather effective and often preferable to topical steroids [30, 43, 45, 61]. For lichenified lesions, 3% ichthyol in Lassar's paste is usually mild enough to be well tolerated and is quite effective. Zinc oxide paste applied thickly over an acute eczema help dry and soothe weeping lesions.

For children ammonium-tumenol preparations (2%–5% ichthammol in pastes or ointments) can be prescribed, while in adults coal tar (e.g., liquor carbonis detergens or pix lithanthracis in pastes and ointments) is also recommended as producing favorable antiakanthotic and antieczematous effects. Low-concentration tar solution added to tub water often provides immediate relief from itch. However, tar preparations must be avoided with exudative or superinfected eczematous lesions. Sunlight exposure after tar application must also be strictly avoided. Other agents suitable to soothe pruritus are thymol (0.5%–2%) and crotamiton (10%) in ointments or lotions.

For subacute and chronic phases of AE topical tar preparations in paste or ointment may be justified alone or alternately with topical steroids, the latter being used by day and tar preparations bandaged on for overnight. This modality often minimizes overnight scratching attacks. Tar-steroid combinations are not rarely less effective than this alternating regimen.

Since sodium cromoglycate (SCG) has been administered orally with some success in AE, it has also been applied topically. In a double-blind trial a cream containing 4% SCG showed no benefit in cases of severe AE, but a statistically significant improvement occurred after 9 weeks in the treated group compared with the placebo group [5, 6, 18, 19, 55]. However, it remains doubtful whether SCG is superior to other nonsteroid topicals agents that are effective in AE.

A new approach to topical treatment could be the lowering of excess phosphodiesterase (PDE) levels in both skin and lymphocytes according to Hanifin [20] and Cooper et al. [13] who found increased PDE contents in the leukocytes of AE patients. Preliminary results of a current double-blind and crossover multicenter study with the topical preparation of the PDE-inhibiting imidazolidinone derivative Ro 20-1724 are favorable, however, differences are not statistically significant (personal service information, Hoffmann-La Roche Inc., Basel). A further PDE-inhibiting drug with β-adrenoceptor agonistic effect, caffeine, has also been proposed for topical application in AE [29]. The same holds true for trials to treat AE topically (or orally) with the β_2-adrenoceptor agonist salbutamol (1% salbutamol base in white soft paraffin). Two applications daily for 2 weeks did not result in marked clinical improvement [4]. Caffeine 30% mixed with 0.5% hydrocortisone in hydrophilic ointment has been recommended for therapy of AE by Kaplan et al. [29], yet confirmatory results are lacking so far.

Topical agents (ointment) containing cyclosporin A can also be expected to be effective in AE due to its anti-CD4-suppressive action [14], yet long-term experiences with the topical application of this drug are not yet available.

Topical use of antihistamines and anesthetics should be strictly avoided with regard to their sensitizing potential. Putting arms of babies suffering from AE into plastic tubes to prevent scratching is malpractice. Such procedures may even inhibit the normal development of manual coordination.

Balneotherapeutic Regimens

Daily tub water baths do not only support débridement of oozing and scaly erythroderma but may also provide additional effects when given as a 1.5%–2% sodium chloride solution. However, slightly hyperosmotic seawater baths are indicated only for dry, lackluster skin free of excoriations or crusts and should be administered only twice a week. Hot temperature of baths should be avoided, since tepid water usually provides more soothing on the atopic skin.

The efficacy of combined balneo-heliotherapy in the Dead Sea is well documented, yet the mode of action is not fully understood. Apart from the keratolytic activity of highly concentrated salt solutions, hydration of the stratum corneum can be retained when lipophilic ointments are applied immediately after bathing. Absorption of dissociated as well as nondissociated hydrophilic agents, namely magnesium and calcium salts, may lead to an increase in intracellular cAMP, thus down-regulating the fastened cell cycle of keratinocytes [15].

Photochemotherapy

Since sunlight acts as an external agent to the skin, phototherapeutic measures should be briefly mentioned in this chapter.

As many patients with AE experience a seasonal improvement in their skin condition during the summer, and ultraviolet light is known to deplete epidermal Langerhans cells in AE lesions, gradual exposure to UVB may be beneficial for sufferers from AE. Heliotherapy has been used since midcentury to treat AE particularly in cases with a history of remissions in the summer. Midelfart et al. [37] reported favorable results with combined UVA and UVB treatment of AE patients, and this regimen was superior to phototherapy with UVA or UVB alone [21]. UVA may reach the mast cell pool in the dermis as well as the blood vessels containing immunocompetent lymphocytes and may thus influence some immunological disturbances in AE by reducing the local pool of T suppressor cells. Moreover, some bactericidal effects of ultraviolet light may also contribute to the positive therapeutic effects of phototherapy in AE [31, 41]. Greenwald [17] achieved success by UVB therapy applied in suberythematous doses two or three times a week. Pre-radiation application of emollients may decrease the amount of light reflected by the skin, thus increasing light absorption in the upper skin.

Photochemotherapy by combined ingestion of psoralen and administration of UVA may also be successful in AE [38, 44], but there are some drawbacks of this procedure, in particular with children, due to the risk of undesired late side-effects by PUVA. Because of an enhancement of cutaneous xerosis, exacerbation of pruritus by erythema, and risk of deleterious late effects by long-term phototherapy, this therapy cannot generally be recommended.

Conclusions

Although there exists no perfect treatment for AE, advanced clinical experience with new potent topical steroids and more cautious administration of such drugs enable both efficacy and safety of modern topical therapy in AE. There are an increasing number of nonsteroid topical agents available for AE treatment, yet obviously the crucial point in successful topical treatment is the stage-adapted and intermittently applied therapy with adequate preparations. However, there is no longer any reason for frustration in the treatment of AE, when profiting from the variety of topical agents available and using skilled techniques to avoid undesired side effects of the therapy. Moreover, several therapeutic modalities to combine avoidance of side effects and sparing of costs have been introduced in recent years. All these newer approaches to an effective therapy justify neither pessimism nor polypragmasy when treating patients with AE. However, with regard to the tempting plethora of current therapeutic possibilities in AE, the ethical imperative *primum non nocere* remains binding.

References

1. Allison AC (1979) Effects of glucocorticoids on lymphocytes and macrophages. Clin Exp Dermatol 4:135–138
2. Altmeyer P, Zaun H (1976) Ergebnisse reflexions-photometrischer Bestimmungen der Vasoconstriction nach topischer Steroidapplikation. Arch Dermatol Res 255:51–56
3. Aoyagi T, Umeda K, Isuka H, Miura Y (1981) Effect of hydrocortisone on the adenylate cyclase system of the skin – in vitro explant study. Brit J Dermatol 105:257–266
4. Archer CB, MacDonald DM (1987) Treatment of atopic dermatitis with salbutamol. Clin Exp Dermatol 12
5. Ariyanayagam M, Barlow TJG, Graham P, Hall-Smith SP, Harris JM (1985) Topical sodium cromoglycate in the management of atopic eczema – a controlled trial. Brit J Dermatol 112, 343–348
6. Atherton DJ, Soothill JF, Elvidge J (1982) A controlled trial of oral sodium cromoglycate in atopic eczema. Brit J Dermatol 106, 681
7. Atherton DJ, Carabott F, Glover MT, Hawk JLM (1988) The role of psoralen photochemotherapy (PUVA) in the treatment of severe atopic eczema in adolescents. Brit J Dermatol 118:791–795
8. Braathen LR (1989) Atopic dermatitis. Acta Derm Venereol (Stockh), Suppl 144
9. Braun-Falco O, Ring J (1984) Zur Therapie des atopischen Ekzems. Hautarzt 35:447–454
10. Butler J, Chan SC, Stevens S, Hanifin JM (1983) Increased leukocyte histamine release associated with elevated cAMP phosphodiesterase activity in atopic dermatitis. J Allergy Clin Immunol 71:490–497
11. Cabrera ME (1984) Treatment of severe or resistant corticosteroid responsive dermatoses. J Int Med Res 12:163–169
12. Chan HL, Aly R, Maibach HI (1982) Effect of topical corticosteroid on the microbial flora of human skin. J Am Acad Dermatol 7:346–348
13. Cooper KD, Kang K, Chan SC, Hanifin JM (1985) Phosphodiesterase inhibition by Ro 20-1724 reduces hyper-IgE synthesis by atopic dermatitis cells in vitro. J Invest Dermatol 84:477–482
14. De Prost Y, Bodemer C, Teillac D (1989) Randomised double-blind placebo-controlled trial of local cyclosporin in atopic dermatitis. Acta Derm Venereol (Stockh), Suppl. 144:136–138
15. Drexel H, Dirnagl K, Pratzel H (1970) Experimentelle Befunde zum chemischen Wirkungsmechanismus der Sole- und Seebäder. Z Phys Med 1:201–222
16. Garretts M (1975) Controlled double-blind comparative trial with fluprednylidene acetate cream and its base. Arch Dermatol Forsch 251:165–168
17. Greenwald D (1985) Twice-weekly ultraviolet B said to clear psoriasis, atopic eczema. Skin and Allergy News 16:5
18. Haider SA (1977) Treatment of atopic eczema in children: clinical trial of 10% sodium cromoglycate ointment. Brit Med J 1:1570
19. Haider SA (1979) Treatment of atopic eczema in children: use of topical sodium cromoglycate. In: Pepys J, Edwards AM (eds) The mast cell – its role in health and disease. Pitman Medical, Tunbridge Wells, p 570
20. Hanifin JM (1987) Veränderte Phosphodiesterase-Aktivität der Leukozyten bei atopischem Ekzem. Hautarzt 38: 258–261
21. Hannuksela M, Karvonen J, Husa M (1985) Ultraviolet light therapy in atopic dermatitis. Acta Dermato Venereol (Stockh), Suppl 114, 137–139
22. Heskel N, Lobitz WC (1983) Atopic dermatitis in children: clinical features and management. Sem Dermatol 2:39–44
23. Hopsu-Havu VK, Saarin H (1980) Wirkungen von Glukokortikoiden auf die in vitro-Synthese von Hyaluronsäure, sulfatierten Glukosaminglykanen und Kollagen. Akt Dermatol 6:83–90
24. Hornstein OP, Schell H (1981) Berücksichtigung von Biorhythmen bei der systemischen Dermatotherapie mit Kortikosteroiden. Hautarzt 32:551–557
25. Hornstein OP, Koch E (1985) Pharmakologische Wirkstoffe. In: Hornstein OP, Nürnberg E (eds) Externe Therapie von Hautkrankheiten. Thieme, Stuttgart, New York, pp 102–146
26. Hornstein OP (1985) Wichtige, vorwiegend entzündliche Hautkrankheiten und ihre Therapie. In: Hornstein OP, Nürnberg E (eds) Externe Therapie von Hautkrankheiten. Thieme, Stuttgart, New York, pp 265–375
27. Ippen H (1985) Lokale Ekzembehandlung. In: Mahrle G, Ippen H (eds) Dermatologische Therapie. Interdisziplinäre Aspekte – wissenschaftliche Grundlagen – Praktische Behandlungsmöglichkeiten. Beiträge zur Dermatologie Band 11, Perimed, Erlangen, pp 17–20
28. Ippen H, Bernecker HA (1976) Corticoid-Externa: Wirkungsweise und Wirksamkeit als Ursache von "Nebenwirkungen". Dtsch med Wschr 101:1263–1267
29. Kaplan RJ, Daman L, Rosenberg EW, Feigenbaum S (1978) Topical use of caffeine with hydrocortisone in the treatment of atopic dermatitis. Arch Dermatol 114:60–61
30. Kasten F (1978) Behandlung chronischer Ekzeme mit teerhaltigen Meerwasserbädern. Hautarzt 29:92–93
31. Leung DYM, Rhodes AR, Geha RS (1987) Atopic Dermatitis. In: Fitzpatrick TN, Eisen AZ, Wolff K, Freedberg IM, Austen KF (eds) Dermatology in General Medicine, Third Edition. MacGraw-Hill Book Company, New York, pp. 1385–1408
32. Lever RS, Mackie R (1984) The use of oral sodium cromoglycate in young adults with severe chronic atopic dermatitis. Clin Exp Dermatol 9:143–148
33. Lodolo JC (1984) Diprolene cream in the treatment of severe or resistant corticosteroid-responsive dermatoses. J Int Med Res 12:114–120
34. Maibach HI, Fisher LB, Trancik RJ (1978) Effects of occlusive tape systems on the mitotic activity of epidermis. Arch Dermatol 114:384–386
35. McKenzie AW, Stoughton RB (1962) Method of comparing percutaneous absorption of steroids. Arch Dermatol 86:608–612
36. Melin L, Frederiksen T, Noren P, Swebilius BG (1986) Behavioural treatment of scratching in patients with atopic dermatitis. Brit J Dermatol 115:467–474
37. Midelfart K, Stenvold SE, Volden G (1985) Combined UVB and UVA phototherapy of atopic eczema. Dermatologica 171:95–98
38. Morrison WW, Parrish JA, Fitzpatrick TB (1978) Oral photochemotherapy of atopic eczema. Brit J Dermatol 98:25–28
39. Munro DD (1976) The effect of percutaneously absorbed steroids on hypothalamic-pituitary-adrenal function after intensive use in in-patients. Brit J Dermatol 94:Suppl 12, 67
40. Pflugshaupt CH (1983) Diskontinuierliche topische Kortikoidtherapie (Review). Zentralbl Haut und Geschlkrankh 148:1229–1244
41. Przybilla B, Ring J, Kejzlar-Lisy G (1988) Behandlung des

atopischen Ekzems mit UVAPUR – klinische und immunologische Befunde. Akt Dermatol 14:326–329
42. Queille C, Pommereda R, Saurat JM (1984) Efficacy versus systemic effects of six topical steroids in the treatment of atopic dermatitis of childhood. Pediatr Dermatol 1:246–283
43. Rajka G (1977) Moderne Behandlung des atopischen Ekzems (Neurodermitis diffusa). Hautarzt 28:348–352
44. Rajka G (1981) Therapeutic advances in atopic dermatitis. Acta Derm Venereol (Stockh) (Suppl) 95:33–35
45. Roth HL (1987) Atopic dermatitis revisited. Int J Dermatol 26:139–149
46. Saarin H, Hopsu-Havu VK (1978) The decrease of hyaluronate synthesis by anti-inflammatory steroids in vitro. Brit J Dermatol 98:445–449
47. Särnstrand B, Brattsand R, Malmström A (1982) Effect of glucocorticoids on glycosaminoglycan metabolism in cultured human skin fibroblasts. J Invest Dermatol 79:412–417
48. Sannwald C, Ortonne JP, Thivolet J (1979) La photochimiothérapie orale de l'eczéma atopique. Dermatologica 159:71–77
49. Schell H, Hornstein OP (1980) Endogener Kortisolrhythmus und Epidermisproliferation. Akt Dermatol 6:27–33
50. Schmitz H, Flinzer E (1982) Zur Frage einer periodisierten Anwendung topischer Corticoide. Arzneim Forsch 32:430–437
51. Schmutzler W (1980) Pharmakologische Eigenschaften therapeutisch angewandter Kortikosteroide (unter Berücksichtigung verschiedener Zubereitungen und Kombinationen mit anderen Arzneimitteln). Allergologie 3:187–193
52. Scott M, Malmsten LA, Thelin I (1981) Effect on plasma cortisol level and urinary cortisol excretion in healthy volunteers, after application of three different topical steroid ointments under occlusion. Acta Dermato Vener (Stockh) 61:543–546
53. Sefton J, Kyriakopoulos AW (1983) Comparative efficacy of hydrocortisone valerate 0.2% ointment in the treatment of atopic dermatitis. Cutis 32:89–91
54. Sudilovsky A, Muir JG, Bocobo FC (1981) A comparison of single and multiple applications of halcinonide cream. Int J Dermatol 20:609–613
55. Thirumoothy T, Greaves M (1978) Disodium cromoglycate ointment in atopic eczema. Brit Med J 2:500
56. Veien WK, Hattel T, Justesen O (1984) Hydrocortisone 17-butyrate (Locoid) 0.1% cream versus hydrocortisone (Uniderm) 1% cream in the treatment of children suffering from atopic dermatitis. Int J Dermatol 23:565–566
57. Verbov J (1986) Treatment of atopic eczema. Arch Dis Child 61:518–521
58. Vivier A du, Stoughton RB (1976) Acute tolerance to effects of topical glucocorticosteroids. Brit J Dermatol (Suppl) 12:25–32
59. Waersted A, Hjorth N (1985) *Pityrosporum orbiculare*: a pathogenic factor in atopic dermatitis in the face, scalp and neck. Acta Derm Venereol (Stockh) Suppl 114:146–148
60. Wallace SM, Falkenberg HM, Runikis JO, Stewart WD (1979) Skin levels and vasoconstrictor assay of topical applied hydrocortisone. Arch Dermatol 115:440–441
61. Wüthrich B (1988) Neurodermitis atopica (atopische Dermatitis). In: Fuchs E, Schulz KH (eds.) Manuale allergologicum. Dustri, Deisenhofen, pp 1–34
62. Young E, Koers WJ, Berrens L (1989) Intracutaneous tests with *Pityrosporon* extract in atopic dermatitis. Acta Derm Venereol (Stockh), Suppl 144:122–124

Syndets in the Treatment of Atopic Eczema

O. Braun-Falco and H. C. Korting

Cleansing of Eczematous Skin – The Scope of the Problem

The idea of cleansing human skin is a comparatively old one. In fact cleansing agents of the soap type have been in use for at least 4500 years. We know from a written document from Tello that long before Christ the Mesopotamians managed to prepare soap from oil and wood ash [55]. The need of skin cleansing using some type of cleansing agent nowadays seems to be obvious to a wide majority of people, at least in industrialized countries. Although the need to cleanse the skin also seems to be common knowledge among dermatologists [42], this need is astonishingly ill defined in scientific terms. In fact, recent reviews on skin cleansing agents concentrate by and large on unwanted but not on wanted effects [61–63]. Certainly one has to keep this in mind when it comes to the role of syndets (or soap) in the treatment of atopic eczema. The use of syndets for skin cleansing in general does largely go back to the problem of cleansing eczematous skin [6].

"Most dermatologists agree that the skin of patients with atopic eczema should be kept clean" [68]. This belief is comparatively well substantiated by clinical and experimental findings and especially applies to the removal of endogenous dirt (crusts, scales, etc.) which obviously are always present. Indeed, the aim of skin cleansing is to remove both endogenous and exogenous dirt, especially considering the workplace. Patients with atopic eczema can react to the intracutaneous injection of human dander with an itching wheal reaction and to the occlusive epicutaneous application (48-h patch test) with an itchy eczematous reaction, as has been demonstrated by Uehara and Ofuji [66, 67] thus substantiating older observations [24, 58]. Debris on eczematous skin such as scales, moreover, might promote [68] the growth of *Staphylococcus aureus*, whose role in the aggravation of the disease has been stressed recently [30].

Despite this rationale for thorough cleansing of eczematous skin, as early as in the thirties dermatologists came to the conclusion, in view of the side effects of the cleansing agents available at that time, that patients with eczema should not use soap. In a fundamental paper from 1930 Stauffer [59] writes: "it seems to be justified to draw the conclusion from these results that the type and chemical condition of the various soaps in general does not influence the development of eczema on a large scale. Individuals, however, prone to the development of eczema should best avoid soap because of the enormous risk of eczematous reaction. For this reason I now forbid the use of soap with almost all of my patients with occupational eczema. I have had good experience in doing so." This approach, which in the German-speaking countries is referred to by the widely used term *Seifenverbot* (no soap) later found many proponents.

This is easily understood, considering the irritant effect of soap even on normal skin, an effect which became evident during the following decades [4]. As early as 1937 Rostenberg and Sulzberger [46] were also able to demonstrate using the patch test that soap irritates the skin of patients with atopic eczema more often than others. Thus "no soap on affected areas" has, for example, become part of the holistic approach towards the management of atopic eczema, which in the United States of America (USA) is known as the "Scholtz regimen" [2, 52, 53]. As with most treatment modalities for atopic eczema the concept of prohibiting the use of soap in patients with atopic eczema has not remained unchallenged [60]. In an open trial Uehara and Takada [68] were able to demonstrate improvement of eczema in patients complying to a protocol of conventional topical therapy for atopic eczema when they started having regular shower baths with common toilet soaps after having refrained from skin cleansing before. Today common text books still advise against a deliberate use of soap. Braun-Falco, Plewig, and Wolff [9] put it this way: "The asteatotic skin tends to dry out and itch. Repeated and prolonged baths with the use of alkaline soaps or foam baths should be avoided."

In short, up to the advent of chemical alternatives to conventional soaps the dermatologist treating patients with atopic eczema had to decide for himself either to advocate the regular use of soap in order to prevent the possible adverse effects of dirty skin, accepting the potential risk of severe irritancy, or just the opposite.

The Development of Synthetic Detergents – A Real Option

In chemical terms skin cleansing agents are amphiphilic substances, i.e., substances comprising both hydrophobic and hydrophilic moieties. When added to water such substances disperse in a certain way. In particular they become arranged in an orderly way at surfaces such as water to air. These substances interact with substances which are only slightly soluble in water, e.g. dirt, and solubilize them, making it easier to rinse them off after washing. It is this effect of soaps which is employed both for washing textiles and human skin. In the USA such substances are still sometimes called detergents. Yet there is now almost general agreement to speak of surfactants instead [55]. Up to the beginning of this century soap, i.e. a mixture of alkali salts and fatty acids, was the only surfactant available for cleansing both textiles and skin. In 1928, however, Bertsch and Schrauth for the first time synthetized fat alcohol sulfates [55]. The introduction of such synthetic detergents, or, to put it more correctly, surfactants, soon revolutionized the field of textile cleansing. At the end of the Second World War synthetic surfactants almost completely replaced conventional ones within a single decade [57]. During this time synthetic surfactants were also introduced in Germany in textile cleansing, not least by a Koblenz-based manufacturer called Maurer. And, in fact, his younger brother, who as a pediatrician was confronted with the problem of cleansing eczematous skin, was one of the first to promote the idea of also using the new substaces to cleanse the skin, especially so-called problem skin [6].

Dermatologic evaluation of the new products was primarily performed by Keining [23] at the dermatology clinic in Mainz. While he still used the term syndet in a more general sense, it is largely due to his work that in a stricter sense syndets are now defined as products composed of synthetic surfactants used for cleansing the skin primarily of the hand or foot and face region. Thus, from a chemical standpoint similar products used for showers etc. are excluded [55]. While soap as a rule is available as a bar, the first syndets were liquid, which primarily seemed to prevent widespread acceptance. Therefore syndet bars were also developed. "Rei" was among the first to be developed, by Maurer, and was clinically evaluated by Keining. In a fundamental paper Keining [23] described various properties of the new cleansing agents:

1. Syndets are more efficient than soaps in removing dirt and bacteria from human skin. As this is linked to their emulsifying properties skin lipids necessarily are also removed to a greater extent, and the skin becomes rougher because its water binding properties are influenced.
2. Syndets other than soaps do not sensitize, hence eczema-prone patients can be allowed to use syndets under certain circumstances.
3. Syndets do not bind calcium and magnesium. This would otherwise lead to deposits which cause itch and then give rise to exacerbation in eczema-prone patients, and so these individuals may use syndets.
4. Syndets can be acidified. In particular it is possible to adjust a pH of 5.7 to 6.0 in order to protect the acid mantle of the skin. This also prevents the swelling of the epidermis seen when soap is used.

Keining added a list of various skin diseases to his paper, thus forming the base of the later concept of syndets as basic treatment (in German so-called *Basistherapie*; [7]) in skin diseases. Keining himself, however, did not include atopic eczema here.

Although fat alcohol sulfates still are frequent ingredients of syndet preparations, a variety of different components and compositions has been developed in the meantime. From a chemist's point of view the major advantages of syndets are:

1. They can be used in hard water. Thus chalk soaps do not result and neither the cleansing capacity nor the potential for foam production are debilitated.
2. The pH can be selected and the skin can be cleansed with a neutral or slightly acidic product.
3. Syndets are compatible with many additives. This makes it possible to meet special requirements [55]. Synthetic detergents can either contain anionic, nonionic, or amphoteric ingredients. Anionic surfactants comprise sulfates such as fatty alcohol sulfate and fatty alcohol ether sulfate, sulfonates such as sulfosuccinate and carboxylates such as sarcosinate (as well as soap) and phosphates such as alkyl phosphate. Nonionic surfactants comprise polyglycol ethers as well as polyglycol esters and fatty acid alkanolamides. A typical representative of amphoteric substances is alkyl betaine [51]. For chemical details see Table 1.

As syndets are mixtures of various chemicals, the composition is of utmost importance. Although nowadays general principles are known to the public, and although ingredients are often declared according to the CTFC recommendations, the desirable and undesirable effects of commercial preparations cannot be derived from readily available information. In fact, dermatologic judgement is made even more difficult as commercial preparations are subject to frequent change. The principles of available preparations are described in more detail in a recent review [49].

Table 1. Major representatives of the various types of surfactant used in syndets and their chemical structure [modified from 51].

Type of Surfactant	Congener	Formula
Anionic		
Sulfates	Fatty alcohol sulfate	$R - CH_2 - OSO_3Na$
	Fatty alcohol ether sulfate	$R - CH_2 - O - (CH_2 - CH_2 - O)_n - SO_3Na$
Sulfonates	Sulfosuccinate	$CH(-SO_3Na)(-COONa)$ – $CH_2 - COOR$
	Methyltauride	$R - CO - N(CH_3) - CH_2 - CH_2 - SO_3Na$
Carboxylates/ phosphates	Sarcosinate	$R - CO - N(CH_3) - CH_2 - COONa$
	Alkyl phosphate	$RO - PO_3Na_2$
		$(RO)_2 > PO_2Na$
Nonionic	Polyglycolether	$R - O\,(CH_2 - CH_2 - O)_nH$
	Polyglycolester	$R - COO - (CH_2 - CH_2 - O)_nH$
	Fatty acid alkanolamides	$R - CO - NH - CH_2 - CH_2 - OH$
		$R - CO - N(CH_2 - CH_2 - OH)_2$
Amphoteric	Alkyl betaine	$(CH_3)_2(R) > N^{\oplus} - CH_2 - COO^{\ominus}$
	Alkylamidopropyl betaine	$R - CONH - (CH_2)_3 - N^{\oplus}(CH_3)_2 - CH_2 - COO^{\ominus}$

Desirable and Undesirable Effects of Syndets on Human Skin – the Role of the pH

Commercial syndet preparations still have high cleansing activity compared to soaps. This does not only apply to normal skin but also to the affected parts of the skin of patients suffering from atopic eczema. Seemingly, the differences between the cleansing capacity of a syndet such as Sebamed and a soap such as Lux are even greater when it comes to eczematous skin [71]. This at least can be derived from experiments with a frequently used skin washing machine devised to remove a staining model dirt [54].

As early as in 1928 Schade and Marchionini [48] published the results of determinations of the skin surface pH giving data ranging from 3.0 to 5.0. As early as that they spoke of an acid mantle (*Säuremantel*) and attributed to it a role in the regulation of the bacterial microflora on the skin surface. This concept was further substantiated in three consecutive papers entitled: "*Säuremantel der Haut und Bakterienabwehr*" (Acid mantle of the skin and protection from bacteria) 10 years later [32–34]. This has been the subject of much controversy up to the present time. The older standpoints are well described by the following statements: According to Pillsbury and Rebell [39] "The hypothesis of an 'acid mantle' as a principal factor in making the skin a less favorable area to support the growth of microorganisms has gained wide acceptance. This hypothesis is dependent upon the fact that the surface of normal unabraded skin has been shown by many observers to have a low pH. It has also been shown that intertriginous areas have a somewhat higher pH, and the conclusion was drawn that this higher pH was therefore the principal reason for localization of infection in intertriginous areas." According to Cornbleet [10] "there is no proof in the literature nor do my experiments support the hypothesis that the self-sterilizing powers of the skin are due to the surface acid." During the last decades many independent research workers have found a skin surface pH in the range 5.4–5.9, i.e., a mean value of about 5.5 [8]. Some, however, still hold the belief that the mean skin surface pH is not close to pH 5 but between pH 6.4 and 6.5 [62]. Although Tronnier is still a proponent of this hypothesis, he and Bussius [64] reported a mean value of pH 5.8 in a large field trial. In fact, the debate on the true skin surface pH has in the meantime resulted in the creation of syndets with a pH of 7.0 considered in terms of irritancy to be superior to slightly acidic ones [37].

Marchionini et al. [34] were the first, but not the only ones, to demonstrate a relationship between the pH of the habitat of skin bacteria and their growth. While they were able to demonstrate differences in the growth of *Bacterium prodigiosum* (today called *Serratia marcescens*) on the skin surface of the forearm claimed to be acidic and the skin surface of the axilla claimed to be alkaline, the fungistatic effect of the fatty acids found in human sweat, in particular of undecylenic acid, was found to be the highest at a pH of 5.0 (as compared to 5.6, 6.0, and 7.0) [14], caprylic acid was found to be more active against *Staphylococcus aureus* at a pH of 4 (instead of 5) [35], and the so-called water-soluble components of the stratum corneum were able to kill both *Staphylococcus aureus* and coagulase-negative staphylococci ("*Staphylococcus albus*") at a pH of 5, but not a pH of 7 or 8 [44, 45]. The idea of the influence of the skin surface pH on skin bacteria is further backed by recent findings from in vitro experiments. While *Staphylococcus aureus* distinctly showed optimum growth at pH 7.5, *Propionibacterium acnes* grew best at pH 6.0 and pH 6.5. Thus minor shifts from pH 5.5 to pH 6.0 may markedly promote the growth of *P. acnes* while the same might not be true for staphylococci [26]. In addition, the pH of the external environment seems to influence the enzymatic activity of skin bacteria. At least the lipase activity of *Corynebacterium acnes* (*Propionibacterium acnes*) is said to be double at a pH of 7.0 as compared to 5.1 [15].

As to optimum pH of skin cleansing preparations, an influence on the human skin microflora, however, can only be expected if cleansing agents can in fact influence the skin surface pH for a substantial amount of time. Yet this has been questioned repeatedly up to the present time. Long-term observation of the influence of repeated washing with various agents on the skin surface pH are scanty. It was mainly Pösl and Schirren [40] who in earlier days contributed to the discussion of the problem. They came to the conclusion that even repeated washings with alkaline soap do not influence the skin surface pH in the long run although it is moved towards the alkaline within the first hours following each individual washing procedure. Interestingly, this conclusion is, however, not completely backed by the experimental findings they referred to. In fact, in the morning before the skin was washed again, it was still somewhat more alkaline than before the start of the systematic washing procedures. The idea of just a temporary influence of alkaline cleansing preparations on the skin surface pH most recently has been virtually substantiated by our own experimental findings. Rieger [43] and Proksch [41] quote the short-term results of a controlled trial in normal human volunteers, showing that after the application of (alkaline) soap the skin surface pH first moves from baseline values by about two pH units followed by a return to about the initial value within about 120 min. Yet they do not quote the additional finding that during the trial performed over 8 weeks on the whole the mean pH in the group using the acidic syndet (Sebamed liquid) was lower by 0.3 pH units than in the group using (alkaline) soap (Lux) [27]. This difference, which in other terms means that three times as many free hydrogen ions are available on the skin surface when the acidic syndet is used repeatedly, correlates with a marked difference in the density of propionibacteria but not coagulase-negative staphylococci. As to be expected from the in vitro findings cited above propionibacteria, but not staphylococci, were significantly more abundant when alkaline soap, not acidic syndet, was used regularly. More recently, these findings were substantiated by further trials. When syndets of almost identical chemical composition except for the pH were used, corresponding differences were found comparing a preparation of pH 5.5 with another one of pH 7.0 [28]. The latter investigation clearly demonstrates that it is the pH value of the cleansing preparation, and not the various components, which actually influence the skin surface pH and, hence, its microflora.

This seems to deserve all the more interest as a shift to the alkaline is one of the features of affected and seemingly unaffected skin in patients suffering from generalized eczema [12]. Only the findings concerning the skin roughness after the repeated application of several chemically different syndets with acidic or neutral pH values hinted at a superiority of the neutral ones in terms of irritancy [37]. Therefore most recently both roughness of the skin surface and transepidermal water loss (TEWL) were examined on repeated application of syndet preparations differing only in their pH. In controlled trials the preparation of pH 5.5 was always compared with the more alkaline one either of pH 7.0 or 8.5. Though both parameters always increased during the trial period, there were no definite differences between the various groups while this was again the case with respect to the skin surface pH [29]. The lack of a clear-cut relationship between the pH of the syndet preparation and its potential for irritancy found here corresponds well to earlier findings. As early as in the sixties Tronnier, Schneider, Schuster, and Modde [65] drew the conclusion from pertinent experimental work that: "The side effects (undesired secondary effects of the tensides) are to a very slight degree pH dependent. However, side effects tend to increase with the elevation of pH values." This is in clear contrast to Schneider's [50] earlier belief that syndets should be slightly alkaline in order to be less irritant. Most recent investigations based on 48-h application of sodium lauryl sulfate under occlusion showed that this ionic surfactant, formerly a major ingredient of syndets, does not increase TEWL if the pH of the preparation lies at 5 or 7, while it does so to a certain extent at a pH of 9 [1].

Although the pH of a syndet preparation might not have a major influence on the side effects, there is scientific basis for believing that a chemical preparation could cleanse human skin without compromising its barrier function in any way [41]. The permeability barrier of human skin is primarily composed of cornifying keratinocytes which are rich in protein and the intracellular substance which is rich in lipids. The intercellular lipids are particularly important as they are able to influence both trans- and paracellular permeation. In the keratinocytes which form the stratum spinosum, the lamellar bodies known as keratinosomes are composed of lipids. These bodies are liberated within the stratum granulosum, providing the upper parts of the epidermis with lipids of lamellar arrangement. These lipids, epidermal lipids, are different from sebum lipids [11]. Another major constituent of the upper parts of the epidermis is water. Its concentration in the uppermost parts of the epidermis, however, is much lower than in others. The mixture of epidermal lipids, sebum lipids, water, salt, and organic acids forms a system which has been interpreted as a water-lipid mantle or natural moisturizing factor [41].

As skin cleansing, by definition, means removal of xenobiotics deposited on the skin surface and emulsified by the water-lipid mantle and of body secretions such as sebum or sweat or other body products such as scales, it is harmful to the epidermis. The practical question, however, is to what extent. In fact, syndets are not necessarily less harmful with respect to irritancy. The clinical dermatologist who had become familiar with "soap dermatitis" by the end of the 1940s [21] was confronted with a new type of "detergent dermatitis" at the beginning of the 1950s in various parts of the world. In Sweden this was due to a syndet called "Original X," containing, apart from other ingredients, 6% lauryl sulfate. Irritancy has soon chased back to this anionic surfactant.

During the past decades the irritant potential of various surfactants being considered as possible ingredients of syndets has been evaluated by different methods comprising the Duhring chamber test. In particular these studies have identified the comparatively high irritant potential of sodium lauryl sulfate [22, 72]. Sodium lauryl sulfate increases the TEWL. Increased TEWL, a typical feature of so-called dry skin, is even higher in patients with atopic eczema than in normal individuals [70]. Sodium dodecyl sulfate applied repeatedly also increases skin roughness. This effect is linked to its adsorption to human keratin layers [19]. Decreased stratum corneum hydration and increased roughness of the skin surface are linked to changes in the composition of epidermal lipids. While the total amount of lipids is not altered, the ratio of free cholesterol to cholesterol ester is increased. The total amount of ceramides is not significantly changed either after the application of sodium dodecyl sulfate, yet the amount of one particular ceramide is, i.e. ceramide 3 [17]. In fact, those intercellular lipids which are depleted are able to reconstitute those water-retention properties needed to keep the skin supple when sodium dodecyl sulfate is applied [20].

Fortunately, other surfactants influence TEWL less than sodium lauryl sulfate. This, for example, applies to sodium laurate [70]. Today, it is common knowledge that one has to look both for the irritant potential of any single possible ingredient as well as at that of the complex mixture when it comes to the evaluation of a cleansing product to be made commercially available [69]. It is no longer justified to assume that efficacy and tolerability of a skin cleansing preparation are closely linked. In a recent trial comparing various commercially available soaps and syndets one particular soap, i.e. Purpose, ranked first with respect to its cleansing capacity but only fourth with respect to irritation potential. In the given context, however, it might be more important for a syndet bar to rank first for its low irritation potential though it is the least effective in terms of cleansing the skin [38]. It is obvious today that no general statement can be made as to the safety of syndets or soaps. Due to a chamber test especially devised for the evaluation of skin cleansing preparations one representative of the syndet group, i.e. Dove, ranked first while another syndet preparation, Zest, ranked almost last (16th of 18) [16]. Definite evaluation of a skin cleansing modality also has to be based on results of long-term application under practical conditions, i.e., on in-use properties [47]. According to the results of a recent trial of that type, irritancy is most marked during the first weeks of regular application [31]. Moreover, the relative increase of side effects does not seem to be greater in individuals prone to atopic disease. Yet this does not preclude the occurrence of clear-cut detergent eczema as shown in Fig. 1 even with most recent syndet preparations.

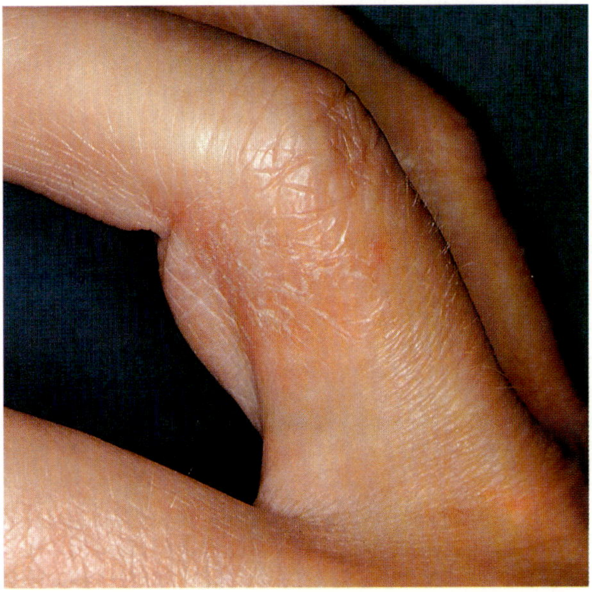

Fig. 1. Irritant dermatitis in an atopic due to the frequent use of a syndet bar representing "detergent eczema"

Syndets and Eczematous Skin – Clinical Assessment

Controlled trials on the desirable and undesirable effects of syndet washings on the normal and affected skin of patients with atopic eczema seemingly do not exist. According to an open trial applying an acidic syndet (pH-5-Eucerin Lotio) twice daily for 14 days to involved or uninvolved skin of 60 patients with eczema, among them 12 with atopic eczema this preparation is well tolerated both on affected and healthy skin [25]. Faulhaber and Lechner [13] found an acidic syndet (i.e., *Sebamed flüssig Waschemulsion*) helpful in 22 of 30 female patients with eczema. Yet the syndet was applied in a bath. Schwarz [56] described a supportive effect of the use of syndets in patients with occupational eczema presumably at least in part linked to atopy. The scanty inconclusive experimental results on the effect of syndets on the skin of patients with atopic eczema compared to soaps corresponds to the lack of definite evidence whether the application of soap to eczematous skin really does major harm. Neither Brain [5] nor Bettly [3] found soap to be injurious when applied regularly to cleanse the eczematous skin of infants.

Hence, further clinical trials of the following design are needed: An adequately large cohort of patients with manifest atopic eczema is graded clinically [18]. Each subject is attributed to one of a total of three subgroups at random. In a modified double-blind fashion each trial participant receives either soap, a syndet, or nothing at all for skin cleansing. The latter group is asked to totally refrain from washing their skin. The other subgroups are asked to use their cleansing agent twice daily before the application of the other treatment modalities for eczema. These treatment modalities are the same for all subgroups. During the entire trial period of 10 days one type of medium-potent glucocorticoid cream is applied in the evening, followed by the corresponding vehicle in the morning. The state of skin is investigated on days 5 and 10 using the same grading scheme as at the start. Corresponding to the usual application of a soap or syndet, the skin areas should be cleansed using a diluted solution for 30 sach and then rinsed with plain tap water. Such a trial would probably clarify whether the inherent harm brought about by the application of a cleansing agent is less than the advantage of removing the dirt from the skin. Moreover, we would know whether soap or syndet is superior if cleansing agents are indeed indicated in the management of atopic eczema.

If this is so, the differential judgement on soap and syndets, respectively, has to take into account that both represent a large variety of compositions of various chemicals substances. This applies even more so to syndets. Thus, for example, the pH of syndet preparations can be selected freely. While at present the ultimate skin cleansing preparation for eczematous skin may not be available, this might be the case in the near future. In fact, it would not astonish us if it were a syndet.

References

1. Antoine JL, Contrieras JL, van Neste DJ (1989) pH influence of surfactant-induced skin irritation. A noninvasive, multiparametric study with sodium lauryl sulphate. Dermatosen 37:96–100
2. Ayres S Jr, Mihan R (1977) Treatment of atopic dermatitis with the Scholtz regimen. Arch Dermatol 113:1616
3. Bettly FR (1972) The irritant effect of detergents. Trans St. John's Hosp Dermatol Soc 58:65–74
4. Bettly FR, Donoghue E (1960) The irritant effect of soap upon normal skin. Br J Dermatol 72:67–76
5. Brain RT (1956) Soap and the skin. Br Med J 2:299–301
6. Braun-Falco O (1990) Vom Seifenverbot zur Hautreinigung von Syndets – präklinische und klinische Aspekte der historischen Entwicklung. In: Braun-Falco O, Korting HC (eds) Hautreinigung mit Syndets. Chemische, ökologische und klinische Aspekte. Springer, Berlin Heidelberg New York, pp 3–10
7 Braun-Falco O, Heilgemeir GP (1981) Syndets zur Reinigung gesunder und erkrankter Haut. Wirkung und dermatotherapeutische Indikationen. Ther Geg 120:1028–1045
8. Braun-Falco O, Korting HC (1986) Der normale pH-Wert der menschlichen Haut. Hautarzt 37:126–129
9. Braun-Falco O, Plewig G, Wolff HH (1990) Dermatology und Venerology. Springer, Berlin Heidelberg New York, p 357
10. Cornbleet T (1933) Self-sterilizing powers of the skin. V. Are they endowed by the surface acid? Arch Dermatol Syphilol 28:526–531
11. Elias PM (1983) Epidermal lipids, barrier function, and desquamation. J Invest Dermatol 80:445–495
12. Epprecht R (1955) Elektrometrische Messungen des pH der Hautoberfläche bei Hautgesunden und Ekzempatienten mit besonderer Berücksichtigung der Säureneutralisation. Dermatologica 111:204–223
13. Faulhaber G, Lechner W (1986) Der Einfluß von sebamed® flüssig Waschemulsion auf die ekzematöse Haut. Ärztl Kosmetol 16:47–54
14. Foley EJ, Hermann F, Lee SW (1947) The effects of pH on the antifungal activity of fatty acids and other agents. Preliminary report. J Invest Dermatol 8:1–2
15. Freinkel RK, Shen Y (1969) The origin of free fatty acids in sebum. II. Assay of the lipases of the cutaneous bacteria and effects of pH. J Invest Dermatol 53:422–427
16. Frosch PJ, Kligman AM (1979) The soap chamber test. A new method for assessing the irritancy of soaps. J Am Acad Dermatol 1:35–41
17. Fulmer HW, Kramer GJ (1986) Stratum corneum lipid abnormalities in surfactant-induced dry scaly skin. J Invest Dermatol 86:598–602
18. Hanifin JM (1989) Standardized grading of subjects for clinical research studies in atopic dermatitis: workshop report. Acta Derm Venereol [Suppl] (Stockh) 144:28–30
19. Imokawa G, Mishima Y (1979) Cumulative effect of surfactants on cutaneous horny layers: absorption onto human keratin layers in vivo. Contact Derm 5:357–366
20. Imokawa G, Akasaki S, Minematsu Y, Kawai M (1989) Importance of intercellular lipids in water-retention properties of the stratum corneum: induction and recovery study of surfactant dry skin. Arch Dermatol Res 281:45–51
21. Jordan JW, Dolce FA, Osborne ED (1940) Dermatitis of the hand in housewives: role of soaps and its etiology, methods of prevention. JAMA 115:1001–1006
22. Kästner W, Frosch PJ (1981) Hautirritationen verschiedener anionaktiver Tenside im Duhring-Kammer-Test am Menschen im Vergleich zu In-vitro- und tierexperimentellen Methoden. Fette Seifen Anstrichm 83:33–46
23. Keining E (1959) Zur Frage der Reinigung gesunder und kranker Haut. Dermatol Wochenschr 140:1245–1251
24. Keller P (1952) Beitrag zu den Beziehungen von Asthma und Ekzem. Arch Dermatol Syph 148:82–97
25. Klaschka F, Flasch CI, Weiland E (1985) Begleitende Behandlung von ekzematösen Erkrankungen und pH-5-Eucerin-Waschlotio. Ergebnisse einer klinischen Studie. Ärztl Kosmetol 15:35–38
26. Korting HC, Bau A, Baldauf P (1987) pH-Abhängigkeit des Wachstumsverhaltens von *Staphylococcus aureus* und *Propionibacterium* acnes. Implikationen einer In-vitro-Studie für den optimalen pH-Wert von Hautwaschmitteln. Arztl Kosmetol 17:41–53
27. Korting HC, Kober M, Mueller M, Braun-Falco O (1987) Influence of repeated washings with soap and synthetic detergents on pH and resident flora of the skin of forehead and forearm. Results of a cross-over trial in healthy probitioners. Acta Derm Venereol (Stockh) 67:41–47
28. Korting HC, Hübner K, Greiner H, Hamm G (in press) Differences in skin surface pH and bacterial microflora due to the long-term application of synthetic detergent preparations of pH 5.5 and pH 7.0. Results of a crossovetrial healthy volunteers. Acta Derm Venereol (Stockh)
29. Korting HC Megele M, Mehringer L, Vieluf D, Zienicke H, Hamm G, Braun-Falco O (in press) Influence of skin cleansing preparation acidity on skin surface property. Int J Cosmet Sci but not its roughness and transepidermal waterloss
30. Lever R, Hadley K, Downey D, McKie R (1988) Staphylococcal colonization in atopic dermatitis and the effect of topical mupirocin therapy. Br J Dermatol 119:189–198
31. Lukacs A, Korting HC (1990) Nebenwirkungen eines neuen sauren Syndet-Waschstücks. Art und Ausmaß bei regelmäßiger Anwendung unter Praxisbedingungen. TW Dermatol 20:416–423
32. Marchionini A, Hausknecht W (1938) Säuremantel der Haut und Bakterienabwehr. I. Mitteilung. Die regionäre Verschiedenheit der Wasserstoffionenkonzentration der Hautoberfläche. Klin Wochenschr 17:663–666
33. Marchionini A, Schmidt R, Kiefer J (1938) Säuremantel der Haut und Bakterienabwehr. II. Mitteilung. Über die regionäre Verschiedenheit der Bakterienabwehr und Desinfektionskraft der Hautoberfläche. Klin Wochenschr 17:736–739
34. Marchionini A, Schmidt R (1938) Säuremantel der Haut und Bakterienabwehr. III. Mitteilung. Über die regionäre Verschiedenheit des Bakterienwachstums auf der Hautoberfläche. Klin Wochenschr 170:773–775
35. Miescher G (1955) Diskussionsbemerkung. Arch Dermatol Syph 200:53–58
36. Nilzen A (1958) Some aspects of synthetic detergents and skin reaction. Acta Derm Venereol (Stockh) 38:104–111
37. Nissen HP, Kreysel HW (1985) Flüssige Waschsyndets verschiedener pH-Wert-Einstellungen. Vergleichende Untersuchung. Ärztl Kosmetol 15:304–313
38. Ortho Pharmaceuticals (1986) Evaluation of the cleansing and the irritating potential of Purpose soap. Purpose Medical Report 86-035. Ortho, Raritan
39. Pillsbury DM, Rebell G (1952) The bacterial flora of the skin. Factors influencing the growth of resident and transient organisms. J Invest Dermatol 18:173–186
40. Pösl H, Schirren CG (1968) Beeinflussung des pH-Wertes

der Hautoberfläche durch Seifen, Waschmittel und synthetische Detergentien. Hautarzt 17:37–40

41. Proksch E (1989) Die Permeabilitätsbarriere der Epidermis und ihre Beeinflussung durch Detergentien und Lokaltherapeutika. Arztl Kosmetol 19:424–443
42. Raab W (1987) Zur Reinigung gesunder und kranker Haut. Ärztl Kosmetol 17:354–359
43. Rieger M (1989) The apparent pH on the skin. Careful quantitative chemical measurements are needed to draw conclusions of this acid-base phenomenon. Cosmet Toilet 104:53–60
44. Röckl H, Pascher G (1960) Der Einfluß wasserlöslicher Bestandteile der Hornschicht auf Bakterien. II. Mitteilung. Arch Klin Exp Dermatol 210:531–536
45. Röckl H, Spier HB, Pascher G (1957) Der Einfluß wasserlöslicher Bestandteile der Hornschicht auf Bakterien. I. Mitteilung. Arch Klin Exp Dermatol 205:420–434
46. Röstenberg A, Sulzberger MB (1937) Some results of patch tests. A compilation and a discussion of cutaneous reactions to about 500 different substances, as elicited by over 10 000 tests in approximately 1000 patients. Arch Dermatol Syphilol 35:433–454
47. Sauermann G, Doerschner A, Hoppe U, Wittern P (1986) Comparative study of skin care efficacy and in-use properties of soap and surfactant bars. J Soc Cosmet Chem 37: 309–327
48. Schade H, Marchionini A (1928) Der Säuremantel der Haut (nach Gaskettenmessungen). Klin Wochenschr 7:12–14
49. Schadenböck W (1990) Zusammensetzung marktüblicher Syndet-Zubereitungen zur Hautreinigung. In: Braun-Falco O, Korting HC (eds) Hautreinigung mit Syndets. Chemische, ökologische und klinische Aspekte. Springer, Berlin Heidelberg New York, pp 31–38
50. Schneider W (1965) Experimentelle Untersuchungen zur Frage der Reinigung, Pflege und externen Therapie der Haut. Dermatol Wochenschr 151:505–514
51. Schneider W (1990) Syndets: chemische Bestandteile. In: Braun-Falco O, Korting HC (eds) Hautreinigung mit Syndets. Chemische, ökologische und klinische Aspekte. Springer, Berlin Heidelberg New York, pp 24–30
52. Scholtz JR (1964) Management of atopic dermatitis: a preliminary report. Calif Med 100:103
53. Scholtz JR (1965) Management of atopic dermatitis. Calif Med 102:210–216
54. Schrader K (1990) Reinigungswirkung von Syndetzubereitungen – methodische Grundlagen ihrer Erfassung. In: Braun-Falco O, Korting HC (eds) Hautreinigung mit Syndets. Chemische, ökologische und klinische Aspekte. Springer, Berlin Heidelberg New York, pp 92–97
55. Schumann K (1990) Der Syndet-Begriff. In: Braun-Falco O, Korting HC (eds) Hautreinigung mit Syndets. Chemische, ökologische und klinische Aspekte. Springer, Berlin Heidelberg New York, pp 13–17
56 Schwarz HG (1964) Zur Frage des Einsatzes von Syndets anstelle von Fettseifen. Fette Seifen Anstrichm 66:1006–1011
57. Schweinsheimer (1959) Cited according to: Keining E (1959) Zur Frage der Reinigung gesunder und kranker Haut. Dermatol Wochenschr 140:1245–1251
58. Simon FA (1945) Cutaneous reactions of persons with atopic eczema to human dander. Arch Dermatol Syphilol 51:402–404
59. Stauffer H (1930) Die Ekzemproben. (Methodik und Ergebnisse). Arch Dermatol Syph 162:562–576
60. Stoughton RB, Potts LE, Clendenning W, Fisher S, Kress M (1960) Management of patients with eczematous diseases. JAMA 73:1196–1198
61. Strube DD, Nicoll G (1987) The irritancy of soaps and syndets. Cutis 39:544–545
62. Tronnier H (1985) Seifen und Syndets in der Hautpflege und -therapie. Arztl Kosmetol 15:19–30
63. Tronnier H (1987) Dermatologische Bewertung von Kosmetika und Körperpflegemittel. Arztl Kosmetol 17:374–398
64. Tronnier H, Bussius H (1961) Über die Zusammenhänge zwischen dem pH-Wert der Haut und ihrer Alkalineutralisationsfähigkeit. Z Haut Geschlechtskr 30:177–195
65. Tronnier H, Schneider W, Schuster G, Modde H (1967) Untersuchungen über den Effekt waschaktiver Tenside unterschiedlicher pH-Werte auf die menschliche Haut. Arch Klin Exp Dermatol 229:40–53
66. Uehara M, Ofuji S (1969) Delayed skin reaction to human dander in atopic dermatitis. Acta Derm Venereol (Stockh) 49:294–298
67. Uehara M, Ofuji S (1976) Patch test reaction to human dander in atopic dermatitis. Arch Dermatol 112:151–154
68. Uehara M, Takada K (1985) Use of soap in the management of atopic dermatitis. Clin Exp Dermatol 10:419–425
69. van der Valk PGM, Crijns MC, Nater JP, Bleumink E (1984) Skin irritancy of commercially available soap and detergent bars as measured by water vapour loss. Dermatosen 32:87–90
70. van der Valk PGM, Nater JP, Bleuming KE (1985) Vulnerability of the skin to surfactants in different groups of eczema patients and controls as measured by water vapour loss. Clin Exp Dermatol 10:98–103
71. Weber G (1987) A new method for measuring the skin cleaning effect of soaps and detergents. Acta Derm Venereol [Suppl] (Stockh) 134:33–34
72. Werner Y, Lindberg M (1985) Transepidermal waterloss in dry and clinically normal skin in patients with atopic dermatitis. Acta Derm Venereol (Stockh) 65:102–105

Topical Vehicles: Composition, Principles of Application and Action

K. Thoma

Introduction

The following aspects of topical vehicles should be considered in their therapeutic application:

- Indication for vehicles in terms of the type of skin
- Choice of vehicles in terms of acuity of the disease
- Effect of different vehicles on the skin
- Properties and composition of vehicles
- Relationships between the composition of vehicles and the biological availability of drugs

Healthy skin also requires an adaptation of the vehicle to the type of skin. As shown in Fig. 1, fatty-free vehicles such as aqueous solutions, lotions, and powders are in general better tolerated by the fatty seborrhoic skin [36]. Usually pastes and o/w creams can be applied for both types of skin. Especially for dry sebostatic skin, greasing vehicles such as fatty ointments and w/o emulsion ointments are useful. Therefore the patient's skin type should be determined for the application of suitable vehicles [39, 53, 54, 56].

As shown in Table 1, external vehicles can be classified according to the acuity of the stage of the disease and the therapeutic effects which they exert on skin. For topical application, the physical effects of vehicles in the skin are decisive for different stages of disease. In the acute stage the cooling, drying, and antiinflammatory effects are of importance; in the chronic stage an activating effect via maceration and heat accumulation is necessary [5, 34, 45, 47].

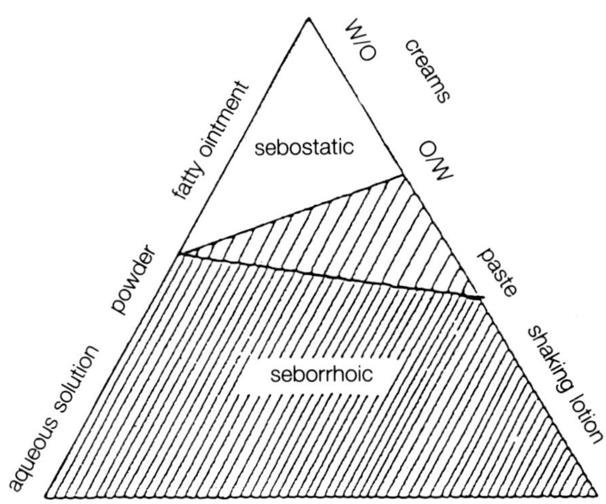

Fig. 1. Relationship of vehicle to type of skin. (From [36])

Table 1. Application and effect of dermal vehicles

Vehicle	Disease stage	Effect	Depth effect
Moist dressing	↑	↑	
Powder	Acute	Cooling,	
shaking lotion		drying,	
Paste		antiinflammatory	
Solution			
Hydrogel			|
o/w Lotion	Subacute		increasing
o/w Cream			↓
Cold cream			
w/o Ointment		Heat accumulation,	
Lipogel ointment	Chronic	macerating,	
Plaster	↓	activating	
Occlusion		↓	

Moist Dressings

Moist dressings using aqueous or aqueous-alcoholic solutions exert antiinflammatory actions in acute, exudative eczema. According to the dermatological rule of "wet on wet" the dressings exert cooling and drying effects and reduce swelling due to the capillary forces of the open gauze dressing (Fig. 2). These must be changed repeatedly, and occlusive dressing must be strictly avoided. The cooling effect can be intensified by adding alcohol, which can be tolerated up to a concentration of 10% [47]. The concentrations of active ingredients should be 0.1%–1% [48].

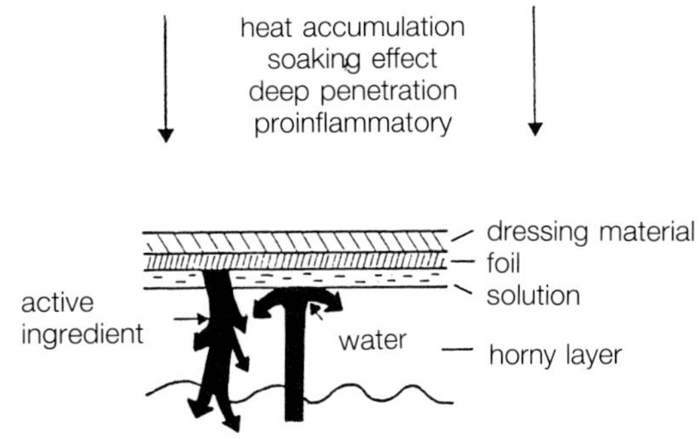

Fig. 2. Effect of a wet dressing in acute exudative inflammatory conditions. (From [56])

Powders

Powders increase the surface of the skin and exert a cooling effect as a consequence of increased heat loss. Various properties can be achieved according to the additives used (Table 2). Besides their function as an inert, cooling vehicle for active compounds, dermatological powders are also useful for their drying and draining effects. They are used mainly for the interval therapy of dermatoses. Powders are contraindicated in exudative dermatoses due to the formation of lumps and reduced heat loss with the increased risk of superinfections [56]. With body powders a marked absorbing effect is desired in addition to the lubricating and smoothing properties.

Table 2. Properties of powder excipients

Properties	Excipients
Cooling effect	Different types of starch; Al-stearates
Absorptive capacity	Colloidal silicic acid (Aerosil); bolus alba; microcristalline cellulose; starch
Absorption without swelling	Etherified starch types (ANM; Nalcip)
Lubrication	Talcum; Zn-, Mg-, Al-stearates
Adhesive properties	Talcum; colloidal silicic acid; starch; lipids; Al hydroxide
Dispersion ability	Colloidal silicic acid; talcum
Camouflage	Titanium dioxide; zinc oxide; Ca carbonate
Absorption ability	Lactose

Shaking Lotions

By evaporation of the liquid portion over the large surface of the powder component, shaking lotions exert a cooling, desiccating, adstringent, and antiinflammatory effect (Table 3). Their use is indicated in widespread, inflammatory, dry, or slightly exudative dermatoses such as sunburn. Shaking lotions are also indicated in irritable skin sensitive to ointments as well as in seborrhoic individuals [36, 48]. Shaking lotions are liquid powders which are applied with a brush. They are usually composed of equal parts of a powdery component, such as zinc oxide, talcum, or titanium dioxide, and an aqueous component. An increase in the cooling effect can be achieved by the addition of alcohol (lotio alba spirituosa). Glycerol or another moisturizer such as solution of sorbitol or propylene glycol causes adhesion of the powder component onto skin surface.

Lotio alba aquosa has been taken over in the revised German formula [37] in unchanged form as zinc oxide shaking lotion; this consists of 20 g zinc oxide, 20 g talcum, 30 g glycerol 85%, and 30 g purified water. The commercial shaking lotion Lotio Cordes contains propylene glycol 20 g, as moisturizer, stabilizers, titanium dioxide 14 g, corn starch 5 g, and purified water ad 100 g. Pure suspension-type shaking lotions can be transferred into

Table 3. Functions of shaking lotions

Functions
Powder components
Cooling, draining
Desiccating, covering
Liquid portion
Cooling, adhering
Facultative excipients
Improvement of the shaking properties
Physical stability
Adhesive effect, microbial stability

emulsion-type suspensions by the use of stabilizers in the form of emulsifier complexes. Additives such as bentonite or carboxymethylcellulose can be used as viscosity-increasing stabilizers in shaking lotions. In a shaking lotion often used by dermatologists, the formation of an o/w emulsion-suspension is achieved with emulgating cetostearyl alcohol; in addition to Lanette N 3g, this consists of zinc oxide, talcum, glycerol 85%, alcohol 70% āā 18g, and purified water ad 100g. The commercial preparation Lotio Hermal is also an emulsion-type shaking lotion and consists of: 20 g zinc oxide, 15 g talcum, 6 g glycerol, 1 g plant lecithin, 0,3 g *p*-hydroxybenzoic acid methylester, sodium carragenate, colloidal silicic dioxide, cetostearyl polyglycolphosphate, isopropyl alcohol, and purified water ad 100 g. Numerous active ingredients such as Ichthyol, liquor carbonis detergens, and Thesit can be used in shaking lotions [56].

Pastes

Pastes are suspension-type ointments with a high content of powdery components. Anhydrous lipophilic preparations are used more frequently as vehicles than emulsions. The application and effects of pastes in skin are markedly influenced by the rate of solid components of the preparation (Fig. 3). Hard pastes act by virtue of their high powder content in a drying, absorbing, and covering manner and are indicated mainly in oily skin and intertriginous areas, while in soft pastes the properties of the ointment component predominate. German formulas prescribe the following zinc paste compositions: for pasta zinci [12]: 25 g zinc oxide, 25 g corn starch, 50 g white petrolatum; for pasta zinci mollis [12]: 30 g zinc oxide, 20 g medium chain length triglycerides, 50 g unguentum alcoholum lanae (in the case of pasta zinci mollis, some recommend using an alternative to unguentum alcoholum lanae because of possible allergic hypersensitivity reactions) (M. Gloor, personal information); for oleum zinci [10]: 50 g zinc oxide, 50 g olive oil. The preparation of Pasta Cordes contains 30% powder with equal parts of titanium dioxide and talcum. Easier to apply and with a stronger drying effect is the liquid paste zinc oil, which is also indicated in petrolatum sensitive dermatoses. It has been included in the revised German formulas [37]. For the production of absorbing pastes the careful removal of water remnants from starch is of great importance (see description of pasta zinci, above).

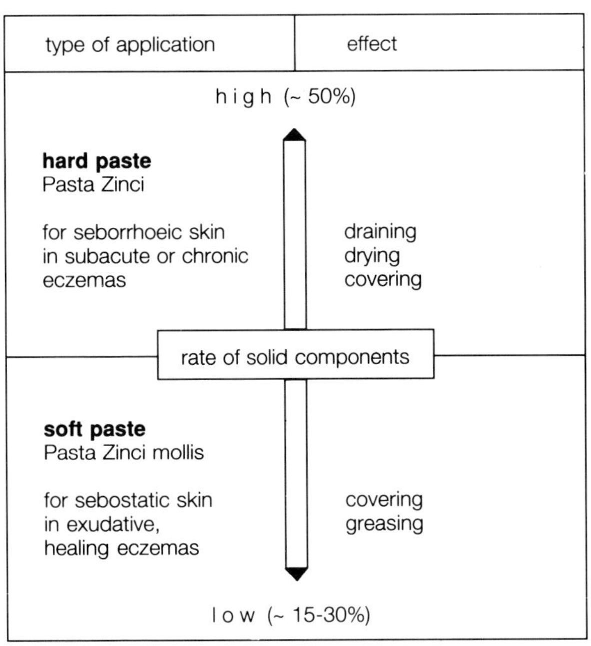

Fig. 3. Function of different types of pastes

Solutions

Alcoholic aqueous solutions which serve as vehicles for antimycotics, corticosteroids, and other paints show properties which depend on the relative proportions of their vehicle components. A higher percentage of ethanol or isopropanol intensifies drying and depth effects. Moisturizers such as glycerol shorten the time needed for drying. Excessive drying can be prevented by the use of castor oil or similar oily additives. The application properties of paints can be modified by the use of cellulose derivatives or polyacrylates increasing viscosity, solvents such as polyethylene glycols, or surfactants.

Hydrophilic Ointments

Hydrophilic ointments include particularly the wash-off ointments, usually anhydrous polyethylene glycol ointments. These have a good resolving power for hydrophilic and lipophilic drugs due to the ether oxygen, alcoholic hydroxy groups, and structural properties of the molecule (Fig. 4). Polyethylen glycol ointments (1 part 300, 1 part 1500) show pronounced hydrophilia and hygroscopicity and possess osmotic activities with regard to wound secretions. They are useful in antiseptic and antimycotic ointments due to the reduction of swelling, good diffusion, and releasing capacity for incorporated, dissolved ingredients [54].

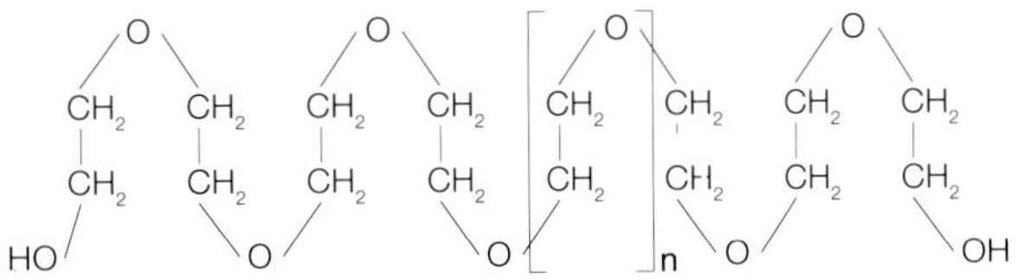

Fig. 4. Molecular structure of polyethylene glycols (n >10)

Hydrogels

Hydrogels and their macromolecular additives can be formally classified as dermatological preparations with film-forming contents (e.g., tinctures containing collodium); they are also designated as varnishes. In contrast to these, however, hydrogels are extremely hydrophilic preparations with a high water or water soluble liquid content of 90%–98% ("water in solid form"). Table 4 shows the German hydrogel formulas. Hydrogels are lipid-free, wash-off vehicles, which are cooling due to evaporation. Since they contain approximately 1%–6% macromolecular hydrogel-forming compounds such as cellulose derivatives, they produce a drying, covering film on the skin surface. Due to the presence of hydrophilic moisturizers (softeners), an elastic wound closure is formed which is used, for example, in wound gels with chemotherapeutics or antiseptic preparations. The properties of these hydrogels are determined by the type of the hydrogel former as well as the components of the water phase (amount of moisturizer, addition of alcohol). Hydrogels with polyacrylates can be rubbed into the skin and allow depth and systemic therapeutic effects amplified by the addition of alcohol. If liposomes with drug substances or cosmetic ingredients [42] are used in topical dosage forms, hydrogels are compatible as vehicles.

Table 4. Gels as dermatological vehicles

Carboxymethylcellulose gel [12]	
Carboxymethylcellulose sodium 600	5.0 g
Glycerol 85%	10.0 g
Purified water	85.0 g
Preservation: 0.1% sorbic acid + 0.1% potassium sorbate; or, if necessary for galenic or therapeutic reasons, 0.1% methyl-4-hydroxybenzoate + 0.04% propyl-4-hydroxybenzoate	
Hydroxyethylcellulose gel [12]	
Hydroxyethylcellulose 30 000	2.5 g
Glycerol 85%	10.0 g
Purified water	87.5 g
Preservation: 0.1% sorbic acid + 0.1% potassium sorbate; or, if necessary for galenic or therapeutic reasons, 0.1% methyl-4-hydroxybenzoate + 0.04% propyl-4-hydroxybenzoate	
Glycerol gel [10]	
Hydroxyethylcellulose 300	4.5 g
Glycerol 85%	30.0 g
Purified water	65.5 g
Aqueous polyacrylate gel	
Polyacrylic acid	0.5 g
Sodium hydroxide solution 5%	3.0 g
Purified water	96.5 g
Preservation: 0.1% sorbic acid + 0.1% potassium sorbate; or, if necessary for galenic or therapeutic reasons, 0.07% methyl-4-hydroxybenzoate + 0.03% propyl-4-hydroxybenzoate	
Isopropylalcoholic polyacrylate gel	
Polyacrylic acid	0.5 g
Sodium hydroxide solution 5%	1.0 g
Isopropyl alcohol	25.0 g
Purified water	73.5 g

o/w Lotions

The o/w emulsions of "skin milk" (lotion) type possess cooling effects and show actions similar to creams in the skin. Due to their liquid consistency they can be more easily applied than creams to certain areas of the body (hairy, intertriginous, other areas difficult to reach, face and ears for cosmetic reasons). They usually contain only a very small percentage of lipophilic components, such as heavy-liquid paraffin, and are useful for subacute and subchronic processes, particularly in seborrhoeic skin. Both anionic complex emulsifiers such as sodium lauryl sulphate/cetostearyl alcohol and nonionic ones such as polyethylene glycol stearate/cetyl alcohol/glycerol monostearate can be used. The composition of the "skin milk" type of lotion is: emulsifier complex 1%–5%, lipophilic component 0%–5%, moisturizer 5%–15%, preservative (qs), and purified water 80%–90%. The o/w lotions act in principle as diluted o/w creams; the following prescription [44] is illustrative: chloramphenicol 1 g, 1,2-propylene glycol 10 g, aqua destillata 15 g, and unguentum emulsificans aquosum 24 g.

Hydrophilic Creams

Hydrophilic creams (o/w creams) are frequently used in commercial preparations but less often in prescriptions made by pharmacists. Their widespread use is due to a number of favorable properties, particularly good tolerance in all stages of eczema [47]. When used as vehicles for active ingredients, creams show a high release rate and good penetration into skin, thus providing high availability [19, 20, 25, 28, 40, 51, 58]. On the skin hydrophilic creams have a cooling effect due to the high content of 50%–70% water in the external phase (Fig. 5) [59]. Cream vehicles are used for normal to fatty skin but may also desiccate depending on their structure [52]. For compatible manufacturing with pharmaceuticals, cream prescriptions must be available with both, anionic and nonionic complex emulsifiers depending on their chemical structure [55]. Table 5 presents the German formulas of hydrophilic creams.

The properties of the lipid phase, which usually consists of petrolatum and liquid paraffins for dermal preparations can be improved by the use of spreading, nonirritating substances such as the ester of oleic acid with oleyl alcohol. Moisturizers prevent drying out [14]. Preservation is also necessary for short-term storage.

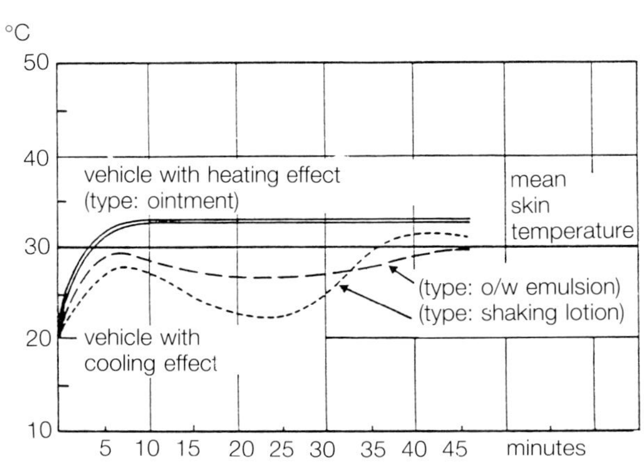

Fig. 5. Effect of dermatological vehicles on skin temperature. (From [23])

Table 5. o/w Emulsion vehicles (hydrophilic creams) as dermatological vehicles

Nonionic hydrophilic cream [12]	
Polysorbate 60	5.0 g
Cetostearyl alcohol	10.0 g
Glycerol 85%	10.0 g
White petrolatum	25.0 g
Purified water	50.0 g
Preservation: 0.1% sorbic acid; or, if necessary for galenic or therapeutic reasons, 0.1% methyl-4-hydroxybenzoate + 0.04% propyl-4-hydroxybenzoate	
Basis cream [10]	
Glyceryl monostearate	4.0 g
Cetyl alcohol	6.0 g
Medium chain length triglycerides	7.5 g
White petrolatum	25.5 g
Polyoxyethylene glycerol monostearate	7.0 g
Propylene glycol	10.0 g
Purified water	40.0 g
Hydrophilic ointment [12]	
Emulgating cetostearyl alcohol	30.0 g
Heavy-liquid paraffin	35.0 g
White petrolatum	35.0 g
Aqueous hydrophilic ointment [12]	
Hydrophilic ointment	30.0 g
Purified water	70.0 g
Preservation: 0.1% sorbic acid; or, if necessary for galenic or therapeutic reasons, 0.06% methyl-4-hydroxybenzoate + 0.04% propyl-4-hydroxybenzoate	
Nonionic hydrophilic ointment [9]	
Polyoxyethylene glycerol monostearate	10.0 g
Light-liquid paraffin	15.0 g
Cetostearyl alcohol	20.0 g
Glycerol 85%	20.0 g
White petrolatum	35.0 g
Aqueous nonionic hydrophilic ointment [9]	
Nonionic hydrophilic ointment	50.0 g
Purified water	50.0 g

Since o/w creams cause no fatty shine in skin and are easily applied and vanishing, they are also important as vehicles for cosmetics. They are used predominantly in day creams, moisturizing creams, and in skin protection and sun protection preparations [55]. The skin care properties of such day creams can be varied according to their liquid content, spreading ability, and skin affinity [38].

Ambiphilic creams should be mentioned as a particular type of hydrophilic creams. These represent an intermediate type with diluting properties toward both hydrophilic water phases and lipid phases. An example is the basis cream [10] (Table 5). Due to basis cream's propylene glycol content of 10%, there is no need for an additional preservative [41].

Microemulsions are transparent vehicles of o/w or w/o type. The emulsion particles are extremely finely dispersed (100–500 A). Their contents are water-, lipoid-, and "inter" phase (amphiphilic alcohols) with relatively high concentrations of excipients [29, 26, 46]. The drug release is remarkable [64], but it is not often used in dermatology.

Important Additives for Hydrophilic Creams, o/w Lotions, and Hydrogels

With regard to moisturizers, the bi-, tri-, and hexavalent alcohols or compounds such as sodium lactate and mixtures of amino acids act by binding water remnants and thus maintain the suppleness of the hydrophilic surface films (Fig. 6). In a comparable manner, these additives protect o/w emulsions from drying out and improve their spreading properties ("softeners").

The use of preservatives in dermatological preparations is usually restricted to hydrogels and hydrophilic creams and lotions. Since their external phase contains water, storage of these preparations requires preservation, i.e., inhibition of microbial growth. The use of phenolic compounds is usually restricted to the widely used *p*-hydroxybenzoic acid esters, less frequently to chlorocresol. Besides the more frequently used substances sorbic acid and benzyl alcohol, other compounds are frequently used particularly in cosmetics (Fig. 7) [55]. Preservatives occasionally cause allergic contact eczema in certain cases due to esters of *p*-hydroxybenzoic acid. Sorbic acid and other compounds may also cause allergic contact dermatitis, albeit less frequently [6, 49, 55]. The German Pharmacopoeia [12] prescribes two alternative methods of preservation.

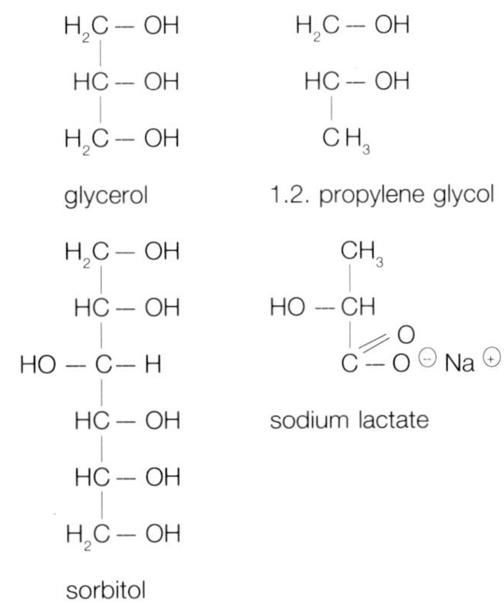

Fig. 6. Moisturizers for hydrophilic creams and hydrogels

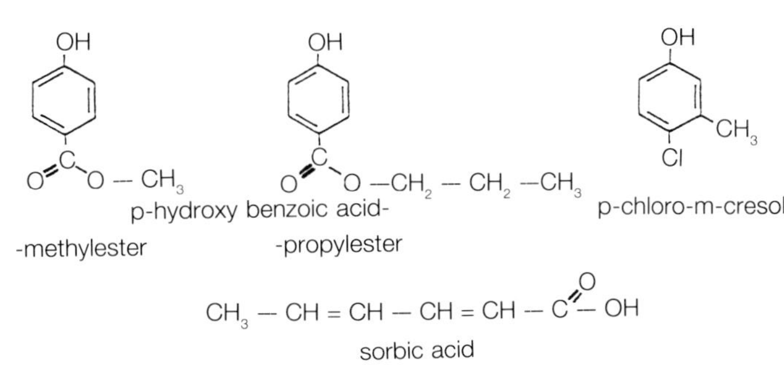

Fig. 7. Preservatives for dermatological preparations

Cold Cream

Cold cream (unguentum leniens [12]) exerts in skin an intermediate effect between that of a hydrophilic and that of a hydrophobic cream. Its properties in skin correspond to those of a weak fatty ointment. It is less occlusive and less greasy, softening, macerating, and penetrating. It is indicated in dry skin and subacute, macerating disorders. The cooling effect of this emulsifier-free w/o quasiemulsion is dependent upon melting and instability of the emulsion after application to skin and warming (15). Cold cream is therefore physically only moderately stable on storage, because it does not contain an emulsifier. In a former edition of the German Pharmacopoeia, "stabilization" was prescribed with the use of the w/o emulsifier glycerol monostearate. This led to a stable, true w/o emulsion with loss of the cooling effect in skin. Therefore, the additive has been now abandoned.

The cooling effect of cold cream is today surpassed by hydrophilic cream vehicles. The dermatologist Unna observed in 1884 that cold cream was tolerated much better than fatty ointments in eczemas and erythemas. Since then this well-defined vehicle has been useful in certain indications due to the lack of irritation in prescriptions made by pharmacists. Since it becomes easily rancid, it should be prepared freshly and stored for less than 1 month if stabilization with an antioxidant is avoided.

Additives for the Hydrophobic Components of Creams and Ointments against Rancidity: Antioxidants

Lipids and other unsaturated bases and additives used in topical preparations, particularly commercial ones, must be protected on longer storage against rancidity by antioxidants. Antioxidants are lipophilic, phenolic compounds. In use are mainly α-tocopherol, propyl gallate, butyhydroxytoluene, butylhydroxyanisole, and nordihydroguaiaretic acid. These phenols cause a break in the radical chain of the fatty acid cleavage reaction and thus inhibit further transformations [3, 55]. The effect of these inhibitors can be further enhanced by the use of so-called secondary antioxidants (synergists), for example, organic acids such as ascorbic or citric acid or the anorganic phosphoric acid. In individual cases, allergic hypersensitivity reactions may also occur with certain antioxidants [55].

Hydrophobic Creams

Due to their lipophilic external phase, these w/o emulsion ointments exert fattening effects even with higher water content and are therefore indicated primarily in dry skin. They prevent insensible water loss and thus return the moisture flow direction in skin to the inside, in analogy to the water-free lipogels. They cannot be washed off, produce the typical oily shine, and represent a transition to the pure lipogels. However, they differ from these, for example, by their releasing properties for active components. Table 6 presents the German Pharmacopoeia and Codex [10, 12] formulae for hydrophobic creams.

Wool wax alcohols and wool wax are most frequently used as w/o emulsifiers; further compounds include sorbitol fatty acid ester, pentaerythritol fatty acid ester, citric acid fatty alcohol ester, propylene glycol, or glycerol fatty acid esters, and fatty alcohols. The lipid phase, containing in general petrolatum and heavy-liquid paraffin, can be structured by bleached wax,

Table 6. w/o Emulsion vehicles (hydrophobic creams) as dermatological vehicles

Aqueous lanolin [12]	
Anhydrous lanolin	75.0 g
Purified water	25.0 g
Lanolin [12]	
Heavy-liquid paraffin	15.0 g
Purified water	20.0 g
Anhydrous lanolin	65.0 g
Unguentum alcoholum lanae aquosum [12]	
Unguentum alcoholum lanae	50.0 g
Purified water	50.0 g
Lanae alcoholum unguentum aquosum pH 5 [37]	
Citric acid	0.75 g
Ammonia solution 10%	0.90 g
Medium chainlength triglycerides	5.0 g
Unguentum alcoholum lanae	40.0 g
Purified water	53.35 g

cetylpalmitate or microcrystalline wax. To improve the greasing properties and skin affinity, substances such as isopropyl myristate or triglycerides can be used. The w/o emulsion ointments frequently contain antioxidants to improve storage capacity. They may, but need not, contain preservatives. The vehicle unguentum molle (prescribed in the German Pharmacopoeia, 6th edition, but still in use today) contains equal parts of lanolin and yellow petrolatum. In cosmetics w/o emulsion ointments are used as night creams and creams for sebostatic skin. Skin care preparations, cold creams, and baby creams are also frequently developed as w/o emulsions.

Water-Emulsifying Ointments

Absorption vehicles are anhydrous hydrocarbon gels or lipogels containing emulsifiers. These emulsifiers improve the product properties of anhydrous preparations, such as skin affinity or release of active components. Wool wax and wool wax alcohols are therefore often used. According to the German Pharmacopoeia (9th edition), unguentum alcoholum lanae is to be used as the vehicle in all cases without further specification; this contains 0.5 g cetostearyl alcohol, 6.0 g wool wax alcohols, and 93.5 g white petrolatum. In some cases, for example, when improved wash-off property of an ointment for use on the scalp is desired, nonionic o/w emulsifiers may be used. Other components serve to improve skin affinity or, as in the case of propylene glycol, to enhance penetration of the active compound.

Hydrophobic Ointments

Monophasic, lipophilic ointments cause occlusion of skin and thus prevent perspiratio insensibilis. Heat and moisture accumulation cause a maceration of the skin and lead to soaking and swelling of the keratins and horny layer. In chronic skin disesases, these vehicles thus allow an enhanced penetration of incorporated active compounds into deeper layers of the skin.

Hydrocarbon Gels. Petrolatum, discovered 1871 by Chesborough, is used as white petrolatum for all vehicles of the Pharmacopoeia which contain petrolatum. As a nonaqueous vehicle, petrolatum shows high storage capacity, chemical inertness, and therefore stability of the incorporated active compounds. Its consistency can be adapted to the respective indication by the use of heavy- or light-liquid paraffin, wax, or fatty alcohols. From liquid skin paraffin and 5% polyethylene MW 21 000 as a backbone, a hydrocarbon gel can be produced (Plastibase). Ointment gels can also be produced from microcrystalline wax and liquid paraffin.

Lipogels. Lipogels are vehicles composed of fatty acid triglycerides or lipophilic compounds such as liquid wax. They show pronounced greasing properties. Lipogel vehicles such as pork lard or hydrated peanut oil are generally avoided in commercial preparations, as these are subjects to rancidity and must usually be stabilized with antioxidants. Topical preparations designated as fatty ointments are usually composed of hydrocarbon vehicles with a certain proportion of fatty acid triglycerides, e.g., hydrated castor oil.

Occlusive Dressings

Occlusive dressings are produced with softener-free plastic foils after the drug has been applied to skin as alcoholic solution or as ointment. As a consequence of covering the skin, there is an accumulation of skin moisture and swelling and loosening of the stratum corneum. The penetration and permeation of active compounds is thus markedly enhanced (Fig. 8). For corticosteroids, there is about a 100-fold increase in penetration and permeation [33]. Irritation effects on

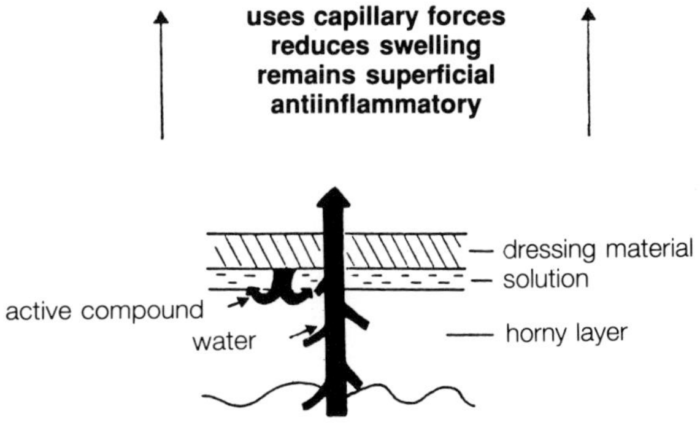

Fig. 8. Effect of an occlusive dressing against chronic dermatosis. (From [56])

skin are possible [4]. The proinflammatory effect is useful in deep-seated chronic processes accompanied by lichenification or hyperkeratosis. Besides self-adhesive corticosteroid foils, there are also self-adhesive or non-adhesive foils without active compounds, which are used in connection with topically applied drugs.

Composition of Topical Vehicles and Biological Availability of Drugs

The therapeutic effect of dermatological preparations depends not only on interactions between vehicle and skin but also on the possible interaction between vehicles and incorporated drugs and on the interaction between drugs and skin (Fig. 9) [2, 25, 51, 54, 56, 61, 62]. Every drug is available in the skin to only a certain degree, if it is liberated in a sufficient quantity and time from the vehicle. Drug delivery from topical vehicles occurs in three steps. Chemical and physical problems of drug stability must therefore be prevented, because every loss of active substance lowers the degree of availability. For example, hydrolysis and oxidative processes that take place in various antibiotics and corticosteroids are particularly liable to occur in hydrophilic creams [8, 22]. Corticosteroid crystal formation in such vehicles, a manifestation of physical instability, also influences bioavailability [24] (Fig. 10). The first step is the release from the vehicle to the surface of the skin [54]; the second the penetration into the skin [53]. Under certain conditions permeation of the horny layer occurs with transdermal absorption and systemic effects, as a dermatologically generally undesired third step.

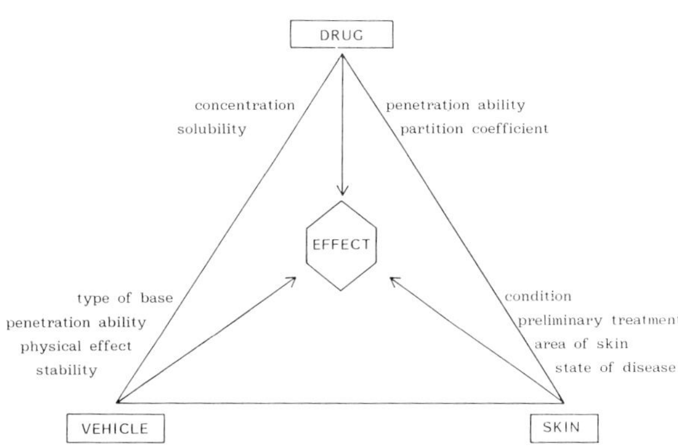

Fig. 9. Effect of dermal preparations as interaction of drug, vehicle, and skin. (From [57])

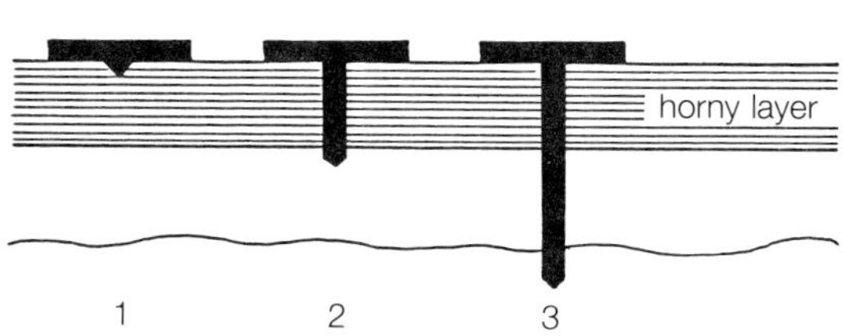

Fig. 10. Dermal and transdermal drug delivery. *1*, Release from the vehicle; *2*, penetration into the skin; *3*, permeation and transdermal absorption

Drug release from the vehicle to the skin is influenced by various parameters which are very important for bioavailability:

- Dissolution properties of the vehicle for the drug: solubility, particle size of unsolved drugs and chemical compatibility of vehicle and drug [18, 19, 20, 54]
- Diffusion of drugs in the vehicle: consistency of the vehicle, absence of physicochemical interactions between vehicle and drug [60]
- Partition relations of drugs between vehicle and skin: partition coefficient of the drug, spreading agents, other dermal excipients [52, 63]

Penetration of drugs into the skin is influenced by [27, 31, 52]:

- Properties of the skin, such as state of disease, condition, application area, thickness of the horny layer as well as age or drug metabolism
- Properties of the drug, such as partition coefficient, molecular size, and concentration
- Affinity and influence of the vehicle, such as spreadability or hydration effects

Changes of penetration behavior by the use of liposomal carriers are currently being investigated [21, 13, 43].

Transdermal absorption occurs when the factors that improve penetration cause permeation of the horny layer [1, 30, 50]. This is influenced by:

- Application area and time [32]
- Decrease in barrier properties such as those caused by occlusive effects or penetration enhancers [35, 16, 7]

Transdermal systems are used in systemic drug therapy [17]. In the case of dermatological preparations, transdermal permeation of drugs, caused by the drug itself or by the influence of vehicles and excipients is a generally undesired effect in dermal therapy.

References

1. Barr M (1962) Percutaneous absorption. J Pharm Sci 51: 395–409
2. Barrett CW, Hadgraft JW, Sarkany I (1964) The influence of vehicles on skin penetration. J Pharm Pharmacol 16:104–107
3. Belitz H-D, Grosch W (1987) Lehrbuch der Lebensmittelchemie, 3rd edn. Springer, Berlin Heidelberg New York Tokyo
4. Bergstresser PR, Eaglstein WH (1973) Irritation by hydrophilic ointment under occlusion. Arch Dermatol 108:218–219
5. Brehm G (1969) Was der Apotheker von der Haut und der Dermato-Therapie wissen muß. Informationsdienst APV 15 (2/3):55–62
6. Brehm K (1973) Nebenwirkungen von Salben- und Cremegrundlagen und deren Konservierungsmitteln. Fette Seifen Anstrichmittel 75:443–445
7. Chien YW (1982) Novel drug delivery systems. Dekker, New York
8. Das Gupta V (1978) Effect of vehicles and other active ingredients on stability of hydrocortisone. J Pharm Sci 67: 299–302
9. Deutscher Arzneimittel-Codex (1979) Govi, Frankfurt aM and Deutscher Apotheker, Stuttgart
10. Deutscher Arzneimittel-Codex (1986) Govi, Frankfurt aM, and Deutscher Apotheker, Stuttgart
11. Deutsches Arzneibuch 8th edn. (1978) Deutscher Apotheker, Stuttgart and Govi, Frankfurt aM
12. Deutsches Arzneibuch 9th edn. (1986) Deutscher Apotheker, Stuttgart and Govi, Frankfurt aM
13. Gesztes A, Mezei M (1988) Topical anesthesia of the skin by liposome-encapsulated tetracaine. Anesth Analg. 67:1079–1081
14. Gloor M (1982) Pharmakologie dermatologischer Externa. Springer, Berlin Heidelberg New York
15. Graf E, Hoheisel H (1975) Zur Objektivierung der Kühlwirkung von Kühlsalben, -gelen und Lotionen. Arch Pharm 308:2–11
16. Guy R, Hadgraft J (1987) The effect of penetration enhancers on the kinetics of percutaneous absorption. J Contr Rel 5:43–51
17. Heilmann K (1984) Therapeutische Systeme, 4th edn. Enke, Stuttgart
18. Horsch W (1984) Transportmechanismen und Einflußfaktoren in den Systemen Salbe/Haut und Arzneistoff/Salbengrundlage. Pharmazie 39:598–605
19 Horsch W, Mette B (1974) In-vitro-Liberation von Hydroxychinolinsulfat aus verschiedenen Dermatica. Pharmazie 29:546–548
20. Horsch W, Kögel J, Teich C, Wendrich M (1973) Beiträge zur Löslichkeit von Arzneistoffen in Salben und zum Verteilungsverhalten zwischen Lipoid- und Wasserphasen. Pharmazie 28:669–673
21. Jacobs M, Martin GP, Marriott C (1988) Effects of phosphatidyl choline on the topical bioavailability of corticosteroids assessed by the human skin blanching assay. J Pharm Pharmacol 40:829–833
22. Kenley RA, Lee MO, Sukumar L, Powell MF (1987) Temperature and pH-dependence of fluocinolone actonide degradation in a topical cream formulation. Pharm Res 4:342–347
23. Kleine-Natrop HE (1961) In: Gottron HA, Schönfeld W (eds) Dermatologie und Venerologie, vol I. Thieme, Stuttgart
24. Kögel J, Horsch W (1978) Untersuchungen zur Dispersität von Arzneistoffen unter besonderer Berücksichtigung von Suspensionssalben. Pharmazie 33:738–746
25. Kotwas J, Schaefer H, Zesch A (1979) Zur Verfügbarkeit von Wirkstoffen an und in der Haut. Arzneimittelforschung 29:562–568
26. Lagues M, Santerey C (1980) Percolation transition in water in oil microemulsions. J Phys Chem 84:3503
27. Lippold BC (1981) Kutane Resorption – Möglichkeiten, Modelle, Beeinflussung. Acta Pharm Technol 27:1–9
28. Lippold BC (1981) Wirkstoffresorption aus Dermatika. Dtsch Apoth Ztg 121:2585–2589
29. Lissant KJ (1974) Emulsions and emulsion technology. Decker, New York
30. Loth H (1987) Grundlagen des intra- und transdermalen Transportes von Arzneistoffen II. Acta Pharm Technol 33: 3–14
31. Loth H, Hailer M (1983) Einfluß einiger experimenteller Parameter auf die Penetration von Arzneistoffen in exzidierte, menschliche Haut. Acta Pharm Technol 29:181–186
32. Mauvais-Jarvis P, Vickers CFH, Wepierre J (1980) Percutaneous absorption of steroids. Academic, London
33. McKenzie AW, Stoughton RB (1962) Method for comparing percutaneous absorption of steroids. Arch Dermatol 86:608–610
34. Merz W (1969) Dermato-pharmazeutische Gesichtspunkte zur Salbentherapie. Informationsdienst APV 15 (1):63–76
35. Montagna W, Van Scott EJ, Stonghton R (1969) Pharmacology and the skin (publ no 511). ACT Meredith, New York
36. Nasemann T, Sauerbrey W (1981) Lehrbuch der Hauterkrankungen und venerischen Infektionen. Springer, Berlin Heidelberg New York
37. Neues Rezeptur-Formularium (NRF) (1987) Deutscher Apotheker, Stuttgart and Govi, Frankfurt aM
38. Neuwald F, Fetting KE, Szakall A (1962) Untersuchungen über die Fähigkeit der Spreitung von Lipoiden und der Permeation von Wasserdampf durch die lebende Haut. Fette Seifen Anstrichmittel 64:465–467
39. Nürnberg E (1978) Welche galenischen Grundlagen werden heute für die Hautbehandlung eingesetzt? Hautarzt 29:61–67
40. Nürnberg E (1986) Aspekte der Entwicklung von Emulsionssystemen. Arzneimittelforschung 18:11–15
41. Nürnberg E, Muckenschnabel R (1982) Hydrophile und ambiphile Cremesysteme. Dtsch Apoth Ztg 122:2093–2106
42. Raab W (1988) Liposomen – eine neue Form dermatologischer Wirkstoffträger. Ärztl Kosmetol 18:213–224
43. Ramachandran KEC, Kittayanond D, Weiner N (1990) Topical delivery of liposomally encapsulated interferon evaluated by in vitro diffusions studies. Antimicrob Agents Chemother 34:107–110
44. Rezeptformeln (1964) Volk und Gesundheit, Berlin (East)
45. Ritschel WA (1968) Biopharmazeutische Aspekte für die cutane Therapie. Dtsch Apoth Ztg 108:1029–1035
46. Prince LM (1977) Microemulsions, theory and practice. Academic, New York, p 57
47. Schneider W (1975) Grundsätzliche Gesichtspunkte in der modernen Ekzemtherapie. Hautarzt 26:88–91
48. Schönfeld W (1969) Lehrbuch der Haut- und Geschlechtskrankheiten, 10th edn. Thieme, Stuttgart
49. Siemer E, Elmahdi K (1987) Empfindliche Haut: Probleme – Pflege – Beratung. Pharm Ztg 132:2135–2141
50. Stricker H, Winter G, Leber A (1987) Galenische Faktoren der kutanen Wirkstoffpenetration in vivo. Acta Pharm Technol 33:80–88

51. Stüttgen G (1981) Pharmakokinetik und Effektivität von Hauttherapeutika. Hautarzt 31:199–207
52. Stüttgen G, Schaefer H (1974) Funktionelle Dermatologie. Springer, Berlin Heidelberg New York
53. Thoma K (1973) Pharmazeutische Technologie und Biopharmazie der Salben. Schriftenreihe der Bundesapothekerkammer zur wissenschaftlichen Fortbildung, Davos, vol. III. Deutscher Apotheker, Frankfurt a. M., pp 133–161
54. Thoma K (1983) Dermatika, 2nd edn. Deutscher Apotheker, Frankfurt aM
55. Thoma K (1989) Apothekenrezeptur und -defektur. Deutscher Apotheker, Stuttgart
56. Tronnier H (1968) Zur Bedeutung der Grundlagen in der dermatologischen Therapie. Z Haut Geschl Kr 44:155–168
57. Tronnier H (1977) Arzneitherapie an der Haut. Pharm Ztg 122:2021–2027
58. Voigt R, Dröseler W (1969) Zur Arzneistoffverteilung in Emulsionssystemen. Pharmazie 24:622–625
59. Werchan D, Ludwig R (1972) Die Kühlwirkung gebräuchlicher dermatologischer Externa. Pharmazie 27:670–672
60. Whitworth CW, Becker CH (1965) Study of diffusion of two sulfonamides from ointment bases. J Pharm Sci 54:569–573
61. Zesch A, Schaefer H (1973) Penetrationskinetik von radiomarkiertem Hydrocortison aus verschiedenen Salbengrundlagen in die menschliche Haut – in vitro. Arch Derm Forsch 246:335–354
62. Zesch A, Schaefer H (1975) Externe Therapie unter biopharmazeutischem Aspekt. Pharm Ztg 120:1460–1464
63. Zesch A, Hoffmann W-D, Schaefer H (1974) Verteilung eines radiomarkierten Pharmakons in der menschlichen Hornschicht aus vier Salbengrundlagen. Pharmazie 29: 198–203
64. Ziegenmeyer J, Führer C (1980) Mikroemulsionen als topische Arzneiform. Acta Pharm Technol 26(4):273–275

Topical Treatment with Corticosteroids

G. Goerz and P. Lehmann

History and Introduction

No other drug has changed the treatment of several diseases in such a succesful manner like cortisol and its derivatives (here called corticosteroids and abbreviated as CS). Perhaps penicillin is a comparable substance, but as it cannot be used as a topical drug it has not achieved such a significance in dermatology.

H. J. Maibach (cited in [74]) has differentiated the history of dermatology in the era *before* and *after* CS therapy. According to Schaefer et al. [74] 95% of all topically applied drugs in skin diseases contain CS derivatives. This fact was correct in 1984; today, however, the great public horror against the side effects has caused a restriction of CS therapy.

40 years ago Hench et al. [39] first reported the therapeutic benefit of an adrenal cortical hormone; compound E (17-hydroxy-11-dehydrocorticosterone) in the treatment of rheumatoid arthritis. For the first time the antiphlogistic effect of CS was observed, which initiated a new era in the treatment of inflammatory diseases and in many other disorders of unknown pathogenesis.

Three years later in 1952 Sulzberger and Witten reported about experiences with topically applied CS [82]. Their trials were stimulated by the findings of Goldman et al. [32], who could partially inhibit positive patch tests in allergic patients after a previous intradermal injection of compound F (17-hydroxycorticosterone-21-acetate). Sulzberger and Witten [82] treated 19 patients with a 2.5% 17-hdroxycorticosterone-21-acetate ointment (lanolin 15%, liquid petrolatum 10%, white petrolatum qs) who suffered from atopic eczema (AE) (n = 7), discoid lupus erythematosus, psoriasis, alopecia areata, etc. With AE no response was seen in 2, was “slightly better” in 4 and “much better” in 1 patient.

These results were the signal for a new development in the treatment of skin diseases with topically applied CS.

Development of Potent Corticosteroids

There have been four main steps in the development of potent CS concerning the modification of the cortisol molecule, which is the physiologically occurring adrenal steroid in humans (fig. 1) [57].

Esterification

Several organic acids, such as propionic or acetic acid, are used to form esters with the hydroxyl groups of cortisol: 17α-and 21-ester (and after hydroxylation in 16α-position, an additional 16α-ester can be formed). A very new trend to potentiate the effectivity of topically applied CS preparations is the formation of diester compounds of corticosteroids.

Dehydrogenation

The introduction of a double bond in position C1–C2 (Δ^1–Δ^2) led to a fivefold increase in the antiphlogistic effect of cortisol, and this modification was the first important progress in the treatment of human diseases with CS. Δ^1–Δ^2-cortisol or prednisolone is a drug which is today one of the best known and most frequently used CS in systemic treatment.

Alcylation

Alkylation – preferentially methylation – at certain positions of the cyclopentanoperhydrophenanthrene ring leads to an additional improvement. Methylation in ring B in 6β-position and in ring D in 16β- and 16α-position initiated a significant increase of the anti-inflammatory effects of prednisolone.

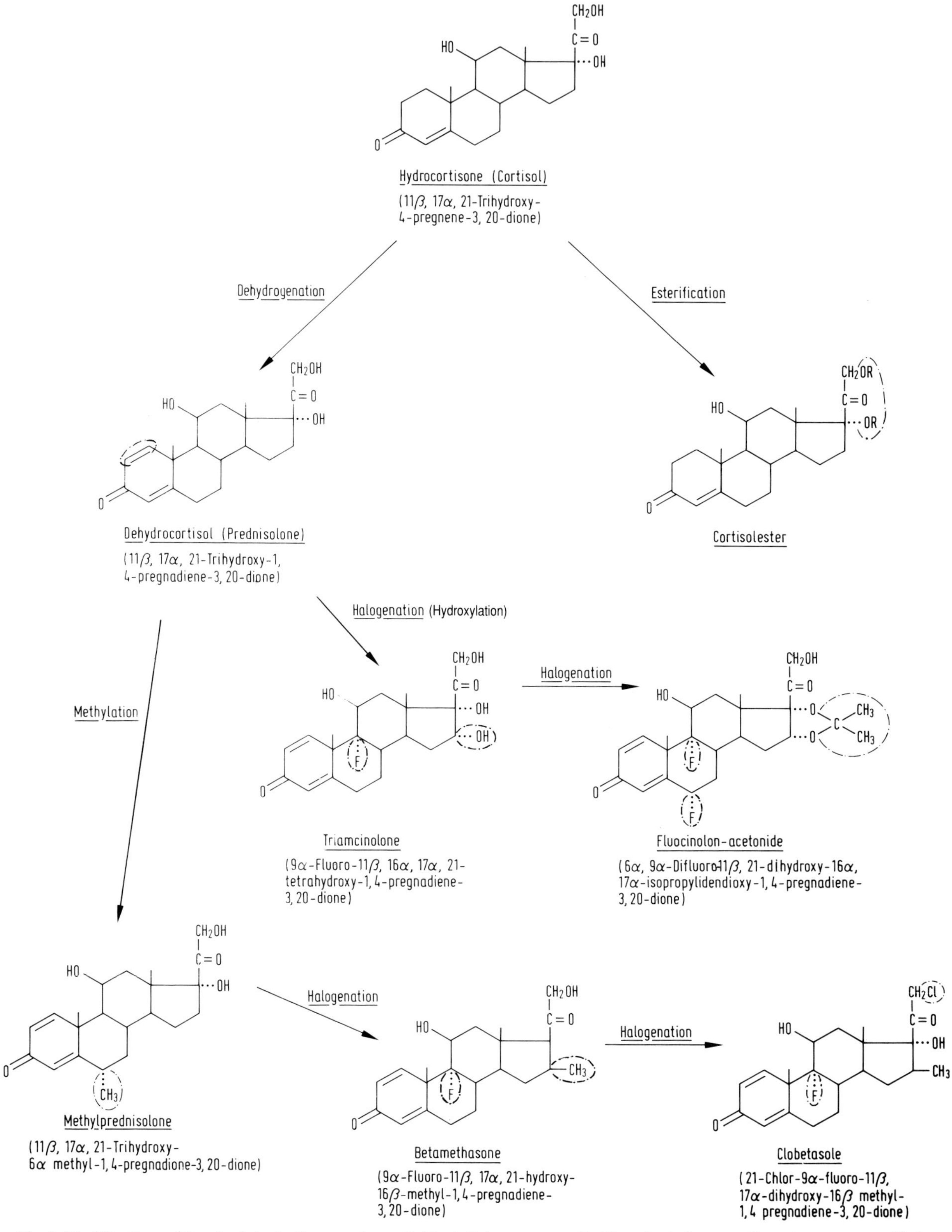

Fig. 1. Modifications of the physiologically occurring antiphlogistic hormone cortisol in order to increase the potency occurred in four main steps:
(1) double blond $\Delta^1 - \Delta^2$; (2) alkylation at steroid ring: 16α-methylation; (3) halogenation: e.g. or 6α For at the side chain C_{21}: Cl and: (4) esterification at the side chain: e.g. 17α-Propionic acid

Halogenation

Substitution with halogens predominantly in ring B increased the efficacy fivefold in comparison with cortisol. The introduction of fluoride (F) in position 6α and/or 9α was very effective. In addition, halogenation and especially the chlorination of the side chains (C_{21}) increased the effect. The combination of these modifications in the cortisol molecule led – especially in topical treatment – to extremely effective preparations, like clobetasol-17-propionate (Dermoxin):

- Double bond: Δ^1–Δ^2
- Alkylation (e.g. methylation): 16α
- Halogenation: 9α-; F; 21-: Cl
- Esterification: 17α-propionic acid

A special development seems to be fluocortinbutylester (6α-fluoro-11β-hydroxy-16α-methyl-3,20-dioxo-1,4-pergnadiene-21-acid-butylester), e.g. Vaspit. This recent introduction represents a new development among CS. In several models it was demonstrated that the preparation has no suppressive effect on the adrenal gland and does not induce undesired local or systemic effects of CS [96]. The C_{21}-butyl-ester is cleaved by esterases which occur ubiquitously in the body, including the epidermis and dermis. Whereas the ester is bound to the cytosolic glucocorticoid receptors and after interaction with DNA induces the various CS effects, the acid of fluocortine is unable to interact with the receptor (see Fig. 2 [96]). From the theoretical point of view fluocortinbutylester seems to be the ideal glucocorticoid preparation, since it should be effective without side effects. However, rigid atrophy models should be used with this drug in order to demonstrate that it has no atrophogenic potential [30].

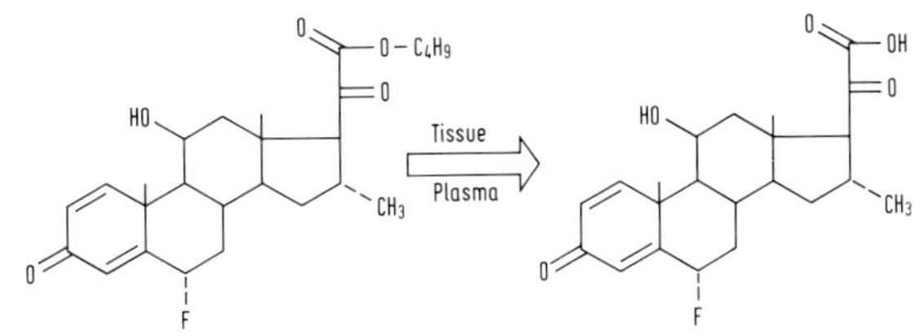

Fig. 2. Attempt to reduce the side effects of corticosteroid therapy. After treatment with fluocortinbutylester, a free acid is formed in the tissue which does not bind to the cytosolic glucocorticoid receptor. Therefore, a reduction of side effects can be expected [96]

Mode of Action of Corticosteroids

According to Cornell and Stoughton [18] (see Fig. 3) we have to differentiate three main effects of glucocorticoids: vasoconstriction, anti-inflammatory effect and anti-proliferative effect.

Vasoconstriction

Constriction of blood vessels leads to blanching of the skin after application of CS ointments. There is a correlation between the intensity of the pharmacodynamic effect of a CS preparation and the blanching of the skin [73, 74, 90]. With the vasoconstriction test it is possible to determine the therapeutic effect of a CS preparation. The vasoconstriction test was first introduced

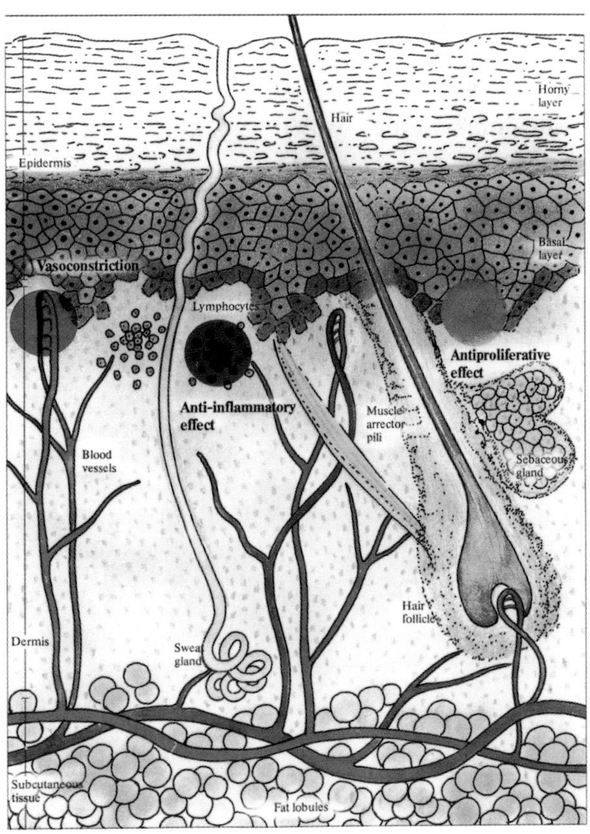

Fig. 3. Mechanism of action of topically applied corticosteroid preparations [18]:
(1) anti-proliferative effect with atrophy of dermis and epidermis after long-term treatment; (2) vasoconstriction as part of the anti-inflammatory effects of the drug, with which it is often clearly correlated; (3) anti-inflammatory effects via direct action on the cells, e.g. on granulocytes and through biochemical effects on membrane-bound phospholipase A2

by McKenzie and Stoughton [60] in dermatology and modified in various ways [57, 74, 90, 97]. Apart from the estimation of CS concentrations in the skin, the blanching or vasoconstriction test is the best method for estimating the potency of a CS preparation. A problem, however, is the reduction and finally the abolishment of the CS effect after long-term application, so-called tachyphylaxis (Fig. 4 [26]). The exact mechanism of CS-induced vasoconstriction is not known. Increased sensitivity against norepinephrine inhibition of histamine-induced vasodilation besides a direct mechanism of CS have been discussed [18].

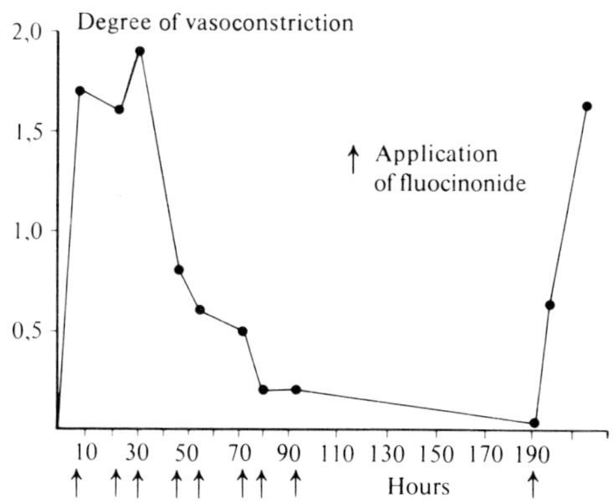

Fig. 4. Tachyphylaxis induced by topically applied fluocinonide (twice daily). Dramatic decrease of efficacy of the corticosteroid preparation measured by blanching test (vasoconstriction) 100 h after the last application [26]

Anti-inflammatory Effects

The molecular basis of the CS actions mainly concerns the inhibition of phospholipase A2, which influences many membrane-mediated reactions in the cell, preferentially those of arachidonic acid metabolism. In addition, various effects on cells such as granulocytes, lymphocytes and mast cells modulate the inflammatory reaction in several ways, leading to an inhibition of inflammation independently of the underlying mechanisms [47].

Anti-proliferative Effects

The inhibition of mitosis in the basal layer and of fibroblasts in the dermis is an obligatory effect of potent CS which is of significance in the treatment of psoriasis whereas in most other CS-treated dermatoses, such as AE, this is an undesired effect. In the past many patients paid for the benefit of long-term CS treatment (of AE) with a pronounced atrophy of the dermis and epidermis and/or striae.

Corticosteroid Preparations

The most frequently used preparations in the USA (see Table 1 [18]) and those used in Europe (see Table 2 [75]) are summarized in this synopsis without any claim of completeness.

Table 1. Potency ranking of some commonly used topical corticosteroids in the USA [18]

	Generic name	Brand name		Concentration (%)
I.	Betamethasone diopropionate	Diprolone[a]	(O)	0.05
II.	Amcinonide	Cyclocort	(O)	0.1
	Betamethasone dipropionate	Diprosone	(O)	0.05
	Desoximetasone	Topicort	(C)	0.25
			(G)	0.05
			(O)	0.25
	Diflorasone diacetate	Florone	(O)	0.05
		Maxiflor	(O)	
	Fluocinonide	Lidex	(C)	0.05
			(G)	0.05
			(O)	0.05
	Halcinonide	Halog	(C)	0.1
III.	Betamethasone dipropionate	Diprosone	(C)	0.05
	Betamethasone valerate	Valisone	(O)	0.1
	Diflorasone diacetate	Florone	(C)	0.05
		Maxiflor	(C)	
	Triamcinolone acetonide	Aristocort	(C)	0.5
IV.	Betamethasone benzoate	Benisone	(O)	0.25
	Desoximetasone	Topicort LP	(C)	0.05
	Fluocinolone acetonide	Synalar	(C)	0.2
		Synalar	(O)	0.25
	Flurandrenolide	Cordran	(O)	0.05
	Hydrocortisone valerate	Westcort	(O)	0.2
	Triamcinolone acetonide	Aristocort	(O)	0.1
		Kenalog	(O)	
V.	Betamethasone benzoate	Benisone	(C)	0.025
	Betamethasone dipropionate	Diprosone	(L)	0.02
	Betamethasone valerate	Valisone	(C)	0.1
			(L)	0.1
	Fluocinolone acetonide	Synalar	(C)	0.25
	Flurandrenolide	Cordran	(C)	0.05
	Hydrocortisone butyrate	Locoid	(C)	0.1
	Hydrocortisone valerate	Westcort	(C)	0.2
	Triamcinolone acetonide	Kenalog	(C)	0.1
			(L)	0.1
VI.	Desonide	Tridesilone	(G)	0.05
	Fluocinolone acetonide	Synalar	(S)	0.01
	Flumethasone pivalate	Lucorten	(C)	0.03
VII.	Topicals with hydrocortisone, flumethasone, prednisolone and methylprednisolone			

O, ointment; C, cream; G, gel; L, lotion; S, solution
Group I is most and VII, least potent (I, II, III = potent steroids; IV, V = mid-strength steroids; VI, VII = mild steroids).
[a] Optimised vehicle

Table 2. Potency ranking of some commonly used topical steroids in Europa [75].

Generic name	Brand name		Concentration (%)
I. Very mild			
Hydrocortisone	Hydrocort dermale	(S)	0.25
	Hydrocort	(S)	0.5
	Ficortril mite	(L/O)	
	Ficortril	(O)	1
	Ficortril spray		
	Hydrocort forte	(S)	2
	Ficortril	(O)	2.5
Hydrocortisone-acetate	Litroderm	(C)	0.2
	Cordes H	(C/O)	1
	Scheroson F	(O)	
Dexamethasone	Sokaral	(L)	0.01
	Dexalocal	(S/C/O)	0.1
II. Mild			
Clobetasone butyrate	Emovate	(C/O)	0.05
Fludroxycortide	Sermaka 1/2	(C/O)	0.025
	Sermaka	(L/C/O)	0.05
Flumetasone pivalate	Locacorten	(L/C/O)	0.02
Flucortinbutylester	Vaspit	(C/L/O)	0.75
Fluocortolone	Syracort	(C/O)	0.2
	Ultralan	(L/C/O)	0.25
Fluocortolone nexanoate			0.25
Fluocortolone pivalate	Ultracur	(C/O)	0.1
+Fluocortolone hexanoate			0.1
Fluprednyliden-acetate	Etacortin	(T/C/O)	0.15
Triamcinolone acetonide	Solodelf	(C)	0.01
III. Medium			
Desonide	Tridesilon	(C/O)	0.05
	Sterax	(C)	0.1
Desoximetasone	Topisolon mite	(C)	0.05
Fludroxycortisol	Sermaka-Folie		$4 \mu g/cm^2$
Fluocinolone acetonide	Jellin gamma s.N.	(C)	0.01
	Jellin	(S/G)	0.025
	Jellin s.N.	(C/O)	
Fluocinonid	Topsymin	(O)	0.01
Fluprednyliden acetate	Decoderm	(O)	0.05
		(L/C)	0.1
Halcinonide	Halcimat	(C)	0.025
Hydrocortisone butyrate	Alfason	(O/C/S)	0.1
Triamcinolone acetonide	Extracort	(C)	0.025
	Volonimat	(C)	
	Delphicort	(C/O)	0.1
	Kortikoid-ratiopharm	(O)	
	Volon A	(C/O)	
IV. Potent			
Betamethasone benzoate	Euvaderm	(C)	0.025
Betamethasone dipropionate	Diprosone	(S/C/O)	0.05
Betamethasone valerate	Betnesol V crinalite	(S)	0.05
	Betnesol V mite	(C/O)	
	Betnesol V	(S/L/C/O)	0.1
	Celestan V	(S/L/C/O)	
Desoximetasone	Topisolon	(L/O)	0.25
Diflorasone diacetate	Florone	(C/O)	0.05
Difluocortolone valerate	Nerisona	(C/O)	0.1
	Temetex	(C/O)	
	Nerisona forte	(O)	0.3
	Temetex forte	(O)	
Fluocinolone acetonide	Jellin ultra	(C)	0.2
Fluocinonide	Topsym	(T/S fettfrei)	0.05
	Topsym F	(O)	
Halcinonide	Halog	(T/O)	0.1
V. Very potent			
Clobetasol propionate	Dermoxinale	(L)	0.05
	Dermoxin	(C/O)	

C, cream; G, gel; L, lotion; O, ointment; P, paste; S, solution

Undesired Effects or Side Effects of Topical CS Treatment (see Table 3)

Short-Term Application

One of the most dangerous effects during treatment with CS – systemic as well as topical – is the increased susceptibility to infections of the skin or internal organs. In AE infections caused by fungi, bacteria or viruses are more often observed than in most other skin diseases or in normal controls. Nearly all these infections can be treated today with corresponding drugs (e.g. fungicidal azoles in tinea, antibiotics in pyoderma or acyclovir in herpes). There is generally no need for antibiotic or antimycotic additives in CS preparations with some exceptions (for details, see below).

Table 3. Some side effects or undesired effets of topically applied corticosteroids (CS)

Epidermal atrophy

Atrophy of the epithelium
Disturbances of pigmentation
Increased light sensitivity

Dermal atrophy

Striae distensae
Purpura and ecchymosis
Pseudo-anetoderma
Cutis linearis punctata colli
Teleangiectasia
Rubeosis faciei
Milia
Fatty tissue atrophy (particularly after intradermal or intralesional application of cristalline CS preparations)
Additional complications of cristalline CS preparations: embolia medicamentosa cutis, embolia arteriae centralis retinae
Disturbed wound healing
Distal phalangeal atrophy

Interactions with skin appendages

Acne ("steroid acne")
Rosacea
Hair loss
Hypertrichosis
Perioral dermatitis (?)

Cutaneous infections

Pyoderma and folliculitis
Tinea (especially *Candida intertrigo*)

Allergic reactions

Allergic contact dermatitis
Photoallergic contact dermatitis

Systemic effects

(Absorption of CS doses greater than the Cushing doses i.e. >7.5 mg prednisolone equivalent per day in adults)

Unknown mechanisms

Granuloma gluteale infantum
Perioral dermatitis
Increased light sensitivity

Long-Term Application

The excellent therapeutic effect of CS in the form of an ointment led to the consequence that CS preparations were without any real competitor and were used in the beginning without criticism for a long time. Subsequently, the undesired effects – most often called side effects – became well-known to the general public, so that today many patients reject topical CS treatment. In table 3 the side effects are summarized. Some rare events, however, have been published recently, such as milia preferentially in the neck and on the supraclavicular region [84], distal phalangeal atrophy [22] and photocontact dermatitis to desoximetasone emollient cream [78].

Most of the side effects are local problems, which include various types of skin damage (epidermis or dermis). In contrast, systemic dysregulation in the form of hypercorticism (Cushing syndrome) or adrenal insufficiency is rarely seen [18, 79]. The penetration of the CS is primarily dependent on the structure of its molecule (see Fig. 1), on the type of vehicle and on the anatomical region treated (see Fig. 5). In addition, interindividual absorption of the same CS preparation in the identical anatomical region can vary by a factor of more than 10 (see Fig. 6) according to Maibach [54].

Apart from the rare findings of clinically clear-cut hypercorticism induced after long-term application of potent topical CS preparations, most frequently under occlusive conditions (R. C. Cornell 1981, cited in [18]), a disturbance of the pituitary adrenal axis is mainly diagnosed by decreased plasma cortisol levels and a cessation of the circadian rhythm of cortisol secretion.

Some 2.25 mg triamcinolone acetonide under occlusive conditions or 0.1% halcinonide cream (15 g over 50% of the skin surface), 0.05% betamethasone dipropionate (90 g weekly over 3 weeks) or 0.05% clobetasol proprionate (25 g weekly) are able to influence the plasma cortisol levels [18]. In contrast, fluocortinbutinylester (Vaspit) applied in amounts comparable to hydrocortisone does not influence adrenal function since the metabolite, the free acid of fluocortin, cannot be bound and is without significant effect on the adrenal gland, the target organs or other cells [96]. In the interpretation of the above-cited findings one should be cautious: a reduction

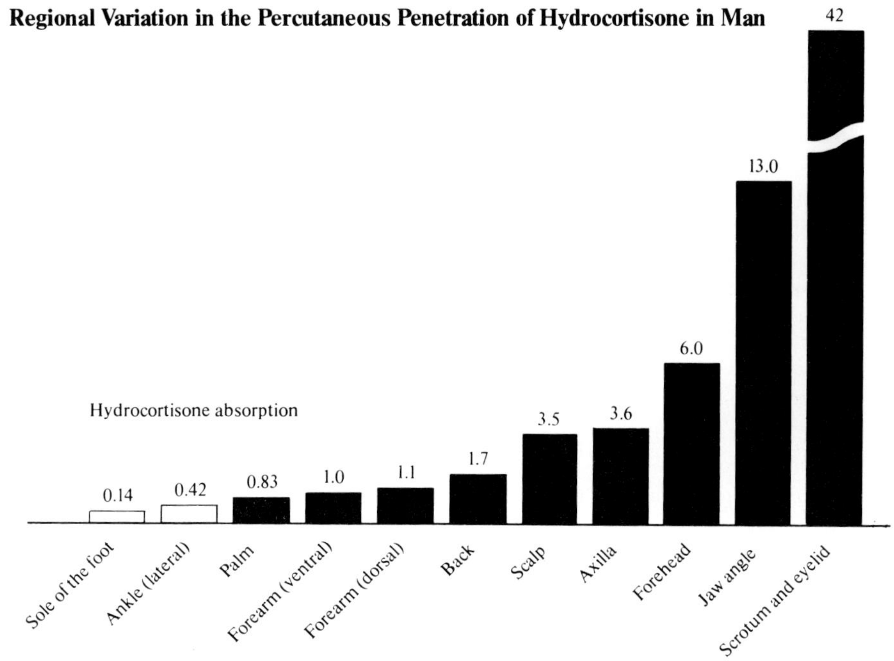

Fig. 5. A small dose of hydrocortisone was applied to each anatomical site and urinary recovery of hydrocortisone and its metabolites quantitated. Data are relative to penetration on the forearm from which approximately 1% of the applied dose is absorbed [55]

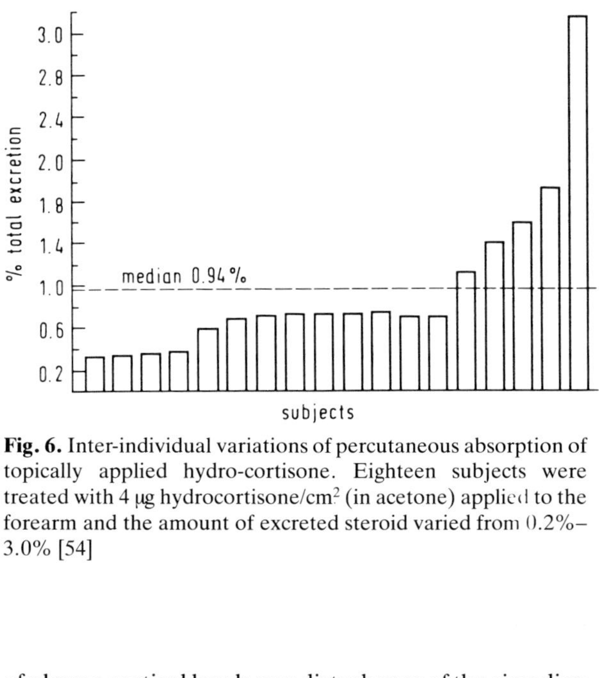

Fig. 6. Inter-individual variations of percutaneous absorption of topically applied hydro-cortisone. Eighteen subjects were treated with 4 μg hydrocortisone/cm^2 (in acetone) applied to the forearm and the amount of excreted steroid varied from 0.2%–3.0% [54]

of plasma cortisol levels or a disturbance of the circadian rhythm does not necessarily mean hypocorticism. Systemic treatment with CS beyond the Cushing level can reduce plasma cortisol levels without any real significance for adrenal function or without a disturbance of the regulation of the pituitary-adrenal axis. Therefore, a small reduction of cortisol plasma level or a shift of the circadian peaks in the blood do not always mean a marked disturbance of adrenal function. In conclusion, it is important to avoid each influence on the adrenal function or its regulation via pituitary hormones by CS treatment. In general, however, especially in adults after CS application (without occlusive conditions) the possibility of inducing such damage is small.

Allergy to Topically Applied Corticosteroids

One problem concerning the application of CS and especially CS-containing ointments has been neglected during the past years (Table 4): allergic reactions, preferentially type IV reactions such as allergic contact dermatitis – against the steroid molecule after application in external preparations. *However,* it is obvious that CS preparations can contain, apart from the steroid molecule, numerous additives, such as antibiotics, antimycotics, stabilizers, antiseptics, antioxidants, emulgators and above all the constituents of the vehicle. Apart from the molecule these constituents can be the cause of an allergic contact dermatitis or rarely a contact urticaria [59, 66, 71].

In addition, the steroid structure cyclopentanoperhydrophenanthrene is obviously a very weak allergen. It is used in rather different modifications of the molecule with numerous indications in medicine: anti-inflammatory glucocorticosteroids (as in AE), androgens, antiandrogens, anabolics, oestrogens, gestagens, cardiaca (digitalis glycosides) or vitamin D. Only exceptionally allergic reactions are described after systemic applica-

Table 4. Allergic reactions caused by topically applied corticosteroids (modified according to [59])

Corticosteroid (CS)	Symptoms	References
Amcinonide	CD	Boujnah-Khoudja et al. (1984) [6] Lozinski and Mitchell (1988) [53] in addition 10 other CS; D3: +)
Betamethasone	CD	Alani and Alani (1972) [2]
Betamethasone-17,21-dipropionate	CD	Reitamo et al. (1986) [71]
Betamethasone-17-valerate	CD	Förström et al. (1982) [28] Reitamo et al. (1986) [71]
Budesonide	CD	Hausen and Kulenkamp (1985) [38]
Clobetasol-17-propionate	CD	Boyle and Peachey (1984) [8] Cox (1988) [21] Dooms-Goossens et al. (1983) [25] Förström et al. (1982) [28] Reitamo et al. (1986) [71] van Ketel and Swain (1981) [86]
	CU	Gottmann-Lückerath (1982) [33]
Clobetasone butyrate	CD	Boyle and Peachey (1984) [8] Dooms-Goossens et al. (1983) [25]
Desonid	CD	Coskey (1978) [19] Sturtz and Rau (1983) [81]
Desoximetasone	CD	Junghans (1985) [42]
Dexamethasone (1980)	CD	van Hecke and Temmermann [85]
Difluocortolone-21-valerate	CD	Junghans (1985) [42] Reitamo et al. (1986) [71]
Fluocinolone-acetonid	CD	Coskey (1978) [19]
Fludroxycortid	CD	Hausen and Kulenkamp (1985) [38]
Fluocortolone	CD	Menne and Andersen (1977) [63]
Fluocortolone caproate	CD	Menne and Andersen (1977) [63]
Fluocortolone monohydrate	CD	Junghans (1985) [42]
Fluocortolone pivalate	CD	Menne and Andersen (1977) [63]
Halcinonide	CD	Coskey (1978) [19] Reitamo et al. (1986) [71]
Hydrocortisone	CD	Alani and Alani (1972) [2] Boyle and Kennedy (1984) [7] Förström et al. (1982) [28]
Hydrocortisone	CD	Reitamo et al. (1986) [71] Sönnichsen (1962) [77] Wilkinson et al. (1967) [93]
	CD + U	O'Garra (1962) [65]
	AR	Mendelson et al. (1974) [62]
Hydrocortisone-17-acetate	CD	Alani and Alani (1972) [2] Burckhardt (1959) [12] Church (1960) [17]
Hydrocortisone-17-butyrate	CD	Brandao and Camarasa (1979) [9] Förström et al. (1982) [28] Reitamo et al. (1986) [71]
Hydrocortisone-17,21-diacetate	CD	Church (1960) [17] Tegner (1976) [83]
Hydrocortisone succinate	CD	Kooij (1959) [45] Coskey and Bryan (1967) [20]
Methylprednisolone	CD	van Hecke and Temmermann (1980) [85] Coskey and Bryan (1967) [20]
	AR	Mendelson et al. (1974) [62]
Methylprednisolone hemisuccinate	AR	Freeman et al. (1981) [29]
Methylprednisolone succinate	AR	Mendelson et al. (1974) [62]
	AR	Rao et al. (1982) [70]
Prednisolone acetate	CD	Gutzwiller (1974) [34]
Prednisone	CD	Gutzwiller (1974) [34]
Tixocortole pivalate	CD	Boujnah-Khoudja et al. (1974) [6] Dooms-Goossens (1988) [23] (12 of 13 patients reacted in addition to other CS-preparations) Dooms-Goossens and Degreef (1989) [24] (19 patients – 16 patients reacted to Tixocortol-pivalate) Hausen and Fousserau (1987) [37]
Triamcinolone	CD	Alani and Alani (1972) [2]
	CD	Coskey (1978) [19]
	CD	Wulf (1967) [94]
Triamcinolone acetonide	CD	Bandmann et al. (1966) [3] Wiegel (1968) [92] Wulf (1967) [94]

AR, anaphylactic reaction; CD, contact dermatitis; CU, contact urticaria; U, urticaria

tions such as progesterone urticaria or drug eruption after digitalis glycosides [5, 98]. Erythema nodosum is sometimes observed after the intake of an oral contraceptive steroid and is perhaps an exception; however, its exact pathogenesis is not clear. Most frequently, allergic reactions to CS are seen after topical CS application. Since the first observations of allergic contact dermatitis after CS therapy by Burckhardt [12], Kooij [45], Church [17], Sönnichsen [77], O'Garra [65] and Bandmann et al. [3], more than 100 patients with such allergic reactions to CS were described [71]. We have summarized the main observations in Table 4 according to Maucher et al. [59]. We assume that allergic contact dermatitis is more frequent than generally expected. It is perhaps true as assumed by Dooms-Goosens [23] for Belgium that allergic skin reactions induced by CS are as frequent as allergic reactions against PABA (*p*-aminobenzoic acid) and its esters. Since CS suppresses allergic contact dermatitis, it is often difficult to interpret correctly the patch test reactions. Overall in relation to the very frequent application of CS-containing preparations, an allergic reaction is still a rare occurrence. This is remarkable since the cortisol molecule has been modified in the past 40 years in such a manner (see Fig. 1) that only the ring structure of the parent substance is identical. In this connection it is important that a new, exclusively topically applied CS; tixocortole pivalate (pregn-4-ene-3,20-dione-21-thiol-11β,17α-dihydroxy-21-pivalate) (Fig. 7) seems to be an exception. Hausen and Foussereau [37] demonstrated that tixocortole pivalate is a potent allergen in guinea pigs. It is interesting that allergic patch test reactions were found in patients who had never been treated with tixocortole pivalate before. Which steroid, which concentration and which vehicle should be used for patch tests with CS preparations is discussed controversially in the literature [23–25, 37, 71]. We now prefer 1% tixocortole pivalate and 1% hydrocortisone-21-acetate in petrolatum in addition to the preparation suspected to be the cause of the contact dermatitis in the patient.

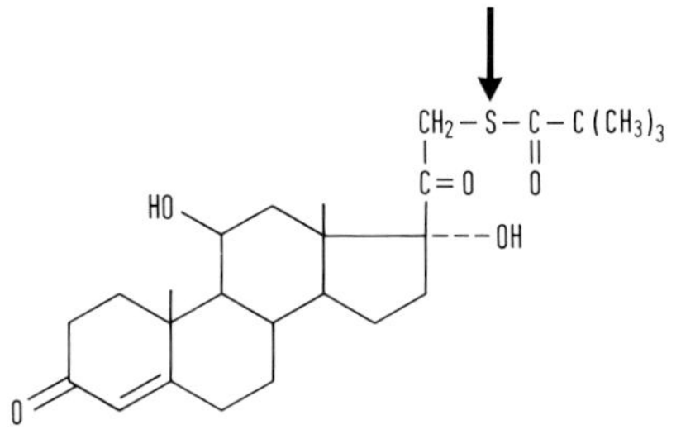

Fig. 7. Structure of tixocortole pivalate (pregn-4-ene-3,20-dione-21-thiol-11β17α-dihydroxy-21-pivalate)

In addition it seems reasonable to perform an usage test with the steroids in the antecubital fossa for several days to evaluate allergic contact dermatitis against these preparations.

Significance of Vehicle for the Effects of Topically Applied Corticosteroid

The affinity between the CS and the vehicle is a determining factor of the efficacy and of the penetration into the skin if the barrier function of the horny layer is intact [50–52, 68, 74]. The higher the degreee of CS saturation in a vehicle, the greater its therapeutic effect. This is correct if the drug is in solution. If the CS, however, is suspended in the base – suspension type of ointment – the maximal effect is independent of the ointment base [40, 67]. This is true in the case of a sufficient CS concentration to guarantee a constant flux and a fast GC liberation without changes of the skin barrier [50, 51, 57, 58, 69].

Malzfeldt et al. [58] could demonstrate that identical concentrations of betamethasone-17-benzoate (5.6 mg

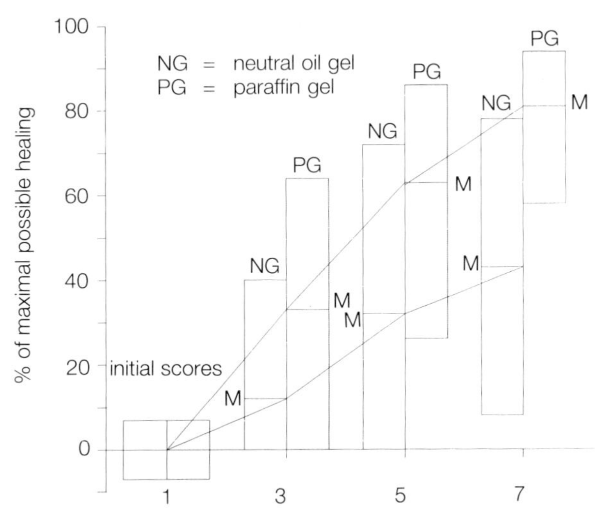

Fig. 8. Comparison of the therapeutic effect of identical concentrations of betamethasone-17-benzoate (5.6 mg/100 g base) in a solution-type ointment (neutral oil, *NG*) or a suspension-type ointment (paraffin, *PG*). Some 31 patients with atopic eczema were treated in a double-blind, bilateral comparative study using a score with 5 clinical symptoms (erythema, scaling, infiltration, lichenification, excoriation) and a 0–3+ scale. They were treated over a period of the least 7 days, and the amelioration was estimated with a healing scale after 3, 5 and 7 days of application. Betamethasone-17-benzoate proved to be more effective in a suspension-type ointment than in a solution-type ointment as evaluated by the development of healing on each body side with time in percentage of maximal possible healing [58]

per 100 g ointment) in a solution-type ointment, e.g. neutral oil gel (neutral oil: 76.5, paraffin: 3.5 and polyethylene glycol 10 000:10.0), was less effective than a suspension-type ointment, e.g. paraffin gel (neutral oil: 9.0, paraffin 81.0 and polyethylene glycol 10 000:10.0), in the treatment of atopic and allergic contact dermatitis. This is in good agreement with findings that CS liberation and skin blanching are more intensive after the application of the same betamethasone-17-benzoate concentration in a suspension-type ointment (paraffin gel) in comparison with a solution-type ointment (neutral oil gel) (Fig. 8) [50–52, 58]. Without exact knowledge of the degree of saturation, solubility and liberation of the CS from the ointment base into the skin, the therapeutic effects of the applied ingredients cannot be predicted. Gibson et al. [31] could not demonstrate significant differences in the blanching activity of clobetasol after a 10-fold dilution. This finding can only be understood by assuming that only a solution-type ointment can be used as vehicle [58]. In addition, the results of Watson and Findlay [89] showing nearly identical liberation of clobetasol from a propylene glycol or a paraffin ointment can be interpreted as that in the concentration used clobetasol must be suspended. In these experiments it was also demonstrated that a very high amount (90%) of the drug was found in the gauze which covered the skin after application of the ointments. Additional constituents such as skin moisturisers [35] and other drugs, e.g. salicylic acid [14], are able to influence the penetration of the CS and thereby the effect of the drug in a barely predictable manner (Fig. 9).

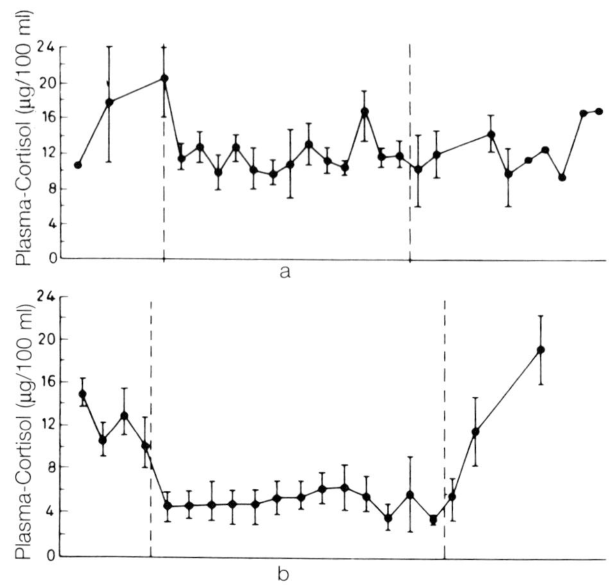

Fig. 9a, b. Influence of salicylic acid on the absorption of corticosteroids (flumethasone pivalate). **a**. Application of 30 g flumethasone pivalate ointment under occlusive dressing; **b.** treatment with flumethasone pivalate in combination with 2% salicylic acid. Topical treatment was performed in the period between the *two dashed lines*. Depression of cortisol plasma level was significatly greater in the flumethasone pivalate-salicylic acid preparation [14]

Therefore, one should be cautious and not use ointments without measuring the liberation and penetration of the CS. It is possible that a dilution of the CS in certain ointment bases does not reduce its potency [31, 58], and as a consequence the preparation may induce unexpected side effects.

Topically Applied Corticosteroids in Atopic Eczema

The first application of local CS was in the treatment of AE [82]. Several international congresses of dermatology (such as London, Munich, Mexico City, Berlin), numerous workshops and nearly uncountable publications have been engaged in this problem. Calnan [13] put forth 25 years after the introduction of this treatment and more than 10 years ago a statement which is still correct:

The value of a drug or of topically applied CS can be measured by three main requisites:

1) Effectiveness (Efficacy)
2) Harmlessness
3) Acceptance

We must state today that there are *no more effective drugs than CS* in the treatment of AE. However, we must be cautious in the estimation of their harmlessness and side effects (undesired effects). We can distinguish the history of topical treatment of AE with CS into three periods:

- First, it was assumed that topical CS therapy would be without side effects
- Second, a period in which side effects or undesired influences of topical steroids on human skin (and/or the organism) became known
- Third, a period of fear in which some physicians and many patients (especially parents of young patients) are against any treatment with topical CS in AE (and/or other skin diseases)

In summary, one has to consider today that any effective preparation may be harmful; moreover, we must expect that it will have specific and/or undesired effects on the skin.

Since the first description in 1952 by Sulzberger and Witten it is correct to state that the acceptance of these preparations has been excellent [82]. In comparison with other preparations used in the treatment of AE such as coal tar, the patient is not troubled by unpleasant smell or coloration of the skin. Although in the past 10 years many new and different preparations have been developed, the statement of Calnan [13] is still valid today.

The main problem today is the fact that we have an effective drug in the form of CS – either topically or systemically applied – which induces, relative to the amount applied per unit time, variably reversible or irreversible damage to the skin or internal organs. The treatment of AE with oral or parenteral CS preparations is further complicated by the fact that very often a reduction of the CS dosage or especially interruption of therapy induces a relapse which is harder to treat and requires often higher and higher doses of CS to ameliorate the dermatitis. (The same phenomenon is well-known in the treatment of psoriasis or other chronic disorders which need high doses of CS to clear up the lesions.) Therefore, oral or parenteral CS administration is only indicated if severe complications are present.

In contrast to the undesired effects after oral or parenteral CS treatment, the topical application of CS is only exceptionally accompanied by systemic damage [18]. Negative consequences of topical CS treatment mainly concern the skin (see Table 3).

Additives in Corticosteroid Preparations for Local Therapy

Many additives such as tar derivatives, salicylic acid, antihistamines (H1-receptor blockers), antiseptics, antibiotics or fungicides have been incorporated into CS preparations for the treatment of skin disorders, especially for the therapy of AE. It can be stated today that the effect of these preparations is mainly or exclusively caused by the efficacy and potency of the CS. Since unpredictable interactions between CS and additives are possible, caution must be exerted, especially when the prescription is composed by the prescribing physician. One problem in AE is the frequency of infectious skin diseases, especially those caused by bacteria. Thus, we have to consider the risks of allergic reactions and the development of resistance against topically applied antibiotics. Neomycine is used as an antibiotic additive, since it is not given systemically. However, an allergy against neomycin can induce allergic cross-reactions against other aminoglycoside antibiotics, such as gentamycin, a very important drug for systemic use. It has been shown [88] that a preparation consisting of gentamycin and betamethasone valerate was more effective than either compound alone. We think, however, that one should be careful with the use of such preparations for the above reasons.

If a severe bacterial infection or superinfection exists, then systemic antibiotic treatment is preferable, either according to the antibiogram or with a broad spectrum antibiotic preparation against those bacteria most often found in infectious skin disorders.

Mupirocin (Eismycin) is a recently developed preparation exclusively for topical use. As far as we know, there is no other drug with a comparable chemical structure in use in human medicine. Therefore, the danger of antibiotic cross-resistance against a potent drug needed to treat systemic infections is unlikely when mupirocin is used. In addition, there is no danger of cross-reactions if an allergic reaction against mupirocin has developed. Combinations of mupirocin and CS for topical use do not exist, and personal prescriptions consisting of a commercial CS preparation and mupirocin could be harmful. Therefore, in AE with pyoderma we apply Eismycin ointment for several hours and thereafter for the rest of the day a CS preparation. In the case of severe pyoderma or especially in systemic infections, we prefer systemic treatment with penicillin derivatives, erythromycin or gyrase inhibitors.

Principles of Treatment with Corticosteroid Preparations

The constituents of the preparations used by us are summarized in Table 5. The principles of the treatment of AE with CS preparations are identical to the principles of local therapy of other skin diseases (10, 11, 13, 15, 16, 36, 43, 46, 49, 61, 76, 87].

The acuity of the dermatitis determines the vehicle of the drug preparation. In the acute phase, a CS preparation in a cream or milk base is used. The CS incorporated should be a potent steroid, such as clobetasol-17-propionate (0.05%). Sometimes we prefer a less potent CS preparation, such as triamcinolone acetonide (0.1%), since the initial treatment may take so long that undesired effects on the skin may appear when such potent steroids as clobetasol-17-propionate are used. Schalla 1985 [75] discussed the possibility of applying initially a weak steroid, such as a hydrocortisone ester, because a disturbance of the barrier function of the epidermis may exist in the acute inflammatory phase of AE. Increased absorption through the skin and increased interaction with the epidermis and dermis could invite side effects with potent steroids at this time. From the findings of Malzfeldt et al. [58], however, it is evident that differences in the barrier function in the acute inflammatory phase of AE do not influence the efficacy

Table 5. Corticosteroid preparations used in treatment of atopic eczema. In our department, there are three CS of various potency

Drug	Manufacturer	Constitutents
I. *High potency*		
Clobetasole-17-propionate		
Dermoxine		
ointment (0.05%)	Glaxo Pharmazeutika GmbH, Bad Oldesloe, FRG	1,2-propylene glycol, sorbitansesquioleate, pretolatium
Dermoxincream (0.05%)		p-chloro-*m*-cresol, glycerol monostearate, cetyl-stearyl-alcohol, polyethylene glycol-glycerol, wax, sodium citrate, citric acid, 1,2-propylene
II. *Triamcinolone acetonide*		
Triamcinolone ointment (0.1%)	von Heyden GmbH, Munich, FRG	Paraffine, polyethylene glycol
Triamcinolone cream (0.1%)		1,2-propylene glycol, sorbitol, petrolatum, emulgator, water
Triamcinolone milk (0.1%)		Lanette, cetiol, water
Triamcinolone lotion (0.1%) aquosa		Lotio alba
III. *Hydrocortisone-21-acetate*		
Hydrocortisone ointment (1.0%)		as triamcinolone ointment
Hydrocortisone cream (1%)		as triamcinolone cream
Hydrocortisone milk (1.0%)		as triamcinolone milk
Hydrocortisone lotion (1.0%)		Lotio alba aquosa

of the CS preparations since the healing potency of a preparation in which the CS is suspended was more pronounced in comparison with the drug in a solution-type preparation (see Fig. 8). In addition, so-called tachyphylaxis must be considered in local CS therapy (see Fig. 4). Tachyphylaxis does mean that a drug, for instance a CS, is less effective after repeated applications [26, 44, 54]. Therefore, it is reasonable to start the therapy with a potent CS preparation to induce an extensive remission.

After 1–4 days' treatment with triamcinolone acetonide (0.1%) cream, remission is usually achieved, and the acute inflammatory signs of the dermatitis disappear. After remission of the acute phase, the skin becomes dry and scaly, and an ointment containing more lipophilic and less hydrophilic constituents must be employed. In this phase the potent steroid can be changed to a less potent one such as hydrocortisone-21-acetate in a corresponding base (see Table 5). In the next 1–4 days the treatment must stabilize the skin, which implies a total treatment with CS-containing preparations of 2–8 days. Thereafter, other principles such as salicylic acid, tannic acid or tar preparations can be used in the external therapy. The purposes of the treatment are to reduce the pathological signs and to provide the patient with skin care which can maintain a "healthy skin" as long as possible. Of course, symptomatic treatment in AE should never consist of the application of topical CS exclusively. In addition H1-receptor blockers or other orally or topically applied anti-pruritic drugs should assist. The problem of systemic treatment with corticosteroids is not included in our discussion. Bathing with various additives should be used in addition to topical treatment.

Development of New Corticosteroid Preparations

Since the introduction of the first preparation (compound F or 17-hydroxycorticosterone-21-acetate) by Sulzberger and Witten in 1952 [82] the periods between the introduction of new preparations became shorter and shorter (the tendency of chemical development is outlined in Fig. 1). The newest trend is the formation of various esters of hydrocortisone such as its diester hydrocortisone-21-acetate-17-propionate (Retef), for which it is assumed that the therapeutic potency is higher than its propensity to induce undesired effects [27]. The reduction of side effects is the main aim of all new developments of CS-containing topical preparations. As pointed out above concerning fluocortinbutylester, one must be cautious in the judgement of these new preparations [96]. Only long-term treatment with them unequivocally show their superiority with respect to undesired side effects.

In the past few years many publications have pointed out that new preparations are better than those used before. Akers [1] has summarised the risk of unoccluded treatment with CS-containing preparations in an overview of 2849 patients in a 14-paired comparison study using seven steroid preparations (betamethasone-benzoate, -dipropionate, -valerate, fluocinolone, halcinonide, hydrocortisone and triamcinolone acetonide) in six different corticosteroid-sensitive skin disorders including AE. In summary, after 5698 treatments 249 adverse reactions were demonstrated corresponding to a frequency of 4.40%: irritation 1.30%, itching 0.95%, burning 0.81%, dryness 0.46%, scaling 0.30% and vesicle-formation 0.16%. In 6.7% the adverse reaction was initiated by the vehicle alone. The benefit: risk ratio from these findings was 28:1 in AE. These values must be taken into account if new preparations are considered.

Some examples show the advantages of the newer preparations: Rosenberg [72] demonstrated that 0.05% fluocinolone cream (6α, 9α-difluoro-11β-21-dihydroxy-16α,17α-isopropyliden-dioxy-1,4-pregnadien-3,20-dione-21-acetate) is more potent than 0.1% betamethasone-21-valerate (9α-fluoro-16β-methyl-11β, 17α-21-trihydroxy-1,4-pregnadiene-3,20-dione-21-valerate). Leibsohn and Bagatell [48] could show that 0.1% halcinonide cream (9α-fluoro-21-chloro-11β-16α,17α-trihydroxy-4-pregnene-3,20-dione-16α,17α-isopropylidene) was more effective in the treatment of AE and other steroid-sensitive skin disorders than 0.1% Valisone cream (betamethasone-17-valerate). On the other hand, Mali [56] pointed out the 0.2% betamethasone dipropionate cream (9α-fluoro-16β-methyl-11β,17α,21-trihydroxy-1,4-pregnadiene-3, 20-dione-21,acetate) was more potent than the dihalogenated 0.02% locacorten pivalate (flumethasone; 6α,9α-difluore-11β, 17α, 21-trihydroxy-16α-methyl-1, 4-pregnadiene,3,20-dione). Jablonska et al. [41] demonstrated, however, that flumethasone is a more potent inducer of skin atrophy in comparison with fluocinolone acetonide (6α-9α-difluoro-11β,17α,21-trihydroxy-16α,17α-isopropylidenedioxy-1,4-pregnadiene-3,20-dione). Betamethasone dipropionate (9α-fluoro-16β-methyl-11β, 17α, 21-trihydroxy-1, 4-pregnadiene-3, 20-dione-17,21-dipropionate) as 0.05% cream was less effective in comparison with 0.25% ointment Desoximetasone (9α-fluoro-11β,21-dihydroxy-16α-methyl-1,4-pregnadiene-3,20-dione; [64]). Yasuda [95] demonstrated in a double-blind study that 0.1% Locoid cream (11β,17α,21-trihydroxy-4-pregnene-3,20-dione-17-butyrate) was more effective than placebo. In addition, 1.0% hydrocortisone-21-acetate was as effective as 0.1% triamcinolone acetonide applied in a hydrophilic plastibase, a base which is also preferred by us. The effect of 0.3% of Nerisona forte ointment (difluocortolone; 6α9α-difluoro-11β, 21-dihydroxy-16α-methyl-1, 4-pregnadiene-3,20-dione-21-valerate) is comparable to that of 0.05% clobetasol-propionate ointment (21-chloro-9α-fluoro-11β, 17α-dihydroxy-16β-methyl-1, 4-pregnadiene-3, 20-dione-propionate) [91]. The latter is thought to be one of the most potent topical steroids. This is in good agreement with the findings of Blum et al. [4]: in a double-blind study, they compared BP 0.05% Dermovate ointment (clobetasol propionate) with 0.05% Diprosone (betamethasone dipropionate) applied as ointment twice daily and demonstrated a better effect of the betamethasone dipropionate ointment if its bioavailability was improved by the addition of propylene glycol.

Table 6. Comparison of trade name corticosteroid formulations with their generic equivalents containing the same corticosteroid in identical concentrations. The trade name formulation most effective in all tests is here set at 100% (according to Stoughton [80])

Corticosteroid	*Trade name*	*Generic name*	*Effect (%)*
Triamcinolone acetonide (0.1% cream)			
	Kenalog		11
		Fougera	100
		Geneva	38
		Goldline	66
		Rugby	57
		URL	68
Triamcinolone acetonide (0.1% ointment)			
	Aristocort A		100
		Goldline	26
		Rugby	47
Betamethasone valerate (0.1% cream)			
	Valisone		100
		Fougera	62
		Geneva	62
		Goldline	65
		Rugby	77
		URL	73
Betamethasone valerate (0.1% ointments)			
	Valisone		100
		Fougera	96
		URL	94
Fluocinolone acetonide (0.025% cream)			
	Synalar		100
		Fougera	94
		Geneva	85
		Goldline	79
		Rugby	50

Conclusions

The main problem in the treatment with CS-containing preparations today is to choose the most effective one and decide how often a well-known preparation should be replaced by a recent development.

First, since an increase of efficacy must always be paid for with an increase of side effects, one should use the most potent CS preparations only exceptionally. Whether the new trends in the development of better preparations will provide new aspects remains to be seen. Skin atrophy and other undesired effects were often seen only after long-term treatment.

Second, numerous factors, such as type of vehicle and additives, influence the effect of the preparation in an unpredictable manner. Therefore, one should change a well-established treatment (see Table 5) only when the superiority of a new preparation is proven. In addition we must consider the phenomenon explored by Stoughton [80] that identical steroids produced by various companies had different therapeutic effects (Tables 6 and 7). Therefore, only after long-term trials which substantiate the improvement brought about by a new preparation, should the switch from well-known preparations be considered.

Table 7. Comparison of the effect of the same corticosteroid preparation (triamcinolone acetonide) in *different* concentrations. Parameter for the determination of the effect was blanching using a vasoconstriction score (according to Stoughton [80])

Trade name	Concentration	Effect (%)
Kenalog	0.025%	100
	0.100%	104
	0.500%	100

References

1. Akers W (1980) Risks of unoccluded topical steroids in clinical trials. Arch Dermatol 116:786–788
2. Alani MD, Alani SD (1972) Allergic contact dermatitis to corticosteroids. Ann Allergy 30:181–185
3. Bandmann HJ, Huber-Riffeser G, Woyton A (1966) Kontaktallergie gegen Triamcinolonacetonid. Hautarzt 17:183–185
4. Blum G, Kröpfli P, Küng D, Suter H (1984) Ergebnisse einer multizentrischen Doppelblindstudie bei Patienten mit resistenter Psoriasis und mit atopischer Dermatitis Diprolon®-Salbe vs. Dermovate®-Salbe. Ther Umsch 41:420–424
5. Bork K (1985) Kutane Arzneimittelnebenwirkungen. Schattauer, Stuttgart
6. Boujnah-Khouadja A, Brändle J, Reuter G, Foussereau J (1984) Allergy to 2 new corticoid molecules. Contact Dermatitis 11:83–87
7. Boyle J, Kennedy CT (1984) Contact urticaria and dermatitis to Alphaderm®. Contact Dermatitis 10:178–190
8. Boyle J, Peachey RDG (1984) Allergic contact dermatitis to Cermovate® and Eumovate®. Contact Dermatitis 11:50–51
9. Brandao FM, Camarasa FM (1979) Contact allergy to hydrocortisone 17-butyrate. Contact Dermatitis 5:354–356
10. Braun-Falco O, Ring J (1984) Zur Therapie des atopischen Ekzems. Hautarzt 35:447–454
11. Braun-Falco O, Plewig G, Wolff HH (1984) Dermatologie und Venerologie, 3rd rev edn. Springer, Berlin Heidelberg New York, p 310
12. Burckhardt W (1959) Kontaktekzem durch Hydrocortison. Hautarzt 10:42–43
13. Calnan CD (1976) Use and abuse of topical steroids. Dermatologica 152 [Suppl 1]:247–251
14. Carruthers JA, August PJ, Stoughton RCS (1975) Observations on the systemic effect of topical clobetasol propionate (Demovate). Br Med J 4:203
15. Champion RH, Parish WE (1979) Atopic dermatitis. In: Rook A, Wilkinson DS, Ebling FJG (eds) Textbooks of dermatology, vol. 1. Blackwell, Oxford, pp 349–361
16. Chapman RS (1979) Treatment of atopic dermatitis. Practitioner 223:713–716
17. Church R (1960) Sensitivity to hydrocortisone acetate ointment. Br J Dermatol 72:341–344
18. Cornell RC, Stoughton RB (1985) Topical corticosteroids: guidelines of therapy. Hoechst (Hoechst medication update)
19. Coskey RJ (1978) Contact dermatitis due to multiple corticosteroid creams. Arch Dermatol 114:115
20. Coskey RJ, Bryan HG (1967) Contact dermatitis due to methylprednisolone. JAMA 199:136
21. Cox NH (1988) Contact allergy to clobetasol propionate. Arch Dermatol 124:911–913
22. Deffer TA, Goette DK (1987) Distal phalangeal atrophy secondary to topical steroid therapy. Arch Dermatol 123:571–572
23. Dooms-Goossens A (1988) Identification of undetected corticosteroid allergy. Contact Dermatitis 18:124–125
24. Dooms-Goossens A, Degreef H, Coopmann S (1989) Corticosteroid contact allergy: a reality. In: Frosch PJ, Dooms-Goossens A, Lachapelle JM, Rycroft RJG, Scheper RJ (eds) Current topics in contact dermatitis. Springer, Berlin Heidelberg New York, pp 233–237
25. Dooms-Goossens A, Vanhee J, Vanderheyden D, Gevers D, Willems L, Degreef H (1983) Allergic contact dermatitis to topical corticosteroides: clobetasol propionate and clobetasol butyrate. Contact Dermatitis 9:470–478
26. Du Vivier A, Stoughton RB (1975) Tachyphylaxistothe action of topically applied corticosteroids. Arch Dermatol 111:581–583
27. Flasch CI, Klaschka F (1986) Therapeutisches Profil des ersten Hydrocortisondiesters in lipophiler Grundlage – Ergebnisse zweier multizentrischer Halbseitenvergleiche. D Dermatol 34:806–828
28. Förström L, Lassus A, Salde L, Niemi KM (1982) Allergic contact eczema from topical corticosteroid. Contact Dermatitis 8:128–133
29. Freeman MD, Schocket AL, Chapel N, Gerber JG (1981) Anaphylaxis after intravenous methylprednisolone administration. JAMA 245:607–608
30. Frosch PJ (1982) Methods for quantifying the cutaneous adverse effects of topical corticosteroids. Safety and efficacy of topical drugs and cosmetics. In: Kligman AM, Leyden JJ (eds) Grune and Stratton, New York, pp 119–134
31. Gibson JR, Darley C, Kirsch J, Saihin EM, Neiiild V (1982) The dilution of proprietary corticosteroid ointments – an attempt to evaluate relative clinical potencues. Br J Dermatol 106:445–448
32. Goldman L, Preston R, Rockwell E (1952) The local effect of 17-hydroxycorticosterone-21-acetate (compound F) on the diagnostic patch test reaction. J Invest Dermatol 18:89–90
33. Gottmann-Lückerath J (1982) Kontakturticaria nach Dermoxin. Derm Beruf Umwelt 30:124
34. Gutzwiller P (1974) Zum Problem der Kortikosteroid-Allergie. Dermatologica 148:253–256
35. Hackemüller D (1988) Einfluß von Feuchthaltemitteln auf Hautmodelle und Wirkstoffpenetration in vivo. Thesis, University Düsseldorf

36. Hanifin JM (1983) Atopic dermatitis. Postgrad Med 74:188–199
37. Hausen BM, Foussereau J (1987) The sensitizing capacity of tixocortol pivalate. Contact Dermatitis 17:63–64
38. Hausen BM, Kulenkamp D (1985) Kontaktallergie auf Fludroxycortid und Cetylalkohol. Dermatosen 33:27–28
39. Hench PS, Kendall EC, Slocumb CH, Polley HF (1949) The effect of a hormone of the adrenal cortex 17-hydroxy-11-dehydrocortocosterone compound E) and of pituitary adrenocorticotreopic hormone on rheumatoid arthritis. Proc Staff Meet Mayo Clin 24:181–197
40. Higuchi T (1960) Physical chemical analysis of percutaneous absorption process from creams and ointments. J Soc Cosmet Chem 11:85–97
41. Jablonska S, Groniowska M, Dabrowski J (1979) Comparative evaluation of skin atrophy in man induced by topical corticoids. Br J Dermatol 100:193–205
42. Junghans C (1985) Allergische Kontaktdermatitis gegen drei verschiedene topische Corticosteroide. Derm Kosmet 26:92–95, 126–129
43. Kaplan RJ, Rosenberg EW (1978) Atopic dermatitis. Postgrad Med 64:52–56
44. Koch E, Hornstein OP (1985) Corticosteroids. In: Hornstein OP, Nürnberber E (eds) Externe Therapie von Hautkrankheiten. Thieme, Stuttgart, pp 103–125
45. Kooij R (1959) Hypersensitivity to hydrocortisone. Br J Dermatol 71:392–394
46. Landes E, Wolf A (1984) Drei-Phasen-Therapie. Z Hautkr 59:157–159
47. Lehmann P, Zheng P, Lavker RM, Kligman AM (1983) Corticosteroid atrophy in human skin. A study by light, scanning and transmission electron microscopy. J Invest Dermatol 81:169–176
48. Leibsohn E, Bagatell FK (1974) Halcinoide in the treatment of corticosteroid responsive dermatoses. Br J Dermatol 90:435–440
49. Leung DYM, Rhodes AR, Geha RS (1987) Atopic dermatitis. In: Fitzpatrick TB, Eisen AZ, Wolff K, Freedberg IM, Austen KF (eds) Dermatology in general medicine 3rd edn. McGraw Hill, New York, pp 1385–1408
50. Lippold BC (1984) Biopharmazie, 2nd edn. Wissenschaftliche Verlagsgesellschaft, Stuttgart
51. Lippold BC (1984) Selection of the vehicle for topical administration of drugs. Pharm Acta Helv 59:166–171
52. Lippold BC, Schneemann H (1984) The influence of vehicles on the local bioavailability of betamethasone-17-benzoate from solution and suspension type ointment. Int J Pharm (Amst) 22:31–43
53. Lozinski AZ, Mitchell JC (1988) Allergic contact dermatitis from multiple topical corticosteroids. Contact Dermatitis 18:244–245
54. Maibach HI (1976) In vivo percutaneous penetration of corticoids in man and unresolved problems in their efficacy. Dermatologica 152 [Suppl 1]:11–25
55. Maibach HI, Stoughton RB (1973) Topical Corticosteroids. Med Clin North Am 57(5):1253–1264
56. Mali JW (1976) An avaluation of betamethasone dipropionate (Diprosone) versus locacorten 0.02% cream. Dermatologica 153:177–178
57. Malzfeldt E (1988) Klinische Wirksamkeit von Betamethason-17-benzoat-Salben in Abhängigkeit von der Wirkstofflöslichkeit in der Salbengrundlage. Thesis, University Düsseldorf
58. Malzfeldt E, Lehmann P, Goerz G, Lippold BC (1989) Drug solubility in vehicle and efficacy of ointments. Arch Dermatol Res 281:193–197
59. Maucher OM, Faber M, Knipper H, Kirchner S, Schöpf E (1987) Kortikoidallergie. Hautarzt 38:577–582
60. McKenzie AW, Stoughton RB (1962) Method for comparing percutaneous absorption of steroids. Arch Dermatol 88:608–611
61. Meigel W (1986) Wie behandle ich Neurodermitis atopica. Treatment of atopic dermatitis. Z Hautkr 61:473–478
62. Mendelson LM, Melzer ED, Hamburger RN (1974) Anaphylaxis-like reactions to corticosteroid therapy. J Allergy Clin Immunol 54:125–131
63. Menne T, Andersen KE (1977) Allergic contact dermatitis from fluocortolone, fluocortolone pivalate and fluocortolone caproate. Contact Dermatitis 3:337–340
64. Nolting S (1985) Behandlung mit Kortikosteroid-Externa bei schweren oder resistenten Dermatosen. Dermatosen 33:140–144
65. O'Garra JA (1962) Anaphylactic reactions to hydrocortisone injections. Br Med J 1:615
66. Oleffe JA, Blondeel A, de Coninck A (1979) Allergy to chlorocresol and propylene glycol in a steroid cream. Contact Dermatitis 5:53–54
67. Ostrenga J, Steinmetz C, Poulsen B (1971) Significance of vehicle composition I: relationship between topicle vehicle composition, skin penetrability, and clinical efficac. J Pharm Sci 60:1175–1179
68. Polano MK, Ponec M (1976) Dependence of corticosteroid penetration on the vehicle. Arch Dermatol 112:675–680
69. Poulsen BJ (1972) Diffusion of drugs from topical vehicles an analysis of vehicle effects. Adv Biol Skin 12:495–509
70. Rao KV, Andersen RC, O'Brien TJ (1982) Successful renal transplantation in a patient with anaphylactic reaction
71. Reitamo S, Lauerma AI, Stubb S, Käyhkö K, Visa K, Förström L (1986) Delayed hypersensitivity to topical corticosteroids. J Am Acad Dermatol 14:582–589
72. Rosenberg EW (1971) Fluocinonide. Arch Dermatol 104: 632–633
73. Schaefer H, Zesch A, Stüttgen G (1982) Skin permeability. Springer, Berlin Heidelberg New York
74. Schaefer H, Zesch A, Schalla W, Stüttgen G (1984) Pharmakokinetik externer Glucocorticoide. Allergologie 3:194–198
75. Schalla W (1985) Lokaltherapie mit Kortikoiden. Z Hautkr 60:609–618
76. Solomon LM (1975) Atopic dermatitis. In: Moschella SL, Pillsbury DM, Hurley HJ (eds) Dermatology, vol 1. Saunders, Philadelphia, pp 258–278
77. Sönnichsen N (1962) Beitrag zur Hypercortison-Überempfindlichkeit. Hautarzt 13:226–227
78. Stierstorfer MB, Baughman RD (1988) Photosensitivity to desoximetasone emollient cream. Arch Dermatol 124:1870–1871
79. Stoppoloni G, Prisco F, Santinelli R, Sicuranza C, Giordano C (1983) Potential hazards of topical steroid therapy. Am J Dis Child 137:1130–1131
80. Stoughton RB (1987) Are generic formulations equivalent to trade name topical glucocorticoids? Arch Dermatol 123:1312–1314
81. Sturtz RP, Rau RC (1983) Contact dermatitis to desonide. Arch Dermatol 119:1023
82. Sulzberger MB, Witten VH (1952) The effect of topically applied compound F in selected dermatoses. J Invest Dermatol 19:101–102
83. Tegner E (1976) Contact dermatitis to corticosteroids. Int J Dermatol 15:250
84. Tsuji T, Kadoya A, Tanaka R, Kono T, Hamada T (1986) Milia induced by corticosteroids. Arch Dermatol 122:139–140

85. Van Hecke E, Temmermann L (1980) Contact allergy to the corticosteroid budesonide. Contact Dermatitis 6:509
86. van Ketel WG, Swain AF (1981) Allergy to clobetasol-17-propionate (Dermovate®). Contact Dermatitis 7:278–279
87. Verbov J (1984) Modern management of atopic eczema. Practitioner 228:1013–1017
88. Wachs GN, Maibach HI (1976) Co-operative double-blind trial of an antibiotic corticoid combination in impetiginized atopic dermatitis. Br J Dermatol 95:323–328
89. Watson WS, Findlay AY (1988) The effect of the vehicle formulation on the stratum corneum penetration characteristics of clobetasol-17-propionate in vivo. Br J Dermatol 118:523–530
90. Wendt H, Frosch PJ (1982) Klinisch-pharmakologische Modelle zur Prüfung von Corticodexterna. Karger, Basel
91. Wendt H, Mugglestone CJ, Wiseman RA (1978) A study of the comparative efficacy of diflucortolone valerate 0.3% ointment and clobetasol propionate 0.05% ointment. Br J Dermatol 99:411–416
92. Wiegel O (1968) Kontaktallergie durch Kortikosteroidhaltige Externa. Med Welt 13:828–829
93. Wilkinson RD, McGarry EM, Solomon S (1967) Allergie contact dermatitis to hydrocortisone. J Invest Dermatol 48:295
94. Wulf K (1967) Beitrag zur Triamcinolon-Kontaktallergie. Z Haut Geschlechtskr 42:765–768
95. Yasuda T (1976) Clinical experiences with hydrocortisone 17-butyrate. Dermatologica 152:221–229
96. Zaumseil RP, Töpert M (1989) Vaspit® – eine risikofreie topische Kortikoidtherapie? In: Macher E, Knop J, Bröcker EB (eds) Jahrbuch der Dermatologie. Biermann, Zülpich, p 197
97. Zaun H, Altmeyer P (1973) Ergebnisse refleksphotometrischer Bestimmungen der Vasoconstriktion nach topischer Steroidapplikation. Arch Dermatol Forsch 247:379–386
98. Zürcher K, Krebs A (1980) Hautnebenwirkungen interner Arzneimittel. Karger, Basel

Antimicrobial Agents in the Treatment of Atopic Eczema

M. V. Dahl

Atopic eczema (AE) is an intensely pruritic, eczematous skin disease. Although the basis for the disorder may be inherited, its appearance and severity are highly dependent upon environmental factors called flare factors [1]. These include irritation, dryness, sweating, tickle and prickle, allergy, anxiety, sudden temperature change, coexistent pruritic skin disease, and scratching. Bacteria on the skin surface may also be a flare factor and elicit or exacerbate dermatitis in at least some atopic individuals at some times.

Role of Staphylococcus aureus

The skin of patients with AE is usually heavily colonized with *Staphylococcus aureus* [2–4]. Leyden et al. [5] obtained aerobic bacterial cultures from the skin of 50 patients with chronic lichenified AE and of 20 patients with exudative AE. *S. aureus* was invariably recovered from the exudative lesions, and the numbers of bacteria in these areas ranges as high as 14×10^6 organisms per cm^2. In nonexudative lesions, *S. aureus* was identified in more than 90% of isolates and in numbers that usually exceeded 1×10^6 bacteria per cm^2. Even on the clinically uninvolved skin of these patients, *S. aureus* was recovered 70% of the time.

Aly et al. [6] confirmed these results in 39 patients with AE. *S. aureus* was recovered from lesions in 93% of patients and constituted 91% of the total aerobic bacterial flora. In uninvolved skin, *S. aureus* was recovered in 76% of patients. Often coagulase-negative staphylococci dominated cultures here, but *S. aureus* still constituted 30% of the total isolated aerobic bacterial population.

What Is Infected Eczema?

A microbiologist would say patients were infected if bacteria had been isolated from the skin surface in high numbers, or if pathogens such as *S. aureus* were found. A diagnostic dermatologist would say infection was present if exudate and crust were present. A therapeutic dermatologist would conclude infection had been present if the dermatitis improved following treatment with systemic antibiotics.

Infection vs Colonization

The crusted lesions of AE resemble impetigo. Following treatment, the crusting slows or stops and the underlying dermatitis improves. This improvement is associated with a decrease in the concentration of *S. aureus* on the skin surface [5]. However, many patients with nonexudative, noncrusted, scaling AE also improve when treated with systemic antimicrobial agents. In other words, it is difficult to know whether AE is infected, and it is even more difficult to discern whether colonization by *S. aureus* is acting as a flare factor.

David and Cambridge [7] followed 190 children with AE prospectively for 2.5 years. They concluded that infection had been present if there was a response to antiinfective treatment. They treated patients with phenoxymethylpenicillin, flucloxacillin, fusidic acid, or erythromycin at a dose of 125 mg q.i.d. if the child was under 10 years of age and 250 mg q.i.d. if the child was over 10 years of age. They also used cefadroxil 250 mg b.i.d. for children under 5 years of age and 500 mg b.i.d. for children over 5 years of age. Some 76 children had among them 164 exacerbations of eczema due to bacterial infection as defined by improvement. In 52 of these children, infection recurred within 3 months. *S. aureus* was recovered from the skin in 97% of the exacerbating episodes, often in combination with β-hemolytic streptococci (recovered in 62%).

Mechanisms of Injury

Colonization with bacteria can act as a flare factor for AE [8]. Elimination or reduction of colonization can improve dermatitis in at least some patients. How do these bacteria aggravate the eruption? I will propose several speculative explanations.

Direct Toxic Injury

S. aureus could directly injure the epidermis by itself or by secreting a toxin. For example, certain strains of *S. aureus* secrete exfoliatin which causes dyshesion between the stratum corneum and the epidermis, while others secrete a toxin which causes toxic shock syndrome. These or other exo-or endotoxins could play a role in exacerbating dermatitis in at least some patients. The typical erythrogenic response of skin affected by these toxins, including staphylococcal scarlatina or even mild local varients of staphylococcal scalded skin syndromes [9], may be masked by severe generalized eczema.

Indirect Injury from Nonspecific Inflammation

S. aureus could indirectly injure the epidermis by provoking inflammation. Intense spongiosis, weeping, and excoriations from scratching leave crusted serum on the skin surface. This offers an ideal culture milieu for *S. aureus* and favors heavy bacterial colonization. In addition, the interaction of staphylococci with serum or plasma generates chemotactic factors such as C5a that foster the migration of neutrophils into the epidermis. Pustules may even form [10]. These neutrophils could possibly damage the epidermis as they pass through it. Alternatively, neutrophils may actively release toxic oxygen intermediates and enzymes into the epidermis in an abortive attempt to destroy those bacteria they cannot engulf. These enzymes and mediators could damage or irritate the epidermis, eliciting eczematous dermatitis.

Indirect Injury from Specific Immune Reactions

At least a small number of patients with AE has high serum levels of IgE antibodies that react with *S. aureus* [11–14]. In these patients and perhaps others, colonization of the skin could induce mast cell degranulation, particularly when *S. aureus* is inoculated into the dermis by scratching. The interaction of *S. aureus* with IgE on the surfaces of mast cells triggers mast cell degranulation and mediator release [15]. Protein A in the staphylococcal cell wall can also degranulate mast cells by its nonspecific interaction with the F_c end of IgE on mast cell surfaces. Histamine and leukotrienes released by mast cells could elicit marked itching and contact urticaria. Scratching could convert this itching, reddened, edematous skin into eczema. Contact urticaria might not be obvious since its erythema might be masked by the erythema of the dermatitis, or mistaken for a dermatographic response to the trauma of scratching. If bacteria colonized fissures in the epidermis, mast cell release would be even more insidious.

Mitchell and Chapman [16] demonstrated a novel mechanism which produces eczema involving the *chronic* interaction of antigen with specific IgE. Eczema could be elicited if an allergen was applied to abraded skin continously for 48 h. Using specific antigen to ragweed, eczematous dermatitis was produced only in patients with immediate urticarial prick test reactions to ragweed. Apparently, the *chronic* interaction of antigens with specific IgE in the skin can evoke eczematous dermatitis, perhaps by eliciting a so-called "late phase reaction". If patients had IgE antibodies to *S. aureus* and if antigens from *S. aureus* diffused through the skin and interacted with these IgE antibodies, AE could be produced or aggravated. Since the barrier might already be disrupted by the eczema, and since most patients rub and scratch, antigens of *S. aureus* could easily find their way to the dermis, mast cells, and specific IgE.

Eosinophils are not usually observed in the inflammatory infiltrate of skin biopsies but are often present in high numbers in the circulating blood of patients with AE. Despite the paucity of eosinophils in the skin, major basic protein (MBP) is plentiful [17]. Seemingly, eosinophils readily discharge their contents into the skin. Since MBP is a major toxin of eosinophils and can kill helminths, it could possibly also damage skin or induce mediators which lead to eczema. There is little experimental evidence to support this concept at this time.

Cell-mediated immune reactions to staphylococci can also occur. Although delayed hypersensitivity reactions to injected antigen are blunted, in vitro the immune responses to antigens of *S. aureus* are increased [18]. Allergic contact dermatitis is a prototype for an eczematous dermatitis elicited by cell-mediated immunity. The histology of allergic contact dermatitis mimics that of AE. An immunological reaction of *S. aureus* or its products with specifically sensitized lymphocytes could conceivably produce an atopic-like dermatitis [19].

Treatment

Regardless of the mechanism, bacteria *aggravate* AE [1]. At present it seems prudent to regard the colonization by *S. aureus* as a flare factor rather than a cause. Antimicrobial agents do not eliminate dermatitis; they only improve it.

Systemic Antibiotics

Administration of systemic antibiotics is indicated in many patients with AE, particularly when the dermatitis is exudative, extensive, or exacerbating.

Erythromycin. Probably the most common antibacterial agent used to treat patients with AE is erythromycin. It is frequently effective and has a lower incidence of allergy than penicillin, particularly in atopic patients. Up to 30% of isolates of *S. aureus* for atopic patients show resistance to erythromycin [2, 7, 8] so one might predict that erythromycin will be of no benefit in at least a third of patients in whom infection is acting as a flare factor. There are no controlled studies addressing this point. Curiously, in my experience, erythromycin seems to help at least some groups of patients with AE even when the bacteria on the skin show relative resistance to the agent.

Many patients with AE have coexisting asthma and are taking theophylline or aminophylline. Erythromycin raises the blood level of theophylline and can lead to theophylline toxicity. In some patients, erythromycin may therefore be contraindicated or may require an adjustment of the dose of theophyline.

Penicillin and Its Derivatives. Remission is also frequently induced by penicillin or its derivatives. Like erythromycin, they have antistreptococcal activity as well as antistaphylococcal activity. Since many isolates of *S. aureus* from atopic patients show resistance to penicillin [2], a semisynthetic penicillin may be the treatment of choice. David and Cambridge [5] used flucloxacillin but indicated that it often has poor coverage for streptococci and recommended that it be used in conjunction with phenoxymethylpenicillin. I have used dicloxacillin extensively in patients with AE and believe it is the treatment of choice for those with severe infections or in whom erythromycin is contraindicated for other reasons such as asthma. I often employ it for patients with extensive and exudative AE who have not responded to erythromycin. I have also used it to treat patients with the hyperimmunoglobulinemia E-staphylococcal abscess syndrome over long periods of time without notable untoward effects. I have not attempted to treat for prolonged periods patients with ordinary, uncomplicated AE, preferring instead to treat intermittently during exacerbations.

Cephalosporine. My experience with cephalosporins in treating patients with AE is limited, but the drugs of this class do seem quite effective in adults. I have preferred either cephalothin 250 mg q.i.d. or cephadroxil 500 mg twice daily. I have not used these drugs for prolonged periods in patients with AE as maintenance therapy.

Topical Antibiotics

Because the skin of patients with AE is often heavily fissured, because many patients are children who absorb topical medications quite readily, and because extensive areas may need to be treated, I have not routinely used topical antibiotics to treat widespread AE. I worry about expense, absorption, or development of an allergy.

Chlorhexadine. Bacteria do not easily develop resistance to this agent. To be effective though, the drug must be applied to the skin in a fairly concentrated state. Mixing several ounces of chlorhexadine with the usual amount of water in a bath dilutes the agent below bacteriocidal concentrations. I recommend that the commercial product be applied to the affected areas of skin and washed off thoroughly with water after 1 min, usually in a shower or bath. The response of the dermatitis to such treatment is usually not as dramatic as the treatment with systemic antimicrobial agents, in my experience. On the other hand, the material seems to be well tolerated when used in this way and does not seem to irritate.

Mupirocin. This drug is available as an ointment. It has great activity against *S. aureus*. Numerous studies have demonstrated its efficacy in improving the eczema of patients with AE and also with other eczematous dermatitides [9, 20]. If absorbed, it is rapidly inactivated. It should be safe to apply the drug to large areas of skin. Unfortunately mupirocin ointment is relatively expensive.

Gentamycin. Wachs and Maibach et al. [219] evaluated the response of AE in a three quadrant experiment using a combination cream containing gentamycin/betamethasone, gentamycin alone, or betamethasone alone. The steroid and steroid/antibiotic combination were most effective and caused the dermatitis to resolve. Gentamycin cream alone improved but did not eliminate the dermatitis.

Neomycin. Polano and DeVries [22] found that the combination of neomycin and prednisolone in petrolatum was superior to either constituent alone for treating AE. Neomycin has a tendency to induce allergic contact dermatitis, especially in eczematous skin. I personally have used topical neomycin only on very rare occasions for the treatment of patients with localized atopic hand dermatitis.

Erythromycin. Unfortunately, a cosmetically elegant preparation of erythromycin in an ointment base is not available in the USA. When such a preparation was available, a combination of this with a topical steroid was often more effective than steroid alone in improving dermatitis, especially atopic hand dermatitis, in my experience. Erythromycin has a high safety profile if absorbed. Topical applications could induce the resistance of bacteria. Then systemic erythromycin might be less effective.

Conclusions

AE is a common eczematous skin disease. Patients are often colonized with *S. aureus*. In at least a subset of patients, extensive or heavy colonization can act as a flare factor for AE. For this reason and because the role of *S. aureus* as a flare factor cannot always be judged from the clinical appearance of the skin, a trial of systemic antistaphylococcal antibiotics is often indicated in patients with widespread AE who do not improve promptly with the usual treatment or who experience a sudden flare-up while using appropriate topical treatments.

Some patients repeatedly respond to systemic antibiotics and flare-up when they are discontinued. A subgroup of them may be candidates for long-term treatment. In such cases appropriate cultures and antibiograms may occasionally need to be carried out, particularly if the dermatitis is poorly controlled. The search for a safe, inexpensive, nonsensitizing, nonirritating, effective, topical antibiotic continues.

References

1. Dahl MV (1977) Atopic dermatitis: the concept of flare factors. South Med J 70:453–455
2. White MI, Nobel WC (1986) Consequences of colonization and infection by *Staphylococcus aureus* in atopic dermatitis. Clin Exp Dermatol 11:34–40
3. Hauser C, Saurat JH (1985) Die Bedeutung der Hautbesiedelung durch Staphylococcus aureus bei der atopischen Dermatitis. Hautarzt 36:605–607
4. Hay RJ (1985) The role of bacteria in eczema. In: Dobson RL, Leyden JJ, Noble WC et al. (eds) Bactroban (mupirocin). Excerpta Medica, Amsterdam pp 166–169
5. Leyden JJ, Marples RR, Kligman AM (1974) *Staphylococcus aureus* in the lesins of atopic dermatitis. Br J Dermatol 90:525–530
6. Aly R, Maibach HI, Shinefield HR (1977) Microbial flora of atopic dermatitis. Arch Dermatol 113:780–782
7. David TJ, Cambridge GC (1986) Bacterial infection and atopic eczema. Arch Dis Child 61:20–3
8. Dahl MV (1983) *Staphylococcus aureus* and atopic dermatitis. Arch Dermatol 119:840–846
9. Lever R, Hadley K, Downey D et al. (1988) Staphylococcal colonization in atopic dermatitis and the effect of topical mupirocin therapy. Br J Dermatol 119:189–198
10. Hanifin JM, Rogge JL (1977) The character of staphylococcal infections in patients with atopic dermatitis. Arch Dermatol 113:1383–1386
11. Abrahamson JS, Dahl MV, Walsh G et al. (1982) Anti-staphylococcal IgE in patients with atopic dermatitis. J Am Acad Dermatol 7:105–110
12. Motala C, Potter PC, Weinberg FCP et al. (1986) Anti-staphylococcus aureus – specific IgE in atopic dermatitis. J Allergy Clin Immunol 78:583–389
13. Friedman SJ, Schroeter AL, Hamburger HA (1985) IgE antibodies to *Staphylococcus aureus*: prevalence in patients with atopic dermatitis. Arch Dermatol 121:869–872
14. Henocq E, Hewitt B, Guerin B (1982) Staphylococcal and human dander IgE antibodies in superinfected atopic dermatitis. Clin Allergy 12:113–120
15. Jorgensen J, Bach-Mortensen N, Koch C et al. (1987) Bacteria and endotoxin release of basophil histamine in

patients with atopic dermatitis: in vitro experiments with *S. aureus*, techoic acid, *E. coli*: and *E. coli* LPS. Allergy 42: 395–397
16. Mitchell EB, Crow J, Chapman MD et al. (1982) Basophils in allergen-induced patch test sites in atopic dermatitis. Lancet i:127–128
17. Lieferman KM, Ackerman SJ, Sampson HA et al. (1985) Dermal deposition of eosinophil granule major basic protein in atopic dermatitis: comparison with onchocerciasis. N Engl J Med 313:282–285
18. Higaki Y, Hauser C, Rilliet A (1986) Increased in vitro cell-mediated immune response to staphylococcal antigens in atopic dermatitis. J Am Acad Dermatol 15:1204–1209
19. Uehara M, Ofuji S (1980) Atopic dermatitis: a discussion of theories concerning its pathogenesis. J Dermatol 7:231–328
20. Dobson DL, Leyden JJ, Noble WC, Price JD (1985) In: Dobson RL, Leyden JJ, Noble WC et al. (eds) Bactroban E (mupirocin). Excerpta Medica Elsevier, Amsterdam, pp 183–189
21. Wachs GN, Maibach HI (1976) Cooperative double-blind trail on an antibiotic/corticoid combination in impetiginized atopic dermatitis. Br J Dermatol 95:323–328
22. Polano MK, DeVries HR (1960) Analysis of results obtained in the treatment of atopic dermatitis with corticosteroid and neomycin containing ointments. Dermatologica 120:191–199

Antihistamines

W. Schmutzler

Histamine is generated by decarboxylation of the amino acid L-(+)-histidine in mast cells and basophil granulocytes which store it in their granules as a complex with protein and heparin. Synthesis of histamine outside those cells has been postulated but never proved. Histamine was first discovered in animal tissues in 1911 [8]. The tissues content depends on the number, subtypes, and maturity of the tissue mast cells and varies considerably in different organs, even in the same species [12, 70, 118].

Histamine exists in two tautomeric forms, the 4-or 5 (2-aminoethyl)imidazole. In the human organism, histamine is inactivated mainly (40%–50%) by methylation of a ring nitrogen and to a lesser degree by oxidative deamination of the side chain nitrogen. This relationship is reversed during pregnancy as a consequence of the high diamine oxidase content of the placenta. Heparin releases substantial quantities of diamine oxidase from the liver or intestinal mucosa into the blood. This effect of heparin is, however, not efficient enough to be used therapeutically [59, 138].

The mediator function of histamine in allergic reactions was demonstrated first in 1932 [10, 40] and – for the model of guinea pig anaphylaxis – finally established in 1963 [137]. In 1937, Staub and Bovet [151] reported the synthesis of the first competitive histamine antagonist and 10 years later antergan was introduced into therapy [20, 45]. It soon became evident that these anthistamines could not inhibit all allergic reactions and not even all histamine effects. This disappointment led to the discovery of a whole range of different mediators of allergy and inflammation and to the claim for several distinct histamine receptors on the one hand and to the development of most modern drugs used in the treatment of psychiatric disorders, on the other hand [94]. Some of the latest antihistamines have been recently redeveloped from the latter group, e.g., terfenadine (from haloperidol) and cetirizine (from hydroxyzine).

The Histamine Receptors

The effects of histamine are mediated by different receptors, which are presently classified as H_1, H_2 or H_3 receptors (Table 1). In allergy and inflammation, particularly atopy, mainly H_1 receptors are involved, although under certain circumstances H_2 or even H_3 receptors might contribute to the syndrome. Other reactions which present typical features of allergy, although specific immunological mechanisms are not involved, are termed pseudoallergic or anaphylactoid.

As far as those reactions can be inhibited by H_1 blockers (under certain circumstances combined with H_2 blockers), the conclusion is justified that histamine is the main mediator involved [32, 33]. In other reactions such as endotoxin shock, burns, and traumatic shock, only during the initial phase can an effect of H-blockers be expected.

Table 1. Effects of histamine classified according to the receptors mediating them.

Receptor		
H_1	H_2	H_3
Bronchoconstriction	Bronchodilation (sheep)	Inhibition of histamine and 5-hydroxytryptamine release via autoreceptors (CNS) and heteroreceptors (periphery)
Endothelial contraction (increase in capillary permeability)	Tachycardia	
Pulmonary artery contraction	Pulmonary artery relaxation (guinea pig)	
Uterus contraction (guinea pig)	Uterus relaxation (rat)	
Epinephrine release	Gastric acid secretion	
Intestinal spasm		
Arteriolar constriction		

Pharmacology of Antihistamines

H_1 Blockers

Many basic compounds that – at concentrations of $<10^{-4}$ M – antagonize histamine at the H_1 receptor have the β-aminoethyl side chain in common with histamine, although there are also antihistamines with different structures [54]. H_1 blockers act as competitive inhibitors of histamine as can be demonstrated clearly in smooth muscles and in the capillary permeability. The effects of histamine on the circulation are entirely (heart) or partially (blood vessels in striated muscles) transmitted via H_2 receptors and can be suppressed only partially or not at all by H_1 blockers.

Most H_1 blockers *inhibit* the histamine release from peritoneal rat mast cells in small concentrations but *cause* a release of histamine at high concentrations. Typical examples are ketotifen and oxatomide. In human mast cells, this effect could only be detected for azelastine and astemizole and has presumably to do rather with calmodulin antagonism than with the H_1 receptor blocking properties of these drugs [139].

In addition, at higher concentrations most H_1 blockers inhibit the histamine *N*-methyltransferase and, therefore, the metabolism of histamine.

The older H_1 blockers exert distinct CNS effects, ranging from sedation to sleep induction in man and laboratory animals [88, 141, 142]. These effects were taken as undesirable for a long time, e.g., in the therapy of hay fever or asthma, but recently the hypnotic effects have been used therapeutically since,in contrast to the usual hypnotics, they cause either none or a different type of drug dependence. This has increased the frequency of antihistamine intoxication, which is particularly hazardous in children (central stimulation with convulsions).

Some of the recent H_1 blockers such as terfenadine, cetirizine, loratadine, azelastine, and astemizole exert either no or only rather weak sedating effects because they themselves or their active metabolites do not pass the blood-brain barrier [109, 167]. Almost all H_1 blockers possess local anesthestic properties which seem to contribute to the therapeutic effects of antihistamines in sunburns or insect stings. The specificity of H_1 blockers varies. Some, particularly the phenothiazines, also possess antiadrenergic, anticholinergic, and anti-tryptaminergic effects.

Generally, H_1 blockers are readily absorbed from the intestine and distributed rapidly within the body. It is doubtful whether they can be absorbed through the intact skin [58, 105, 133, 157, 171]. Table 2 presents the elimination halftimes. Some H_1 blockers, e.g., terfenadine, loratadine, astemizole, undergo a definite first-pass effect leading to metabolites which have a much slower half-time than their parent compound. In addition, some of the recent H_1 blockers stick very fast, some even irreversibly, to the receptor (e.g., azelastine, astemizole). Their effects last, therefore, much longer than one would expect from their elimination half-time.

H_2 Blockers

The first H_2 blockers possessing satisfactory activity still exhibited the hydrophile imidazole ring of histamine and a side chain in which the amino group was replaced by thiourea (burimamide), guanidine (metiamide), or cyoguanidine (cimetidine) [16]. Further variations led to the development of ranitidine, roxatidine, famotidine and nizatidine. These very recently developed variations

Table 2. Elimination half times of H_1 and H_2 blockers including their respective active metabolites

Generic Name	Registered Trade Name	Recommended Daily Dose for Adults (mg)		Elimination Half Time (hrs)
H_1-Blockers (sedative)				
Azatadine	Optimine	2x	1	9
Chlor-pheniramine	Chlor-Trimeton	2x	4–8	20
Clemastine	Tavegil	2x	2	8
Dimetindene	Fenistil	3x	1–2	6
Diphen-hydramine	Benadryl	2x	25–50	8,5
Hydroxyzine	Atarax		25–75	14
Ketotifen	Zaditen	2x	1	20
Meclozine	Postafen	1–2x	25	2 – 3
Oxatomide	Tinset	2x	30	18
H_1-Blockers (non-sedative)				
Acrivastine	–	3x	8	4
Astemizole	Hismanal	1x	10	450
Azelastine	Azeptin	2x	1–2	25 – 35
Cetirizine	Zyrtec	1–2x	10	7 – 10 (–21)
Loratidine	Lisino	1x	10	19
Terfena-dine	Seldane, Teldane	2x	60	17
H_2-Blockers				
Cimetidine	Tagamet		800	1,5 – 2
Famotidine	Pepdul		40	2,5 – 4
Nizatidine	Gastrax, Nizax		300	1 – 1,5
Ranitidine	Sostril, Zantic		300	2 – 3
Roxatidine	Roxit		150	4 – 6

differ from cimetidine in their increased efficacy and/or fewer side effects.

H_2 blockers inhibit effects of histamine on gastric acid secretion, which might be increased in systemic mastocytosis, and also the H_2 effects in the heart and blood vessels. Adverse reactions are infrequent (up to 1%) and include, for example, leukopenia, thrombopenia, cholestasis, fever, interstitial nephritis, diarrhoea, dizziness (particularly in the elderly) gynecomastia, and loss of libido and fertility. Cimetidine, but not ranitidine or famotidine, blocks the P_{450} in the liver. This might cause a diminished metabolism of drugs such as lidocain, phenytoin, or theophylline.

The oral absorption rate is 40%–45% for famotidine and 50%–60% for ranitidine 78%–93% for roxatidine, 98% for nizatidine. Roxatidine is also available as a substained release formulation. If the combined administration of an H_1 and an H_2 blocker is to be considered, care should be taken to choose an H_1 blocker with a comparable elimination half-time to the H_2-blocker used.

H_3 Receptors Active Substances

The class of H_3 receptors was discovered first in histaminergic presynaptic nerve endings in the rat brain, and later in the human brain [3, 5]. They mediate as auto- or heteroreceptors the inhibition of histamine or 5-hydroxytryptamine release at rather low agonist concentrations ($\approx 10^{-8}\,M$).

In the meantime, a specific agonist, *R*-(α)-methylhistamine, and a specific antagonist, thioperamide, have been developed [4]. With their help, H_3 receptors were also discovered in postganglionic cholinergic nerves in the airways [76], in the gastrointestinal tract [154], in perivascular nerve endings of the mesenteric artery [77], and on the muscle cells themselves [42]. Their existence means that at low concentrations histamine via H_3 receptors elicits the opposite effects of those seen at higher concentrations via H_1 or H_2 receptors. In human adenoidal mast cells *R*-(α)-methylhistamine was found to be devoid of any effect. Thioperamide, however, caused a dose-dependent histamine release in concentrations of $10^{-4}\,M$ and above [13, 44]. There is no information yet about the existence of H_3 receptors in the mast cells or blood vessels of the skin.

Therapeutic Use of H_1 Blockers

General Aspects

High expectations were projected when the first H_1 blockers became available for therapeutic purposes, but were then diasppointed when most allergic reactions in which the main mediator function of histamine was suspected did not respond satisfactorily or over a longer period of time to such treatment [63, 109]. Nevertheless, the H_1 blockers are used for the palliative treatment of allergic reactions, particularly type I reactions (Table 3). H_1 blockers are effective in relieving the symptoms of seasonal or perennial allergic rhinitis. They relieve sneezing, rhinorrhea, nasal itching, and conjunctivitis, but have no effect on nasal congestion [136]. For the optimally effective treatment of hay fever, it is necessary to start treatment before the start of the pollen season [155].

Antihistamines have been regarded as of little value in bronchial asthma due to the involvement of mediators other than histamine [56, 64, 69, 86]. Recent studies with new H_1 blockers indicate, however, that this question might depend rather on pharmacokinetic parameters and on appropriate dosage [71, 72]. The modern H_1 blockers themselves (e.g., cetirizine) or their active metabolites (e.g., terfenadine) do not pass the blood-brain barrier and are, therefore, almost entirely free of sedative side effects. They can be administered at higher doses than the old, sedative substances. In addi-

Table 3. Therapeutic use of H_1-antihistamines

Treatment of	Comments
Allergic reactions	Histamine antagonism and other actions
Urticaria	Pruritus > edema > number of lesions
Hay fever	Especially milder states, sedative side effects might be beneficial at night
Asthma	Milder states, long-acting antihistamines
Angioneurotic edema	
Serum sickness	Especially concomitant urticaria and skin irritations
Other hypersensitivity reactions	
Vasomotor rhinitis	Nasal irritation and watery discharge; little effect on nasal obstruction
Emesis	Some antihistamines
irradiation sickness	
postoperative vomiting	
nausea and vomiting in pregnancy	
Local anesthesia	Topical application
Common cold	No effect
Mastocytosis	Combination of H_1 and H_2 antihistamines
Anaphylactoid reactions caused by plasma substitutes	

tion, the new H_1 blockers stick much faster to the H_1 receptors and exert a prolonged action [28]. Other pharmacological properties, e.g., anti-inflammatory or anticholinergic effects, might add to the antiasthmatic action [9, 21, 25, 26, 27, 34, 43, 48, 106].

These aspects might turn out to be relevant also for other types of allergies, although H_1 antihistamines may be used in the treatment of systemic allergic reactions only as adjuncts. H_1 blockers are effective in treating allergic skin diseases including urticaria, pruritus, insect bites, dermographism, and some drug allergies and contact allergies to plants. In serum sickness, H_1 blockers effectively alleviate urticaria and skin irritations, although fever and joint symptoms are little affected.

Therapeutic Effects in Atopic Eczema

The pathogenesis of atopic eczema is still obscure ([158, 173, 174]; see chapter Ring et al., pp. 330-335). Experimental and clinical evidence point to the involvement of activated complement and histamine, although definite proof for a mediator function of histamine is lacking.

In view of their therapeutic efficacy in various forms of urticaria, H_1 blockers have been used for a long time to combat the most tormenting symptom, namely, the itching [23, 41, 47, 49, 79–81, 101, 105, 110, 115, 130, 143, 168, 169]. It was soon realized that the antipruriginous effect of the antihistamines obviously had little to do with the H_1 blocking properties, but rather with their sedative or other centrally acting side effects [1, 18]. Consequently, in addition to the antihistamines, a number of tranquilizers, antidepressants, and neuroleptic drugs have also been used, though with limited success [38, 93]. A number of reports stress the antipruriginous efficacy of hydroxyzine, which exerts strong sedative and relatively weak H_1 blocking effects [165]. A discussion about the existence of H_2-receptors led to the combined administration of an H_1 and an H_2 blocker, e.g., chlorpheniramine and cimetidine [35, 50, 53, 113, 146] in atopic eczema. These attempts failed to show any therapeutic effects and cast doubts on the overall usefulness of H_2 blockers (Table 3).

Very little is yet known about the efficacy of the modern, non sedating H_1 blockers in atopic eczema. They are discussed below in more detail, along with two sedating H_1-blockers, dimetindene and Ketotifen. Their efficacy might be particularly interesting because CNS effects should contribute very little to a possible therapeutic effect [57, 131].

Table 4. Adverse reactions to H_1 antihistamines

Reaction	*Type*	*Drug(s)*
Sedation (may diminish after a few days)	Including loss of concentration, lassitude, dizziness, hypotension, muscular weakness, incoordination	Diphenhydramine Oxatomide
Affection of Mental state –Abuse –Addiction		Brompheniramine Oxatomide Tripelenamine Cyclizine Diphenhydramine
Extrapyramidal symptoms	Neuroleptic type, usually benign	Brompheniramine Chlorpheniramine Cinnarizine Flunarizine Diphenhydramine Oxatomide (in adults phenindamine)
Cerebral stimulation	Overdosage, especially in children: convulsions, hyperpyrexia, insomnia, nervousness, tachycardia, tremor, muscle twitching	
Epileptic seizures	Large doses	
Other effects in the central or peripheral nervous system	Sense of smell and taste affected, headache, anorexia, tinnitus, irritability, nightmares, difficulty in micturition, dryness of the mouth, tightness of the chest and tingling, heaviness, weakness of hands, blurred color vision	
Gastrointestinal disturbances	Nausea, vomiting, diarrhoea or constipation, epigastric pain	
Photosensitivity		Promethazine
Skin sensitization	Local but also oral applications	
Eczematous eruptions		Terfenadine
Alopecia		
Allergy and anaphylaxis		
Blood dyscrasias		Brompheniramine
Agranulocytosis	Rare	Mebhydroline Antazoline
Hemolytic anemias	Rare	Chlorpheniramine Diphenhydramine
Porphyria	Enhancement	Cinnarizine Clemastine Hydroxyzine Promethazine Terfenadine
Cardiac disorders		Astemizole
Venous thrombosis		Promethazine
Fetal abnormalities	Respiratory malformation, urogenital malformation, inguinal hernia	Pheniramine Diphenhydramine Meclozine Chlorcyclizine Cyclizine

Terfenadine

After ingestion of 60 mg terfenadine, the plasma concentration is maximal after about 1.5 h. The elimination half-time is about 4.5–9 hrs [112]. About 60% of the dose is excreted with the feces, i.e., only about 40% is absorbed [55]. A total of 97% is bound to plasma proteins, 99.5% of the absorbed drug is metabolized by first-pass effect through the liver. Two major metabolites have been found: one of these possesses about 30% of the antihistamine activity of terfenadine. Both metabolites are hydrophilic and are ionized at physiological pH. They cannot, therefore, pass the blood-brain barrier. Under the condition of overdosage unmetabolized terfenadine can enter the CNS and can exert CNS (sedative) effects.

Extensive studies revealed a therapeutic efficacy in acute allergic rhinitis [15, 87, 134, 161] asthma [72, 126, 127, 156], chronic urticaria [24, 46, 51, 52, 90, 116, 117, 135, 148]. In atopic eczema terfenadine could be observed to have therapeutic effects on pruritus, and also on other symptoms [37, 46, 62, 159].

Astemizole

Peak plasma concentrations were measured 1–4 h after oral administration of 10 mg astemizole (Janssen, unpublished results). The distribution phase lasts 1–3 days, and a steady state is reached after about 1 week. Astemizole is strongly bound to plasma proteins (about 61%) and to blood cells (about 36%), but also to food components which can reduce absorption from the intestine (down to 60%) [11, 95]. Astemizole is metabolized with a half-time of 1–3 days to desmethyl or 6-hydroxydesmethyl astemizole and some minor metabolites. The hydroxymetabolites possess antihistamine activity. Taken together, the elimination half-life of astemizole plus its active metabolites is about 19 days. After administration of high doses, astemizole passes the blood-brain barrier and the placenta and enters the breast milk (Janssen, unpublished results). Astemizole and its active metabolites bind with high affinity and, de facto, irreversibly to the H_1 receptors in vitro and in vitro (Janssen; Bürger and Schmutzler, unpublished results; [139]). At high concentration (10^{-5} *M*), astemizole inhibits the stimulated histamine release from human adenoidal mast cells [139].

Under the recommended dosage of 10 mg daily, no significant sedative or other side effects except a weight gain in about 1% of patients have been observed [30]. In various types of urticaria, astemizole exerted an antiwhealing and antipruritus effect [75, 91, 116, 162]. No data are available on the efficacy of astemizole in atopic eczema. For allergic rhinitis, a therapeutic effect of astemizole in conjunctivitis, sneezing, and watery secretion is well documented [17, 74] and also for bronchial asthma [72].

Loratadine

Loratadine is rapidly absorbed after oral administration, and peak plasma concentrations are reached within 1–1.5 h. It undergoes rapid metabolism, the major metabolite descarboethoxy-loratadine (DCL) being pharmacologically active [65]. About 98% of loratadine and about 75% of DCL and bound to plasma proteins. The elimination half-lives are 8–11 h for loratadine and 17–24 h for DCL [65]. Loratadine and DCL are secreted into the breast milk [66, 67, 125]. Loratadine has no appreciable anticholinergic but a potent antiserotonin activity [92, 166]. Loratadine was found to be therapeutically effective in allergic rhinitis and perennial rhinitis. It equalled terfenadine with respect to overall efficacy and side effects and had a more rapid onset of action than astemizole [19, 22, 61, 73, 83, 111, 114].

Loratadine has been found to be about as equally effective in chronic urticaria as terfenadine [14, 108, 115, 120, 122, 149]. No studies in patients with atopic eczema have yet been published.

Loratadine is said to have a small incidence rate of side effects consisting of sedation (2% higher than in the placebo group and much lower than in the traditional antihistamine group). Drug allergy (urticaria and angioedema) was observed in one patient.

Cetirizine

Cetirizine, the carboxylic analogue of hydroxyzine, has recently been developed. It is rapidly and extensively absorbed from the gastrointestine, undergoes no substantial first-pass effect, and is slowly metabolized. Its plasma half-time is 7 – 10 h, in renal insufficiency up to 21 h [96, 102, 144, 145, 172]. Cetirizine is effective in suppressing peripheral wheal and flare responses to histamine, etc. [163, 164], but has no appreciable effects on the CNS [119, 131, 147]. Cetirizine exerts certain anti-inflammatory effects, e.g., eosinophil migration in vivo [43, 97]. Cetirizine was found to be effective in chronic urticaria [29, 80]; its efficacy in atopic eczema is not yet sufficiently established.

Azelastine

Azelastine is rapidly and to about 95% absorbed from the intestine. In healthy and asthmatic subjects, peak plasma concentrations were achieved 4–5 h after single doses of azelastine of 2–16 mg. They were approximately doubled in geriatric compared with younger volunteers [103].

In animal studies, radiolabeled azelastine was found to be distributed mainly to the liver, lung, kidney, adrenal glands, pancreas, and spleen and concentrations were particularly high here after continuous oral dosing over 21 days, indicating some accumulation in the body. Azelastine concentrations in the brain were found to be consistently low. From studies in rats, placental transfer f azelastine has to be assumed. In healthy volunteers the mean elimination half-time of azelastine after a single dose of 4 mg was 25 h; this increased to about 35 h after multiple dosing.

In man, azelastine undergoes hydroxylation, demethylation, and zwitterion formation. Demethylazelastine is the major pharmacologically active metabolite and presumably contributes to the overall pharmacological activity of azelastine. After administration of 4 mg orally or 0.5 mg intravenously, about 25% of radioactivity was recovered in urine and 50% in the faeces. In all, 90% was recovered within 240 h. Azelastine may undergo enterohepatic recirculation, although this is not yet entirely clear.

Placebo-controlled studies revealed a significant improvement in bronchial asthma [60, 128, 129, 160]. Some studies indicated comparable therapeutic efficacy to normal therapeutic doses of theophylline, salbumatol, or ketotifen [2, 87, 99, 100, 121, 150, 152]. Oral azelastine in daily dosages of 1–8 mg was found to improve the symptoms of seasonal and perennial rhinitis [170].

Two noncomparative clinical studies have investigated the efficacy of oral azelastine administered in a dosage of 1–2 mg twice daily for 2–6 weeks in 23 patients whith atopic eczema, 22 with eczema and 4 with other dermatological disorders. Azelastine was judged to be useful in 80%–86% of patients with eczema and in 54% of patients with atopic eczema. However, no appropriate controls could be carried out. Therefore, the results still require substantiation [6, 68, 175].

Adverse effects were reported from 19%–42% of patients after a 4-mg daily azelastine dose consisting of altered taste perception and drowsiness or fatigue (3%–18%). After intranasal administration, about 5% of patients felt a burning sensation at the site of application and an altered taste perception.

Ketotifen

Ketotifen is rapidly and to more than 80% absorbed from the intestine. In healthy subjects, peak plasma concentrations were achieved 2–4 h after oral administration of 2 mg. In animal studies ketotifen was found to bind to about 75% to serum proteins. The highest concentrations were discovered in the liver, kidney, and lung. Ketotifen passes the blood-brain and the placenta barriers and enters the breast milk to a substantial degree. In healthy volunteers, the elimination half-time was found to be about 20 h. No information is available about changes of elimination half-time in elderly patients, particularly in those with decreased liver or renal function (Sandoz, internal reports).

Ketotifen is rapidly metabolized in the body. In the blood plasma, relatively high concentrations of the 10-hydroxy derivatives of the parent compound and of the metabolite nonketotifen have been found [82]. Some of the metabolites seem to be pharmacologically active. About 30% of the dose appear in urine in conjugated form as *N*-glucuronide. A multitude of studies have been devoted to the establishment of ketotifen as an antiasthmatic, particularly in children and when given prophylactically.

It is a matter of controversy whether ketotifen acts solely as an H_1 antihistamine or also through other mechanisms. Since the market strategy focused mainly on these alternative mechanisms, relatively little attention was paid to its therapeutic efficacy in other allergic reactions such as rhinitis or skin disorders including atopic eczema [107].

Dimetindene Maleate

After ingestion of 5 mg dimetindene maleate, peak plasma concentrations were reached within the first and second hour. Most of the radiolabeled compound was eliminated with the urine within 24 h [7]. A pilosebacial absorption of dimetidine through the skin has been demonstrated in the rat [36]. Topical application to the skin of patients allergic to insect venom had, however, no preventive or curative effect [133].

Dimetindene was found to be equally effective in rhinitis vasomotorica, pollinosis, and hay fever as other antihistamines, e.g., dextrochlorpheniramine maleate [123].

In bronchial asthma, dimetindene was not sufficiently effective, but has been extensively used in combination with cimetidene to prevent anaphylactoid reactions to muscle relaxants, X-ray contrast media, and plasma expanders [39, 98, 140].

Dimetindene was found to be effective in preventing

or diminishing pruritus in chronic urticaria, urticaria factitia, Hodgkin's disease, leukemia, diabetes, liver disease, or pruritus without any specific underlying disease. Chronic types of eczema, however, did not respond to dimetindene treatment.

There are only scanty reports about the efficacy of dimetindene in atopic eczema. Korossy [89] found it to be effective in about 76% ot patients suffering from different types of pruritus including atopic eczema. May and Nelemans [104] found an effect in a double-blind study in about 50% of patients (against 28% placebo) although the small number of patients suffering from atopic eczema obviously did not benefit from that treatment.

Conclusions

Obviously no effective basic treatment of atopic eczema exists. In about half of patients, sufficiently high doses of H_1 antihistamines seem to offer more or less pronounced relief from the most tormenting symptom pruritus. However, this relief presumably only partially stems from the H_1 effects in the strict sense, but equally from the tranquilizing side effects on the CNS of the antihistamines, as represented by hydroxyzine. Unfortunately, there are too few properly controlled clinical studies in a sufficiently great number of patients to substantiate such a notion.

References

1. Advenier C, Queille-Roussel C (1989) Rational use of antihistamines in allergic dermatological conditions. Drugs 38: 634-644
2. Ambrosi L, Bariffi F, Carino M, Catena E, Ceccarelli G, Ciampini M, Condoluci M, Crimi N, Ferretti G, Gambaro G et al. (1989) Azelastine in the prophylactic treatment of bronchial asthma: an Italian multicenter comparison with ketotifen. J Int Med Res 17:218–225
3. Arrang JM, Garbarg M, Schwartz JC (1983) Auto-inhibition of brain histamine release mediated by a novel class (H_3) of histamine receptor. Nature 302:832–837
4. Arrang JM, Garbarg M, Lancelot JC, Lecomte JM, Pollard H, Robba M, Schunack W, Schwartz JC (1987) Highly potent and selective ligands for histamine H_3-receptors. Nature 327:117–123
5. Arrang JM, Devaux B, Chodkiewicz JP, Schwartz JC (1988) H_3-receptors control histamine release in human brain. J Neurochem 51:105–108
6. Atkins P, Merton H, Karpink P, Weliky I, Zweiman B (1985) Azelastine inhibition of skin test reactivity in humans. J Allergy Clin Immunol 75:167
7. Balant L, Wermeille M, Huber G, Gumma A, Golden G (1981) In: Aiache JM, Hirtz I (Eds) Dimethindene half-life estimation in urine. First Europ Congr Biopharmaceutics and Pharmacokinetics 2: 403-406
8. Barger G, Dale HH (1911) β-Iminazolyl ethylamine a depressor constituent of intestinal mucosa. J Physiol (Lond) 41:499–503
9. Baroody F, Proud D, Kagey-Sobotka A, Freidhoff L, Norman PS, Lichtenstein LM, Naclerio RM (1989) The effects of H_1 antihistamines on the early allergic response. Ann Allergy 63:551–555
10. Bartosch R, Feldberg W, Nagel E (1932) Das Freiwerden eines histamin-ähnlichen Stoffes bei der Anaphylaxie des Meerschweinchens. Pflügers Arch Gesamte Physiol 230: 129–153
11. Bateman DN, Chapman PH, Rawlins MD (1983) Lack of effect of astemizole on ethanol dynamics or kinetics. Eur J Clin Pharmacol 25:567–568
12. Behrendt H, Bachert C, Magnussen H, Goerz G (1989) Mast cell heterogeneity: morphological aspects in humans. Allergologie 12:101–108
13. Bent S, Fehling U, Braam U, Schunack W, Schmutzler W (1991) The influence of H_1-, H_2- and H_3-receptors on the spontaneous and Con A induced histamine release from human adenoidal mast cells. Agents and Actions 33: 67–70
14. Bernstein IL, Bernstein DI (1988) The efficacy and safety of loratidine in the management of chronic idiopathic urticaria. J Allergy Clin Immunol 81:211
15. Bertrand B, Clement P, Daele J, Halloy JL, Michel O, Piessens M (1990) Double-blind parallel-group comparison of once a dax terfenadine and loratadine in seasonal allergic rhinitis. A multicentre study. Acta Ther 16: 351-362
16. Black JW, Duncan WAM, Durant CJ, Gauellin CR, Parsons EM (1972) Definition and antagonism of histamine H_2 receptors. Nature 236: 385–390
17. Boland N (1988) A double blind study of astemizole and terfenadine in the treatment of perennial rhinitis. Ann Allergy 61:18–24
18. Borelli S, Schellert P (1967) Zur Wirksamkeit von Psychopharmaka bei atopischer Neurodermitis. Vergleichende Untersuchung von Diazepam (Valium), Promethazin (Phenergan) und Placebo. Dermatologica 135:485–496
19. Bousquet J, Chanal I, Skassa-Brociet W, Lemonier C, Michel FB (1990) Lack of subsensitivity to loratadine during long-term dosing during 12 weeks. J Allergy Clin Immmunol 86: 248-253
20. Bovet D (1950) Introduction to antihistamine agents and antergan derivatives. Ann NY Acad Sci 50:1089–1126

21. Brik A, Tashkin DP, Gong jr H, Dauphinee B, Lee E (1987) Effect of cetirizine, a new histamine H_1 antagonist, on airway dynamics and responsiveness to inhaled histamine in mild asthma. J Allergy Clin Immunol 80:51–56
22. Bruttmann G, Arendt C, Bernheim J (1989) Double-blind, placebo controlled comparison of cetirizine 2HCl and terfenadine in atopic perennial rhinitis. Acta Therap 15: 99-109
23. Cap JP, Schwanitz HJ, Czarnetzki BM (1985) Die Wirkung von Ketotifen bei der Urticaria factitia und der Urtikaria cholinergica im gekreuzten Doppelblindversuch. Hautarzt 36:509–511
24. Cerio R, Lessof MH (1984) Treatment of chronic idiopathic urticaria with terfenadine. Clin Allergy 14:139–141
25. Chand N, Nolan K, Diamantis W, Perhach jr JL, Sofia RD (1983) Inhibition of leukotriene (SRS-A)-mediated allergic bronchospasm by azelastine, a novel orally effective drug. J Allergy Clin Immunol 71:149
26. Chand N, Pillar J, Nolan K, Diamantis W, Sofia RD (1989) Inhibition of allergic and non-allergic leukotriene C4 formation and histamine secretion by azelastine: implication for its mechanism of action. Int Arch Allergy Appl Immunol 90:67–70
27. Charlesworth EN, Kagey-Sobotka A, Norman PS, Lichtenstein LM (1989) Effect of cetirizine on mast cell-mediator release and cellular traffic during the cutaneous late-phase reaction. J Allergy Clin Immunol 83:905–912
28. Cheng HC, Woodward JK (1982) A kinetic study of the antihistamine effect of terfenadine. Arzneimittelforschung 32:1160–1166
29. Coulie P, Wery M, Ghys L, Rihoux JP (1989) Pharmacologic modulation by cetirizine – 2HCl of cutaneous reactions and pruritus in man. Skin Pharmacol 2:38–40
30. Craft TM (1986) Torsade de pointes after astemizole overdose. Br Med J [Clin Res] 292:660
31. Carruthers SG, Shoeman DW, Hignite CE, Azarnoff DL (1978) Clin Pharmacol Ther 23:375–382
32. Dale HH (1933) Progress in autopharmacology. Bull Johns Hopkins Hosp 53:297–347
33. Dale HH (1948) Antihistamine substances. Br Med J [Clin Res] 2:281–283
34. de Vos C, Joseph M, Leprevost C, Vorng H, Tomassini M, Capron M, Capron A (1989) Inhibition of human eosinophil chemotaxis and of the IgE-dependent stimulation of human blood platelets by cetirizine. Int Arch Allerg Appl Immunol 88:212–215
35. Diller G, Orfanos CE (1982) H_2-Antagonisten und Möglichkeiten ihrer therapeutischen Anwendung in der Dermatologie. Hautarzt 33:521–528
36. Dobozy A (1973) Die Resorption des Dimetindenum maleicum in der Rattenhaut. Z f Hautkrh 48: 787-789
37. Dockx P, Lambert J, Arendt C, Darte D (1987) Comparison of cetirizine and terfenadine in idiopathic urticaria. Revista Espan Allergol Immunol Clin 2:113
38. Dodson ME, Eastley RJ (1978) Comparative study of two long-acting tranquillizers for oral premedication. Br J Anaesth 50:1059–1064
39. Doenicke A, Lorenz W (1982) Histamine release in anaesthesia and surgery. Predication with H_1- and H_2-receptor antagonists: Indications, benefits and possible problems. Klin Wochenschr 60: 1039-1045
40. Dragstedt CA, Gebauer-Fuelnegg E (1932) Studies in anaphylaxis. I. The appearance of physiologically active substance during anaphylactic shock. Am J Physiol 102:512–519
41. Duncan JS, Kennedy HJ, Triger DR (1984) Treatment of pruritus due to chronic obstructive liver disease. Br Med J [Clin Res] 289:22
42. Ea-Kim L, Oudart N (1988) A highly potent and selective H_3 agonist relaxes rabbit middle cerebral artery in vitro. Eur J Pharmacol 150:393–396
43. Fadel R, Herpin-Richard N, Rihoux JP, Henocq E (1987) Inhibitory effect of cetirizine 2HCl on eosinophil migration in vivo. Clin Allergy 17:373–379
44. Fehling U, Bent St, Schmutzler W (1990) Influence of H_3-receptors on the histamine release from human adenoidal mast cells. XIX Meeting EHRS, Kuopio, Abstr. 96
45. Feinberg SM (1947) The antihistaminic drugs. Pharmacology and therapeutic effects. Am J Med 3:560–570
46. Ferguson J, McDonald KJS, Kenicer KJA (1985) Terfenadine and placebo compared in the treatment of chronic idiopathic urticaria: a randomized double-blind study. Br J Clin Pharmacol 20:639–641
47. Filderman RB (1988) Inhibition of skin reactivity by antihistamines. Cutis 42:19–21
48. Finnerty JP, Holgate ST, Rihoux JP (1990) The effect of 2 weeks treatment with cetirizine on bronchial reactivity to metacholine in asthma. Br J Clin Pharmacol 29:79–84
49. Fitzsimons EJ, Dagg JH, McAllister EJ (1981) Pruritus of polycythemia vera: a place for pizotifen? Br Med J [Clin Res] 283:277
50. Foulds IS, Mackie RM (1981) A double-blind trial of the H_2 receptor antagonist cimetidine, and the H_1 receptor antagonist promethazine hydrochloride in the treatment of atopic dermatitis. Clin Allergy 11:319–323
51. Frederiksson T, Hersle K, Hjorth N, Mobacken H, Salo O, Schmidt H, Thomsen K (1985) Ann Allergy 55:285
52. Frederiksson T, Hersle K, Hjorth N, Mobacken H, Persson T, Salde L Salo O, Schmidt H, Thomsen K (1986) Terfenadine in chronic urticaria: a comparison with clemastine and placebo. Cutis 38:128–130
53. Frosch PJ, Schwanitz HJ, Macher E (1984) A double blind trial of H_1 and H_2 receptor antagonists in the treatment of atopic dermatitis. Arch Dermatol Res 276:36–40
54. Ganellin CR (1978) Chemistry and Structure-Activity Relationships of H_2-Receptor Antagonists. In: Rocha e Silva M (ed) Histamine II and anti-histaminics. Chemistry, metabolism, and physiological and pharmacological action. Springer, Berlin Heidelberg New York, pp 251–294 (Handbook of experimental pharmacology, vol 18, part 2)
55. Garteiz DA, Hook RH, Walker BJ, Okerholm RA (1982) Pharmacokinetics and biotransformation studies of terfenadine in man. Arzneimittelforschung 32:1185–1190
56. Geddes DM (1984) Chronic airflow obstruction. Postgrad Med J 60:194–200
57. Ghys L, Rihoux JP (1989) Pharmacological modulation of cutaneous reactivity to histamine: a double-blind acute comparative study between cetirizine, terfenadine and astemizole. J Int Med Res 17:24–27
58. Gibbs CJ, Coutts II, Jackson SM, White RJ (1983) Skin test wheal size and erythema not reduced by topical antihistamine. Br Med J [Clin Res] 287:1427–1428
59. Giertz H, Hahn F, Seseke G, Schmutzler W (1967) Über die Wirkung von Heparin und Aminoguanidin auf den anaphylaktischen, Anaphylatoxin- und Histamin-Schock des Meerschweinchens. Arch Pharmacol Exp Pathol 256: 26–39
60. Gould CAL, Ollier S, Aurich R, Davies RJ (1988) A study of the clinical efficacy of azelastine in patients with

extrinsic asthma, and its effect on airway responsiveness. Br J Clin Pharmacol 26:515–525

61. Gutkowski A, Bedard P, Del Carpio J, Hebert J, Prevost M, Schulz J, Turenne Y, Yeadon C (1988) Comparison of the efficacy and safety of loratadine, terfenadine, and placebo in the treatent of seasonal allergic rhinitis. J Allergy Clin Immunol: 902-907
62. Gütling M, Wüthrich B,Dieterich HA, Henauer S (1986) Atopische Dermatitis im Kindesalter. Inform Arzt 7:56–62
63. Hahn F (1978) Antianaphylactic and Antiallergic Effects. In: Rocha e Silva M (ed) Histamine II and antihistaminics-Chemistry, metabolism, and physiological and pharmacological action. Springer, Berlin Heidelberg New York, pp 439–504 (Handbook of experimental pharmacology, vol 18, part 2).
64. Henry RL, Hodges IG, Milner AD, Stokes GM (1983) Bronchodilator effects of the H_1 receptor antagonist clemastine. Arch Dis Child 58:304–305
65. Hilbert J, Radwanski E, Weglein R, Luc V, Perentesis G, Symchowicz S, Zampaglione N (1987) Pharmacokinetics and dose proportionality of loratidine. J Clin Pharmacol 27:694–698
66. Hilbert J, Moritzen V, Parks A, Radwanski E, Perentesis G, Symchowicz S, Zampaglione N (1988) The pharmacokinetics of loratidine in normal geriatric volunteers. J Int Med Res 16:50–60
67. Hilbert J, Radwanski E, Affrime MB, Perentesis G, Symchowicz S, Zampaglione N (1988) Excretion of loratidine in human breast milk. J Clin Pharmacol 28:234–239
68. Hinogaki Y, Hidano N (1988) Efficacy of E-0659 (azelastine) in atopic dermatitis, eczema and contact dermatitis. Medical Consult News Remedies 25: 581-586
69. Hlouskova Z,Gutova M, Hlousek Z (1980) A comparison between the efficacy of ketotifen and clemastine in children. J Int Med Res 8:408–412
70. Holgate ST, Church MK (1989) Mast cell heterogeneity and its clinical implications. Allergologie 12:109–113
71. Holgate ST, Finnerty JP (1989) Antihistamines in asthma. J Allergy Clin Immunol 83:537–547
72. Holgate ST, Emanuel MB, Howarth PH (1985) Astemizole and other H_1-antihistaminic drug treatment in asthma. J Allergy Clin Immunol 76:375–380
73. Horak F, Bruttmann G, Pedrali P, Weeke B, Frolund L, Wolff HH, Christophers E (1988) A multicentric study of loratadine, terfenadine and placebo in patients with seasonal allergic rhinitis. Drug Res 38: 124–128
74. Howarth PH, Emanuel MB, Holgate ST (1984) Astemizole, a potent histamine Hsub 1-receptor antagonist: Effekt in allergic rhinoconjunctivitis, on antigen and histamine induced skin weal responses and relationship to serum levels. Br J Clin Pharmacol 18: 1–8
75. Huerter CJ, Bergfeld WF, Wagner WO, Dijkstra JW (1989) Treatment of chronic idiopathic urticaria with astemizole. Cleve Clin J Med 56:263–266
76. Ichinose M, Barnes PJ (1989) Inhibitory histamine H_3 receptors on cholinergic nerves in human air ways. Eur J Pharmacol 163:383–386
77. Ishikawa S, Sperelakis N (1987) A novel class (H_3) of histamine receptors on perivascular nerve terminals. Nature 327:158–160
78. Johnson HH, De Orco GA, Lascheid OP, Mitchell F (1960) Skin histamine levels in chronic atopic eczema. J Invest Dermatol 34:237–241
79. Jolliffe DS, Sim-Davis D, Templeton JS (1985) A placebo-controlled comparative study of sustained-release brompheniramine maleate against clemastine fumarate in the treatment of chronic urticaria. Curr Med Res Opin 9:394–399
80. Juhlin L, Arendt C (1988) Treatment of chronic urticaria with cetirizine dihydrochloride a non-sedating antihistamine. Br J Dermatol 119:67–72
81. Juhlin L, de Vos C, Rihoux JP (1987) Inhibition by cetirizine of histamine and 48/80 induced wheals and flares, experimental dermographism and cold induced urticaria. J Allergy Clin Immunol 80:599–602
82. Julien-Larose C, Guerret M, Lavene D, Kiechel JR (1983) Quantitation of Ketotifen and its metabolites in human plasma by gas chromatography mass spectrometry. Biomed Mass Spectrom 10:136–142
83. Kaminszczik I, Soto-Roman L, Kutwak A, Rodriguez L, Cataldo J (1986) Loratidine vs astemizole: Onset of allergy symptoms relief. XIIIth Congr Europ Acad Allergology Clin Immonol, Budapest
84. Kapp A, Wokalek H, Schöpf E (1985) Involvement of complement in psoriasis and atopic dermatitis – Measurement of C3a and C5a, C_3, C_4 and C_1 inactivator. Arch Dermatol Res 277:359–361
85. Kapp A, Kemper A, Schöpf E, Deicher H (1986) Detection of circularing immune complexes in patients with atopic dermatitis and psoriasis. Acta Derm Venereol (Stockh) 66:121–126
86. Karlin JM (1972) The use of antihistamines in asthma. Ann Allergy 30:342–347
87. Kemp JP, Meltzer EO, Orgel HA, Welch MJ, Bucholtz GA, Middleton E Jr, Spector SL, Newton JJ, Perhach JL Jr (1987) A dose-response study of the bronchodilator action of azelastine in asthma. J Allergy Clin Immunol 79:893–899
88. Kok TH, Taitz LS, Bennett MJ, Holt DW (1982) Drowsiness due to clemastine transmitted in breast milk (letter). Lancet 1:914–915
89. Korrossy S (1977) Fenistil und Pruritus. Arch Arzneither I:259–262
90. Krause LB, Shuster S (1984) The effect of terfenadine on dermographic wealing. Br J Dermatol 110:73–79
91. Krause LB, Shuster S (1985) A comparison of astemizole and chlorpheniramine in dermographic urticaria. Br J Dermatol 112:447–453
92. Kreutner W, Chapman RW, Gulbenkian A, Siegel MI (1987) Antiallergic activity of loratidine, a non-sedating antihistamine. Allergy 42:57–63
93. Kris MG, Tyson LB, Gralla RJ, Clark RA, Allen JC, Reilly LK (1983) Extrapyramidal reactions with high-dose metoclopramide (letter). N Engl J Med 309:433–434
94. Laborit H, Huguenard P, Alluaume R (1952) Un nouveau stabilisateur vegetatif, le 4560 RP. Presse Med 60:206–208
95. Laduron PM, Janssen PFM, Gommeren W, Leysen J (1982) In vitro and in vivo binding characteristics of a new long-acting histamine H_1 antagonist, astemizole. Mol Pharmacol 21:294–300
96. Lefebvre RA, Rosseel MT, Bernheim J (1988) Single dose pharmacokinetics of cetirizine in young and elderly volunteers. Int J Clin Pharmacol Res 8:463–470
97. Leprevost C, Capron M, de Vos C, Tomassini M, Capron A (1988) Inhibition of eosinophil chemotaxis by a new antiallergic compound (cetirzine). Int Arch Allergy Appl Immunol 87: 9-13
98. Lorenz W, Doenicke A, Schöning B, Mamorski J, Weber D,

Hinterlang E, Schwarz B, Neugebauer E (1980) Histamine release; $H_1 + H_2$-receptor antagonists for premedication in anaesthesia and surgery: a critical view based on randomized clinical trials with haemaccel and various antiallergic drugs. Agents and Actions 10: 114–124

99. Magnussen H, Reuss G, Joerres R, Aurich R (1988) The effect of azelastine on exerzise-induced asthma. Chest 93: 937–940
100. Magnussen H, Reuss G, Jörres R, Aurich R (1989) Duration of the effect of a single dose of azelastine on histamine-induced bronchoconstriction. J Allergy Clin Immunol 83:467–470
101. Mathews KP (1985) The urticarias. Current concepts in pathogenesis and treatment. Drugs 30:552–560
102. Matzke GR, Yeh J, Awni WM, Halstenson CE, Chung M (1987) Pharmacokinetics of ceterizine in the elderly and patients with renal insufficiency. Ann Allergy 59:25–30
103. McTavish D, Sorkin EM (1989) Azelastine. A review of its pharmacodynamic and pharmacokinetics properties. Drugs 38:778–800
104. May KL, Nelemans FA (1966) The antipruritic effect of fenistil (dimethpyrindene) in allergic conditions. Double blind clinical study. Acta Allergologica 21:337–342
105. Menzel I, Nasemann T, Pfister R (1978) Erfahrung mit Tavegil Gel bei juckenden Dermatosen. Z Allgemeinmed 54:1763–1764
106. Michel L, de Vos C, Rihoux JP, Burtin C, Benveniste J, Dubertret L (1988) Inhibitory effect of oral cetirizine on in vivo antigen induced histamine and paf-acether release and eosinophil recruitment in human skin. J Allergy Clin Immunol 82:101–109
107. Molkhous P, Dupont C (1989) Ketotifen treatment of atopic dermatitis and other food allergy diseases. Allergy 44 [Suppl 9]:117–123
108. Monroe EW, Fox RW, Green AW, Izmo GT, Bernstein DJ (1988) Efficacy and safety of loratidine in the management of idiopathic chronic urticaria. J Am Acad Dermatol 19:138–139
109. Norman PS (1985) Modulation of the mast cell and inhibition of its modulators. J Allergy Clin Immunol 76:366
110. Nykamp D (1986) Comparison of H_1-antihistamines for pruritus in end-stage renal dosage. Drug Intell Clin Pharm 20:806–807
111. Oei HD, Verheij E, Schwab D, Lherminier M, Bruynzeel PLB (1987) A comparative study of the efficacy of loratadine (L) and astemizole (A). J Allergy Clin Immunol 79: 190
112. Okerholm RA, Weiner DL, Hook RH, Walker BJ, Leeson GA, Biederbach SA, Cawein MJ, Dusebout TD, Wright GJ (1981) Bioavailability of terfenadine in man. Biopharm Drug Dispos 2:185–190
113. Paslin D (1978) The proposed use of H_2-receptor antagonists in urticaria and atopic dermatitis. Arch Dermatol 114:1855–1856
114. Passaleva A, Ricci M (1988) Loratidine, a new antihistaminic drug in seasonal allergic rhinitis. Allergy 43 (Suppl 7): 111
115. Paul E (1988) Loratidine and terfenadine in the treatment of chronic urticaria. Allergy 43 [Suppl 7]:122
116. Paul E, Bödeker RH (1985) Vergleich von Astemizol u. Terfenadin in der Behandlung der chronischen Urtikaria. Eine randomisierte Doppelblind-Studie an 40 Patienten. Z Hautkr 60 [Suppl 1]:50–55
117. Paul E, Bödeker RH (1989) Comparative study of astemizole and terfenadine in the treatment of chronic idopathic urticaria. A randomized double-blind study of 40 patients. Ann Allergy 62:318–320
118. Pearce FL (1986) On the heterogeneity of mast cells. Pharmacology 32:61–71
119. Pechadre JC, Vernay D, Trolese JF, Bloom M, Dupont P, Rihoux JP (1988) Comparison of the central and periphere effects of cetirizine and terfenadine. Eur J Clin Pharmacal 35:255–259
120. Pedrali P, Bruttmann G(1986) Efficacy of loratadine in the management of idiopathic chronic urticaria. XIIIth Congress of the Eur Acad Allergology Clin Imunology, Budapest
121. Piacenza G, Ciampini M, Mantellini E, Ferretti G (1987) Preventive effectiveness of azelastine in broncial asthma. Double-blind comparison with ketotifen. Riv Patol Clin 42: 275–284
122. Pleskow WW (1987) Studies of a new antihistamine in the management of perennial allergic rhinitis and chronic idiopathic urticaria. 44th Ann Congr Amer Coll Allergists, Boston Nov.
123. Poisson A, Brunet CM (1984) Essai en simple insu d'un nouvel antihistaminique: Le Maleate de Dimetindene dans la Pollinose. Gaz Med Fr 91: 65–70
124. Porter J, Jick H (1977) Drug-induced anaphylaxis, convulsions, deafness, and extrapyramidal symptoms. Lancet 1:587–588
125. Radwanski E, Hilbert J, Symchowicz S, Zampaglione N (1987) Loratidine: multiple-dose pharmacokinetics. J Clin Pharmacol 27:530–533
126. Rafferty D, Holgate ST (1987) Terfenadine (Seldane) is a potent and selective histamine receptor antagonist in airways. Am Rev Respir Dis 135:181–184
127. Rafferty P (1989) The european experience with antihistamines in asthma. Ann Allergy 63:389–391
128. Rafferty P, Harrison PJ, Aurich R, Holgate ST (1988) The in vivo potency and selectivity of azelastine as an H_1 histamine-receptor antagonist in human airways and skin. J Allergy Clin Immunol 82:1113–1118
129. Rafferty P, Ng WH, Phillips G, Clough J, Church MK, Aurich R, Ollier S, Holgate ST (1989) The inhibitory actions of azelastine hydrochloride on the early and late bronchoconstrictor responses to inhaled allergen in atopic asthma. J Allergy Clin Immunol 84:649–657
130. Rajka G (1968) Evaluation of drug influence on the itch duration in the skin of patients with atopic dermatitis, various eczemas and psoriasis. I. Experiments in involved skin. Comparison with itch threshold technique. Acta Derm Venereol (Stockh) 48:93–97
131. Rihoux JP, Dupont P (1987) Comparative study of the peripheral and central effects of terfenadine and cetirizine 2HCl. Ann Allergy 59:235–238
132. Ring J, Senter T, Arroyare CM, Cornell R, Tan EM (1979) Plasma complement and histamine changes in atopic dermatitis. Br J Dermatol 100:521–530
133. Rohdewald P, Milsmann E (1985) Zur Effektivität einer externen Therapie mit Antihistaminika. Allergologie 8: 231–236
134. Sabbah A, Bonneau JC, Arendt C (1987) Comparison of cetirizine and terfenadine in perennial allergic rhinitis. Allergol Immunol Clin 2:322
135. Salisbury J, Bor S, Blair C (1987) A double-blind placebo controlled study of terfenadine in the treatment of chronic idiopathic urticaria. Br J Clin Pract 41:859–861
136. Schaaf L, Hendeles L, Weinberger M (1979) Suppression of seasonal allergic rhinitis symptoms with daily hydroxyzine. J Allergy Clin Immunol 63:129–133

137. Schmutzler W, Giertz H, Hahn F (1963) Neue Untersuchungen über die Rolle des Histamins bei der Meerschweinchenanaphylaxie. Int Arch Allergy 22:69–76
138. Schmutzler W, Hahn F, Seseke G, Bernauer W (1966) Über die Herkunft der Plasmahistaminase im anaphylaktischen Schock des Meerschweinchens. Arch exp Path Pharmak 252:332–338
139. Schmutzler W, Glück St, Riesener KP, Frings M (1989) Histamine and other mediators in asthma. In: Pichler WJ, Stadler BM, Dahinden CA, Pécond AR, Frei P, Schneider CH, de Weck AL (eds) Progress in allergy and clinical immunology. Hogrefe and Huber, Bern, pp 209–212
140. Schöning B, Lorenz W, Doenicke A (1982) Prophylaxis of anaphylactoid reactions to a polypeptidal plasma substitute by H_1-plus H_2-receptor antagonists: Synopsis of three randomized controlled trials. Klin Wochenschr 60: 1048–1055
141. Schwinghammer TL, Kroboth FJ, Juhl RP (1984) Extrapyramidal reaction secondary to oral promethazine. Clin Pharm 3:83–85
142. Shawn DH, McGuigan MA (1984) Poisoning from dermal absorption of promethazine. Can Med Assoc J 130:1460–1461
143. Shuster S (1988) Antihistamines in the treatment of urticarial disorders. Cutis 42:26–28
144. Simons FE, Simons KJ, Chung M, Yeh J (1987) The comparative pharmacokinetics of H_1-receptor antagonists. Ann Allergy 59:20–24
145. Simons KJ, Watson WT, Chen XY, Simons FE (1989) Pharmacokinetic and pharmacodynamic studies of the H_1-receptor antagonist hydroxyzine in the elderly. Clin Pharmacol Ther 45:9–14
146. Singh G (1984) H_2-blockers in chronic urticaria. Int J Dermatol 23:627–628
147. Snyder SH, Snowman AM (1987) Receptor effects of cetirizine. Ann Allergy 59:4–8
148. Sorkin EM, Heel RC (1985) Terfenadine. A review of its pharmacodynamic properties and therapeutic efficacy. Drugs 29:34–56
149. Soto LD, Falabella R, Hojyo T, Múzquiz D (1987) Estudio multicéntrico comparativo entre dos antihistaminicos anti H_1 en el manejo de dermatosis crónicas pruriginosas. Dermatologica Revista Mexicana 31: 9–14
150. Spector SL, Perhach JL, Rohr AS, Rachelefsky GS, Katz RM, Siegel SC (1987) Pharmacodynamic evaluation of azelastine in subjects with asthma. J Allergy Clin Immunol 80:75–80
151. Staub AM, Bovet D (1937) Action de la thymoxy éthyl-dié thylamine (929 F.) et de éthers phénoliques sur le choc anaphylactique du cobaye. C R Soc Biol (Paris) 125:818–821
152. Storms W, Middleton E, Dvorin D, Kemp J, Spector S et al (1985) Azelastine in the treatment of asthma. J Allergy Clin Immunol 75: 167
153. Sutherland DC (1989) Antihistamine agents: new options or just more drugs? Med J Aust 151:159–162
154. Tamura K, Palmer JM, Wood JD (1988) Presynaptic inhibition produced by histamine at nicotinic synapses in enteric ganglia. Neuroscience 25: 171–179
155. Taudorf E, Moseholm L (1988) Pollen count, symptoms and medicine score in birch pollinosis. Int Arch Allergy Appl Immunol 86:225–233
156. Taytard A, Beaumont D, Pujet JC, Sapene M, Lewis PJ (1987) Treatment of bronchial asthma with terfenadine; a randomised controlled trial. Br J Clin Pharmacol 24:743–746
157. Tham R, Norlander B, Haegermark O, Fransson L (1978) Gaschromatography of clemastine. A study of plasma kinetics and biological effect. Arzneimittelforschung 28: 1017–1020
158. Thiers BH (1989) Topical steroid therapy of atopic skin diseases. Allergy Proc 10:413–416
159. Tholen S, Dieterich HA (1989) Terfenadin versus Ketotifen bei Kindern mit atopischer Dermatitis. Allergologie 12:60–63
160. Tinkelmann DG, Bucholtz GA, Kemp JP, Koepcke JW, Repsher LH, Spector SL, Storms WW, van As A (1990) Evaluation of the safety and efficacy of multiple doses of azelastine to adult patients with bronchial asthma over time. Am Rev Respir Dis 141:569–574
161. Troise C, Voltolini S, Cilli P, Negrini AC (1989) A double-blind comparative trial of astemizole and terfenadine for the treatment of hay fever. Allerg Immunol (Paris) 21:396–398
162. Tyoelahti H, Lahti A (1989) Start and end of the effects of terfenadine and astemizole on histamine-induced wheals in human skin. Acta Derm Venereol 69:269–271
163. van Neste D, Rihoux JP (1988) Inhibition of the cutaneous response to histamine by H_1-blocking agents. Quantitative evaluation of micro-vascular changes in the skin after histamine challenge and a comparison of the effects of a single intake of cetirizine and terfenadine. Skin Pharmacol 1:192–199
164. van Neste D, Ghys L, Antoine JL, Rihoux JP (1989) Pharmacological modulation by cetirizine and atropine of the histamine- and metacholine-induced wheals and flares in human skin. Skin Pharmacol 2:93–102
165. Verbov J (1984) Modern management of atopic eczema. Practitioner 28:1013–1017
166. Villani FJ, Magatti CV, Vashi DB, Wong J, Popper TL (1986) N-substituted 11-(4-piperidylene)-5,6-dihydro-11-11-benzo-[5,6] cyclohepta [1,2] pyridines. Arzneimittelforschung 36:1311–1314
167. Vincent J, Liminana R, Meredith PA, Reid JL (1988) The pharmacokinetics, antihistamine and concentration-effect relationship of ebastine in healthy subjects. Br J Clin Pharmacol 26:497–501
168. Wahlgren CF, Haegermark O, Bergstroem R, Hedin B (1988) Evaluation of a new method of assessing pruritus and antipruritic drugs. Skin Pharmacol 1:3–13
169. Warin RP (1984) The effect of large doses of H_1 antagonists in urticaria (letter). Br J Dermatol 111:121
170. Weiler JM, Donnelly A, Campbell BH, Connell JT, Diamond L, Hamilton LH, Rosenthal RR, Hemsworth GR, Perhach JL Jr (1988) Multicenter, double-blind, multiple-dose, parallel-groups efficacy and safety trial of azelastine, chlorpheniramine, and placebo in the treatment of spring allergic rhinitis. J Allergy Clin Immunol 82:801–811
171. Witte PK, Irmisch R, Hajdu P (1985) Pharmacokinetics of pheniramine (Avil) and metabolites in healthy subjects after oral and intravenous administration. Int J Clin Pharmacol Ther Toxicol 23:59–62
172. Wood SG, John BA, Chasseaud LF, Yeh J, Chung M (1987) The metabolism and pharmacokinetics of ^{14}C-cetirizine in humans. Ann Allergy 59:31–34
173. Wüthrich B (1988) Neurodermitis atopica (atopische Dermatitis). In: Fuchs E, Schulz KH (eds) Manuale allergologicum, V. 14. Dustri, Deisenhofen, pp 1–34
174. Wüthrich B (1989) Therapie der akuten und chronischen Urtikaria und des Quincke-Ödems. Schweiz Rundsch Med Prax 78:576–581
175. Yoshida M, Tezuka T (1988) Clinical efficacy of azelastine in eczema and dermatitis. J New Remed and Clin 37: 171-174

Mast Cell Blockers and Atopic Eczema

L. Businco and A. Cantani

Introduction

The concept of foods which are forbidden and should not be eaten goes back to the Garden of Eden and subsequently to suggestions of Hippocrates and Lucretius. Cow's milk could cause gastric upset and hives according to Hippocrates. Furthermore, the Roman poet Lucretius stated "one man's meat is another man's poison" [1].

The role of dietary factors in atopic eczema (AE) has long been a subject of controversy. However, it has been shown that food allergy (FA) plays a role in some children with AE, a multifaceted disorder which should be examined from various points of view and requires all the skill a physician can gather. Therefore, the management of AE is a challenge for pediatricians, dermatologists and allergists [2].

It has long been known that elimination of the offending allergens is the treatment of choice for childhood FA. At variance with inhalant allergens which are omnipresent in every environment, both outdoor and indoor, and therefore unlikely to be avoided effectively, food allergens can frequently be successfully excluded from the diet. An effective elimination diet is easily prescribed (and the compliance is good) when the offending items are not widely diffused in the daily diet, including peaches, beans, pork, lentils, citrus fruit and strawberries or when the offending items are not necessary nutrients, such as seafoods, nuts, chocolate, pepper, etc. Problems arise if the child is allergic to several foods, or when the triggering agents are foods such as cow's milk, egg and wheat, which are common items in the child's diet, widespread and incorporated into many baby foods. In this case, their exclusion can be impractical and problematic, and nutritional derangements can easily start, especially if the restricted diet is too protracted. For a 2-year-old child, 500 ml of cow's milk provides 100% of the daily requirement of Ca, 50% of that of protein, 100% of that of riboflavin and 24% of the energy. Moreover, even minimal nutritional deficiencies have been reported to induce changes in the immune response, especially in cell-mediated immunity. It would be preposterous if a nutritional derangement provoked in the effort of treating allergy could in turn aggravate the allergic disease. Therefore, before embarking on a strict avoidance diet in children, one should know that derangements are very frequent when the sensitisation is to foods such as cow's milk and egg, which are contained not only in everyday servings or courses but also in a large variety of foodstuffs, including biscuits, cakes, snacks and ice creams, especially appreciated by children [3].

It is believed that food allergens stimulate the release of mediators from the superficial mast cells located in the gut, thus inducing an increased permeability of the gastrointestinal (GI) tract. The resulting absorption of food proteins into the blood is followed by various manifestations at distant sites, including asthma, angioedema, urticaria, AE as well as GI symptoms which are induced by the effects on the gut itself [4].

Pharmacological agents which are able to prevent mast-cell degranulation should be considered as the ideal medication for patients with FA. Their use is indicated when symptoms continue despite efforts to maintain an elimination diet. Such problems may depend upon an incorrect or incomplete diagnosis, unavoidable exposure or intentional departures.

Herein we will review the studies on the use of sodium cromoglycate (SCG) and ketotifen, drugs which are considered as mast-cell blockers in AE.

Studies on Sodium Cromoglycate

SCG, which is the salt of a bis-chromone carboxylic acid, has been shown to be of proven efficacy in the prophylaxis of bronchial asthma, allergic rhinitis and other disorders associated with mast-cell degranulation. The drug has different modes of action, such as inhibition of rat passive cutaneous anaphylaxis and the antigen-induced histamine release (HR) from passively sensitised peritoneal cells. Recently, clinical studies indicated that SCG has a direct effect on inflammatory cells, inhibiting either various leukocyte functions (membrane receptor expression, cytotoxic capacity) or in vitro activation of human neutrophils, eosinophils and monocytes [5, 6].

Since SCG is generally believed to inhibit HR from tissue mast cells, studies have tried to ascertain how this action takes place. The concept of mast cell heterogeneity, first proposed in 1966 by Enerbäck, is therefore of great relevance [7]. His studies, in demonstrating fixation differences between the connective tissue and GI mast cell, suggested that their granule content was not the same, showing the existence of functional differences. Subsequent in vitro comparisons of rat peritoneal and intestinal mast cells supported the concept of heterogeneity by demonstrating striking differences in their responses to certain pharmacological agents. Also in humans, two types of mast cells have been described. One which is present predominantly in the lung and GI mucosa contains only tryptase (T mast cell) and seems most similar to the rodent MMC (mucosal mast cell). The other type contains both tryptase and chymase (TC mast cell), is present predominantly in the skin and GI submucosa and appears most similar to the rodent peritoneal mast cell. SCG appears to inhibit HR only in rat peritoneal mast cells, and in addition human mast cells can vary in their response to the drug [8]. Several studies examined the possibility that human mast cell populations could be distinguished by their responses to pharmacological manipulations of HR in the same manner as in the rat. An effect of SCG on human intestinal MMC was demonstrated that elicited a maximal inhibition of 20% HR, but this event could also be caused by an effect on a small contaminating connective tissue mast cell population. In addition, there was a marked difference between the effect of SCG on bronchoalveolar lavage-derived mast cells and those obtained from dispersed lung, the latter being poorly inhibited by SCG [8]. In a recent study [9] no significant functional or pharmacological differences were found between the human lung and GI mast cells, and this agrees with indications that both tissues may contain a mix of cells with a variety of granule contents. It is therefore possible that cells in different stages of activation or maturity may express different cell products or sensitivity to pharmacological agents [9]. This variability can explain different results of studies employing SCG and not a non-existent "functional heterogeneity". Clinical studies in patients with systemic mastocytosis and successfully treated with SCG [10] may support the theory according to which the drug acts by inhibiting HR from mast cells.

Laboratory Data

Clinical studies have shown that SCG is able to reduce significantly the absorption of macromolecules, apparently inhibiting mediator release from the sensitised mast cells in the GI mucosa. Six patients slightly sensitive to egg were challenged with oral ovalbumin (100 mg/kg) without and with SCG treatment, 400 mg daily in four doses for 7 days. After the first challenge, the patients exhibited symptoms such as urticaria, itching, diarrhoea, pain and swelling of the joints and/or detectable amounts of serum ovalbumin. After SCG treatment, the second challenge induced weaker symptoms in two patients, and less albumin was detected in the serum. Several studies have reported the use of SCG in FA patients, in whom food produces immune complexes (IC). In all these studies, oral SCG prior to food challenge prevented both the symptoms and IC formation. To evaluate the GI permeability in 22 children, half of whom were allergic and half healthy, the 6-h urinary recovery of different-sized polyethylene glycols was measured before and after SCG administration. While no difference was noted between the two groups before the trial, after SCG was given a significant decrease in uptake was observed in the FA children. These results implied that after SCG treatment the permeability properties of the intestine of the affected children returned to normal. Recently, sugar absorption has been employed as a diagnostic tool in different GI disorders. Normally, lactulose is not absorbed by the GI mucosa, whereas mannitol crosses its barrier. Because of these properties, measurements of urine mannitol and lactulose have been performed as noninvasive means of evaluating the state of the GI mucosa in celiac disease and of diagnosing FA. In FA patients, a reduction in mannitol absorption and an increase in lactulose absorption have been demonstrated after challenge tests. In addition, SCG in water solution at a dose of 300 mg 15 min before challenge with the offending food is able to reduce significantly the absorption of lactulose and to increase the absorption of mannitol [11].

Put together, these data suggest that SCG acts by inhibiting mast cell degranulation in the gut, thus reducing the gut permeability for food allergens.

Table 1. Clinical trials with sodium cromoglycate in the management of atopic eczema in children

Author	Year	*n*	Age (years)	Study	Dose/day (mg)	duration of therapy	ST	RAST	Challenge	Eval.	Effic.
Shaw [17]	75	1	6	o	nr	nr	nd	nd	o	cha	yes
Molkhou and Waguet [18]	79	39	0.5–12	o	100–600	1–3 mo	nd	+	o	cha	yes
Cavagni et al. [19]	81	13	1–9	o	800	1.5 mo	+	+	o	cl	yes
Atherton et al. [13]	82	30	2–10	ddb	400	1 mo	nd	nd	o	cha	no
Molkhou and Waguet [20]	82	40	nr	db	200–800	2 mo	nd	nd	o	cha	yes
Harris et al. [14]	83	29	7	o	100–200	1 wk	+	+	db	cl	?
Giannetti et al. [15]	84	11	1–14	db	40	1.5 mo	nd	nd	nd	cl	yes
Graham et al. [21]	84	29	3–12	db	nr	1.5 mo	–	+	nd	cl	no
Corrias et al. [23]	85	20	0.5–10	b	40	1.5 mo	+	+	o	cl	yes
Boner et al. [22]	85	28	0.5–9	o	200–1600	1.5 mo	nd	nd	o	cl	yes
Businco et al. [12]	86	31	0.5–10	db	400–1600	2 mo	+	+	o	cha	yes
Burks and Sampson [16]	88	10	3–15	db	40	1 wk	+	nd	db	cha	no

st, skin tests; o, open; b, blind; db, double-blind; nd, not done; nr, not reported; cha, challenge

Clinical Data

Although SCG has been widely used for the management of respiratory allergy, conflicting results of FA treatment have been reported by several investigators since the first report in which it was shown that SCG pretreatment of a soy-allergic patient gave no protection when the drug was inhaled, whereas oral treatment with 400 mg blocked either the immediate or the late reaction. Twelve papers on the use of SCG in the management of children with FA have been reviewed. They included 281 children aged 0.5–15 years affected by AE (Table 1) [11].

The analysis of the 12 studies shows that 5 were carried out in open, 1 in single-blind and 6 in double-blind fashion. The children were selected as follows: in 6 skin tests were done (5 yielded positive results and 1 negative) and in 6, RAST (positive in all cases); the clinical efficiency of SCG was evaluated in 6 with challenge tests, and in the remaining 6 the evaluation was clinical. The dosage of SCG employed in the trial was not reported by 5 studies. Of the 13 remaining trials, one employed a dosage of 100 mg/day, one of 150, one of 200, one between 100 and 200, one between 100 and 600, one 400, one 600, one 800, one between 200 and 800 and one between 200 and 1600 mg. The remaining studies employed a dosage based on body weight (30–40 mg/kg bw). The duration of the trial was not reported by 3 studies. It was less than 1 month in 5, varied betweeen 1 and 3 months in 7, between 3 and 6 months in 2. In another one the duration was longer than 1 year. Four out of five studies in the open fashion yielded positive results, that is, SCG was effective in the management of AE. The double-blind studies were positive in 3 and negative in 3. The only trial with doubtful results was conducted in the open fashion [12–23] (Table 1).

Figures 1–6 show the result of a double-blind crossover trial with oral SCG in 31 children with AE due to FA [12]. The children under study were divided into two groups: those receiving SCG first, followed by placebo, and those receiving placebo first. Analysis of the different groups showed marked variations.

Figures 1 and 2 show the severity of AE (scale 0 to 240) assessed by the clinician at each clinic visit using body diagrams. Figure 1 indicates the patients who received the treatments in the oral SCG-placebo order: there is not any significant difference between treatments although there was a trend in favour of SCG at the end of the challenge period. Figure 2 indicates the patients who received the treatment in the placebo-oral SCG order: at the end of the diet period there was a significant difference in favour of oral SCG ($P < 0.05$). This difference between the two treatment order groups could be due to a carry-over therapeutic effect of oral SCG.

Figures 3 and 4 show the mean total daily diary card scores (scale 0 to 12) for each treatment phase as assessed

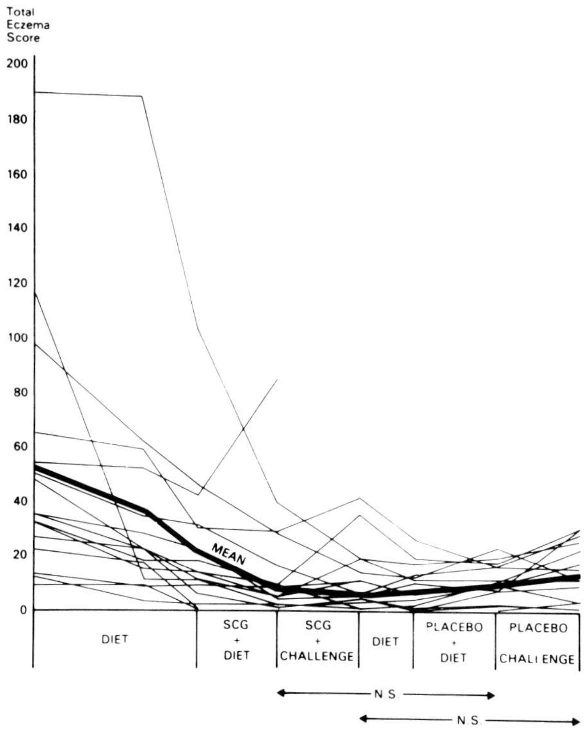

Fig. 1. Mean of total symptom scores assessed by clinician (body diagrams) in the oral SCG-placebo order group

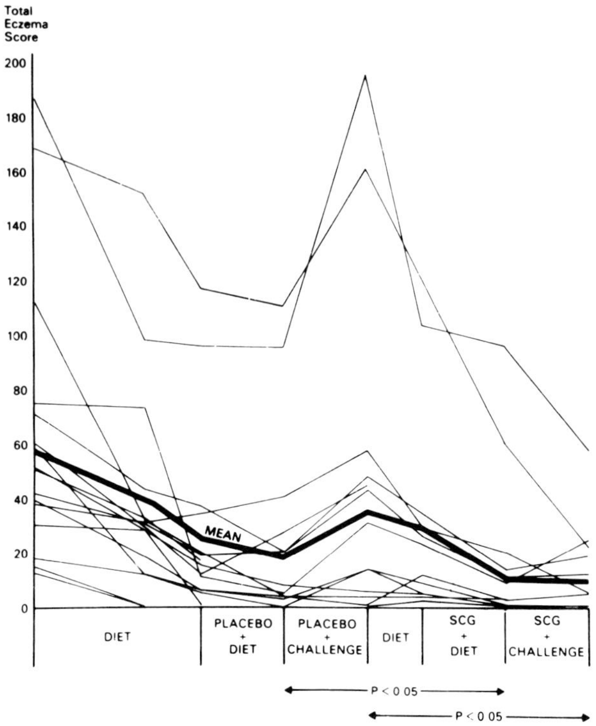

Fig. 2. Mean of total symptom scores assessed by clinician (body diagrams) in the placebo-oral SCG order group

by the parents. Figure 3 shows the oral SCG-placebo order group: there is no significant difference between treatments. Figure 4 shows the placebo-oral SCG order group: at the end of the elimination diet period there was a significant difference in favour of SCG ($P < 0.01$). At the end of the challenge period there was also a significant difference in favour of SCG ($P < 0.01$).

Considering all patients as a whole and using either the clinician assessment by body diagrams or the parent assessment by diary cards, there is an overall significant difference between oral SCG and placebo during both the diet and the challenge phase of the trial. The best overall clinical assessment of the eczema was at the end of the treatment period of oral SCG with an elimination diet (mean value = 9.5), which was significantly better ($P < 0.05$) than the one at the end of placebo and elimination diet period (mean value = 13.3). At the end of the challenge phase, oral SCG had proved to be significantly better (mean = 7.7) than placebo (mean = 22.5) in preventing the symptom exacerbation caused by food reintroduction ($P < 0.01$) (Fig. 5). The same situation applies to the analysis of parents' daily diary cards. Overall, oral SCG and elimination diet were significantly ($P < 0.05$) better (mean value = 1.19) than placebo and elimination diet (mean = 1.9) in giving the lowest symptom score (Fig. 6). For the other parameters (use of test medications, antihistamine usage, other symptoms) there were no significant differences between the two treatments.

At the end of the trial and before the code was broken, both parents and clinicians recorded their opinions as to which treatment was considered by them to be more effective. In the parent/patient's opinions, there was a significant difference in favour of SCG for the placebo-SCG order group. In the clinician's opinion, there was a significant difference in favour of SCG both for individual order groups and overall, the difference being highly significant ($P < 0.001$) for the placebo-SCG order group and overall [12].

There have been a number of publications on the use of oral SCG in children with AE and/or FA. The data in the present study have shown that it is effective in the prevention of IgE-mediated FA. However, several studies yielded doubtful or negative results [13–16].

As already reported by previous studies, there are several explanations for the conflicting results of SCG in FA. The discrepancy of observations may be dependent upon several factors such as different selection criteria of patients, the wide variations in daily dosage of SCG used by various investigators, the different amount of food antigens ingested by the patients during the trials depending upon the varying diet followed, the diversity in the evaluation of SCG efficacy, problems regarding patient compliance and side effects.

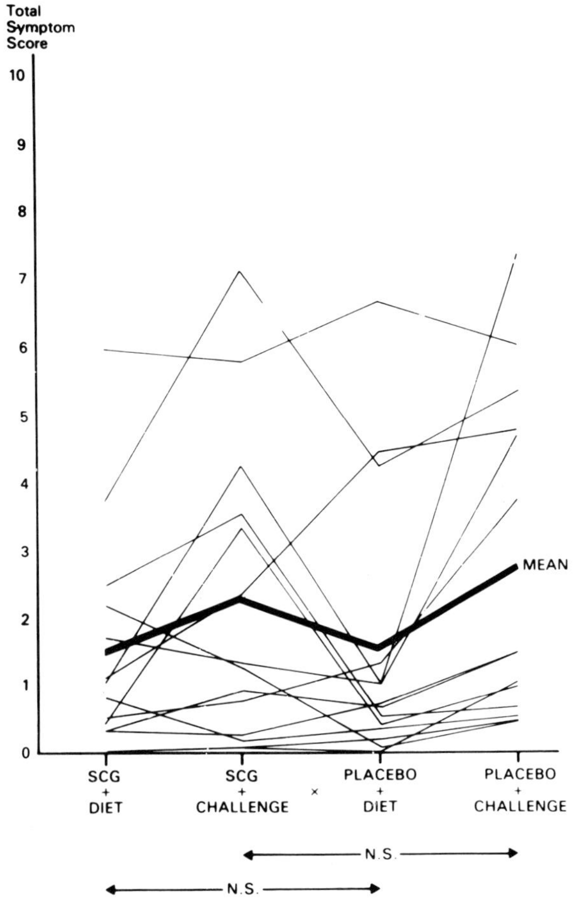

Fig. 3. Mean of daily symptom scores assessed by parents (diary cards) in the oral SCG-placebo order group

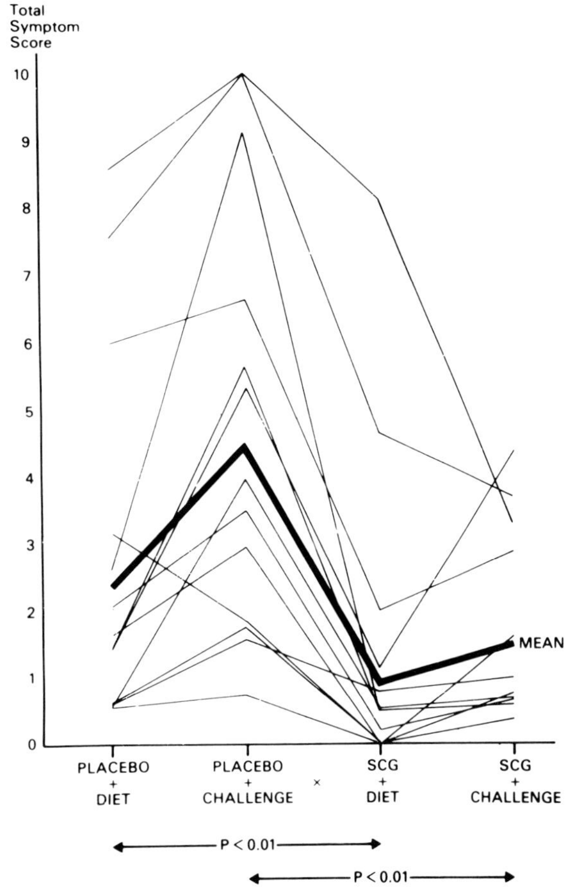

Fig. 4. Mean of daily symptom scores assessed by parents (diary cards) in the placebo-oral SCG order group

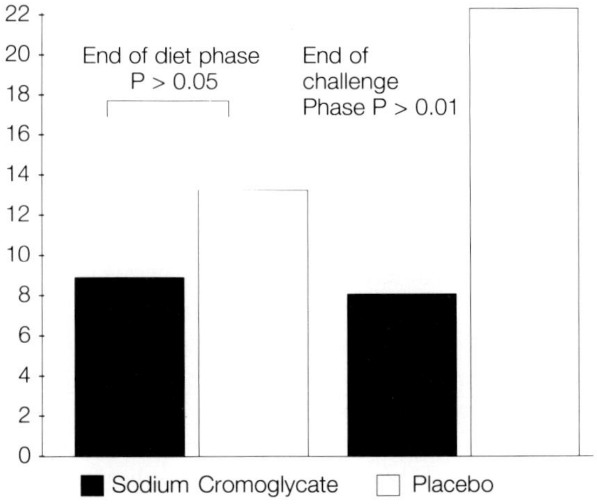

Fig. 5. Mean of total symptom scores assessed by clinicians at the end of the diet and challenge periods, while children were receiving either placebo or SCG

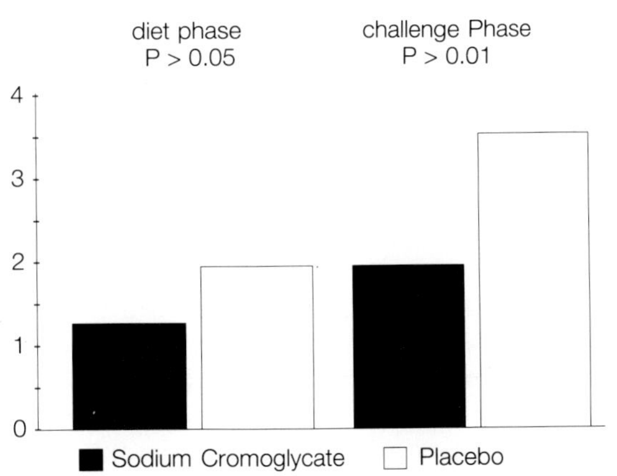

Fig. 6. Mean of daily symptom scores assessed by the parents at the end of the diet and challenge periods, while children were receiving either placebo or SCG

We stress that children to be treated with SCG should be strictly selected according to well-defined criteria. This should initially be done in order to assess whether they have definitive clinical and immunological findings of IgE-mediated FA. As regards the clinical findings, Burks and Sampson in a very elegant study [16] recently failed to confirm SCG efficacy in 10 children with AE and egg hypersensitivity. However, two patients had no symptoms of AE at the time of the study, and one only slight signs (symptom score = 3). It seems to be very difficult to draw conclusions from a study including 7 children treated only for 7 days.

Another cause of conflicting results regards the different study designs. Many studies, for example, have employed widely varying SCG dosages. However, the dosage in the range of 30–50 mg/kg daily seems to be most effective. Several studies yielding doubtful or negative results employed much lower SCG dosages, which could have prevented a (more) positive result.

As far as the treatment schedules are concerned, SCG was administered during some trials when patients were following an elimination diet, during other studies when they were on a normal, unrestricted diet. Since it is already known that SCG exerts its action only in the sense of prevention, its use in patients given widely differing diets may meet with varying success. In this sense, it may be clear why Atherton et al. [13] failed to obtain positive results, since we cannot evaluate the amount of food antigens ingested by children on a normal diet.

Differing evaluations of SCG efficacy may also yield controversial data. An evaluation based upon a challenge test is more objective than a clinical evaluation of the severity score.

Conflicting results can also arise when the compliance of either the parents or the children is required. When SCG is available in the form of capsules, children may object that they find them difficult to swallow. However, the alternative is to dissolve the capsules in a little hot water and dilute this to ½ cupful with cold water or another suitable liquid, and the resulting drink must be swilled around the mouth, so that the buccal mucous membrane is coated before the drug is swallowed, and this procedure must be repeated four times a day before meals. Moreover, most children attend daycare nurseries from the age of 2–4, and the institution cannot ensure special therapies. Tea parties and picnics are also good occasions for such omissions.

Studies on Ketotifen

Laboratory Data

Clinical and immunological investigations tend to demonstrate that ketotifen, a tricyclic benzocycloheptathiophene derivative with anti-anaphylactic and antihistamine activities, is a drug able to play a role in IgE-dependent as well as in non-IgE-mediated mechanisms [24].

The compound protects against IgE-mediated passive anaphylactic reactions in guinea pigs, inhibits the increase in lung resistance in sensitised rats and guinea pigs challenged with antigen, prevents 48/80-induced HR from peritoneal mast cells and inhibits anti-IgE-induced release of both histamine and slow reacting substance of anaphylaxis (SRS-A) from human basophils. The most important functional property of ketotifen relies on the blocking of slow calcium channels and restoration of tachyphylaxis. It has also been studied as a possible inhibitor of human neutrophil activation induced by platelet-activating factor (PAF)-acether [25, 26].

Recently, ketotifen has been reported to inhibit the PAF-induced increase in bronhical responsiveness in the guinea pig model [27]. In addition, ketotifen treatment significantly inhibited the flare areas and the wheal volumes induced either by PAF or histamine [27].

In vitro studies have demonstrated that one of the novel modes of ketotifen action is the inhibition of eosinophil degranulation attributable to the release of cytotoxic major basic protein as observed in a CMA patient, manifested as bronchial asthma. In addition, ketotifen is able to inhibit in vitro direct and antibody-dependent allergic autocytotoxicity (ACT) induced by challenge with food antigens in patients sensitive to corn, wheat and cow's milk. The observed dose-dependent linear inhibition in ACT suggests the existence of a ketotifen cellular binding protein [28].

Further investigation of human neutrophils elicited that ketotifen is a potent inhibitor of leukotriene production and release from leukocytes. In 15 patients suffering from FA and food intolerance, ketotifen showed after treatment a significant inhibitory effect on autologous mixed lymphocyte reaction [29].

Miyasato [30] by demonstrating that ketotifen decreases peripheral eosinophils and that this effect is directly related to the improvement of allergic manifestations, attempted to elucidate the clinical significance of the increased blood eosinophils in atopic diseases by determining quantitative dynamic changes in this cell population. The author measured the density distribution in the peripheral blood and evaluated the eosinophil morphology. Ten patients with AE received 2 mg of ketotifen for 2 weeks. The results showed that following clinical improvement the number of peripheral eosinophils was significantly decreased compared with controls. After the measurement of density distribution by Nicodenz density gradient, it was found that the rate of decrease of hypodense eosinophils was notable. Consequently, the author suggested that if ketotifen is able to decrease hypodense eosinophils, which are activated eosinophils, and can also inhibit the eosinophil activation in vivo, one could also suppose that this inhibitory effect of the drug may be a factor of the ketotifen-induced clinical improvement.

Clinical Data

Several investigators in open and double-blind studies have confirmed the efficacy of ketotifen in patients sensitised to a spectrum of foods and suffering after ingestion from various skin, nasal, conjunctival, respiratory and GI disorders [28]

In adults, ketotifen was shown to protect atopic patients from FA after 5 days of treatment in one open, uncontrolled [31] after 14 days in one double-blind, placebo-controlled [32] and after 1 month in a randomised, double-blind, placebo-controlled study [33].

Molkou and Dupont [28] studied 16 children aged 3.5 months – 15 years, of whom 10 suffered from AE, 3 from asthma, 3 from urticaria, 1 from allergic rhinitis, 1 from angioedema and 2 from GI symptoms. In this open, uncontrolled study, ketotifen was administred for 2–20 months. In children with AE, 70% were greatly improved and 30% remained unchanged, while all children suffering from other atopic disorders were completely protected.

In a second, open, uncontrolled study, 17 children with a median age of 4.6 ± 0.9 years with severe AE unresponding to diet were treated for 12 weeks with ketotifen. Symptoms were effectively decreased by treatment, the improvement being statistically significant by the 2nd month of treatment [34].

In another, open, uncontrolled study we evaluated 21 children (aged 10 months–12 years) with AE after a 3-month treatment with ketotifen. Patients were selected on the basis of FA being a causative factor of AE exacerbations, and the offending food(s) were identified during the diagnostic period. During the first 3 weeks of treatment children were given ketotifen while on an elimination diet. During the second and third month of therapy they consumed offending food(s) in the same amounts which induced AE exacerbations during the diagnostic period. Ketotifen significantly reduced the severity of AE exacerbations following the ingestion of offending foods, therefore allowing a less restricted diet for 14 of 21 children (66,6%) [35].

In conclusion, the management of children with AE is a challenge for pediatricians, dermatologists and allergists. The multifactorial origin of the disease makes its management very difficult. As reported in the present paper, the results obtained by different authors using either SCG or ketotifen are rather controversial. However, a short course (1–2 months) of these drugs should be tried in childen with AE associated with FA.

References

1. Businco L, Benincori N, Cantani A (1984) Epidemiology, incidence and clinical aspects of food allergy. In: Reinhardt MC, Bellanti JA, Rossi E (eds) Food allergies and intolerances: a Nestlé Foundation workshop. Lausanne, 7–9 Sept 1983. Ann Allergy 53:615
2. Sampson HA (1988) Immunologically mediated food allergy: the importance of food challenge procedures. Ann Allergy 60:262
3. Businco L, Benincori N, Cantani A (1986) The spectrum of food allergy in infancy and childhood. Ann Allergy 57:213
4. Businco L, Cantani A, Monteleone AM, Ziruolo MG (1988) Atopic dermatitis in children: an update. Folia Allergol Immunol Clin 35:41
5. Kay AB, Walsh GM, Moqbel R et al. (1987) Disodium cromoglycate inhibits activation of human inflammatory cells in vitro. J Allergy Clin Immunol 80:1
6. Skedinger MC, Augustine NH, Morris EZ et al. (1987) Effect of disodium cromoglycate on neutrophil movement and intracellular calcium mobilization. J Allergy Immunol 80:573
7. Enerbäck L (1966) Mast cells in rat gastrointestinal mucosa. II. Dye binding and metachromatic properties. Acta Pathol Microbial Scand A 66:303
8. Bienenstock J (1988) An update on mast cell heterogeneity. J Allergy Clin Immunol 81:763
9. Fox CC, Wolf EJ, Kagey-Sobotka A, Lichtenstein LM (1988) Comparison of human lung and intestinal mast cells. J Allergy Clin Immunol 81:89
10. Businco L, Cantani A, Businco E, Pepys J (1984) Systemic mastocytosis in a 5-year-old child: Successful treatment with disodium cromoglycate. Clin Allergy 14:147
11. Businco L, Cantani A, Meglio P, Giampietro PG (1990) Sodium cromoglycate in the management of food allergy in children. In: Harms HK, Wahn U (eds) Food allergy in infancy and childhood. Springer, Berlin Heidelberg New York

12. Businco L, Benincori N, Cantani A et al. (1986) Double-blind crossover trial with oral sodium cromoglycate in children with atopic dermatitis due to food allergy. Ann Allergy 57:433
13. Atherton DJ, Soothill JF, Elvidge J (1982) A controlled trial of oral sodium cromoglycate in atopic eczema. Br J Dermatol 126:681–685
14. Harris JM, Graham P, Hall-Smith SP et al. (1983) The use of sodium cromoglycate and exclusion diets in childhood atopic eczema. Proceedings of the 2nd Fisons Food Allergy Workshop. Harrogate, 19–21 Jan 1983. Medicine Publishing Foundation, Oxford, p 111
15. Giannetti A, Lembo G,Zanoletti T et al. (1984) Il disodiocromoglicato nella dermatite atopica. G Ital Dermatol Venereol 119:365
16. Burks AW, Sampson HA (1988) Double-blind placebo-controlled trial of oral cromolyn in children with atopic dermatitis and documented food hypersensitivity. J Allergy Clin Immunol 81:471
17. Shaw RF (1975) Cromolyn therapy in chronic infantile eczema. Arch Dermatol 3:1537
18. Molkhou P, Waguet JC (1979) Oral disodium cromoglycate in the treatment of atopic eczema in children. In: Pepys J, Edwards AM (eds) The mast cell: its role in health and disease. Pitman Medical, Bath, p 617
19. Cavagni G, Paganelli R, Rigoli E (1985) SCG effect on macromolecular absorption of food antigens in atopic dermatitis (AD). Pediatr Res 19:1119
20. Molkhou P, Waguet JC (1982) Atopic dermatitis in children and food allergy. Mechanisms of action of oral sodium cromoglycate. Communication 2nd International Symposium on Immunological and Clinical Problems of Food Allergy. Milan, Italy, Oct 1982
21. Graham P, Hall-Smith SP, Harris JM et al (1984) A study of hypoallergenic diets and oral sodium cromoglycate in the management of atopic eczema. Br J Dermatol 110:457
22. Boner AL, Valletta EA, Antolini I et al (1985) Trattamento della dermatite atopica con sodiocromoglicato in bambini non selezionati per allergia alimentare. Minerva Pediatr 37:263
23. Corrias A, Rossi G, Orani S et al (1985) Terapia con DSCG nell'allergia alimentare dell'infanzia. Minerva Pediatr 37: 453
24. Oehling A, Ona J, Wierna G et al. (1985) The inhibitory effect of ketotifen on in vitro histamine release in allergic patients. Allergol Immunopathol (Madr) 13:475
25. Craps LP (1985) Immunologic and therapeutic aspects of ketotifen. J Allergy Clin Immunol 76:389
26. Morley J, Page CP, Mazzoni L et al. (1986) Effects of ketotifen upon responser to platelet activating factor. A basis for asthma prophylaxis. Ann Allergy 56:335
27. Chung KF, Minette P, McCusker M, Barnes PJ (1988) Ketotifen inhibits the cutaneous but not the airway responses to platelet-activating factor in man. J Allerg Clin Immunol 81:1192
28. Molkou P, Dupont C (1987) Ketotifen in prevention and therapy of food allergy. Ann Allergy 59:187
29. André C (1986) Allergie alimentaire. Diagnostic objectif et test de l'efficacité thérapeutique par mesure de la perméabilité intestinale. Presse Méd 15:105
30. Miyasoto M (1988) Effect of ketotifen on density distribution of eosinophils in patients with atopic dermatitis. Inflammation 8:260
31. Neffen H, Oehling A, Subira ML (1980) A study of the protective effect of ketotifen in food allergy. Allergol Immunopathol (Madr) 8:97
32. Romanski B, Kurek M, Swiatkowski M (1982) Study of the protective action of Zaditen in cases of allergic disorders provoked by food allergy. In: Fuchs E, Halm D (eds) Asthma bronchiale, bronchiale Übererregbarkeit, Asthma Prophylaxe. Schattauer, Stuttgart, p 111
33. Boner AL, Richelli C, Antolini I et al. (1986) The efficacy of ketotifen in a controlled double-blind food challenge study in patients with food allergy. Ann Allergy 57:61
34. Fiocchi A, Riva E, Borella E et al (1985) Ketotifen treatment of atopic dermatitis in childhood. Curr Ther Res 37:1113
35. Benincori L, Ferrara M, Cantani A et al. (1988) Valutazione dell'efficacia del chetotifene nella prevenzione dell' esacerbazione della dermatite atopica da intolleranza alimentare del bambino. Folia Allergol Immunol 35:399

Significance of Climatic Factors in the Treatment of Atopic Eczema (Atopic Constitutional Neurodermatitis)

T. Steiger and S. Borelli

Historical Development of Climatotherapy

The description of bioclimatic influences and their therapeutic use may be traced back as far as the Sumerian-Babylonian era around 2000 BC. References to the favourable effects of sunbathing already exist in the writings of pre-Socratic philosophers. This natural philosophical disposition is the guiding principle to the epidemic books of Hippocrates (460–377 BC), which present empirical findings concerning the influence of seasons and atmospheric conditions. As well as case histories, volumes I and III of "epidemiorum" describe the relationship between disease and atmospheric conditions on the island Thasos over a 3-year period and give a brief report on the same topic following a 4-year study carried out elsewhere.

The experiences concerning the influence of climatic factors on health and disease collected during his various travels are outlined in περὶ ἀέρων, ὑδάτων, τόπων (de aere, aquis, locis) [66]. A change of climate accompanied by pharmaco-balneo-therapy was also customary under the ancient Romans. In cases of phthisis, Celsius (c. 30 BC–c. 50 AD), recommended such a change, e.g. from Italy to Alexandria. At the beginning of the second century AD, the theory that all diseases were basically due to excessive laxity ("status laxus") or tension ("status strictus") found expression in the writings of Soranus from Ephesus [36]. Here we have the first reference to μετασύνκρισις, the transforming effect of sea water on both "status laxus" and "status strictus" [87].

Galenos from Pergamon (129–c. 200 AD) took up the Hippocratic dogma concerning the omnipotence of phthisis, as expressed in his famous maxim: Ἰητρὸς γάρ ἐστιν ὑπηρέτης τῆς φύσεως (A doctor is the servant of Nature) [66].

After the long spell of the Middle Ages, the impetus for basic science research brought a revived interest in climatotherapy as the "ultimum refugium" especially for chronically ill patients. The English physician Russel (1700–1771) described the healing quality of sea water in his publication, "Dissertatio de tabe glandulari, sive de usu aquae marinae in morbis glandularum". The so-called Russel cure prescribes three dips in the sea, with the aid of a dipper. He transformed a small fishing village into the famous seaside resort, Brighton [40, 91]. The London doctor, Lettsom (1744–1815), born on a sugar plantation on the West Indian island, Tortola, laid the foundation stone for the building of the first sea hospital in Margate (Southern England) in 1792 [39]. On 20 July 1796, the Royal Sea Bathing Infirmary for the Relief of the Scrofulous Poor of London and All England was opened. It contained 30 beds. Following this example, sea hospices and sanatoriums for children sprang up along almost every European coast.

In 1794, von Vogel (1750–1830) incorporated sea bathing into therapy for the first time [91]. On 17 May 1797, the North sea health resort, Norderney, was founded, which together with Doberan near Rostock is the oldest German sea bathing resort. Other well-known sea bathing spots are Helgoland (1826), Borkum (1850) and Westerland auf Sylt (1855). Beneke (1824–1882), the pioneer of thalassotherapy in Germany, carried out the first climatotherapeutic investigations in Norderney during the winter of 1881/1882 [91]. In 1819 the oldest seaside resort, Wyk on Föhr, was founded among the north Fresian islands. A sea hospice sanatorium under the directorship of Drs. R. and F. Felten-Stoltzenberg was established in St. Peter-Ording in 1913. At this time, the indications for climatotherapy were tuberculosis and scrofulosis [see also 31].

The significance of natural heliotherapy had been described by Edwards in 1824 [33]. In 1856, Moleschott [65] studied the influence of light on nerve sensitivity. The healing quality of sunlight was confirmed in 1867 by the Englishman, Winslow [99].

The following years witnessed an interest in the topic climatotherapy in skin diseases. Figures 1 and 2 may serve to demonstrate the type of publications written by non-dermatologists such as Mehl [60], who developed the Mehlian Sun Therapy in 1894 and founded the heliosanatorium in Oranienburg near Berlin for skin and lupus disorders.

The scientifically based knowledge favoured mainly climates with a strong, stimulating effect, i.e. North sea islands or high mountainous climates (over 1500 m above sea level). This led to the founding of the first dermatological clinic in Norderney by Hartung in May 1953 [42, 67, 77].

The "Symposium Primum Dermatologicum Bulgariae", initiated by Popchristov and exclusively dedicated to

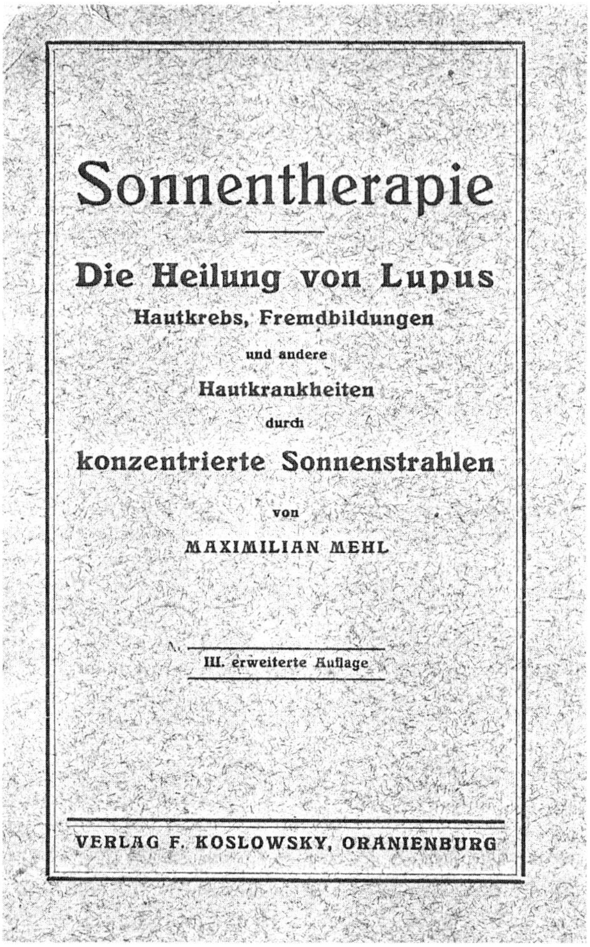
Sonnentherapie

Die Heilung von Lupus
Hautkrebs, Fremdbildungen
und andere
Hautkrankheiten
durch
konzentrierte Sonnenstrahlen
von
MAXIMILIAN MEHL

III. erweiterte Auflage

VERLAG F. KOSLOWSKY, ORANIENBURG

Fig. 1. Front cover of Mehl's (1896) publication on "sun therapy"

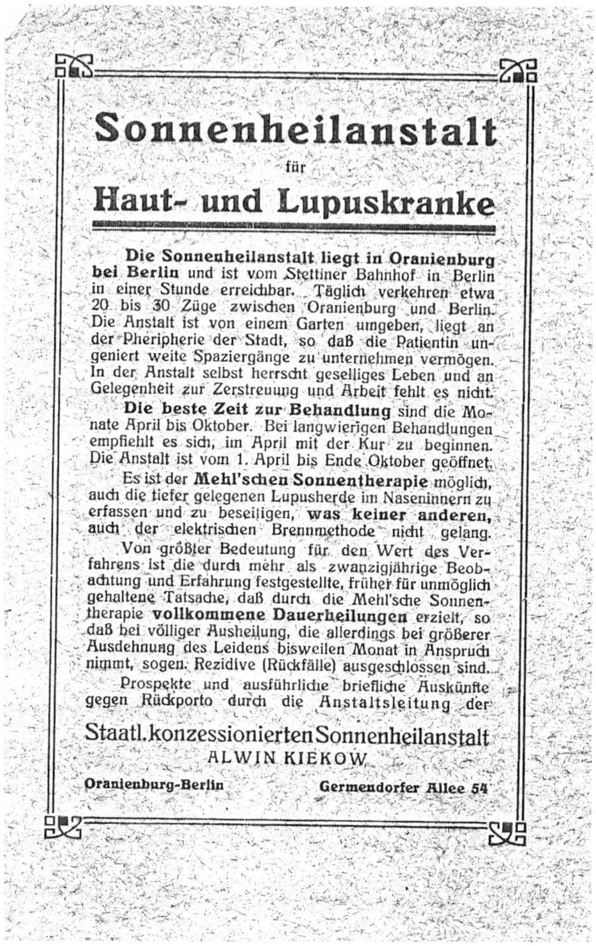
Sonnenheilanstalt
für
Haut- und Lupuskranke

Die Sonnenheilanstalt liegt in Oranienburg bei Berlin und ist vom Stettiner Bahnhof in Berlin in einer Stunde erreichbar. Täglich verkehren etwa 20 bis 30 Züge zwischen Oranienburg und Berlin. Die Anstalt ist von einem Garten umgeben, liegt an der Pheripherie der Stadt, so daß die Patientin ungeniert weite Spaziergänge zu unternehmen vermögen. In der Anstalt selbst herrscht geselliges Leben und an Gelegenheit zur Zerstreuung und Arbeit fehlt es nicht.

Die beste Zeit zur Behandlung sind die Monate April bis Oktober. Bei langwierigen Behandlungen empfiehlt es sich, im April mit der Kur zu beginnen. Die Anstalt ist vom 1. April bis Ende Oktober geöffnet.

Es ist der Mehl'schen Sonnentherapie möglich, auch die tiefer gelegenen Lupusherde im Naseninnern zu erfassen und zu beseitigen, was keiner anderen, auch der elektrischen Brennmethode nicht gelang.

Von größter Bedeutung für den Wert des Verfahrens ist die durch mehr als zwanzigjährige Beobachtung und Erfahrung festgestellte, früher für unmöglich gehaltene Tatsache, daß durch die Mehl'sche Sonnentherapie vollkommene Dauerheilungen erzielt, so daß bei völliger Ausheilung, die allerdings bei größerer Ausdehnung des Leidens bisweilen Monat in Anspruch nimmt, sogen. Rezidive (Rückfälle) ausgeschlossen sind.

Prospekte und ausführliche briefliche Auskünfte gegen Rückporto durch die Anstaltsleitung der

Staatl. konzessionierten Sonnenheilanstalt
ALWIN KIEKOW
Oranienburg-Berlin Germendorfer Allee 54

Fig. 2. Back cover of "sun therapy"

dermatological climatotherapy, took place in Sofia in 1962 [sea also 56]. This conference was the occasion for the first directive resolution concerning the significance of climatotherapy and its value for suitable indications.

Marchionini and Borelli [58] carried out preinvestigations with neurodermatitic patients from Istanbul, prescribing climatotherapy at an altitude of 1800 m in a hotel in the Bythinic Olymp. On his return to Germany, further investigations in collaboration with Borelli [58, 59] were done, first from Hamburg to the North Sea, later from Munich to the Bavarian Alpine regions, the Austrian Alps and Switzerland (Samedan at St. Morritz), and on 1 April 1961 the German Dermatological Department (now Clinic for Dermatology and Allergy, Davos; Alexanderhaus Klinik) was established in the German state-owned Sanatorium Valbella, in Davos, Graubuenden/Switzerland (1560 m high) [12, 13, 21, 58, 59].

"This was the first opportunity for German patients suffering from chronic skin diseases and allergies to undergo hospitalised high Alpine therapy in such a region as Davos – since such favourable conditions do not exist in Germany – irrespective of health insurance [12, 13]".

Treatment Through Climate

Climatotherapy differentiates between therapy through climate and therapy in climate [29, 53].

Definition of Terms

The word "climate" can be traced back to Aristoteles (384–322 BC), who used the word to describe the propensity of the surface of the earth towards the sun's rays (το κλίμα = region, district; κλίνω = I tend) [66]. In *Cosmos*, A. v. Humboldt (1769–1859) defines climate as "all atmospheric changes having a noticeable effect on our organs" [24, 49].

This definition was still attributed to humans at the beginning of the twentieth century. For Rubner [86] "climate" means "all environmental influences on the health", whilst Loewy [57] defines climate as "the sum of all atmospheric and terrestrial conditions typical of a location, through which our state of health is immediately influenced".

The generally held current definition of climate is "the entire meteorological phenomena which defines the mean state of the atmosphere in any given place of the earth over a long period of time" [56].

The so-called climatic factors, or weather factors, are present in measurable quantities for the characterisation of the climate. Basically, one differentiates between natural and anthropogenous climatological influencing factors. The first to be calculated are:

- Air pressure (oxygen partial pressure)
- Air temperature
- Humidity
- Depression (rain, snow, hail, fog)
- Wind (force, direction, speed)
- Heat and radiation (ultraviolet rays, visible light, diffuse celestial light, infrared light)
- Aerosol

These climatic factors are mostly place-related, i.e. there is a dependence on the respective geographical degree of latitude, altitude and orography. Additionally, the nature of the ground, distribution of land and water and the season are all significant [88].

In contrast to the countryside, anthropogenous climatic factors represent the extremely variable climate of cities and crowded areas, industrial and transportation installations emanating exhaust fumes, waste heat and dust as well as forestry measures, clearance, irrigation and drainage.

A climatic assessment of a place will depend on the aforementioned meteorological factors, especially temperature. Accordingly, the classification into tropical (mean annual temperature 20°–30°C), moderate (0°–20°C) and polar (+2°C) climates is in accordance with the geographical zones [71]. This may be explained as the dependency of the temperature of a place on its geographical situation.

The differentiation between spatial climate and compact climate is useful for determining the climatic dependence of AE. Spatial climate includes interior, marine, coastal, moderately high and high mountainous climate. The degree of stimulus produced by one or several of these will largely depend on the type of disease responding to a particular stimulus.

Compact climate is significant insofar as it can exert an unfavourable influence on the favourable effects of spatial climate. Orography and vegetation and also the infrastructure of a city (industrial plants, etc.) are largely characteristic of a compact climate.

The systematic investigations of Marchionini and Borelli [58] demonstrated the effects of a change of climate. Inhabitants living in flat areas are strongly stimulated by mountainous regions and vice versa. The deciding factor is a radical change of climate.

Stimulating or protective climate may be used to refer to the original climate of the patient (analogous to mountain sickness or low plane sickness as extreme variants of a climatic stimulus). Every climate has a stimulating effect on the organism. It has therefore proved appropriate to classify the various climatic regions according to medically effective degrees of stimulus. The Team for Climatic Issues, engaged by the Internal Department of Switzerland in 1951 and affiliated to the Federal Health Department, determined the degrees of climatic stimulation and classification of climatic health resorts (or, as in Germany curative climatic health resorts) in the context of medical bioclimatology. They are hereafter defined as

> localities, parts of such and in special circumstances individual sanatoriums, where climatic curative factors obtain. These factors must exert a suitably transforming effect on the human organism, thus influencing a disease or disposition towards disease or promote recovery and strength so that regeneration or improvement of health, performance and working ability can be expected.

Individual climatic health resorts are classified according to mean annual protective and stimulating factors as follows: grade 0 (protective climate) to 3 (stimulating climate).

Grade 0. This climatic health resort has protective climate with general effects as follows: sedative, protective; calming and stimulation of the sympathetic and parasympathetic nervous systems, respectively; maximal protection of the heart and circulation; convalescent treatment for breathing; reduction of metabolic processes; modest demand for heat production; modest demand for blood supply and secretion of mucus membrane; sedative effect on the nervous system.

Stimulation Grade 1. This climatic health resort has mild stimulating factors with general effects as follows: sedative, mildly stimulating; mild to moderate stimulation of the sympathetic nervous system and mainly stimulation of the parasympathetic nervous system; protective adjustment and – depending on altitude – moderate to complete stimulation of the organism; heart, circulation, breathing and metabolism are subjected to less strain and simultaneously stimulated; there is less demand on heat production; has a calming effect on the nervous system.

Stimulation Grade 2. This climatic health resort has moderate to powerful stimulating factors with general effects as follows: moderate to vigorously stimulating; marked stimulation of the sympathetic nervous system and simultaneous stimulation of the parasympathetic nervous system; stimulation of circulation and respiration; change in metabolic processes and endocrine system; moderate to powerful stimulation of the nervous system; stimulation of blood production; increase in functional capacity.

Stimulation Grade 3. This climatic health resort has intensive stimulating factors and often bracing winds, with general effects as follows: vigorously stimulating; intensive stimulation of the sympathetic nervous system and simultaneously moderate to non-existent stimulation of the parasympathetic nervous system; intensive stimulation of organic resistance; invigoration of circulation, breathing and metabolism; stimulation of blood production; increase in functional capacity [95].

Inspection of the climatic resort by a medical practitioner is recommended for grade 2 and is obligatory in grade 3.

Significance of Meteorlogical Factors

In view of the overall effect of the various climatic factors and the difficulty in assigning a specific effect to individual factors, a broad classification of complexes of effects has proved useful, in accordance with Wiedemann [98]:

- Thermohygric complex of effects
- Photo-actinic complex of effects
- Atmospheric/air chemical complex of effects

Thermohygric Complex of Effects

The thermohygric complex of effects includes climatic factors such as air temperature, humidity, wind speed (convection) and heat rays (solar and diffuse celestial rays). The temperature changes transmitted via thermoreceptors to the thermal regulatory centres in the hypothalamus and formatio reticularis can trigger off a circulatory reaction.

The climatic therapeutic significance of the thermohygric complex of effect in atopic constitutional neurodermatitis lies in the stabilisation of the circulatory regulation and functional improvement of the circulation in the capillaries of the skin. The circadian rhythm of heat regulation is also significant. A constant heat supply produces maximum perspiration at night and a minimum quantity in the morning.

Photo-actinic Complex of Effects

The photo-actinic complex of effects includes cosmic radiation, gamma radiation, X-radiation, ultraviolet radiation (UV-A, UV-B, UV-C), visible light, infrared radiation and long-wave high-frequency radiation (wave length 6–100 km). A central position collects the ultraviolet radiation of the wavelengths 280–315 nm (UV-B) and 315–400 nm (UV-A). The boundary between ultraviolet light (UV-A) and ultraviolet radiation (UV-B) lies at 315 nm according to DIN and CIE (Commission Internationale d'Eclairage). In the American literature, this boundary is extended to 320 nm. Attempts are being made to extend the UV-B area to 340 nm since the waves between 315 and 340 nm could produce further biological reactions. In the USA, ultraviolet light is subdivided into UV-A_1 (340–400 nm) and UV-A_2 (320–340 nm). Short wave UV-C (200–280 nm) is absorbed by the ozone layer of the stratosphere. According to current information, this layer is endangered through halogenated fuel gases (fluoric-chloric-carburetted hydrogen gas). There is a dual effect: heat is held in the lower layers of the atmosphere whilst the protection against life-threatening ultraviolet radiation diminishes. According to the latest reports from the Federal Commission of Enquiry, the fading of the ozone layer over the Antarctic has meanwhile attained a dimension which covers an area the size of the USA. At a height of 15–20 km the degree of destruction amounts to about 95% at certain times.

The influence of UV light depends on the wavelength, exposure, geographical latitude, situation of the sun, time of day and year as well as height above sea level. Immunosuppression, stimulation of haemopoiesis and hypophysis as well as increased phagocytic index are its known effects on the organism.

About two-thirds of UV-B rays are absorbed or reflected in the stratum corneum, and 16% reach the stratum granulosum of the epidermis [1]. There they are absorbed by the nucleic acids of the cell nucleus, exerting an inhibiting effect on DNA, RNA, protein synthesis and mitosis. Above all, UV-B is responsible for the development of skin cancer and sunburn.

UV-A rays penetrate more deeply into the skin, to about 1% of the epidermis. Due to their limited energy content, they are less biologically active and are mainly responsible for skin tan. From the so-called photo-addition (photoaugmentation) effect, they are likely to aggravate UV-B-induced skin damage [48].

The latest investigations reveal that infrared radiation has a carcinogenic effect. Extensive exposure to infrared rays causes an immediate reddening of the skin (erythema ab igne), which over a long period of time can lead to chronic heat rash and skin cancer (known as Kang cancer in China, caused by sleeping on hot tiles). Above all, due to the effect of photoaugmentation, infrared radiation intensifies the effect of other radiation on the skin [83].

Air Chemical Complex of Effects

Elements of the air chemical complex of effects include the major atmospheric gases (nitrogen, oxygen and carbon dioxide), trace gases (inert gases, hydrogen, iodine, ammonia), water vapour, impurities such as aerosols, condensation particles and pollutive gases, the most significant of which are sulphur dioxide, nitric oxide and carbon monoxide.

It is well-known that with increasing altitude the oxygen partial pressure decreases by approximately 21% when the oxygen component of the air remains constant. This is one of the specific climatic factors of high mountainous regions. Plants produce oxygen by means of assimilation. The distribution of respiratory gases therefore depends not only on the altitude but also on the vegetation.

Aerosols form a further significant climatic factor. This is generally conceived of a gas in which liquid or solid particles are finely distributed (dispersed). These floating particles, also known as condensation nuclei, are hygroscopic and swell in the moisturised respiratory air of the bronchii to twice their diameter on average. Aerosols are also present in pollen and spores of plants. Since they function as inhalational allergens, they can induce asthma and hay fever.

The production of aerosol in maritime surfing zones is a significant therapeutic factor in that aerosol comes in with the tide and is deposited on the sand. Depending on the natural differences in the size of its particles (heterodispersive aerosol), it may reach the small bronchi and alveoli. A spell in a surfing zone will improve the muco-ciliary transport and secretolysis in the bronchial system. On the island of Norderney, numerous investigations using the Tiffeneau (lung function) test in children and adults with obstructive respiratory disease demonstrated forced expectoration and freer breathing, resulting in improved lung ventilation [63].

The increasing concentration of pollutive gases is a consequence of combustion processes (industry, heating, motor cars) and is frequently typical of cities or crowded areas with high populations [23]. Pollution of the atmosphere has a damaging effect on the mucous membrane of the respiratory tract and inhibits gas exchange, i.e. the intake of oxygen and expulsion of carbon dioxide.

Season and Weather Dependence of Atopic Constitutional Neurodermatitis

Season-dependent reactions on the human organism have long been known as "biorhythms". In medical climatology, endogenous seasonal fluctuations are an important consideration in the classification of meteotropic behaviour according to biological seasons: winter (December to February), spring (March to May), summer (June to August), autumn (September to November). An ergotropic stimulus during the first half of the year produces an intensification and subsequent preponderence of the sympathicotonia. Mid-August witnesses a vegetative change whereby the increasing trophotropic reaction situation causes an increase in sympathicotonia [56].

The literature abounds in frequently contradictory theories concerning the seasonal dependence of atopic constitutional neurodermatitis [37, 50, 89]. According to Korting [54], a higher morbidity frequently occurs during the winter months and is closely related to seasonal variations in skin moisturisation. The disease reaches its statistically proven maximum in spring and autumn. In this case, weather fluctuations exclusively influence the disease or recurrence quota. The combination of higher outdoor temperature and humidity and simultaneously the slightly lower convection typical of cities on sunny summer days depresses the evaporation of perspiration on the surface of the skin, causing intensive itching. The North Sea climate, with its high pressure weather zones (optimal sunshine periods) and westerly weather zones (invigorating sea breezes) has a mostly positive effect, whereas dull and cloudy weather conditions are more likely to induce severe itching. During the winter months in high mountainous regions, there is a greater potential for biotropic influence on pruritus in neurodermatitic patients than in summer.

Therapy in Climate

Therapy in climate involves the curative climates of both maritime and mountainous zones.

Mountain Climatotherapy

In languages other than German, "middle" and "high" mountainous regions defy differentiation. One speaks of "high mountains" and "hautes montagnes", but it is difficult to translate "Mittelgebirge" into either English or French. The phrase "petites montagnes" is a poor translation for "Mittelgebirge" whilst "moderately high mountains" is a very free translation.

High Mountainous Climate

It is difficult to determine how high a mountain must be before it can be referred to as a high mountain, owing to worldwide discrepancies in the various climatic zones. Geographers classify according to relative height (relief energy). According to Krebs [55], a moderately high mountainous climate reaches a relief energy of 1000 m, whilst alpine relief represents greater relief energy. For high mountainous regions, however, a relative height of 1500 m was taken for clear differentiation. Meanwhile, high mountainous regions are generally defined as those situated in temperate zones with a relative altitude difference of 1500 m.

High mountainous region relates not only to a singular orographic, climatic or morphological factor, but to the whole character of the landscape which incorporates all the climatic, geomorphological, ecological and biological activity.

Increasing altitude produces climatic changes in the following factors (stimulating factors):

- Air pressure (decrease of c. 12%/1000 m)
- Oxygen partial pressure (decrease of c. 12%/1000 m)
- Temperature (decrease of 6°C/1000 m)
- Water vapour pressure (decrease of c. 25%/1000 m)
- UV radiation (increase of 20%–30%/1000 m)
- Global radiation (incrase of 10%–20%/1000 m)

Global radiation represents the sum of direct solar radiation and diffuse celestial radiation [38]. By comparison with single climatic regions in central Europe, Daubert and Aichinger [28] discovered a preference of global radiation for high mountainous regions (Davos / Switzerland-Zugspitze / Germany) followed by maritime regions (Wyk/Föhr) rather than urban climates (Karlsruhe, Bochum).

The climatic stimulation produced by global radiation and UV radiation is even more intense when the ground is covered with snow which – especially freshly fallen snow – reflects about 80% of the UV light. The situation of the region above the inversion layer constitutes a further thermophysiological advantage as there is permanent high pressure.

The specific stimulating factor in mountainous regions is the reduction of oxygen partial pressure, which induces an increase in erythrocytes and haematocrit. The purity of the air and low allergenic activity are protective factors. Regions above 1500 m are practically allergen-free. Humidity is prevented by low temperatures and water pressure.

Moderately High Mountain Climate

The moderately high mountain climate produces stimulating effects which are similar to but less intense than those of high mountainous regions [98], due to the difference in altitude [64]. Mountainous regions of 800–1000 m have a proven curative effect with increased erythropoiesis. Reversal of atmospheric conditions over 400 m is practically unknown. The prevailing westerly weather conditions on the low Atlantic coastlines generate cloudier weather with increased rain. In the sheltered region (leeside) of the mountains, there is less depression and more sunshine.

Because of the forestation typical of highland regions, allergens, pollen and aetheric oils such as terpene (pine woods) abound. Forestry climate protects against wind and noise and shades from radiation. The water produced by assimilation condenses, thereby regulating temperature and water balance [1].

Thalassotherapy

Thalassotherapy (ἡ θάλασσα = the sea) means treatment with the curative elements of the sea. This involves the entire meteorogical influences existing in maritime and coastal regions.

Coastal Climate

Local climate, wind conditions and orographic factors determine the maritime or continental character of the coastal climate. Seawater is warmed by the same solar radiation as the continent, but at a slower pace (lower thermal conduction property) and, as a result of its greater heat capacity, retains the heat for a longer period of time. Sudden temperature variations are seldom. At the same latitude, spring and summer are therefore cooler around the coast than on the continent, and autumn and winter tend to be warmer. The transition from one season to another is also less noticeable. Under the additional influence of the Gulf Stream, which transports warm water from the north and south equatorial streams northwards via the Gulf of Mexico, the North Sea is bestowed with a mild climate, contrary to the continental influences governing the Baltic Sea.

The variation between land and sea temperature rise, with the resulting drop in pressure, produces a daily rhythm between maritime and continental winds. The constancy of winds, their strength and direction are criteria to be considered when selecting a climatic seaside resort [85]. Wind speed generates a strong stimulating factor and is employed therapeutically as a "regimen refrigerans" for additional strength.

In general, the island resorts of the North Sea (Helgoland, Borkum, Sylt, Amrum, Wyk auf Föhr) are preferred due to the prevailing sea winds during the summer months. The frequently prevailing continental winds of the Baltic Sea generate a therapeutically negative cooling of the water.

Aerosol, another significant climatic factor, depends on the wind direction and geographical situation. Sea winds blow particles of brine into the air, which in maritime surfing zones may be inhaled for therapeutic purposes, whereas the coastal air, influenced by continental winds, contains no seawater aerosol. In relatively cool sea coastal climates, the recondensation effect of the respiratory air generates increased moisturisation of the mucus membrane in the upper respiratory tract, resulting in increased secretolysis [35, 92–94].

Another advantage of sea air compared with continental air is its purity and low allergenic activity. The slight fluctuations in temperature and constant air humidity (no sultry periods) are further protective factors.

In the photo-actinic complex of effect, UV radiation over the coastal shores and sand acts as a stimulus. Because of the broad horizon and absence of land obstacles, the celestial radiation can penetrate the organism freely. Most of the ultraviolet radiation is reflected by dry, light drift sand (17%), whilst the reflection from the seawater at 5% is comparatively insignificant (47). A suntan is acquired more quickly in the dunes than at the water's edge.

Radiation measurements carried out on Sylt demonstrated that posture influences UV radiation [100]. In upright postures, certain areas of the body (scalp, shoulder level, lower lips) are considerably more exposed to the sun than the arms and legs [6, 83].

Deep Sea Climate

The strongest climatic stimulation is to be expected in the deep sea climate, where the following climatic factors prevail:

- Absence of allergens
- Far-reaching constancy of humidity and temperature
- More intensive photo-actinic complex of effects

In 1965, Linser and Kleinsorge organised a deep sea climatic cure on the passenger ship MS "Voelkerfreundschaft" [cf. 52]. During a cruise of just under 4 weeks over the North Baltic Canal and Gulf of Biscay to the Canary Isles and back, 82% of the patients suffering from atopic constitutional neurodermatitis were either symptomless or showed a marked improvement of the disorder.

Practical Execution of Clinical Climatic Therapy

Climatic therapy is practiced in regions especially selected for their first-class climatic factors. The category of climatic regions corresponds to the medically effective stimulation grades 0–3 according to standard indications. This facilitates the choice for both patient and doctor. Change of climatic stimulation through controlled exposure and place-related climatic factors is necessary for optimal exploitation of climatotherapy. The following types of cure are available:

The *open air rest cure* is suited to both the high mountainous climate and the dunes. Provided the patient has adequate thermal protection, this cure may take place in winter, without any adverse effects from temperature changes.

Aerotherapy is a modification of the open air rest cure in that the body is exposed to the local climate. In appropriate temperatures, it is possible to combine both therapies. Specially designed application improves the blood circulation in the cutaneous vessels. Additionally, aerotherapy offers more active physical therapy (gymnastics, sport).

Solar therapy (heliotherapy), as natural light therapy, may be practiced in high mountainous regions (e.g. Davos) practically throughout the year. Due to maximum annual global radiation, a high mountainous climate is preferred to northern coastal climates, where heliotherapy is in any case limited to the summer months [18].

Marinotherapy in the North and Baltic seas is available only in summer due to the relatively low water temperature. Sylt, Wyk and Amrum offer cures from mid-June to mid-September. In Helgoland, Norderney and Borkum, marinotherapy starts at the beginning of July, since the water is tolerably warm right up to the end of

September. In the Baltic sea, the cure can begin in mid-June, but it usually ends at the beginning of September.

Marinotherapy consists of mild to moderately cool brine baths which promote hyperaemia and tonicise the sympathetic nervous system [61, 62]. The mechanical friction produced by the impact of the waves and whirling grains of sand is manifested in the reddening of the skin and is a comfortable feeling for the bather. Above all, the motion of the waves promotes muscular activity, generating a fitness training effect. Additional options include inhalation with sea water, warm seawater baths (especially during the winter months) and mud packs applied at a low temperature (32°C) for patients with atopic constitutional neurodermatitis [32].

In the practical application of the various techniques, a slow increase in stimulation and individual dosage is the proven golden rule. The acclimatisation process lasts 4 weeks. With respect to individual disposition, age and severity of disease, a climatic cure should be carried out for at least 6 weeks.

The *absolute contraindications* for climatic therapy are:

- Photodermatosis (phototoxic or photo-allergic reactions, photourticaria, polymorphous photodermatosis, lupus erythematosus, porphyrinopathy, xeroderma pigmentosum)
- Severe cardiovascular disease
- florid infectious diseases
- Cerebral attacks (epilepsy) and apoplectic seizures
- Poorly attuned diabetes mellitus
- Bleeding mucosal ulcers

Relative contraindications include varicose syndromes, bullous dermatoses, collagenoses or dermatoses in an advanced stage of pregnancy, and especially all acute or chronic dermatoses beyond current climatotherapeutic experience [17].

Climatic Terrain Cure

A correct amount of exercise is an important feature of climatic treatment. It is due to Beckmann [7] that the broad-based physical therapy practiced in the climatic cures of the previous century has been reintegrated into the so-called climatic terrain therapy. Special stretching exercises are repeated through a complete range of walks and mountain hikes. Regular active spells in the open air can be undertaken according to the severity of disease, adaptation, prevailing weather conditions and physical capacity.

The potential process of adaptation to regular activity and greater exposure to the cold, diminished oxygen partial pressure and intensive UV radiation necessitates an individually appropriate amount of climatic exposure.

Correct measures promote appropriate functional and structural reactions, improving general functional capacity. Together with an increase in cardiopulmonally function, exercise-oriented climatic treatment cultivates a so-called crossed adaptation, i.e. faster and more intensive vasoconstriction to a low-temperature stimulus (low-temperature adaptation). The vegetative nervous system demonstrates an increased functional capacity due to the training effect of physical therapy and considerable parasympathetic adjustment.

Schuh et al. [90] discovered that compared with control groups, atopic patients demonstrate significantly increased stamina and improved thermoregulatory adaptation following a terrain cure in the high mountainous region of Davos under low-temperature conditions. The adaptation phenomena are statistically proven even 3 months after climatic treatment.

Terrain cures provide the favourable climatic conditions which influence the organism and accelerate mountain acclimatisation. They are the non plus ultra for those patients requiring more exercise.

Reactions of the Skin under Climatotherapeutic Conditions

Reactions of the skin under climatotherapeutic conditions are difficult to determine. Assessment is purely empirical and will depend on the absence of further attacks in the course of the disease. Moreover, there are very few suitable methods for investigating the pathogenesis of atopic constitutional neurodermatitis at the cutaneous target organ.

Atopic Constitutional Neurodermatitis Reaction Patterns and Distribution of Frequency

Polymorphous patterns of development and singular findings under various different methods of treatment yield several pathogenetic entities for the clinical picture of atopic constitutional neurodermatitis. Borelli and Schnyder [19] described three reaction patterns ("réactions cutanées" according to Brocq): lichenoid reaction pattern, pruriginous reaction pattern and eczematous reaction pattern.

All types may present alternatively, simultaneously or consecutively.

According to Puerschel [73–76], there are four specific patterns of development:

- Neurodermatitic pattern of development. This presents in 38% of all cases and is identified by its lichenoid lesions, lichenification and excoriations. In 23%, there is a connection with bronchial asthma and in 6%, with rhinitis atopica. Leptosome habitus with schizothymic features is frequently seen.
- Prurigo pattern. This occurs least frequently, only in 3%, and is characterised by a monomorphic picture of prurigo efflorescences.
- Seborrhoid pattern of reaction. This has a 10% frequency of occurrence and displays erythematous patterns. It mostly affects the pyknic-athletic type of constitution. Organic coupling is seldom seen.
- Mixed form. This occurs most frequently in 49% of cases. Lichenoid, pruriginous, eczematoid and seborrhoid patterns appear concurrently. Organic coupling is seldom seen; it mostly affects patients of athletic or pyknic constitution.

Typical results were attained following climatotherapy in the stimulating climate of the North sea ($n = 3240$) (Table 1). From 1 April 1961 to 31 December 1986, a total of 16 330 patients with atopic constitutional neurodermatitis (with/without bronchial asthma; with/without rhinitis) were treated in the German Clinic for Dermatology and Allergy in Davos (Alexanderhausklinik). Some 94% returned completely free of symptoms or with considerable improvement [30].

Table 1. Results of climatotherapy in North sea climate. [According to 76]

	Symptom-less	Improvement (residual foci)
Neurodermatitic pattern of development	91%	9%
Prurigo pattern	89%	11%
Seborrhoid pattern	95%	5%
Mixed pattern	92%	8%

Degree of Severity and the Effect-Time Factor

The changes to be expected (cure effect) by the end of the cure will largely depend on the degree of severity of the disease [97]. According to Hildebrandt et al. [46], phasic reaction patterns are usually observed in the course of a cure:

- Early reactive pattern is characterised by a 7-day (circaseptan) period with an early state of maximum reaction.
- Maximum reaction of later reactive patterns occurs at the end of the 3rd week of therapy.

Both patterns are a result of an unspecific vegetative change of the organism and are subject to hormonal control. The reaction patterns show that the resulting reactive processes – especially in late-reacting types with more severe symptoms – still persist after the 4–6 weeks' treatment.

The duration of climatotherapy usually falls just under 6 weeks. In such a short time, the patient may witness a period of atypical weather. The short period of treatment cannot be compensated by forced treatment, since the reactive periodical development pattern of climatotherapy – as implied above – is determined by biological rhythms. For this reason, patients with an earlier reactive pattern of development require a cure of at least 6 weeks' duration [9, 10, 34]. This should be extended to 8 weeks for patients with late-reactive patterns of development and initial ergotropic condition.

Late-reacting patterns of development often present during the biological winter. Since higher than average exacerbations occur at this time of the year, an extension of the cure is particularly recommended for seasonal-dependent diseases such as atopic constitutional neurodermatitis.

In a vast number of cases, it may be assumed that patients who are positively influenced by the cure will also enjoy long-term effects. Although a temporary exacerbation might be experienced on returning home and to work, additional constant deterioration is seldom. Moreover, there is much discrepancy between subjective and objective assessments of the curative success, frequently due to the doubtful adequacy of the criteria. Longitudinal research has confirmed a high correlation between subjective long-term success and objective cure effect [45].

In the literature, there is unanimous agreement that the earliest possible date for the evaluation of curative success is 3 months after the cure. The crucial factor in determining curative success is not merely the status at the end of the cure but the effect on the entire development of the disease. Along with the interval for assessment, individual factors such as severity of disease, age, duration of eczema and biological annual rhythm all play an important role.

Climatic Stress, Climatic Effect and Skin Reactivity: Experimental Investigations

The term "climatic stress", analogous to the theories of Selye [96], pioneer of stress research, may be attributed to physical or chemical stimulations working as stress factors. The stress reactions produced by climatic change influence the pituitary-adrenocortical system causing an increase in corticosterone release through ACTH stimulation [43]. Closely related is the sympathicus-adrenal system, which influences peripheral organic systems through the release of catecholamines.

Borelli et al. [20] reporting on the hyposensitising, mediatorial effect of alpine climatic stress in 1967 determined comparable measurements of urticarial dimension after intracutaneous testing with histamine, serotonin, acetylcholine and bradykinin on a large group of atopic patients. Climatic stress reduces the raised reactivity, diminishes histamine deposits and other mediators and reduces allergic hypersensitivity [22]. Following high mountainous climatic therapy, atopic patients display an alteration of histamine and sympathicus reactivity from raised to normal values [15, 16]. A higher normalisation tendency was also shown to correlate with longer periods in a high mountainous climate.

A further indication of the success of high alpine climatic therapy is manifested in the normalisation of the mechanically and chemically induced dermographism in atopic constitutional neurodermatitis. Regarding pruritus, alternating phases of intensity associated with daily/annual time periods were confirmed [79]. Current findings on atopic constitutional neurodermatitis reveal that pruritus is due to an alteration in the cortisol rhythm, which in turn is a result of overregulated hypothalamic or subcortical centres [44].

At the 1962 "Symposium Primum Dermatologicum Bulgariae", Popchristov et al. [69, 70] and Popchristov and Balevska [68] reported on high mountainous climatic therapy in the Pirin mountains and in the Rhodops as well as the Black sea and Warna. The seaside resorts (Sonnenstrand, Burgas and Nessebar) provide excellent facilities for climatic, helio- and thalassotherapy. The favourable climatic conditions of the Bulgarian Black sea coast are also conducive for winter cures [3–5].

During hospitalised treatment in the North Sea climate, Puerschel and Pahl [80, 81] confirmed a significant reduction of absolute eosinophil granulocytes, with partial normalisation. The total IgE, as well as allergen-specific antibodies, showed a marked reduction compared with respective pathological values at the outset. Thermal conductivity measurements [72] confirmed a considerable reduction in thermal conductivity in neurodermatitic disease, accompanied by a marked improvement towards normalisation in cutaneous blood circulation [82].

Measurements of skin moisturisation, by determining the water content of the cutaneous layer, revealed no basic difference between neurodermatitic patients in maritime climatic zones and persons with healthy skin [51]. A reduction of pathological total IgE and instances of pruritus was confirmed in atopic patients in sea climates. An improved functional capacity of the adrenal cortex was reflected in a greater 17-hydroxycorticosteroid excretion in the urine during the adaptation phase in the 1st and 3rd weeks with subsequent reactive diminution of hormone excretion in the urine during the 7th week [26, 27].

Investigation of the endogenous corticol secretion in neurodermatitic patients during thalassotherapy yielded a normalisation of the highly pathologically diminished values at the outset [78].

Clinical/chemical laboratory tests with red blood count, ESR, serum lability, transaminase and electrophoresis showed values which lay within the normal variation. Histological findings during climatotherapy correlate microscopically with macroscopic improvement [41].

Sociomedical Aspects of Climatotherapy

Rehabilitation of constitutional eczematic patients involves not only successful climatic treatment of the acute condition but also various measures to ensure occupational and social rehabilitation, i.e. long-term success with absence of relapses and restored fitness for work.

Questions Concerning Rehabilitation, Profitability and Working Ability

The term "rehabilitation" implies all measures affecting the optimal restoration of physical, mental and emotional functions of a patient following a disease or suffering from a disease. The following statutory authorities are involved: for legal health insurance, for pension, for legal accident insurance, for supplementary benefits, for social compensation of health impairment (pension offices) and federal employment office.

Introducing rehabilitation measures for patients with AE at the earliest possible period is the generally accepted aim today [2, 8, 14, 25, 84]. A significant criterion for success is the patient's ability to work following the cure. This depends on the state of relapse or duration of symptomless intervals. Catamnestic control in neurodermatitic patients regarding their inability and ability to work before and after mountain climatotherapy, respectively, yielded a 55% decline in those unfit for work, an 80% decline of the total period of working incapacity and a decline of 55.8% in the average period of working inability [11].

Relapse Frequency Following In-patient Climatotherapy

Mountain Climate. In the German Clinic for Dermatology and Allergy in Davos (Alexanderhausklinik), 94% of a total of 16 330 constitutional eczematous patients were discharged symptomless or with considerably improved conditions during the period 1961–1986 [30].

Sea Climate. Comparably favourable results were attained during climatic cures at the North sea. Approximately 90% of the patients were symptomless.

It goes without saying that a constitutionally induced dermatosis such as atopic constitutional neurodermatitis cannot be completely cured by a 6–8 week stay in the high mountains or at the seaside. Comprehensive catamnestic studies nevertheless confirmed reduced or at least milder relapses following repeated climatotherapy. There is a clear, statistically proven significance between the first and third cure and the first and all other cures; a pronounced significance between the first and sixth, second and sixth and even between the third or fourth and sixth climatic cure [41].

There were also fewer complaints concerning bronchial asthma and rhinitis allergica. Symptomless periods of up to several years and permanent cure by moving to a curative climate are quite frequent [42, 58].

The so-called back home effect, which is mostly connected with a decrease in vitality and temporary exacerbation is a result of a return to the home climate and life style. Since this phase usually lasts for 2–3 weeks, the patient with constitutional eczema is advised to apply for a 2-week protective period (sick leave).

Economic Comparison with Hospitalised Treatment

Atopic constitutional neurodermatitis represents one of the most frequent skin diseases, affecting roughly 2%–5% of the population. In the scientific literature, there is unanimous agreement upon the success of climatotherapy. Even in children with similar stigmata (infant eczema, flexural eczema), further development of atopic constitutional neurodermatitis is favourably influenced through repeated bioclimatic cures.

Basically, one may differentiate between clinical care (with hospital certificate of admission) in a special clinic or treatment at a special clinic according to paragraph 184 RVO (German Reich Insurance Code); treatment in a special or rehabilitation clinic according to paragraph 184a RVO, which is approved by state insurances; and paediatric curative practice in sanatoriums or rehabilitation centres according to paragraph 1305 RVO or paragraph 84 AVG (employment insurance), which is approved by the statutory pension authority. According to paragraph 184a of the Reich Insurance Code[1], the national insurance system authorises treatment with accommodation and care in curative and special centres, if these are the only means for curing, improving or checking the disease.

In comparing the cost/benefit ratio for special or local clinics, one might consider the more economical daily nursing care during climatotherapy as well as the bonus effect of curative climates and specialist treatment of the disease. During climatic therapy, the consumption of

1 The health reform law which was implemented on 1 January 1989 is analogous in principle.

internal and external steroids and other medicaments for differential treatment are drastically reduced, since the skin of neurodermatitic patients is usually treated with neutral oils [34]. The costs are thereby considerably reduced. These economical and sociopolitical advantages – at a time of cost-conscious health authorities – once again reflects the efficacy of climatotherapy in atopic constitutional neurodermatitis.

Conclusions

Climatic therapy in the form of high mountainous climatic treatment or thalassotherapy currently provides an additional opportunity for therapeutic and social rehabilitation of patients with chronic skin disorders. (Truly effective high mountain climatotherapy can be practised only in the high mountainous conditions that exist in the Swiss regions of 1500 m or more, e.g. in the high mountainous valley of Davos at 1560 m.) Atopic constitutional neurodermatitis is at the top of the list for dermatological indications.

The available space allocated for this presentation cannot incorporate all that may be found in the literature on the subject of climatotherapy.

References

1. Amelung W, Hildebrandt G (eds) (1986) Medizinische Klimatologie Praxis der Balneo- und Klimatherapie. Springer, Berlin Heidelberg New York (Balneologie und medizinische Klimatologie, vol 3)
2. Arbeitsgemeinschaft Allergiekrankes Kind (1987) Heilverfahren oder Klimabehandlung für asthma- und allergiekranke Kinder. Wo? Wann? Wie? Arbeitsgemeinschaft Allergiekrankes Kind – Hilfen für Kinder mit Asthma, Ekzem oder Heuschnupfen e.V., Herborn
3. Balewska N, Petkow IL, Iowew S, Mustakow G (1964) Klima-, Helio- und Thalassotherapie der disseminierten Neurodermitis im Schwarzmeerkurort "Sonnenstrand". Symposium Primum Dermatologicum Bulgariae, 1962: excerpta lectiorum. Medicina i Fizkultura, Sofia
4. Balewska N, Petkow IL, Mustakow G, Iowew S (1964) Probebehandlung von Hautkranken an der Meeresküste im Winter. Symposium Primum Dermatologicum Bulgariae 1962: excerpta lectiorum, Medicina i Fizkultura, Sofia
5. Balewska N, Petkow IL, Mustakow G, Iowew S (1964) Ergebnisse der Thalassotherapie von Kranken mit Neurodermitis, Ekzem, chronischer Urticaria und anderen Hautkrankheiten an der Meeresküste bei Warna. Symposium Primum Dermatologicum Bulgariae, 1962: excerpta lectiorum. Medicina i Fizkultura, Sofia
6. Becker-Casademont R (1988) Phototherapie: In: Drexel H, Becker-Casademont R, Seichert N (eds) Elektro- und Lichttherapie. Hippokrates, Stuttgart, pp 147–154 (Physikalische Medizin, vol 4)
7. Beckmann P (1958) Rehabiliation und Frühheilverfahren des Kreislaufgeschädigten. Münch Med Woschenschr 100:426–428
8. Borelli S (1961) Das psychische Verhalten der an konstitutioneller Neurodermitis Erkrankten und die volkswirtschaftliche Bedeutung des Leidens. Dtsch Gesundheitswes 16 (3/4):122–127
9. Borelli S (1969) Probleme der Klimatherapie bei Dermatosen. Münch Med Wochenschr 35:1709–1716
10. Borelli S (1972) Zur Klimatherapie von Hautkrankheiten. Ther Umsch 29 (10):610–616
11. Borelli S (1976) Medizinische Rehabilitation und Heilverfahren bei Hautkranken und Allergikern aus arbeits- und sozialmedizinischer Sicht. Arbeitsmed Sozialmed Präventivmed 11 (3):70–87
12. Borelli S (1979) Zur Hochgebirgsklimatherapie bei Allergien, Atopien und Dermatosen. In: Report of the Clinic Dermatology and Allergy in Davos based on the seminar on Allergy and Dermatology, Davos, 12–16 Sept 1979
13. Borelli S (1979) Zur Bedeutung der Klimatherapie. In: Böhlau V (ed) Altern und Balneologie. Schattauer, Stuttgart, pp 50–71
14. Borelli S, Brenn H (1969) Zur Rehabilitation der atopischen Neurodermitis. Z Haut- Geschlechtskr 44 (18):819–826
15. Borelli S, Chlebarov ST (1966) Änderungen der neurovegetativen Reagibilität der Haut nach Hochgebirgs-Klimabehandlung. Münch Med Wochenschr 108 (11):589–592
16. Borelli S, Chlebarov ST (1966) Änderungen der Histaminreagibilität der Haut nach Hochgebirgs-Klimabehandlung. Münch Med Wochenschr 108 (11):592–596
17. Borelli S, Chlebarov ST (1969) Indikationen und Erfolgsaussichten der Hochgebirgsklimabehandlung bei Hautkrankheiten. Arch Phys Ther 21 (6):406–417
18. Borelli S, Fries P (1986) Hautkrankheiten und Allergien. In: Amelung W, Hildebrandt G (eds) Medizinische Klimatologie. Praxis der Balneo- und Klimatherapie. Springer, Berlin Heidelberg New York, pp 115–120 (Balneologie und medizinische Klimatologie, vol 3)
19. Borelli S, Schnyder UW (1962) Neurodermitis constitutionalis sive atopica. In: Miescher G, Storck H (eds) Entzündliche Dermatosen. Springer, Berlin Göttingen, Heidelberg, pp 228–319 (Handbuch der Haut- und Geschlechtskrankheiten, vol 2(1))
20. Borelli S, Michailov P, Ene-Popescu C (1967) Die Veränderungen der allergisch-mediatorischen Reaktivität bei Neurodermitis-constitutionalis-Kranken nach Höhenklimatherapie. Hautarzt 18 (10):456–458
21. Borelli S, Brenn H, Chlebarov ST, Ene-Popescu C, Gehrken H, Kopecka B, Michailov P, Vossieck H (1968) Zur Wirkung des hochalpinen Klimas bei der atopischen kon-

stitutionellen Neurodermitis. In: Jadassohn W, Schirren CG (eds) XIII. Congressus Internationalis Dermatologiae. München 1967. Springer, Berlin Heidelberg New York, pp 1395–1397

22. Brenn H (1969) Dermatologie und Klimatherapie mit besonderer Berücksichtigung des Davoser Klimas. Dermatologica 139:278–285
23. Bründl W, Mayer H, Baumgartner A (1986) Untersuchung des Einflusses von Bebauung und Bewuchs auf das Klima und die lufthygienischen Verhältnisse in bayerischen Großstädten – Abschlußbericht zum Teilprogramm "Klimamessungen München". In: Bayrisches Staatsministerium für Landesentwicklung und Umweltfragen: Klimamessungen in München. Materialien 43
24. Bucher K, Mohr M, Staiger H, Trenkle H (1986) Medizinmeteorologische Information. In: Faust V (ed) Wetter-Klima-menschliche Gesundheit. Hippokrates, Stuttgart, pp 132–150
25. Bundesarbeitsgemeinschaft für Rehabilitation (ed) (1984) Die Rehabilitation Behinderter. Deutscher Ärzte-Verlag, Cologne
26. Chlebarov ST (1974) Klinische und klimaphysiologische Untersuchungen beim atopischen Symptomenkomplex im Kindesalter an der Nordsee (Norderney). Habilitationsschrift, Technical University of Munich
27. Chlebarov ST (1977) Atopischer Symptomenkomplex im Kindesalter. Fortschr Med 95 (23):1527–1532
28. Daubert K, Aichinger F (1958) Wetter-Klima-Haut. In: Gottron HA, Schönfeld W (eds) Dermatologie und Venerologie, vol I/2. Thieme, Stuttgart, pp 905–954
29. Dschwanden KS (1972) Klima in der Therapie. Bioklimatische Forschungsstation, Adelboden
30. Deutsche Klinik für Dermatologie und Allergie (1987) Jahresstatistik 1986. Davos
31. Deutscher Bäderverband (ed) (1973) Deutscher Bäderkalender. Flöttmann, Gütersloh
32. Deutscher Bäderverband (ed) (1987) Grundlagen der Kurortmedizin und ihr Stellenwert im Gesundheitswesen der Bundesrepublik Deutschland. Meister, Kassel
33. Edwards WF (1824) De l'influence des agens physiques sur la vie. Paris
34. Engst R (1977) Ergebnisse hochalpiner stationärer Klimatherapie bei chronisch Hautkranken und Allergikern aus der Klinik für Dermatologie und Allergie, Davos. Dtsch Dermatol 25:283–292
35. Fink E, Rieken M (1987) Die Inhalationsfibel. Plantorgan Werk KG, Bad Zwischenahn
36. Fischer-Homberger E (1977) Geschichte der Medizin. Springer, Berlin Heidelberg New York
37. Gloor M (1983) Neurodermitis atopica. Klinik-Pathophysiologie-Therapie. Fortschr Med 101 (20):919–923
38. Gühring H (1988) Klimatherapie unter besonderer Berücksichtigung des Davoser Hochgebirges. Z Hautnah 5: 69–72
39. Haberling W, Vierordt H (1931) Biographisches Lexikon der hervorragenden Ärzte aller Zeiten und Völker, vol 3. Urban and Schwarzenberg, Berlin
40. Haberling W, Vierordt H (1932) Biographisches Lexikon der hervorragenden Ärzte aller Zeiten und Völker, vol 4. Urban and Schwarzenberg, Berlin
41. Harnack K (1966) Klinische und experimentelle Untersuchungen zur Klimatherapie des endogenen Ekzems. Habilitationsschrift, Humboldt University, Berlin
42. Hartung J (1962) Klimatherapie. In: Gottron HA, Schönfeld W (eds) Dermatologie und Venerologie, vol II/1. Thieme, Stuttgart, pp 250–276
43. Helle S (1968) Pharmacorticolspiegel-Bestimmungen bei Neurodermitikern während der Behandlung in der Bonner Klimakammer. Hautarzt 20 (3):132–134
44. Heubeck B, Schönberger A, Hornstein OP (1988) Sind Verschiebungen des zirkadianen Cortisolrhythmus ein endokrines Symptom des atopischen Ekzems? Hautarzt 39:12–17
45. Hildebrandt G (1985) Therapeutische Physiologie, Grundlagen der Kurortbehandlung. In: Amelung W, Hildebrand G (eds) Therapeutische Physiologie Grundlagen der Kurortbehandlung. Springer, Berlin Heidelberg New York (Balneologie und medizinische Klimatologie, vol 1)
46. Hildebrandt G, Geyer F, Brüning W (1982) Circaseptan adaptive periodicity and weekly rhythm. In: Hildebrandt G, Hensel H (eds) Biological adaptation. Thieme, Stuttgart, pp 113–116
47. Holtmeier HJ (1983) Gesundheit aus dem Meer. Molden, Munich
48. Hönigsmann H (1981) Dermatologische Effekte und Konsequenzen der erhöhten UV-Intensität in Höhenlagen. In: Deetjen P, Humpeler E (eds) Medizinische Aspekte der Höhe. Thieme, Stuttgart, pp 117–122
49. Humboldt AV (1845) Cosmos, Entwurf einer physischen Weltbeschreibung, vol 1. Cotta, Stuttgart, p 340
50. Imai S, Takeuchi S, Mashiko T (1987) Jahreszeitliche Änderungen im Verlauf des atopischen Ekzems. Hautarzt 38:599–602
51. Keilhauer A, Wienert V, Pürschel W (1982) Die Hautfeuchtigkeit bei Neurodermitikern in maritimer Klimazone. Z Hautkr 57 (20):1477–1486
52. Kleinsorge H, Lazarus P (1966) Erster Bericht über die Hochseeklimakur mit MS "Völkerfreundschaft". Allerg Asthma 12 (4):220–225
53. Kneist W, Rakoski J (1987) Neurodermitis atopica – Klimatherapie im Hochgebirge. Allergologie 10 (12):531–535
54. Korting GW (1959) Das endogene Ekzem. In: Gottron HA, Schönfeld W (eds) Dermatologie und Venerologie, vol III/1. Thieme, Stuttgart, pp 549–593
55. Krebs N (1922) Die Karte der Reliefenergie Süddeutschlands. Haack, Gotha (Petermanns Geographische Mitteilungen)
56. Linser K (1967) Der wetterbedingte Biotropismus im Blickfeld der Dermatologie und die Klimatherapie bei Hautkrankheiten. In: Gottron HA (ed) Grundlagen und Grenzgebiete der Dermatologie. Springer, Berlin Heidelberg New York, pp 722–887
57. Loewy A (1931) Physiologie des Höhenklimas. Springer, Berlin
58. Marchionini A, Borelli S (1956) Klimabehandlung der Neurodermitis disseminata. Dtsch Med Wochenschr 81 (21):811–816
59. Marchionini A, Borelli S (1957) Zur Klimabehandlung der atopischen Dermatitis, Neurodermitis constitutionalis sive atopica. 11th International Congress of Dermatology. Acta Derm Venereol 3:18–23
60. Mehl M (1896) Sonnentherapie, 3rd edn. Koslowsky, Oranienburg
61. Menger W (1984) Klimatherapie – aber richtig dosiert. In: Forschungsgemeinschaft für Meersheilkunde (ed) Beiträge zur Meeresheilkunde, vol 10. Forschungsgemeinschaft für Meeresheilkunde, Oldenburg, pp 3–14
62. Menger W (1984) Wirkungen kalter Seebäder. In: Schriftenreihe der Forschungsgemeinschaft für Meeresheilkunde e.V., Oldenburg, vol 10, pp 23–27

63. Menger W, Schellhaas J (1980) Telemetrische Untersuchungen zum Nachweis des sekretolytischen Effektes der Brandungszone bei Kindern mit Asthma bronchiale. Prax Pneumol 34:746
64. Mohring D (1971) Klimaeinflüsse. In: Mohring D (ed) Touristikmedizin. Thieme, Stuttgart, pp 34–59
65. Moleschott J (1856) Über den Einfluß des Lichtes auf die Reizbarkeit der Nerven. Würzburg
66. Neuberger M, Pagel J (eds) (1971) Handbuch der Geschichte der Medizin, vol 1, 2. Ohms, Hildesheim
67. Pahl O, Pürschel W (1973) Nordseeklima und Hautkrankheiten. 20 Jahre dermatologische Klimatherapie an der Nordsee. Z Hautkr 48 (21):871–879
68. Popchristov P, Balevska N (1966) Hochgebirgsklimatherapie und Thalassotherapie Hautkranker in Bulgarien. Medicina i Fiskultura, Sofia
69 Popchristov P, Botew ST, Chlebarow ST, Kapnilow ST, Welew N, Michailow P, Konstantinow AL (1964) Beobachtungen über die Hochgebirgskur bei Gruppen Hautkranken im Piringebirge. Symposium Primum Dermatologicum Bulgariae, 1962: excerpta lectiorum. Medicina i Fiskultura, Sofia
70. Popchristov P, Konstantinow AL, Kapnilow ST, Michailow P, Chlebarow ST, Botew ST (1964) Beobachtungen über die hochgebirgsklimatische Behandlung von Hautkranken in den Rhodopen. Symposium Primum Dermatologicum Bulgariae, 1962: excerpta lectiorum. Medicina i Fiskultura, Sofia
71. Prausnitz W (1912) Grundzüge der Hygiene. Lehmanns, Munich
72. Pürschel W (1968) Zur Klimatherapie und Katamnese der Neurodermitis. Arch Dermatol Forsch 244:357–362
73. Pürschel W (1968) Klimatherapie von Hautkrankheiten an der Nordsee. 13 Konr Int Dermatol, Munich. Springer, Berlin Heidelberg New York, pp 1397–1400
74. Pürschel W (1973) Dermatologische Klimatherapie an der Nordsee – klinisch-analytische Untersuchung am konstitutionellen Ekzematoid. Dermatologica 146 [Suppl 1]: 1–98
75. Pürschel W (1977) Neurodermitis im Erwachsenenalter. Z Hautkr 2 [Suppl]:81–91
76. Pürschel W (1982) Klimatherapie der Neurodermitis atopica an der Nordsee. Allergol 5:64–69
77. Pürschel W (1986) Wie behandele ich die Neurodermitis atopica. Z Hautkr 61 (10):731–734
78. Pürschel W (1987) Neurodermitis atopica – Klimabehandlung am Meer. Allergol 10 (12):526–530
79. Pürschel W, Pahl O (1956) Pruritus chronischer Ekzematiker und seine Witterungsabhängigkeit im Nordseeklima. Hautarzt 7:27–31
80. Pürschel W, Pahl O (1968) Das Verhalten eosinophiler Granulozyten beim konstitutionellen Ekzem mit/ohne Asthma bronchiale während dermatologischer Klimatherapie an der Nordsee. Z Haut-Geschlechtskr 43 (23):953–962
81. Pürschel W, Pahl O (1985) Verhalten von eosinophilen Granulozyten, Gesamt-IgE und allergen-spezifischen Ig-E Antikörpern bei Neurodermitis atopica während stationärer Behandlung im Nordseeklima. Z Hautkr 60 (8):661–670
82. Pürschel W, Pahl O, Aljounied A (1982) Fluvographische Untersuchungen bei Neurodermitis während Klimatherapie an der Nordsee. Z Hautkr 57 (1):38–46
83. Raab W (1987) Lichtfibel. Fischer, Stuttgart
84. Rakoski J, Borelli S (1987) Hinweise für Beratungsdienste zur Rehabilitation Behinderter. Blatt 44: Zur Beratung von Patienten mit Neurodermititis constitutionalis atopica. Rehabilitation 26:XVII–XX
85. Reinke R, Swantes HJ (1984) Der Einfluß von Wetter und Klima auf Rehabilitation und Erholung. Schriftenreihe der Forschungsgemeinschaft für Meeresheilkunde e.V. 11:53–64
86. Rubner M, von Gruber M, Ficker M (eds) (1911) Handbuch der Hygiene, vols 1, 2. Leipzig
87. Schadewaldt H (1987) Zur Geschichte des römischen Bäderwesens. Ärztl Kosmet:302–321
88. Schirmer H, Buschner W, Cappel A, Matthäus G, Schlegel M (1987) Meyers kleines Lexikon Meteorologie. Meyers Lexikon, Mannheim
89. Schudel P, Wüthrich B (1985) Klinische Verlaufsbeobachtungen bei Neurodermitis atopica nach dem Kleinkindesalter. Z Hautkr 60 (6):479–486
90. Schuh A, Kneist W, Schnizer W, Schobel G, Streicher U, Fischer A (1988) Training und Abhärtung bei Atopikern nach Hochgebirgsklimatherapie. Z Hautkr 63 (4):108–110
91. Schultze EG (1973) Meeresheilkunde. Urban and Schwarzenberg, Munich
92. Schultze EG (1987) Warum Klimatherapie bei Hautkrankheiten. Z Hautnah 3:45–48
93. Schultze EG (1988) Klimatologische Aspekte zur Neurodermitis-Therapie. Z Hautnah 1:70–79
94. Schultze EG (1988) Welchen Einfluß hat das Brandungsaerosol auf den Heuschnupfen. Z Hautnah 4:41–44
95. Schweizerische Verkehrszentrale, Schweizerische Vereinigung der Klimakurorte (1979) Das Klimabuch der Schweiz. Zürich
96. Selye H (1953) Einführung in die Lehre vom Adaptationssyndrom. Thieme, Stuttgart
97. Serowy C, Klinker L (1974) Saisonrhythmisches Verhalten von Morbidität, Kureffektivität und Kurerfolg beim endogenen Ekzem. Dermatol Monatsschr 10:735–741
98. Wiedemann E (1987) Physikalische Therapie. de Gruyter, Berlin
99. Winslow G (1867) Light: its influence on life and health. London
100. Witzleb E (19829 Kurgastbezogene Strahlenmessungen an der See. Z Phys Med 11:163–171

Unsaturated Fatty Acids in the Treatment of Atopic Eczema

J. Ring and B. Kunz

Introduction

The ongoing debate on the role of dietary factors in atopic eczema dates back to the beginning of this century. In recent years two aspects have mainly been the focus of interest: (1) the role of food allergy or pseudo-allergy and (2) the possible benefit of unsaturated fatty acids. The latter has gained strong support, motivated especially by the tremendous amount of research going on in cardiovascular medicine, in which polyunsaturated fatty acids, mostly of marine origin, have been documented to decrease the incidence of several pathological conditions such as hypertension, hypertriglyceridemia, elevated cholesterol levels, etc. [6, 15, 26, 40, 55, 58]. The "fish oil debate" originated from the observation that Eskimos and other fish-eating populations seemed to suffer from a lower incidence of heart disease than meat-eating people. Similarly, a decreased incidence of psoriasis and other inflammatory skin diseases has been reported [4, 29].

Today the use of unsaturated fatty acids in inflammatory skin diseases is put forward for two main reasons. Firstly, certain unsaturated fatty acids seem to be important in restoring the barrier function of the skin, acting as parts of critical lipid molecules ([6, 12, 31] and see the chapter by Melnik, this volume). Secondly, unsaturated fatty acids have been shown to exert antiinflammatory effects in various in vitro and in vivo models [14, 17, 19, 24, 32, 34, 41, 48, 57, 61].

In the following, after a short discussion of the theoretical background, clinical experiences with unsaturated fatty acids in atopic eczema shall be discussed. Since mainly two approaches have been used, it seems justified to regard γ-*linolenic* acid (GLA) and derivatives and *eicosapentaenoic acid* (EPA) separately.

Theoretical Background

There is substantial evidence that unsaturated fatty acids play an important role in the lipid barrier function of the epidermis. Linoleic acid, part of the glycosphingosin Ceramide A, deserves particular mention ([12] and see the chapter by Melnik, this volume).

Since the first description of skin symptoms, e.g., dry skin, scaling, hyperproliferation, and hyperkeratosis, in essential fatty acid deficiency [21], the role of unsaturated fatty acids in certain inflammatory skin diseases has been thoroughly discussed. Among the first diseases mentioned was atopic eczema [21], which was ameliorated by a diet rich in unsaturated fatty acids.

Animals such as rats and guinea pigs with essential fatty acid deficiencies have been used as models for various abnormal skin conditions [31, 36, 63]. Clinical conditions of essential fatty acid deficiencies have also been observed in patients under total parenteral nutrition, bowel bypass surgery, or severely restricted diets (e.g, children with malabsorption problems or the excessive consumption of skim milk). Due to the introduction of intravenous lipid emulsions these conditions are now observed much less frequently.

Essential fatty acids such as linoleic acid and its derivatives are either derived from plants, vegetable oils, (evening primrose, etc.), or fish (EPA). Linoleic acid is transformed via δ-6-desaturase to GLA, dihomo-γ-lino-

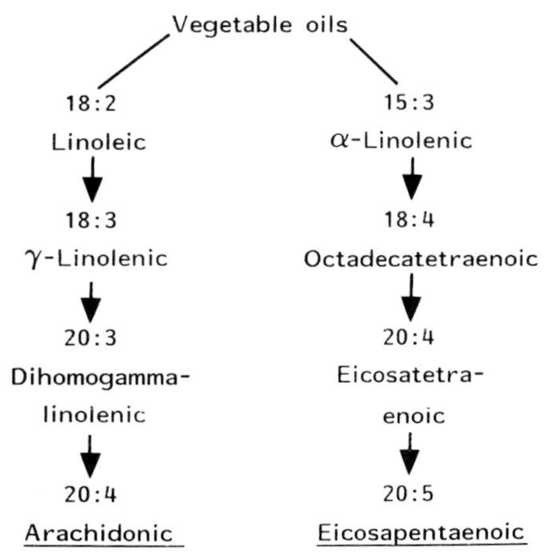

Fig. 1. Main sources of essential fatty acids and their derivatives

lenic acid (DGLA), and finally to arachidonic acid (AA) (Fig. 1). The addition of GLA to the normal diet is thought to lead to increased amounts of prostaglandin (PG) E and prostacyclin ([57] and see the chapter by Melnik, this volume).

EPA is an Ω-3 unsaturated fatty acid (20:5) which is transformed by lipoxygenase to leukotriene (LT) A5 and LTB5 or by cyclooxygenase to PGE5, PGI3 and thromboxane (TX) TXA3. These latter compounds have been shown to have distinctly lower inflammatory activity than the PGs of the 2 or the LTs of the 4 series, respectively [32, 34] (Fig. 2). Metabolites of linoleic acid, e.g., 15-hydroxy-8,11,13-eicosatrienoic acid (15-OH-20:3 n-6) and EPA, e.g., 15-hydroxy-5,8,11,13,17-EPA (15-OH-20:3n-3), belong to the most potent inhibitors of the LTB4 series [62, 63].

A lupus-like disease in mice can be considerably improved by addition of EPA [24].

Linoleic acid has been found to exert a variety of immunoregulatory functions. These include not only antiinflammatory effects [41], but also immunosuppression as shown by prolonged survival of skin allografts in rats [48].

EPA has been shown to inhibit a variety of leukocyte functions such as neutrophil activity (chemotaxis, etc.) [32, 34], B cell proliferation in response to mitogens and expression of interleukin-2 receptors [56], in vitro production of interleukin-1 and tumor necrosis factor by peripheral blood lymphocytes [13], and synthesis of endothelial cell-derived growth factors [16]. Furthermore, EPA inhibits LT4 generation significantly [35]. However, in a rat model there was no significant effect of EPA either on inflammatory changes in the skin or on antibody production; there was a slight effect on delayed-type hypersensitivity reactions [61].

Clinical investigations in patients with atopic eczema have found different lipid mediator abnormalities [47, 49] (Ruzicka and Ring, this volume). One hypothesis postulates a desaturase deficiency [38] as the basis of a deficiency in GLA and its metabolites together with increased levels of linoleic acid. This was strengthened by Strannegard et al., who reported that in serum lecithin of children with atopic eczema, increased amounts of linoleic acid were found together with decreased levels of GLA [53].

Although the problem of absorption of unsaturated fatty acids in humans is important [44], application of linoleic acid has been found valuable by some authors in a variety of studies [42].

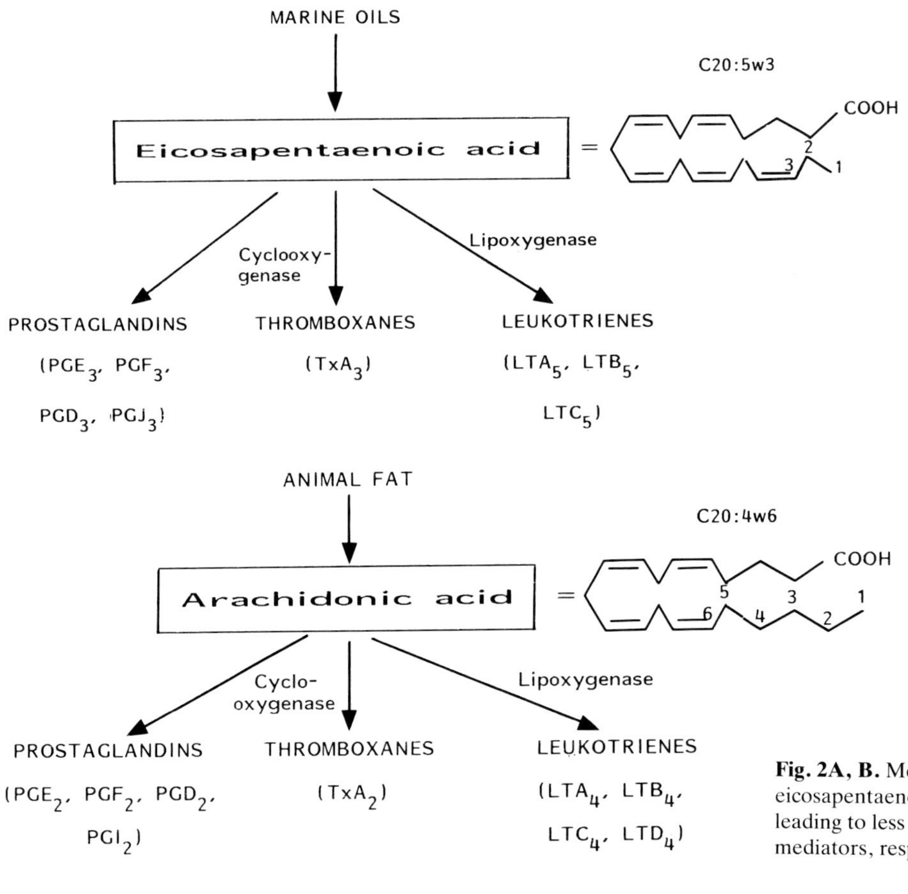

Fig. 2A, B. Metabolic pathways of eicosapentaenoic (EPA) and arachidonic acid leading to less and more active inflammatory mediators, respectively

It seems interesting that objective measurements of unsaturated fatty acid concentrations in blood or tissues of patients with inflammatory skin diseases undergoing clinical trials have not shown in all cases profound changes compatible with the clinical results. Moreover, things are not as simple as one might speculate on the basis of the various schemes. This was shown in an animal experiment by Lee and Arm [33], who were able to protect animals treated with EPA from bronchial symptoms after inhaled allergen challenge. However, EPA had an enhancing effect on the intensity of clinical symptoms of systemic anaphylaxis after intravenous antigen application.

Clinical Studies

Since the observation of Hansen [21] in the 1930s that children with atopic eczema improved after dietary addition of unsaturated fatty acids from corn or linseed, this issue has been debated vehemently [20]. It gained new interest when the study of Wright and Burton [60], using oral evening primrose oil, was published. In this double-blind, controlled cross-over study the effect of various doses of oral evening primrose oil was investigated in nearly 100 patients with atopic eczema; a significant clinical improvement following administration of a high dose (12 capsules containing 360 mg linoleic acid and 45 mg GLA) was observed [60]. Other authors also found partly beneficial effects in treating psoriasis [28]. While there was no effect on psoriasis vulgaris, one patient with psoriasis pustulosa improved in the pilot study of Kettler et al. [25]. No effect of evening primrose oil was found in the studies by Bamford et al. [3], Skogh [52] and Wehrmann et al. [59].

In a meta-analysis of nine clinical, partly placebo-controlled trials, a general efficacy of evening primrose oil in atopic eczema was found [42]. Schalin-Karrila et al. [50] observed, in a double-blind trial, some statistically significant improvement, the clinical relevance of which, however, may be regarded as small. We have treated three patients with evening primrose oil (according to Wright and Burton's study) without obvious clinical improvement (unpublished work). The observation of Guenther, who described some benefit of evening primrose oil against a concomitant hyperactivity syndrome in some children with atopic eczema is also of interest [18].

In a study with EPA, Bjorneboe et al. [8] found no significant effect on psoriasis, while there was a mild improvement, especially with regard to scaling and itch, in a double-blind study using EPA to treat atopic eczema [7]. A modest improvement of atopic eczema was also observed in a study by Maurice et al. [39]. When EPA was used not as a monotherapy but in addition to UVB treatment there was a significant effect on psoriasis [19].

Results of Our Own Double-Blind Study with EPA

We studied the effect of oral EPA on the clinical course of atopic eczema in a double-blind, placebo-controlled trial [30]. After a survey period of 1 month, 20 patients suffering from severe atopic eczema received EPA in gelatin capsules (initially 25 mg/kg/day over 4 weeks, then 12 mg/kg daily for 3 months) or a mixture of saturated fatty acids as a placebo. After treatment patients were followed for another month. During the study, symptomatic treatment with fluprednidene acetate cream and dimetindene maleate tablets was allowed as a "rescue" regimen together with standard emollients. The therapeutic effect was evaluated subjectively by symptom diaries, objectively by quantitation of the body surface involved, and by dermatological assessment of characteristic skin lesions using a severity score. At the end of the observation time, all parameters showed significant improvement both in the EPA and placebo groups. Some parameters (dryness, erythema, desquamation) even showed a more pronounced amelioration in the placebo group (Fig. 3). EPA treatment did not modify the amount of topical steroids or systemic antihistamines used as rescue therapy. In vitro studies with basophils showed no effect of EPA treatment on anti-IgE, Ca-ionophore, or C5a-induced histamine release. We conclude that it is the regular, intensive, and careful dermatologic guidance in an optimal patient-physician relationship rather than the effect of EPA that accounts for successful management of patients with atopic eczema.

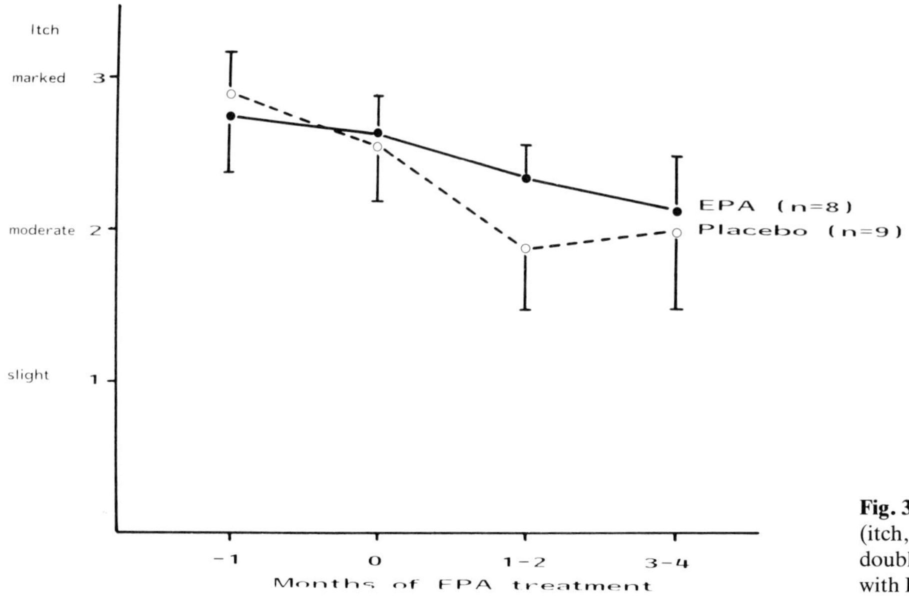

Fig. 3. Intensity of clinical symptoms (itch, subjectively evaluated) during a double-blind, placebo-controlled trial with EPA in severe atopic eczema

Conclusions

Taken together it seems fair to state that the clinical efficacy of unsaturated fatty acids in the treatment of atopic eczema still remains a matter of scientific controversy, awaiting further studies with possibly more purified or enriched lipid fractions. Since some studies clearly demonstrated improvement of some patients or a trend towards improvement, it seems justified to try this kind of therapy in patients with severe disease for a certain period (2–3 months) and thereafter assess the results critically. It is obvious that unsaturated fatty acids in the context of epidermal lipid formation and skin inflammation are a highly interesting area of research.

References

1. Arm JP, Horton C, Mencia-Huerta JM, House F, Eiser NM, Clarc TJH, Spur BW, Lee TH (1988) Effect of dietary supplementation with fish oil lipids on mild asthma. Thorax 43:84–92
2. Ashley JM, Lowe NJ, Borok ME, Alfin-Slater RB (1988) Fish oil supplementation results in decreased hypertriglyceridemia in patients with psoriasis. J Am Acad Dermatol 19:76–82
3. Bamford JT, Gibson RW, Renier CM (1985) Atopic eczema unresponsive to evening primrose oil (linoleic and γ-linoleic acids) J Am Acad Dermatol 13:959–965
4. Bang HO, Dyerberg J (1980) The composition of Eskimo food in northeast Greenland. Am J Clin Nutr 33:2657–615
5. Bégin ME, Das UN (1986) A deficiency in dietary gamma-linoleic and/or eicosapentaenoic acids may determine individual susceptibility to AIDS. Med Hypotheses 20:1–8
6. Bibel DJ, Miller SJ, Brown BE, Pandey BB, Elias PM, Shinefield HR, Aly R (1989) Antimicrobial activity of stratum corneum lipids from normal and essential fatty acid-deficient mice. J Invest Dermatol 92:632–638
7. Bjorneboe A, Soyland E, Bjorneboe GA, Rajka G, Drevon CA (1987) Effect of dietary supplementation with eicosapentaenoic acid in the treatment of atopic dermatitis. Br J Dermatol 117:463–469
8. Bjorneboe A, Klemeyer Smith A, Bjorneboe GA, Thune PO, Drevon CA (1988) Effect of dietary supplementation with n-3 fatty acids on clinical manifestations of psoriasis. Br J Dermatol 118:77–83
9. Braun-Falco O, Ring J (1984) Zur Therapie des atopischen Ekzems. Hautarzt 35:447–454
10. Burr GO, Burr MM (1929) A new deficiency disease produced by the rigid exclusion of fat from the diet. J Biol Chem 82:345–367
11. Burton JL (1989) Dietary fatty acids and inflammatory skin disease. Lancet I:27–32
12. Elias PM, Brown PE, Ziboh VA (1980) Permeability barrier in essential fatty acid deficiency: evidence for a direct role for linoleic acid in epidermal barrier function. J Invest Dermatol 74:230–233
13. Endres S, Ghorbany R, Kelley VE, Georgilis K, Lonnemann G, van der Meer JWM, Cannon JG, Rogers TS, Klempner MS, Weber PC, Schaefer EJ, Wolff SM, Dinarello CA (1989) The effect of dietary supplementation with n-3 polyunsaturated fatty acid on the Synthesis of interleukin-1 and tumor necrosis factor by mononuclear cells. N Engl J Med 320:265–271
14. Erickson KL (1986) Dietary fat modulation of the immune response. Int J Immunopharmacol 8:529–543

15. Fischer S, Weber PC (1984) Prostaglandin I_3 is formed in vivo in man after dietary eicosapentaenoic acid. Nature 307:165–168
16. Fox PL, Cicorleto PE (1988) Fish oils inhibit endothelial cell production of platelet-derived growth factor-like protein. Science 241:453–456
17. Gonnerman WA, Mortensen RF, Tebo JM, Conte JM, Leslie CA, Cathcart ES (1988) Dietary fish oil modulation of macrophage amyloid P component responses in mice. J Dermatol 140:796–799
18. Guenther L, Wexler D (1987) Efamol in the treatment of atopic dermatitis. J Am Acad Dermatol 17:860
19. Gupta AK, Ellis CN, Tellner DC, Anderson TF, Voorhees JJ (1989) Double-blind, placebo-controlled study to evaluate the efficacy of fish oil and low-dose UVB in the treatment of psoriasis. Br J Dermatol 120:801–807
20. Hanifin JM (1983) Diet, nutrition and allergy in atopic dermatitis. J Am Acad Dermatol 8:729–731
21. Hansen AE (1937) Serum lipids in eczema and other pathological conditions. Am J Dis Child 53:933–946
22. Hughes D, Caspary EA, Wisniewski HM (1975) Immunosuppression by linoleic acid. Lancet I:501
23. Isseroff RR, Davis CA (1988) Fish again for dinner! The role of fish and other dietary oils in the therapy of skin disease. J Am Acad Dermatol 19:1073–1080
24. Kelly VE, Itzior S (1983) Enriched lipid diet aceelerates lupus nephritis in NZB x W mice. Am J Pathol 111:288–297
25. Kettler AH, Baughn RE, Orengo IF, Black H, Wolff JE (1988) The effect of dietary fish oil supplementation on psoriasis. J Am Acad Dermatol 18:1267–1273
26. Knapp HR, Garret AF (1989) The antihypertensive effects of fish oil. N Engl J Med 320:1037–1043
27. Kort WJ, Hulsmann LO, Weijma IM, Zondervan PE, Westbroek DL (1986) Influence of the linoleic acid content of the diet in tumor growth in transplantable rat tumor models. Ann Nutr Metab 30:120–128
28. Kragballe K, Fogh K (1989) A low-fat diet supplemented with dietary fish oil (Max-EPA) results in improvement of psoriasis and in formation of leukotrine B_5. Acta Derm Venereol (Stockh) 69:23–28
29. Kromann N, Green A (1980) Epidemiological studies in the Upernnavik district, Greenland. Acta Med Scand 200:401–406
30. Kunz B, Ring J, Braun-Falco O (1989) Eicosapantaenoic acid (EPA) treatment in atopic eczema (AE): a prospective double-blind trial. J Allergy Clin Immunol 83:196
31. Lambrey, Schalla W, Kail N, Lahmy JP, Schaefer H (1987) Influence of an essential fatty acid deficient diet on absorption of topical hydrocortisone in the rat. Br J Dermatol 117:607–615
32. Leaf A, Weber PC (1988) Cardiovascular effects of n-3 fatty acids. N Engl J Med 318:549–557
33. Lee TH, Arm JP (1986) Prospects for modifying the allergic response by fish oil diets. Clin Allergy 16:89–100
34. Lee TH, Hoover RL, Williams JD, Sperling RI, Ravalese J, Spur BW, Robinson DR, Corey EJ, Lewis RA, Austen FK (1985) Effect on dietary enrichment with eicosapentaenoic and docosahexaenoic acids on in vivo neutrophil and monocyte leukotriene generation and neutrophil function. N Engl J Med 312:1217–1224
35. Lefkowith JB (1988) Essential fatty acid deficiency inhibits the in vivo generation of leukotriene B_4 and suppresses levels of resident and elicited leukocytes in acute inflammation. J Immunol 140:228–233
36. Lowe NJ, DeQuoy PR (1978) Linoleic acid effects on epidermal DNA synthesis and cutaneous prostaglandin levels in essential fatty acid deficiency. J Invest Dermatol 70:200–203
37. Mackie BS, Curtin LD, Bourne DJ (1987) Melanoma and dietary lipids. Nutr Cancer 9:219–226
38. Manku MS, Horrobin DF, Morse NL, Wright S, Burton JL (1984) Essential fatty acids in the plasma phospholipids of patients with atopic eczema. Br J Dermatol 110:643–648
39. Maurice PDL, Allen BR, Barkley AS, Cockbill SR, Stammers J, Bather PC (1987) The effects of a dietary supplementation with fish oil in patients with psoriasis. Br J Dermatol 17:599–606
40. Mensink RP, Katan MB (1989) Effect of a diet enriched with monounsaturated or polyunsaturated fatty acids on levels of low-density and high-density lipoprotein cholesterol in healthy women and men. N Engl J Med 321:436–441
41. Mertin J, Stackpole A, Shumway S (1985) Nutrition and immunity: the immunregulatory effect of n-6 essential fatty acids is mediated through prostaglandin E. Int Arch Allergy Appl Immunol 77:390–395
42. Morse PF, Horrobin DF, Manku MS, Stewart RA, Littlewood S, Wright S, Burton J, Gould DJ, Holt PJ, Jansen CT, Mattila L, Meigel W, Dettke T, Wexler D, Guenther L, Bordon A, Patrizi A (1989) Meta-analysis of placebo-controlled studies of the efficacy of Epogam in the treatment of atopic eczema. Relationship between plasma essential fatty acid changes and clinical response. Br J Dermatol 121:75–90
43. Mustakallio KK, Kiistala U, Piha HJ, Nieminen E (1967) Epidermal lipids in Besnier's prurigo (atopic eczema). Ann Med Exp Fenn 45:323–325
44. Olubajo O, Marshall MW, Judd JT, Adkins JT (1986) Effects of high- and low-fat diets on the bioavailability of selected fatty acids, including linoleic acid, in adult men. Nutr Res 6:931–955
45. Reis GJ, Boucher TM, Sipperly ME, Silverman DI, McCabe CH, Baim DS, Sacks FM, Grossman W, Pasternak RC (1989) Randomised trial of fish oil for prevention of restenosis after coronary angioplasty. Lancet I:177–181
46. Ring J (1988) Angewandte Allergologie, 2nd edn. MMV-Vieweg, Munich
47. Ring J, Dorsch W (1985) Altered releasability of vasoactive mediator secreting cells in atopic eczema. Acta Derm Venereol (Stockh), Suppl 114:9–23
48. Ring J, Seifert J, Mertin J, Brendel W (1974) Prolongation of skin allografts in rats by treatment with linoleic acid. Lancet 2:1331
49. Ruzicka T, Simmet T, Peskar BA, Ring J (1986) Skin levels of arachidonic acid-derived inflammatory mediators and histamine in atopic dermatitis and psoriasis. J Invest Dermatol 86:105–108
50. Schalin-Karrila M, Mattila L, Jansen CT, Uotila P (1987) Evening primrose oil in the treatment of atopic eczema: effect on clinical status, plasma phospholipid fatty acids and circulating blood prostaglandins. Br J Dermatol 117: 11–19
51. Sherertz EF (1988) Improved acanthosis nigricans with lipodystrophic diabetes during dietary fish oil supplementation. Arch Dermatol 124:1094–1096
52. Skogh M (1986) Atopic eczema unresponsive to evening primrose oil (linoleic and γ-linolenic acid). J Am Acad Dermatol 5:114–115
53. Strannegard IL, Svennerholm A, Strannegard O (1987) Essential fatty acids in serum lecitin of children with atopic dermatitis and in umbilical cord serum of infants with high or low IgE levels. Int Arch Allergy Appl Immunol 82:422–423

54. Strasser T, Fischer S, Weber PC (1985) Leukotriene B_5 is formed in human neutrophils after dietary supplementation with eicosapentaenoic acid. Proc Natl Acad Sci USA 82:1540–1543
55. Trucheret E, Brändle I, Grosshans E (1987) Hautveränderungen, Pathophysiologie und Therapie bei Mangel an essentiellen Fettsäuren. Z Hautkr 63:290–301
56. Virella G, Kilpatrick JM, Rugeles MT, Hyman B, Russell R (1989) Depression of humoral responses and phagocytic functions in vivo and in vitro by fish oil and eicosapentaenoic acid. Clin Immun Immunopathol 52:257–270
57. Voorhees JJ (1983) Leukotrienes and other lipoxygenase products in the pathogenesis and therapy of psoriasis and other dermatoses. Arch Dermatol 119:541–547
58. Weber PC, Scherer B, Held E, Witzgall H, Lorenz R (1982) Arachidonic acid metabolites, hypertension and arteriosclerosis. Klin Wochenschr 60:479
59. Wehrmann W, Nissen HP, Kreysel HW (1989) Beeinflussung des Fettsäuremetabolismus bei atopischer Dermatitis. Ärztl Kosmetol 19:79–81
60. Wright S, Burton JL (1982) Oral evening-primrose-seed oil improves atopic eczema. Lancet 2:1120–1122
61. Yoshino S, Ellis EF (1987) Effect of a fish-oil-supplemented diet on inflammation and immunological processes in rats. Int Arch Allergy Appl Immunol 84:233–240
62. Ziboh VA (1989) Implications of dietary oils and polyunsaturated fatty acids in the management of cutaneous disorders. Arch Dermatol 125:241–245
63. Ziboh VA, Cohen KA, Ellis CN, Miller C, Hamilton TA, Kragballe K, Hydrick CR, Voorhees JJ (1986) Effects of dietary supplemenation of fish oil on neutrophil and epidermal fatty acids. Arch Dermatol 122:1277–1282

Dietary Management in Atopic Eczema

A. Giannetti and S. Seidenari

Numerous aggravating factors and possible etiological agents have been proposed as triggers for atopic eczema lesions. The importance of dietary factors as emerged in earlier clinical practice has been confirmed in recent years with data derived from more accurate observations and controlled experiments. From a qualitative point of view the diet can be adapted to eliminate foods which are thought or proven to play a pathogenic role in inducing the dermatitis or to correct with supplementary factors possible or supposed metabolic defects. Dietary treatment is suggested in atopic eczema either for diagnostic reasons to establish the presence of food allergies, for therapy, or as a preventative measure in the newborn at risk.

Elimination or Hypoallergenic Diet

Elimination diet is a dietary management that, in the first phase, excludes those foods which are statistically most likely to be allergizing. It seeks to resolve symptoms or to obtain a baseline symptom level that allows a correct interpretation of dermatitis exacerbation during food challenges (diagnostic diet). In the final phase the patient follows a diet which eliminates only those foods which provoke the eczema (therapeutic maintainance diet).

Many authors have reported benefit from elimination diets in atopic eczema, although few studies have been adequately controlled. In a double-blind crossover trial of a milk- and egg-free diet, Atherton et al. [1] overcame the problem of a control diet by using a milk substitute for the excluded cow's milk comprising dried soy or a mixture of dried eggs and cow's milk. The authors observed a significant improvement in the dermatitis in two-thirds of children under the age of 8 years. In 1978, in an open study, Juto et al. [2] treated 20 infants with a strict elimination diet comprising casein hydrolysate or soy milk formula and obtained good results. Hill and Lynch in 1982 [3] and Graham et al. in 1984 [4] instituted dietary management based, respectively, on elemental diet and a hypoallergenic diet in children affected by chronic eczema; both described encouraging results. A double-blind placebo-controlled crossover trial performed by Neild et al. [5] on children and young adults with an egg and milk exclusion diet showed only a 25% response rate, although younger patients benefited to a greater extent. Recently, Sampson [6] has described the clinical course of 34 children who were followed for 3–4 years. One group consisted of 17 children with food hypersensitivity who were maintained with appropriate elimination diets; the other group comprised children in whom no food hypersensitivity could be detected by food challenges. The first group demonstrated a highly significant improvement in clinical scores, both at the midpoint and at the end of the study period.

Indications for Dietary Prescriptions

Although the majority of authors agree that dietary restrictions in atopic eczema are worth trying, they also consider the selection of subjects for treatment to be extremely important, both to save patients unnecessary inconvenience and to avoid uselessly prolonging the diagnostic and therapeutic procedure.

It is generally felt that subjects with only slight dermatitis limited to a few skin sites should not be subjected to dietary treatment. Many authors draw attention to the fact that dietary restrictions constitute a great personal and organizational sacrifice and are a potential risk to health [7, 8]. The American Task Force on Pediatric Dermatology [9] recommends not instituting dietary management if the patient shows a limited dermatitis which responds to basic therapy; it also underlines that severe and prolonged dietary restriction should not be introduced without full consideration of its impact on the patient's general health.

Clinical history is rarely useful in indicating the presence of food allergies or in identifying the food or foods responsible for the symptoms. In our case study 30% of the subjects who responded positively to the elimination diet reported anamnestic indications which were useful for the choice of prescribed foods, and which coincided with the result of the challenge test.

It is advisable to carry out prick tests for the main food allergens before starting a hypoallergenic diet. Positivity may suggest a food allergy and justify subsequent, more complex diagnostic procedures. Indeed, it has been shown that foods selected by positive prick test results are those most likely to cause reactions to food challenges [10–12]. On the other hand, the majority of children over 3 years of age and adults with negative skin test reactions would not have adverse reactions to foods during a properly performed challenge [13]. A negative prick test, however, is no guarantee of the absence of food allergy. The least reliable results are those from prick tests carried out with cow's milk proteins [14]. Of the subjects with atopic eczema in our case study who were negative to the milk allergens in the prick test, 20% showed adverse reactions after challenge with milk and milk products.

Results of the radioallergosorbent test correlate well with prick puncture skin test and can be used to select patients following the same criteria. Table 1 shows prick test results in our case study. The percentages of prick test positivity to the main food allergens are grouped by age of patient at the time of examination. As regards the age of subjects undergoing treatment, it is known that food allergy is rarer in adult atopic eczema. Many subjects who show adverse reactions to foods in infancy overcome the allergy in childhood [15–19]. Munkvad et al. [20] studied the efficacy of an antigen-free diet on dermatitis activity in a double-blind study of 33 adults given an elemental or normal diet; they found no significant differences between the groups. Therefore, positive results from dietary management are more probable in infants and children rather than in adults.

Table 1. Percentage of positive prick tests results to food allergens according to age

	Age of execution of prick test		
Allergen	6–12 months	12–24 months	>2 years
Casein	40.7	15.3	9.6
Wheat	33	7.7	11.7
Whole milk	26.9	11.5	4.6
α-Lactalbumin	25	11.1	7.5
Egg yolk	22.7	15.4	9.1
Pear	22.7	3.8	11.2
Codfish	20.8	11.6	7.4
Orange	19	7.7	11.2
Pork	15	7.7	6
Chicken	14.3	3.8	6
Apple	13.6	0	6.5
Rice	12.5	3.8	9.6
Soy	12.5	16.7	25
Egg white	4.1	42.3	11.8

The Choice of Diagnostic Diet

Obviously, in the diagnostic phase the diet cannot be considered completely anallergic, as each patient can be allergic to any food, including one permitted in the most rigid diets. In most cases the foods responsible for skin symptoms are ingested several times a week. For this reason it is good practice to prescribe a diagnostic diet containing relatively unusual foods.

McEwen's [21] classic diet (Table 2) permits the patient a relatively large list of foods for at least 3 weeks. If this diet fails, the patient must change to a much more rigid one which is continued for a further week. Milk and eggs are the most common allergizing foods, as is evident from the results of diets which eliminate them and, above all, from provocation tests. Sampson [22] observed that 90% of children undergoing blind challenges reacted to 6 food antigens – egg, peanut, milk, wheat, fish, and soy – whereas Atherton [23] found that two-thirds of children

Table 2. The McEwen diet

Diet sheet no. 1
You can eat:

Carnation brand milk, only ½ pint per day maximum. Dilute with water.

Cornflakes and other cereals, porridge, oats, rice, cornflour.

Tea and instant coffee.

Sugar.

Bread, pastry, cakes, biscuits (avoid cream cakes and ones with much egg in them).

Butter (in small quantities), corn oil, or cooking lard.

Beef, salt beef, beef sausage, mince (mutton may be allowed).

Green vegetables, lettuce, carrots (no cauliflower), mushrooms (not more than ¼ lb. per week, and not all at once), potatoes.

Apples, pears, bananas (avoid cores, and don't eat too many), rhubarb, pineapple.

Diet sheet no. 2
Additional diet
If the past three weeks dieting has not helped you, it is advisable to spend the next week on an even more restrictive diet, which completely avoids milk, wheat flour and fruit.
You can eat only:

Sugar.

Porridge and treacle or syrup, rice.

Beef, mince, beef sausages.

Green vegetables and lettuce.

Potatoes.

Butter (in small quantities), cooking lard.

Oat cakes (obtainable at health food stores and big grocers).

You will have to drink water and tea without milk or lemon.

Rhubarb.

under the age of 8 years may benefit from an egg- and milk-free diet. The initial choice of diet can therefore be one which eliminates only milk and eggs and causes relatively little discomfort. If prick tests are positive for other foods, it may be useful to eliminate the main ones among these as well as eggs and milk.

The clinical cross-reactivity between eggs and chicken and milk and veal has been described but not sufficiently controlled with blind challenges. Nevertheless, it is thought to be useful to exclude chicken and veal during a milk- and egg-free diet. If many foods are suspected, an elimination diet with severe restrictions may be tried first. An example is to choose one food in each group of grain, fruit, vegetable, and meat and to allow only these four foods. This oligoantigenic diet is nutritionally inadequate and should be used only for a short period [24]. However, allergy to cereals is frequent, above all in children but also in adults, and it is often necessary to substitute wheat through other cereals. Rice, which is considered less antigenic than wheat, can cause skin symptoms in subjects allergic to wheat, and clinical cross-reactivity between several cereals of the Gramineae family is occasionally observed. Furthermore, in some geographic areas where rice is consumed in very large quantities, for example, Japan and Lombardy in Italy, the percentage of subjects allergic to rice is close to or above that allergic to wheat [25]. In our opinion, therefore, it is more reasonable to substitute simultaneously cereals of the Gramineae family with foods such as buckwheat, white potatoes, sweat potatoes, chestnut meals, sesame seeds, linseed and linseed meal, soya flour and legumes, and bananas.

Especially in adults is sensitization to legumes frequent. Of subjects older than 5 years in our case study, 20% showed specific IgE in prick tests for peanuts, beans, and peas, and 10% had positive exposure tests for one or more legumes. Furthermore, soy is present in many processed foods. Bernhisel-Broadbent and Sampson [26] demonstrated positive oral challenges in 41 of 69 children who showed positive prick test results to legumes. As a result of some degree of cross-reactivity between antigens in various foods of the same family, many authors suggest that it is necessary to reduce or completely avoid the intake of other members of that food family (Table 3). However, results of oral food challenges demonstrate that clinically important cross-reactivity to legumes in children is very rare and that clinical hypersensitivity to one legume does not always warrant dietary elimination of all of them [6, 26, 27]. Patients who are allergic to common foods that are often used in many food preparations should be provided with advice and with special recipes (Table 4) [28–31].

The ultimate avoidance diet is an elemental diet composed of preparations containing crystalline amino acids, dextrose, simple fats derived from oils, vitamins, and minerals. This diet is used particularly if symptoms are severe, there has been no therapeutic response to the previous elimination diet, but there exists a strong suspicion of food allergy.

The therapeutic importance in atopic eczema of additive-free diets is not known. Indeed, food intolerance is an aspect of this illness which has still been little studied.

Table 4. Soya-free diet

Avoid: soy beans, soy milk, soy flour, vegetable oils, margarines, soy lecithin, soy sauces, processed meats, tofu, soy bean sprouts. (Read labels!)

Milk and egg free diet
Avoid: milk, yoghurt, cream, cheese, ice cream, butter, margarines that include milk, sauces that include milk, chocolate, processed meats, other prepacked foods containing milk or milk powder, eggs, cakes and puddings containing eggs, processed meats, pasta, other prepacked foods containing eggs. (Read labels!)

Suggestions for substitution of cow's milk
Cow's milk may be substituted by: soy milk, protein hydrolysates, elemental formula, mixture of water with ground almonds, sesame seeds, or coconut (almond, sesame seed, and coconut milk), herbal tea and fruit juice.
Cheese may be substituted by tofu.

Table 3. Some examples of families of cross-reacting foods

Legumes	Parsley	Potatoes	Cereals	Fruit	Citrusfruits	Nuts
Beans	Carrots	Potatoes	Barley	Almonds	Grapefruit	Brazilnuts
Cocoa beans	Celery	Tomatoes	Corn	Apricots	Lemons	Walnuts
Lentils	Parsley	Aubergines	Oat	Cherries	Tangerines	
Peanuts			Rice	Peaches	Oranges	
Peas			Rye	Plums		
Soy beans			Wheat			

Choice of Infant Formulas

Atopic eczema in infants presents particular diet problems. Given the characteristics of the diet of a baby aged only a few months, there are certainly only a few foods which can be responsible for the eczema, but the dietary alternatives are equally few. Cow's milk can be replaced by soy milk, which contains a proteinic component made up exclusively of the protein of purified soy. However, after about 2 weeks one-third of the patients experience a relapse caused by allergization to soy, probably resulting from absorbtion of undigested soy proteins during the first days of the diet when the intestinal mucosa was still damaged. Replacing the milk with formulas based on hydrolysates gives greater guarantees, although the cost is higher.

Protein hydrolysates are produced by treating a highly nutritional protein, generally casein, with enzymatic hydrolysis. This process makes nitrogen available as amino acids and peptides. A hydrolysate with low immunogenic strength does not contain peptides with a molecular weight greater than 1500 [32, 33]. On the other hand, there are also references in the literature to intolerance of protein hydrolysates [34–36]. Probably polypeptides which are generally too small to induce an immunological response are nevertheless able to provoke such a response in subjects who are already allergic to milk proteins. These subjects can be sensitized not only to the proteins as a whole but also to the peptide products of their digestion. The allergizing strength of formulas made up of a mixture of amino acids is, in contrast, zero, if the theoretical possibility of a recomposition of immunogenic oligopeptides during milk preparation or digestion is excluded. The nutritional value is, however, less than that of the hydrolysates.

Breast-fed infants who develop atopic eczema may be intolerant to a food ingested by the lactating mother. This frequent observation has also been confirmed by Cant et al. [37] who studied 19 breast-fed infants with eczema taking part with their mothers in a double-blind crossover trial excluding eggs and cow's milk. The authors were able to confirm the relationship between ingestion of eggs and milk by the lactating mother and appearance of eczema in six infants. Thus, in breast-fed infants, restriction of the mother's diet is worth trying, and weaning is not recommended as the initial step.

An elimination diet does not require nutritional supplementation unless it continues for more than 1 month. In this case a daily multivitamin with iron supplement should be recommended. During a milk-free diet a calcium supplementation is necessary, for example, 600–800 mg calcium carbonate for children and male adults, 1200 mg for adolescents, and 1000 mg for premenopausal women. For long-term diets it is advisable to refer the family to a trained nutritionist for instruction [24, 31].

Open Food Challenges

Apart from failure to adhere to the diet, a lack of improvement with the dietary therapy could be the result of the limited pathogenetic importance of the food allergy in the particular subject or the choice of allergizing foods in the particular case. Recovery or improvement of the dermatitis may indicate that the clinical picture is at least partially conditioned by food intolerance and also allows a number of tolerated foods to be identified. At this point it is possible to reintroduce the eliminated foods one at a time at 1 week intervals, watching for any recurrence of symptoms, which may appear within 2 h or 1–3 days after initial administration. As a result of the relative nutritional inadequacy of the base diet, initial challenges should be performed with foods chosen to improve the nutritional content of the diet. However, where an adverse reaction to a food is strongly suspected, it is advisable not to use this food in the first phase of food reintroduction. Although the reappearance of the dermatitis may confirm the correlation between the food and the eczema, it may also discourage the patient and impede continuation of the diet. It may therefore be useful to begin adding foods to the diet which are only slightly suspected, so that a more varied and palatable diet may be provided quickly. As foods are incriminated by open challenge, they should be eliminated from the diet. If a food has been added without apparent problems, it should be left in the diet. Such therapeutic diets should be followed for some months, up to the next challenge tests.

Open food challenges can be undertaken at home. However, it is very important to directly check subjects who carry out food reintroductions at intervals equal to the length of exposure to each food (generally 1 week). Assessment is performed by the physician and patient together in terms of objective and subjective improvement in the symptoms. In most cases the systematic assessment of the foods excluded from the diet takes 2–3 months. Open food challenges are easy to administer and in many instances are useful in demonstrating an absence of relationship between ingested food and symptoms. However, not all authors are convinced that these tests provide scientifically valid indications in cases of positivity, since the means of assessment do not exclude the subjective element on the part of the physician and the patient [22, 38, 39]. On the other hand, other authors insist that food reactions can be verified only by repeating administration and observation of the patients for some days during the exposure tests [14, 23].

Hammer [40] performed oral provocation tests in 81 children with atopic eczema, testing them with 100 g cow's milk and 100 g cereals daily for 3 consecutive days and recording skin symptoms. Fifteen children showed positive reactions, which did not appear until the 2nd or 3rd day. Erythema and pruritus were present as primary symptoms mostly on old sites, and these were followed the next day by scaling and/or papular dermatitis which was sometimes disseminated. Juto et al. [2] challenged 19 children with atopic eczema and under 2 years of age by repeated administration of cow's milk after a period of elimination diet. Eczematous delayed reactions were reported in 12 of them.

Blind Challenges

While in the open challenge both the patient and the physician are aware of the contents of the challenge, in the single-blind challenge the patient does not know the challenging food. Some authors believe that only the double-blind challenge with placebo control, where neither the patient nor the physician are aware of the content of the challenge, can guarantee reliable results and control psychogenic factors and physician bias [22, 38, 39]. Foods selected for challenge may be based upon historical information or results of skin prick tests and radioallergosorbent test. Dehydrated foods can be put in opaque capsules or camouflaged in shakes, juices, or preparations of amino acids for elemental diets. The challenge is begun with an amount of food less than the smallest amount thought to produce the reaction. Incremental challenges should be undertaken at 15-min intervals to reach a total dose of 8–10 g dehydrated food. All patients should be observed for a minimum of 2 h after the challenge. If the symptoms have not been reproduced with the blind challenge, the food should be introduced openly to confirm that the patient is not sensitive, and that the food can be consumed without difficulty.

Sampson [6] studied 160 patients with atopic eczema, ranging in age from 3 to 24 years, with double-blind placebo-controlled food challenges. After intensive topical treatment, he performed challenges with up to 10 g dehydrated food in opaque capsules or camouflaged in juice. Egg, peanut, and milk accounted for the majority of the hypersensitivity reactions. He observed all reactions occurring within 3 h of initiating the challenge. Many patients experiencing immediate skin symptoms developed pruritus and, less frequently, a macular pruritic rash in reaction sites 6–8 h after the initial response. The author did not observe isolated late reactions. Symptoms confined to the skin occurred in only 29% of the reactions, gastrointestinal symptoms were observed in 43% and respiratory symptoms in 28%. Patients experiencing symptoms after food challenge were found to have a significant rise in plasma histamine [41]. Sampson [6] believes that food hypersensitivity can provoke pruritus and erythema, which subsequently lead to scratching and eczematous changes.

On reviewing the literature concerning food challenges, the differences in study design often make comparison of results between one study and another difficult. Many important criteria used in the selection of patients and method of food challenge vary markedly from one study to another. The most important controversial area is the timing of reactions. Many authors have divided onset of reactions into prompt or immediate, intermediate and delayed (after 24 h or more), based on the number of minutes, hours, or days since the food challenge began. Authors who perform double-blind placebo-controlled challenges never observe delayed reactions. On the other hand, those who carry out programmed reintroductions of 1 week for each food, believe that single challenges are inadequate because they fail to elicit an exacerbation of eczema in patients in whom repeated challenges on successive days can succeed in doing so [14]. Atherton [23] believes that an item may have to be ingested on several occasions over a period of time or in large amounts to induce detectable exacerbations, and that the interval between ingestion and exacerbation may be on the order of several days. Bock [38] tries to explain the discrepancies between these observations, stating that when an offending food is first administered in a small amount, a reaction (either immunological or nonimmunological) may begin in the gut, but that it may take numerous doses for a biological threshold to be exceeded and for clinical symptoms to be produced. Also, the reaction observed may be due to the last dose.

In reality patients receive several exposures to allergens with normal food intake each day. Such exposure is similar to that realized by programmed successive challenges, both in the quantity of food administered and in the association to other foods such as alcohol or fats which may alter the absorption rates. Moreover, it is not excluded that in the same subject a particular food can induce different reactions (immediate or delayed) acting with different pathogenetic mechanisms. This may also happen as the result of different methods of administration: singly as with blind challenge or repeatedly, as is the case with programmed food reintroductions.

Most children with food allergy and adverse reactions to foods grow out of their sensitivities. The changed reactivity may be due to a decreased absorption of immunogenic food proteins caused by maturation of the intestinal mucosa and the secretory immune system or perhaps to a decreased sensitivity of the target organs.

The particular food which causes the symptoms influences the prognosis of food allergy. While most children outgrow their cow's milk and egg allergy after some years, clinical reactivity to other allergens tends to persist [6]. Bock and Atkins [27] observed that none of 32 children with positive challenges to peanut were seen to have lost their reactivity 2–14 years after the first observation.

Therefore, it is necessary to perform food reintroductions periodically to avoid useless and prolonged dietary restrictions in patients with food allergy.

Preventive Aspects of Dietary Therapy

The expression of allergic illness results from complicated interrelationships between the atopic genetic constitution and the encountered environment. Sensitization against food allergens may occur in the uterus or during breast feeding and may be influenced by the time of onset and type of early solid feeding, by exposure to inhalant allergens, drugs and tobacco smoke, and by viral infections [42–45].

Prenatal Sensitization

IgE have been documented in infant cord blood by Paper Radio Immuno-Sorbent Test in 13% to 82% of term pregnancies depending in part on atopic status of parents, maternal IgE, and other pharmacological and infectious factors [46–48]. Specific prenatal sensitization across the placenta to food (egg, milk) and inhalant allergens seems to occur in fewer than 1% of human newborns [47, 49, 50]. Skin prick positivity has been demonstrated in newborn babies [51], and in a few cases the occurrence of specific IgE antibodies to food in cord sera have been reported [42, 52]. To prevent the transplacental passage of antigens with possible fetal sensitization some authors have instituted maternal avoidance diets and have studied the effect of these on at risk babies.

Dietary Management in Pregnancy

In a prospective randomized study Fälth et al. [53] monitored the effect of maternal abstention from cow's milk and egg from week 28 of pregnancy to delivery on the development of atopy in 213 babies. At 18 months of age the occurrence of allergies, assessed by skin prick testing, determination of serum IgE, questionnaires, and blinded physical examination did not differ significantly in the two groups of babies whose mothers did or did not receive the diet during pregnancy. These authors also observed no protective effect of high levels of maternal IgG antibodies to foods at delivery and high food antibody levels against development of atopy in cord blood [54, 55]. Moreover, the cord blood IgG levels did not differ between babies whose mothers were on diet during pregnancy and babies whose mothers had a normal exposure to egg and cow's milk. Lilja et al. [56] found no differences in total cord blood IgE levels, the presence of cord blood IgE antibodies to egg and milk, or IgE antibody levels to milk and egg in infants of atopic women whose diets were either high or low in egg or cow's milk in the third trimester in pregnancy. The abovedata do not support a diet during pregnancy as the only preventative measure against the development of atopic eczema.

Postnatal Sensitization

Postnatal sensitization to food allergens may occur either directly by exposure or indirectly by dietary antigens consumed by the mother and transferred into the breast milk [57, 58]. The passage of egg [59, 60], milk [61], and wheat [62] antigens consumed by the mother into breast milk has been well documented. Postnatal sensitization to food antigens in breast milk has been reported as causing food allergy reactions in about 6% of breast-fed infants, with symptoms often occurring during initial direct food exposure [63, 64]. However, the real frequency of human postnatal sensitization through breast milk of presumably exclusively breast-fed infants is difficult to evaluate, as the majority of the studies on this subject fail to rule out the possibility that some infants developing IgE antibodies may have inadvertently or occasionally been given the foodstuffs directly, a practice which, according to some authors, would constitute the most frequent cause of sensitization to cow's milk proteins in newborns at risk [65, 66]. In breast-fed infants, subsequent exposure to the minute amounts of cow's milk proteins in human milk may act as booster doses eliciting allergic manifestations. This hypothesis is supported by studies that have reported that infants with cow's milk allergy were given cow's milk formula significantly more often than controls during the first 4 weeks of life, and that the frequency of cow's milk allergy is higher among newborns who have ingested cow's milk formula supplements than among newborns exclusively breast-fed as infants [65, 66]. Possibly occasional administration of small quantities of cow's milk is more deleterious than regular feeding, as is evident in animal studies, where continuous exposure to the antigen has been considered as a way of promoting the development of immunological competence in young rats. A "low-antigen diet," with trace amounts of antigens, may thus also induce an IgE response in human newborns [67–69].

Breast Feeding

Breast feeding may decrease allergic sensitization by reducing exposure and inducing an earlier maturation of the intestinal barrier or by passively providing factors that promote such a barrier thus limiting intestinal absorption of food antigens.

In a study of 9-month-old infants in 1936, Grulee and Sanford [70] documented a reduction in the incidence of eczema in breast-fed infants compared to those fed with cow's milk. Since then many prospective infant feeding studies have been performed, but these have produced conflicting results. Two common factors emerging from the studies which suggest that breast feeding may reduce allergic disease are prolonged breast feeding (over 4 months) and delayed solid food introduction. Inversely, from the negative studies one can conclude that very brief breast feeding with early solid food introduction most likely provides no overall benefit for the reduction of allergies compared with cow's milk feeding and early solid food feeding [48]. Zeiger et al. [64] studied the effect of maternal avoidance of cow's milk, eggs, and peanuts during the third trimester of pregnancy and lactation and infant use of casein hydrolysate for supplementation or weaning, associated with late introduction of solid foods on the development of allergic diseases in infants of atopic parents. They demonstrated that a strict food allergen avoidance regimen resulted in a significant reduction of food-related atopic eczema during the 1st year and of food-specific IgE sensitization. At 24 months, however, the cumulative prevalence of allergic disease was similar in the prophylactically treated and control groups. Chandra et al. [71] found that a maternal diet excluding milk, eggs, peanuts, fish, and beef during pregnancy and lactation, coupled with breast feeding and delaying solid food introduction for 6 months, reduced the incidence of eczema from 31% to 14% in infants at risk for atopy.

Studies on the effect of soy feeding on the development of allergy in infancy provide conflicting results. Some authors found no protective effect of soy versus cow's milk feeding on the prevalence of allergy in the first 3 years of life [72, 73], whereas according to other authors the association of soy milk supplementation with breast feeding and a maternal avoidance regimen seemed to reduce the percentage of infants developing atopic manifestations [74].

Modulation of Cutaneous Arachidonic Acid Metabolism by Dietary Essential Fatty Acids

In 1933 it was reported that eczematous children had decreased levels of unsaturated fatty acids in the blood. Since then, several studies have been performed with the introduction of vegetable oils into the diet of atopic eczema patients. Results have been conflicting.

In 1981 Lovell and Burton [75] reported that administration of capsules of primrose seed oil produce a small but significant improvement in patients with atopic eczema. Subsequently, Whright and Burton [76] found a 43% improvement in the clinical signs of atopic eczema in children given evening primrose oil. In similarly affected adults, they found a progressively better response, particularly with regard to severity of itching, as the dose was raised. Bamford et al. [77] used evening primrose oil in amounts similar to those employed by Whright and Burton [2–8g] but observed no significant effect on skin symptoms. Recently, Schalin-Karrila et al. [78] treated 25 adults with atopic eczema in a double-blind trial with evening primrose oil or placebo and observed a statistically significant improvement, particularly in the severity and grade of inflammation of the dermatitis. The data of Morse et al. [79] comprise nine controlled trials of evening primrose oil performed in eight centers. Four of the trials were parallel and five crossover. In all studies there was a highly significant improvement, with a striking effect on itching.

The evening primrose plant is a rich source of linoleic acid and γ-linolenic acid, two polyunsaturated fatty acids of the n-3-series. The clinical improvement of atopic eczema during administration of evening primrose oil correlates with a rise in plasma fatty acids [78–80]. Ziboh [80] speculated that the possible mechanisms for the reported beneficial effects of linolenic acid in some cutaneous disorders could result in the in vivo epidermal generation of 15-hydroxy acids, the local increase of which inhibit the production of proinflammatory arachidonic acid metabolites generated by the 5-lipoxygenase pathway, particularly leukotriene B_4. Manku et al. [81, 82] suggest that the alterations in fatty acid composition of plasma phospholipids, in particular the decrease in γ-linolenic acid, indicate defective functioning of the converting enzyme Δ6-desaturase in atopic eczema patients.

Oral administration of γ-linolenic acid bypasses the Δ6-desaturase block in atopic eczema patients [83]. γ-Linolenic acid is converted into dihomo-γ-linolenic acid, which serves as a precursor for PGE_1 synthesis. PGE_1 activates adenylate cyclase, which increases the cAMP levels of mast cells and basophils, thereby leading to dose-dependent inhibition of histamine release [84–86]. Melnik and Plewig [83] hypothesize that the significantly reduced pruritus in patients supplemented with evening primrose oil might be explained by a PGE_1-mediated inhibition of histamine release from mast cells and basophils. They state that the deficiency of Δ6-desaturase activity is the primary genetically transmitted defect in atopy and leads to deficient formation of PGE_1 and subsequently to deficient T-cell function and uncontrolled B-cell responses, in other words, the atopic state. The same authors recommend oral administration of γ-linolenic acid to the nursing mother and her baby for at least 3 months after birth, that is, during a period of high PGE_1 responsiveness of the newborn's T-cell system.

The assumption about defective functioning of Δ6-desaturase in atopics is not shared by all authors. Schalin-Karrila et al. [78] found no difference in the fatty acid composition of plasma phospholipids from patients with atopic eczema as compared to that of healthy subjects. They also observed a significant increase in the level of dihomo-γ-linolenic acid, but not that of PGE_1, in the plasma of atopic eczema patients after treatment with primrose oil. Eicosapentaenoic acid, a major polyunsaturated fatty acid in fish oil, is metabolized, like γ-linolenic acid, by epidermal 15-lipoxygenase into 15-hydroxyeicosapentaenoic acid, a potent in vitro inhibitor of leukotriene B_4 generation. The effect of the administration of fish oil to psoriatic patients has been studied by many authors, but with conflicting results [87–89]. Soyland et al. [90] investigated the effects of a dietary supplementation with *n*-3 fatty acids in patients with atopic eczema in a double-blind study and observed favorable results.

References

1. Atherton DJ, Sewell M, Soothill JF, Wells RS, Chilvers CED (1978) A double-blind controlled crossover trial of an antigen avoidance diet in atopic eczema. Lancet i:401–403
2. Juto P, Engberg S, Winberg J (1978) Treatment of infantile atopic dermatitis with a strict elimination diet. Clin Allergy 8:493–500
3. Hill DJ, Lynch BC (1982) Elemental diet in the management of severe eczema in childhood. Clin Allergy 12:3133–3135
4. Graham P, Hall-Smith SP, Harris JM, Price ML (1984) A study of hypoallergenic diets and oral sodium cromoglycate in the management of atopic eczema. Br J Dermatol 110: 457–467
5. Neild VS, Marsden RA, Bailes JA, Bland JM (1986) Egg and milk exclusion diets in atopic eczema. Br J Dermatol 114:117–123
6. Sampson HA (1988) The role of food allergy and mediator release in atopic dermatitis. J Allergy Clin Immunol 81: 635–645
7. Webber SA, Graham-Brown RAC, Hutchinson PE, Burns DA (1989) Dietary manipulation in childhood atopic dermatitis. Br J Dermatol 121:91–98
8. David TJ, Waddington E, Stanton RHJ (1984) Nutritional hazards of elimination diets in children with atopic eczema. Arch Dis Child 59:323–325
9. Caputo RV, Frieden I, Krafchik BR, Lane AT, Lucky A, Paller A et al. (1986) Diet and atopic dermatitis. J Am Acad Dermatol 15:543–545
10. Hannuksela M (1987) Diagnosis of dermatologic food allergy. Ann Allergy 59:153–156
11. Sampson HA, Albergo R (1984) Comparison of results of skin tests, RAST, and double-blind, placebo-controlled food challenges in children with atopic dermatitis. J Allergy Clin Immunol 74:26–33
12. Sampson HA (1987) Immunologically mediated reactions to foods: IgE in eczema. Ann Allergy 59:71–76
13. Hanifin JM (1986) Significance of food hypersensitivity in children with atopic dermatitis. Pediatr Dermatol 3:163–165
14. Atherton DJ (1986) Significance of food hypersensitivity in children with atopic dermatitis. Pediatr Dermatol 3:161–163
15. Bock SA (1985) Natural history of severe reactions to foods in young children. J Pediatr 107:676–680
16. Eggleston PA (1987) Prospective studies in the natural history of food allergy. Ann Allergy 59:179–182
17. Ford RPK, Taylor B (1982) Natural history of egg hypersensitivity. Arch Dis Child 57:649
18. Bock SA (1982) The natural history of food sensitivity. J Allergy Clin Immunol. 69:173–177
19. Sampson HA (1985) Persistence of food hypersensitivity in children with atopic dermatitis. J Allergy Clin Immunol 75:179
20. Munkvard M, Danielsen L, Hoj L, Povlsen CO, Secher L, Svejgaard E, Bundgaard A, Larsen PO (1984) Antigen-free diet in adult patients with atopic dermatitis. Acta Derm-Venereol (Stockh) 64:524–528
21. McEwen LM (1970) The use of a dietary and antibacterial regimen in the management of intrinsic allergy. Ann Allergy 28:256
22. Sampson HA (1988) Immunologically mediated food allergy: the importance of food challenge procedures. Ann Allergy 60:262–269
23. Atherton DJ (1981) Allergy and atopic eczema II. Clin Exper Dermatol 6:317–325
24. Mahan LK, Furukawa CT (1988) General nutritional considerations and diet for adverse food reactions. In: Bierman CW, Pearlman DS (eds) Allergic diseases from infancy to adulthood. Saunders Philadelphia: 367–376
25. Ikezawa Z, Miyakawa J, Komatsu H, Sugiyama A, Suga C, Miyakawa K et al (1989) Analysis of rice allergen in atopic dermatitis and preparation of hypoallergenic rice. Abstracts of the ESDR-JSID-SID Tricontinental Meeting Washington, CD. April 26–30, 1989

26. Bernhisel-Broadbent J, Sampson HA (1989) Cross-allergenicity in the legume botanical family in children with food hypersensitivity. J Allergy Clin Immunol 83:435–440
27. Bock SA, Atkins FM (1989) The natural history of peanut allergy. J Allergy Clin Immunol 83:900–904
28. Hamrick B, Wiesenfeld SL (1981) The eggfree, milkfree, wheatfree cookbook. Cygnus Midland, TX
29. American Dietetic Association (1971) Allergy Recipes. American Dietetic Association, Chicago
30. US Department of Agriculture (1975) Baking for people with food allergies. Home and Garden Bulletin No. 147. US Government Printing Office, Washington DC
31. Krause MV, Mahan LK (1984) Food, nutrition and diet therapy, 7th edn. Saunders, Philadelphia
32. Knights RJ, Manes JD (1987) Composition, molecular weight, and antigenicity of casein hydrolysates used in a formula for food allergic and malabsorptive infants. In: Chandra RK (ed) Food allergy, pp 273–285
33. Singh B, Lee KC, Fraga E, Wilkinson A, Wong M, Marton MA (1980) Minimum peptide sequences necessary for priming and triggering of humoral and cell-mediated immune responses in mice. Use of synthetic peptide antigens of defined structure. J Immunol 124:1336–1343
34. Takase M, Fukuwatari Y, Kawasi K, Kiyosawa I, Ogasa K, Suzuki S, Kuroume T (1979) Antigenicity of casein enzymatic hydrolysate. J Dairy Sci 62:1570–1576
35. Verkasalo M, Kuintuven P, Savilahti E (1981) Changing pattern of cow's milk intolerance. Acta Paediatr Scand 70:289
36. Schwartz HR, Neururakar LS, Spies JR et al (1980) Milk hypersensitivity: RAST studies using new antigens generated by pepsin hydrolysis of betalactoglobulin. Ann Allergy 45:242
37. Cant AJ, Bailes JA, Marsden RA, Hewitt D (1986) Effect of maternal dietary exclusion on breast fed infants with eczema: two controlled studies. Br Med J 293:231–233
38. Bock SA (1986) A critical evaluation of clinical trials in adverse reactions to foods in children. J Allergy Clin Immunol 78:165–174
39. Bock SA (1988) Evaluation of patients with adverse reactions to foods. In: Bierman CW, Pearlman DS (eds) Allergic diseases from infancy to adulthood. Saunders Philadelphia: 359–365
40. Hammar H (1977) Provocation with cow's milk and cereals in atopic dermatitis. Acta Derm-Venereol (Stockh) 57:159–163
41. Sampson HA, Jolie PA (1984) Increased plasma histamine concentrations after food challenges in children with atopic dermatitis. N Engl J Med 311:372
42. Kjellman NIM (1981) Effect of parental smoking on IgE levels in children. Lancet i:993
43. Settipane RJ, Hagy GW (1979) Effect of atmospheric pollen on the newborn. RI Med J 62:477
44. Bjorksten F, Suoniemi I (1979) Dependence of immediate hypersensitivity on the month of birth. Clin Allergy 6:165
45. Frick OL, German DF, Mills J (1979) Development of allergy in children. I. Association with virus infections. J Allergy Clin Immunol 63:228
46. Businco L, Marchetti F, Pelligrini G, Berlini R (1983) Predictive value of cord blood IgE levels in "at risk" newborn babies and influence of type of feeding. Clin Allergy 13:503–508
47. Kjellmann NM, Croner S (1984) Cord blood IgE determination for allergy prediction-a follow-up to seven years of age in 1,651 children. Ann Allergy 53:167–171
48. Zeiger RS, Heller S, Mellon M, O'Connor R, Hamburger RN (1986) Effectiveness of dietary manipulation in the prevention of food allergy in infants. J Allergy Clin Immunol 78:224–238
49. Kjellman NIM, Johansson SGO (1976) IgE and atopic allergy in newborn and infants with a family history of atopic disease. Acta Paediatr Scand 65:495
50. Croner S, Kjellman NIM, Eriksson B, Roth A (1982) IgE screening in 1701 newborn infants and the development of atopic disease during infancy. Arch Dis Child 57:364
51. Kaufman HS (1971) Allergy in the newborn: skin test reactions confirmed by the Prausnitz-Küstner test at birth. Clin Allergy 1:363–367
52. Michel FB, Bousquet J, Greillier P, Robinet-Levy M, Coulomb Y (1980) Comparison of cord blood IgE concentrations and maternal allergy for the prediction of atopic disease in infancy. J Allergy Clin Immunol 65:422–430
53. Fälth-Magnusson K, Kjellman N-IM (1987) Development of atopic disease in babies whose mothers were receiving exclusion diet during pregnancy – a randomized study. J Allergy Clin Immunol 80:868–875
54. Fälth-Magnusson K, Oman H, Kjellman NIM (1987) Maternal abstention from cow's milk and egg in allergy-risk pregnancies: effect on antibody production in the mother and the newborn. Allergy 42:64–73
55. Fälth-Magnusson K, Kjellman NIM, Magnusson K-E (1988) Antibodies IgG, IgA, and IgM to food antigens during the first 18 months of life in relation to feeding and development of atopic disease. J Allergy Clin Immunol 81: 743–749
56. Lilja G, Dannaeus A, Magnusson KF et al. Immune response of the atopic woman and foetus: effects of high- and low-dose food allergen intake during late pregnancy. Clin Allergy 18:131–142
57. Kilshaw PJ, Cant AJ (1984) The passage of maternal dietary proteins into human breast milk. Int Arch Allergy Appl Immunol 75:8–15
58. Jacobsson I, Lindberg T, Benediktsson B, Hansson BG (1985) Dietary bovine β-lactoglobulin is transferred to human milk. Acta Paediatr Scand 74:342–345
59. Shannon WR (1921) Demonstration of food proteins in human breast milk by anaphylactic experiments on guinea pigs. Am J. Dis Child 22:223
60. Donnally HH (1930) The question of elimination of foreign protein (egg white) in woman's milk. J Immunol 19:15
61. Stuart CA, Twiselton R, Nicholas MF, Hide DW (1984) Passage of cow's milk protein in breast milk. Clin Allergy 14:533
62. Hemmings WA, Kulangara AC (1978) Dietary antigens in breast milk. Lancet 2:575
63. Van Asperen PP, Kemop AS, Mellis CM (1983) Immediate food hypersensitivity reactions on the first known exposure to the food. Arch Dis Child 58:253
64. Zeiger RS, Heller S, Mellon MH, Forsythe AB, O'Connor RD, Hamburger RN, Schatz M (1989) Effect of combined maternal and infant food-allergen avoidance on development of atopy in early infancy: a randomized study. J Allergy Clin Immunol 84:72–89
65. Host A, Husby S, Osterballe O (1988) A prospective study of cow's milk allergy in exclusively breast-fed infants. Acta paediatr Scand 77:663–670
66. Stintzing G, Zetterstrom R (1978) Cow's milk allergy incidence and pathogenetic role of early exposure to cow's milk formula. Acta Paediatr Scand 68:383–387
67. Jacobsson I, Lindberg T (1979) A prospective study of cow's milk protein intolerance in Swedish infants. Acta Paediatr Scand 68:853–859

68. Jarrett EE (1984) Perinatal influences on IgE responses. Lancet ii:797–799
69. Jarrett EE, Hall E (1984) The development of IgE-suppressive immunocompetence in young animals: influence of exposure to antigen in the presence or absence of maternal immunity. Immunology 53:365–373
70. Grulee CG, Sanford HN (1936) The influence of breast and artificial feeding on infantile eczema. J Pediatr 9:223–226
71. Chandra RK, Puri S, Suraiya C, Cheema PS (1986) Influence of maternal food antigen avoidance during pregnancy and lactation on incidence of atopic eczema in infants. Clin Allergy 16:563–571
72. Brown EB, Josephson BM, Levine HS, Rosen M (1969) A prospective study of allergy in a pediatric population. Am J Dis Child 117:693
73. Kjellman NIM, Johansson SGO (1979) Soy versus cow's milk in infants with a biparenteral history of atopic disease: development of atopic disease and immunoglobulins from birth to 4 years of age. Clin Allergy 9:347
74. Businco L, Cantani A, Meglio P, Bruno G (1987) Prevention of atopy: results of a long-term (7 months to 8 years) follow-up. Ann Allergy 59:183–186
75. Lovell CR, Burton JL, Horrobin DF (1981) Treatment of atopic eczema with evening primrose oil. Lancet i:278
76. Wright S, Burton JL (1982) Oral evening-primrose-seed oil improves atopic eczema. Lancet ii:1120–1122
77. Bamford JTM, Gibson RW, Renier CM (1985) Atopic eczema unresponsive to evening primrose oil (linoleic and γ-linolenic acids). J Am Acad Dermatol 13:959–965
78. Schalin-Karrila M, Mattila L, Jansen CT et al (1987) Evening primrose oil in the treatment of atopic eczema: effect on clinical status, plasma phospholipid fatty acids and circulating blood prostaglandins. Br J Dermatol 117:11–19
79. Morse PF, Horrobin DF, Manku MS, Stewart JCM, Allen R, Littlewood S et al (1989) Meta-analysis of placebo-controlled studies of the efficacy of Epogam in the treatment of atopic eczema. Relationship between plasma essential fatty acid changes and clinical response. Br J Dermatol 121:75–90
80. Ziboh VA (1989) Implications of dietary oils and polyunsaturated fatty acids in the management of cutaneous disorders. Arch Dermatol 125:241–245
81. Manku MS, Horrobin DF, Morse N et al (1982) Reduced levels of prostaglandin precursors in the blood of atopic patients: defective delta-6-desaturase function as a biochemical basis for atopy. Prostaglandins Leukotrienes Med 9:615–628
82. Manku MS, Horrobin DF, Morse NL et al (1984) Essential fatty acids in the plasma phospholipids of patients with atopic eczema. Br J Dermatol 110:643–648
83. Melnik BC, Plewig G (1989) Is the origin of atopy linked to deficient conversion of ω-6-fatty acids to prostaglandin E_1? J Am Acad Dermatol. 21:557–563
84. Samuelsson B, Goldyne M, Granström E et al (1978) Prostaglandins and thromboxanes. Ann Rev Biochem 47:997–1029
85. Hanifin JM (1983) Clinical and basic aspects of atopic dermatitis. Semin Dermatol 2:5–13
86. Bourne HR, Lichtenstein LM, Melmon KL (1972) Pharmacologic control of allergic histamine release in vitro: evidence for an inhibitory role of 3', 5'-adenosine monophosphate in human leukocytes. J Immunol 108:695–705
87. Ziboh VA, Miller C, Kragballe K et al (1986) Effects of dietary supplementation of fish oil on neutrophil and epidermal fatty acids: modulation of the clinical course of psoriatic subjects. Arch Dermatol 122:1277–1282
88. Burton JL (1989) Dietary fatty acids and inflammatory skin disease. Lancet i:27–31
89. Bjørneboe A, Smith AK, Bjørneboe GE, Thune PO, Drevon CA (1988) Effect of dietary supplementation with n-3 fatty acids on clinical manifestations of psoriasis. Br J Dermatol 118:77–83
90. Soyland E, Rajka G, Bjørneboe A, Bjørneboe GE, Drevon CA. Effect of dietary supplementation with eicosapentaenoic acid in the treatment of atopic dermatitis. Abstracts of the third international symposium on atopic dermatitis, 29 May–1 Jun, 1988, Oslo

Immunomodulation in the Treatment of Atopic Eczema

H. Zachariae

Introduction

The mechanisms leading to the symptoms of allergic rhinitis and allergic asthma are today well characterised, while the pathophysiology of atopic eczema (AE) is still to a high degree obscure [16]. There is, however, no doubt concerning the close association between the different atopic diseases, and this clinical association suggests a possible pathogenic role for reaginic antibodies. Concomitant respiratory allergy and AE have also long been recognized, and it has been suggested by several authors that inhaled allergens, e.g. house dust mites [13, 43], algae [6] and fungi [34], may contribute to allergy, exacerbating the dermatitis.

Some 80% of patients with AE show positive skin tests reacting to one or more environmental allergens [34], and serum IgE levels are elevated in approximately the same percentage with the highest values occurring in patients with extensive dermatitis [26]. The levels in these patients are higher than in patients with asthma or allergic rhinitis [16], and patients with high levels of IgE are likely to have a poor prognosis. Hanifin [16] agrees that all this information suggests a special pathogenic role for IgE, but he also shows that other evidence tends to gainsay this role. This evidence against a causal relationship includes: typical flexural eczema in patients with agammaglobulinaemia, normal IgE levels in 20% of patients, high levels of IgE in some conditions without dermatitis such as parasitosis and high IgE levels sometimes persisting during remissions. It is also stated that persons who were cured and free of classic signs of AE for a year had normal IgE levels even if they had persistent or recurrent eczema of the hands or nummular eczema.

Patients with AE also show other signs of lack of immunological balance such as unusual susceptibility to skin infections [10, 25] and reduced delayed-type hypersensitivity [12]. There are reduced circulating T lymphocytes, especially reduced T-gamma T lymphocytes [23], low responses in vitro to mitogens and antigens [39], a reduced antibody-dependent cellular toxicity of mononuclear cells and monocytes [28], reduced natural killer cell activity [24] and a defective, non-specific, suppressor cell capacity [23]. The lowered natural killer cell activity has been related to low IL-2 production, and both factors correlate inversely with the concentration of IgE in the serum [14]. Synthesis of IgE in vitro by unstimulated peripheral blood leukocytes from patients with AE is increased, suggesting that the deficient T-suppressor cell accounts for the over-production of IgE [16]. Another finding was of complexed IgE in AE [30].

The lack of immunological balance and especially the high IgE levels in the most severe patients have led to trials with non-specific immunomodulation as well as to the use of specific immunotherapy. The reported effect of psoralens together with UVA-light (PUVA) on AE [29] is not discussed in this chapter, but the possibility cannot be ruled out that it is an effect of immunomodulation.

Plasma Separation

The reduction of IgE or IgE immune complexes by plasma separation has been reported in one patient with AE with increased serum IgE and asthma [15] and in one patient with hyper IgE syndrome [20]. In both instances clinical improvement was observed.

The effect of intensive plasma separation has also been studied in four patients with AE, bronchial asthma and elevated levels of IgE [30]. Plasma separation was performed eight times within 5 weeks. IgE immune complexes were demonstrated in three of the patients prior to treatment. Shortly after eight separations IgE was reduced in all patients to a mean level of 46%, and the IgE immune complexes disappeared. After 3 weeks, however, serum IgE rose to 80% in three patients, and in one the serum IgE exceeded the initial level. Two of the patients again had IgE immune complexes. A questionable clinical improvement of the dermatitis was reported, which was short lasting. These investigators concluded that as plasma separation is both expensive and time consuming, and as the effect is not lasting, for the time being this procedure could not be recommended.

Transfer Factor

Transfer factor (TF) is a low molecular weight extract from human leukocytes, with the ability to increase cutaneous cell-mediated immune reactions [17]. TF has been given as treatment to patients with immunodeficiency diseases and has been used to intensify cell-mediated immunity in patients with relative immunological defects, among them patients suffering from neoplastic disorders. TF has previously been found to decrease serum IgE in mycosis fungoides [42]. It is able to induce a significant increase in cAMP in T-gamma lymphocytes [17] and could therefore be of value in AE by an effect on non-specific suppressor cells for IgE.

TF has been claimed to have been used with success in two children with severe AE [1, 37], while other workers [18] tried TF for weeks in adult patients in a double-blind, crossover study without effect.

I treated ten patients with AE with TF (from 2 x 10^9 leukocytes given intramuscularly every other week) (sterile isotonic saline) or placebo for 1 year [43]. The same physician gave a clinical evaluation before treatment, each month during treatment and 1 month after treatment. The extent and severity of the disease was quantitated, and the use of topical steroids calculated monthly.

A number of in vivo and in vitro tests were performed both before, during and after the treatment period such as a Danish standard series of prick tests, RAST tests for *Dermatophagoides pteronyssinus*, estimation of serum IgE, enumeration of T and B lymphocytes, subpopulations of T lymphocytes, mitogen reactivity of lymphocytes, antibody-dependent cytotoxicity of monocytes and isoproterenol stimulation of cAMP in monocytes.

I found no evidence for an improvement in the dermatitis during therapy. Nor were there any significant differences between the two groups or any significant change in the immunological parameters. Table 1 shows the results of IgE in serum.

As observations by Jarisch et al. [22] indicated that daily injections of TF in children with high levels of IgE lead to a very pronounced reduction of this antibody in serum, I also tried TF 2 i.u. per day for 7 days. The treatment was given to 4 adult patients with severe AE in order to see whether such intensive therapy could change the IgE concentration [43], but there was no convincing effect. The conclusion is that TF, as given in this study, was not able to influence the clinical course or immunoreactivity in adult patients with AE.

Table 1. IgE in serum (IU/ml) in 10 patients with atopic eczema treated with placebo or transfer factor (TF) for 1 year

No.	Before	3 months	6 months	12 months
Placebo				
I	897	867	1 460	1 560
II	2 560	3 380	2 400	1 610
III	2 080	1 910	1 950	1 690
IV	3 350	3 180	2 260	1 850
VI	8 880	16 100	11 100	11 700
Mean	3 589	5 087	3 834	3 682
TF				
VIII	633	1 160	689	1 230
IX	2 240	2 130	2 660	1 790
X	2 020	1 520	1 430	1 790
XI	1 840	4 550	4 490	1 950
XII	4 250	4 330	3 660	4 750
Mean	2 197	2 738	2 586	2 302

Colchicine

Colchicine has for many years been used in gout. The drug inhibits chemotaxis of polymorphonuclear leukocytes [5], blocks leukocyte adhesiveness [32] and stabilises lysosomal membranes [33]. Suppression of inflammatory responses by it has been shown in animal experiments, and DNCB-induced irritant dermatitis has been markedly inhibited. Colchicine has been tried in cutaneous vascular diseases as well as in familial Mediterranean fever [11]. In 1982 Ilfeld and Kuperman [19] reported the correction of a deficient Con A-activated suppressor cell function by colchicine in four patients. This led me to try the drug in ten patients with severe AE and high values of serum IgE.

Colchicine was given as tablets 1 mg twice daily for 4 weeks. All patients were treated simultaneously during the spring. The clinical evaluation was carried out after 2 and 4 weeks by the same physician. All patients were allowed to continue with topical treatment, a group II steroid. Serum IgE was investigated before and at each control visit. In seven patients polymorphonuclear leukocyte chemotaxis was also studied.

Although chemotaxis was reduced in all seven patients, thus establishing the activity of the drug, no one improved clinically, and the serum IgE level did not change during the study. The laboratory data can be seen in Tables 2 and 3. Under the circumstances of this investigation, colchicine was found to be of no clinical value in AE.

Table 2. Chemotactic index (CI) in atopics before and after 2 weeks colchicine 2 mg daily

Patient no.	CI Before	After
1	4.4	1.2
2	3.4	1.6
3	3.5	1.4
4	3.4	1.7
5	2.2	1.3
6	2.6	1.9
7	2.6	1.6

Table 3. Serum IgE in nine atopics prior to and after 2 weeks' colchicine 2 mg daily

Patient no.	IgE (units) Before	After
1	2 740	3 430
2	9 370	7 780
3	17 300	17 160
4	1 320	1 640
5	24 000	20 000
6	3 910	1 990
7	7 160	6 400
8	11 100	13 300
9	15 000	11 400

Bestatin and Fanetizole Mesylate

Bestatin [(2S, 3R)-3-amino-2-hydroxy-4-phenyl-butanoylL-leucocine], a competitive inhibitor of aminopeptidase B and leucine aminopeptidase, augments various immune responses [4] and has been found to induce a transient reduction in IgE concentration in the sera of healthy, non-atopic persons [3]. We have therefore tried bestatin therapy in ten adult patients with severe AE [40].

Bestatin was given as tablets 20 mg twice daily for 3 months. The study was conducted over a 1-year period with 2 or 3 participants every 4 month in order to avoid a bias from seasonal variation. The clinical evaluation was carried out by the same physician, giving points for disease activity in 5 different regions. Five of the patients participated in an immunological assessment before and during the treatment period.

The clinical evaluation showed that bestatin was not able to change the course of the dermatitis, and no statistically significant changes occurred in the laboratory data (Table 4). Our conclusion is that bestatin seems to be of no value in the therapy of patients with AE. Rocklin et al. [36] studied the effect of fanetizole mesylate or CP-48810, an experimental immunostimulating drug, on suppressor cell function and IgE synthesis in vitro in atopic patients with allergic rhinitis and/or asthma and eczema. In the absence of the drug, histamine ($10^{-3}M$) stimulated blood mononuclear cells from 23 atopic patients and suppressed Con A-induced lymphocyte proliferation by a mean of 9.3% ± 3.5% compared with 25.1% ± 2.7% of cells from non-atopic controls. The addition of the drug in vitro significantly increased histamine suppressor cell activity of atopic patients to 26.6% ± 3.9% in the presence of the drug. This study indicates that fanetizole mesylate could be a drug of value for correction of immunoregulation of AE. As yet there seems, however, to have been no clinical trials with the drug.

Table 4. Bestatin therapy of patients with atopic dermatitis: serum IgE concentrations (IU/ml)

Patients	Age	0	1 month	2 months	3 months
Woman	24	2100	1890	1990	3970
Woman	28	3430	1990	1860	2090
Woman	35	993	1130	1190	1570
Woman	40	4720	4900	4920	4680
Woman	38	7620	7670	5290	6590
Woman	35	4700	4160	3180	3480
Woman	35	1690	1860	1940	1740
Woman	61	9160	9000	9450	10900
Woman	32	12900	12000	12600	16000
Man	27	5960	5600	4990	5075
Median value		4710	4480	4050	4325

Specific Immunotherapy

Specific immunotherapy (SIT) involves repeated injections of increasing doses of the relevant immunogen [21]. There is normally a rise of IgG "blocking" antibodies, whereas the corresponding IgE antibodies initially increase and then slowly decrease [9]. The IgG antibodies belong to the subclass IgG4, but IgG1 and IgG2 may also possibly interfere with the reaction between allergen and mast cell-bound IgE. Repeated injections of antigen increase the number of suppressor T cells [4]. It was long believed that successful SIT (hyposensitization) depended upon the formation of the blocking antibodies. More recently, it has been found likely that the stimulus to form T-suppressor cells is the important factor. Besides induction of specific suppressor T cells, SIT also seems to lead to an allergen non-specific production of lymphokines with a more general suppressive effect on IgE production (suppressor factor of anaphylaxis or SFA). After hyposensitization a significant decrease of anti-IgE and specific antigen-induced histamine release from the basophils occurs [8]. The aim of the therapy is clinical protection, but no simple parameter for this has been established yet.

Absolute contraindications for SIT include serious immunopathological conditions, malignancies, poor compliance, severe psychological disorders, coronary heart disease and treatments with β-blockers. SIT should not be started during pregnancy [38]. It should be taken into consideration that allergic side-effects may occur since material to which the patient is allergic is injected. These reactions may be immediate or delayed, local reactions or general symptoms such as urticaria, angioedema, asthma and rhinitis, or multiple symptoms ending up with anaphylactic shock. Most schedules involve giving incremental doses at 1–2 week intervals followed by maintenance injections at monthly intervals. The optimal duration of treatment in an individual patient is not known, but in patients in whom efficacy has been demonstrated, the duration of treatment is at least 3 years. All patients should be warned that at the beginning of treatment their dermatitis will usually be aggravated. The immunotherapy subcommittee of the European Academy of Allergology and Clinical Immunology have published a position paper on SIT [38]. This paper includes recommendations for practice, safety monitoring, and prevention and treatment of side effects. The subcommittee does not include AE in their recommendations for treatment for SIT.

It is generally accepted that SIT plays a limited part in the management of AE even when an allergic factor has been firmly established [7]. Such therapy is effective in allergic rhinitis and in insect sting anaphylaxis and less so in allergic asthma. There are, however, occasionally patients who may benefit; they have severe widespread AE, often showing extensive erythema, severe lichenification and widespread prurigo papules. The allergen must be one which is constantly in the patient's surroundings and cannot be eliminated. House dust mite is the most important of these.

The effect of SIT has been studied on AE in dogs by Willemse et al. [41]. In a double-blind study, 51 dogs with clinically defined AE were injected with either alum-precipitated allergen solutions or placebo. Comparing the treatment results of both groups on the basis of scores for clinical symptoms, a significant difference in improvement was established in favour of the allergen-treated dogs ($P < 0.01$). Of 27 dogs treated with an allergen solution 16 (59%) showed an improvement of 51% or more. In the placebo group 5 of 25 dogs (20%) reached this value.

Due to conflicting data on the results of SIT in human AE [7], we felt in reasonable to re-study this approach in patients with severe disease and established allergy to house dust mites, an allergen which is constantly in their surroundings. It has been found [2] that the amount of house dust mites in dust from the homes of patients with severe AE is significantly higher when compared with that in dust from homes of asthma patients not allergic to house dust mites, and that the amount of mites in our homes not only depends on relative air humidity but also on the production of human dander.

Twelve adult patients sensitive to house dust mites were treated with specific immunotherapy. Three also suffered from asthma, three from rhinitis, and two displayed all three main atopic diseases. The major problem was, however, in all patients AE, and this was the only purpose for treatment. Injections were given in increasing dosages with intervals lengthening from 1 to 8 weeks. All patients were allowed to use a medium-strength topical steroid according to their needs. The cream was delivered by us, and the amounts used were measured in nine patients.

Six patients improved (Table 5), three showed slight improvement, while two were unchanged, and one worsened after the observation period, which lasted from 1.5 to 5 years. Most but not all patients exhibited the pattern of an increase in serum IgE followed by a decrease (Fig. 1). There were similar but less pronounced changes in specific antibody activity as measured by RAST. However, no significant change in RAST class was observed. Two patients were reduced from class 4 to class 3, while two went from class 2 to class 3 or 4. Urinary histamine was studied in seven patients and was unchanged following 6 months of treatment and generally within normal values. The consumption of topical

Table 5. IgE in serum (IU/ml) in 12 patients sensitive to house dust mites treated with specific immunotherapy

		IgE (IU)					
Age/sex	Treatment period	Before	Highest	After	Status 1983	Clinical response	Status 1983
29/M	1977–1980	3430	6650	3370	1000	Improved	In remission
40/F	1976–1978 +since 1980	3470	3973	2220	3130	Improved	Slightly improved
24/F	1977–1978 +since 1979	7860	13000	1900	2300	Improved	Improved
29/F	1976–1978	10900	27800	14150	4870	Improved	In remission
36/F	1977–1980 +since 1980	6370	7500	3580	2900	Improved	Improved
62/F	1976–1980 +since 1980	11300	22900	3600	11900	Improved	Unchanged
48/F	1977–1980	1790	3440	2190	–	Slightly improved	Slightly improved
37/F	1977–1980 +since 1980	2550	7200	2340	3680	Slightly improved	Improved
37/F	1977–1982	1580	1860	1350	–	Slightly improved	Slightly improved
29/F	1976–1980	4930	7490	3230	2110	Unchanged	Improved
27/M	1977–1980	4418	9450	6570	8470	Unchanged	Improved
47/M	1978–1979	4261	10400	6540	–	Worse	Not seen

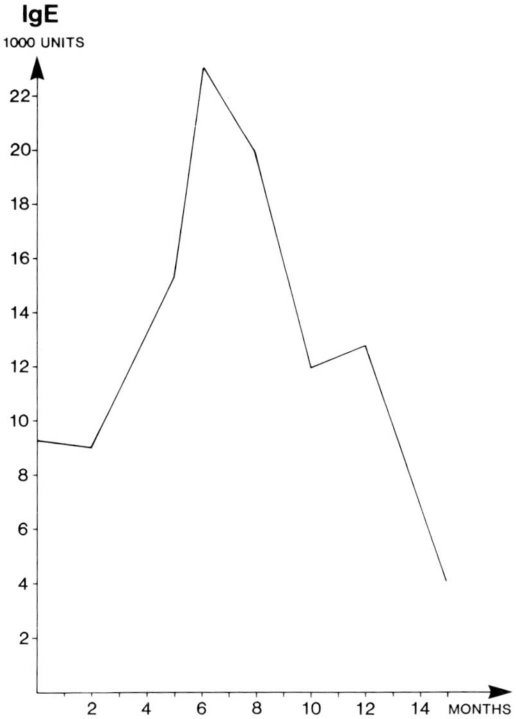

Fig. 1. Serum IgE in a patient sensitive to house dust mites during the first 15 months of specific immunotherapy

steroids was found to be reduced during treatment. When evaluated from 4 to 7 years after initiation of therapy, 8 of 11 declared that their present condition was significantly better than that prior to treatment.

Based upon this investigation [43] as well as on other reports [27, 35], hyposensitisation seems to be worthwhile in these patients with severe AE and an established allergy to an allergen which is constantly found in their environment.

The general unpopularity of SIT is probably based upon the lack of controlled studies and the fact that in most patients the disease worsens during start of therapy. This aggravation is the reason why the European Academy of Allergology and Clinical Immunology reckon AE as a relative contraindication to SIT [38].

The two reports in favour of SIT [27, 35] are mentioned here for special reasons. One [27] was a placebo-controlled study. Kaufman and Roth studied 26 patients with chronic AE in a blind study lasting for more than 24 months. Thirteen of 16 treated with antigen improved, while only 4 of 10 treated with buffered saline improved. There was a significant difference in improvement between the two groups.

Ring's study [35] is a report of a trial in monozygotic twins. The two sisters, suffering from severe AE with pronounced seasonal exacerbation during spring and early summer were treated with subcutaneous injections of either grass pollen extract or saline. After 2 years of preseasonal treatment in the skin symptoms improved significantly in the patient treated with grass pollen extract, while the placebo produced minimal change in her twin (Fig. 2). The therapeutic effect was paralled by a decrease in total serum IgE from 4200 to 1370 IU/l in the pollen-treated patient compared with 3500 to 2580 IU/l in the control twin.

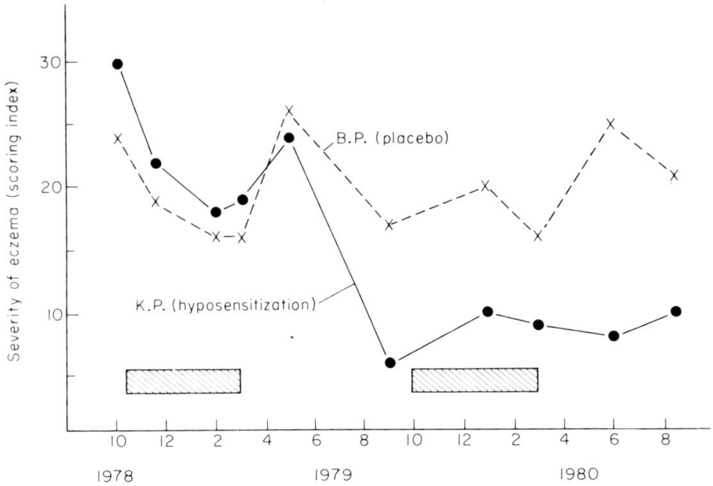

Fig. 2. Symptom score of intensity of atopic eczema (AE) in patiens *K.P.* (grass pollen extract) and *B.P.* (placebo) over an observation period of 2 years. Note the seasonal dependence of skin symptoms and the remarkable amelioration in both patients after a vacation at the North sea in summer 1979. Hatched boxes represent treatment periods

Conclusions

None of the experimental trials using non-specific immunotherapy may at present be considered promising for the practical treatment of AE, while SIT may be suggested in selected cases. The allergen must, as stated, be one which cannot be eliminated, and the patient should have a notion that exposure to the allergen causes intensification of the itching and inflammatory changes. The patient should also be prepared to accept that during the start of therapy a temporary worsening can take place. House dust mite is the most important allergen.

References

1. Allonso A (1976) Transfer factor in severe atopic dermatitis. Lancet i:1352
2. Beck H-I, Bjerring P (1987) House dust mites and human dander. Allergy 42:471–472
3. Blomgren H, Forsgren M, Nordberg R, von Stedingk L-V, Wasserman J (1981) Influence of Bestatin, a new immunomodulator on Ig secretion by human lymphocytes in vitro and in vivo. Int Arch Allergy Appl Immunol 64:338–344
4. Bruley-Rosset M, Florentin I, Kiger N, Schultz J, Mathé G (1979) Restoration of impaired immune functions of aged animals by chronic Bestatin treatment. Immunology 38:75–83
5. Caner J (1965) Colchicine inhibition of chemotaxis Arthritis Rheum 8:757–760
6. Champion R (1971) Atopic sensitivity to algae and lichens. Br J Dermatol 85:551–557
7. Champion R, Parish W (1986) Atopic dermatitis. In: Rook A, Wilkinson D, Ebling F, Champion R, Burton J (eds) Textbook of dermatology. Blackwell, London, p 433
8. Chyrek-Borowska S, Kuczewska B, Royalewska A, Hofman J (1986) Immunologic histamine release from isolated basophils during specific immunotherapy. Agents Actions 18:176–177
9. Clayton W, Reisman R, Georgitis J, Wypyck J, Arbesman C (1983) Effect of prolonged venom immunotherapy on serum venom-specific IgE and IgG. Clin Allergy 13:301–307
10. Copeman P, Wallis H (1964) Eczema vaccinatum. Br Med J 2:906–908
11. Dinarello CV, Wolff S, Goldfinger S, Dale D, Alling D (1974) Colchicine therapy for familial Mediterranean fever. N Engl J Med 291:934–937
12. Elliot S, Hannifen J (1979) Delayed cutaneous hypersensitivity and lymphocyte transformation: disassociation in atopic dermatitis. Arch Dermatol 115:36–39
13. Elliston W, Heise E, Huntley C (1982) Cell-mediated hypersensivity to mite antigens in atopic dermatitis. Arch Dermatol 118:26–29
14. Frajman M, Gonzales L, Alvarado A, Yock J (1987) Cellular immunity and IgE levels in atopic patients. Allergy 42:81–84
15. Gartmann J, Grob P, Frey M (1978) Plasmapheresis in severe asthma. Lancet ii:40
16. Hanifin J (1984) Pathophysiology of atopic dermatitis. In: Soter N, Baden H (eds) Pathophysiology of dermatologic diseases. McGraw-Hill, New York, p 135
17. Herlin T, Jensen J, Thestrup-Pedersen K, Zachariae H (1981) Dialyzable leukocyte extract stimulates CMP in T-gamma-lymphocytes. Allergy 36:337–343
18. Hovmark A, Ekre H (1978) Failure of transfer factor therapy in atopic dermatitis. Acta Derm Venereol (Stockh) 58:497–500
19. Ilfeld D, Kuperman O (1982) Correction of a suppressor cell deficiency in 4 patients with familial Mediterranean fever by in vitro and in vivo colchicine. Clin Exp Immunol 50:99–106
20. Ishikawa I, Fukudo Y, Kitada H, Yuri T, Shinoda A,

Hyakawa Y, Sawano K, Usui T (1982) Plasma exchange in a patient with hyper-IgE syndrome. Ann Allergy 49:295–297
21. Ishizaka K (1978) Hyposensitization. In: Bach E (ed) Immediate hypersensitivity. Dekker, New York, p 127
22. Jarisch R, Eibl M, Sandor I, Boltz A (1981) Influence of dialyzable transfer factor on IgE concentrations in patients with atopic dermatitis. Allergy 36:99–105
23. Jensen J, Cramers M, Thestrup-Pedersen K (1981) Subpopulations of T-lymphocytes and non-specific cell activity in patients with atopic dermatitis. Clin Exp Immunol 45:118–123
24. Jensen J, Jørgensen A, Thestrup-Pedersen K (1984) Modulation of natural killer cell activity in patients with atopic dermatitis. J Invest Dermatol 82:30–34
25. Jones H, Reinhardt J, Rinaldi M (1973) A clinical, mycological and immunological survey for dermatophytosis. Arch Dermatol 108:61–65
26. Juhlin L, Johannsson S, Bennich H, Högmann C, Thyresson N (1969) Immunoglobulin in dermatoses: levels in atopic dermatitis and urticaria. Arch Dermatol 100:12–16
27. Kaufman H, Roth H (1974) Hyposensitization with alum-precipitated extracts in atopic dermatitis – a placebo-controlled study. Ann Allergy 32:321–327
28. Kragballe K, Herlin T, Jensen J (1980) Impaired monocyte toxicity in atopic dermatitis. Arch Dermatol Res 269:21–29
29. Morrison W, Parrish J, Fitzpatrick T (1978) Oral psoralen photochemotherapy of atopic eczema. Br J Dermatol 98: 25–30
30 Nielsen H, Thomson B, Djurup R, Søndergaard I, Kabbelgaard E, Berkowicz A, Kjersen H, Dahlager J, Szpirt W, Ullman S, Valerius N, Weeke B (1984) Plasma separation in patients with bronchial asthma, atopic dermatitis and hyperimmunoglobulinemia E. Allergy 39:329–337
31. Norman P (1978) A review of immunotherapy. Allergy 33: 62–70
32. Penny R, Galton D, Scott J (1966) Studies on neutrophil function. Br J Haematol 12:623–632
33. Rajan K (1969) Lysosomes and gout. Nature 210:959–960
34. Rajka G (1961) Prurigo Besnier (atopic dermatitis) with special reference to the role of allergic factors: II. The evaluation of the results of skin reactions. Acta Derm Venereol (Stockh) 41:1–39
35. Ring J (1982) Successful hyposensitization treatment in atopic dermatitis: results of a trial in monozygotic twins. Br J Dermatol 107:597–602
36. Rocklin R, Hemady Z, Matloff S, Kiselis I, Lina M (1984) Correction of an in vitro immunoregulatory defect in atopic subjects by the immunostimulating drug fanetizole mesylate (CP48810). Int J Immunopharmacol 6:1–8
37. Strannegaard I-L, Hansson L, Mobacken H, Strannegaard O (1975) Transfer factor in severe atopic disease. Lancet ii: 702
38. Subcommittee for Immunotherapy of EAACI (1988) Immunotherapy – position paper. Allergy 43 [Suppl 6]:1–33
39. Thestrup-Pedersen K, Ellegaard J, Thulin H, Zachariae H (1977) Mitogen and PPD responsiveness in severe atopic dermatitis. Clin Exp Immunol 27:118–126
40. Thestrup-Pedersen K, Cramers M, Kongsholm H, Zachariae H (1983) Bestatin therapy of patients with atopic dermatitis. Acta Derm Venereol (Stockh) 63:549–552
41. Willemse A, van den Brom W, Rijnberk A (1984) Effect of hyposensitization on atopic dermatitis in dogs. J Am Vet Med Assoc 184:1277–1280
42. Zachariae H, Ellegaard J, Grunnet E, Thestrup-Pedersen K (1980) Transfer factor in mycosis fungoides: three years experience. Dermatologica 160:1–6
43. Zachariae H, Cramers M, Herlin T, Jensen J, Kragballe K, Ternowitz T, Thestrup-Pedersen K (1985) Non-specific immunotherapy and specific hyposensitization in severe atopic dermatitis. Acta Derm Venereol [Suppl] (Stockh) 114:48–54

ADDENDUM

Since this chapter was completed two other types non-specific immunomodulation have been tried. Recombinant gamma interferon which in vitro inhibits IgE synthesis was studied in AE over an up to six week period, and although there was no significant reduction in serum IgE, there was a reduction in clinical seventy (Boguniewicz M et al. (1990) Am J Med 88: 365– 370). Cyclosporin A, although its activity is mainly an inhibition of T-lymphocytefunctions, has also been tried in AE with encouraging results (Ross J, Camp R (1990) Br J Dermat 122 Suppl 36: 41–45). Both treatments should, however, still be considered experimental. Specific immunomodulation has been tried with injection of allergen-antibody complexes with a significant clinical improvement after 3–4 months and maintained through 9 months (Leroy B et al. (1991). Dermatologica 182: 98–106). Also this study suggested that the immune response to wards house dust mites is a relevant factor in AE.

Ultraviolet Radiation Therapy of Atopic Eczema

W. L. Morison

Introduction

Ultraviolet (UV) radiation has been used as a therapeutic modality in the treatment of atopic eczema for many decades, but only in the past decade have there been attempts at controlled evaluation of this treatment. Thus, we are beginning to move towards a position of knowing whether UV radiation is useful in atopic eczema, but before reaching that point, several considerations must be kept in mind. First, atopic eczema is not a uniform disease, it presents as a spectrum of pathology from acute vesiculation through to chronic lichenification, so that a treatment might be effective in one phase of the disorder and not another. Second, different parts of the body may pose varied therapeutic and photobiologic problems. For example, eczema on the palms and soles may respond differently to that at other locations. Finally, there have been few controlled observations of the effect of UV radiation. For example, there appears to have been only one bilateral, paired-comparison study, although this type of investigation is essential in a disease that is renowned for its psychological overtones. Thus, many more controlled studies utilizing crisp endpoints are required before the remaining questions are correctly answered.

Many different types of UV radiation have been used to treat atopic eczema. However, since published studies have been restricted to an evaluation of methoxsalen/UV-A radiation (PUVA) therapy and UV phototherapy, most attention will focus on these modalities.

Oral Psoralen Photochemotherapy

Generalized Atopic Eczema

The first study of PUVA therapy in the management of atopic eczema was published in 1978 [1] soon after this treatment had been found effective in psoriasis [2]. Fifteen patients with widespread atopic eczema were treated three times a week using the standard PUVA protocol for psoriasis. The clinical picture in those patients is summarized in Table 1. Ten of the patients were initially treated in a half-body, bilateral comparison study and then received whole-body PUVA, while the other five received whole-body treatment with a control patch on the buttock kept covered during exposure to UV-A radiation. All patients were outpatients, and topical and oral corticosteroids were stopped before treatment or gradually removed in the early phase of therapy.

The results of the study are summarized in Tables 2–4. The controlled phase of the study demonstrated that PUVA therapy could clear eczema in most patients and

Table 1. Clinical picture in patients with atopic eczema treated by standard PUVA psoriasis

Number of patients	15
Surface area involved	30%–100% (mean: 80%)
Type of lesions present:	
Acute and subacute eczema	15
Lichenification	6
Nail dystrophy	3
Scalp involvement	4
Chronic blepharitis	4

Table 2. Treatment response in three groups of patients

Whole-body PUVA	99% clearance of eczema (5/5 patients)
Control site	Increased eczema (5/5 patients)
PUVA half-body	95% clearance of eczema (5/5 patients)
No treatment half-body	No change (5/5 patients)
PUVA half-body	95% clearance of eczema (5/5 patients)
UV-B half-body	Eczema increased in 4, no change in 1

Table 3. Treatment requirements in 15 patients to achieve clearance to 1% eczema

Number of treatments	18–59 (mean:36)
Number of days	50–202 (mean: 101)
Final cleareance dose of UV-A	7–24 J/cm^2 (mean: 13 J/cm^2)

Table 4. Five-year follow-up of 15 patients

Maintenance therapy	No. of patients
Weekly	5
Every other week	5
Ceased treatment	
Complete remission	2
Poor control	1
Dermatitis artefacta	2

that this effect is local at the site of exposure to radiation. However, as is evident from Table 3, more treatment is required to clear atopic eczema than psoriasis. A lessening of pruritus was usually the first sign of improvement, and this symptom had almost stopped at the time of clearance of eczema. In addition, there was no apparent correlation between the type of eczema and response to treatment. Maintenance therapy was given to all patients, but despite this, during the short-term follow-up of 9 months, ten patients had moderate (5% body surface) or major (60% body surface) exacerbations of their disease; however, these were controlled by resumption of treatment 2 or 3 times each week. The patients were again evaluated 5 years after initially commencing treatment, and their maintenance requirements are often high for retaining control of the eczema; some patients cannot be controlled with a reasonable amount of treatment, and psychological factors can be important in determining the outcome of therapy. The two patients with dermatitis artefacta needed a skin disease as an emotional prop, and both requested cessation of treatment.

Since this first study, experience with PUVA therapy in atopic eczema has considerably expanded in our centers, and about 30–40 patients are receiving treatment at any one time. Most patients are referred for treatment because of a failure of topical therapy, dependency on oral steroids or adverse effects from these treatments; striae and growth retardation during adolescence are the most common problems in the last group. Psychological factors are carefully evaluated, particularly with respect to motivation for treatment and adjustment to disease. If emotional factors are playing a major role, it is likely that the patient will show a poor response or have recurrent exacerbations after initial clearance. A key factor in the success is initial and continued education of the patient about what to expect from the treatment. Improvement is rarely seen in less than ten treatments and often requires twenty or more treatments. During this time the eczema will fluctuate in severity, and exacerbations should not be interpreted as a failure of treatment, instead they are an indication for more treatment. This is very different to the use of PUVA therapy in psoriasis where early and consistent improvement is usual. Furthermore, patients with atopic eczema are more questioning, anxious, and introverted as compared with those with psoriasis, and, as a consequence, they require more support and time from the physician.

The principal change in the approach to PUVA therapy in atopic eczema concerns the use of adjunctive corticosteroid treatment. In the initial study this medication was stopped at the start of treatment to provide a clear evaluation of PUVA therapy. Nowadays, such treatment is gradually phased out when the eczema has been controlled, since this avoids the necessity of having to suppress a poststeroid exacerbation at the same time as the underlying disease. In addition, if a patient is slow to respond, complains of irritation of the skin from the treatment, or is having a severe exacerbation in the early phase of clearance therapy, a brief course of prednisone will often permit the dose of UV-A radiation to be quickly raised to a level sufficient to control the disease. The dose of prednisone will vary with the circumstances, but it should be sufficient to suppress the patient's eczema totally.

Maintenance therapy is essential and must be more aggressive and rigid than in the case of psoriasis. If a patient with psoriasis misses a few treatments, a couple of spots might return, but if a patient with eczema does this, whole-body exacerbation is a likely consequence. Treatment is initially given weekly, but after a few months of good control, treatment every other week can be attempted. The main adjunctive treatment during maintenance is oral antibiotics to control folliculitis. This is a common problem, and the lesions are pruritic, so if it is left untreated it may cause an exacerbation of the eczema. Some patients require long-term rotating antibiotics to control folliculitis, and tetracycline and erythromycin are suitable in these cases. During both the clearance and maintenance phases of treatment, lubricants are an essential requirement. Patients with atopic eczema have dry skin, and this is accentuated by any type of phototherapy.

Three areas of the body require some special attention during PUVA therapy: nails, eyelids, and scalp. Nail dystrophy is not uncommon if the dorsa of the hands are involved with eczema, and it responds to treatment, although complete clearance usually takes several months. Additional exposure to UV-A radiation should be given to the dorsa in a hand treatment unit after each whole-body exposure to ensure rapid and complete clearance. Chronic blepharitis is also a problem often seen and when present should be treated by exposing the eyelids with the eyes closed during the whole-body treatment. The eyelids block transmission of UV-A radiation, and this is a safe procedure in an intelligent and cooperative patient. Involvement of the scalp is treated with a medicated shampoo plus a topical corticosteroid lotion since little UV-A radiation will penetrate hair. However, an interesting finding is that most patients can stop this treatment once eczema of the rest of the body is controlled.

The results of my initial study have been confirmed in a few subsequent studies. Sannwald et al. [3] achieved from 80% improvement to complete clearance in 9 of 11 patients, but recurrences occurred while the patients were on maintenance therapy, so that only 3 patients were considered to have a very good result. Rajka [4] observed that eczematous lesions responded better than areas of lichenification and that maintenance therapy was essential. Salo et al. [5] reported clearance of eczema in 48 of 56 patients treated with PUVA therapy while Soppi et al. [6] produced "considerable improvement" in 22 adult patients. Most recently, Atherton et al. [7] published a detailed account of treating 15 children and adolescents. These patients were selected because they had exceptionally severe disease, and in addition, many of them had marked retardation of growth. Such growth retardation is common in young atopic patients and is presumably partly due to the disease plus a large contribution from therapy with topical and oral corticosteroids. They achieved clearance of eczema in 14 children, and the treatment was associated with normal or accelerated growth. All the patients were given initial maintenance therapy after clearance. After the mean follow-up period of 1 year, 9 of the 14 patients were in remission (off treatment), 2 were on maintenance therapy, and 3 had relapsed and stopped treatment. Thus, the overall conclusions from these studies appears to be that PUVA therapy can control eczema in a majority of patients. However, as observed again in this recent study [7], aggressive treatment, often with fairly high doses of UV-A radiation, is required in the clearance phase, and maintenance treatment is essential, at least initially.

Palmar and Plantar Eczema

There have been no specific studies of the treatment of eczema of the palms and soles in atopic patients. However, chronic eczema at this sites responded well to local irradiation in two bilateral comparison studies [8, 9] and one open study [10], and undoubtedly some atopic patients were included in these investigations. Eczema confined to the hands and feet is a common manifestation of atopy and often shows a poor response to topical therapy, leading to considerable disability because of the important functions of these body parts. Fortunately, it shows an excellent response to PUVA therapy in almost all patients, clearing in 20–30 treatments of the hands and 30–40 treatments of the feet. However, as with generalized eczema, long-term maintenance treatment is usually essential, and this proviso particularly applies to people engaged in traumatic occupations such as hairdressing, mechanical work, and the culinary profession.

Variants of Atopic Eczema

Pityriasis alba, whether associated with atopic eczema or occurring as an isolated phenomenon, shows an excellent response to PUVA treatment [11]. Clearance is usually achieved in less than 20 treatments, and maintenance therapy is unnecessary in most cases. This condition, when present in a generalized form, causes considerable emotional disturbance to dark-skinned individuals and is usually unresponsive to other treatments. Thus, its clearance is a very rewarding experience for both the patient and the doctor.

Photosensitivity in association with atopy [12] is another indication for PUVA therapy since, again, it is usually unresponsive to any other treatment and can cause considerable limitations of lifestyle. Most patients are very sensitive to UV-A radiation and have photosensitivity year-round, but some more mildly afflicted patients are only affected during the summer months. The approach to treatment is similar to that for other UV-A-sensitive photodermatoses [13], namely, high doses of prednisone combined with PUVA therapy. After about 10 treatments, prednisone can be rapidly reduced in dosage and stopped after about 20 treatments. A maintenance schedule of weekly PUVA treatment during the summer and treatment every other week during winter is required to maintain control of the condition. Most patients lose their photosensitivity over the course of 2 or 3 years.

Mechanism of Treatment

The pathogenesis of atopic eczema still remains a mystery, and likewise the mechanism by which PUVA therapy induces a beneficial effect in this condition is unknown. A few observations have been made. Serum IgE levels and qualitative cultures of bacterial skin flora did not change significantly during treatment [1]. Alterations in the mitogenic responses of lymphocytes and nonspecific suppressor cell activity were observed during PUVA therapy in one study [6], but these changes were probably epiphenomena; the distribution of lymphocyte subpopulations and leukocyte migration inhibitory factor production were not altered by treatment.

PUVA therapy is effective in a very diverse group of disorders. A plausible hypothesis to explain these many effects might be that the treatment is therapeutic whenever an activated cell, responsible for mediating the disease, exhibits selective sensitivity to the cytotoxic effects of the treatment. For example, if atopic eczema is mediated in the skin by a population of activated lymphocytes, selective killing of those cells could result in suppression of the disease.

Adverse Effects

The carcinogenic and cataractogenic effects of PUVA therapy are the most serious long-term sequelae of the treatment and must always be considered when starting a patient on a course of therapy; these adverse effects have been documented elsewhere and will not be discussed here in any detail. However, the elements that contribute to the risk: benefit ratio of using PUVA therapy in atopic eczema should be carefully considered. Regarding skin cancer, there is a risk for nonmelanoma skin cancer [14], which is usually easily treated and mainly confined to fair-skinned individuals. There is no reason to believe that cataracts could arise provided eye protection is used [15]. Second, corticosteroids which are the main alternative treatment, are not themselves altogether safe, and some of their side effects, such as collapsed vertebrae, growth retardation, and striae, are not reversible. The potential risks of some newer suggested treatments, such as cyclosporin A, make the side effects of PUVA therapy pale in comparison. Finally, for the patient, having extensive eczema represents a considerable burden on his mental and physical well-being.

There are two short-term problems specific to using PUVA therapy in atopic eczema. Postinflammatory depigmenation is a common problem when lichenified areas are cleared. This is mainly a problem for dosimetry since the areas become erythematous as a result of treatment; application of a broad-spectrum sunscreen to affected areas prior to irradiation usually solves this problem. Repigmentation is slow but often occurs over 1–2 years of treatment. Recurrent herpes labialis is common, as in all patients treated with PUVA therapy. Herpes infection of the eye occurred in two patients in the first study [1], but this complication has not been observed since.

Ultraviolet Phototherapy

Generalized Atopic Eczema

If the number of published reports of studies evaluating a treatment are a measure of its popularity, UV phototherapy for atopic eczema has suddenly become a favorite treatment, at least in Europe. Four of the five studies assessing its efficacy have been published in the past 5 years. Most of them have compared the effect of UV-B phototherapy to that of mixed UV-A/UV-B phototherapy, and the overall conclusion is that the latter is somewhat superior. In a study from Finland [16], 107 patients with severe atopic eczema were treated with UV-B radiation. They were hospitalized and received daily phototherapy and adjunctive topical corticosteroids, and a good result was achieved in 93%. An average course of treatment lasted 9 days with half the patients requiring only one course and a third requiring three courses of treatment. A comparably affected group of 89 atopic patients treated with UV-A/UV-B radiation achieved a good result in 94%. They were outpatients and were treated 3–5 times each week, and, when their eczema was controlled, they received maintenance treatment 1–2 times each week for up to 45 weeks. It was noted that lichenification did not diminish very much with either protocol. Treatment was fairly aggressive since 25% of all the patients developed erythema.

In a study reported from Tromsø, Norway [17], 106 patients with atopic eczema were treated as outpatients 5 days a week. Of 52 patients treated with UV-B radiation, 84% were completely cured after an average of 23 treatments while 94% of the 54 patients treated with UV-A/UV-B radiation reached this endpoint in an average of 18 treatments. Adjunctive corticosteroid treatment was not used, and phototherapy was suberythemal in most patients with only a few of those receiving UV-B irradiation showing any erythema. Most had mild or moderate disease, only 20 patients were classified as having severe involvement; it was noted that the latter patients required more treatment and more frequently relapsed. Maintenance treatment was not given initially, but later it was found that 1 or 2 treatments each week were necessary for those who relapsed.

A third study, also from Tromsø, Norway [18], reported the results of phototherapy in 56 patients with severe atopic eczema. Of 23 patients treated with combined UV-A/UV-B radiation 48% were cleared and 48% achieved a good result, while of 33 patients treated with UV-B radiation alone 27% were cleared and 58% obtained a good result. Treatment was suberythemal, and adjunctive corticosteroids were used. No comment was made as to whether the treatments were ambulatory or in hospital, and maintenance treatment was apparently not used.

Finally, a study from Helsinki [5] compared PUVA therapy and selective UV phototherapy; the lamp used for the latter treatment emits mainly UV-A radiation with a small amount of UV-B. These two treatments were found to be comparable. The status of the patients regarding hospitalization and adjunctive treatment was not mentioned.

At the time of the initial evaluation of PUVA therapy in atopic eczema, much anecdotal comment was provided by my colleagues as to the "known" efficacy of UV-B phototherapy in this condition. For that reason one portion of the bilateral comparison study included UV-B phototherapy to one-half of the patient's body while PUVA therapy was given to the other half [1]. Only 5 patients, all with severe atopic eczema, were treated, but over the course of 13–19 treatments with UV-B radiation, 4 patients had an increase of eczema on the side treated with that modality while in 1 the eczema was unchanged. The conclusion reached at the time, perhaps prematurely, was that UV-B phototherapy was not efficacious in atopic eczema, and no further controlled investigation was made. There are several possible explanations for the discrepancy between these results and more recent studies. First, the number of patients was small and may by chance have included only nonresponders since such patients have been seen in more recent studies. Second, they were outpatients who did not receive topical corticosteroids. A combination of inpatient treatment, adjunctive steroids, and phototherapy may be effective whereas phototherapy alone is not. Third, these patients had very severe atopic eczema, and UV phototherapy may only be beneficial in lesser degrees of affliction. Finally, of course, the explanation may involve a mixture of all these elements.

Three recent studies have demonstrated that UV phototherapy may have a place in the treatment of atopic eczema. What is now required is a controlled evaluation to confirm this observation, define whether it is effective in all degrees and types of disease, and establish whether or not maintenance treatment is necessary. Other variables, such as the psychological impact of hospitalization and the beneficial effect of corticosteroids, should be eliminated until phototherapy alone is proven effective. A paired, bilateral comparison of UV-B alone versus UV-A/UV-B mixed radiation would probably be most interesting in advancing our knowledge in this area.

Hand Eczema

The effect of UV-B phototherapy on hand eczema in association with atopy has not been evaluated. One study [19] found this treatment to be beneficial in other forms of eczema of the hands, but many months of therapy were required to clear the disease. Since UV-A is more penetrating than UV-B radiation, PUVA is probably the treatment of choice for eczema involving the palms and soles.

Adverse Effects

UV-B phototherapy is generally considered to be a very safe modality. An increased risk of nonmelanoma skin cancer has been considered as a long-term adverse effect of this treatment in patients with psoriasis, but conflicting results of an increased risk [20] and a decreased risk [21] suggest, that the effect is probably small. However, before accepting this finding as proven, at least two considerations should be kept in mind. These studies used retrospective data, and no prospective study of patients treated with UV phototherapy has ever been published. Retrospective studies can be misleading and should be regarded as preliminary findings prior to initiating a good prospective study. Furthermore, phototherapy for psoriasis during the period of time covered by these studies was usually an intermittent treatment given as one or sometimes two courses each year. Phototherapy for psoriasis has now changed in many centers to utilize routine maintenance therapy. Similarly, it is very likely that long-term maintenance therapy is also necessary in phototherapy for atopic eczema. The recent European studies and experience with PUVA therapy support this possibility. Maintenance therapy greatly increases the cumulative exposure dose and consequently is likely to increase the risk of nonmelanoma skin cancer. Recent projections [22] from analysis of exposure doses suggest this increased risk could be considerable.

Heliotherapy

Exposure to sunlight is often thought to be beneficial in some patients with atopic eczema; however, no studies have evaluated this treatment. Some atopic patients, probably about a third, state they are better in summer, while a third claim to be worse during that season, and the remainder do not observe any difference. When treating patients with atopic eczema by PUVA therapy, one is soon struck by the lack of correlation between the presence or absence of a particular seasonal effect and subsequent response to treatment. Once patients with photosensitivity have been excluded, it appears irrelevant as to whether the patient is better in summer or winter or fails to notice a difference between the seasons. This suggests that improvement in some patients during the summer is probably not due to ambient UV radiation. Sunlight is a very complex treatment modality due to such variables as vacations, relaxation, exposure to salt water, and increased temperature. The temperature rise is quite possibly responsible for the deterioration of some patients in summer because of excessive perspiration and folliculitis leading to increased pruritus and eczema.

References

1. Morison WL, Parrish JA, Fitzpatrick TB (1978) Oral Psoralen photochemotherapy of atopic eczema. Br J Dermatol 98:25–30
2. Parrish JA, Fitzpatrick TB, Tanenbaum L, Pathak MA (1974) Photochemotherapy of psoriasis with oral methoxsalen and longwave ultraviolet light. N Engl J Med 291:1207
3. Sannwald C, Ortonne J, Thivolet JP (1979) La photochimiotherapie orale de l'eczema atopique. Dermatologica 159:71–77
4. Rajka G (1980) Recent therapeutic events: cimetidine and PUVA. Acta Derm Venereol [Suppl] (Stockh) 92:117–118
5. Salo VO, Lassus A, Juvakoski T, Kanerva L, Lauharanta J (1983) Behandlung der Dermatitis atopica und der Dermatitis seborrhoica mit selektiver UV-Phototherapie and PUVA. Dermatol Monatsschr 169:371–375
6. Soppi E, Viander M, Soppi AM, Jansen CT (1982) Cell-mediated immunity in untreated and PUVA treated atopic dermatitis. J Invest Dermatol 79:213–217
7. Atherton DJ, Carabott F, Glover MT, Hawk JLM (1988) The role of psoralen photochemotherapy (PUVA) in the treatment of severe atopic eczema in adolescents. Br J Dermatol 118:791–795
8. Morison WL, Parrish JA, Fitzpatrick TB (1978) Oral methoxsalen photochemotherapy of recalcitrant dermatoses of the palms and soles. Br J Dermatol 99:297–302
9. LeVine MJ, Parrish JA, Fitzpatrick TB (1981) Oral methoxsalen photochemotherapy (PUVA) of dyshidrotic eczema. Acta Derm Venereol (Stockh) 61:570–571
10. Tegner E, Thelin I (1985) PUVA treatment of chronic eczematous dermatitis of the palms and soles. Acta Derm Venereol (Stockh) 65:451–453
11. Zaynoun S, Jaber LAA, Kurban AK (1986) Oral methoxsalen photochemotherapy of extensive pityriasis alba. J Am Acad Dermatol 15:61–65
12. Frain-Bell W, Scatchard M (1971) The association of photosensitivity and atopy in the child. Br J Dermatol 85: 105–110
13. Morison WL, White HAD, Gonzalez E, Parrish JA, Fitzpatrick TB (1979) Oral methoxsalen photochemotherapy of uncommon photodermatoses. Acta Derm Venereol (Stockh) 59:366–367
14. Stern RS, Lange R (1988) Non-melanoma skin cancer occurring in patients treated with PUVA five to ten years after first treatment. J Invest Dermatol 91:120–124
15. Stern RS, Parrish JA, Fitzpatrick TB (1985) Ocular findings in patients treated with PUVA. J Invest Dermatol 85:269–273
16. Hannuksela M, Karvonen J, Husa M, Jokela R, Katajamaki L, Leppisaari M (1985) Ultraviolet light therapy in atopic dermatitis. Acta Derm Venereol (Stockh) 114:137–139
17. Falk S (1985) UV-light therapies in atopic dermatitis. Photodermatol 2:241–246
18. Midelfart K, Stenvold SE, Volden G (1985) Combined UVB and UVA phototherapy of atopic eczema. Dermatologica 171:95–98
19. Mork NJ, Austad J (1983) Short-wave ultraviolet light (UVB) treatment of allergic contact dermatitis of the hands. Acta Dermatol 63:87–99
20. Stern RS, Zierler S, Parrish JA (1980) Skin carcinoma in patients with psoriasis treated with topical tar and artificial ultraviolet radiation. Lancet i:732–735
21. Larko O, Swanbeck G (1982) Is UVB treatment of psoriasis safe? A study of extensively UVB-treated psoriasis patients compared with a matched control group. Acta Derm Venereol (Stockh) 62:507–512
22. Schothorst AA, Slaper H, Schouten R, Suurmond D (1985) UVB doses in maintenance psoriasis phototherapy versus solar UVB exposure. Photodermatol 2:213–220

Addendum

Since this chapter was written two excellent studies that evaluated UV phototherapy for atopic eczema have been published [1,2]. In a paired comparison study of the effect of UVB radiation versus visuble light, UVB was clearly superior to the placebo and cleared eczema in most of the patients treated. Interestingly, most of the patients had mild to moderate eczema and the few with severe atopic eczema did not respond to treatment. In a second paired comparison study a combination of UVA plus UVB was found to be superior to UVB alone. Thus further study is necessary to define the therapeutic action spectrum.

The conclusion to be drawn from these and previous studies is that UV phototherapy is an effective treatment in mild to moderate atopic eczema and PUVA therapy is more effective in patients with extensive, severe disease.

References

1. Jekler J, Larko O (1988) UVB phototherapy of atopic dermatitis. Brit J Derm 119:697–705
2. Jekler J, Larko O (1990) Combined UVA-UVB versus UVB phototherapy for atopic dermatitis: A paired-comparison study. J Am Acad Dermatol 22:49–53

Psychotherapeutic Approaches in the Treatment of Atopic Eczema

J. A. Cotterill

Introduction

> The essential unit of medical practice is the occasion when, in the intimacy of the consulting room, or the sick room, the person who is ill, or believes himself to be ill, seeks the advice of a doctor whom he trusts. This is a consultation and all else in the practice of medicine derives from it [17].

The dermatological consultation is the focal point of management in patients with atopic eczema, yet the consultation with a child with atopic eczema is unlike any other. For instance, the atopic child will almost always be accompanied by both parents whereas this is unusual, certainly in the UK, for most other dermatological problems, e.g. psoriasis, in which the skin may be involved to an equal extent. The mother is usually first into the consulting room, followed by a reluctant child and an even more reluctant and relatively passive father. It is the mother who does all the talking, turning occasionally to the father to corroborate her statements. Whilst the history is being taken the atopic child charges around the consulting room disrupting everything in sight. This hyperkinetic behaviour is very characteristic of the child with atopic eczema and is not usually seen in other dermatological situations. Within 5 min the whole consulting room can be completely disrupted and instruments and well-loved momentoes shattered. The mother rises repeatedly from her chair to try and minimise the damage done to the consulting room. When the time comes for the child to be examined there is usually some reluctance and in many instances a temper tantrum develops, often rendering adequate examination impossible. The child refuses to be calmed verbally, but it is unusual for the atopic parents to chastise the child, despite considerable provocation. Conducting a reasonable conversation with the parents whilst all this is going on becomes an impossibility and only a very limited transfer of information is possible. In many instances it appears just as important to treat the parents, and the mother in particular, as the index patient. However, often an uneasy compromise with a more mechanistic approach using ointments, creams, emollient oils, optimism and reassurance will lead to a happy resolution. Frank psychotherapeutic approaches are rarely required but will often be utilised almost unconsciously by many dermatologists during their consultations with the family.

The Dermatological Consultation – A View Utilising Game Analysis

There have been many papers published recently leading to the conclusion that doctor/patient relationships in medicine may be unsatisfactory from the patient's point of view. Factors which can affect the doctor/patient relationship in dermatology in general were explored by Savin [16], whilst Jobling [10] from a survey of psoriatic patients described doctors as "prescribers" who did not recognise or accept the many other medical, social and psychological problems experienced by their patients. The formation of self-help societies, for instance for eczema, may in fact be a reaction of sufferers to a non-understanding of the disease by physicians and the problems this creates [19]. Patients with atopic eczema pose particular problems for the dermatological consultation, and a mechanistic approach with ointments and creams and other measures, such as oral antihistamines, may not always be appropriate.

There are many ways of analysing the dermatological consultation. The most suitable method is to use that of game analysis [3, 8]. Berne [3] proposed that human beings structure their time in three main ways: with pastimes which have no ulterior motive, with games which always have an ulterior motive and with an ultimate search for intimacy which is desirable but rarely possible because absolute truth is usually incompatible with the social pressures of life [4]. Berne [4] defined a "game" thus:

> Games are played by people who are afraid of intimacy either in general or with each other. They are a way of getting close to others and having meaningful transactions without the surrender that intimacy requires.

Thus, games can be exploited, particularly in doctor/patient relationships and as a way of reaching a patient without becoming emotionally involved. During the consultation a number of games evolve, so that the physician will play games with the patient and the patient and his family will play games with the physician. An analysis of this situation and a recognition of the games involved can lead to much more effective doctor/patient relationships.

Games Likely to Be Played By Patients with Atopic Eczema or Their Families During the Dermatological Consultation

Reassurance

Reassurance is one of the most common games played during a consultation, not only in the dermatological consultation but in medicine in general. Physicians learn to play this game unconsciously during their training, and reassurance may come to be used as a ploy by the physician in the face of therapeutic impotence. However, the patient or the family of the child with atopic eczema come to the dermatologist genuinely looking for reassurance. These patients and their families need to know that the eczema is not infectious, but they should also be told that the condition may be made worse by infections such as herpes simplex. Some older, depressed patients with eczema need reassurance that they have not got skin cancer. The family with the atopic child comes along looking for reassurance about the future and for reassurance that local steroids being used on the child's skin are safe.

Prognosis

Prognosis flows on naturally from reassurance. The family with an atopic child can be reassured that in many instances the child will outgrow the eczema but often not until the teenage years. During the Prognosis Game it should be explained that there may be symptom shifts from eczema into asthma or hay fever. The opportunity may also be taken at this time to explain that stress can make the eczema worse.

Another aspect of the Prognosis Game is acceptance. Some patients with eczema and some families with an atopic child find it difficult to come to terms with the problems. In short, they will not accept this blight on the family. Persuading such a family to cope with the atopic eczema can pose many problems in advocacy, but once acceptance of the situation has occurred, a happier status quo usually evolves.

Tests

Many patients or their families will come to dermatologists asking for investigations to try and find out what is triggering exacerbations of the eczema in a particular patient. In the UK there is a great interest in the possibility that diet may be important in initiating the exacerbating eczema, and many families have often tried quite elaborate and sometimes dangerous dietary regimes before consulting a dermatologist. It may be that patch tests will be important in trying to eliminate contact factors as an exacerbating cause, and occasionally RAST tests my be helpful. However, some patients and their families and some physicians come to equate management of the patient with eczema with tests. This can have disastrous results, ultimately leading to the media-invented total allergy syndrome, when the families of the patients and eventually the patients themselves come to believe that they are allergic to almost everything in their environment. This type of patient is unlikely to accept conventional medical treatment and requires an almost saintly degree of tolerance on the part of the unfortunate medical advisers.

Diagnosis

The diagnosis of atopic eczema is usually not in doubt. However, this is only a starting point to management. The site of the eczema is often of crucial importance. The sight of a small child with a severe atopic eczema of the face, produced with consummate ease following a few minutes of scratching, is clearly alarming to the parents and to the medical advisers. The young adult with severe atopic eczema involving the face is quite likely to have severe depression of body image, self-esteem and a resulting reactive depression. Relatively trivial dermatological problems in areas of crucial importance with regard to body image can produce very grave depression. Important body image areas include the face, nose, scalp, genital area and breasts in women. Thus, it is important not to miss significant depression in these patients.

Treatment Games

New

'New' is one of the most common therapy games played by physicians, often aided and abetted by patients, the advertising media and the pharmaceutical industry. In the UK the typical patient is referred by the family physician to a specialist, who usually does not disappoint either the family or the referring physician and prescribes something 'new' from the pharmacopoeia. All of us in hospital-based medicine are likely to prescribe, for instance, a different local steroid or antihistamine than the primary referring physician's initial choice.

Folklore and Archaeology

Whilst most patients like to try new therapies, there are those families who are suspicious of anything new, and this type of personality will be evident during the consultation. It is a mistake to try and prescribe new products for this type of rather rigid, obsessional patient, and much greater success may accrue from prescribing a rather more conservative, old-fashioned, well-trusted and safe remedy. Such patients may do better with old-fashioned tar therapy, for instance, than the latest local and potent corticosteroid.

It may be true that it matters little what is prescribed, but how it is prescribed is vital.

Allergy

'Allergy' is a game played most often by patients, but to a lesser extent also by physicians and specialists. It may be played very strongly from time to time by the media. The concept of allergy provides a fairly easy explanation for patients of their problems. Paramedical personnel and beauticians may be very difficult to deal with and may play a very hard Allergy Game during the consultation with the dermatologist. Those patients who see their problems in terms of allergy are usually happy to accept a treatment regimen which involves the elimination of house dust mites and dietary privations.

Numbers

The Numbers Game is played by rather cunning dermatologists, who will tell their patients that "perhaps 7 out of 10 will get better with treatment X." This sort of game, like a mutation for a geneticist, always provides a convenient let-out should the physician's treatment fail.

Placebo

The concept of a drug as a placebo should never be forgotten. It is occasionally important to keep bored patients busy, and one method is to ritualise the therapy so that quite complicated treatment regimes involving two or even three different ointments being used in strict rotation for certain periods of time may be prescribed. Lack of success can again be blamed on the patient who does not adhere rigidly to the ritual which is being laid down. There are even patients who blossom when the colour of their urine is altered by the professional placebo expert. Some patients, however, will develop symptoms on placebos (the nocebo response). This type of patient is likely to be refractory to almost any form of therapy and is often severely depressed.

Follow-up Games

There are several ways of following up a patient with atopic eczema. One is to give him or her a regular appointment at perhaps monthly or 6 weekly intervals. Usually, however, in such instances the patients come into the consultation saying that they were a lot worse last week but now they are much better. I prefer to leave it to the patients to contact me when they feel they need new advice about their skin.

Hate

Dermatologists have to deal with large numbers of patients with chronic and often severely debilitating disease. This can result in prolonged and often stressful doctor/patient relationships. In a recent study of patients with systemic lupus erythematosus Goodwin et al. [9] showed that the patients whom the attending physicians disliked most were either suicidal or had organic brain damage. These workers concluded that active dislike on the part of the physician may be a clue to serious psychiatric disturbances in the patient. I think this can be extrapolated quite easily to the difficult patient with atopic eczema.

Admission Games

Patients with atopic eczema may suffer severe exacerbations from time to time. As a generalisation, patients with atopic eczema do not like to be admitted to hospital and prefer to remain at work despite the most appalling cutaneous disabilities. Patients in such situations often require oral steroids and a review appointment if their skin has not settled. They can be told that if their condition has not improved by the time of the review appointment in a week or 10 days, then they will need to be admitted to hospital. I refer to this Admission Game as "Gauntlet". The gauntlet is thrown down on the floor for the patient either to grasp or to reject. Admission of a patient with infantile eczema to a dermatological unit can have both positive and negative results. Those patients who find it difficult to accept their problem may be helped by seeing others in similar circumstances or even worse circumstances than themselves. On the other hand, admission to a ward parts the patient from work and family. Kemp writes,

> Confronted with real illness, our reflex action is to stop the patient working; this gets rid of any ideas he might have about his personal importance. Then we take away his clothes and put him in a horizontal, subservient position; this strips him of his physical dignity, making it clear he is ill and at our mercy [11].

One advantage of admission from the physician's point of view is that a close eye can be kept on compliance, because lack of compliance is a common cause of therapeutic failure. Mothers anxious particularly about corticosteroids may at times prefer to have their children afflicted with severe eczema rather than risk what to them seems to be the most terrible of side effects.

Once within the confines of the hospital, most patients' only desire is to get out. The dermatologist in charge and the patient will usually agree about the date of discharge, but occasionally difficult patients may be denied their liberty by the physician as a therapeutic ploy to make the patients less demanding in the long term.

Another advantage of admission to a hospital unit is that of collusion. The patient can be seen by other colleagues, and this often shares the clinical load and takes away some of the threat of the clinical situation.

Collusion

Collusion is a game played by a specialist in hospital. Its aims are laudable in that a second opinion is required to reassure both the patient and the referring physician. On the other hand, such collusion can be seen as a retreat from the threat of the clinical situation. It is very important to avoid management by committee, because this usually adds up to no management at all. However, a psychiatric opinion or that of a clinical psychologist can be sometimes very useful in a patient with atopic eczema and resulting body image disturbance and depression.

Touching

It is important to touch patients with skin disease. Touching a fellow human being is one of the simplest ways of indicating concern. Touching a patient with skin disease may also indicate to the patient the physician's lack of concern about contagion (the leper complex).

Other Psychotherapeutic Approaches

Whilst most of the information presented above may be required at one time or another in the management of a patient with infantile eczema, some patients fail to respond to these reasonable approaches and require other, more sophisticated techniques. These include psychotherapy and behaviour therapy.

Psychological Profile of Patients with Atopic Eczema

Hyperkinesis of children with atopic eczema has been mentioned above. This state of affairs can produce severe exhaustion in one or both parents. It can also disrupt completely nocturnal marital life, in that the child seeks to come into the parents' bed each night, severely affecting a normal relationship. Al-Ahmar and Kurban [1] investigated a group of patients with atopic eczema and another group of patients with other dermatological disorders together with a control group of normal subjects. Variables studied included anxiety, neurosis, extroversion, depression, hypochondriasis and hysteria. These workers showed that patients with atopic eczema responded significantly differently from the other two groups. The patient with atopic eczema tended to be in a state of high manifest anxiety, depressed, neurotic and hypochondriacal. These workers felt that the findings pointed to a homogenicity and uniformity of the personality in atopic patients which indicated that they belonged to a different and specific population. In short, the patient with atopic eczema is an introverted, depressed and highly anxious individual. Unfortunately, in this study there were no data given of the extent of the atopic eczema or of the body site involved.

Psychiatric Referral

The potential benefit of referring a patient with difficult eczema to an interested psychiatrist has been stressed by Brown and Bettley [5]. Those patients who are keen to be referred to the interested psychiatrist and those in whom anxiety or depression or both are found were all treated with antidepressants or tranquillisers. They did well, and much better than the control group. The most important prognostic factors in determining an outcome was the motivation of the patient and the overtness of the emotional disturbance. There is no point referring an unwilling and unmotivated patient to a psychiatrist because when eczema is part of a reaction to stress in a patient who does not want the real nature of his or her problem to be explored, the prognosis is likely to be poor.

Family-Oriented Referral

Koblenzer and Koblenzer [12] regard chronic, intractable atopic eczema as a physical sign of impaired parent/child relationships and psychological developmental arrest, although only a very small proportion of patients with atopic eczema fall into this group. Improvement in the parent/child relationships are a vital part of therapy; this can follow giving parents insight into their conflictual feelings of love and hate.

Koblenzer and Koblenzer point out that the itchy atopic infant has very specific tactile needs and that problems will occur if the mother is "out of touch" [12]. They found that the parents of the atopic child tended to deal with their conflict by offering unrestrained cutaneous stimulation, whilst the children responded intuitively to the unconscious parental hostility with heightened anxiety, heightened undirected motor activity and delayed psychosocial development [12]. The child then learns to become manipulative and becomes hyperkinetic, with an inability to tolerate any frustration. This further strains intrafamily relationships and magnifies parental resentment. Koblenzer and Koblenzer helped their patients' parents to recognise the difficulties in their relationships with the atopic child and the disruptive effect these relationships were having on intrafamily relations. A starting point with this type of therapy is to concentrate during the consultation on the mother's feeling towards the child [12].

Group Psychotherapy

Cole et al. [7] described a group of 10 adult patients with eczema who were given group psychotherapy as a supplement to their regular medical regimen. The group training programme consisted of 10 components, namely, relaxation training, behavioral ratings, sensational discrimination, identification of behavioural triggers, alternative behaviour response training, attitude discrimination, attitude modification training, pairing of behavioural and attitudinal alternatives, generalisation and post-evaluation. The patients were asked to spend 1 h each day practising the relaxation technique and to use a pocket manual counter to keep track of the number of times they scratched per day. In the subsequent week, patients were asked to assess itching intensity as well as the number of times scratched and subsequently to describe possible trigger events. Finally, patients were asked to assess the degree of pleasure generated by scratching. The records kept by the patients were examined in detail so that they could see how life events associated with anger, frustration or anxiety led to increased scratching behaviour. The group were also initiated in some behavioural techniques aimed at moderating itching, such as rubbing or slapping, or using a cold slushy mixture on the skin. Cole et al. encouraged patients to share their experiences with the rest of the group [7].

Behaviour Therapy in Dermatological Practice

The role of behaviour therapy in dermatological practice has been reviewed by Bär and Kuypers [2]. Many techniques are available, and these may be classified into four main groups, namely, systematic desensitisation, aversion therapy, operant techniques and assertive training. Systematic desensitisation is employed mainly in neurotic disorders where anxiety is the main typical feature. An attempt is made to induce inhibition of anxiety following repeated exposures to weak anxiety-arising stimuli, after which progressively stronger stimuli can be introduced. Aversion therapy can be useful in patients with persistent behaviour disorders such as compulsive scratching. The patient can be given an unpleasant stimulus, e.g. an electric shock, whenever the undesirable habit is demonstrated or displayed. Operant techniques are used to modify compulsive habits: rewards are given to reinforce adaptive behaviour while unadaptive behaviour is neglected or punished. A token economy system may be used in which the patient receives a token after a short fixed interval of good (non-scratching) behaviour. This technique is said to be very useful in treating children, especially those with compulsive scratching.

Cataldo et al. [6] used an operant technique to try and modify the scratching behaviour of an individual who had a long history of severe dermatitis and excoriations which had defied all traditional medical therapy. Their 37-year-old patient had a 3.5-year history of exfoliative dermatitis. The treatment procedures consisted of the therapist ceasing his social interaction with the patient for 1 min whenever the patient began to scratch. As soon as the patient was observed scratching he was told he was scratching and then asked to fold his arms and think of something pleasant. Some patients with atopic eczema are not aware of the frequency with which they scratch, so it is important to point this out to them, and the simple expedient of folding the arms meant scratching was impossible. The withdrawal of normal social attention from the patient provided a mild punishment for the scratching behaviour. This simple modification of the itch/scratch cycle in this patient led to clinical improvement, whilst the rest of his skin therapy was left unchanged.

Melin et al. [14] described the behavioural method of habit reversal to try and modify scratching in patients with atopic eczema. Initially, the patients were asked to describe and demonstrate their scratching and subsequently were taught to recognise when they were bringing their hands towards the itchy areas. The patients were then taught situation awareness, there is, to recognise situations in which they usually scratched, and the unpleasant aspects of scratching were also discussed.

With regard to habit reversal, the patients were told to put their hands firmly on the itching area and keep them there for 1 min before moving them to the sides of their thighs or to grasp some other object. Subsequently, the patients were taught to move their hands directly to their thighs or to grasp an object rather than scratch. A strong correlation was demonstrated between a reduction in scratching and improvement in skin status in the patients studied.

Finally, Miller and Coger [15] described skin conductance conditioning in 33 patients with dyshidrotic eczema. Their patients were trained either to increase or decrease the electrical conductivity of the skin. Most patients trained to decrease skin conductance showed clinical improvement more often than controls and also showed a significant decrease in anxiety.

References

1. Al-Ahmar HF, Kurban AK (1976) Psychological profile of patients with atopic dermatitis. Br J Dermatol 95:373–377
2. Bär LHJ, Kuypers BRM (1973) Behaviour therapy in dermatological practice. Br J Dermatol 88:591–598
3. Berne E (1964) Games People Play. Penguin, London
4. Berne E (1973) Sex in human loving. Penguin, London
5. Brown DG, Bettley FR (1971) Psychiatric treatment of eczema: a controlled trial. Br Med J 1:729–734
6. Cataldo MF, Varni JW, Russo DC, Estes SA (1980) Behaviour therapy techniques in treatment of exfoliative dermatitis. Arch Dermatol 116:919–922
7. Cole WC, Roth HL, Sachs LB (1988) Group psychotherapy as an aid in the medical treatment of eczema. J Am Acad Dermatol 18:286–291
8. Cotterill JA (1981) Dermatological games. Br J Dermatol 105:311–320
9. Goodwin JM, Goodwin JS, Kellner R (1979) Psychiatric symptoms in disliked medical patients. JAMA 241:1117–1120
10. Jobling RG (1976) Psoriasis – a preliminary questionnaire of sufferers. Subject experience. Clin Exp Dermatol 1:233–236
11. Kemp R (1964) The golden bed. Lancet ii:1025–1027
12. Koblenzer CS, Koblenzer PJ (1988) Chronic intractable atopic eczema. Its occurrence as a physical sign of impaired parent-child relationships and psychologic developmental arrest: improvement through parent insight and education. Arch Dermatol 124:1673–1677
13. Launer J (1976) Self-help society for eczema sufferers and their families. Br Med J 2:1494–1495
14. Melin L, Frederiksen T, Noren P, Swebilus BG (1986) Behavioural treatment of scratching in patients with atopic dermatitis. Br J Dermatol 115:467–474
15. Miller RM, Coger RW (1979) Skin conductance conditioning with dyshidrotic eczema patients. Br J Dermatol 101:435–440
16. Savin J (1970) Patients' beliefs about psoriasis. Trans St John's Hosp Dermatol Soc 56:139–142
17. Spence J (1960) The need for understanding the individual as part of the training of doctors and nurses. In: The purpose and practice of medicine. Oxford University Press, Oxford

Therapy of Atopic Eczema: Synopsis

T. Ruzicka, J. Ring and B. Przybilla

Introduction

Atopic eczema is a disease of unknown etiology. Causally directed therapy is thus not available. Furthermore, the disease is characterized by a complex interplay of numerous pathophysiological factors culminating in manifest skin disease (see the chapter by Ring et al., this volume). The multifactorial nature of exacerbating, so-called flare factors contributing to the development of atopic eczema makes it self-evident that treatment directed only at one of them should prove a failure. Similarly, orientation at only one pathogenetic model resulting in fixation on a single therapeutic concept is a sign of a lack of understanding of the complexity of the disease – or ideologic, almost religious belief in a unifying, simplistic theory whose proponents may frequently pursue economic benefits.

A serious approach to the individual patient with atopic eczema must take into consideration at least some of the pathogenetic and clinical features of the disease listed in Table 1 and take the corresponding therapeutic measures [4, 13, 14].

Table 1. Pathogenetic factors in atopic eczema: consequences for treatment

Factor	*Therapy*
Dry skin	Elimination of exacerbating factors, prevention of skin irritation, skin care (emollients, oil baths)
Inflammation	Antiinflammatory drugs (glucocorticoids, tar), ultraviolet, cyclosporin (?)
Infection	Antibiotics, antiviral agents
IgE	Environmental control, hyposensitization (?), climatic change (high mountains, sea), interferons (?), cyclosporine (?)
Mediators, itch	Antihistamines, antiinflammatory agents, mast cell blockers (?) ultraviolet, phosphodiesterase inhibitors, diet
Psychosomatic factors	Psychotherapy, sedative drugs
Immune deficiency	Immunomodulators (?)
Food allergy, intolerance	Diet, mast cell blockers (?)
Occupational influences	Occupational hygiene measures, avoidance of irritants, contact allergens, proteins inducing contact urticaria, stress

Besides considering individual flare factors, therapeutic decisions must relate to the stage of the disease and be adapted to the clinical symptoms and severity (Table 2).

Choice of the correct topical vehicle and skin care according to the type of eczema (acute exudative vs chronic lichenified) is an art requiring extensive dermatological experience (see the chapters by Hornstein and by Thoma, this volume). Basic management of all patients with atopic eczema includes dermatological skin care, avoidance of skin irritation, intelligent and responsible use of topical glucocorticoids, antihistamines, and antimicrobial treatment as indicated. It is estimated that in about 90% of atopic eczema patients, the disease can be kept under control using these simple measures. The second stage of management, reserved for severe disease unresponsive to the basic treatment modalities, may include environmental control, empirical elimination diet, and ultraviolet therapy. In selected patients, individual restricted diets, climatic measures, immunosuppresssive treatment modalities, and psychotherapy may be indicated.

Table 2. Stage-adapted treatment plan in atopic eczema

Stage	*Treatment*
I asymptomatic	Emollients, avoidance of skin irritation
II slight, localized	Glucocorticoids, tar preparations
III moderate, widespread	Antihistamines, ultraviolet
IV severe	Hospitalization, wet dressings, allergological evaluation, elimination diet, antibiotics
V severe, unresponsive to standard measures	Restricted diets, DSCG (?), environmental control measures, hyposensitization (?), PUVA, psychotherapy
VI extreme, unresponsive to above	Glucocorticoids systemically, immunosuppressants, (azathioprine, cyclophosphamide, cyclosporine), immunomodulators (interferons) (?), climatic therapy

Skin Care

Dermatological management of atopic individuals should be based on treatment of dry, irritable skin which results in disturbed epidermal barrier function, itch, eczema, and superinfection. Care of the sebostatic skin should include liberal use of topical emollients (see the chapter by Hornstein, this volume). The choice of the emollient should, in our opinion, follow the principle "the fatter, the better," particularly in winter. Patients should be instructed in changing bathing habits and using regular oil baths and syndets for cleansing (see the chapter by Braun-Falco and Korting, this volume).

Glucocorticoids

Glucocorticoids are and remain the best and standard regimen for symptomatic treatment of atopic eczema (see the chapter by Goerz and Lehmann, this volume). Their introduction into dermatological therapy has dramatically changed the quality of life of atopic eczema patients. When applied by experienced dermatologists, these drugs hardly ever lead to serious side effects, which usually result from their inconsiderate use. In this respect, glucocorticoids resemble most other highly useful drugs in medicine. Inappropriate use of insulin or digitalis can kill a patient, but nobody would doubt their therapeutic usefulness when correctly applied.

Choosing the correct glucocorticoid preparation means considering the potency of the drug and the vehicle, both of which should be adapted to the stage of disease. We prefer the short-term use of intermediate to high potency steroids in lotions or creams in the acute exudative stage, which must be followed by the use of low potency drugs. Glucocorticoids can also be applied intermittently with base creams and ointments. Chronic, lichenified lesions require the application of fatty ointments, pastes, or occlusive dressings with the addition of tar preparations and/or glucocorticoids. Generally, the long-term use of intermediate to potent steroids does not have a greater antiinflammatory effect than hydrocortisone, but puts the patient at risk of unwanted and serious side effects.

Antihistamines

The symptomatic relief of itch provided by antihistamines helps to interrupt the itch-scratch-eczema-itch vicious cycle and greatly improves the quality of life of atopic eczema patients (see the chapter by Schmutzler, this volume). The paucity of serious side effects, even after long-term use, should reinforce the readiness of physicians to use antihistamines in the management of eczema patients. The dose should be individually titrated, insufficient dosage being a frequently observed mistake. Even high doses usually lack toxicity except for sedation in some, but not all, individuals. Many patients observe an adaptation to the sedative effect of classical antihistamines. The advent of new, nonsedating antihistamines may be an advantage to some patients, but the sedation provided by classical antihistamines can offer an additional therapeutic principle in addition to the antihistamine effect per se. At least in hospitalized atopic eczema patients, there is little rationale for using new antihistamine preparations.

Antiinfectious Treatment

Colonization and impetiginization of eczematous skin with *Staphylococcus aureus* or other infectious agents may represent a provoking factor in atopic eczema [5]. When indicated, appropriate antimicrobial treatment should be instituted. Deliberate, general use of antimicrobials may not be recommended due to the emergence of resistant organisms and the sensitizing potential of many antibiotic preparations. New antibiotic agents such as mupirocin with high activity against *Staphylococcus aureus* may be useful in the treatment of patients with atopic eczema. New antiviral drugs represent a great advance in the treatment of infectious complications, particularly eczema herpeticum (see the chapter by Vieluf and Ruzicka, this volume).

Ultraviolet Treatment

Many patients experience improvement of atopic eczema by sun exposure. Although this may be due to a number of circumstantial factors, numerous therapeutic reports attest to the efficacy of ultraviolet irradiation in atopic eczema (see the chapter by Morison, this volume). The combination of UVA and UVB seems to be particularly suited for treatment of moderate to severe eczema [9]. In patients with unresponsive disease, psoralen and UVA (PUVA) treatment should prove useful. UV treatment offers the additional advantage of regular supervision of the patient with improved skin care, psychological sense of well-being, etc.

The rationale for ultraviolet treatment in atopic eczema is based not only on empirical experience, but also on experimental findings which show that UV rays exert an influence on Langerhans cells, contact sensitization, releasability of inflammatory mediators, release of neuropeptides from skin, and many other effects. However, when considering UV treatment in an individual patient,the possibility of UV-sensitive eczema should be kept in mind.

Diet

Generally, two types of diets can be distinguished in the management of atopic eczema: elimination diets based on food intolerance and supplementation diets based on a deficiency of, e.g., essential fatty acids.

The role of food allergy and the resulting dietary regimens are highly controversal [1, 17, 22]. The discussion carried out by the medical and general public is sometimes obscured by ideological argumentation, lack of knowledge of even basic principles of allergy, and lack of scientific evidence for many of the proposed dietary regimens. An increasing number of children are being admitted to university hospitals suffering from inconsiderate use of dangerous restriction diets leading to deficiency of vital nutrients.

However, recent scientific evidence, resulting from careful work by Sampson (see the chapter in this volume and [19]), Atherton [1] and others, provides a sound basis for dietary management of a highly selected patient population (see the chapter by Gianetti and Seidenari, this volume). The selection of patients for dietary measures should include some of the following considerations: The disease should be sufficiently severe since it makes no sense to put a child with minimal flexural eczema, which primarily disturbs his mother, on a severe restricted diet; the diet should not be worse than the eczema; the diet should not disrupt the normal life of the patient and his family thus causing psychosocial problems as a replacement for the allergological ones; dietary measures are usually more effective in younger than in older children and adults; and the simple elimination diets, excluding only a few nutrients such as milk, eggs, etc., should be considered first.

Individual restricted diets must be based upon thorough allergological evaluation, which is often tedious and difficult [18]. Therapeutic decisions based only on prick tests and RAST results are a frequently committed mistake. Correct interpretation of the clinical relevance of positive allergological test results is obligatory. Nonetheless, since food intolerance need not necessarily be IgE mediated, provocation tests are absolutely necessary.

In some food intolerant patients, disodium cromoglycate (DSCG) treatment may be useful, although controlled studies generally show only a marginal effect ([21] Businco and Cantani, this volume).

The usefulness of prophylactic breast feeding of infants at risk for developing atopic eczema and the role of hypoallergenic elimination diets for the lactating mother are still unsettled (see the chapter by Björksten, this volume).

Another matter of controversy is the use of supplementation diets with essential fatty acids. Although based on scientific evidence suggesting a role for essential fatty acids in the pathogenesis of atopic eczema, trials with supplementation of γ-linolenic and eicosapentaenoic acids showed in most cases only slight benefits ([3, 24] and see the chapter by Kunz and Ring, Ring and Ruzicka, this volume).

Environmental Control

Environmental control is aimed at the elimination of flare factors responsible for the provocation and exacerbation of atopic eczema in a genetically predisposed individual. Numerous measures can be summarized, which must be individualized for each patient. These include: elimination of irritating clothing, e.g., wool; elimination of allergenic foods; elimination of housedust mites by appropriate bedding and housing conditions and new insecticidal agents (Platts-Mills et al., this volume); reduction of pet contacts; elimination of contact allergens, irritants, and substances causing contact urticaria from household and occupation; occupational counseling regarding the choice or a change of occupation and work protection (see the chapter by Rystaedt, this volume); hospitalization; climatotherapy at high altitude or seaside (see the chapter by Steiger and Borelli, this volume); and elimination of stress (family, occupation).

In cases where elimination of inhalation allergens is not possible, hyposensitization may be considered (e.g., with pollen or housedust mite extracts) [20]. In a double-blind study in a pair of twins, hyposensitization with grass pollen extract led to improvement of eczema in the treated vs the placebo-treated twin [15]. However, hyposensitization carries the risk of exacerbation of disease. Although difficult to perform, large scale, placebo-controlled, double-blind studies should provide further information on the value of specific hyposensitization in the managment of atopic eczema.

Psychotherapeutic Approaches

The psychosomatic interplay in atopic eczema is a self-evident phenomenon to every physician involved in the management of patients with this disease [7] (Bosse, this volume). The influence of psychological factors thus requires education and stabilization of patients and family members. In selected patients, psychotherapeutic treatment (Cotterill, this volume), family or group therapy, and/or use of sedative drugs which additionally exert antihistamine effects (e.g., opipramol, hydroxyzine) may be needed. Behavioral treatment and autogenic therapy may be directed at reduction of scratching.

Immunomodulators and Immunosuppressive Drugs

The pathophysiology of atopic eczema is characterized both by immunodeficiency and hyperimmunity. Thus, the physician is confronted with the perplexing question whether to treat the severely affected patient with immunostimulating or immunosuppressive drugs.

Several immunomodulators have been used in atopic eczema with varying, but generally disappointing, results: levamisole, thymopoietin and TP5, thymosin, transfer factor, and others ([4] and Zachariae, this volume). At present, they can be regarded as experimental drugs at best.

Drugs aimed at reduction of IgE production hold greater promise in the treatment of atopic eczema. Of particular interest to dermatopharmacology is cyclosporine, which has been shown to reduce IgE synthesis and exert therapeutic effects in severe atopic eczema [8, 11, 23]. It is questionable whether its efficiency is due solely to inhibition of IgE synthesis, since the drug exerts rather unrelated antiinflammatory actions, as evidenced by its efficacy in psoriasis and other inflammatory dermatoses. Due to the lack of extensive, long-term experience with cyclosporine and its side effects, the drug should be used at present only in experimental settings and with great caution. It is indicated only in treating extreme, intractable diease. Another approach aimed at reducing IgE synthesis and immunostimulation is the use of interferons α and γ [2, 12]. Experimental evidence has justified their use in controlled trials. Although the results of these trials have not been reported to date, they should clarify whether the theoretical usefulness of interferons is reflected by clinical efficacy.

Pharmacological interventions into the disturbed phosphodiesterase-cyclic adenosine monophosphate system (Hanifin, this volume) may also correct immunopharmacological abnormalities of atopic eczema. Similarly, manipulations of disturbed eicosanoid metabolism in atopic eczema should prove both antiinflammatory and immunomodulating. In particular, the protective and immunosuppressive effects of prostaglandin [12, 16] (Ruzicka and Ring, this volume) deserve further interest. Systematic evaluation of drugs interfering with arachidonic acid metabolism has not yet taken place with respect to atopic eczema.

In rare, desperate cases in which patients are unresponsive to standard therapeutic regimens, immunosuppressive treatment with oral glucocorticoids, azathioprine, or cyclophosphamide may be necessary [10]. In our institution, these therapeutic modalities represent the last resort and are very rarely used. In the future, cyclosporine may replace cytotoxic drugs in the treatment of extreme, intractable disease, but sufficient experience with this drug in atopic eczema is lacking.

Summary and Outlook

Symptomatic therapy in atopic eczema must be individualized and consider the multifactorial pathogenesis of the disease. It is based upon the use of emollients, glucocorticoids, and antihistamines. Individual flare factors should be eliminated whenever possible. New therapeutic approaches are emerging, but future progress will decisively depend upon better understanding of the etiology and complex pathophysiology of the disease [6] (Ring et al., this volume).

References

1. Atherton DJ (1983) The role of food in atopic eczema. Clin Exp Dermatol 8:227–232
2. Bieber T, Rieger A, Neuchrist C et al. (1989) Induction of Fc$^{\varepsilon}$R2/CD23 on human epidermal Langerhans cells by human recombinant interleukin 4 and γ interferon J Exp Med 70:309–314
3. Bjorneboe A, Soyland E, Bjorneboe GEA, Rajka G, Drevon CA (1987) Effect of dietary supplementation with eicosapentaenoic acid in the treatment of atopic dermatitis. Br J Dermatol 117:463–469
4. Braun-Falco O, Ring J (1984) Zur Therapie des atopischen Ekzems. Hautarzt 35:447–454
5. Dahl MV (1983) *Staphylococcus aureus* in atopic dermatitis. Arch Dermatol 119:840–844
6. Hanifin JM (1982) Atopic dermatitis. J Am Acad Dermatol 6:1–13
7. Jordan JM, Whitlock PA (1974) Atopic dermatitis, anxiety and conditional scratch responses. J Psychosom Res 18:297–304
8. King CL, Gallin JI, Malech HL, Abramson SL, Nutman TB (1989) Regulation of immunoglobulin production in hyperimmunoglobulin E recurrent-infection syndrome by interferon γ. Proc Natl Acad Sci USA 86:10085–10089
9. Midelfart K, Stenvold SE, Volden G (1985) Combined UVB and UVA phototherapy of atopic eczema. Dermatologica 171:95–98
10. Morrison GL, Schulz EJ (1978) Treatment of eczema with cyclophosphamide and azathioprine. Br J Dermatol 98: 203–206
11. Okudaira H, Sakurai Y, Tereda K (1986) Cyclosporin A-induced suppression of ongoing IgE-antibody formation in the mouse. Int Arch Allergy Appl Immunol 79:164–168
12. Pène J, Rousset F, Brière F, Chrètien I, Bonnefoy T, Arai N, Arai KI, Banchereau I, de Vries IE (1988) IgE production by normal human lymphocytes is induced by interleukin 4 and suppressed by interferons γ and α and prostaglandin E_2. Proc Natl Acad Sci USA 85:6880–6884
13. Rajka G (1989) Essential aspects of atopic dermatitis. Springer, Berlin Heidelberg New York
14. Rasmussen IE (1984) Recent developments in the management of patients with atopic dermatitis. J Allergy Clin Immunol 74:771–776
15. Ring J (1982) Successful hyposensitization treatment in a pair of monozygotic twins suffering from atopic eczema. Br J Dermatol 10:597–602
16. Ruzicka T (1980) The physiology and pathophysiology of eicosanoids in the skin. Eicosanoids 1:59–72
17. Ruzicka T (1987) Ernährung und atopisches Ekzem. Z Hautkr [Suppl] 62:96–99
18. Ruzicka T (1987) Diagnostik von Nahrungsmittelallergien. Hautarzt 38:510–515
19. Sampson HA (1983) Role of immediate food hypersensitivity in the pathogenesis of atopic dermatitis. J Allergy Clin Immunol 7:473–480
20. Seidenari S, Mosca M, Taglietti M (1986) Specific hyposensitization in atopic dermatitis. Dermatologica 172: 229–232
21. Sondergaard J, Kassis V, Knudsen L, Wadskov S, Wanscher B, Weismann K (1980) Cromones in atopic dermatitis. Arch Dermatol Res 267:223–228
22. Special Symposium (1986) Significance of food hypersensitivity in children with atopic dermatitis. Pediatr Dermatol 36:161–174
23. Van Joost T, Stolz E, Henle D (1987) Efficacy of low-dose cyclosporine in severe atopic skin disease. Acta Dermatol 123:166–167
24. Wright S, Burton IL (1982) Oral evening-primrose-seed oil improves atopic eczema. Lancet 2:1120–1122

Subject Index